Dacie and Lewis
Practical Haematology

Commissioning Editor: Michael Houston
Development Editor: Nani Clansey
Editorial Assistant: Kirsten Lowson
Project Manager: Alan Nicholson
Design: Charles Gray
Illustration Manager: Bruce Hogarth
Marketing Manager: Helena Mutak

Dacie and Lewis
Practical Haematology

Eleventh Edition

Barbara J. Bain FRACP, FRCPath

Professor in Diagnostic Haematology, Imperial College Faculty of Medicine, St. Mary's Hospital, London, UK

Imelda Bates MD, FRCP, FRCPath

Professor of Tropical Haematology, Liverpool School of Tropical Medicine, Liverpool, UK

Michael A. Laffan DM, FRCP, FRCPath

Professor of Haemostasis and Thrombosis, Honorary Consultant in Haematology, Imperial College Faculty of Medicine, Hammersmith Hospital, London, UK

S. Mitchell Lewis MD, FRCPath, DCP FIBMS

Emeritus Reader in Haematology, Imperial College Faculty of Medicine, Hammersmith Hospital, London, UK

ELSEVIER
CHURCHILL
LIVINGSTONE

ELSEVIER
CHURCHILL
LIVINGSTONE

CHURCHILL LIVINGSTONE an imprint of Elsevier Limited

© 2012 Elsevier Ltd. All rights reserved.

First edition 1950	Seventh edition 1991
Second edition 1956	Eighth edition 1995
Third edition 1963	Ninth edition 2001
Fourth edition 1968	Tenth edition 2006
Fifth edition 1975	Eleventh edition 2012
Sixth edition 1984	

The right of Barbara J. Bain, Imelda Bates, Michael A. Laffan, and S. Mitchell Lewis to be identified as authors of this work has been asserted by them in accordance with the Copyright, Designs and Patents Act 1988.

Notices

Knowledge and best practice in this field are constantly changing. As new research and experience broaden our understanding, changes in research methods, professional practices, or medical treatment may become necessary.

Practitioners and researchers must always rely on their own experience and knowledge in evaluating and using any information, methods, compounds, or experiments described herein. In using such information or methods they should be mindful of their own safety and the safety of others, including parties for whom they have a professional responsibility.

With respect to any drug or pharmaceutical products identified, readers are advised to check the most current information provided (i) on procedures featured or (ii) by the manufacturer of each product to be administered, to verify the recommended dose or formula, the method and duration of administration, and contraindications. It is the responsibility of practitioners, relying on their own experience and knowledge of their patients, to make diagnoses, to determine dosages and the best treatment for each individual patient, and to take all appropriate safety precautions.

To the fullest extent of the law, neither the Publisher nor the authors, contributors, or editors, assume any liability for any injury and/or damage to persons or property as a matter of products liability, negligence or otherwise, or from any use or operation of any methods, products, instructions, or ideas contained in the material herein.

Churchill Livingstone

British Library Cataloguing in Publication Data

Dacie and Lewis practical haematology. – 11th ed.
  1. Blood–Examination. 2. Blood–Analysis.
  3. Hematology–Technique.
  I. Practical haematology II. Bain, Barbara J. III. Dacie,
  John V. (John Vivian), Sir. Practical haematology.
616′.07561-dc22

ISBN: 9780702034084
International ISBN: 9780702034077

Printed in China

Last digit is the print number: 9 8 7 6 5 4 3 2 1

Contents

v

Contents

Preface

This 11th edition celebrates the 61st year of *Practical Haematology*. The first edition by J.V. Dacie was published in 1950. This work, and subsequent editions with Mitchell Lewis as co-author, were based on the haematology course for the London University Diploma of Clinical Pathology (DCP) and subsequently the MSc in Haematology at the then Royal Postgraduate Medical School.

Medical science has expanded exponentially in the last half century, but no discipline has expanded more than haematology, which has often led the way in applying new techniques. This exponential rise is reflected in the parallel increase in the size of this book and in the complexity of the tests described. In this edition we have sought to encompass the full range of tests carried out in a modern haematology laboratory, but recognizing the increasing utilization of commercial ready-to-use kits and point-of-care testing and not neglecting quality control and laboratory organization and management. The role of the internet is acknowledged and we have indicated important websites that are relevant to haematology. We recognize that many of the more sophisticated tests are not readily available in all laboratories, and a chapter is devoted to the essential tests in under-resourced laboratories.

Biomedical scientists are increasingly responsible for laboratory practice as medically qualified haematologists become more concerned with clinical care of patients. Both groups need an understanding of the clinical relevance of haematological investigations and this is clearly expounded. The principles of good laboratory practice were established by Dacie in his first edition, when he wrote that, 'all those concerned with laboratory work should understand what is the significance of the tests that they carry out, the relative value of haematological investigations and the order in which they should be undertaken.' We have attempted to maintain his approach, albeit appropriately updated to meet present-day practices.

During the preparation of this edition we were grieved by the deaths of three of our contributors. Dr Noriyuki Tatsumi (co-author of Chapter 1) died on 18 November 2010. He was recognized as one of the most distinguished haematologists in Japan and had made major contributions in Asia and also worldwide, notably to advances in haematology technology, automation and quality assurance. These initiatives were reflected by his membership on the Board of the International Council for Standardization in Haematology and his impact on the work of their Expert Panels. Dr David Swirsky (co-author of Chapter 15) was a noted British haematologist who died on 23 January 2011. His contribution to *Practical Haematology* commenced with the 8th edition, 17 years ago, and is evidence of his long-term interest in diagnostic haematology, commencing at Cambridge and continuing at Hammersmith Hospital and later at the Leeds Haematological Malignancy Diagnostic Service. He was a popular teacher as well as an expert morphologist and gave wise advice. He was held in affectionate regard by the UK haematology community and abroad. Corrine Jury who died on 7th May 2011 was at the time of her death a senior biomedical scientist and a key member of the haematology department at Hammersmith Hospital. She was a loyal member of the department, having started work there as a trainee 25 years earlier. Despite her serious illness she participated enthusiastically in writing for this book.

Sir John V. Dacie, MD, FRCPath, FRS 1912–2005

S. Mitchell Lewis, BSc, MD, DCP(London), FRCPath, FIBMS 1924–

As a 61-year tribute, this edition is dedicated to Sir John Dacie and to Mitchell Lewis. Sir John was one of the pre-eminent British haematologists of the second half of the 20th century; he established haematology as a distinct discipline and his books on haemolytic anaemia have become modern classics. Mitchell Lewis was a founder member of the International Committee (subsequently Council) for Standardization in Haematology, and subsequently its Chairman; he was also the founder of the UK National External Quality Assessment Scheme and the British Committee for Standards in Haematology. He is internationally renowned for his work with the ICSH and was a member of the WHO International Expert Advisory Panel on Health Laboratory Services. Together they made major contributions to the training of haematologists; their ex-trainees are dispersed throught the world.

Barbara J. Bain
Imelda Bates
Michael A. Laffan

Contributors

Barbara J. Bain, MB BS, FRACP, FRCPath
Professor in Diagnostic Haematology,
Department of Haematology,
St Mary's Hospital,
London, UK

Imelda Bates, MD, FRCP, FRCPath
Professor of Tropical Haematology,
Liverpool School of Tropical Medicine,
Liverpool, UK

Sheena Blackmore, FIBMS
UK NEQAS Haematinics Scheme Manager,
Haematology Department,
Good Hope Hospital,
Heart of England Foundation Trust,
Birmingham, UK

Anne E. Bradshaw, BSc, FIBMS, DMLM
Divisional Manager,
Department of Haematology,
Charing Cross Hospital,
London, UK

Carol Briggs, BSc FIBMS
Head of Haematology Evaluation Unit,
Department of Haematology Evaluations,
University College London Hospital,
London, UK

John Burthem, PhD, FRCP, FRCPath
Clinical Senior Lecturer and Honorary Consultant
Haematologist,
Department of Clinical Haematology,
Manchester Royal Infirmary,
Manchester, UK

Carol Cantwell, CSci, FIBMS, DMS
Blood Transfusion Laboratory,
St Mary's Hospital,
Imperial College NHS Trust,
London, UK

Jane Y. Carter, MBBS, FRCPC
Director, Clinical and Diagnostics,
African Medical and Research Foundation (AMREF),
Kenya Country Office,
Nairobi, Kenya

Peter Charles Cotton, AIBMS
Senior Biomedical Scientist,
Radioisotopes Department,
Haematology Department,
Imperial College Healthcare NHS Trust,
Hammersmith Hospital,
London, UK

Letizia Foroni, MD, PhD, FRCPath
Consultant Clinical Scientist,
Haematology Department,
Hammersmith Hospital,
London, UK

Malcolm S. Hamilton, MBChB, FRCP, FRCPath
Consultant Haematologist,
Dept Haematology,
Royal Devon and Exeter Hospital,
Exeter, UK

Corrine L. Jury, * FIBMS
Senior Biomedical Scientist,
Diagnostic Haematology Laboratory,
Imperial College Healthcare NHS Trust,
Hammersmith Hospital,
London, UK

Jaspal Kaeda, PhD, FRCPath
Charite Virchow-Klinikum,
Hämatologie/Onkologie,
Berlin, Germany

Michael A. Laffan, DM FRCP FRCPath
Professor of Haemostasis and Thrombosis,
Honorary Consultant in Haematology,
Faculty of Medicine,
Imperial College,
Hammersmith Hospital,
London, UK

*Deceased

Contributors

Mark Layton, FRCP, FRCPCH
St Mary's Hospital, Imperial College,
Healthcare NHS Trust,
London, UK

S. Mitchell Lewis, BSc, MD, FRCPath, DCP, FIBMS
Emeritus Reader in Haematology,
Imperial College Faculty of Medicine,
Department of Haematology,
Hammersmith Hospital,
London, UK

Richard A. Manning, BSc, CSci, FIBMS
Chief Biomedical Scientist,
Diagnostic Haematology,
Imperial College Healthcare NHS Trust,
Hammersmith Hospital,
London, UK

Estella Matutes, MD, PhD, FRCPath
Reader in Haemato-Oncology,
Consultant Haematologist,
Haemato-Oncology unit,
Royal Marsden Hospital,
London, UK

Alison May, PhD
Senior Research Fellow,
Department of Haematology,
Cardiff University School of Medicine,
Cardiff, UK

Clare Milkins, BSc CSci FIBMS
UK NEQAS (BTLP),
Watford General Hospital,
Watford, Herts, UK

Ricardo Morilla, MSc, FRMS
Clinical Scientist,
Haemato-Oncology Section,
Institute Cancer Research,
Royal Marsden Hospital,
Sutton, Surrey, UK

Alison M. Morilla, BSc
Clinical Scientist,
Section of Haemato-Oncology,
Institute of Cancer Research,
Royal Marsden Hospital,
Sutton, Surrey, UK

Yutaka Nagai, PhD
Guest Researcher,
Research Institute for Science and Engineering,
Faculty of Science and Engineering,
Institution for Advanced Biomedical Sciences,
Waseda University,
Nakano, Tokyo, Japan

Kuldip S. Nijran, BSc, MSc, DMS, PhD, MIPEM, CSci
Head of Nuclear Medicine Physics,
Radiological Sciences Unit,
Imperial College Healthcare NHS Trust,
Hammersmith Hospital,
London, UK

Andrew Osei-Bimpong, MSc, CSci, FIBMS, MIHM
Chief Biomedical Scientist,
Diagnostic Haematology,
Imperial College Healthcare NHS Trust,
Hammersmith Hospital,
London, UK

Fiona A.M. Regan, MBBS, FRCP, FRCPath
Consultant Haematologist,
NHS Blood and Transplant (North London)
and Imperial College Healthcare NHS Trust,
London Hammersmith Hospital,
London, UK

David Roper, MSc, CSci, FIBMS
Principal Biomedical Scientist,
Diagnostic Haematology,
Imperial College Healthcare NHS Trust,
Hammersmith Hospital,
London, UK

Megan Rowley, FRCP, FRCPath
Consultant in Haematology and Transfusion Medicine,
St Mary's Hospital,
Imperial College Healthcare NHS Trust,
London, UK

David Swirsky,* FRCP, FRCPath
Consultant Haematologist,
Haematological Malignancy Diagnostic Service,
St. James's University Hospital,
Leeds, UK

Noriyuki Tatsumi,* MD, PhD
Professor Emeritus,
Osaka City University,
Nakano, Tokyo, Japan

Joan-Lluis Vives-Corrons, MD, PhD
Professor of Haematology,
Red Cell Pathology Unit,
Hospital Clinic i Provincial,
University of Barcelona,
Barcelona, Spain

---

*Deceased

Thomas J. Vulliamy, BA(Hons), PhD, FRCPath
Senior Lecturer in Molecular Biology,
Centre for Paediatrics,
Institute of Cell and Molecular Science,
Barts and The London School of Medicine and Dentistry,
London, UK

Mary A. West, DBMS, MSc, FIBMS, CSci
International External Quality Assessment Scheme for
Haematology Coordinator,
UK NEQAS (H),
Watford General Hospital,
Watford, UK

Barbara J. Wild, PhD, FIBMS
Department of Haematology,
King's College Hospital,
London, UK

Nay Win, MBBS, FRCP, FRCPath, CTM(Edin)
Consultant Haematologist,
Red Cell Immunohaematology,
NHS Blood and Transplant (Tooting),
London, UK

Mark Worwood, PhD, FRCPath, FMedSci
Emeritus Professor,
Department of Haematology,
Cardiff University School of Medicine,
Cardiff, UK

Thomas J. Vulliamy, BA(Hons), PhD, FRCPath
Senior Lecturer in Molecular Biology,
Centre for Paediatrics,
Institute of Cell and Molecular Science,
Barts and The London School of Medicine and Dentistry,
London, UK

Mary A. West, DBMS, MSc, FIBMS, CSci
International External Quality Assessment Scheme for
Haematology Coordinator,
UK NEQAS (H),
Watford General Hospital,
Watford, UK

Barbara J. Wild, PhD, FIBMS
Department of Haematology,
King's College Hospital,
London, UK

Nay Win, MBBS, FRCP, FRCPath, CTM(Edin)
Consultant Haematologist,
Red Cell Immunohaematology,
NHS Blood and Transplant (Tooting),
London, UK

Mark Worwood, PhD, FRCPath, FMedSci
Emeritus Professor,
Department of Haematology,
Cardiff University School of Medicine,
Cardiff, UK

Chapter | 1 |

Collection and handling of blood

Corrine Jury, Yutaka Nagai, Noriyuki Tatsumi

In investigating physiological function and malfunction of blood, accurate and precise methodology is essential to ensure, as far as possible, that tests do not give misleading information because of technical errors. Obtaining the specimen is the first step towards analytic procedures. It is important to use appropriate blood containers and to avoid faults in specimen collection, storage and transport to the laboratory. Venous blood is generally used for most haematological examinations and for chemistry tests; capillary skin puncture samples can be almost as satisfactory for some purposes if a free flow of blood is obtained (see p. 4), but in general this procedure should be restricted to children and to some 'point-of-care' screening tests which require only a drop or two of blood. Bone marrow aspirates are described in Chapter 7.

BIOHAZARD PRECAUTIONS

Special care must be taken to avoid risk of infection from various pathogens during all aspects of laboratory practice, and the safety procedures described in Chapter 24 must be followed as far as possible when collecting blood. The operator should wear disposable plastic or thin rubber gloves. It is also desirable to wear a protective apron or gown, as well as glasses or goggles, if necessary. Care must be taken to prevent injuries, especially when handling syringes, needles and lancets.

Disposable sterilized syringes, needles and lancets should be used if at all possible, and they should never be re-used. Re-usable items must always be sterilized after use (see Chapter 24).

STANDARDIZED PROCEDURE

The constituents of the blood may be altered by a number of factors which are listed in Box 1.1. It is important to have a standard procedure for the collecting and handling of blood specimens. Recommendations for standardizing the procedure have been published.[1-3]

VENOUS BLOOD

It is now common practice for specimen collection to be undertaken by specially trained phlebotomists, and there are published guidelines which set out an appropriate training programme.[1,4]

Phlebotomy Tray

It is convenient to have a tray which contains all the requirements for blood collection (Box 1.2).

Disposable Plastic Syringes and Disposable Needles

The needles should not be too fine, too large, or too long; those of 19 or 21G* are suitable for most adults. 23G are suitable for children and ideally should have a short shaft (about 15 mm). It may be helpful to collect the blood by means of a winged ('*butterfly*') needle connected to a

length of plastic tubing which can be attached to the nozzle of the syringe or to a needle for entering the cap of an evacuated container (see below).

Specimen Containers

The common containers for haematology tests are available commercially with dipotassium, tripotassium, or disodium ethylenediaminetetra-acetic acid (EDTA) as an anticoagulant, and they are marked at a level to indicate the correct amount of blood to be added. Containers are also available containing trisodium citrate, heparin or acid-citrate-dextrose, as well as containers with no additive which are used when serum is required. Design requirements and other specifications for specimen collection containers have been described in a number of national and international standards, e.g. that of the International Council for Standardization in Haematology,[5] and there is also a European standard (EN 14820). Unfortunately, there is not yet universal agreement regarding the colours for identifying containers with different additives; phlebotomists should familiarize themselves with the colours used by their own suppliers.

Evacuated tube systems which are now in common use consist of a glass or plastic tube/container (with or without anticoagulant) under defined vacuum, a needle, and a needle holder which secures the needle to the tube. The main advantage is that the cap can be pierced, so that it is not necessary to remove it either to fill the tube, or subsequently to withdraw samples for analysis, thus minimizing the risk of aerosol discharge of the contents. An evacuated system is useful when multiple samples in different anticoagulants are required. The vacuum controls the amount of blood which enters the tube, ensuring an adequate specimen for the subsequent tests and the correct proportion of anticoagulant, when this is present. Silicone-coated evacuated tubes can be used for routine coagulation screening tests.

---

*The International Organization for Standardization has established a ~~dard~~ (ISO 7864), which relates the following diameters for the ~~gauges~~: 19G = 1.1 mm; 21G = 0.8 mm; 23G = 0.6 mm.

Phlebotomy Procedure

The phlebotomist should first check the patient's identity, making sure that it corresponds to the details on the request form, and also ensure that the phlebotomy tray contains all the required specimen containers.

Blood is best withdrawn from an antecubital vein or other visible veins in the forearm by means of either an evacuated tube or a syringe. It is usually recommended that the skin should be cleaned with 70% alcohol (e.g. isopropanol) or 0.5% chlorhexidine, and allowed to dry spontaneously before being punctured; however, some doubts have been expressed on the utility of this practice for preventing infection at the venepuncture site.[6] Care must also be taken when using a tourniquet to avoid contaminating it with blood because infection risks have been reported during blood collection.[7] The tourniquet should be applied just above the venepuncture site and released as soon as the blood begins to flow into the syringe or evacuated tube – delay in releasing it leads to fluid shift and haemoconcentration as a result of venous blood stagnation.[4] Except for very young children, it should be possible with practice to obtain venous blood even from patients with difficult veins. A butterfly needle is especially useful when a series of samples is required.

Successful venepuncture may be facilitated by keeping the subject's arm warm, applying to the upper arm a sphygmomanometer cuff kept at approximately diastolic pressure and tapping the skin over the site of the vein a few times. After cleaning and drying the site and applying a tourniquet, ask the patient to make a fist a few times. Veins suitable for puncture will usually become apparent. If the veins are very small, a butterfly needle or 23G needle should enable at least 2 ml of blood to be obtained satisfactorily. In obese patients, it may be easier to use a vein on the dorsum of the hand, after warming it by immersion in warm water; however, this site is not generally recommended as vein punctures tend to bleed into surrounding tissues more readily than at other sites. Venepuncture should not be attempted over a site of scarring or haematoma.

If a syringe is used for blood collection, the piston of the syringe should be withdrawn slowly and no attempt made to withdraw blood faster than the vein is filling. Anticoagulated specimens must be mixed by inverting the containers several times. Haemolysis can be avoided or minimized by using clean apparatus, withdrawing the blood slowly, not using too fine a needle, delivering the blood gently into the receiver and avoiding frothing during the withdrawal of the blood and subsequent mixing with the anticoagulant. If the blood is drawn too slowly or inadequately mixed with the anticoagulant some coagulation may occur. After collection, the containers must be firmly capped to minimize the risk of leakage.

If blood collection fails, it is important to remain calm and consider the possible cause of the failure. This includes poor technique, especially stabbing, rather than holding the needle parallel to the surface of the skin as it enters, as this may result in the needle passing through the vein. After two or three unsuccessful attempts, it may be wise to refer the patient to another operator after a short rest.

After obtaining the blood and releasing the tourniquet, remove the needle and then press a sterile swab over the puncture site. The arm should be elevated after withdrawal of the needle and pressure should continue to be applied to the swab with the arm elevated for a minute or two before checking that bleeding has completely ceased. Then cover the puncture site with a small adhesive dressing.

Obtaining blood from an indwelling line or catheter is a potential source of error. As it is common practice to flush lines with heparin, they must be flushed free from heparin and the first 5 ml of blood discarded before any blood is collected for laboratory tests. If intravenous fluids are being transfused into an arm, the blood sample should not be collected from that arm.

Post-phlebotomy Procedure

The phlebotomist should again check the patient's identity and must make sure that it corresponds to the details on the request form. It is essential that every specimen, as well as the request form, is labelled with adequate patient identification immediately after the samples have been obtained. On the labels this should include at least surname and forename or initials, hospital number, date of birth and date and time of specimen collection. The same information must be given on the request form, together with ward or department, name of requesting clinician and test(s) requested. When relevant, a biohazard warning must also be affixed to the container and to the request form. If automated patient identification is available both the label and the request form should be bar-coded with the relevant data unless the sample is to be used for blood transfusion tests, in which case the label should be handwritten, with the name in full (see Chapter 21).

Specimens should be sent in individual plastic bags separated from the request forms to prevent contamination of the forms in the event of leakage. Alternatively, the specimen tubes must be set upright in a holder or rack and placed in a carrier together with the request forms for transport to the laboratory.

Waste Disposal

Without separating the needle from the syringe, place both, together with the used swab and any other dressings, in a puncture-resistant container, for disposal (see Chapter 24). If it is essential to dispose of the needle separately it should be detached from the syringe only with forceps or a similar tool. Alternatively, the needle can be destroyed *in situ* with a special device, e.g. *Sharp-X* (Biomedical Disposal Inc: www.biodisposal.com)

CAPILLARY BLOOD

Skin puncture can be used for obtaining a small amount of blood either for direct use in an analytic process or for collecting into capillary tubes coated with heparin for packed cell volume or into a special anticoagulated microcollection device. These methods are mostly used when it is not possible to obtain venous blood (e.g. in infants under 1 year, in gross obesity) or for point-of-care blood tests.

Collection of Capillary Blood

Skin puncture is carried out with a needle or lancet. In adults and older children, blood can be obtained from a finger; the recommended site is the distal digit of the third or fourth finger on its palmar surface, about 3–5 mm lateral from the nail bed. Formerly the ear lobe was commonly used, but it is no longer recommended because reduced blood flow renders it unrepresentative of the circulating blood.[1] In infants, satisfactory samples can be obtained by a deep puncture of the plantar surface of the heel in the area shown in Figure 1.1. As the heel should be really warm, it may be necessary to bathe it in hot water. The central plantar area and the posterior curvature should not be punctured in small infants to avoid the risk of injury and possible infection to the underlying tarsal bones, especially in newborns.

Clean the area with 70% alcohol (e.g. isopropanol) and allow to dry. Puncture the skin to a depth of 2–3 mm with a sterile disposable lancet. Wipe away the first drop of blood with dry sterile gauze. If necessary, squeeze very gently to encourage a free flow of blood. Collect the second and following drops directly onto a reagent strip or by a 10 ml or 20 ml micropipette for immediate dispensing into diluent. A free flow of blood is essential, and only the very gentlest squeezing is permissible; ideally, large drops of blood should exude slowly but spontaneously. If it is necessary to squeeze firmly in order to obtain blood, the results are unreliable. If the poor flow is due to the sampling site being cold and cyanosed, too high figures for haemoglobin concentration, red cell count, and leucocyte count are usually obtained.

There are methods for collecting the blood into a capillary tube fixed into the cap of a microcontainer to allow the blood to pass by capillary action into the container (e.g. *Microtainer**).[8] In another system (*Unopette**), a

Figure 1.1 Skin puncture in infants. Puncture must be restricted to the outer medial and lateral portions of the plantar surface of the foot where indicated by the shaded area.

calibrated capillary is completely filled with blood and linked to a pre-measured volume of diluent.[9] An adequate puncture with a free flow of blood can also enable a larger volume to be collected, drop by drop, into a plastic or glass container.[10]

After use, lancets (and needles) should be placed in a puncture-resistant container for subsequent waste disposal, and they must never be re-used on another individual.

BLOOD FILM PREPARATION

Ideally, blood films should be made immediately the blood has been collected. As blood samples are usually sent to the laboratory after a variable delay there are advantages in preparing blood films when the phlebotomy is carried out. The phlebotomy tray might include some clean glass slides and spreaders, and phlebotomists should be given appropriate training for film preparation as described in Chapter 4. An automated device for making smears is also available.[11] When films are not made on site they should be made in the laboratory without delay as soon as the specimens have been received.

*BD Ltd.

DIFFERENCES BETWEEN CAPILLARY AND VENOUS BLOOD

Venous blood and capillary blood are not quite the same. Blood from a skin puncture is a mixture of blood from arterioles, veins and capillaries, and it contains some interstitial and intracellular fluid.[1,4,12] Although some studies have suggested that there are negligible differences when a free flow of blood has been obtained,[13] others have shown definite differences in composition between skin puncture and venous blood samples in neonates,[14] children[15] and adults.[16] The differences may be exaggerated by cold with resulting slow capillary blood flow.[4]

The packed cell volume (PCV), red cell count (RBC) and haemoglobin concentration (Hb) of capillary blood are slightly greater than in venous blood. The total leucocyte and neutrophil counts are higher by about 8%, the monocyte count by about 12%, and in some cases by as much as 100%, especially in children. Conversely, the platelet count appears to be higher in venous than in capillary blood; this is on average by about 9% and in some cases by as much as 32%.[14-16] This may be due to adhesion of platelets to the site of the skin puncture.

SAMPLE HOMOGENEITY

In order to ensure even dispersal of the blood cells it is essential that specimens are mixed effectively immediately prior to taking a sample for testing. Place the specimen tube on a mechanical rotating mixer for at least 2 min or invert the tube 8–10 times by hand. If the specimen has been stored at 4°C, it will be viscid and the blood should be allowed to warm up to room temperature before mixing.

SERUM

The difference between plasma and serum is that the latter lacks fibrinogen and some of the coagulation factors. Blood collected in order to obtain serum should be delivered into sterile tubes with caps or commercially available plain (non-anticoagulant) evacuated collection tubes and allowed to clot undisturbed for about 1 h at room temperature.* Then loosen the clot gently from the container wall by means of a wooden stick, or a thin plastic or glass rod. Rough handling will cause lysis. Close the tube with a cap/stopper. Some products contain a clot activator combined with a gel for accelerated separation of serum, e.g. *Serum separator tubes* (BD Ltd).

---

*Room temperature is usually taken as 18–25°C.

The tubes, whether with or without a serum separator, are centrifuged for 10 min at about 1200 rpm. Pipette the supernatant serum into another tube and centrifuge again for 10 min at about 1200 rpm. Transfer the supernatant serum to tubes for tests or for storage. For most tests, serum should be kept at 4°C until used, but if testing is delayed, serum can be stored at −20°C for up to 3 months and at −40°C or lower for long-term storage. Frozen specimens should be thawed in a water-bath or in a 37°C incubator, then inverted several times to ensure homogeneity before use for a test. Do not refreeze thawed specimens.

Defibrinating Whole Blood

When the red cells are required, as in the investigation of certain types of haemolytic anaemia, the sample can be defibrinated. The morphology of the red cells and the leucocytes is well preserved. This can be performed by placing the blood in a conical flask containing a central glass rod on to which small pieces of glass capillary have been fused (Fig. 1.2). The blood is whisked

Figure 1.2 Flask for defibrinating 10–50 ml of blood. The glass rod has had some small pieces of drawn-out glass capillary fused to its lower end.

around the central rod by moderately rapid rotation of the flask. Coagulation is usually complete within about 5 min, with most of the fibrin collecting on the central rod. When fibrin formation seems complete, the glass rod should be removed from the flask. If serum is required, the blood may be centrifuged and the serum can be obtained quickly and in relatively large volumes.

COLD AGGLUTININS

If cold agglutinins are to be titrated, the blood must be kept at 37°C until the serum has separated, and if cold agglutinins are known to be present in high concentration, it is best to bring the patient to a suitable location close to the laboratory and to collect blood into a previously warmed syringe and then to deliver the blood into containers which have been kept warm at 37°C. When filled, the containers should be promptly replaced in the 37°C water-bath. In this way, it is possible to obtain serum free from haemoglobin, even when cold antibodies are present capable of causing agglutination at temperatures as high as 30°C. A practical way of warming the syringe is to place it in its container for 10 min in an oven at approximately 50°C or for 30 min or so in a 37°C incubator. When the clot has retracted in the sample and clear serum has been expressed, the serum is removed by a Pasteur pipette and transferred to a tube which has been warmed by being allowed to stand in a water-bath. It is then rapidly centrifuged so as to rid it of any suspended red cells.

ANTICOAGULANTS

EDTA and sodium citrate remove calcium which is essential for coagulation. Calcium is either precipitated as insoluble oxalate (crystals of which may be seen in oxalated blood) or bound in a non-ionized form. Heparin binds to antithrombin, thus inhibiting the interaction of several clotting factors.

EDTA is used for blood counts; sodium citrate is used for coagulation testing and the erythrocyte sedimentation rate. For better long-term preservation of red cells for certain tests and for transfusion purposes, citrate is used in combination with dextrose in the form of acid-citrate-dextrose (*ACD*), citrate-phosphate-dextrose (*CPD*) or Alsever's solution. Anticoagulant mixtures are also used to compensate for disadvantages in each and to meet the needs of the analytic process;[18,19] these include ACD, CPD or heparin combined with EDTA and EDTA, citrate, or heparin combined with sodium fluoride. Any anticoagulant can be used for collecting blood for flow cytometry.[17,19]

Ethylenediaminetetra-acetic Acid (EDTA)

The sodium and potassium salts of EDTA are powerful anticoagulants and they are especially suitable for routine haematological work. EDTA acts by its chelating effect on the calcium molecules in blood. To achieve this requires a concentration of 1.2 mg of the anhydrous salt per ml of blood (*c* 4 mmol). The dipotassium salt is very soluble (1650 g/l) and is to be preferred on this account to the disodium salt which is considerably less soluble (108 g/l).[20] Coating the inside surface of the blood collection tube with a thin layer of EDTA improves the speed of its uptake by the blood.

The dilithium salt of EDTA is equally effective as an anticoagulant,[21] and its use has the advantage that the same sample of blood can be used for chemical investigation. However, it is less soluble than the dipotassium salt (160 g/l).

The tripotassium salt dispensed in liquid form has been recommended in the USA by NCCLS.[3] However, blood delivered into this solution will be slightly diluted, and the tripotassium salt produces some shrinkage of red cells which results in a 2–3% decrease in PCV within 4 hours of collection, followed by a gradual increase in mean cell volume (MCV). By contrast, there are negligible changes when the dipotassium salt is used.[1,4] Accordingly, the International Council for Standardization in Haematology recommends the dipotassium salt at a concentration of 1.50–2.2 mg/ml of blood; the tripotassium salt may be accepted as an alternative.[22] Na_3-EDTA is not recommended because of its high pH.

Excess of EDTA, irrespective of which salt, affects both red cells and leucocytes, causing shrinkage and degenerative changes. EDTA in excess of 2 mg/ml of blood may result in a significant decrease in PCV by centrifugation and increase in mean cell haemoglobin concentration (MCHC).[4] The platelets are also affected; excess of EDTA causes them to swell and then disintegrate, causing an artificially high platelet count, as the fragments are large enough to be counted as normal platelets. Care must therefore be taken to ensure that the correct amount of blood is added, and that by repeated inversions of the container the anticoagulant is thoroughly mixed in the blood added to it. Blood films made from EDTA blood may fail to demonstrate basophilic stippling of the red cells in lead poisoning. EDTA has also been shown to cause leuco-agglutination affecting both neutrophils and lymphocytes,[23] and it is responsible for the activity of a naturally occurring antiplatelet auto-antibody which may sometimes cause platelet adherence to neutrophils in blood films. Monocyte activation measured by release of tissue factor and tumour necrosis factor activity has been reported as being lower with EDTA than with citrate and heparin. Similarly, neutrophil activation measured by lipopolysaccharide-induced release of lactoferrin is low with EDTA. EDTA also appears to suppress platelet degranulation.[24]

Trisodium Citrate

For coagulation studies, 9 volumes of blood are added to 1 volume of 109 mmol/l sodium citrate solution (32 g/l of $Na_3C_6H_5O_7.2H_2O$*).[25] This ratio of anticoagulant to blood is critical as osmotic effects and changes in free calcium ion concentration affect coagulation test results. This ratio of citrate to blood may need to be adjusted for samples with a high haematocrit requiring coagulation studies (see Chapter 18).

For the erythrocyte sedimentation rate (ESR), four volumes of blood are added to 1 volume of the sodium citrate solution (109 mmol/l) and immediately well mixed with it. The mixture is taken up in a Westergren tube.[26]

Heparin

Lithium or sodium salt of heparin at a concentration of 10–20 iu/ml of blood is a commonly used anticoagulant for chemistry, gas analysis and emergency tests. It does not alter the size of the red cells and it is recommended when it is important to reduce to a minimum the chance of lysis occurring after blood has been withdrawn. It is thus the best anticoagulant for osmotic fragility tests and is suitable for immunophenotyping.

However, heparin is not suitable for blood counts as it often induces platelet and leucocyte clumping.[4,27,28] Nor should it be used for making blood films as it gives a faint blue coloration to the background when the films are stained by Romanowsky dyes, especially in the presence of abnormal proteins. It inhibits enzyme activity[17] and it should not be used in the study of polymerase chain reaction with restriction enzymes.[29]

EFFECTS OF STORAGE ON THE BLOOD COUNT

Various changes take place in anticoagulated blood when it is stored at room temperature, and these changes occur more rapidly at higher ambient temperatures. These occur regardless of the anticoagulant, although they are less marked in blood in ACD, CPD or Alsever's solution than in EDTA blood and greater in the tripotassium salt than in the dipotassium salt of EDTA. The red cell count, white cell count, platelet count and red cell indices are usually stable for 8 h after blood collection, although as the red cells start to swell the PCV and MCV start to increase,

osmotic fragility increases and the erythrocyte sedimentation rate decreases. When the blood is kept at 4°C the effects on the blood count are not usually significant for up to 24 h. Thus, for many purposes blood may safely be allowed to stand overnight in the refrigerator if precautions against freezing are taken. Nevertheless, it is best to count leucocytes and especially platelets within 2 h and it should be noted that the fall in leucocyte count and a progressive fall in the absolute lymphocyte count may become marked within a few hours, especially if there is an excessive amount of EDTA (>4.5 mg/ml).[19] Storage beyond 24 h at 4°C results in erroneous data for automated white cell differential counts although the extent depends on instrument performance and the manufacturer's recommendation, which should be followed when an automated counting method is employed. One study using an aperture impedance analyser on blood left at room temperature showed WBC and neutrophils to be stable for 2–3 days but other leucocytes were stable for only a few hours.[30]

Reticulocyte counts are unchanged when the blood is kept in either EDTA or ACD anticoagulant for 24 h at 4°C, but at room temperature the count begins to fall within 6 h. Nucleated red cells disappear in the blood specimen within 1–2 days at room temperature.

Haemoglobin concentration remains unchanged for days, provided that the blood does not become infected, as shown by turbidity or discoloration of the specimen. However, within 2–3 days, and especially at high ambient temperatures, the blood begins to lyse, resulting in a decrease in the red cell count and PCV, with an increase in the calculated MCH and MCHC.

Coagulation test stability is critical for diagnosis and treatment of coagulopathies; NCCLS has recommended that tests be carried out within 2 h when the blood or plasma is stored at 22–24°C, 4 h at 4°C, 2 weeks at −20°C, and 6 months when stored at −70°C.[3]

For a serum or plasma test, blood should be centrifuged within 5 h of collection. For vitamin B_{12} and folate assays, the serum or plasma should be kept at 4°C or at −20°C if storage for more than 2–3 weeks is required. For long-term storage specimens should be divided into several aliquots to avoid repeated freezing and thawing.

Inappropriate handling of blood specimens during transfer to the laboratory (e.g. excess shaking) may cause haemolysis, partial coagulation and cell disintegration. Shipping of specimens requires special packaging.

EFFECTS OF STORAGE ON BLOOD CELL MORPHOLOGY

Changes in blood cell morphology of stored samples occur within a few hours of blood collection. The changes are not solely due to the presence of an anticoagulant for

---

*Or 38 g/l of $2Na_3C_6H_5O_7.11H_2O$.

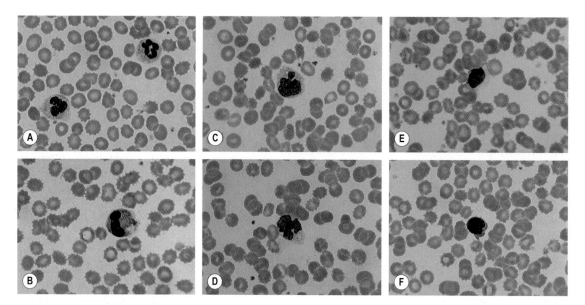

Figure 1.3 Effect of storage on blood cell morphology. Photomicrographs from films made from ethylenediaminetetra-acetic acid (EDTA) blood after 24 h at 20°C. (A,B) Polymorphonuclear neutrophils; (C,D) Monocytes; (E,F) Lymphocytes. Red cell crenation is prominent in all images.

they also occur in defibrinated blood. Irrespective of anticoagulant, films made from blood which has been standing for <1 h at room temperature are not easily distinguished from films made immediately after collection of the blood. By 3 h, changes may be discernible and by 12–18 h these become striking. Some but not all neutrophils are affected; their nuclei may stain more homogeneously than in fresh blood, the nuclear lobes may become separated and the cytoplasmic margin may appear ragged or less well defined; small vacuoles appear in the cytoplasm (Fig. 1.3A,B). Some or many of the large monocytes develop marked changes; small vacuoles appear in the cytoplasm and the nucleus undergoes irregular lobulation which may almost amount to disintegration (Fig. 1.3C). Lymphocytes undergo similar changes: a few vacuoles may be seen in the cytoplasm, nuclei stain more homogeneously than usual and in some the nucleus undergoes budding, giving rise to nuclei with two or three lobes (Fig. 1.3D–F). Normal red cells are little affected by standing for up to 6 h at room temperature. Longer periods lead to progressive crenation and sphering (Fig. 1.3B,E,F). With an excess of EDTA, a marked degree of crenation occurs within a few hours. All the above changes are retarded but not abolished in blood stored at 4°C. Their occurrence underlines the importance of making films as soon as possible after the blood has been collected. But a delay of up to 3 h is permissible.

These artefactual changes must be distinguished from apoptosis which is a controlled process of programmed cell death related to mitochondrial dysfunction in which cytokines and growth factors regulating cell survival are depleted or inhibited,[31,32] Apoptosis is characterized morphologically (Fig. 1.4) by cell shrinkage with cytoplasmic condensation around the nuclear membrane and indentations in the nucleus, followed by its fragmentation; finally the cell remnants form dense basophilic masses (the apoptotic bodies). Apoptotic neutrophils with a single apoptotic body may be confused with nucleated red cells if the cytoplasmic features are not appreciated. The remnants are removed from the circulation by phagocytosis and usually in a film only an occasional apoptotic cell is seen, surrounded by viable cells;[33] more frequent apoptotic cells can be seen in leukaemia.

Figure 1.4 Morphological features of apoptosis.

REFERENCES

1. Tatsumi N, Miwa S, Lewis SM. International Council for Standardization in Haematology/ International Society of Hematology. Specimen collection, storage, and transportation to the laboratory for hematological tests. *Int J Hematol.* 2002;75:261–268.

2. CLSI. *Procedures for the collection of diagnostic blood specimens by venipuncture. Approved standard.* 6th ed. Document H3-A6. Wayne PA: CLSI; 2007.

3. NCCLS. *Tubes and additives for venous blood specimen collection. Approved standard.* 5th ed. Wayne PA: NCCLS; 2003.

4. Van Assendelft OW, Simmons A. Specimen collection, handling, storage and variability. In: Lewis SM, Koepke JA, eds. *Hematology Laboratory Management and Practice.* Oxford: Butterworth-Heinemann; 1995:109–127.

5. Tatsumi N, van Assendelft OW, Naka K. ICSH recommendation for blood specimen collection for hematological analysis. *Lab Hematol.* 2002;8:1–6.

6. Sutton CD, White SA, Edwards R. A prospective controlled trial of the efficacy of isopropyl alcohol wipes before venesection in surgical patients. *Ann R Coll Surg.* 1999;81:183–186.

7. Golder M, Chen CLH, O'Shea S, et al. Potential risk of cross-infection during peripheral-venous access by contaminated tourniquets. *Lancet.* 2000;355:44.

8. Meitis S. Skin puncture and blood collection techniques for infants: updates and problems. *Clin Chem.* 1988;34:1890–1894.

9. Hicks JR, Rowland GL, Buffone GJ. Evaluation of a new blood collection device ('Microtainer') that is suitable for pediatric use. *Clin Chem.* 1976;22:2034–2036.

10. Freudlich MH, Gerarde HW. A new, automatic disposable system for blood count and hemoglobin. *Blood.* 1963;21:648–655.

11. Tatsumi N, Pierre R. Automated image processing; past, present, and future of blood cell morphology identification. *Clin Lab Med.* 2002;22:299–316.

12. Conway AM, Hinchliffe RF, Earland J, et al. Measurement of hemoglobin using single drops of skin puncture blood: is precision acceptable? *J Clin Pathol.* 1998;51:248–250.

13. Yang Z-W, Yang S-H, Chen L, et al. Comparison of blood counts in venous, finger tip and arterial blood and their measurement variation. *Clin Lab Haematol.* 2001;23: 155–159.

14. Kayiran SM, Özbek N, Turan M, et al. Significant differences between capillary and venous complete blood counts in the neonatal period. *Clin Lab Haematol.* 2003;25:9–16.

15. Daae LNW, Hallerud M, Halvorsen S. A comparison between haematological parameters in 'capillary' and venous blood samples from hospitalized children aged 3 months to 14 years. *Scand J Clin Lab Invest.* 1988;51:651–654.

16. Daae LNW, Halvorsen S, Mathison PM, et al. A comparison between haematological parameters in 'capillary' and venous blood from healthy adults. *Scand J Clin Lab Invest.* 1988;48:723–726.

17. Narayanan S. The pre-analytic phase: an important component of laboratory medicine. *Am J Clin Pathol.* 2000;113:429–457.

18. Tatsumi N. Universal anticoagulants. *Japanese Society of Thrombosis and Haemostasis.* 2003;13:158–168.

19. CLSI. *Clinical application of flow cytometry: quality assurance and immunophenotyping of peripheral blood lymphocytes.* Document H43-A2. Wayne PA: CLSI; 2007.

20. Hadley GG, Weiss SP. Further notes on use of salts of ethylene diaminetetraacetic acid (EDTA) as anticoagulants. *Am J Clin Pathol.* 1955;25:1090–1093.

21. Sacker LS, Saunders KE, Page B, et al. Dilithium sequestrene as an anticoagulant. *J Clin Pathol.* 1959;12:254–257.

22. International Council for Standardization in Haematology. Recommendations for ethylenediaminetetra-acetic acid anticoagulation of blood for blood cell counting and sizing. *Am J Clin Pathol.* 1993;100:371–372.

23. Deal I, Hernandez AM, Pierre RV. Ethylenediaminetetra-acetic acid-associated leukoaggulutination. *Am J Clin Pathol.* 1995;103:338–340.

24. Engstad CS, Gutteberg TJ, Osterud B. Modulation of cell activation by four commonly used anticoagulants. *Thromb Haemost.* 1997;77:690–696.

25. Ingram GIC, Hills M. The prothrombin time test; effect of varying citrate concentration. *Thromb Haemost.* 1976;36:230–236.

26. International Committee for Standardization in Haematology. Recommendation for measurement of erythrocyte sedimentation rate of human blood. *Am J Clin Pathol.* 1977;66:505–507.

27. Salzman EW, Rosenberg RD. Effect of heparin and heparin fractions on platelet aggregation. *J Clin Invest.* 1980;65:64–73.

28. Hirsh J, Levine NM. Low molecular weight heparin. *Blood.* 1992;79:1–9.

29. Yokota M, Tatsumi N, Nathalang O, et al. Effects of heparin on polymerase chain reaction for blood white cells. *J Clin Lab Anal.* 1999;13:133–140.

30. Gulati GL, Hyland LJ, Kocher W, et al. Changes in automated complete blood count and differential leucocyte count results induced by storage of blood at room temperature. *Arch Pathol Lab Med.* 2002;126:336–342.

31. Kerr JF, Wylie AH, Curie AR. Apoptosis: a basic biological phenomenon with wide-ranging implications in tissue kinetics. *Br J Cancer.* 1972;26:239–257.

32. Wylie AH, Kerr JFR, Currie AR. Cell death: the significance of apoptosis. *Int Rev Cytol.* 1980;68: 251–306.

33. Lach-Szyrma V, Brito-Babapulle F. The clinical significance of apoptotic cells in peripheral blood smears. *Clin Lab Haematol.* 1999;21: 277–280.

Chapter | 2 |

Reference ranges and normal values

Imelda Bates, S. Mitchell Lewis

A number of factors affect haematological values in apparently healthy individuals. As described in Chapter 1, these include the technique and timing of blood collection, transport and storage of specimens, differences in the subject's posture when the sample is taken, prior physical activity and whether the subject is confined to bed. Variation in the analytic methods used may also affect the measurements. These can all be standardized.

More problematic are the inherent variables as a result of sex, age, occupation, body build, genetic background and adaptation to diet and to environment (especially altitude). These factors must be recognized when establishing physiologically normal values. Furthermore, it is difficult to be certain in any survey of a population for the purposes of obtaining data from which normal ranges may be constructed, that the 'normal' subjects are completely healthy and do not have nutritional deficiencies, mild chronic infections, parasitic infestations or the effects of smoking.

Haematological values for the normal and abnormal will overlap and a value within the recognized normal range may be definitely pathological in a particular subject. For these reasons the concept of 'normal values' and 'normal ranges' has been replaced by *reference values* and the *reference range*, which is defined by *reference limits* and obtained from measurements on the *reference population* for a particular test. The reference range is also termed the *reference interval*.[1,2] Ideally, each laboratory should establish a databank of reference values that take account of the variables mentioned earlier and the test method, so that an individual's result can be expressed and interpreted relative to a comparable apparently normal population, insofar as normal can be defined.

Recently new haematological parameters such as immature forms of cells, red cell fragments and detection of functional iron deficiency or malarial infection have become available. Currently these parameters are only used for research and, as internal quality control or external quality assessments are not yet available for some of these tests, their use in clinical decision making is not recommended.[3]

REFERENCE RANGES

A reference range for a specified population can be established from measurements on a relatively small number of subjects (discussed later) if they are assumed to be representative of the population as a whole.[2] The conditions for obtaining samples from the individuals and the analytic procedures must be standardized, whereas data should be analysed separately for different variables such as individuals who are in bed or ambulant, smokers or non-smokers and so on. One approach is that specimens are collected at about the same time of day, preferably in the morning before breakfast; the last meal should have been eaten not later than 9 p.m. on the previous evening and at that time alcohol should have been restricted to one bottle of beer or an equivalent amount of other alcoholic drink.[4] An alternative approach is that, unless a test is usually done on a fasting patient, specimens are collected throughout the day on subjects who are not fasting or resting, as this will produce a reference range that is more relevant to results from patients. It is sometimes appropriate that the reference population is defined as having normal results for specific laboratory tests. For example, if determining a reference range for blood count components it may be necessary, in some populations, to exclude iron deficiency and β thalassaemia heterozygosity.

STATISTICAL PROCEDURES

In biological measurements, it is usually assumed that the data will fit a specified type of pattern, either symmetric (Gaussian) or asymmetric with a skewed distribution (non-Gaussian). With a Gaussian distribution, the *arithmetic mean* (×) can be obtained by dividing the sum of all measurements by the number of observations. The *mode* is the value that occurs most frequently and the *median* (m) is the point at which there are an equal number of observations above and below it. In a true Gaussian distribution they should all be the same. The standard deviation (SD) can be calculated as described on p. 625.

If the data fit a Gaussian distribution, when plotted as a frequency histogram the pattern shown in Figure 2.1 is obtained. Taking the mode and the calculated SD as reference points, a Gaussian curve is superimposed on the histogram. From this curve, practical reference limits can be determined even if the original histogram included outlying results from some subjects not belonging to the normal population. Limits representing the 95% reference range are calculated from arithmetic mean ± 2SD (or more accurately ± 1.96SD).

When there is a log normal (skew) distribution of measurements, the range to −2SD may even extend to zero (Fig. 2.2A). To avoid this anomaly, the data should be plotted on semilogarithmic graph paper to obtain a normal distribution histogram (Fig. 2.2B). To calculate the mean and SD the data should be converted to their logarithms. The log-mean value is obtained by adding the logs of all the measurements and dividing by the number of observations. The log SD is calculated by the formula on p. 625 and the results are then converted to their antilogs to express the data in the arithmetic scale. This process is now generally carried out using an appropriate statistical computer program.

When it is not possible to make an assumption about the type of distribution, a non-parametric procedure may be used instead to obtain the median and SD. To obtain an approximation of the SD, the range that comprises the middle 50% spread (i.e. between 25% and 75% of results) is read and divided by 1.35. This represents 1SD.

Confidence Limits

In any of the methods of analysis, a reasonably reliable estimate can be obtained with 40 values, although a larger number (≥120) is preferable (Fig. 2.3).[5] When a large set of reference values is unattainable and precise estimation is impossible, a smaller number of values may still serve as a useful clinical guide. Confidence limits define the reliability (e.g. 95% or 99%) of the established reference values when assessing the significance of a test result, especially when it is on the borderline between normal

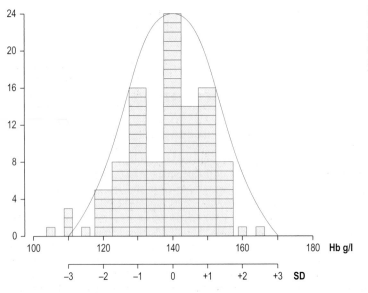

Figure 2.1 Example of establishing a reference range. Histogram of data of Hb measurements in a population, with Gaussian curve superimposed. The ordinate shows the number that occurred at each reference point. The mean was 140 g/l; the reference ranges at 1SD, 2SD and 3SD are indicated.

Figure 2.2 Example of conversion to a log normal distribution. Data of serum vitamin B_{12} measurements in a population.
(A) Arithmetic scale: mean 340; 2SD range calculated as 10–665 pg/ml.
(B) Geometric scale: mean 308; 2SD range calculated as 120–780 pg/ml.

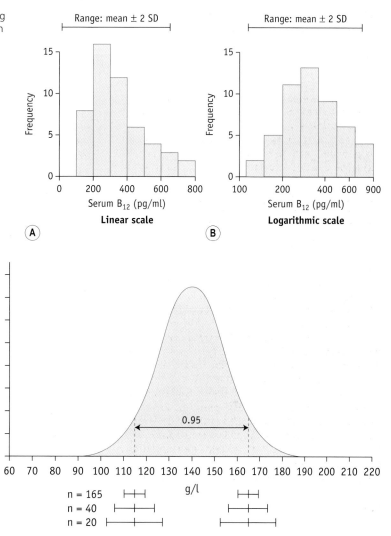

Figure 2.3 Effect of sample size on reference values. A smoothed distribution graph was obtained for Hb measurement from a group of normal women; the ordinate shows the frequency distribution. The 95% reference interval is defined by the lower and higher reference limits, which are 115 and 165 g/l, respectively. The confidence levels for these values are shown for three sample sizes of 20, 40 and 165 values, respectively.

and abnormal. Calculation of confidence limits is described on p. 625. Another important measurement is the coefficient of variation (CV) of the test because a wide CV is likely to influence its clinical utility (see p. 625).

NORMAL REFERENCE VALUES

The data given in Tables 2.1, 2.2 and 2.3 provide general guidance to normal reference values that are applicable to most healthy adults and children, respectively, in industrialized countries. The data have been derived from personal observations as well as various published reports.[6–11] However, slightly different ranges may be found in individual laboratories where different analysers and methods are used. The reference interval, which

comprises a range of ± 2SD from the mean, indicates the limits that should cover 95% of normal subjects; 99% of normal subjects will be included in a range of ± 3SD. Age and sex differences have been taken into account for some values. Even so, the wide ranges that are shown for some tests reflect the influence of various factors, as described below. Narrower ranges would be expected under standardized conditions. Because modern analysers provide a high level of technical precision, even small differences in successive measurements may be significant. It is thus important to establish and understand the limits of physiological variation for various tests. The blood count data and other test results can then provide sensitive indications of minor abnormalities that may be important in clinical interpretation and health screening.

It should be noted that in Table 2.1 the differential white cell count is shown as percentages and in absolute

Table 2.1 Haematological values for normal adults (predominantly from Europe and North America) expressed as a mean $\pm$ 2SD (95% range)

Red blood cell count

Men	$5.0 \pm 0.5 \times 10^{12}$/l
Women	$4.3 \pm 0.5 \times 10^{12}$/l

Haemoglobin concentration[a]

Men	150 ± 20 g/l
Women	135 ± 15 g/l

Packed cell volume (PCV) or Haematocrit (Hct)

Men	0.45 ± 0.05 (l/l)
Women	0.41 ± 0.05 (l/l)

Mean cell volume (MCV)

Men and women	92 ± 9 fl

Mean cell haemoglobin (MCH)

Men and women	29.5 ± 2.5 pg

Mean cell haemoglobin concentration (MCHC)

Men and women	330 ± 15 g/l

Red cell distribution width (RDW)

As coefficient of variation (CV)	$12.8 \pm 1.2\%$
As standard deviation (SD)	42.5 ± 3.5 fl

Red cell diameter (mean values)

Dry films	6.7–7.7 µm
Red cell density	1092–1100 g/l
Reticulocyte count	50–100×10^9/l (0.5–2.5%)
White blood cell count	4.0–10.0×10^9/l

Differential white cell count

Neutrophils	2.0–7.0×10^9/l (40–80%)
Lymphocytes	1.0–3.0×10^9/l (20–40%)
Monocytes	0.2–1.0×10^9/l (2–10%)
Eosinophils	0.02–0.5×10^9/l (1–6%)
Basophils	0.02–0.1×10^9/l (<1–2%)

Lymphocyte subsets (approximations from ranges in published data)

CD3	0.6–2.5×10^9/l (60–85%)
CD4	0.4–1.5×10^9/l (30–50%)
CD8	0.2–1.1×10^9/l (10–35%)
CD4/CD8 ratio	0.7–3.5
Platelet count	$280 \pm 130 \times 10^9$/l

Bleeding time[b]

Ivy's method	2–7 min
Template method	2.5–9.5 min
Thrombin time	15–19 s
Plasma fibrinogen concentration	1.8–3.6 g/l
Euglobulin clot lysis time	90–240 min
Plasminogen concentration[d]	0.75–1.60 u/ml
Antithrombin concentration[d]	0.75–1.25 u/ml

Protein C concentration[d]

Functional	0.70–1.40 u/ml
Antigen	0.61–1.32 u/ml

Protein S concentration[d]

Total antigen	0.78–1.37 u/ml
Free antigen	0.68–1.52 u/ml
Pre-menopausal women[c]	0.55–1.55 u/ml
Function	0.60–1.35 u/ml
Pre-menopausal women	0.55–1.35 u/ml
Heparin cofactor II concentration[d]	0.55–1.45 u/ml

Median red cell fragility (MCF) (g/l NaCl)

Fresh blood	4.0–4.45 g/l NaCl
After 24 h at 37°C	4.65–5.9 g/l NaCl
Cold agglutinin titre (4°C)	<64

Blood volume (normalized to 'ideal weight')
Red cell volume

Men	30 ± 5 ml/kg
Women	25 ± 5 ml/kg
Plasma volume	45 ± 5 ml/kg
Total blood volume	70 ± 10 ml/kg
Red cell lifespan	120 ± 30 days

Serum iron

Men and women	10–30 µmol/l (0.6–1.7 mg/l)
Total iron-binding capacity	47–70 µmol/l (2.5–4.0 mg/l)
Transferrin saturation	16–50%

Serum ferritin concentration

Men	15–300 µg/l (median 100 µg/l)
Women	15–200 µg/l (median 40 µg/l)
Serum vitamin B₁₂ concentration	180–640 ng/l
Serum folate concentration	3–20 µg/l (6.8–45 nmol/l)
Red cell folate concentration	160–640 µg/l (0.36–1.45 µmol/l)
Plasma haemoglobin concentration	10–40 mg/l

Serum haptoglobin concentration

Radial immunodiffusion	0.8–2.7 g/l
Haemoglobin binding capacity	0.3–2.0 g/l
HbA₂	2.2–3.5%
HbF	<1.0%
Methaemoglobin	<2.0%

Sedimentation rate (mm in 1 h at $20 \pm 3°C$)
Men

17–50 years	≤ 10
51–60 years	≤ 12
61–70 years	≤ 14
>70 years	≤ 30

Table 2.1 Haematological values for normal adults (predominantly from Europe and North America) expressed as a mean ± 2SD (95% range) – Cont'd

Women		Plasma viscosity	
17–50 years	≤12	25°C	1.50–1.72 mPa/s
51–60 years	≤19	37°C	1.16–1.33 mPa/s
61–70 years	≤20		
>70 years	≤35		

[a]Haemoglobin concentration may sometimes be reported as g/dl.
[b]Bleeding time is no longer recommended for routine assessment of haemostasis but may be useful in suspected collagen disorders.
[c]From Dykes AC, Walker ID, McMahon AD et al 2001 Protein S antigen levels in 3788 healthy volunteers. *British Journal of Haematology* 113:636–641.
[d]These ranges are for general guidance only as each laboratory should establish its own normal range.

numbers. Automated analysers provide absolute counts for each type of leucocyte and because proportional (percentage) counting is less likely to indicate correctly their absolute increase or decrease, the International Council for Standardization in Haematology has recommended that the differential leucocyte count should always be given as the absolute number of each cell type per unit volume of blood.[12] The neutrophil:lymphocyte ratio obtained from a differential leucocyte count should be regarded only as an approximation.

Reference ranges for pre-term infants vary with gestational age. In infants in the USA between 22 and 41 weeks' gestation, the packed cell volume increased from 40 to 52 l/l, the haemoglobin from 140 to 170 g/l and the platelet count from 200 to 250 × 10^9/l, whereas the MCV and MCH gradually decreased from 121 to 105 fl and 40.5 to 35.5 pg, respectively.[13]

PHYSIOLOGICAL VARIATIONS IN THE BLOOD COUNT

Red Cell Components

There is considerable variation in the red blood cell count (RBC) and haemoglobin concentration (Hb) at different periods of life and there are also transient fluctuations, the significance of which is often difficult to assess. At birth the Hb is higher than at any period subsequently (Table 2.2). The RBC is high immediately after birth,[6] and values for Hb >200 g/l, RBC higher than 6.0 × 10^{12}/l and a haematocrit (Hct) over 0.65 are encountered frequently when cord clamping is delayed and blood from the placenta and umbilical artery re-enter the infant's circulation. After the immediate postnatal period, the Hb falls fairly steeply to a minimum by about the 2nd month (Fig. 2.4). The RBC and Hct also fall, although less steeply, and the cells may become microcytic with the development of iron deficiency. The changes in the mean cell haemoglobin (MCH), mean cell haemoglobin concentration and mean cell volume (MCV) from the neonate through infancy to early childhood are shown in Tables 2.2 and 2.3.

The Hb and RBC increase gradually through childhood to reach almost adult levels by puberty.[7] However, in a health survey of apparently normal men and women in Britain, mean Hb values of 145 g/l for men and 128 g/l for women have been reported;[9] the lower normal limits for Hb (i.e. 2SD below the mean) are usually taken as 130 and 120 g/l, respectively, but in some apparently normal men and women lower limits of 120 and 110 g/l, respectively, have been noted. Statistically, at least 1% of a normal population have levels more than 3SD below the mean, but in some studies there have been considerably larger numbers.[9] It is possible that some have nutritional deficiencies, especially iron deficiency, without clinical effects. The levels in women tend to be significantly lower than those of men.[9] Apart from a hormonal influence on haemopoiesis, iron deficiency is likely to be a factor influencing the difference; the extent to which menstrual blood loss is a significant factor is not clear because a loss of up to 100 ml of blood with each period may lead to iron depletion without causing anaemia.[15] There may be ethnic differences in Hb. A major 6-year survey in the USA has shown that in socially comparable populations the Hb in Black Americans is 5–10 g/l lower than their White counterparts at all ages and as much as 20 g/l lower in the first 2 years of life.[16]

Pregnancy

In normal pregnancy, there is an increase in erythropoietic activity.[17] However, at the same time, an increase in plasma volume occurs,[18] and this results in a progressive decrease in Hb, Hct and RBC (Table 2.4). The level returns to normal about a week after delivery. There is a slight increase in MCV during the 2nd trimester.[19] Serum ferritin decreases in early pregnancy and usually remains low throughout pregnancy, even when supplementary iron is given.[20]

Table 2.2 Haematological values for normal infants (amalgamation of data derived from various sources; expressed as mean ± 2SD or 95% range)[a]

	BIRTH	DAY 3	DAY 7	DAY 14	1 MONTH	2 MONTHS	3-6 MONTHS
Red blood cell count (RBC) (× 10^{12}/l)	6.0 ± 1.0	5.3 ± 1.3	5.1 ± 1.2	4.9 ± 1.3	4.2 ± 1.2	3.7 ± 0.6	4.7 ± 0.6
Haemoglobin concentration (g/l)	180 ± 40	180 ± 30	175 ± 4	165 ± 4	140 ± 25	112 ± 18	126 ± 15
Haematocrit (Hct) (l/l)	0.60 ± 0.15	0.56 ± 0.11	0.54 ± 0.12	0.51 ± 0.2	0.43 ± 0.10	0.35 ± 0.07	0.35 ± 0.05
Mean cell volume (MCV) (fl)	110 ± 10	105 ± 13	107 ± 19	105 ± 19	104 ± 12	95 ± 8	76 ± 8
Mean cell haemoglobin (MCH) (pg)	34 ± 3	34 ± 3	34 ± 3	34 ± 3	33 ± 3	30 ± 3	27 ± 3
Mean cell haemoglobin concentration (MCHC) (g/l)	330 ± 30	330 ± 40	330 ± 50	330 ± 50	330 ± 40	320 ± 35	330 ± 30
Reticulocytes (× 10^9/l)	120-400	50-350	50-100	50-100	20-60	30-50	40-100
White blood cell count (WBC) (× 10^9/l)	18 ± 8	15 ± 8	14 ± 8	14 ± 8	12 ± 7	10 ± 5	12 ± 6
Neutrophils (× 10^9/l)	4-14	3-5	3-6	3-7	3-9	1-5	1-6
Lymphocytes (× 10^9/l)	3-8	2-8	3-9	3-9	3-16	4-10	4-12
Monocytes (× 10^9/l)	0.5-2.0	0.5-1.0	0.1-1.7	0.1-1.7	0.3-1.0	0.4-1.2	0.2-1.2
Eosinophils (× 10^9/l)	0.1-1.0	0.1-2.0	0.1-0.8	0.1-0.9	0.2-1.0	0.1-1.0	0.1-1.0
Lymphocyte subsets (× 10^9/l)[b]							
CD3		3.1-5.6				2.4-6.5	2.0-5.3
CD4		2.2-4.3				1.4-5.6	1.5-3.2
CD8		0.9-1.8				0.7-2.5	0.5-1.6
CD4/CD8 ratio		1.1-4.5				1.1-4.4	1.1-4.2
Platelets (× 10^9/l)	100-450	210-500	160-500	170-500	200-500	210-650	200-550

[a]There have been some reports of WBC and platelet counts being lower in venous blood than in capillary blood samples, although still within these reference ranges. In one study venous blood from a newborn gave lower values for Hb, RBC and WBC than capillary blood but gave higher values for platelets and lymphocytes.[14]
[b]Approximations because of wide variations that have been reported in different studies.

Table 2.3 Haematological values for normal children (amalgamation of data derived from various sources; expressed as mean ± 2SD or 95% range)

	1 YEAR	2–6 YEARS	6–12 YEARS
Red cell count ($\times 10^{12}$/l)	4.5 ± 0.6	4.6 ± 0.6	4.6 ± 0.6
Haemoglobin concentration (g/l)	126 ± 15	125 ± 15	135 ± 20
Haematocrit (Hct) or packed cell volume (PCV) (l/l)	0.34 ± 0.04	0.37 ± 0.03	0.40 ± 0.05
Mean cell volume (MCV) (fl)	78 ± 6	81 ± 6	86 ± 9
Mean cell haemoglobin (MCH) (pg)	27 ± 2	27 ± 3	29 ± 4
Mean cell haemoglobin concentration (MCHC) (g/l)	340 ± 20	340 ± 30	340 ± 30
Reticulocytes ($\times 10^9$/l)	30–100	30–100	30–100
White cell count ($\times 10^9$/l)	11 ± 5	10 ± 5	9 ± 4
Neutrophils ($\times 10^9$/l)	1–7	1.5–8	2–8
Lymphocytes ($\times 10^9$/l)	3.5–11	6–9	1–5
Monocytes ($\times 10^9$/l)	0.2–1.0	0.2–1.0	0.2–1.0
Eosinophils ($\times 10^9$/l)	0.1–1.0	0.1–1.0	0.1–1.0
Lymphocyte subsets ($\times 10^9$/l)[a]			
CD3	1.5–5.4	1.6–4.2	0.9–2.5
CD4	1.0–3.6	0.9–2.9	0.5–1.5
CD8	0.6–2.2	0.6–2.0	0.4–1.2
CD4/CD8 ratio	1.0–3.0	0.9–2.7	1.0–3.0
Platelets ($\times 10^9$/l)	200–550	200–490	170–450

[a]Approximations because wide variations have been reported in different studies.

Figure 2.4 Changes in Hb values in the first 2 years after birth. The perpendicular lines show means and 2SD ranges.

Table 2.4 Haemoglobin concentration values in pregnancy

1st trimester	124–135 g/l
2nd trimester	110–117 g/l
3rd trimester	106–109 g/l[a]
Mean values postpartum	
Day 2	104 g/l
Week 1	107 g/l
Week 3	116 g/l
Month 2	119 g/l

[a]Higher values (120 g/l or higher) may be found when supplementary iron is being given.

athletes may also have decreased levels of serum iron and ferritin, possibly associated with loss of iron in sweat. Conversely, in sprinters who require a short burst of very strenuous muscular activity, there is a transient increase in RBC by 0.5×10^{12}/l and in Hb by 15 g/l, largely because of reduction in plasma volume and to a lesser extent the re-entry into the circulation of cells previously sequestered in the spleen.[30] The effects of exercise must be distinguished from a form of haemolysis known as 'runner's anaemia' or 'march haemoglobinuria', which occurs as a result of pounding of the feet on the ground.[31]

Posture

There is a small but significant alteration in the plasma volume with an increase in haemoglobin and Hct as the posture changes from lying to sitting, especially in women[32]; conversely, changing from walking to lying down results in a 5–10% decrease in the Hb and Hct. Thus, subjects should rest for 5–10 min before their blood is collected. The difference in position of the arm during venous sampling, whether dependent or held at atrial level, can also affect the Hct.

These aspects highlight the relevance of using a standardized method for blood collection, although this is not necessarily practicable in routine practice. This is discussed in Chapter 1 and the differences between venous and capillary blood are described on p. 5.

The Elderly

In healthy men and women, Hb, RBC, Hct and other red cell indices remain remarkably constant until the 6th decade. Anaemia becomes more common in those older than 70–75 years[21,22] and is associated with poor clinical outcomes due to poorer cognitive status, increased frailty and an elevated risk of hospitalization and of complications during hospitalization.[23] In the elderly, the difference in Hb between men and women is less than in younger subjects, so that a difference of 20 g/l in younger age groups is reduced to 10 g/l or less in the elderly. There is a concomitant increase in serum iron in women, although serum ferritin levels remain higher in men than in women. Factors which contribute to the lower Hb in the elderly include renal insufficiency, inflammation, testosterone deficiency, diminished erythropoiesis, stem cell proliferative decline and myelodysplasia.[24,25] Moderate or severe anaemia should never be attributed to ageing *per se* until underlying disease has been excluded; however, a significant number of elderly subjects with anaemia have no identifiable clinical or nutritional causes.

Diurnal and Seasonal Variation

Changes in Hb and RBC during the course of the day are usually slight, about 3%, with negligible changes in the MCV and MCH. However, variation of 20% occurs with reticulocytes.[8] Studies of diurnal variation of serum erythropoietin have shown conflicting results.[33] Pronounced, but variable, diurnal variations are seen in serum iron and ferritin and in patients taking iron-containing supplements.[34,35] It has been suggested that minor seasonal variations also occur, but the evidence for this is conflicting.[36–38]

Exercise

Optimal athletic performance depends on proper function of many organs, including the blood. Several haematological parameters can affect or be influenced by physical activity including blood cells and coagulation mechanisms.[26] For example endurance athletes may develop so-called 'sports anaemia', which is thought to be the result of increased plasma volume.[27,28] Increasing oxygen delivery by raising the haematocrit is a simple acute method to improve athletic performance. Legal means of raising the haematocrit include altitude training and hypoxic tents. Illegal means include blood doping and the administration of erythropoietin (EPO) (see Chapter 6).[29] Endurance

Altitude

The effect of altitude is to reduce plasma volume, increase the Hb and Hct and raise the number of circulating red cells with a lower MCV.[39] The magnitude of the polycythaemia depends on the degree of hypoxaemia. At an altitude of 2000 m (c 6500 ft), Hb is c 8–10 g/l and Hct is 0.025 higher than at sea level; at 3000 m (c 10 000 ft), Hb is c 20 g/l and Hct is 0.060 higher and at 4000 m (c 13 000 ft) Hb is 35 g/l and Hct is 0.110 higher. Corresponding increases occur at intermediate and at higher altitudes.[40] These increases appear to be the result of both increased erythropoiesis which is secondary to the hypoxic stimulus and the decrease in plasma volume that occurs at high altitudes.

Smoking

Cigarette smoking affects Hb, RBC, Hct and MCV (see p. 20).

Leucocyte Count

The effect of age is indicated in Tables 2.1, 2.2 and 2.3; at birth, the total leucocyte count is high; neutrophils predominate, reaching a peak of c $13.0 \times 10^9/l$ within 6–8 h for neonates of >28 weeks' gestation and 24 h for those delivered at <28 weeks.[13] The count then falls to c $4.0 \times 10^9/l$ over the next few weeks and then to a level at which the count remains steady. The lymphocytes decrease during the first 3 days of life often to a low level of c 2.0–2.5 $\times 10^9/l$ and then rise up to the 10th day; after this time, they are the predominant cell (up to about 60%) until the 5th to 7th year, when they give way to the neutrophils. From that age onwards, the levels are the same as for adults.[7] There are also slight sex differences; the total leucocyte count and the neutrophil count may be slightly higher in girls than in boys,[7] and in women than in men.[41] After the menopause, the counts fall in women so that they tend to become lower than in men of similar age.[41]

People differ considerably in their leucocyte counts. Some tend to maintain a relatively constant level over long periods; others have counts that may vary by as much as 100% at different times. In some subjects, there appears to be a rhythm, occurring in cycles of 14–28 days and in women this may be related to the menstrual cycle or to oral contraception.[41] There is no clearcut diurnal variation, but minimum counts are found in the morning with the subject at rest and during the course of a day there may be differences of 14% for the total leucocyte count, 10% for neutrophils, 14% for lymphocytes and 20% for eosinophils;[8] in some cases this may result in a reversed neutrophil:lymphocyte ratio. Random activity may raise the count slightly; strenuous exercise causes increases of up to $30 \times 10^9/l$, partly because of mobilization of marginated neutrophils and changes in cortisol levels.[42] Large numbers of lymphocytes and monocytes also enter the bloodstream during strenuous exercise. However, there have also been reports of neutropenia and lymphopenia in athletes undergoing daily training sessions.[43,44]

Epinephrine (adrenaline) injection causes an increase in the numbers of all major types of leucocytes (and platelets), possibly reflecting the extent of the reservoir of mature blood cells present not only in the bone marrow and spleen but also in other tissues and organs of the body. Emotion may possibly cause an increase in the leucocyte count in a similar way. A transient lymphocytosis with a reversed neutrophil:lymphocyte ratio occurs in adults with physical stress or trauma.[45] The effect of ingestion of food is uncertain. Cigarette smoking has an effect on the leucocyte count (see p. 20).

Table 2.5 [a]Effects of cigarette smoking[53–59]

INCREASED	DECREASED
Haemoglobin concentration (Hb)	Plasma volume
Red cell count (RBC)	Protein S
Haematocrit (Hct)	
Mean cell volume (MCV)	
Mean cell haemoglobin (MCH)	
White cell count (WBC)	
Neutrophil count	
Lymphocyte count	
T cells (CD4-positive)	
Monocyte count	
Carboxyhaemoglobin (>2%)	
Platelet count (transient)	
Mean platelet volume	
Fibrinogen concentration	
β-thromboglobulin concentration	
von Willebrand factor	
Red cell mass	
Haptoglobin concentration	
Plasma viscosity	
Whole blood viscosity	
Erythrocyte sedimentation rate (ESR)	

[a]Extent of change from normal reference values varies with individuals and amount smoked; some effects may occur only during and immediately after smoking. Some effects may be transient and their severity varies between individuals as well as with the number of cigarettes smoked.

A moderate leucocytosis of up to $15 \times 10^9/l$ is common during pregnancy, owing to a neutrophilia, with the peak in the 2nd trimester.[19] The count returns to non-pregnancy levels a week or so after delivery.[46]

In individuals of African ancestry there is a tendency for the neutrophil:lymphocyte ratio to be reversed primarily due to a reduction in neutrophil count. This is thought to be due to genetic rather than environmental factors because significantly lower leucocyte counts, especially neutrophil counts, have also been observed in Africans and Afro-Caribbeans living in Britain.[47] 'Benign ethnic neutropenia' occurs in up to 5% of African Americans and is defined as a neutrophil count $<1.5 \times 10^9$/l without overt cause or complications.[48] A region on chromosome 1, possibly the Duffy Null polymorphism, has recently been associated with the difference in WBC and neutrophil count between African Americans and European Americans.[49] Elderly people receiving influenza vaccination show a lower total leucocyte count owing to a decrease in lymphocytes.[50]

Platelet Count

There is a slight diurnal variation in the platelet count of about 5%;[8] this occurs during the course of a day as well as from day-to-day. Within the wide normal reference range, there are some ethnic differences and in healthy West Indians and Africans platelet counts may on average be 10–20% lower than those in Europeans living in the same environment.[51] There may be a sex difference; thus, in women, the platelet count has been reported to be about 20% higher than in men.[52] A decrease in the platelet count may occur in women at about the time of menstruation. There are no obvious age differences; however, in the 1st year after birth the platelet count tends to be at the higher level of the adult normal reference range. Strenuous exercise causes a 30–40% increase in platelet count;[42] the mechanism is similar to that which occurs with leucocytes.

Other Blood Constituents

As with the blood count, variations from normal reference values occur in respect of sex, age, exercise, stress, diurnal fluctuation and so on. These are described in the relevant chapters.

EFFECTS OF SMOKING

Both active and passive cigarette smoking have a significant effect on many haematological normal reference values.[53,54] Some effects may be transient and their severity varies between individuals as well as by the number of cigarettes smoked. Smoking ≥ 10 cigarettes a day results in slightly higher Hb, Hct and MCV.[38,55] This is probably at least in part a consequence of the accumulation of carboxyhaemoglobin in the blood together with a decrease in plasma volume. After a single cigarette, the carboxyhaemoglobin level increases by about 1%,[56] and in heavy smokers the carboxyhaemoglobin may constitute $c4$–5% of the total Hb. Smoking may be associated with polycythaemia.[57]

The leucocyte count increases, largely as a result of an increase in the neutrophils and neutrophil function may be affected.[53,58] Smoking may also cause an increase in CD4-positive lymphocytes and total lymphocyte count.[53,58,59]

Smokers tend to have higher platelet counts than non-smokers, but the counts decrease rapidly on cessation of smoking.[53] Studies of platelet aggregation and adhesiveness have given equivocal results, but there appears to be a consistent increase in platelet turnover with decreased platelet survival and increased plasma β-thromboglobulin. Elevated fibrinogen concentration (with increased plasma viscosity) and reduced protein S have been reported, but smoking does not seem to have any consistent effects on the fibrinolytic system.[53]

The influence of smoking on the blood is summarized in Table 2.5.

REFERENCES

1. International Committee for Standardization in Haematology. The theory of reference values. *Clin Lab Haematol.* 1981;3:369–373.

2. International Federation of Clinical Chemistry and International Council for Standardization in Haematology. The theory of reference values Part 6: Presentation of observed values related to reference values. *Journal of Clinical Biochemistry.* 1987;25:657–662.

3. Briggs C. Quality counts: new parameters in blood cell counting. *International Journal of Laboratory Hematology.* 2009;31:277–297.

4. International Committee for Standardization in Haematology. Standardization of blood specimen collection procedures for reference values. *Clin Lab Haematol.* 1982;4:83–86.

5. International Federation of Clinical Chemistry and International Council for Standardization in Haematology. The theory of reference values Part 5: Statistical treatment of collected reference values. Determination of reference limits. *J Clin Chem Clin Biochem.* 1987;25:645–656.

6. Lilleyman JS, Hann IM, Blanchette VS. *Pediatric Hematology.* 2nd ed. London: Churchill Livingstone; 1999.

7. Taylor MRH, Holland CV, Spencer R, et al. Haematological reference ranges for school children. *Clin Lab Haematol.* 1997;19:1–15.

8. Richardson Jones A, Twedt D, Swaim W, et al. Diurnal change of blood count analytes in normal subjects. *Am J Clin Pathol.* 1996;106:723–727.

9. White A, Nicolaas G, Foster K, et al. *Health Survey for England: Office of population census and surveys – Social Survey Division.* London: HMSO; 1991.

10. Bellamy GJ, Hinchliffe RF, Crawshaw KC. Total and differential leucocyte counts in infants at 2, 5 and 13 months of age. *Clin Lab Haematol.* 2000;22:81–87.

11. Handin RI, Lux SE, Stossel TP. *Blood – Principles and Practice of Hematology.* 2nd ed. Philadelphia PA: Lippincott Williams and Wilkins; 2003:2219.

12. International Council for Standardization in Haematology: Expert Panel on Cytometry. Recommendation of the International Council for Standardization in Haematology on reporting differential leucocyte counts. *Clin Lab Haematol.* 1995;17:113.

13. Christensen RD, Henry E, Jopling J, et al. The CBC: reference ranges for neonates. *Semin Perinatol.* 2009;33: 3–11.

14. Kayiran SM, Özbek N, Turan M, et al. Significant differences between capillary and venous complete blood counts in the neonatal period. *Clin Lab Haematol.* 2003;25:9–16.

15. Masse PG, Roberge AG. Long-term effect of low-dose combined steroid contraceptives on body iron status. *Contraception.* 1992;46:243–252.

16. Houwen B, van Assendelft OW. Haemoglobinometry: screening and routine practice. In: Rowan RM, van Assendelft OW, Preston FE, eds. *Advanced Laboratory Methods in Haematology.* London: Arnold; 2002:182–190.

17. McMullin MF, White R, Lappin T, et al. Haemoglobin during pregnancy: relationship to erythropoietin and haematinic status. *Eur J Haematol.* 2003;71:44–50.

18. Large RD, Dynesius R. Blood volume changes during normal pregnancy. *Clin Haematol.* 1973;2:433–451.

19. Balloch AJ, Cauchi MN. Reference ranges for haematology parameters in pregnancy derived from patient populations. *Clin Lab Haematol.* 1993;15:7–14.

20. Howells MR, Jones SE, Napier JAF, et al. Erythropoiesis in pregnancy. *Br J Haematol.* 1986;64:595–599.

21. Carmel R. Anemia and aging: an overview of clinical, diagnostic and biological issues. *Blood Rev.* 2001;15:9–18.

22. Nilsson-Ehle H, Jagenburg R, Landahl S, et al. Blood haemoglobin declines in the elderly: implications for reference intervals from age 70 to 85. *Eur J Haematol.* 2000;65: 297–305.

23. Steensma DP, Tefferi A. Anemia in the elderly: how should we define it, when does it matter and what can be done? *Mayo Clin Proc.* 2007;82: 958–966.

24. Makipour S, Kanapuru B, Ershler WB. Unexplained anemia in the elderly. *Semin Hematol.* 2008;45:250–254.

25. Price EA. Aging and erythropoiesis: current state of knowledge. *Blood Cells Mol Dis.* 2008;41: 158–165.

26. Mercer KW, Densmore JJ. Hematologic disorders in the athlete. *Clin Sports Med.* 2005;24:599–621, ix.

27. Smith JA. Exercise, training and red blood cell turnover. *Sports Med.* 1995;19:9–31.

28. Green HJ, Sutton JR, Coates G, et al. Response of red cell and plasma volume to prolonged training in humans. *J Appl Physiol.* 1991;70: 1810–1815.

29. Cooper CE. The biochemistry of drugs and doping methods used to enhance aerobic sport performance. *Essays Biochem.* 2008;44:63–83.

30. Allsop P, Peters AM, Arnot RN, et al. Intrasplenic blood cell kinetics in man before and after brief maximal exercise. *Clin Sci.* 1992;83:47–54.

31. Davidson RJL. March or exertional haemoglobinuria. *Seminars in Haematology.* 1964;6:150–161.

32. Felding P, Tryding N, Hyltoft Petersen P, et al. Effects of posture on concentration of blood constituents in healthy adults: practical application of blood specimen collection procedures recommended by the Scandinavian Committee on Reference Values. *Scand J Clin Lab Invest.* 1980;40: 615–621.

33. Gunga HC, Kirsch KA, Roecker L, et al. Erythropoietin regulations in humans under different environmental and experimental conditions. *Respir Physiol Neurobiol.* 2007;158:287–297.

34. Romslo I, Talstad I. Day-to-day variations in serum iron, serum iron binding capacity, serum ferritin and erythrocyte protoporphyrin concentration in anaemic subjects. *Eur J Haematol.* 1988;40:79.

35. Dale JC, Burritt MF, Zinsmeister AR. Diurnal variation of serum iron, iron-binding capacity, transferrin saturation and ferritin levels. *Am J Clin Pathol.* 2002;117:802–808.

36. Costongs GM, Janson PCW, Bas BM, et al. Short-term and long-term intra-individual variations and critical differences of haematological laboratory parameters. *J Clin Chem Clin Biochem.* 1985;23:69–76.

37. Ross DW, Ayscue LH, Watson J, et al. Stability of hematologic parameters in healthy subjects: intraindividual versus interindividual variation. *Am J Clin Pathol.* 1988;90:262–267.

38. Kristal-Boneh E, Froom P, Harari G, et al. Seasonal differences in blood cell parameters and the association with cigarette smoking. *Clin Lab Haematol.* 1997;19:177–181.

39. Saunders PU, Pyne DB, Gore CJ. Endurance training at altitude. *High Alt Med Biol.* 2009;10:135–148.

40. Myhre LD, Dill DB, Hall FG, et al. Blood volume changes during three week residence at high altitude. *Clin Chem.* 1970;16:7–14.

41. England JM, Bain BJ. Total and differential leucocyte count. *Br J Haematol.* 1976;33:1–7.

42. Avloniti AA, Douda HT, Tokmakidis SP, et al. Acute effects of soccer training on white blood cell count in elite female players. *International Journal of Sports Physiology & Performance.* 2007;2: 239–249.

43. Watson HG, Meiklejohn DJ. Leucopenia in professional football players. *Br J Haematol.* 2001;112:824–827.

44. Bain BJ, Phillips D, Thomson K, et al. Investigation of the effect of marathon running on leucocyte counts of subjects of different ethnic origins: relevance to the aetiology of ethnic neutropenia. *Br J Haematol.* 2000;108:483–487.

45. Karandikar NJ, Hotchkiss EC, McKenna RW. Transient stress lymphocytosis: an immunophenotypic characterization of the most common cause of newly identified adult lymphocytosis in a tertiary hospital. *Am J Clin Pathol.* 2002;117:819–825.

46. Cruickshank JM. The effects of parity on the leucocyte count in pregnant and non-pregnant women. *Br J Haematol.* 1970;18:531–540.

47. Bain BJ, Seed M, Godsland I. Normal values for peripheral blood white cell counts in women of four different ethnic origins. *J Clin Pathol.* 1984;37:188–193.

48. Hsieh MM, Everhart JE, Byrd-Holt DD, et al. Prevalence of neutropenia in the U.S. population: age, sex, smoking status and ethnic differences. *Ann Intern Med.* 2007;146:486–492.

49. Reich D, Nalls MA, Kao WH, et al. Reduced neutrophil count in people of African descent is due to a regulatory variant in the Duffy antigen receptor for chemokines gene. *PLoS Genet.* 2009;5:e1000360.

50. Cummins D, Wilson ME, Foulger KJ, et al. Haematological changes associated with influenza vaccination in people aged over 65: case report and prospective study.

51. Bain BJ, Seed M. Platelet count and platelet size in healthy Africans and West Indians. *Clin Lab Haematol.* 1986;8:43–48.

52. Stevens RF, Alexander MK. A sex difference in the platelet count. *Br J Haematol.* 1977;37:295–300.

53. Bain BJ. The haematological effects of smoking. *Journal of Smoking-related Diseases.* 1992;3:99–108.

54. Andrews JO, Tingen MS. The effect of smoking, smoking cessation and passive smoke exposure on common laboratory values in clinical settings: a review of the evidence. *Crit Care Nurs Clin North Am.* 2006;18: 63–69, xii.

55. Whitehead TP, Robinson D, Allaway SL, et al. The effects of cigarette smoking and alcohol *Clin Lab Haematol.* 1998;20: 285–287.

consumption on blood haemoglobin, erythrocytes and leucocytes: a dose related study on male subjects. *Clin Lab Haematol.* 1995;17:131–138.

56. Russell MA, Wilson C, Cole PV, et al. Comparison of increases in carboxyhaemoglobin after smoking 'extramild' and 'non mild' cigarettes. *Lancet.* 1973;2: 687–690.

57. Smith JR, Landaw SA. Smoker's polycythemia. *N Engl J Med.* 1978;298:6–10.

58. Parry H, Cohen S, Schlarb J. Smoking, alcohol consumption and leukocyte counts. *Am J Clin Pathol.* 1997;107:64–67.

59. Bain BJ, Rothwell M, Feher MD, et al. Acute changes in haematological parameters on cessation of smoking. *J R Soc Med.* 1992;85:80–82.

Chapter 3

Basic haematological techniques

Carol Briggs, Barbara J. Bain

It is possible to use manual, semiautomated or automated techniques to determine the various components of the full blood count (FBC). Manual techniques are generally low cost with regard to equipment and reagents but are labour intensive; automated techniques entail high capital costs but permit rapid performance of a large number of blood counts by a smaller number of laboratory workers. Automated techniques are more precise, but their accuracy depends on correct calibration and the use of reagents that are usually specific for the particular analyser. Many laboratories now use automated techniques almost exclusively, but certain manual techniques are necessary as reference methods for standardization. Manual methods may also be needed to deal with samples that have unusual characteristics that may give discrepant results with automated analysers.

All the tests discussed in this chapter can be performed on venous or free-flowing capillary blood that has been anticoagulated with ethylenediaminetetra-acetic acid (EDTA) (see p. 6). Thorough mixing of the blood specimen before sampling is essential for accurate test results. Ideally, tests should be performed within 6 h of obtaining the blood specimen because some test results are altered by longer periods of storage. However, results that are sufficiently reliable for clinical purposes can usually be obtained on blood stored for up to 24 h at 4°C (see p. 7).

HAEMOGLOBINOMETRY

The haemoglobin concentration (Hb) of a solution may be estimated by measurement of its colour, by its power of combining with oxygen or carbon monoxide or by its iron content. The methods to be described are all colour or light-intensity matching techniques, which also measure, to a varying extent, any methaemoglobin (Hi) or sulphaemoglobin (SHb) that may be present. The oxygen-combining capacity of blood is 1.34 ml O_2 per g haemoglobin. Ideally, for assessing *clinical* anaemia, a functional estimation of Hb should be carried out by measurement of oxygen capacity, but this is hardly practical in the routine haematology laboratory. It gives results that are at least 2% lower than those given by the other methods, probably because a small proportion of inert pigment is always present. The iron content of haemoglobin can be estimated accurately,[1] but again the method is impractical for routine purposes. Estimations based on iron content are generally taken as authentic, but iron bound to inactive pigment is included. Iron content is converted into haemoglobin by assuming the following relationship: 0.347 g iron = 100 g haemoglobin.[2]

MEASUREMENT OF HAEMOGLOBIN CONCENTRATION USING A SPECTROMETER (SPECTROPHOTOMETER) OR PHOTOELECTRIC COLORIMETER

Two methods are in common use: (1) haemiglobincyanide (HiCN; cyanmethaemoglobin) method and (2) oxyhaemoglobin (HbO_2) method. There is little to choose in accuracy between these methods, although a major advantage of the HiCN method is the availability of a stable and reliable reference preparation.

Although the HiCN reagent contains cyanide, there is only 50 mg of potassium cyanide per litre and 600–1000 ml would have to be swallowed to produce serious effects. However, the use of potassium cyanide has been viewed as a potential hazard; alternative nonhazardous reagents that have been proposed are sodium azide[3] and sodium lauryl sulphate,[4,5] which convert haemoglobin to haemiglobinazide and haemiglobinsulphate, respectively. They are used in some automated systems, but no stable standards are available and they, too, are toxic substances that must be handled with care.

Other methods that have been used include Sahli's acid-haematin method, which is less accurate because the colour develops slowly, is unstable and begins to fade almost immediately after it reaches its peak. The alkaline-haematin method gives a true estimate of total Hb even if carboxyhaemoglobin (HbCO), Hi or SHb is present; plasma proteins and lipids have little effect on the development of colour, although they cause turbidity. The original method was more cumbersome and less accurate than the HiCN or HbO_2 methods, but a modified method has been developed in which blood is diluted in an alkaline solution with non-ionic detergent and read in a spectrometer at an absorbance of 575 nm against a standard solution of chlorohaemin.[6,7] One evaluation has given encouraging results,[8] although another study has shown a bias of 2.6% when compared with the reference method, with non-linearity in the relationship between haemoglobin concentration and absorbance at high and low haemoglobins.[9]

HAEMIGLOBINCYANIDE (CYANMETHAEMOGLOBIN) METHOD

The haemiglobincyanide (cyanmethaemoglobin) method is the internationally recommended method[2] for determining the haemoglobin concentration of blood. In some countries cyanide reagents are no longer available. The basis of the method is dilution of blood in a solution containing potassium cyanide and potassium ferricyanide. Haemoglobin, Hi and HbCO, but not SHb, are converted to HiCN. The absorbance of the solution is then measured in a spectrometer at a wavelength of 540 nm or a photoelectric colorimeter with a yellow-green filter (e.g. Ilford 625, Wratten 74, Chance 0 Gr1).

Diluent

The original (Drabkin's) reagent had a pH of 8.6. The following modified solution listed in Table 3.1, Drabkin-type reagent, as recommended by the International Committee for Standardization in Haematology (ICSH),[2] has a pH of 7.0–7.4. It is less likely to cause turbidity from precipitation of plasma proteins and requires a shorter conversion time (3–5 min) than the original Drabkin's solution, but it has the disadvantage that the detergent causes some frothing.

The pH should be 7.0–7.4 and must be checked with a pH meter at least once a month. The diluent should be clear and pale yellow in colour. When measured against water as a blank in a spectrometer at a wavelength of 540 nm, absorbance must be zero. If stored at room temperature in a brown borosilicate glass bottle, the solution keeps for several months. If the ambient temperature is

Table 3.1 Drabkin-type reagent

Potassium ferricyanide (0.607 mmol/l)	200 mg
Potassium cyanide (0.768 mmol/l)	50 mg
Potassium dihydrogen phosphate (1.029 mmol/l)	140 mg
Non-ionic detergent[a]	1 ml
Distilled or deionized water	To 1 litre

[a]Suitable non-ionic detergents include Nonidet P40 (VWR International, Merck, Eurolab) and Triton X-100 (Aldrich).

higher than 30°C, the solution should be stored in the refrigerator but brought to room temperature before use. It must not be allowed to freeze. The reagent must be discarded if it becomes turbid, if the pH is found to be outside the 7.0–7.4 range or if it has an absorbance other than zero at 540 nm against a water blank.

Haemiglobincyanide Reference Standard

With the advent of HiCN solution, which is stable for many years, other standards have become outmoded.[10] The International Committee for Standardization in Haematology[2] has defined specifications on the basis of a relative molecular mass (molecular weight) of human haemoglobin of 64 458 (i.e. 16 114 as the monomer) and a millimolar area absorbance (coefficient extinction) of 11.0 (that is, the absorbance at 540 nm of a solution containing 55.8 mg of haemoglobin iron per litre).

Some standards are prepared from ox blood, which has the same coefficient extinction but a molecular weight of 64 532 (16 133 as the monomer). These specifications have been widely adopted; a World Health Organization (WHO) International Standard has been established and a comparable reference material is available from the ICSH. A new lot of the haemoglobincyanide or haemoglobin standard was released in 2008.[11] This newly released standard replaces the previous lot and was produced using the same methodology previously specified by ICSH.[2] The current standard has an assigned concentration value of 574.2 ($\pm$ 5.1) mg/l or 35.63 ($\pm$ 0.32) µmol/l; the exact concentration is indicated on the label. The stability expectation of this standard is 15 years[11] but it will continue to be monitored on a twice-yearly basis over the lifetime of this lot of reference material. The haemoglobin standard provides a reference material from which both laboratory-based cell counters and point-of-care instruments calibrate their haemoglobin methods.[2]

The HiCN solution is dispensed in 10 ml sealed ampoules and is regarded as a dilution of whole blood.

The original Hb that it represents is obtained by multiplying the figure stated on the label by the dilution to be applied to the blood sample. Thus, if the standard solution contains 800 mg (0.8 g) of haemoglobin per litre, it will have the same optical density as a blood sample containing 160 g/l of haemoglobin if diluted 1 to 200 or as one containing 200 g/l of haemoglobin if diluted 1 to 250. Within the SI system, haemoglobin may be expressed in terms of substance concentration as $\mu mol/l$ or in mass concentration as g/l (or g/dl) or $\mu mol/l = g/l \times 0.062$. For clinical purposes, there are practical advantages in expressing haemoglobin in mass concentration per litre or per decilitre (dl).

The HiCN reference preparation is intended primarily for direct comparison with blood that is converted to HiCN. It can also be used for the standardization of a whole-blood standard in the HbO_2 method (discussed later).

Method

Make a 1 in 201 dilution of blood by adding 20 μl of blood to 4 ml of diluent. Stopper the tube containing the solution and invert it several times. Let the test sample stand at room temperature for at least 5 min (to ensure the complete conversion of haemoglobin to haemiglobincyanide) and then pour it into a cuvette and read the absorbance in a spectrometer at 540 nm or in a photoelectric colorimeter with a suitable filter (e.g. Ilford 625, Wratten 74, Chance 0 Gr1) against a reagent blank. The absorbance of the test sample must be measured within 6 h of its initial dilution. The absorbance of a commercially available HiCN standard (brought to room temperature if previously stored in a refrigerator) should also be compared to a reagent blank in the same spectrometer or photoelectric colorimeter as the patient sample. The standard should be kept in the dark and, to ensure that contamination is avoided, any unused solution should be discarded at the end of the day on which the ampoule is opened.

Calculation of Haemoglobin Concentration

$$\frac{Hb}{(g/l)} = \frac{*A^{540} \text{ of test sample}}{A^{540} \text{ of standard}} \times \text{Conc. of standard} \times \frac{\text{Dilution factor } (201)^{\dagger}}{1000}$$

---

*Absorbance of a solution containing 5.8 mg of haemoglobin iron per litre at 540 mm.

†Or 251 if initial dilution is 1 in 250 (i.e. 20 μl blood to 5 ml reagent).

Preparation of Standard Graph and Standard Table

When many blood samples are to be tested, it is convenient to read the results from a standard graph or table relating absorbance readings to haemoglobin in g/l for the individual instrument. This graph should be prepared each time a new photometer is put into use or when a bulb or other component is replaced. It can be prepared as follows.

Prepare five dilutions of the HiCN reference standard (or equivalent preparation) (brought to room temperature) with the cyanide-ferricyanide reagent according to Table 3.2. Because the graph will be used to determine the haemoglobin measurements, it is essential that the dilutions are performed accurately.

The haemoglobin concentration of the reference preparation in each tube should be plotted against the absorbance measurement. For example, if the label on the reference preparation states that it contains 800 mg/l (i.e. 0.8 g/l) and the method for haemoglobin measurement uses a dilution of 1:201, the respective haemoglobin concentrations of tubes 1–5 would be 160 g/l, 120 g/l, 80 g/l, 40 g/l and zero.

Using linear graph paper, plot the absorbance values on the vertical axis and the haemoglobin values (absorbance; formerly called optical density) on the horizontal axis. (If the readings are in percentage transmittance, use semilogarithmic paper with the transmittance recorded on the vertical or log scale.) The points should fit a straight line that passes through the origin. Providing that the standard has been correctly diluted, this provides a check that the calibration of the photometer is linear. From the graph, it is possible to construct a table of readings and corresponding haemoglobin values. This is more convenient than reading values from a graph when large numbers of measurements are made. It is important that

Table 3.2 Dilutions of haemiglobincyanide (HiCN) reference solution for preparation of standard graph

TUBE	HAEMOGLOBIN[a] (%)	HiCN volume (ml)	REAGENT VOLUME (ml)
1	100 (full strength)	4.0 (neat)	None
2	75	3.0	1.0
3	50	2.0	2.0
4	25	1.0	3.0
5	0	None	4.0 (neat)

[a]As percentage of haemoglobin in reference solution.

the performance of the instrument does not vary and that its calibration remains constant in relation to haemoglobin measurements. To ensure this, the reference preparation should be measured at frequent intervals, preferably with each batch of blood samples.

The main advantages of the HiCN method for haemoglobin determination are that it allows direct comparison with the reference standard and that the readings need not be made immediately after dilution so batching of samples is possible. It also has the advantage that all forms of haemoglobin, except SHb, are readily converted to HiCN.

The rate of conversion of blood containing HbCO is markedly slow. This difficulty can be overcome by prolonging the reaction time to 30 min before reading.[12] The difference between the 5 and 30 min readings can be used as a semiquantitative method for estimating the percentage of HbCO in the blood.

As referred to earlier, lauryl sulphate[5] or sodium azide[3] can be used as non-hazardous substitutes for potassium cyanide. However, no stable standards are available for these methods so a sample of blood that has first had a haemoglobin value assigned by the HiCN method needs to be used as a secondary standard.

Abnormal plasma proteins or a high leucocyte count may result in turbidity when the blood is diluted in the Drabkin-type reagent. The turbidity can be avoided by centrifuging the diluted sample or by increasing the concentration of potassium dihydrogen phosphate to 33 mmol/l (4.0 g/l).[13]

OXYHAEMOGLOBIN METHOD

The HbO_2 method is the simplest and quickest method for general use with a photometer. Its disadvantage is that it is not possible to prepare a stable HbO_2 standard, so the calibration of these instruments should be checked regularly using HiCN reference solutions or a secondary standard of preserved blood or lysate (see p. 25). The reliability of the method is not affected by a moderate increase in plasma bilirubin, but it is not satisfactory in the presence of HbCO, Hi or SHb.

Method

Wash 20 ml of blood into a tube containing 4 ml of 0.4 ml/l ammonia (specific gravity 0.88) to give a ×201 dilution. Use a tightly fitting stopper and mix by inverting the tube several times. The solution of HbO_2 is then ready for matching against a standard in a spectrometer at 540 nm or a photometer with a yellow-green filter (e.g. Ilford 625) against a water blank. If the absorbance of the haemoglobin solution exceeds 0.7, dilute the blood further with an equal volume of water and read again. Fresh ammonia solution must be made up each week. Once diluted, the blood sample is stable at 20°C for about 2 days.

Standard

A standard should be prepared from a specimen of normal anticoagulated whole blood. Its haemoglobin concentration is first determined by the HiCN method (see p. 25). The blood is then diluted 1:201 by pipetting 20 ml of the well-mixed blood into 4 ml of ammonia; sequential dilutions are made in ammonia and absorbance is read in a spectrometer at 540 nm or photometer using a yellow-green filter (Ilford 625, Wratten 74 or Chance 0 Gr 1). The readings are plotted on arithmetic graph paper. Linearity of response is checked and absorbance is related to haemoglobin from the measurement obtained in the original sample by the HiCN method.

Colorimeters and light filters unfortunately, differ sufficiently to make it essential to check the chosen standard at frequent intervals against a HiCN reference preparation in the photometer in which it is going to be used. It is probably preferable to use a new fresh whole-blood sample each day as a secondary standard after measuring its haemoglobin concentration by the HiCN method. Preserved blood (see p. 599) or lysate (see p. 599) can be used instead.

Direct calculation from a standard:

$$Hb\ (g/l) = \frac{A^{540}\text{test sample}}{A^{540}\text{standard}} \times \frac{\text{Conc. of}}{\text{standard}} \times \frac{\begin{array}{c}\text{Dilution}\\\text{factor}\end{array}}{1000}$$

If the HiCN method is not available, a neutral grey filter of 0.475 density (Ilford or Chance) can be used as a calibration standard. This corresponds to a 1:201 dilution of blood with 146 g/l haemoglobin concentration in a 1 cm cuvette at a wavelength of 540 nm.

DIRECT SPECTROMETRY

The haemoglobin concentration of a diluted blood sample can be determined by spectrometry without the need for a standard, provided that the spectrometer has been correctly calibrated. The blood is diluted 1:201 (or 1:251) with cyanide-ferricyanide reagent (see p. 25) and the absorbance is measured at 540 nm. Haemoglobin concentration is calculated as follows:

$$Hb\ (g/l) = \frac{A^{540}HiCN \times 16\ 114 \times \text{Dilution factor}}{11.0 \times d \times 1000}$$

$$\text{or } Hb\ (\mu mol/l) = \frac{A^{540}HiCN \times \text{Dilution factor}}{11.0 \times d \times 1000}$$

where A^{540} = absorbance of solution at 540 nm; 16 114 = monomeric molecular weight of haemoglobin; dilution = 201 when 20 ml of blood are diluted in 4 ml of reagent; 11.0 = millimolar coefficient extinction; d = layer thickness in cm; and 1000 = conversion of mg to g.

When assigning a value to a haemoglobin solution that may be used as a reference preparation, it is necessary first to calibrate the spectrometer. This requires checking wavelength with a holmium oxide filter, absorbance with a set of calibrated neutral density filters and stray light with a neutral density filter at 220 nm (National Physical Laboratory, Teddington, UK). Matched optical or quartz glass cuvettes with a transmission difference of <1% at 200 nm should be used. Subsequently, the calibration of the spectrophotometer can be checked by verifying that it gives an accurate reading of the HiCN standard. Slight deviations from the expected A^{540} HiCN value for the standard may be used to correct the results of test samples for a bias in measurement.[2]

DIRECT READING PORTABLE HAEMOGLOBINOMETERS

Colour Comparators

These are simple clinical devices that compare the colour of blood against a range of colours representing haemoglobin concentrations. They are intended for anaemia screening in the absence of laboratory facilities and are described in Chapter 26.

Portable Haemoglobinometers

Portable haemoglobinometers have a built-in filter and a scale calibrated for direct reading of haemoglobin concentration in g/dl or g/l. They are generally based on the HbO_2 method. A number of instruments are now available that use a light-emitting diode of appropriate wavelength and are standardized to give the same results as with the HiCN method.

The HemoCue system (HemoCue AB, Ängelsholm, Sweden) is a well-established method for haemoglobinometry. It consists of a precalibrated, portable, battery-operated spectrometer; no dilution is necessary because blood is run by capillary action directly into a cuvette containing sodium nitrite and sodium azide, which convert the haemoglobin to azidemethaemoglobin. The absorbance is measured at wavelengths of 565 and 880 nm. Measurements are not affected by high levels of bilirubin, lipids or white cells and it is sufficiently reliable for use as a laboratory instrument; it is easy for non-technical personnel to operate and is thus also suitable for use at point-of-care. The cuvettes must be stored in a container with a drying agent and kept within the temperature range of 15–30°C. Some devices are now available that use reagent-free cuvettes that will not deteriorate in adverse climatic conditions.[14] HemoCue have recently released a portable system that measures both haemoglobin and the white blood cell count (WBC), the HemoCue WBC.[15]

Chempaq (Chempaq A/S, Hirsemarken 1B, Farum, Denmark) produce two different portable multiplatform haematology analysers that use impedance cell counting and measurement of haemoglobin by a spectrophotometric method on 20 μl of blood. The Chempaq XBC uses a disposable cartridge to measure three different test profiles, Hb alone or WBC, with three-part differential, plus Hb or Hb with red blood cell count (RBC), haematocrit (Hct), mean cell volume (MCV), mean cell haemoglobin (MCH) and mean cell haemoglobin concentration (MCHC). The Chempaq XDM701 uses the same principles but also reports a platelet count.

The DiaSpect Haemoglobinometry system is a newly developed technology for measuring haemoglobin concentration in unaltered whole blood in a special plastic cuvette that also serves as the sampling device.[16] The instrument is a portable spectrophotometer powered by 3.6 V integrated lithium-ion rechargeable batteries or 100–240 V adaptor. As the cuvettes do not contain any reagents, they are not affected by temperature or humidity and no special storage conditions are required. They have a shelf life of at least 2 years. Haemoglobin fractions are measured from absorbance wavelengths between 400 and 800 nm. A patented method eliminates the impact of scattering from the blood cells while possible background turbidity from interfering substances is measured and compensated for at high wavelength. The results are displayed in <5 seconds. Preliminary studies have shown an accuracy within ± 3 g/l for measurements between 10 and 200 g/l.

Non-invasive Screening Tests

Methods are being developed for using near infrared spectroscopy at body sites, mainly a finger, to identify the spectral pattern of haemoglobin in an underlying blood vessel and derive a measurement of haemoglobin concentration. Early studies have shown an approximate correlation with blood haemoglobinometry.[17,18]

RANGE OF HAEMOGLOBIN CONCENTRATION IN HEALTH

See Chapter 2, Tables 2.1, 2.2 and 2.3. It should be noted that there are sex differences, diurnal variations and environmental and physiological factors that must also be taken into account.

PACKED CELL VOLUME OR HAEMATOCRIT

The packed cell volume (PCV) can be used as a simple screening test for anaemia, as a reference method for calibrating automated blood count systems and as a rough guide to the accuracy of haemoglobin measurements. The PCV × 1000 is about three times the Hb expressed in g/l. In conjunction with estimations of Hb and RBC, it can be used in the calculation of red cell indices. However, its use in under-resourced laboratories may be limited by the need for a specialized centrifuge and a reliable supply of capillary tubes.

Microhaematocrit Method

The microhaematocrit method[19] is carried out on blood contained in capillary tubes 75 mm in length and having an internal diameter of about 1 mm. The tubes may be plain for use with anticoagulated blood samples or coated inside with 1 iu of heparin for the direct collection of capillary blood. The centrifuge used for the capillary tubes provides a centrifugal force of $c12\,000\,g$ and 5 min centrifugation results in a constant PCV. When the PCV is >0.5, it may be necessary to centrifuge for a further 5 min.

Allow blood from a well-mixed specimen, or from a free flow of blood by skin puncture, to enter the tube by capillarity, leaving at least 15 mm unfilled. Then seal the tube by a plastic seal (e.g. Cristaseal, Hawksley, Lancing, Sussex). Sealing the tube by heating is not recommended because the seals tend to be tapered and there is the likelihood of lysis. After centrifugation for 5 min, measure the proportion of cells to the whole column (i.e. the PCV) using a reading device.

Accuracy of Microhaematocrit

The microhaematocrit method has an adequate level of accuracy and precision for clinical utility.[20] However, attention must be paid to a number of factors that may produce an inaccurate result.

Anticoagulant

K_2-EDTA is recommended, because K_3-EDTA causes shrinking of the red cells, reducing the PCV by about 2%. Anticoagulant concentration in excess of 2.2 mg/ml may also cause a falsely low PCV as a result of cell shrinkage.

Blood Sample

Because the PCV gradually increases with storage, the test should be performed within 6 h of collecting the blood sample, but a delay of up to 24 h is acceptable if the blood is kept at 4°C.

Failure to mix the blood sample adequately will produce an inaccurate result. The degree of oxygenation of the blood also affects the result because the PCV of venous blood is ≈2% higher than that of fully aerated blood (which has lost CO_2 and taken up O_2).[21] To ensure adequate oxygenation and sample mixing, the free air space above the sample should be >20% of the container volume.

Capillary Tubes

Variation of the bore of the tubes may cause serious errors if they are not within the narrow limits of defined specifications that should be met by manufacturers: length 75 ± 0.5 mm; internal diameter 1.07–1.25 mm; wall thickness 0.18–0.23 mm; and bore taper not exceeding 2% of the internal diameter over the entire length of the tube.[20]

Centrifuge

Centrifuges should be checked at intervals (at least annually) by a tachometer for speed and by a stopwatch for timer accuracy. Efficiency of packing should also be tested by centrifuging samples of normal and polycythaemic blood for varying times from 5 to 10 min to determine the minimum time for complete packing of the red cells.

Reading

The test should be read as soon as possible after centrifugation because the red cells begin to swell and the interface becomes progressively more indistinct. To avoid errors in reading with the special reading device, a magnifying glass should be used. White cells and platelets (the buffy coat) must be excluded as far as possible from the reading of the packed red cell volume. If a special reading device is not available, the ratio of red cell column to whole column can be calculated from measurements obtained by placing the tube against arithmetic graph paper or against a ruler.

Plasma Trapping

The amount of plasma trapped between red cells, especially in the lower end of the red cell column, and red cell dehydration during centrifugation generally counterbalance each other and the error caused by trapped plasma is usually not more than 0.01 PCV units. Thus, in routine practice, it is unnecessary to correct for trapped plasma, but if the PCV is required for calibrating a blood cell analyser or for calculating blood volume, the observed PCV should be reduced by a 2% correction factor after it has been centrifuged for 5 min or for 10 min with polycythaemic blood.[22] It is, however, preferable to use the surrogate reference method.[23] Plasma trapping is increased in macrocytic anaemias,[24] spherocytosis, thalassaemia, hypochromic anaemias and sickle cell anaemia;[25] it may be as high as 20% in sickle cell anaemia if all the cells are sickled.[24]

International Council for Standardization in Haematology Reference Method

Haemoglobin concentration is measured by the routine method on blood specimens with a range of haemoglobin concentrations. Samples of the same specimens are then taken into special borosilicate glass capillary tubes, which are centrifuged for 5 min or longer to achieve full red cell packing. The tubes are then broken at the midpoint of the packed red cells, blood is extracted with a micropipette and its haemoglobin concentration is measured. PCV is calculated as the ratio of the Hb of whole blood to that of the packed cells. This method[26] is appropriate for instrument and reagent manufacturers, but it is time-consuming and requires significant expertise, which makes it impractical for occasional use in routine laboratories. Accordingly, the International Council for Standardization in Haematology (ICSH) has developed a 'surrogate reference method'.[23]

Surrogate Reference Method

Equipment

Standard microhaematocrit centrifuge.
Borosilicate glass capillary tubes with the following specifications: length 75 ± 0.5 mm; inner diameter 1.55 ± 0.085 mm; outer diameter 1.9 ± 0.085 mm (Drummond Scientific, Broomall PA 19008: Catalogue #1–000–751C).
Capillary tube holder consisting of a 75×25 mm glass slide mounted on a 75×50 mm slide.
Microscope fitted with a vernier scale and ocular crossbar.

Method

1. Take up duplicate samples of well-mixed blood into the specified capillary tubes and centrifuge as described on p. 29.
2. Promptly remove the tubes from the centrifuge, position each in turn against the edge of the 25 mm slide and place this on the stage of the microscope.
3. Ensure that the capillary tube is aligned in a true horizontal position relative to the field of view and, using low power, note on the vernier scale the lengths of the tube at the interfaces of (a) red cells and seal, (b) red cells and leucocytes and (c) plasma and air.
4. Calculate the spun PCV = (B–A)/(C–A). Determine the acceptability of paired measurements – duplicates must agree within 0.007 units; if they do not, the paired tests must be repeated.
5. Calculate the surrogate reference PCV from the formula:

$$\frac{\text{Spun PCV} - 0.0119}{0.9736}$$

This formula applies only to the specified capillary tubes; other tubes require specific validation by the ICSH reference method[22] so that an appropriate formula can be derived. If the surrogate reference measurements are to be used to validate equipment or methods, a minimum of six different blood samples are required, at least two in each of the ranges of PCV 0.20–0.25, 0.40–0.45 and 0.60–0.65. If necessary, the PCV of normal samples may be adjusted by the appropriate addition or removal of autologous plasma.

Range of Packed Cell Volume in Health

See Chapter 2, Tables 2.1, 2.2 and 2.3.

MANUAL CELL COUNTS AND RED CELL INDICES

The principles of manual cell counts, the use of the haemocytometer counting chamber for manually counting white cells and platelets and the limitations of these measurements are described in Chapter 26.

An accurate RBC enables the MCV and MCH to be calculated. In well-equipped laboratories, where these indices are provided by an automated system (see p. 41), they are of considerable clinical importance and are widely used in the classification of anaemia. Where automated analysers are not used, manual RBCs (and consequently, calculations of these red cell indices) are so inaccurate and time-consuming that they have become obsolete.

The only measurement that can be obtained with reasonable accuracy by manual methods is MCHC because this is derived from Hb and PCV from the following formula:

$$\text{MCHC (g/l)} = \text{Hb (g/l)} \div \text{PCV (l/l)}.$$

Range of MCHC in Health

See Chapter 2, Tables 2.1, 2.2 and 2.3.

MANUAL DIFFERENTIAL LEUCOCYTE COUNT

Differential leucocyte counts are usually performed by visual examination of blood films that are prepared on slides by the spread or 'wedge' technique. Unfortunately, even in well-spread films, the distribution of the various cell types is not totally random (see below).

For a reliable differential count on films spread on slides, the film must not be too thin and the tail of the film should be smooth. To achieve this, the film should be made with a rapid movement using a smooth glass spreader. This should result in a film in which there is some overlap of the red cells, diminishing to separation near the tail, and in which the white cells in the body of the film are not too badly shrunken. If the film is too thin or if a rough-edged spreader is used, many of the white cells, perhaps even 50% of them, accumulate at the edges and in the tail (Fig. 3.1). Moreover, a gross qualitative irregularity in distribution is the rule: polymorphonuclear neutrophils and monocytes predominate at the margins and the tail; lymphocytes predominate in the middle of the film (Fig. 3.2). This separation probably depends on differences in stickiness, size and specific gravity of the different types of cells.

Differences in distribution of the various types of cells are probably always present to a small extent even in

Figure 3.2 Schematic drawing of a blood film made on a slide. The film has been spread from left to right. An indication is given of the way the white blood cells are distributed.

well-made films. Various systems for performing the differential count have been advocated, but none can compensate for the gross irregularities in distribution in a badly made film. On well-made films, the following technique of counting is recommended.

Method

Count the cells using a ×40 objective in a strip running the whole length of the film. Avoid the lateral edges of the film. Inspect the film from the head to the tail and if fewer than 100 cells are encountered in a single narrow strip, examine one or more additional strips until at least 100 cells have been counted. Each longitudinal strip represents the blood drawn out from a small part of the original drop of blood when it has spread out between the slide and spreader (Fig. 3.3). If all the cells are counted in such a strip, the differential totals will closely approximate the true differential count. This technique is liable to error if cells in the thick part of the film cannot be identified; also, it does not allow for any excess of neutrophils and monocytes at the edges of the film, but this preponderance is slight in a well-made film and in practice makes little difference to the result.

This technique is easy to carry out; with high counts ($10-30 \times 10^9$/l) a short, 2–3 cm, film is desirable. In

Direction of spreading

Figure 3.3 Schematic drawing illustrating the longitudinal method of performing differential leucocyte counts. The original drop of blood spreads out between spreader and slide (D–D_1). The film is made in such a way that representative strips of films, such as A–A_1 and B–B_1, are formed from blood originally at A and B, respectively. To perform an accurate differential count, all the leucocytes in one or more strips, such as A–A_1 and B–B_1, should be inspected and classified.

Figure 3.1 Badly spread film. Two areas of a badly spread film from a patient with a white blood cell count of 20×10^9/l showing (A) many leucocytes in the tail and (B) very few leucocytes in body of film.

patients with very high counts (as in leukaemia), the method has to be abandoned and the cells should be counted in any well-spread area where the cell types are easy to identify. Other systems of counting, such as the 'battlement' count, are more elaborate but may minimize error owing to variation of distribution of cells between the centre and the edge of the film. The results of the differential count can be recorded using a multiple manual register or they can be directly entered onto a computer.

The variance of the differential count depends not only on artefactual differences in distribution owing to the process of spreading but also on 'random' distribution; together they are by far the most important cause of unreliable differential counts. The random distribution means that, if a total of 100 cells are counted, with a true neutrophil proportion of 50%, the range ($\pm$ 2SD) within which 95% of the counts will fall is of the order of $\pm$ 14% (i.e. 36–64%) neutrophils. A 200-cell count can provide a more accurate estimate; in the previous example, the $\pm$ 2SD range will be about 40–60%. In a 500-cell count, the range would be reduced to 44–56% neutrophils. In practice, a 100- or 200-cell count is recommended as a routine procedure. However, if abnormal cells are present in small numbers, they are more likely to be detected when 200–500-cell counts are performed than with a 100-cell count.

BASOPHIL AND EOSINOPHIL COUNTS

A manual basophil or eosinophil count may be necessary to validate an automated count or when abnormal characteristics of the cells render an automated count unreliable, e.g. with degranulated eosinophils. Count the percentage of eosinophils or basophils in a differential count of all the leucocytes on a stained blood film. If the cells of interest are infrequent, a 500-cell differential count should be performed. If fewer than 500 cells are seen in the film, continue the count on a second film. However, if the eosinophil count is markedly elevated a conventional 100-cell count will suffice for most purposes. Calculate the eosinophil or basophil count per litre from the total leucocyte count. It is essential to have thin, preferably short, films with the leucocytes evenly distributed throughout the film and readily identified (see p. 31).

Range of Eosinophil Count in Health

See Chapter 2, Tables 2.1, 2.2 and 2.3.

There is normally considerable diurnal variation in the eosinophil count and differences amounting to as much as 100% have been recorded. The lowest counts are found in the morning (10 a.m. to noon) and the highest at night (midnight to 4 a.m.).[27,28] For a review of the causes of eosinophilia, see Brito-Babapulle.[29]

Range of Basophil Count in Health

See Chapter 2, Table 2.1.

Gilbert and Ornstein[30] reported a 95% distribution in normal subjects of $0.01–0.08 \times 10^9$/l. There are no age or sex differences, although serial counts have shown lower levels during ovulation.[31]

REPORTING THE DIFFERENTIAL LEUCOCYTE COUNT

The differential count, expressed as the percentage of each type of cell, should be related to the total leucocyte count and the results should be reported in absolute numbers ($\times 10^9$/l). Myelocytes and metamyelocytes, if present, are recorded separately from neutrophils. Band (stab) cells are generally counted as neutrophils, but it may be useful to record them separately. They normally constitute <6% of the neutrophils; an increase may point to an inflammatory process even in the absence of an absolute leucocytosis.[32] However, the band cell count is imprecise and, although it is sometimes recommended in infants, it has been found to be unhelpful in predicting occult bacteraemia in this group.[33]

Correcting the Count for Nucleated Red Blood Cells

When nucleated red blood cells (NRBCs) are present, they will be included in the total WBC, which is really a 'total nucleated cell count' (TNCC). They should also be included in the differential count, as a percentage of the TNCC and reported in absolute numbers ($\times 10^9$/l) in the same way as the different types of leucocytes. If they are present in significant numbers, the TNCC should be corrected to obtain the true total WBC. Thus, for example, if total WBC is 8.0×10^9/l and the percentage of NRBCs on the differential count is 25%, then

$$\text{Corrected WBC} = 8 - (8 \times 25/100) = 6 \times 10^9/\text{l}.$$

Care should be taken to differentiate small lymphocytes from nucleated red blood cells (e.g. Chapter 5, Fig. 5.64).

Reference Differential White Cell Count

A reference method is required to validate the accuracy of automated systems[34] (described later). The method that has been used widely for this purpose is essentially similar to the routine manual procedure on stained blood films, but to ensure adequate precision a 200-cell count is carried out by two independent observers, each on two films prepared from the same sample. However, this is still too imprecise for cells with a low frequency; attempts have been made to establish a reference method using flow cytometry with specific monoclonal-antibody labelling of the specific cell types including immature leucocytes.[35,36] More recent flow cytometric protocols also include blast cells, reactive lymphocytes, differentiation between B and T lymphocytes and nucleated red cells.[37,38]

Range of Differential White Cells in Health

See Chapter 2, Tables 2.1, 2.2 and 2.3.

PLATELET COUNT

The method for manual counting of platelets using a counting chamber is described on p. 610. If an RBC by a semiautomated counter is available, it is possible to obtain an approximation of the platelet count by counting the proportion of platelets to red cells in a thin part of a film made from an EDTA-anticoagulated blood sample, using the $\times 100$ oil-immersion objective and, if possible, eyepieces provided with an adjustable diaphragm, as for a reticulocyte count.

Range of Platelet Count in Health

See Chapter 2, Tables 2.1, 2.2 and 2.3.

RETICULOCYTE COUNT

Reticulocytes are juvenile red cells; they contain remnants of the ribosomal ribonucleic acid (RNA) that was present in larger amounts in the cytoplasm of the nucleated precursors from which they were derived. Ribosomes have the property of reacting with certain basic dyes such as azure B, brilliant cresyl blue or New methylene blue (see below) to form a blue or purple precipitate of granules or filaments.

This reaction takes place only in vitally stained unfixed preparations. Stages of maturation can be identified by their morphological features. The most immature reticulocytes are those with the largest amount of precipitable material; in the least immature, only a few dots or short strands are seen. Reticulocytes can be classified into four groups, ranging from the most immature reticulocytes, with a large clump of reticulin (group I), to the most mature, with a few granules of reticulin (group IV) (Fig. 3.4).

If a blood film is allowed to dry and is afterwards fixed with methanol, reticulocytes appear as polychromatic red cells staining diffusely basophilic if the film is stained with one of the basic dyes.

Complete loss of basophilic material probably occurs in the bloodstream and, particularly, in the spleen after the

cells have left the bone marrow.[39] This maturation is thought to take 2–3 days, of which about 24 h are spent in the circulation.

The number of reticulocytes in the peripheral blood is a fairly accurate reflection of erythropoietic activity, assuming that the reticulocytes are released normally from the bone marrow and that they remain in circulation for the normal time period. These assumptions are not always valid because an increased erythropoietic stimulus leads to premature release into the circulation. The average maturation time of these so-called 'stress' or stimulated reticulocytes may be as long as 3 days. In such cases, a higher than normal proportion of immature reticulocytes will be found in circulation. A more precise assessment of reticulocyte maturation is possible by quantitative flow cytometry of their RNA content. Nevertheless, adequate information is usually obtained from a simple reticulocyte count recorded either as a percentage of the red cells or, preferably, when the RBC is known, as an absolute number per litre. When there is severe anaemia, the reticulocyte count should be corrected for the anaemia and expressed as a reticulocyte index.[40]

$$\text{Reticulocyte index} = \text{Observed reticulocyte}\%$$
$$\times \frac{\text{Measured Hb or PCV}}{\text{Appropriate normal Hb or PCV}}$$

Reticulocyte Stains and Count

Better and more reliable results are obtained with New methylene blue than with brilliant cresyl blue. New methylene blue is chemically different from methylene blue, which is a poor reticulocyte stain. New methylene blue stains the reticulofilamentous material in reticulocytes more deeply and more uniformly than does brilliant cresyl blue, which varies from sample to sample in its staining ability. Azure B is a satisfactory substitute for New methylene blue; it has the advantage that the dye does not precipitate and it is available in pure form.[41] It is used in the same concentration and the staining procedure is the same as with New methylene blue.

Staining Solution

Dissolve 1.0 g of brilliant cresyl blue (CI 51010) or 1.0 g of New methylene blue (CI 52030) or azure B (CI 52010) in 100 ml of 3% trisodium citrate-saline solution (30 g sodium citrate in 1 l saline). Filter once the dye has been dissolved.

Method

Deliver 2 or 3 drops of the dye solution into a 75×10 mm plastic tube by means of a plastic Pasteur pipette. Add 2–4 volumes of the patient's EDTA-anticoagulated blood to the dye solution and mix. Keep the mixture at 37°C for

Figure 3.4 Photomicrographs of reticulocytes showing stages of maturation. (A,B) Most immature (group I); (C,D) intermediate (group II); (E,F) later-stage intermediate (group III); (G) most mature (group IV); and (H) haemolytic anaemia, stained supravitally by New methylene blue.

15–20 min. Resuspend the red cells by gentle mixing and make films on glass slides in the usual way. When dry, examine the films without fixing or counterstaining.

The exact volume of blood to be added to the dye solution for optimal staining depends on the RBC. A larger proportion of anaemic blood, and a smaller proportion of polycythaemic blood, should be added than of normal blood. In a successful preparation, the reticulofilamentous material should be stained deep blue and the non-reticulated cells should be stained diffuse shades of pale greenish blue. Films should not be counterstained. The reticulofilamentous material is not better defined after counterstaining and precipitated stain overlying cells may cause confusion. Moreover, Heinz bodies will not be visible in fixed and counterstained preparations. If the stained preparation is examined under phase contrast, both the mature red cells and reticulocytes are well defined. By this technique, late reticulocytes characterized by the presence of remnants of filaments or threads are readily distinguished from cells containing inclusion bodies. Satisfactory counts may be made on blood that has been allowed to stand (unstained) for as long as 24 h, although the count will tend to decrease after 6–8 h unless the blood is kept at 4°C.

Counting Reticulocytes

An area of film should be chosen for the count where the cells are undistorted and where the staining is good. A common fault is to make the film too thin; however, the cells should not overlap. To count the cells, use the ×100 oil-immersion objective and, if possible, eyepieces provided with an adjustable diaphragm. If eyepieces with an adjustable diaphragm are not available, a paper or cardboard diaphragm, in the centre of which has been cut a small square with sides about 4 mm in length, can be inserted into an eyepiece and used as a less convenient substitute.

The counting procedure should be appropriate to the number of reticulocytes present. Very large numbers of cells have to be surveyed if a reasonably precise count is to be obtained when only small numbers of reticulocytes are present. When the count is <10%, a convenient method is to survey successive fields until at least 100 reticulocytes have been counted and to count the total red cells in at least 10 fields to determine the average number of red cells per field.

Calculation

Number of reticulocytes in n fields = x
Average number of red cells per field = y
Total number of red cells in n fields = $n \times$ y
Reticulocyte percentage = $[x \div (n \times y)] \times 100\%$
Absolute reticulocyte count = % × RBC.

Thus, when the reticulocyte percentage is 3.3 and the RBC is 5×10^{12}/l, the absolute reticulocyte count per litre is as follows: $[3.3/100] \times 5 \times 10^{12} = 165 \times 10^{9}$

It is essential that the reticulocyte preparation be well spread to ensure an even distribution of cells in successive fields.

When the reticulocyte count exceeds 10%, only a relatively small number of cells will have to be surveyed to obtain a standard error of 10%.

An alternative method is based on the principle of balanced sampling, using a Miller ocular (Graticules Ltd, Morley Road, Tonbridge, UK). This is an eyepiece giving a square field, in the corner of which is a smaller ruled square, one-ninth the area of the total square (Fig. 3.5). Reticulocytes are counted in the large square and the total number of red cells is counted in the small square.

The number of fields that should be surveyed to obtain a desired degree of precision depends on the proportion of reticulocytes (Table 3.3).

It is essential that the reticulocyte preparation be well spread and well stained. Other important factors that affect the accuracy of the count are the visual acuity and patience of the observer and the quality and resolving power of the microscope. The most accurate counts are carried out by a conscientious observer who has no knowledge of the supposed reticulocyte level, thus eliminating the effect of conscious or unconscious bias.

Differentiating between Reticulocytes and Other Red Cell Inclusions

The decision as to what is and what is not a reticulocyte may be difficult because the most mature reticulocytes contain only a few dots or threads of reticulofilamentous material. Fortunately, in well-stained preparations viewed under the light microscope, the Pappenheimer (iron-containing) type of granular material – usually present as a single small dot, less commonly as multiple dots – stains

Figure 3.5 Miller ocular.

Table 3.3 Accuracy of reticulocyte counts with Miller ocular

RETICULOCYTES		STANDARD ERROR (σ)		
Percentage	Proportion (p)	2%	5%	10%
1	0.01	27 500	4400	1100
2	0.02	13 600	2180	550
5	0.05	5280	845	210
10	0.10	2500	400	100
25	0.25	835	135	35

Columns 3–5 indicate the total number of red cells to be counted *in the small squares* so as to give the required standard error at different reticulocyte levels. It is derived from the following:

$$\sigma = \sqrt{p(1-p)/\lambda}$$

where p = number of reticulocytes in n large squares ÷ (number of red cells in n small squares × f); f = ratio of large to small squares (i.e. 9); and λ = approximate total number of cells in n large squares.

a darker shade of blue than does the reticulofilamentous material of the reticulocyte. As described earlier, phase contrast will help to distinguish them. If there is any doubt, Pappenheimer bodies can be identified by overstaining the film for iron by Perls' reaction.

Haemoglobin H undergoes denaturation in the presence of brilliant cresyl blue or New methylene blue, resulting in round inclusion bodies that stain greenish-blue (see Chapter 15, Figs 15.6, 15.7). These can be easily differentiated from reticulofilamentous material (Fig. 15.8).

Heinz bodies are also stained by New methylene blue, but they stain a lighter shade of blue than the reticulofilamentous material of reticulocytes and stain well with methyl violet (Figs 15.5, 15.6).

Fluorescence Methods for Performing a Reticulocyte Count

Reticulocytes can be counted manually by fluorescence microscopy on appropriately stained films.[42] Add 1 volume of acridine orange solution (50 mg/100 ml of 9 g/l NaCl) to 1 volume of blood. Mix gently for 2 min; make films on glass slides, dry rapidly and examine with a fluorescent microscope. RNA gives an orange–red fluorescence, whereas nuclear material (DNA) fluoresces yellow. Although the amount of fluorescence is proportional to the amount of RNA, the brightness and colour of the fluorescence fluctuates and the preparation quickly fades when exposed to light; also, it requires a special fluorescence microscope. It is thus not suitable for routine use for reticulocyte counting.

Fluorescent staining combined with flow cytometry has been developed as a method for automated reticulocyte counting (see p. 48).

Manual Reference Method

The manual reference method[43,44] is essentially the same procedure as for the routine method, the supravitally stained films being examined by bright field or phase contrast-microscopy. Reticulocytes are identified as non-nucleated red cells that contain at least two blue staining particles or one particle linked to a filamentous thread; every non-nucleated cell in each field must be classified as a red cell or a reticulocyte. Three suitable blood films must be selected for each sample and counting is performed by moving from field to field in a battlement pattern until sufficient red cells have been counted to satisfy precision requirement (Table 3.3). An objective is a variance of 2%, but this is impractical when the reticulocyte proportion is in the range 0.01–0.02.

Range of Reticulocyte Count in Health

The range of reticulocyte counts in adults and children is $50–100 \times 10^9/l$ (0.5–2.5%). At birth or in cord blood, it is $120–400 \times 10^9/l$ (2–5%).

AUTOMATED BLOOD COUNT TECHNIQUES

A variety of automated instruments for performing blood counts are in widespread use. Semiautomated instruments require some steps (e.g. dilution of a blood sample) to be carried out by the operator. Fully automated instruments require only that an appropriate blood sample is presented to the instrument. Semiautomated instruments often measure a small number of components (e.g. WBC and Hb). Fully automated multichannel instruments usually measure from 8 to 20 components for the basic FBC and white blood cell differential, including some variables that have no equivalent in manual techniques. Automated instruments usually have a high level of precision, which, for cell counting and cell-sizing techniques, is greatly superior to that achievable with manual techniques. If instruments are carefully calibrated and their correct operation is ensured by quality control procedures, they produce test results that are generally accurate. When blood has abnormal characteristics, the results for one or more parameters may be aberrant; instruments are designed so that such inconsistent results are 'flagged' for subsequent review. The abnormal characteristics that lead to inaccurate counts vary between instruments, so it is important for instrument operators to be familiar with the types of factitious results to which their instruments are prone.

Blood cell counters may have automated procedures for sample recognition (e.g. by bar-coding), for ensuring that adequate sample mixing occurs, for taking up the test sample automatically and for detection of clots or inadequately sized samples. Ideally, blood sampling is carried out by piercing the cap of a closed tube so that samples that carry an infection hazard can be handled with maximum safety.

Laboratories performing large numbers of blood counts each day require fully automated blood counters capable of the rapid production of accurate and precise blood counts, including platelet counts and differential counts, either three-part or five- to seven-part. The sample throughput required varies with the workload and the timing of arrival of blood specimens in the laboratory, but for most large laboratories, a throughput of 100 or more samples per hour is required. Sample size and the availability of a 'predilute' mode are particularly relevant if the laboratory receives many paediatric specimens.

Choice of an instrument for an individual laboratory, as well as for point-of-care sites outside the laboratory (see p. 574), should take account of capital expenditure and running costs, including maintenance and reagents; size of instrument; requirements of services such as water, compressed air, drainage and an electricity supply with stable voltage; environmental disturbance by generation of heat, vibration and noise; any influence on performance by the ambient temperature and humidity; storage requirements for the often bulky reagents; ease of operation; and the likely level of support that can be expected from the manufacturer.

A practical guide on the principles of the various systems has been published,[45] and there are guidelines to help in the choice of an instrument suitable for the needs of an individual laboratory and also to assess its performance, as compared with the claims of the manufacturer, when it has been installed and is being used in routine practice.[46] Choice of instrument may be aided by reference to published reports of instrument evaluations and related monographs.[45,47–49] Some semiautomated instruments aspirate a sample of accurately determined volume and so can perform absolute cell counts and accurate estimations of Hb. Most automated instruments, however, count for a specified period of time rather than measure an exact volume of blood; they therefore require calibration by means of the direct counts derived from instruments counting cells in a defined volume of diluted blood. For some variables, instruments are calibrated by the manufacturer, but others require calibration in the laboratory. Performance characteristics of an instrument vary over time, so periodic recalibration is needed: both when quality control procedures indicate the necessity and when certain components are replaced.

HAEMOGLOBIN CONCENTRATION

Many automated counters still measure haemoglobin concentration by a modification of the manual HiCN method with cyanide reagent; however manufacturers are changing their methods to allow the use of a non-hazardous chemical, such as sodium lauryl sulphate, imidazole, sodium dodecyl sulphate or dimethyl laurylamine oxide, which avoids possible environmental hazards from disposal of large volumes of cyanide-containing waste. Modifications include alterations in the concentration of reagents and in the temperature and pH of the reaction. A non-ionic detergent is included to ensure rapid cell lysis and to reduce turbidity caused by cell membranes and plasma lipids. Measurements of absorbance are made for haemoglobin measurement at various wavelengths depending on the final stable haemochromogen, cyanmethaemoglobin, oxyhaemoglobin, methaemoglobin or monohydroxyferriporphyrin and at a set time interval after mixing of blood and the active reagents but before the reaction is completed.

RED BLOOD CELL COUNT

Red cells and other blood cells can be counted in systems based on either aperture impedance or light-scattering technology. Because large numbers of cells can be counted rapidly, there is a high level of precision. Consequently, electronic counts have rendered the RBC and the red cell indices derived from it (the MCV and the MCH) of much greater clinical relevance than was possible when only a slow and imprecise manual RBC was available.

COUNTING SYSTEMS

Impedance Counting

Impedance counting, first described by Wallace Coulter in 1956,[50] depends on the fact that red cells are poor conductors of electricity, whereas certain diluents are good conductors; this difference forms the basis of the counting systems used in Beckman Coulter, Sysmex, Abbott, Horiba Medical and a number of other instruments.

For a cell count, blood is highly diluted in a buffered electrolyte solution. The flow rate of this diluted sample is controlled by a mercury siphon (as in the original Coulter system) or by displacement of a tightly fitting piston. This results in a measured volume of the sample passing through an aperture tube of specific dimensions (e.g. 100 mm in diameter and 70 mm in length). By means of a constant source of electricity, a direct current is maintained between two electrodes, one in the sample beaker or the chamber surrounding the aperture tube and another inside the aperture tube. As a blood cell is carried through the aperture, it displaces some of the conducting fluid and increases the electrical resistance. This produces a corresponding change in potential between the electrodes, which lasts as long as the red cell takes to pass though the aperture; the height of the pulses produced indicates the volume of the cells passing through. The pulses can be displayed on an oscillograph screen. The pulses are led to a threshold circuit provided with an amplitude discriminator for selecting the minimal pulse height, which will be counted (Fig. 3.6). The height of the pulses is used to determine the volume of the red cells.

Light Scattering

Red cells and other blood cells may be counted by means of electro-optical detectors.[51] A diluted cell suspension flows through an aperture so that the cells pass, in single file, in front of a light source; light is scattered by the cells passing through the light beam. The scattered light is detected by a photomultiplier or photodiode, which converts it into electrical impulses that are accumulated and counted. The amount of light scattered is proportional to the surface area and therefore the volume of the cell so that the height of the electrical pulses can be used to estimate the cell volume. The high-intensity coherent laser beams used in current instruments have superior optical qualities to the non-coherent tungsten light of earlier instruments. Sheathed flow allows cells to flow in an axial stream with a diameter not much greater than that of a red cell; light can be precisely focused on this stream of cells. Electro-optical detectors are used for red cell sizing and counting in Siemens (previously Bayer-Technicon) systems and for white cell differential counting in a number of other instruments.

RELIABILITY OF ELECTRONIC COUNTERS

Electronic counts are precise, but care needs to be taken so that they are also accurate. The recorded count on the same sample may vary from instrument to instrument and even between different models of the same instrument. Inaccuracy may be introduced by coincidence (i.e. by two cells passing through an orifice simultaneously and being counted as one cell or by a pulse being generated during the electronic dead time of the circuit); by recirculation of cells that have already been counted; by red cell agglutination (which causes a clump of cells to be counted as one cell); and by the counting of bubbles, lipid droplets, microorganisms or extraneous particles as cells. Faulty maintenance may lead to variation in the volume aspirated or the flow rate. Single-channel instruments may have their thresholds set incorrectly and multichannel instruments may be incorrectly calibrated.

A statistical correction may be applied for coincidence (coincidence correction); in some instruments, this is done automatically by electronic editing. Errors of coincidence can be detected by carrying out a series of measurements at various dilutions of the same specimen, plotting the data on graph paper and then extrapolating the graph to the baseline for the true value. Alternatively, the need for coincidence correction can be avoided by having the dimensions and flow characteristics of the aperture through which the cells pass such that cells can only pass in single file; this may be achieved by sheathed flow or hydrodynamic focusing in which diluted blood is injected into a sheath of fluid as it flows into the sensing zone. This induces the cells to pass through the centre of the sensing zone in single file and free of distortion. Coincidence can be more effectively reduced with sheathed flow

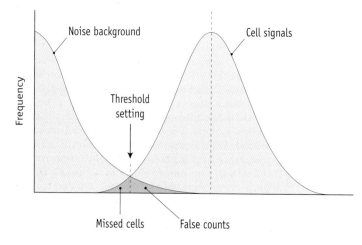

Figure 3.6 Effect of threshold discrimination (horizontal axis) in separating cell signals from background noise.

and precisely focused light in an electro-optical detector than in an impedance counter so that less dilution of the blood sample is needed.[46] Electrical impulses generated by recirculation of cells can be eliminated by electronic editing; alternatively, recirculation of cells in the region of the aperture can be prevented by 'sweep flow' in which a directed stream of diluent sweeps cells and debris away from the aperture, thus preventing cells from being recounted and debris from being counted as cells.

Inaccurate counts consequent on red cell agglutination are usually the result of cold agglutinins. They are recognized as erroneous because of an associated marked factitious elevation of the MCV. A correct count can be achieved by prewarming the blood sample and, if necessary, also prewarming the diluent.

A correct RBC and, particularly, a correct measurement of the MCV is dependent on the use of an appropriate diluent. For impedance counters, pH, temperature and rate of ionization have to be standardized and remain constant because changes alter the electrical field and may lead to artefactual alterations in the size, shape and stability of the blood cells in the diluent. Diluents must be free of particles and give a background count of <50 particles in the measured volume. The correct diluent for each individual instrument must be used; other diluents, even those made by the same manufacturer, may not be interchangeable. Any laboratories using diluents other than those recommended by the manufacturer of the instrument must satisfy themselves that no error is being introduced.

For red cell counting in simple single-channel counters a suitable diluent requires a pH of 7.0–7.5 and osmolality of 340 ± 10 mmol. Physiological saline (9 g/l NaCl) or phosphate-buffered saline, which have the advantages of simplicity and ready availability, can be used as a red cell diluent, provided that the counts are performed immediately after dilution to avoid errors owing to sphering. Commercial solutions of saline (for intravenous use) are usually particle-free. Other solutions may require filtration through a 0.22 or 0.45 mm micropore filter to remove dust.

Setting Discrimination Thresholds

An accurate RBC requires that thresholds be set so that all red cells, but a minimum of other cells, are included in the count. Some counters have a lower threshold but no upper threshold so that white cells are included in the 'RBC'. Because the WBC is usually very low in relation to the RBC, this is not usually of practical importance; however, an appreciable error can be introduced if the WBC is greatly elevated, particularly if the patient is also anaemic. The setting of the lower threshold is of considerable importance because it is necessary to ensure that microcytic red cells are included in the count without also counting large platelets.

Current multichannel instruments, both impedance counters and counters using light-scattering technology, have thresholds that are either precalibrated by the manufacturer or are automatically adjusted, depending on the characteristics of individual blood samples. Single-channel impedance instruments capable of performing a direct RBC require setting of thresholds so as to separate pulses generated by red cells from background noise and from pulses generated by platelets. This is done by adjusting the aperture current and the pulse amplification. A simple method is to dilute a fresh blood sample and carry out successive counts on the suspension, while the lower threshold control is moved incrementally from its maximum to its minimum position. At the maximum position, the count should be zero or close to zero and the counts will increase as the amplitude is reduced. The counts at each setting are plotted on arithmetic graph paper (Fig. 3.7). The correct threshold setting is at the left of the horizontal part of the graph before the line begins to slope. It is important to check that the setting selected is valid for microcytic cells. The threshold can be defined more precisely for an individual sample by means of a pulse height analyser linked to the counting system. The lower threshold is correctly set if beyond this point there are <0.5% of the counts at the peak (mode) of the pulse size distribution curve (Fig. 3.6).

PACKED CELL VOLUME AND MEAN CELL VOLUME

Modern automated blood cell counters estimate PCV/haematocrit by technology that has little connection with packing red cells by centrifugation. It is sometimes convenient to use different terms to distinguish the manual and automated tests and for this reason the International Council for Standardization in Haematology has suggested that the term 'haematocrit' (Hct) rather than PCV should be used for the automated measurement. However, it should be noted that, in the past, the terms 'packed cell volume' and 'haematocrit' have been used interchangeably for the manual procedure.

With automated instruments, the derivations of the RBC, PCV and MCV are closely interrelated. The passage of a cell through the aperture of an impedance counter or through the beam of light of a light-scattering instrument leads to the generation of an electrical pulse, the height of which is proportional to cell volume. The number of pulses generated allows the RBC to be determined, as discussed earlier. Pulse height analysis allows either the MCV or the Hct to be determined. If the average pulse height is computed, this is indicative of the MCV and the Hct can be derived by multiplying the estimated MCV by the RBC. Similarly, if the pulse heights are summated, this figure is indicative of the Hct and the MCV can, in turn, be derived by dividing the Hct by the RBC.

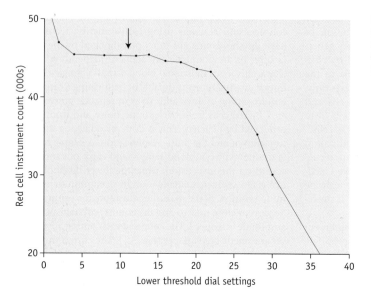

Figure 3.7 Method to establish working conditions of cell counters. The correct setting of the threshold (at arrow) is intended to exclude noise pulses without loss of the signal pulses produced by the blood cells.

Automated instruments require calibration before the Hct or MCV can be determined. Calibration of the Hct can be based on manual Hct determinations. Alternatively, the MCV can be calibrated by means of the pulse heights generated by latex beads, stabilized cells or some other calibrant containing particles of known size; however, unfixed human red cells that are biconcave and flexible will not necessarily show the same characteristics in a cell counter as latex particles or some other artificial calibrant. BCR Certified preparations are available from the Institute for Reference Materials and Measurements (IRMM) (see p. 588). Aperture-impedance systems measure an apparent volume that is greater than the true volume, being influenced by a 'shape factor';[52] this factor is less than 1.1 for young, flexible red cells; between 1.1 and 1.2 for fixed biconcave cells; and about 1.5 for spheres, whether they be fixed cells or latex spheres.[51,52]

The MCV, and therefore the Hct, as determined by an automated counter, will vary with certain cell characteristics other than volume. As indicated earlier, such characteristics include shape, which in turn is partly determined by flexibility. With impedance counters, the normal disc-shaped red cell becomes elongated into a cigar shape as it passes through the aperture; this is caused by deformation in response to shear force, which occurs in cells of normal flexibility. Cells with a reduced haemoglobin concentration undergo more elongation than normal cells; this leads to a reduced 'shape factor', a reduced pulse height in relation to the true size of the cell and underestimation of the MCV. Conversely, cells with abnormally rigid membranes and cells such as spherocytes with a high haemoglobin concentration will undergo less deformation than normal and the MCV will be overestimated. Earlier light-scattering instruments also underestimated the volume of red cells with a reduced haemoglobin concentration because light scattering was affected by the haemoglobin concentration.[53] These artefacts are seen even with normal red cells of varying haemoglobin concentration but are more apparent with red cells from patients with defects in haemoglobin synthesis such as those from patients with iron deficiency. Light-scattering instruments have been developed to avoid artefacts of this type. Cells are isovolumetrically sphered; light-scattering characteristics of sphered red cells are predictable and permit the computation of both individual cell volume and intracellular haemoglobin concentration using a calibrated Mie map that describes the scatter and refraction characteristics of spherical particles in a monochromatic light source.[54] Light scattering by each individual cell is measured at two angles: low angle at 2–3° and high angle scatter at 5–15°, which permits computation of both cell volume and haemoglobin concentration.[53] The measure of cellular haemoglobin is designated as the cellular haemoglobin concentration mean (CHCM) to distinguish it from the traditional MCHC derived from the Hb and the PCV. If all measurements are accurate, the CHCM and the MCHC should give the same results, thus providing an internal quality control mechanism.

The automated MCV and Hct are prone to certain errors that do not occur or are less of a problem with manual methods. These include those resulting from microclots or partial clotting of the specimen, extreme microcytosis and the presence of cryoglobulins or cold agglutinins; the last is a relatively common cause of factitious elevation of the MCV because clumps of cells are sized as if they were single cells. Because the RBC is underestimated, the Hct is less affected, although it is also inaccurate. It is rare for warm agglutinins to cause a similar problem. Sickling may cause a factitious increase in MCV and Hct, whereas alterations in plasma osmolarity occurring, for example, in severe hyperglycaemia, also cause factitious elevation of the MCV and Hct.[49,55,56]

RED CELL INDICES

Red cell indices traditionally have been the derived parameters of MCV, MCH and MCHC; more recently, red cell distribution width (RDW) has also been included and, for some instruments, haemoglobin distribution width (HDW). These indices can provide a basis for classifying anaemias and in various combinations they have been used to aid in the distinction between iron deficiency and thalassaemias.[57–59] It is important to note, however, that these formulae may not be consistent between different instruments and their use provides only a guide to the most likely diagnosis. When diagnosis is important, as in preconceptual or antenatal screening for thalassaemia, definitive tests are required, even in patients whose red cell indices are more suggestive of iron deficiency.

Mean Cell Volume

As described earlier, in most automated systems, MCV is measured directly, but in semiautomated counters MCV is calculated by dividing the Hct by RBC.

Thus, for example, if the Hct is 0.45 (i.e. 0.45 l of red cells per litre of blood) and the RBC is 5×10^{12} per litre,

$$\text{Volume of 1 cell} = 0.45 \div 5 \times 10^{12}$$
$$= 90 \text{ femtolitres (fl)}$$

Mean Cell Haemoglobin and Mean Cell Haemoglobin Concentration

MCH is derived from the Hb divided by RBC.

Thus, for example, if there are 150 g of Hb and 5×10^{12} red cells per litre,

$$\text{MCH} = 150 \div 5 \times 10^{12} = 3 \div 10^{11} \text{ g}$$
$$= 30 \text{ picograms (pg)}$$

The MCHC is derived in the traditional manner (see p. 30) from the Hb and the Hct with instruments that measure the Hct and calculate the MCV, whereas when the MCV is measured directly and the Hct is calculated, the MCHC is derived from the Hb, MCV and RBC according to the following formula:

$$\text{MCHC (g/l)} = \frac{\text{Hb (g/l)} \times 1000}{\text{MCV (fl)} \times \text{RBC} \times 10^{-12}/l}$$

For example, if Hb is 150 g/l, MCV is 90 fl and RBC is $5 \times 10^{12}/l$,

$$\text{MCHC} = 150 \times \frac{1000}{90 \times 5}$$
$$= 333 \text{ g/l}$$

As automated counters were developed and introduced, it was noted that the reduced MCHC, which with manual methods had been a useful indicator of hypochromia in early iron deficiency, was a less sensitive indicator of developing iron deficiency. The explanation of this is complex. In iron deficiency, there is not only true hypochromia but also increased plasma trapping within the column of red cells in a microhaematocrit tube that increases the PCV and exaggerates the decrease in the MCHC. The lowered MCHC is thus partly a true reflection of hypochromia and partly an artefact. When the MCHC is derived by automated counters, the artefact of increased plasma trapping is no longer present, but the instruments are also less sensitive to a true reduction of the MCHC because of the underestimation of the size of hypochromic red cells described earlier. Because the MCHC is calculated from the formula given earlier, the underestimation of the MCV leads to an overestimation of the MCHC. The MCHC thus shows little alteration as cells become hypochromic. Where CHCM is available, it is a more directly measured equivalent of the MCHC. This provides improved sensitivity to iron deficiency because true MCHC and the CHCM decrease as hypochromia develops.[60]

VARIATIONS IN RED CELL VOLUMES: RED CELL DISTRIBUTION WIDTH

Automated instruments produce volume distribution histograms that allow the presence of more than one population of cells to be identified. Instruments may also assess the percentage of cells falling above and below given MCV thresholds and 'flag' the presence of an increased number of microcytes or macrocytes. Such measurements may indicate the presence of a small but significant increase in the percentage of either microcytes or macrocytes before there has been any change in the MCV.

Most instruments also produce a quantitative measurement of the variation in cell volume, an equivalent of the microscopic assessment of the degree of anisocytosis. This parameter has been named the 'red cell distribution width'. The RDW is derived from pulse height analysis and can be expressed either as the standard deviation (SD) in fl or as the coefficient of variation (CV) (%) of the measurements of the red cell volume. The RDW SD is measured by calculating the width in fl at the 20% height level of the red cell size distribution histogram and the RDW CV is calculated mathematically as the coefficient of variation, i.e. RDW (CV)% = 1SD/MCV × 100%.

Most instruments express the RDW as the SD, but Sysmex instruments and the Beckman Coulter instrument the DxH express it as both SD and CV. The normal reference range is in the order of $12.8 \pm 1.2\%$ as CV and 42.5 ± 3.5 fl as SD. However, widely different ranges have been reported; therefore it is important for laboratories to determine their own reference ranges. The RDW expressed as the CV has been found of some value in distinguishing between iron deficiency (RDW usually increased) and thalassaemia trait (RDW usually normal) and between megaloblastic anaemia (RDW often increased) and other causes of macrocytosis (RDW more often normal).

PERCENTAGE HYPOCHROMIC RED CELLS AND VARIATION IN RED CELL HAEMOGLOBINIZATION: HAEMOGLOBIN DISTRIBUTION WIDTH

Instruments that determine the haemoglobin concentration of individual red cells provide the percentage of hypochromic red cells, with distribution curves of the haemoglobin concentration, and are able to 'flag' the presence of increased numbers of hypochromic or hyperchromic cells. The percentage of hypochromic red cells depends on the concentration of haemoglobin in individual cells rather than being a mean, such as MCH or MCHC. It is a more sensitive marker of the availability of iron for erythropoiesis because small changes in the number of red cells with inadequate haemoglobin can be measured before there is any change in the MCHC. Hypochromic red cells are defined as cells with a haemoglobin concentration of less than 28 g/dl (280 g/l).[61] In the healthy population the percentage of hypochromic red cells does not exceed 2.5% and values greater than this are indicative of iron deficient erythropoiesis.[62] It has been reported to be a useful indicator of functional iron deficiency (where reticuloendothelial iron stores are normal or even high, but the iron is not delivered to erythroblasts and is therefore unavailable for erythropoiesis) in haemodialysis patients. Other manufacturers' instruments have other parameters reported to be equivalent to percentage hypochromic red cells, such as low haemoglobin density (LHD%) on some Beckman Coulter instruments.[63] LHD% is derived from a sigmoid transformation of the MCHC and has been proposed as a parameter to assess the available iron stores for erythropoiesis.

The degree of variation in red cell haemoglobinization is quantified as the haemoglobin distribution width or HDW; this is the CV of the measurements of haemoglobin concentration of individual cells. The normal 95% range is 1.82–2.64. Because the volume of individual red cells is determined, it is possible to distinguish between hypochromic microcytes, which are indicative of a defect in haemoglobin synthesis and hypochromic macrocytes, which often represent reticulocytes.[64] The identification of an increased percentage of hyperchromic cells may be caused by the presence of spherocytes, irregularly contracted cells or sickled cells.

TOTAL WHITE BLOOD CELL COUNT

The WBC is determined in whole blood in which red cells have been lysed. The lytic agent is required to destroy the red cells and reduce the red cell stroma to a residue that causes no detectable response in the counting system without affecting leucocytes in such a manner that the ability of the system to count them is altered. Various manufacturers recommend specific reagents and for multichannel instruments that also perform an automated differential count use of the recommended reagent is essential. For a simple single-channel impedance counter, the following fluid is satisfactory:

Cetrimide 20 g
10% formaldehyde (in 9 g/l NaCl) 2 ml
Glacial acetic acid 16 ml
NaCl 6 g
Water to 1 litre.

Relatively simple instruments are also available that determine the Hb and the WBC by consecutive measurements on a single blood sample. The diluent contains a reagent to lyse the red cells and another to convert haemoglobin to haemiglobincyanide. Hb is measured by a modified HiCN method and white cells are counted by impedance technology. Apart from the reagents specified by the manufacturers, a diluent containing potassium cyanide and potassium ferricyanide together with ethylhexadecyldimethyl-ammonium bromide can be used.[65,66]

Fully automated multichannel instruments perform WBCs by impedance or light-scattering technology or both. Residual particles in a diluted blood sample are counted after red cell lysis or, in the case of some light-scattering instruments, after the red cells have been rendered transparent. Thresholds are set to exclude normal platelets from the count, although giant platelets are included. Some or all of any nucleated red cells present are usually included, so that when nucleated red cells are present the count approximates more to the TNCC than to the WBC.

Factitiously low automated WBCs occasionally occur as a consequence of leucocyte agglutination, prolonged sample storage or abnormally fragile cells (e.g. in leukaemia). Factitiously high counts are more common and usually result from failure of lysis of red cells. With certain instruments this may occur with the cells of neonates or be consequent on uraemia or on the presence of an abnormal haemoglobin such as haemoglobin S or haemoglobin C; high counts may also be the result of microclots, platelet clumping or the presence of a cryoglobulin.

AUTOMATED DIFFERENTIAL COUNT

Most automated differential counters that are now available use flow cytometry incorporated into a full blood counter rather than being stand-alone differential counters. Increasingly, automated blood cell counters have a differential counting capacity, providing either a three-part or a five- to seven-part differential count. Counts are performed on diluted whole blood in which red cells are either lysed or are rendered transparent. A three-part differential count assigns cells to categories usually designated: (1) 'granulocytes' or 'large cells'; (2) 'lymphocytes' or 'small cells'; and (3) 'monocytes', 'mononuclear cells', or 'middle cells'. In theory, the granulocyte category includes eosinophils and basophils, but in practice it is common for an appreciable proportion of cells of these types to be excluded from the granulocyte category and to be counted instead in the monocyte category.[67] Some other three-part differentials categorize leucocytes as WBC-small cell ratio (equivalent to lymphocytes), WBC-middle cell ratio (equivalent to monocytes, eosinophils and basophils) and WBC-large cell ratio (equivalent to neutrophils).[68]

Five- to seven-part differential counts classify cells as neutrophils, eosinophils, basophils, lymphocytes and monocytes and in an extended differential count may also include immature granulocytes or large immature cells (composed of blasts and immature granulocytes) and atypical lymphocytes (including small blasts). Automated instruments performing differential counts (that do not enumerate immature granulocytes or nucleated red cells separately) are able to 'flag' or reject counts from the majority of samples with nucleated red cells, myelocytes, promyelocytes, blasts or atypical lymphocytes. To a lesser extent, instruments incorporating a three-part differential count, although not capable of enumerating eosinophils or basophils as individual categories of cells, are able to flag a significant proportion of samples that have an increased number of one of these cell types.

Both impedance counters and light-scattering instruments are capable of producing three-part differential counts from a single channel; the categorization is based on the different volume of various types of cell following partial lysis and cytoplasmic shrinkage. Most five- to seven-part differential counts require two or more channels in which cell volume and other characteristics are analysed by various modalities (Table 3.4). Analysis may be dependent only on volume and other physical characteristics of the cell or also on binding of certain dyes to granules or activity of cellular enzymes such as peroxidase. Technologies used to study cell characteristics include light scattering and absorbance and impedance measurements with low- and high-frequency electromagnetic current or radiofrequency current. Cells may have been exposed to lytic agents or a cytochemical reaction may have occurred before cell characteristics are studied. Two-parameter analysis or more complex discriminant functions divide cells into clusters that can be matched with the position of the various white cell clusters in normal blood. Thresholds, some fixed and some variable, divide clusters from one another, permitting cells in each cluster to be counted.

Automated differential counters using flow cytometry count a far greater number of cells than is possible with a manual differential count. Automated counts are consequently much more precise than manual counts. The accuracy of automated counters is less impressive than their precision. With all types of counters, unusual cell characteristics or ageing of a blood specimen can lead to

Table 3.4 Automated full blood counters with a five-part or more differential counting capacity[a]

INSTRUMENT AND MANUFACTURER	TECHNOLOGY USED FOR DIFFERENTIAL COUNT
Beckman Coulter GEN-S, LH series, DxH	Impedance with low-frequency electromagnetic current Impedance with high-frequency electromagnetic current Laser light scattering
Sysmex SE, X-series	Impedance with low-frequency direct current Impedance with radiofrequency current Fluorescence flow cytometry
Siemens Technicon H series, Advia series	Light scattering and absorbance following peroxidase reaction Two-angle light scatter following differential cytoplasmic stripping
Abbott Cell-Dyn 3500, 4000, Sapphire	Four light-scattering parameters: forward light scatter, orthogonal light scatter, narrow-angle light scatter and depolarized orthogonal light scatter
Horiba Medical Pentra series	Electrical impedance with intact cells and following differential cytoplasmic stripping Light absorbance

[a]In addition to the blood counters listed here, there are an increasing number of instruments, some designed for point-of-care testing, on the market that are capable of providing full differential or partial differential counts using various technologies.

misclassification of cells. Although the majority of samples containing abnormal cells are 'flagged', this is not invariably so; the presence of nucleated red cells, immature granulocytes, atypical lymphocytes and blasts (even occasionally quite large numbers of blasts) may not give rise to a 'flag'. However, human observers performing a 100-cell manual differential count also miss significant abnormalities. In general, automated counts have compared favourably with routine manual counts, especially if the instruments are assigned only two functions, performing differential counts on normal samples and 'flagging' abnormal samples. If morphological abnormalities are flagged, microscopic examination of a stained blood film should always be undertaken.

THE AUTOMATED IMMATURE GRANULOCYTE COUNT

Most fully automated analysers now report an immature granulocyte count. Promyelocytes, myelocytes and metamyelocytes are all included in the automated immature granulocyte count and are not identified as separate classes of cells. The presence of low numbers of immature granulocytes is more reliably detected on automated haematology analysers than by manual microscopy, due to the higher number of cells counted. Often low numbers of immature granulocytes, particularly in leucopenic samples or when small percentages are present, are missed in a 100-cell differential count or film review. Immature granulocytes may be identified either by a combination of light absorbance (after staining of the cells) and impedance or by flow cytometry to detect side-scattered light and fluorescence of cells stained with a fluorescent dye. Measurement of immature granulocytes may be clinically relevant. The percentage of immature granulocytes as measured by the Sysmex XE-2100 has, for example, been found to be predictive of infection, although it should be noted that it is no more predictive than the absolute neutrophil count.[69]

Some instruments do not quantitate immature granulocytes and still rely on an abnormal white cell flag generated by the analyser to indicate their possible presence in the blood sample.

For instruments that do not report a separate automated count for nucleated red blood cells (NRBC), automated differential counts often include some, but not all, NRBC in the total 'WBC'; thus, in the presence of a significant number of NRBC, the total count is neither a true 'WBC' nor a true 'TNCC' and the absolute WBC counts calculated from the total will necessarily be somewhat erroneous. This differs from the situation with earlier instruments that included any NRBC in the 'WBC'. It may be possible to make some assessment of the proportion of the NRBCs included in the total count

by studying the graphic output of the instrument; otherwise, if accurate absolute counts of different leucocyte types are needed, it is necessary to revert to earlier instruments to provide the TNCC and to correct it to a WBC by means of a differential count.

THE AUTOMATED NUCLEATED RED BLOOD CELL COUNT

The ability of haematology instruments to perform precise and accurate automated NRBC counts over the entire concentration range in peripheral blood offers advantages to the diagnostic laboratory. Enumeration of NRBC is important because their presence can have a direct effect on the accuracy of the WBC on some blood cell counters. The correct WBC was previously only obtained by examination of a peripheral blood film. The NRBC are reported as the number per 100 white blood cells and subtraction of the number of NRBC from the total nucleated count gives the correct WBC. The morphological correction of the WBC can be inaccurate since if the nuclear size of an NRBC falls below the white blood cell threshold of the instrument, these cells are not included in the automated WBC in the first place. Instruments currently in use that automatically count NRBC and correct the WBC for NRBC interference include the Abbott Sapphire, the Sysmex XE-2100 and XE-5000, the Beckman Coulter LH750 and DxH, the Horiba Medical Pentra DX120 and the Siemens Advia 2120.

Instruments determine NRBC by staining them with a nuclear dye and using either fluorescence laser light scatter or flow cytometry to separate them from WBC or a combination of impedance and cell volume. Beckman Coulter instruments use cell volume conductivity and scatter measurements. The Siemens Advia 2120 utilizes nuclear density and degree of peroxidase staining to identify NRBC. The white cell count and differential are corrected for the presence of nucleated red blood cells where necessary.

The NRBC counting method on some instruments is not a direct measure of the cells and there is the possibility of other interfering substances in blood occupying the NRBC signature position and producing false-positive results.

AUTOMATED DIGITAL IMAGING ANALYSIS OF BLOOD CELLS

Over the last 20 years automated imaging processes have started to be introduced where stained blood films are scanned by a computer-driven microscope and leucocytes classified; early methods were slow and had difficulty in classifying abnormal cells and, as only a small number of cells were counted in a reasonable time, the precision of the automated count was no better than that of a manual count.[70] However, with improved computing technology and with the use of artificial neural networks, such instruments, e.g. CellaVision DM96 AB, Lund, Sweden and HemoFAXS, Tissuegnostics GmbH, Tabarstasse 10/12/8, A-1020, Wein, Austria, are now capable of providing a useful differential count on blood samples, even those containing abnormal cells.[71] The DM96 is composed of a slide scanning unit and a computer. The scanning unit consists of a motorized microscope and a digital charge-coupled device (CCD) camera. The instrument scans the stained blood film, identifies potential white cells, takes digital images of them and uses artificial neural network-based software to analyse the cells. Up to 30 films an hour can be processed. Digital images of pre-classified cells are presented to the operator on a computer screen for conformation or re-classification. The operator of the instrument needs to be skilled in blood cell morphology in order to accept or re-classify accurately the cells presented.[72]

NEW WHITE CELL PARAMETERS

Many instruments are able to 'flag' the presence of abnormal leucocytes by features such as an alteration in cell size, nuclear size or cell granularity which causes changes in impedance or light-scattering characteristics. Automated white cell counters can also analyse cell characteristics by novel technologies and identify cell types by features that differ greatly from those used when a blood film is examined visually. It is possible, for example, to identify eosinophils by the ability of their granules to polarize light[73] or to detect a left shift or the presence of blasts by the reduced light scattering of the nuclei of more immature granulocytes. There is also the potential to produce information that is not directly analogous with that available from a manual differential count. Recently white blood cell differential parameters have been reported to demonstrate clinical utility in the diagnosis of some diseases. Abnormal cell populations that have previously only triggered an abnormal flag, on some instruments, can now be quantitated.

Numerical data (coordinates) generated by analysers that use volume, conductivity and scatter (VCS) are now available. These coordinates indicating the position and size of the cell cluster in the VCS differential plot are available for neutrophils, lymphocytes, monocytes and eosinophils and cells of each cell type have normal values. Any deviations away from normal are thought to reflect differences in cell size and complexity and may be indicative of a potential disease process or specific to a morphological characteristic. These parameters are still for laboratory use only but it may be possible to use them as advanced flags for specific diseases or conditions in certain clinical circumstances. Lymphocyte positional parameters can be used to distinguish between different lymphoproliferative disorders and viral infections.[74] Neutrophil conductivity and neutrophil scatter can be used in the detection of dysplastic neutrophils,[75] with low values for these parameters correlating with neutrophil hypogranulation.

Sepsis-associated neutrophil left shift can be identified by a change from normal values of neutrophil volume and may be used as an indicator of acute bacterial infections.[76]

It has been suggested that VCS and other instrument parameters used for defining leucocyte types might also allow detection of the presence of malaria pigment in white blood cells or larger than normal monocytes and may be used as a screening test for malaria.[77,78]

In a similar way, using forward scattered light and fluorescence, new parameters have been developed on the basis of abnormal leucocyte positions in the differential scattergram. Plasma cells appear in a high fluorescence area of the lymphocyte cluster in the differential channel of the XE-2100 and are flagged as atypical lymphocytes; they can now be quantitated.[79] On the same instrument, NEUT-X is the mean value for side scatter diffraction of the neutrophil population; it represents the internal structure of the neutrophils. It correlates with hypogranularity of neutrophils and when taken into consideration with anaemia is suggestive of a myelodysplastic syndrome.[80] Instruments such as Siemens Advia analysers that incorporate a cytochemical reaction give information on enzyme activity expressed as the mean peroxidase activity index (MPXI). An increased MPXI has been observed in infections, in some myelodysplastic syndromes and leukaemias, in the acquired immune deficiency syndrome (AIDS) and in megaloblastic anaemia, whereas a reduced MPXI occurs in inherited and acquired neutrophil peroxidase deficiency.[60,81,82] These new parameters provide numerical values for the changes that can be seen in the instruments' scatter plots by an experienced operator. Such measurements have the potential for clinical usefulness and may allow the development of specific disease flags and new indicators of abnormality.

AUTOMATED INSTRUMENT GRAPHICS

Fully automated instruments produce a graphic display of much of the data produced. This is displayed on a colour monitor and can be printed, either in black and white or in colour. Inspection of the graphic display can give further information beyond that which is available from assessment of the numeric data. Displays usually include histograms of red cell, white cell and platelet size and sometimes histograms of red cell haemoglobin concentration and scatter plots of size versus haemoglobin concentration. Differential counts are graphically represented as scatter plots of two variables or scatter plots of discriminant functions derived from more than two variables.

Typical printouts of histograms or scatter plots of current automated instruments are shown in Figure 3.8.

Figure 3.8 Patterns of blood count printout of some automated systems. (A) Beckman Coulter DxH; (B) Sysmex XE-2100; (C) Siemens Advia; (D) Abbot Cell-Dyn 4000.

PLATELET COUNT

Platelets can be counted in whole blood using the same techniques of electrical or electro-optical detection as are used for counting red cells. An upper threshold is needed to separate platelets from red cells and a lower threshold is needed to separate platelets from debris and electronic noise. Recirculation of red cells near the aperture should be prevented, as pulses produced may simulate those generated by platelets. Three techniques for setting thresholds have been used: (1) platelets can be counted between two fixed thresholds (e.g. between 2 and 20 fl); (2) pulses between fixed thresholds can be counted with subsequent fitting of a curve and extrapolation so that platelets falling outside the fixed thresholds are included in the computed count; and (3) thresholds can vary automatically, depending on the characteristics of individual blood samples, to make allowance for microcytic or fragmented red cells or for giant platelets. Factitiously low impedance platelet counts may be the result of giant platelets being identified as red cells or of EDTA-induced platelet clumping or satellitism (see p. 98). Misleadingly, high platelet counts may be due to markedly microcytic or fragmented red cells, to white cell fragments in leukaemia[83] or to bacteria or fungi.

An optical fluorescence platelet count has been introduced on some Sysmex analysers, in addition to the traditional impedance count.[84] A dye is used to stain the RNA/DNA of reticulocytes and platelet membranes and granules. The fluorescent staining of the platelets allows the exclusion of non-platelet particles from the count and also allows the inclusion of large or giant platelets. However, for samples from patients undergoing cytotoxic chemotherapy, the impedance count is sometimes more accurate. This is probably due to the erroneous staining of white cell fragments following apoptosis.[83] A switching algorithm has been designed on the instrument to report the most accurate platelet count, either optical or impedance.

An immunofluorescent method for platelet counting by flow cytometry has also been developed.[85] Platelets in a blood sample are labelled fluorescently with a specific monoclonal antibody or combination of antibodies and by measuring the RBC:platelet ratio the platelet count can be calculated. Suitable antibodies to platelet antigens are CD41, CD42 and CD61. This method using CD41 and CD61 has been adopted by the International Council for Standardization in Haematology as the reference method.[86] The Abbott Cell-Dyn and Sapphire instruments provide an automated immunological platelet count for diagnostic use. Although instruments can count platelets down to levels of 10×10^9/l or less, it should be noted that precision at these levels is often poor with CVs of 22–66% being observed[87] and with counts below 10×10^9/l differing appreciably between instruments

and from the International Council for Standardization in Haematology reference method.[88]

Platelet Count in Health

In health, there are approximately $150–400 \times 10^9$ platelets per litre of blood. The counts are somewhat higher in women than in men,[89] and there is a cycling, with slightly lower count at about the time of menstruation.[90] Lower platelet counts have been observed in apparently healthy West Indians and Africans than in Caucasians.[91]

Mean Platelet Volume

The same techniques that are used to size red cells can be applied to platelets. The mean platelet volume (MPV) is derived from the impedance platelet size distribution curve. The MPV is very dependent on the technique of measurement and on length and conditions of storage prior to testing the blood. When MPV is measured by impedance technology, it has been found to vary inversely with the platelet count in normal subjects. If this curve is extrapolated, it has been found that data fit the extrapolated curve when thrombocytopenia is caused by peripheral platelet destruction; however, the MPV is lower than predicted when thrombocytopenia is caused by megaloblastic anaemia or bone marrow failure.[92,93] Large platelets are haemostatically more active than smaller platelets and may be more important functionally than smaller platelets. An increase in MPV has been observed in patients at risk of and following myocardial infarction[94] and cerebral infarction.[95] A high MPV can provide important evidence of an inherited macrothrombocytopenia. The MPV is generally greater than predicted in myeloproliferative neoplasms, but differentiating essential thrombocythaemia from reactive thrombocytosis on this basis has not been very successful.

Other platelet parameters that can be computed by automated counters include the platelet distribution width (PDW), which is a measure of platelet anisocytosis and the 'plateletcrit', which is the product of the MPV and platelet count and, by analogy with the haematocrit, may be seen as indicative of the volume of circulating platelets in a unit volume of blood. The platelet large cell ratio (P-LCR), reported by some instruments is the number of platelets falling above the 12 fl threshold on the platelet size histogram divided by the total number of platelets. A high P-LCR or PDW may indicate peripheral immune destruction of platelets.[96] The PDW has been found to be of some use in distinguishing essential thrombocythaemia (PDW increased) from reactive thrombocytosis (PDW normal). The plateletcrit does not appear to provide any information of clinical value. All derived platelet parameters are highly specific to the individual technologies, with different analysers having different normal ranges.

Reticulated Platelets and Immature Platelet Fraction

After labelling with specific immunological markers and a fluorescent dye that binds RNA, it is possible to identify young platelets with a higher RNA content by flow cytometry.[86,97–99] By analogy with the reticulocyte count, these have been called 'reticulated platelets', and it has been suggested that an increased number in the circulation is a sensitive and early indication of recovery of thrombopoiesis in aplastic anaemia. However, because there is a constant exchange of platelets between the circulation and the spleen, it is not clear whether their presence in the blood has the same significance as reticulocytes

A new automated method to quantitate reticulated platelets, expressed as the immature platelet fraction (IPF), has been developed on some Sysmex instruments. The measurement of the IPF uses a fluorescent dye containing polymethine and oxazine. These two dyes penetrate the cell membrane, staining any RNA in red cells and platelets, and the stained cells are then passed through a semiconductor diode laser beam. The resulting forward scatter light (cell volume) and fluorescence intensity (RNA content) are measured and reticulocytes and reticulated platelets are identified. The IPF is raised in patients with peripheral consumption/destruction of platelets (idiopathic thrombocytopenic purpura and thrombotic thrombocytopenia purpura) and is normal or low in patients with marrow failure.[100] Following a peripheral blood stem cell transplant the IPF has been reported to increase 1–2 days prior to the platelet count increasing.[101,102]

RETICULOCYTE COUNT

Automated reticulocyte counts have been developed by using the fact that various dyes and fluorochromes combine with the RNA of reticulocytes.[40,103] Following binding of the dye, fluorescent cells can be enumerated using a flow cytometer. Most fully automated blood counters now incorporate a reticulocyte counting capacity so that use of a stand-alone reticulocyte counter is no longer necessary and use of a general purpose flow cytometer is no longer appropriate. An international standard for this method has been published by the Clinical and Laboratory Standards Institute (CLSI) in collaboration with ICSH.[44] The dyes used in the different systems include auramine O or polymethine with oxazine (Sysmex), thiazole orange (ABX), CD4K 530 (Abbott), as well as nonfluorescent dyes such as oxazine 750 (Siemens) and the traditional New methylene blue (Beckman Coulter, Abbott).

After staining, it is necessary to separate the reticulocytes from unstained red cells and, because the dyes also combine with DNA of nucleated cells, these cells must also be excluded. The threshold for this exclusion is determined by the intensity of fluorescence and particle sizing. Although the separation of reticulocytes from mature red cells is not always clear cut, automated reticulocyte counts correlate well with manual reticulocyte counts; however, absolute counts may differ because automated counts are dependent on the conditions of incubation and the method of calibrating the instrument.[103] Precision is much superior to that of the manual count because many more cells are counted, which has allowed reliable flagging of reticulocytopenia and the subjective element inherent in recognizing late reticulocytes is eliminated. Potential sources of inaccuracy are the inclusion of some leucocytes and platelets and, less often, Howell-Jolly bodies or malarial parasites in the 'reticulocyte' count.

Automated reticulocyte counts are fairly stable in blood that has been stored for 1–2 days at room temperature or up to 3–5 days at 4°C.

Immature Reticulocyte Fraction

Fully automated instruments provide a measure of the various degrees of reticulocyte maturation because the most immature reticulocytes, produced when erythropoietin levels are high, have more RNA and fluoresce more strongly than the mature reticulocytes normally present in the peripheral blood. An assessment of reticulocyte maturation can be important for diagnosing the cause of anaemia and assessing the degree of effective erythropoiesis.

For example, an increase in mean fluorescence intensity indicative of the presence of immature reticulocytes has been noted as an early sign of engraftment following bone marrow transplantation.

The characteristics of reticulocyte output in different types of anaemias can be especially appreciated from an output bivariate graph relating fluorescent intensity to reticulocyte count.[40] As described earlier, low total count with a relatively high immature reticulocyte fraction (IRF) is indicative of a repopulating marrow, whereas a reticulocytopenia with low IRF is typical of severe aplastic anaemia or renal failure A high total count with high IRF occurs in acute haemolysis and blood loss, whereas a low to normal total count with a high IRF occurs in dyserythropoiesis and in early response to haematinics.[104–106] The appearance of reticulocytes with high fluorescence also heralds response when severe aplastic anaemia is being treated with immunosuppressive therapy,[104] and is a reliable indication of haemopoietic regeneration after marrow ablative chemotherapy. A high IRF has also been found to be useful in predicting the optimal time for stem cell harvests in some but not all studies.[107] A normal total count with an unexpectedly high IRF in athletes has been suggested as a method to detect 'doping' with erythropoietin.[108] It may also be useful in deciding whether a macrocytic anaemia is megaloblastic or non-megaloblastic.[109]

Reticulocyte Counts in Health

The normal reticulocyte count in men or women is: $50-100 \times 10^9/l$ (0.5-2.5%).

However, reference ranges reported for automated reticulocyte counts vary considerably between different automated methods and it is important to use instrument-specific normal ranges and for laboratories to establish their own values.

Measurement of Reticulocyte Haemoglobin

The reticulocyte count provides a quantitative measure of erythropoiesis but no information on the quality of erythropoiesis. With the development of flow cell haematology analysers it is now possible to measure the volume and haemoglobin content of reticulocytes. The parameter from Siemens is termed CHr (mean reticulocyte haemoglobin content) and from Sysmex the Ret-H$_e$, (the reticulocyte haemoglobin concentration). CHr is measured in the stained reticulocytes using two angle light scatter and Ret-H$_e$, is a measure of the forward scatter of stained reticulocytes and has a curvilinear relationship with CHr.[110] The reticulocyte haemoglobin content provides an indirect measure of the functional iron available for new red blood cell production over the previous 3-4 days. More recently, other instruments have developed parameters that may give information equivalent to reticulocyte haemoglobin; these are based on a measure of mean reticulocyte volume (MRV). Reticulocyte haemoglobin and reticulocyte volume may have similar clinical utility, but the MRV produced by different instruments lacks standardization, which means numeric results from different manufacturers are not comparable. Red blood cell size factor (RSf) is a new parameter provided by Beckman Coulter, which relates to the volume of erythrocytes and reticulocytes. Good correlation between CHr and RSf has been reported.[111]

POINT-OF-CARE INSTRUMENTS

There are two types of technology to support point-of-care testing (POCT) (see p. 574), small bench top analysers and hand-held devices. The bench top systems are often smaller versions of laboratory analysers providing an FBC with red cell indices and either a five-part white cell differential or a partial three-part differential. Bench top analysers are equipped with automated calibration and quality control; however, they are too large for use at the patient's bedside and are designed for use in clinics or small laboratories. It is recommended that instruments that employ primary sampling are used, rather than instruments that involve dilution of whole blood in the pre-analytical phase.[112] The most widely used test with a hand-held device is the measurement of haemoglobin concentration, but another device, using a disposable cartridge, has recently been introduced that measures haemoglobin concentration, counts leucocytes and platelets and performs a three-part differential on capillary blood. The range of equipment available will inevitably expand as more POCT is implemented. POCT devices should generate results that are comparable to those of the local reference laboratory. Internal quality control (IQC) must be available for all POCT instruments to detect significant deviations from acceptable performance. The analysis of control material before analysing patient samples can provide reassurance that the system is working correctly. At regular intervals parallel testing of a patient sample may be carried out at the POCT site and the main laboratory to ensure comparable results.

Ideally, there should also be an objective external method of quality assurance, external quality control (EQA). EQA involves the analysis of samples received from an accredited external source with undisclosed values; this could be from the supervising laboratory itself, from a manufacturer or from accredited national schemes. Results are subject to peer group assessment and statistical analysis to compare results across different sites. Local haematologists/pathologists should encourage POCT users to participate in the supervising laboratory's EQA.[112]

Haematologists should be aware of the potential for error if point-of-care blood gas analysers are used for estimation of Hb or Hct. Use of instruments that are based on conductivity measurements is not recommended since discrepancies of 20 g/l in the Hb and 0.04 l/l in the Hct can occur when the plasma protein concentration is low (e.g. if crystalloid has been used for blood replacement) and there is also a downward biases when the haematocrit is less than 0.30 l/l.[112] Furthermore, the reproducibility of Hct measurements can be poor. As long as there is adequate quality control, instruments based on spectrophotometry/co-oximetry agree more closely with laboratory measurements of Hb.[112]

CALIBRATION OF AUTOMATED BLOOD CELL COUNTERS

The following methods are recommended for calibrating an automated blood cell counter:[113,114]

1. By using fresh normal blood specimens to which values have been assigned for Hb, PCV, RBC, WBC and platelet count by standardized reference methods

2. By use of a stable calibrant (either preserved blood or a substitute) to which values appropriate for the instrument in question have been assigned by comparison with fresh normal blood

3. By use of a commercial calibrant with assigned values suitable for the instrument in question.

For reasons of convenience and economy, control materials are commonly used as calibrants; but this practice is not recommended. Such materials are not sufficiently stable to serve as calibrants and their stated values are often approximations that are not assigned by reference methods. They are designed to give test results within a stated range over a stated period rather than a specific result.

The procedure for assigning values to fresh blood samples and indirectly to a stable calibrant is as follows:

1. 4 ml blood specimens are obtained from three haematologically normal volunteers and are anticoagulated with K_2 EDTA.
2. The Hb value is assigned by using the haemiglobincyanide method and the mean of two measurements.
3. The PCV is assigned by the microhaematocrit method, taking the mean of measurements in four microhaematocrit tubes.
4. The RBC is assigned by performing counts on a single-channel aperture-impedance counter capable of performing a direct cell count; the mean of two dilutions, each counted twice, is used.
5. The MCV is assigned by calculation from the RBC and PCV.
6. The WBC is assigned by performing counts on a single-channel aperture-impedance instrument capable of performing direct cell counts; the mean of two dilutions, each counted twice, is used.
7. The platelet count is assigned by using a flow cytometer capable of measuring the ratio of platelets to red cells; the platelet count is calculated from the ratio and an independently measured RBC. Where fluorescent monoclonal antibody labelling is available, the ICSH/ISLH reference method[86] should be used. In preparations intended as a differential leucocyte count or a reticulocyte count calibrant, assign the values by the reference manual methods,[34,43] as described on p. 32 and p. 36, respectively.

To calibrate the automated counter directly from the three fresh blood samples, perform two counts with each sample and take the means. If the measured counts differ from those assigned, recalibrate the counter appropriately.

To calibrate a stable calibrant, perform two counts on the calibrant and on each fresh sample using the automated instrument, A, and take the means. From the ratio of the test results on fresh blood to those on the calibrator, assign corrected values to the calibrator by using the following calculations:

$$\text{Corrected calibrator value} = A_C \times \sqrt[3]{\frac{D_{F1}}{A_{F1}} \times \frac{D_{F2}}{A_{F2}} \times \frac{D_{F3}}{A_{F3}}}$$

where:

A_C = measurement of calibrator by automated counter
A_F = measurement of the fresh bloods (1, 2 and 3) by automated counter
D_F = direct measurement of the fresh bloods (1, 2 and 3).

Considerable care is required to ensure that the initial measurements on the fresh blood are as accurate as possible. Dilutions should be made with individually calibrated pipettes and grade A volumetric flasks. The cell counter should be calibrated as described on p. 39, with a signal-to-noise ratio of >100:1 and the count corrected for coincidence. Details of procedures to be used are described by the International Committee for Standardization in Haematology.[115] Procedures for verification of the performance of multichannel analysers by the users have also been published by ICSH[46] and in the USA, by the National Committee for Clinical Laboratory Standards.[116]

FLAGGING OF AUTOMATED BLOOD COUNTS

'Flagging'[117,118] refers to a signal that the specimen being analysed may have a significant abnormality because one or more of the blood count variables are outside specified limits (usually 2SD) or there is a qualitative abnormality that requires a quality control check and/or additional investigation. Abnormal cells have differing characteristics, such as nuclear size and granule content, from normal cells. The instrument detects a cell population as having an abnormal size or shape by cluster analysis. Under these circumstances, abnormal cell flags are generated to alert the user to the possibility of inaccurate results. Abnormal cells or interfering substances may render the automated differential inaccurate or unreportable. A blood film will need to be examined microscopically to verify the automated count and confirm the presence of abnormal cells. Most point-of-care bench top analysers have the ability to generate flags in the presence of abnormal cells or interfering substances; however, the range of alert flags available on these instruments is limited and their sensitivity and specificity may not be as good as those on more sophisticated laboratory haematology analysers. Although it is theoretically desirable for every blood count to include examination of a stained film, this has become impossible as a result of increasing workloads; time- and cost-effective rationalization has therefore been required. This has been helped by the availability of automated analysers that report differential leucocyte counts on every specimen. Consequently, significantly fewer blood films are now examined microscopically. Thus, a decision of when a blood film should be made, stained and examined should take account of

Box 3.1

Blood count request: Is it a first-time count or repeat count?

First-time count: Is it a routine screening test or special category?

If routine: Analyser report for blood count alone.
Film required if any flags are signalled.

Special category film required:

1. Diagnosed blood disease patients
2. Patients receiving radiotherapy and/or chemotherapy
3. Recent onset of renal disease
4. Neonates
5. Intensive care unit patients
6. If special tests have also been requested for: infectious mononucleosis, haemolytic anaemia, enzymopathy, abnormal haemoglobins
7. If the clinical details on the request form indicate lymphadenopathy, splenomegaly, jaundice or suggest the possibility of leukaemia or lymphoma
8. Specific requests by clinician.

Repeat count film required:

1. Delta check positive when compared with previous record
2. Any flag occurs in present count
3. On each occasion for patients with known blood diseases, for neonates and when specifically requested by clinicians.

Figure 3.9 Cross-section of microscope, showing its components. E, eyepiece; S, stand; O, objective; M, mechanical stage; C, condenser. The broken lines indicate the light path. Note that this shows an external light source being directed into the microscope. In most modern microscopes there is a built-in lamp in the base.

flagging and the need to ensure analytic reliability. This includes a check of any significant changes from a recent previous count (delta check), as well as any specific clinical circumstances. There are previously published guidelines that describe blood film review criteria following FBC and differential analysis,[119] which may be adapted to the individual laboratory's needs. Box 3.1 is a guide to this selection.

MICROSCOPY

Microscope Components

The main components of most routine microscopes are illustrated in Figure 3.9. The objectives are usually marked with their magnifying power, but older lenses may be marked by their focal length instead. The approximate equivalents are in Table 3.5.

The working distance of the objective is the distance between the objective and the object to be visualized. The greater the magnifying power of the objective, the smaller the working distance (Table 3.6).

Table 3.5 Approximate equivalents of focal length to magnifying power

FOCAL LENGTH (mm)	MAGNIFICATION
2	×100
4	×40
16	×10
40	×4

These specifications mean that when a coverslip is used, if it is too thick it will not be possible to focus at high magnification. Thus, the coverslip should be no more than 0.15 mm thick for examination of covered preparations by the ×100 oil-immersion objective. Furthermore, if the glass slide is too thick, this may prevent correct focus of the light path through the condenser to the object, as described later.

Table 3.6 Objective magnifying power and the associated working distance

OBJECTIVE	WORKING DISTANCE
×10	5–6 mm
×40	0.5–1.5 mm
×100	0.15–0.20 mm

Setting Up the Microscope Illumination

1. If the microscope requires an external light source, using the mirror at the base, direct the light into the condenser. If the illumination is built in, make sure that the lamp voltage is turned down before switching on the microscope; then turn up the lamp until it is at *c* 70% of maximum power.
2. Place a slide of a blood film with a coverslip on the stage.
3. Lower the condenser, open the iris diaphragm fully and bring the preparation on the slide into focus with the ×10 objective.
4. Check that the eyepieces are adjusted to the operator's interpupillary width and that the specimen is in focus for each eye by rotating the focusing mechanism on the adjustable eyepiece.
5. Close the diaphragm and raise the condenser slowly until the edge of the circle of light comes into sharp focus and there is a faint blue tinge at the edge of the diaphragm.
6. Using the condenser centering screws, adjust its position so that the circle of light is in the centre of the field.
7. Open the diaphragm completely so that light fills the whole field of view.
8. Remove the eyepieces, so that the upper lens of the objective is seen to be filled with a circle of light. Close the diaphragm slowly until the circle of light occupies about two-thirds of the surface.
9. Replace the eyepieces, refocus the specimen and if necessary readjust the condenser aperture and lamp brightness to obtain the sharpest possible image.

Examination of Slides

Low power (×10). Start with the objective just above the slide preparation. Then raise the objective with the coarse adjustment screw until a clear image is seen in the eyepiece. If there is insufficient illumination, rack up the condenser slightly.

High power (×40). Rack the condenser halfway down; lower the objective until it is just above the slide preparation. Use the coarse adjustment to raise the objective very slowly until a blurred image appears. Then bring into focus using the fine adjustment. If necessary, raise the condenser to obtain sufficient illumination.

Oil immersion (×100). Place a small drop of immersion oil on the part to be examined. Rack up the condenser as far as it will go. Lower the objective until it is in contact with the oil. Bring it as close as possible to the slide, but avoid pressing on the preparation. Look through the eyepiece and turn the fine adjustment very slowly until the image is in focus.

After using the oil-immersion objective, to avoid scratching the lens or coating the ×40 lens with oil, first swing the ×10 objective (or an empty lens space on the nosepiece) into place before removing the slide. As far as possible, use oil only when essential (e.g. for determining malaria species) and examine blood films for morphology or differential leucocyte count with the ×40 lens without oil.

If you cannot focus using the oil-immersion lens, consider that:

The coverslip may be too thick
Two coverslips may have been accidentally applied
You might have inverted the slide.

Routine Maintenance of the Microscope

The microscope is a delicate instrument that must be handled gently. It must be installed in a clean environment away from chemicals, direct sunlight, heating sources or moisture. If the stage is contaminated with saline, it must be cleaned immediately to avoid corrosion. Even in a temperate climate, humidity and high temperatures cause growth of fungus, which can damage optical surfaces. Because storage in a closed compartment encourages fungal growth, do not store the microscope in its wooden box, but keep it standing on the bench protected by a light plastic cover.

After use of the microscope, wipe the oil-immersion objective with lens tissue, absorbent paper, soft cloth or medical cotton wool. If other lenses are smeared with oil, wipe them with a little toluene or a solution of 40% petroleum ether, 40% ethanol and 20% ether.

Lenses must never be soaked in alcohol because this may dissolve the cement.

Clean non-optical parts with mild detergent and remove grease or oil with petroleum ether, followed by 45% ethanol in water. Remove dust from the inside and outside of the eyepieces with a blower or soft camel-hair brush.

Clean the condenser in the same way as the lenses with a soft cloth or tissue moistened with toluene and clean the mirror (if present) with a soft cloth moistened with 5% alcohol. The iris diaphragm is very delicate and if damaged or badly corroded it is usually beyond repair.

Never force the controls. If movement of the focusing screws or mechanical stage becomes difficult, lubricate them with a small drop of machine oil. All accessible moving parts should be cleaned occasionally and given a touch of oil to protect against corrosion. Do not use vegetable oils because they become dry and hard. Always keep the surface of the fixed stage dry because moving wet slides requires increased force, which may damage the mechanical stage.

For care of microscopes in hot humid and hot dry climates, see p. 606.

see p. 606.

REFERENCES

1. Zijlstra WG, van Kampen EJ. Standardization of hemoglobinometry. I. The extinction coefficient of hemiglobincyanide at 1 = 540mm: e540HiCN. *Clin Chim Acta*. 1960;91:719–726.

2. International Committee for Standardization in Haematology. *Recommendations for Reference Method for Haemoglobinometry in Human Blood (ICSH Standard 1995) and Specifications for International Haemiglobincyanide Standard*. 4th ed. *J Clin Pathol*. 1996;49:271–274.

3. Vanzetti G. An azide-methemoglobin method for hemoglobin determination in blood. *J Lab Clin Med*. 1966;67:116–126.

4. Oshiro I, Takenaka T, Maeda J. New method for hemoglobin determination by using sodium lauryl sulfate (SLS). *Clin Biochem*. 1982;15:83–88.

5. Lewis SM, Garvey B, Manning R, et al. Lauryl sulphate haemoglobin: a non-hazardous substitute for HiCN in haemoglobinometry. *Clin Lab Haematol*. 1991;13:279–290.

6. Zander R, Land W, Wolf HU. Alkaline haematin D-575, a new tool for the determination of haemoglobin as an alternative to the cyanhaemiglobin method. I. Description of the method. *Clin Chim Acta*. 1984;136:83–93.

7. Wolf HU, Land W, Zander R. Alkaline haematin D-575, a new tool for the determination of haemoglobin as an alternative to the cyanhaemiglobin method. II. Standardization of the method using pure chlorohaemin. *Clin Chim Acta*. 1984;136:95–104.

8. Lema OE, Carter JY, Arube PA, et al. Evaluation of the alkaline haematin D-575 method for haemoglobin estimation in east Africa. *Bull World Health Organ*. 1994;72:937–941.

9. van Assendelft OW, Zijlstra WG. Observations on the alkaline haematin/detergent complex proposed for measuring haemoglobin concentration. *J Clin Chem Clin Biochem*. 1989;27:191–195.

10. Van Assendelft OW, Buursma A, Zijlstra WG. Stability of haemiglobincyanide standards. *J Clin Pathol*. 1996;49:275–277.

11. Davies B, Jungerius B. International Council for Standardization in Haematology technical report 1–2009: new reference material for haemoglobincyanide for use in standardization of blood haemoglobin measurements. *Int J Hematol*. 2010; E-pub ahead of print.

12. Van Kampen EJ, Zijlstra WG. Spectrophotometry of hemoglobin and hemoglobin derivatives. *Adv Clin Chem*. 1983;23:199–257.

13. Matsubara T, Okuzono H, Senba U. Modification of Van Kampen-Zijlstra's reagent for the hemiglobincyanide method. *Clin Chim Acta*. 1979;93:163–164.

14. Morris LD, Osei-Bimpong A, McKeown D, et al. Evaluation of the utility of the HemoCue 301 haemoglobinometer for blood donor screening. *Vox Sang*. 2007;93:64–69.

15. Osei-Bimpong A, Jury C, McLean R, et al. Point-of-care for total white cell count: an evaluation of the HemoCue WBC device. *Int J Hematol*. 2008;31:657–664.

16. Robertson L, Lewis D, Osei-Bimpong A. *The utility of the DiaSpect Haemoglobinometry System as a point-of-care analyser*. 2010. In press.

17. Kinoshita Y, Yamane T, Takubo T, et al. Measurement of hemoglobin concentrations using the Astrim noninvasive blood vessel monitoring apparatus. *Acta Haematol*. 2002;108:109–110.

18. Rendell M, Anderson E, Schlueter W, et al. Determination of hemoglobin levels in the finger using near infra-red spectroscopy. *Clin Lab Haematol*. 2003;25:93–97.

19. International Council for Standardization in Haematology. Recommendations for reference method for determination by centrifugation of packed cell volume of blood. *J Clin Pathol*. 1980;33:1–2.

20. World Health Organization. *Recommended method for the determination of packed cell volume by centrifugation (Prepared by Expert Panel on Cytometry of the International Council for Standardization in Haematology) Document WHO/DIL/00.2:1–9*. Geneva: WHO; 2000.

21. Bryner MA, Houwen B, Westengard J, et al. The spun haematocrit and mean red cell volume are affected by changes in the oxygenation state of red blood cells. *Clin Lab Haematol*. 1997;19:99–103.

22. International Committee for Standardization in Haematology. Recommended methods for measurement of red-cell and plasma volume. *J Nucl Med*. 1980;21:793–800.

23. Bull BS, Fujimoto K, Houwen B, et al. International Council for Standardization in Haematology (ICSH). Recommendations for 'surrogate reference' method for the packed cell volume. *Lab Hematol*. 2003;9:1–9.

24. England JM, Walford DM, Waters DAW. Reassessment of the reliability of the haematocrit. *Br J Haematol*. 1972;23:247–256.

25. Pearson TC, Guthrie DL. Trapped plasma in microhematocrit. *Am J Clin Pathol*. 1982;78:770–772.

26. Expert Panel on Cytometry of the International Council for Standardization in Haematology. Recommendations for reference method for the packed cell volume

(ICSH Standard). *Lab Hematol.* 2001;7:148–170.

27. Rothenberg ME. Eosinophilia. *N Engl J Med.* 1998;338:1592–1699.

28. Uhrbrand H. The number of circulating eosinophils: normal figures and spontaneous variations. *Acta Med Scand.* 1958;160:99–104.

29. Brito-Babapulle F. The eosinophilias, including the idiopathic hypereosinophilic syndrome. *Br J Haematol.* 2003;121:203–223.

30. Gilbert HS, Ornstein L. Basophil counting with a new staining method using Alcian blue. *Blood.* 1975;46:279–286.

31. Mettler L, Shirwani D. Direct basophil count for timing ovulation. *Fertil Steril.* 1974;25:718–723.

32. Mathy KA, Koepke JA. The clinical usefulness of segmented vs stab neutrophil criteria for differential leucocyte counts. *Am J Clin Pathol.* 1974;61:947–958.

33. Gombos M, Bienkowski R, Gochman R, et al. The absolute neutrophil count: Is it the best indicator for occult bacteraemia in infants? *Am J Clin Pathol.* 1998;109:221–225.

34. Clinical and Laboratory Standards Institute. *Reference leukocyte differential count (proportional) and evaluation of instrument methods. Approved standard.* CLSI document H20-A2. Wayne PA: CLSI; 2007.

35. Hubl W, Wolfbauer G, Andert S, et al. Towards a new reference method for the leukocyte five-part differential. *Cytometry.* 1997;30: 72–84.

36. Fujimoto H, Sakata T, Hamaguchi Y, et al. Flow cytometric method for enumeration and classification of reactive immature granulocyte populations. *Cytometry.* 2000;42: 371–378.

37. Faucher JL, Lacronique-Gazaille C, Frébet E, et al. '6 markers/5 colors' extended white cell differential by flow cytometry. *Cytometry.* 2007;71:934–944.

38. Björnsson S, Wahlström S, Norström E, et al. Total nucleated cell differential for blood and bone marrow using a single tube in a five color flow cytometer. *Cytometry B Clin Cytom.* 2008;74:91–103.

39. Groom AC, Schmidt EE. Microcirculatory blood flow through the spleen. In: Bowdler AJ, ed. *The Spleen: Structure, Function and Clinical Significance.* London: Chapman and Hall; 1990:45–102.

40. D'Onofrio G, Zini G, Rowan RM. Reticulocyte counting: methods and clinical applications. In: Rowan RM, van Assendelft OW, Preston FE, eds. *Advanced Laboratory Methods in Haematology.* London: Arnold; 2002:78–126.

41. Wittekind D, Schulte E. Standardized azure B as a reticulocyte stain. *Clin Lab Haematol.* 1987;9:395–398.

42. Jahanmehr SAH, Hyde K, Geary CG, et al. Simple technique for fluorescence staining of blood cells with acridine orange. *J Clin Pathol.* 1987;40:926–929.

43. International Council for Standardization in Haematology. Proposed reference method for reticulocyte counting based on the determination of the reticulocyte to red cell ratio. *Clin Lab Haematol.* 1998;20:77–79.

44. Clinical and Laboratory Standards Institute and International Council for Standardization in Haematology. *Methods for reticulocyte counting (automated blood cell counters, flow cytometry and supravital dyes): approved guideline.* 2nd ed. Document H44-A2, Vol. 24(8). Wayne PA: CLSI; 2004.

45. Groner W, Simson E. *Practical Guide to Modern Haematology Analysers.* Chichester: Wiley; 1995.

46. International Council for Standardization in Haematology. Guidelines for the evaluation of blood cell analysers including those used for differential leucocyte and reticulocyte counting and cell marker applications. *Clin Lab Haematol.* 1994;16: 157–174.

47. Bain BJ. *Blood Cells: A Practical Guide.* 4th ed. Oxford: Blackwell; 2006.

48. Simson E, Ross DW, Kocher WD. *Atlas of Automated Cytochemical Hematology.* Tarrytown, NY: Technicon; 1988.

49. Houwen B. The blood count. In: Rowan RM, van Assendelft OW, Preston FE, eds. *Advanced Laboratory*

Methods in Haematology. London: Arnold; 2002:19–44.

50. Coulter WH. High speed automatic blood cell counter and cell size analyser. *Proceedings of National Electronics Conference.* 1956;12: 1034–1040.

51. Thom R. Automated red cell analysis. *Baillieres Clin Haematol.* 1990;3:837–850.

52. England JM, van Assendelft OW. 1986: Automated blood counters and their evaluation. In: Rowan RM, England JM, eds. *Automation and Quality Assurance in Haematology.* Oxford: Blackwell Scientific.

53. Mohandas N, Kim YR, Tycko DH, et al. Accurate and independent measurement of volume and hemoglobin concentration of individual red cells by laser scattering. *Blood.* 1986;68:506–513.

54. Tycko DH, Metz MH, Epstein EA, et al. Flow-cytometric light scattering measurement of red blood cell volume and hemoglobin concentration. *Appl Opt.* 1985;24:1355–1366.

55. Evan-Wong L, Davidson RJ. Raised Coulter mean corpuscular volume in diabetic ketoacidosis and its underlying association with marked plasma hyperosmolarity. *J Clin Pathol.* 1983;36:334–336.

56. Holt JT, DeWandler MJ, Arvan DA. Spurious elevation of the electronically determined mean corpuscular volume and hematocrit caused by hyperglycemia. *Am J Clin Pathol.* 1982;77:561–567.

57. Bentley SA, Ayscue LH, Watson JM, et al. The clinical utility of discriminant functions in the differential diagnosis of microcytic anemias. *Blood Cells.* 1989;15: 575–582.

58. Lafferty JD, Crowther MA, Ali MA, et al. The evaluation of various mathematical RBC indices and their efficacy in discriminating between thalassemic and non-thalassemic microcytosis. *Am J Clin Pathol.* 1996;106:201–295.

59. Green R, King R. A new red cell discriminant incorporating volume dispersion for differentiating iron deficiency anemia from thalassemia minor. *Blood Cells.* 1989;15: 481–491.

60. Ross DW, Bentley SA. Evaluation of an automated hematology system (Technicon H-1). *Arch Pathol Lab Med.* 1986;110:803–808.

61. Horl WH, Cavill I, MacDougall IC, et al. How to diagnose and correct iron deficiency during r-huEPO therapy – a consensus report. *Nephrol Dial Transplant.* 1996;11:246–250.

62. Schaefer RM, Schaefer L. The hypochromic red cell: a new parameter for monitoring of iron supplementation during rhEPO therapy. *J Perinat Med.* 1995;23:83–88.

63. Urrechaga E. The new mature red cell parameter, the haemoglobin density of the Beckman-Coulter LH750: clinical utility in the diagnosis of iron deficiency. *International Journal of Laboratory Hematology.* 2010;32:e144–e150.

64. Bain BJ, Cavill I. Hypochromic macrocytes – are they reticulocytes? *J Clin Pathol.* 1993;46:963–964.

65. Ballard BC. Lysing agent for the Coulter S. *J Clin Pathol.* 1972;25:460.

66. Skinnider LF, Musglow E. A stromatolysing and cyanide reagent for use with the Coulter Counter Model S. *Am J Clin Pathol.* 1972;57:537–538.

67. Bain BJ. An assessment of the three population differential count on the Coulter Model S Plus IV. *Clin Lab Haematol.* 1986;8:347–359.

68. Briggs C, Kunka S, Pennaneach C, et al. Performance evaluation of a new compact haematology analyser, the Sysmex pocH-100i. *Lab Hematol.* 2003;9:225–233.

69. Ansari-Lari MA, Kickler TS, Borowitz MJ. Immature granulocyte measurement using the Sysmex XE-2100. *Am J Clin Pathol.* 2003;120:795–799.

70. Bentley SA. Automated differential white cell counts: a critical appraisal. *Baillieres Clin Haematol.* 1990;3:851–869.

71. Ceelie H, Dinkelaar RB, van Gelder W. Examination of peripheral blood films using automated microscopy; evaluation of Diffmaster Octavia and Cellavision DM96. *J Clin Pathol.* 2007;60:72–79.

72. Briggs C, Longair I, Slavik M, et al. Can automated image analysis replace the manual differential? An evaluation of the CellaVision DM96 automated image analysis software. *International Journal of Laboratory Haematology.* 2007;31:48–60.

73. Cornbleet PJ, Myrick D, Judkins S, et al. Evaluation of the CELL-DYN 3000 differential. *Am J Clin Pathol.* 1992;98:603–614.

74. Silva M, Fourcade C, Fartoukh C, et al. Lymphocyte volume and conductivity indices of the haematology analyser Coulter GEN. STM in lymphoproliferative disorders and viral diseases. *Clin Lab Haematol.* 2006;28:1–28.

75. Miguel A, Orero M, Simon R, et al. Automated neutrophil morphology and its utility in the assessment of neutrophil dysplasia. *Lab Haematol.* 2007;13:98–102.

76. Chaves F, Tierno B, Xu D. Quantitative determination of neutrophil VCS parameters by the Coulter automated hematology analyser: new and reliable indicators for acute bacterial infection. *Am J Clin Pathol.* 2005;124:440–444.

77. Fourcade C, Casbas MJ, Belaouni H, et al. Automated detection of malaria by means of the haematology analyser Coulter GEN.S. *Clin Lab Haematol.* 2004;26:367–372.

78. Hänscheid T, Pinto BG, Cristino JM, et al. Malaria diagnosis with the haematology analyser Cell-Dyne 3500: what does the instrument detect? *Clin Lab Haematol.* 2000;22:259–261.

79. Linssen J, Jennissen V, Hildmann J, et al. Identification and quantification of high fluorescence-stained lymphocytes as antibody synthesizing/secreting cells using the automated routine hematology analyser XE-2100. *Cytometry B Clin Cytom.* 2007;72:157–166.

80. Furundarena JR, Araiz M, Uranga M, et al. The utility of the Sysmex XE-2100 analyzer's NEUT-X and NEUT-Y parameters for detecting neutrophil dysplasia in myelodysplastic syndromes. *International Journal of Laboratory Hematology.* 2009;32:360–366.

81. D'Onofrio G, Zini G, Tommasi M, et al. *Anomalie ultramorfoligiche dei granulociti neutrofili nelle infezioni da virus HIV. Atti del V Incontro del Club Utilizzatori Sistemi Ematologici.* Montecatini Terme: Bayer-Technicon; 1992.

82. Taylor C, Bain BJ. Technicon H1 automated white cell parameters in the diagnosis of megaloblastic erythropoiesis. *Eur J Haematol.* 1991;46:248–249.

83. van der Meer W, Mackenzie MA, Dinnissen JW, et al. Pseudoplatelets: A retrospective study of their incidence and interference with platelet counting. *J Clin Pathol.* 2003;56:772–774.

84. Briggs C, Harrison P, Grant D, et al. New quantitative parameters on a recently introduced automated blood cell counter – the XE 2100. *Clin Lab Haematol.* 2000;17:163–172.

85. Ault KA. The clinical utility of flow cytometry in the study of platelets. *Semin Hematol.* 2001;38:160–168.

86. ICSH (Expert Panel on Cytometry) and International Society of Laboratory Hematology (ISLH) . Platelet counting by the PLT/RBC ratio – a reference method. *Am J Clin Pathol.* 2001;115:460–464.

87. Parker-Williams J. Immunoplatelet counting: platelet transfusions. *Br J Haematol.* 2003;123:750–751.

88. Segal HC, Briggs C, Kunka S, et al. Accuracy of platelet counting haematology analysers in severe thrombocytopenia and potential impact on platelet transfusion. *Br J Haematol.* 2005;128:520–525.

89. Bain BJ. Platelet count and platelet size in males and females. *Scand J Haematol.* 1985;35:77–79.

90. Morley A. A platelet cycle in normal individuals. *Australas Ann Med.* 1969;18:127–129.

91. Bain BJ, Seed M. Platelet count and platelet size in Africans and West Indians. *Clin Lab Haematol.* 1986;8:43–48.

92. Bessman JD, Williams LJ, Gilmer PR. Platelet size in health and hematologic disease. *Am J Clin Pathol.* 1982;78:150–153.

93. Bowles KM, Cooke LJ, Richards EM, et al. Platelet size has diagnostic predictive value in patients with thrombocytopenia. *Clin Lab Haematol.* 2005;27:370–373.

94. Khandekar MM, Khurana AS, Deshmukh SD, et al. Platelet volume indices in patients with coronary artery disease and acute myocardial infarction: an Indian scenario. *J Clin Pathol.* 2006;59:146–149.

95. D'Erasmo E, Aliberti G. Platelet count, mean platelet volume and their relation to prognosis in cerebral infarction. *J Intern Med.* 1990;227:11–14.

96. Kaito K, Otsubo H, Usui N, et al. Platelet size deviation width, platelet large cell ratio and mean platelet volume have sufficient sensitivity and specificity in the diagnosis of immune thrombocytopenia. *Br J Haematol.* 2005;128:698–702.

97. Takubo T, Yamane T, Hino M, et al. Usefulness of determining reticulated and large platelets in idiopathic thrombocytopenic purpura. *Acta Haematol.* 1998;99:109–110.

98. Macchi I, Chamlian V, Sadoun A, et al. Comparison of reticulated platelet count and mean platelet volume determination in the evaluation of bone marrow recovery after aplastic chemotherapy. *Eur J Haematol.* 2002;69:152–157.

99. Robinson MSC, Mackie IJ, Machin SJ, et al. Two colour analysis of reticulated platelets. *Clin Lab Haematol.* 2000;22:211–213.

100. Briggs C, Kunka S, Hart D, et al. Assessment of an immature platelet fraction (IPF) in peripheral thrombocytopenia. *Br J Haematol.* 2004;126:93–99.

101. Abe Y, Wada H, Tomatsu H, et al. A simple technique to determine thrombopoiesis level using immature platelet fraction (IPF). *Thromb Res.* 2006;118:463–469.

102. Zucker ML, Murphy CA, Rachel JM, et al. Immature platelet fraction as a predictor of platelet recovery following hematopoietic progenitor cell transplantation. *Lab Hematol.* 2006;12:125–130.

103. Riley RS, Ben-Ezra JM, Tidwell A, et al. Reticulocyte analysis by flow cytometry and other techniques. *Haematol Oncol Clin North Am.* 2002;16:378–420.

104. Sica S, Sora F, Laurenti L, et al. Highly fluorescent reticulocyte count predicts haemopoietic recovery after immunosuppression for severe aplastic anaemia. *Clin Lab Haematol.* 1999;21:387–389.

105. Davies SV, Cavill I, Bentley N, et al. Evaluation of erythropoiesis after bone marrow transplantation: quantitative reticulocyte counting. *Br J Haematol.* 1992;81:12–17.

106. Davis BH, Bigelow N, Ball ED, et al. Utility of flow cytometric reticulocyte quantification as a predictor of engraftment in autologous bone marrow transplantation. *Am J Hematol.* 1989;32:81–87.

107. Gowans ID, Hepburn MD, Clark DM, et al. The role of the Sysmex SE9000 immature myeloid index and Sysmex R2000 reticulocyte parameters in optimizing the timing of peripheral blood cell harvesting in patients with lymphoma and myeloma. *Clin Lab Haematol.* 1999;21:331–336.

108. Parisotto R, Gore CJ, Emslie KR, et al. A novel method utilising markers of altered erythropoiesis for the detection of recombinant human erythropoietin abuse in athletes. *Haematologica.* 2000;85:564–572.

109. Torres Gomez A, Casaño J, et al. Utility of reticulocyte maturation parameters in the differential diagnosis of macrocytic anaemias. *Clin Lab Haematol.* 2003;25:283–288.

110. Thomas L, Franck S, Messinger M, et al. Reticulocyte hemoglobin measurement – comparison of two methods in the diagnosis of iron-restricted erythropoiesis. *Clin Chem Lab Med.* 2005;43:1193–1202.

111. Urrechaga E. Clinical utility of the Beckman Coulter parameter red blood cell size factor in the study of erythropoiesis. *International Journal of Laboratory Hematology.* 2009;31:623–629.

112. Briggs C, Guthrie D, Hyde K, et al. British Committee for Standards in Haematology General Haematology Task Force. Guidelines for point-of-care testing: haematology. *Br J Haematol.* 2008;142:904–915.

113. International Committee for Standardization in Haematology; Expert Panel on Cytometry. The assignment of values to fresh blood used for calibrating automated blood cell counters. *Clin Lab Haematol.* 1988;10:203–212.

114. Lewis SM, England JM, Rowan RM. Current concerns in haematology 3: Blood count calibration. *J Clin Pathol.* 1991;44:881–884.

115. International Council for Standardization in Haematology. Reference method for the enumeration of erythrocytes and leucocytes. *Clin Lab Haematol.* 1994;16:131–138.

116. National Committee for Clinical Laboratory Standards . *Performance goals for the internal quality control of multichannel hematology analysers; approved standard.* Wayne PA: NCCLS; 1996.

117. British Committee for Standards in Haematology . Assessment of the need for blood film examination with blood counts by aperture-impedance systems. In: Roberts B, ed. *Standard Haematology Practice.* Oxford: Blackwell Scientific; 1991:34–42.

118. Koepke JA. Instrument flagging and blood film review. In: Rowan RM, van Assendelft OW, Preston FE, eds. *Advanced Laboratory Methods in Haematology.* London: Arnold; 2002:64–77.

119. Barnes PW, McFadden S, Machin SJ, et al. The international consensus group for hematology review: suggested criteria for action following automated CBC and WBC differential analysis. *Lab Hematol.* 2005;11:83–90.

Chapter | 4 |

Preparation and staining methods for blood and bone marrow films

Barbara J. Bain, S. Mitchell Lewis

PREPARATION OF BLOOD FILMS ON SLIDES

Blood films should be made on clean glass slides. Films made on coverglasses have negligible advantages and are unsuitable for modern laboratory practice. Films may be spread by hand or by means of an automated slide spreader, the latter being either a stand-alone instrument or a component of an automated blood cell counter.

Manual Method

Blood films can be prepared from fresh blood with no anticoagulant added or from ethylenediaminetetra-acetic acid (EDTA)-anticoagulated blood. Heparinized blood should not generally be used because its staining characteristics differ from those of EDTA-anticoagulated blood. Good films can be made in the following manner, using clean slides, if necessary wiped free from dust immediately before use. Slides should measure 75 × 25 mm and be approximately 1 mm thick; ideally, they should be frosted at one end to facilitate labelling, but these are more expensive.

First, make a spreader from a glass slide that has a smooth end. Using a glass cutter, break off one corner of the slide, leaving a width of about 18 mm as the spreader. A spreader can be used repeatedly unless the edge becomes chipped, but it must be thoroughly cleaned and dried between films.

Place a small drop of blood in the centre line of a slide about 1 cm from one end. Then, without delay, place a spreader in front of the drop at an angle of about 30° to the slide and move it back to make contact with the drop. The drop should spread out quickly along the line of contact. With a steady movement of the hand, spread the drop of blood along the slide. The spreader must not be lifted off until the last trace of blood has been spread out; with a correctly sized drop, the film should be about 3 cm in length. It is important that the film of blood finishes at least 1 cm before the end of the slide (Fig. 4.1).

The thickness of the film can be regulated by varying the pressure and speed of spreading and by changing the angle at which the spreader is held. With anaemic blood, the correct thickness is achieved by using a wider angle, and, conversely, with polycythaemic blood, the angle should be narrower.

The ideal thickness is such that on microscopy there is some overlap of red cells throughout much of the film's length (see p. 30). The leucocytes should be easily recognizable throughout most of the film. With poorly made films the leucocytes will be unevenly distributed, with monocytes and other large leucocytes being pushed to the end and the sides of the spread. An irregular streaky film will occur if the slide is greasy, and dust on the surface will cause patchy spots (Fig. 4.1).

The films should be allowed to dry in the air. In humid conditions the films may be exposed to a current of warm air (e.g. from a hairdryer), but this should be in a microbiological safety hood.

Automated Methods

The manufacturer's instructions should be followed unless local experience has demonstrated that variation of the recommended technique achieves better results.

Labelling Blood Films

The film should be labelled immediately after spreading. Write either a laboratory reference number or the name of the patient and the date in pencil on the frosted end of the slide or on the film itself (writing on the thickest part, which is least suitable for microscopic examination). A label written in pencil will not be removed by staining. A paper label should be affixed to the slide later. If blood films are to be stored for future reference, apply the paper label in such a manner that it is easily read when the slides are filed.

In a computerized laboratory, bar-coded specimen identification labels are convenient and preferable. These should have the patient's name, the date and the laboratory number as well as the barcode.

Fixing Blood Films

To preserve the morphology of the cells, films must be fixed as described on p. 59. This must be done without delay, and the films should never be left unfixed for more than a few hours. If films are sent to the laboratory by post, it is essential that, when possible, they are thoroughly dried and fixed before dispatch.

Figure 4.1 Blood films made on slides. (A) A well-made film. (B) An irregular patchy film on a dusty slide. (C) A film that is too thick. (D) A film that has been spread with inconsistent pressure and using an irregularly edged spreader, resulting in long tails. (E) A film made on a very greasy slide.

Bone Marrow Films

The method for preparation of films of aspirated bone marrow is described on p. 126. They should be made without delay. Films must be thoroughly dry before they are fixed or artefactual changes will occur. At least one film should be fixed for a Perls' stain on the initial bone marrow aspirate of each patient, and, if necessary, films should be fixed in the appropriate fixatives for special staining (Chapter 15); others should be fixed and stained with a Romanowsky stain as described later. Crushed bone marrow particles and touch preparations from trephine biopsy specimens can be stained in the same manner.

STAINING BLOOD AND BONE MARROW FILMS

Romanowsky stains are used universally for routine staining of blood films, and satisfactory results can be obtained. The remarkable property of the Romanowsky dyes of making subtle distinctions in shades of staining, and of staining granules differentially, depends on two components: azure B (trimethylthionin) and eosin Y (tetrabromo-fluorescein).[1,2]

The original Romanowsky combination was polychrome methylene blue and eosin. Several of the stains now used routinely that are based on azure B also include methylene blue, but the need for this is debatable. Its presence in the stain is thought by some to enhance the staining of nucleoli and polychromatic red cells; in its absence, normal neutrophil granules tend to stain heavily and may resemble 'toxic granules' in conventionally stained films.[3]

There are a number of causes of variation in staining. One of the main factors is the presence of contaminants in the commercial dyes and a simple combination of pure azure B and eosin Y might be considered preferable to the more complex stains because this ensures consistent results from batch to batch.[1,4,5] However, in practice, absolutely pure dyes are expensive, and it is sufficient to ensure that the stains contain at least 80% of the appropriate dye.[6] Among the Romanowsky stains now in use, Jenner is the simplest and Giemsa is the most complex. Leishman's stain, which occupies an intermediate position, is still widely used in the routine staining of blood films, although the results are inferior to those obtained by the combined May–Grünwald–Giemsa, Jenner–Giemsa, and azure B–eosin Y methods. Wright's stain, which is widely used in North America, gives results that are similar to those obtained with Leishman's stain, whereas Wright–Giemsa is similar to May–Grünwald–Giemsa.

A pH to the alkaline side of neutrality accentuates the azure component at the expense of the eosin and vice versa. A pH of 6.8 is usually recommended for general use, but to some extent this depends on personal preference. (When looking for malaria parasites, a pH of 7.2 is recommended to see Schüffner's dots.) To achieve a uniform pH, 50 ml of 66 mmol/l Sörensen's phosphate buffer (see p. 622) may be added to each litre of the water used in diluting the stains and washing the films.

The mechanism by which certain components of a cell's structure stain with particular dyes and other components fail to do so depends on complex differences in binding of the dyes to chemical structures and interactions between the dye molecules.[7] Azure B is bound to anionic molecules, and eosin Y is bound to cationic sites on proteins.

Thus, the acidic groupings of the nucleic acids and proteins of the cell nuclei and cytoplasm of primitive cells determine their uptake of the basic dye azure B, and, conversely, the presence of basic groupings on the haemoglobin molecule results in its affinity for acidic dyes and its staining by eosin. The granules in the cytoplasm of neutrophil leucocytes are weakly stained by the azure complexes. Eosinophilic granules contain a spermine derivative with an alkaline grouping that stains strongly with the acidic component of the dye, whereas basophilic granules contain heparin, which has an affinity for the basic component of the dye. These effects depend on molar equilibrium between the two dyes in time-dependent reactions.[2] DNA binds rapidly, RNA more slowly, and haemoglobin more slowly still; hence the need to have the correct azure B to eosin ratio to avoid contamination of the dyes and to stain for the right time. Standardized stains and staining method have been proposed (see p. 61).

The colour reactions of the Romanowsky effect are shown in Table 4.1; causes of variation in staining are given in Table 4.2.

Preparation of Solutions of Romanowsky Dyes

May–Grünwald Stain

Weigh out 0.3 g of the powdered dye and transfer to a conical flask of 200–250 ml capacity. Add 100 ml of methanol and warm the mixture to 50°C. Allow the flask to cool to c 20°C and shake several times during the day. After letting it stand for 24 h, filter the solution. It is then ready for use, no 'ripening' being required.

Jenner's Stain

Prepare a 5 g/l solution in methanol in exactly the same way as described earlier for the May–Grünwald stain.

Giemsa's Stain

Weigh 1 g of the powdered dye and transfer to a conical flask of 200–250 ml capacity. Add 100 ml of methanol and warm the mixture to 50°C; keep at this temperature

Table 4.1 Colour responses of blood cells to Romanowsky staining

CELLULAR COMPONENT	COLOUR
Nuclei	
Chromatin	Purple
Nucleoli	Light blue
Cytoplasm	
Erythroblast	Dark blue
Erythrocyte	Dark pink
Reticulocyte	Grey-blue
Lymphocyte	Blue
Metamyelocyte	Pink
Monocyte	Grey-blue
Myelocyte	Pink
Neutrophil	Pink/orange
Promyelocyte	Blue
Basophil	Blue
Granules	
Promyelocyte (primary granules)	Red or purple
Basophil	Purple black
Eosinophil	Red-orange
Neutrophil	Purple
Toxic granules	Dark blue
Platelet	Purple
Other inclusions	
Auer body	Purple
Cabot ring	Purple
Howell–Jolly body	Purple
Döhle body	Light blue

Table 4.2 Factors giving rise to faulty staining

APPEARANCES	CAUSES
Too blue	Incorrect preparation of stock, eosin concentration too low
	Stock stain exposed to bright daylight
	Batch of stain solution overused
	Impure dyes
	Staining time too short
	Staining solution too acid
	Film too thick
	Inadequate time in buffer solution
Too pink	Incorrect proportion of azure B:eosin Y
	Impure dyes
	Buffer pH too low
	Excessive washing in buffer solution
Pale staining	Old staining solution
	Overused staining solution
	Incorrect preparation of stock
	Impure dyes, especially azure A and/or C
	High ambient temperature
Neutrophil granules not stained	Insufficient azure B
Neutrophil granules dark blue/black (pseudo-toxic)	Excess azure B
Other stain anomalies	Various contaminating dyes and metal salts
Stain deposit on film	Stain solution left in uncovered jar
	Stain solution not filtered
Blue background	Inadequate fixation or prolonged storage before fixation
	Blood collected into heparin as anticoagulant

for 15 min with occasional shaking, then filter the solution. It is then ready for use, but it will improve on standing for a few hours.

Azure B–Eosin Y Stock Solution

The stock solution includes azure B, tetrafluoroborate or thiocyanate (Colour index 52010), >80% pure, and eosin Y (Colour index 45380), >80% pure.

Dissolve 0.6 g of azure B in 60 ml dimethyl sulphoxide (DMSO) and 0.2 g of eosin Y in 50 ml DMSO; preheat the DMSO to 37°C before adding the dyes. Stand at 37°C, shaking vigorously for 30 s at 5 min intervals until both dyes are completely dissolved. Add the eosin Y solution to the azure B solution and stir well. This stock solution should remain stable for several months if kept at room temperature in the dark. DMSO will crystallize below 18°C; if necessary, allow it to redissolve before use.

Leishman's Stain

Weigh out 0.2 g of the powdered dye, and transfer it to a conical flask of 200–250 ml capacity. Add 100 ml of methanol and warm the mixture to 50°C for 15 min, occasionally shaking it. Allow the flask to cool and filter the solution. It is then ready for use, but it will improve on standing.

Buffered Water

Make up 50 ml of 66 mmol/l Sörensen's phosphate buffer of the required pH to 1 litre with water at a pH of 6.8 (see p. 622). An alternative buffer may be prepared from buffer tablets, which are available commercially. Solutions of the required pH are obtained by dissolving the tablets in water.

STAINING METHODS

May–Grünwald–Giemsa Stain

Dry the films in the air, then fix by immersing in a jar of methanol for 5–10 min. For bone marrow films, allow a longer time to ensure thorough drying and then leave it for 15–20 min in the methanol. Films should be fixed as soon as possible after they have dried. If they are left unfixed at room temperature it may be found that the background of dried plasma stains a pale blue that is impossible to remove without spoiling the staining of the blood cells. It is important to prevent any contact with water before fixation is complete. Methyl alcohol (methanol) is the fixative of choice, although ethyl alcohol ('absolute alcohol') can also be used. To prevent the alcohol from becoming contaminated with absorbed water, it must be stored in a bottle with a tightly fitting stopper and not left exposed to the atmosphere, especially in humid climates. Methylated spirits must not be used because it contains water.

Transfer the fixed films to a staining jar containing May–Grünwald stain freshly diluted with an equal volume of buffered water. After the films have been allowed to stain for about 15 min, transfer them without washing to a jar containing Giemsa's stain freshly diluted with 9 volumes of buffered water, pH 6.8.

After staining for 10–15 min, transfer the slides to a jar containing buffered water, pH 6.8, rapidly wash in three or four changes of water, and finally allow to stand undisturbed in water for a short time (usually 2–5 min) for differentiation to take place. This may be controlled by inspection of the wet slide under the low power of the microscope; with experience, the naked-eye colour of the film is often a good guide. The slides should be transferred from one staining solution to the other without being allowed to dry. Because the intensity of the staining is affected by any variation in the thickness of a film, it is not easy to obtain uniform staining throughout a film's length.

When differentiation is complete, stand the slides upright to dry. This method is designed for staining a number of films at the same time. Single slides may be stained by flooding the slide with a combined fixative and staining solution (e.g. Leishman's stain, discussed later), but it is important to ensure that the methanol used as fixative is completely water-free. As little as 1% water may affect the appearance of the films, and a higher water content causes gross changes (Fig. 4.2). The red cells will also be affected by traces of detergent on inadequately washed slides (see Fig. 26.5, p. 612).

The diluted stains usually retain their staining powers sufficiently well for several batches of slides to be stained in them. They must be made up freshly each day, and it is probably best to stain the day's films in two batches, morning and afternoon. There is no need to filter the stains before use unless a deposit is present.

Standardized Romanowsky Stain

A standardized Romanowsky stain[2,5] based on a method with pure dyes has been proposed by the International Committee for Standardization in Haematology. It is useful for checking the performance of routine stains. The method is described fully in previous editions.

Jenner–Giemsa Stain

Jenner's stain may be substituted for May–Grünwald stain in the technique described on the previous page. The results are a little less satisfactory. The stain is used with 4 volumes of buffered water and the films, after being fixed in methanol, are immersed in it for approximately 4 min before being transferred to the Giemsa stain. They should be allowed to stain in the latter solution for 7–10 min. Differentiation is carried out as described earlier.

Leishman's Stain

Air dry the film and flood the slide with the stain. After 2 min, add double the volume of water and stain the film for 5–7 min. Then wash it in a stream of buffered water until it has acquired a pinkish tinge (up to 2 min). After the back of the slide has been wiped clean, set it upright to dry.

Automated Staining

Automatic staining machines are available that enable large batches of slides to be handled. They may be either stand-alone staining machines or a part of a large automated blood counting instrument. In many instances, the instrument spreads, fixes and stains blood films. Some automated instruments incorporating staining can only be

Figure 4.2 Blood film appearances following methanol fixation. Photomicrographs of Romanowsky-stained blood films that have been fixed in methanol containing: (A) 1% water; (B) 3% water; (C) 4% water; and (D) 10% water. The red cells and leucocytes are well fixed in (A), reasonably well fixed in (B) but badly fixed in (C) and (D).

programmed to prepare and stain a single film per sample. Others can prepare and stain multiple films from a single blood sample; this is useful for preparing slides for teaching large numbers of students. Some systems apply staining solutions to slides lying horizontally (flat-bed staining), whereas others either immerse a slide or slides in a bath of staining solution ('dip-and-dunk' technique) or spray stain onto slides in a cytocentrifuge. Problems include increased background staining, inadequate staining of neutrophil granules, degranulation of basophils and blue or green rather than pink staining of erythrocytes. These problems are usually related to the specific stains and staining protocols used rather than to the type of instrument, although flat-bed stainers are more likely to cause problems with stain deposit. However, as a rule, staining is satisfactory provided that reliable stains are used and there is careful control of the cycle time and other variables.[8] Flat-bed stainers may not stain an entire film (e.g. a bone marrow film) if the film exceeds the standard length.

Rapid Staining Method

Field's method[9,10] was introduced to provide a quick method for staining thick films for malaria parasites (see below). With some modifications, it can be used fairly satisfactorily for the rapid staining of thin films. The stains are available commercially ready for use, or they can be prepared as follows.

Stains

Stain A (Polychromed Methylene Blue)

Methylene blue	1.3 g
Disodium hydrogen phosphate (Na$_2$HPO$_4$.12H$_2$O)	12.6 g
Potassium dihydrogen phosphate (KH$_2$PO$_4$)	6.25 g
Water	500 ml

Dissolve the methylene blue and the disodium hydrogen phosphate in 50 ml of water. Then boil the solution in a waterbath almost to dryness to 'polychrome' the dye. Add the potassium dihydrogen phosphate and 500 ml of freshly boiled water. After stirring to dissolve the stain, set aside the solution for 24 h before filtering. Filter again before use. The pH is 6.6–6.8.

Alternatively, azure B may be added to the methylene blue in the proportion of 0.5 g of azure B to 0.8 g of methylene blue, and the combined dyes are then dissolved directly in the phosphate buffer solution.

Stain B (Eosin)

Eosin	1.3 g
Disodium hydrogen phosphate (Na$_2$HPO$_4$.12H$_2$O)	12.6 g
Potassium dihydrogen phosphate (KH$_2$PO$_4$)	6.25 g
Water	500 ml

Dissolve the phosphates in warm freshly boiled water and then add the dye. Filter the solution after letting it stand for 24 h.

Method

Fix the film for 10–15 s in methanol. Pour off the methanol and drop on the slide 12 drops of diluted Stain B (1 volume of stain to 4 volumes of water). Immediately, add 12 drops of Stain A. Agitate the slide to mix the stains. After 1 min, rinse the slide in water, then differentiate the film for 5 s in phosphate buffer at pH 6.6, wash the slide in water, and then place it on end to drain and dry. Two-stage stains of this type are also available commercially.

MOUNTING OF COVERGLASS

When thoroughly dry, cover the blood film with a rectangular No. 1 coverglass, using for this purpose a mountant that is miscible with xylol (e.g. DPX Mountant, Merck). For a temporary mount, cedarwood oil may be used.

The coverglass should be large enough to overlie the whole film, so that the edges and the tail of the film can be examined. If a neutral mounting medium is used, the staining should be preserved for many years if kept in the dark. Although it is probable that stained films keep best unmounted, there are objections to this course: it is almost impossible to keep the slides free from dust and from being scratched and, in the absence of a coverglass, the observer is tempted to examine the film solely with the oil-immersion objective, a practice that is to be deprecated because it is important to have a general overview of the film before studying specific cells.

EXAMINATION OF WET BLOOD FILM PREPARATIONS

The examination of a drop of blood sealed between a slide and coverglass is sometimes of considerable value. The preparation may be examined in several ways: by ordinary illumination, by dark-ground or by Nomarski (interference) illumination. Chemically clean slides and coverglasses (see p. 623) should be used,* and the blood should be allowed to spread out thinly between them. If the glass surfaces are free from dust, the blood will spread out spontaneously, and pressure, which is undesirable, should not be necessary. The edges of the preparation may be sealed with a melted mixture of equal parts of petroleum jelly and paraffin wax or with nail varnish.

Red Cells

Rouleaux formation is typically seen in varying degrees in wet preparations of whole blood and must be distinguished from autoagglutination. The distinction is sometimes a matter of considerable difficulty, particularly when, as not infrequently happens, rouleaux formation is superimposed on agglutination. The rouleaux, too, may be notably irregular in haemolytic anaemias characterized by spherocytosis, whereas the clumping caused by massive rouleaux formation of normal type may closely simulate true agglutination. This pseudoagglutination owing to massive rouleaux formation may be distinguished from true agglutination in two ways:

1. By noting that the red cells, although forming parts of larger clumps, are mostly arranged side by side as in typical rouleaux.
2. By adding 3–4 volumes of 9 g/l NaCl to the preparation. Pseudoagglutination owing to massive rouleaux formation should either disperse completely or transform itself into typical rouleaux. The addition of saline to blood that has undergone true agglutination may cause the agglutinates to break up somewhat, but a major degree of it is likely to persist and typical rouleaux will not be seen.

Anisocytosis and *poikilocytosis* can be recognized in 'wet' preparations of blood, but the tendency to crenation and the formation of rouleaux tend to make observations on shape changes rather difficult. Such changes can best be studied in a wet preparation after fixation. For this, dilute a sample of freshly collected heparinized or EDTA-anticoagulated

---

*Pre-cleaned slides and coverglasses are available commercially.

blood in 10 volumes of iso-osmotic phosphate buffer, pH 7.4 (see p. 622) and immediately fix with an equal volume of 0.3% glutaraldehyde in iso-osmotic phosphate buffer, pH 7.4. After standing for 5 min, add 1 drop of this suspension to 4 drops of glycerol and place 1–2 drops on a glass slide that is then sealed.[11]

Pitting occurs normally in less than 2% of the red cells; an increase of more than 4% is an indication of splenic dysfunction. The pits are readily identified by Nomarski illumination or electron microscopy when they have the appearance of small crater-like indentations on the cell surface.[12]

Sickling of red cells in 'wet' preparations of blood is described in Chapter 14.

Crystals of haemoglobin C can be demonstrated by incubating a sample of blood with an equal volume of 30 g/l sodium chloride for 4 h at 37°C.[13] In blood from patients with haemoglobin C disease this induces formation of intracellular haemoglobin C crystals, large, clear structures that are well shown when the preparation is then stained by any Romanowsky stain.[13] They can also be demonstrated in red cells from patients with compound heterozygosity for haemoglobins S and C.

Cryoglobulinaemia

To identify cryoglobulinaemia, put a drop of blood from an EDTA sample that has been kept at room temperature onto a glass slide, cover it with a glass coverslip, and examine it by phase contrast microscopy. The cryoglobulin will be seen as large clear deposits of amorphous material or as refrigent precipitates that disappear when the slide is warmed to 37°C.

This is a useful test when an automated blood count gives anomalous results with spuriously elevated white blood cell and platelet counts.[14]

Leucocytes

The motility of leucocytes can be readily studied in heparinized blood if the microscope stage can be warmed to about 37°C. Usually, only the granulocytes show significant progressive movements. However, the examination of living neutrophils in plasma is not useful in day-to-day routine haematological practice. Specialized microscopy techniques applicable to leucocytes are discussed in the 8th edition of this book.

SEPARATION AND CONCENTRATION OF BLOOD CELLS

A number of methods are available for the concentration of leucocytes or abnormal cells when they are present in only small numbers in the peripheral blood. Concentrates are most simply prepared from the buffy coat of centrifuged blood. However, most methods affect to some extent subsequent staining properties, chemical reactions and viability of the separated cells.

Making a Buffy Coat Preparation

Centrifuge an EDTA blood sample in a plastic tube for 5–10 min at 1200–1500 g. Then remove the supernatant plasma carefully with a fine plastic pipette and with the same pipette deposit the platelet and underlying leucocyte layers onto one or two slides. Mix the buffy coat in a drop of the patient's plasma and then spread the films. Allow them to dry in the air and then fix and stain in the usual way.

When leucocytes are scanty or if many slides are to be made, it is worthwhile centrifuging the blood twice; first, about 5 ml are centrifuged and a second tube is then filled from the upper cell layers of this sample.

As an alternative to centrifugation, the blood may be allowed to sediment by placing the tube vertically on the bench without disturbance, with or without the help of sedimentation-enhancing agents such as fibrinogen, dextran, gum acacia, Ficoll (Pharmacia) or methylcellulose.[15] Bøyum's reagent[16] (methylcellulose and sodium metrizoate) is particularly suitable for obtaining leucocyte preparations with minimal red cell contamination.

Utility of the Buffy Coat

It is well known that atypical or primitive blood cells circulate in small numbers in the peripheral blood in health. Thus, atypical mononuclear cells, metamyelocytes and megakaryocytes may be found. Even promyelocytes, blasts and nucleated red cells may occasionally be seen but only in very small numbers. Efrati and Rozenszajn[17] described a method for the quantitative assessment of the numbers of atypical cells in normal blood and gave figures for the incidence of megakaryocyte fragments (e.g. mean 21.8 per 1 ml of blood) and of atypical mononuclear cells and metamyelocytes and myelocytes. In cord blood, the incidence of all types of primitive cells is considerably greater.[18]

In disease, abnormal cells may be seen in buffy coat preparations in much larger numbers than in films of whole blood (Fig. 4.3). Another example, for instance, is megakaryocytes and immature cells of the granulocyte series found in relatively large numbers in disseminated carcinoma.[19] Megaloblasts, if present, may help in the diagnosis of a megaloblastic anaemia. Ring sideroblasts may be seen in patients with sideroblastic anaemia; their presence can be confirmed with a Perls' stain. Haemophagocytosis, which is more often observed in the bone marrow, may also sometimes be demonstrated in buffy coat preparations.[20] Erythrophagocytosis may be conspicuous in cases of autoimmune haemolytic anaemia (Fig. 4.4). In systemic lupus erythematosus (SLE) a few LE cells may be found, but this is not the best way to demonstrate

Figure 4.3 Buffy coat film. From blood of a patient with pancytopenia showing two hairy cells, an erythroblast and a bare nucleus. Only rare cells resembling hairy cells were seen in the conventional film, whereas the buffy coat film showed many such cells.

Figure 4.4 Film of a buffy coat. Erythrophagocytosis in autoimmune haemolytic anaemia.

LE cells; moreover, the detection of LE cells for the diagnosis of SLE has been supplanted by immunological tests for the detection of antinuclear or anti-DNA antibodies.

Buffy coat films can be useful for the detection of bacteria, fungi or parasites within neutrophils, monocytes or circulating macrophages; they also can help find cells that may be present in very small numbers (e.g. hairy cells in hairy cell leukaemia). With the availability of monoclonal antibodies reactive with epithelial and other tumour cells, immunocytochemical techniques can now be applied for the identification of infrequent neoplastic cells.

Separation of Specific Cell Populations

It is now possible to identify specific cell populations by flow cytometric immunophenotyping, and the need for separation of mononuclear cells from blood has diminished. However, differences in density of cells can also be used to separate individual cell types, using gradient solutions of selected specific gravity.[16,21] This is also a useful method for use in leucocyte imaging with radio-isotope-labelled neutrophils (see p. 388). A simple convenient technique has been described for layering the blood or bone marrow over the density preparations.[22] The median density values for the main haemopoietic cells are as follows:

Erythrocytes	1100
Eosinophils	1090
Neutrophils	1085
Myelocytes	1075
Lymphocytes	1070
Monocytes	1064
Myeloblasts	1062
Platelets	1035

BACTERIA AND FUNGI DETECTABLE IN BLOOD FILMS

Ehrlichiosis is a tick-borne fever in which clusters of small organisms may be seen in Romanowsky-stained blood smears. The detection of organisms within neutrophils or monocytes is important for its diagnosis. Other bacteria and fungi are occasionally detected within neutrophils or monocytes or extracellularly.

PARASITES DETECTABLE IN BLOOD, BONE MARROW OR SPLENIC ASPIRATES

There are now a number of screening tests for diagnosing malaria based on the detection of malarial antigens (see Chapter 6). However, the essential method for a definitive diagnosis remains the finding of parasites in a blood film and the identification of the species by morphology.[23,24] Only brief outlines of the microscopic diagnoses are given in this chapter. For more detailed accounts, readers are referred to a parasitology textbook. In addition to the plasmodia that give rise to malaria, the other important parasites to be found in the blood are leishmaniae, babesiae, trypanosomes and microfilaria.

In addition to standard thin films, thick films are extremely useful when parasites are scanty. These should be prepared and examined as a routine, although identification of the species is less easy than in thin films and mixed infections may be missed. If 5 min are spent examining a thick film, this is equivalent to about 1 h spent in traversing a thin film. Once the presence of parasites has been confirmed, a thin film should be used for determining the species and, in the case of *Plasmodium falciparum*, for assessing the severity of the infection by counting the percentage of parasitized cells (excluding cells containing only gametocytes).

Low levels of parasitaemia detected by immunological tests may be missed by microscopy and proficiency testing studies have demonstrated the need for all laboratories, and especially those lacking expertise, to take part in external quality control programmes and to refer problematic cases to more experienced centres.[25,26]

Thick blood films are also useful for the detection of microfilaria. When they are used for this purpose, it is important to scan the entire film using a low-power objective, or parasites may be missed. Examination of wet preparations of blood can be used for diagnosis of microfilariae and has the advantage that the parasites are easily detected because they are moving. A stained film is necessary for confirmation of species. Wet preparations are also useful for the detection of trypanosomes and the spirochaetes of relapsing fever. The presence of small numbers of trypanosomes or spirochaetes is revealed by occasional slight agitation of groups of red cells. Examination of a stained film confirms their nature.

EXAMINATION OF BLOOD FILMS FOR PARASITES

Making Thick Films

Make a thick film by placing a small drop of blood in the centre of a slide and spreading it out with a corner of another slide to cover an area about four times its original area. The correct thickness for a satisfactory film will have been achieved if, with the slide placed on a piece of newspaper, small print is just visible.

Allow the film to dry thoroughly for at least 30 min at 37°C. If it is necessary to hurry the procedure, the slide can be left near, but not touching, a light bulb where the temperature is 50–60°C, for about 7 min; the quality of the film may deteriorate if it is overheated. Films which are not completely dry may wash off in the stain.

Staining Thick Films

Field's method of staining[9,10] is quick and usually satisfactory for thick films, but the method is not practical for staining large numbers of films; for this purpose the Giemsa, Leishman or azure B–eosin Y methods are more suitable. Careful attention to pH is critical for satisfactory staining of parasites.

Field's Stain

The preparation of the stains is described on p. 62.

1. Dip the slide with the dried film on it into Stain A for 3 s.
2. Dip into a jar of tap water for 3 s with gentle agitation.
3. Dip into Stain B for 3 s.
4. Wash gently in tap water for a few seconds until all excess stain is removed.
5. Drain the slide vertically and leave to dry. Do not blot.

Giemsa's Stain

1. Dry the films thoroughly, as explained previously.
2. Immerse the slides for 20–30 min in a staining jar containing Giemsa's stain freshly diluted with 20 volumes of buffered water (pH 7.2).
3. Wash in buffered water pH 7.2 for 3 min.
4. Stand the slides upright to dry. Do not blot.

Azure B–Eosin Y Stain

1. Prepare a staining solution from the stock stain, as described on p. 60, but using HEPES buffer at pH 7.2.
2. After the films have been dried and treated as described earlier, stain for 10 min in the staining solution.
3. Rinse for 1 min in buffered water, pH 7.2.
4. Stand the slides upright to dry. Do not blot.

Sometimes when thick films are stained, they become overlaid by a residue of stain or spoilt by the envelopes of the lysed red cells. These defects can be minimized by adding 0.1% Triton X-100 to the buffer before diluting the stock stain.[27] An alternative, but more laborious, method is to lyse 1 volume of blood with 3 volumes of 1% saponin in saline for 10 min, then centrifuge for 5 min, decant the supernatant, and make films from the residual pellet.[28]

Staining Thin Films for Parasites

Thin films should be stained with Giemsa's stain or Leishman's stain at pH 7.2, not with a standard May–Grünwald–Giemsa stain.

Leishman's Stain

Use commercially available stain or prepare stain as follows:

1. Add glass beads to 500 ml of methanol.
2. Add 1.5 g of Leishman's powder.
3. Shake well, leave on a rotary shaker during the day, then incubate at 37°C overnight.

There is no need to filter.

Method

1. Make a thin film and air dry rapidly.
2. Place the film on a staining rack, flood with Leishman's stain, and leave for 30 s to 1 min to fix.

3. Add twice as much buffered distilled water (preferably from a plastic wash bottle because this permits better mixing of the solution), pH 7.2.
4. Leave to stain for 10 min.
5. Wash off stain with tap water.

Thick blood films are also useful for the detection of microfilariae. When they are used for this purpose, it is important to scan the entire film using a low-power objective or parasites may be missed. Examination of fresh liquid blood (see below) can also be used for the identification of microfilariae and has the advantage that, because the parasites are moving, they are easily detected. A stained film is necessary for confirmation of species.

REFERENCES

1. Wittekind D. On the nature of Romanowsky dyes and the Romanowsky Giemsa effect. *Clin Lab Haematol.* 1979;1:247–262.
2. Horobin RW, Walter KJ. Understanding Romanowsky staining. I. the Romanowsky-Giemsa effect in blood smears. Azure B-eosin as a substitute for May–Grünwald–Giemsa and Jenner–Giemsa stains. *Microsc Acta.* 1987;79:153–156.
3. Marshall PN. Romanowsky-type stains in haematology. *Histochem J.* 1978;10:1–29.
4. Wittekind DH, Kretschmer V, Sohmer I. Azure B-eosin Y stain as the standard Romanowsky-Giemsa stain. *Br J Haematol.* 1982;5:391–393.
5. International Committee for Standardization in Haematology. ICSH reference method for staining of blood and bone marrow films by azure B and eosin Y (Romanowsky stain). *Br J Haematol.* 1984;57:707–710.
6. Schenk EA, Willis CT. Note from the Biological Stain Commission: certification of Wright stain solution. *Stain Technol.* 1989;64:152–153.
7. Wittekind DH. On the nature of Romanowsky-Giemsa staining and its significance for cytochemistry and histochemistry: an overall view. *Histochem J.* 1983;15:1029–1047.
8. Hayashi M, Gauthier S, Tatsumi N. Evaluation of an automated slide preparation and staining unit. *Sysmex Journal International.* 1996;6:63–69.
9. Field JW. The morphology of malarial parasites in thick blood films. IV. The identification of species and phase. *Trans R Soc Trop Med Hyg.* 1940–1941;34:405–414.
10. Field JW. Further notes on a method of staining malarial parasites in thick films. *Trans R Soc Trop Med Hyg.* 1941–1942;35:35.
11. Zipursky A, Brown E, Palko J, et al. The erythrocyte differential count in newborn infants. *Am J Pediatr Hematol Oncol.* 1983;5:45–51.
12. Sills RH. Hyposplenism. In: Pochedly C, Sills RH, Schwartz AD, eds. *Disorders of the Spleen.* New York: Marcel Dekker; 1989.
13. Nagel RL, Fabry ME, Steinberg MH. The paradox of hemoglobin SC disease. *Blood Rev.* 2003;17:167–178.
14. Fohlen-Walter A, Jacob C, Lacompte T, et al. Laboratory identification of cryoglobulinema from automated blood cell counts, fresh blood samples, and blood films. *Am J Clin Pathol.* 2002;117:606–614.
15. Bloemendal H, ed. *Cell Separation Methods.* Amsterdam: Elsevier-North Holland; 1977.
16. Bøyum A. Separation of lymphocytes, granulocytes and monocytes from human blood using iodinated density gradient media. *Methods Enzymol.* 1984;108:88–102.
17. Efrati P, Rozenszajn L. The morphology of buffy coat in normal human adults. *Blood.* 1960;16:1012–1019.
18. Efrati P, Rozenszajn L, Shapira E. The morphology of buffy coat from cord blood of normal human newborns. *Blood.* 1961;17:497–503.
19. Romsdahl MM, McGrew EA, McGrath RG, et al. Hematopoietic nucleated cells in the peripheral venous blood of patients with carcinoma. *Cancer (Philadelphia).* 1964;17:1400–1404.
20. Linn YC, Tien SL, Lim LC, et al. Haematophagocytosis in bone marrow aspirate: a review of the clinical course of 10 cases. *Acta Haematol.* 1995;94:182–191.
21. Ali FMK. *Separation of Human Blood and Bone Marrow Cells.* Bristol: Wright; 1986.
22. Islam A. A new, fast and convenient method for layering blood or bone marrow over density gradient medium. *J Clin Pathol.* 1995;48:686–688.
23. Hänscheid T. Diagnosis of malaria: a review of alternatives to conventional microscopy. *Clin Lab Haematol.* 1999;21:235–245.
24. Moody AH, Chiodini PL. Methods for the detection of blood parasites. *Clin Lab Haematol.* 2000;22:189–202.
25. Thomson ST, Lohmann RC, Crawford L, et al. External quality assessment in the examination of

blood films for malaria parasites within Ontario, Canada. *Arch Pathol Lab Med.* 2000;124:57–60.

26. Bell D, GO R, Miguel C, et al. Diagnosis of malaria in a remote area of the Philippines: comparison of techniques and their acceptance by health workers and the community. *Bull World Health Organ.* 2001;79:933–941.

27. Melvin DM, Brooke MM. Triton X-100 in Giemsa staining of blood parasites. *Stain Technol.* 1955;30: 269–275.

28. Gleeson RM. An improved method for thick film preparation using saponin as a lysing agent. *Clin Lab Haematol.* 1997;19:249–251.

Chapter | 5 |

Blood cell morphology in health and disease

Barbara J. Bain

Examination of a fixed and stained blood film is an essential part of a haematological investigation, and it cannot be emphasized too strongly that, to obtain maximum information from the examination, the films must be well spread, well stained and examined systematically. Details of the recommended procedure for examination are given later in this chapter.

The most important red cell abnormalities, as seen in fixed and stained films, are described and illustrated, and some notes on their significance and diagnostic importance are added. Leucocyte and platelet abnormalities are also described and, where appropriate, are illustrated. The slides were stained with May–Grünwald–Giemsa. Variations in the colours are due not only to minor variations in the stains but also to whether a daylight blue filter was used in the microscope and to photographic processing.

Figure 5.1 Photomicrograph of a blood film from a healthy adult.

EXAMINATION OF BLOOD FILMS

Blood films should be examined systematically, starting with macroscopic observation of the stained film and then progressing from low-power to high-power microscopic examination. It is useless to place a drop of immersion oil randomly on the film and then to examine it using the high-power ×100 objective.

First, the film should be examined macroscopically to assess whether the spreading technique was satisfactory and to judge its staining characteristics and whether there are any abnormal particles present that may represent large platelet aggregates, cryoglobulin deposits or clumps of tumour cells. Either before or after macroscopic assessment, the film should be covered with a coverglass (coverslip) using a neutral medium as mountant. Next the film should be inspected under a low magnification (with a ×10 or ×20 objective) to: (a) get an idea of the quality of the preparation; (b) assess whether red cell agglutination, excessive rouleaux formation or platelet aggregation is present; (c) assess the number, distribution and staining of the leucocytes; and (d) find an area where the red cells are evenly distributed and are not distorted. A large part of the film should be scanned to detect scanty abnormal cells such as occasional granulocyte precursors or nucleated red blood cells.

Having selected a suitable area, a ×40 or ×50 objective or ×60 oil-immersion objective should then be used. A much better appreciation of variation in red cell size, shape and staining can be obtained with one of these objectives than with the ×100 oil-immersion lens. It should be possible to detect features such as toxic granulation or the presence of Howell–Jolly bodies or Pappenheimer bodies. The major part of the assessment of a blood film is usually done at this power. The ×100 objective in combination with ×6 or ×10 eyepieces should be

used only for the final examination of unusual cells and for looking at fine details such as basophilic stippling (punctate basophilia) or Auer rods. Whether it is necessary to examine a film with a ×100 objective depends on the clinical features, the blood count and the nature of any morphologic abnormality detected at lower power (Fig. 5.1).

Because the diagnosis of the type of anaemia or other abnormality present usually depends on comprehension of the whole picture the film presents, the red cells, leucocytes, and platelets should all be systematically examined. The film examination also serves to validate the automated blood count, distinguishing, for example, between true macrocytosis and factitious macrocytosis caused by the presence of a cold agglutinin and, similarly, between true thrombocytopenia and factitious thrombocytopenia caused by platelet aggregation or satellitism.

RED CELL MORPHOLOGY

In health, the red blood cells vary relatively little in size and shape (Fig. 5.1). In well-spread, dried and stained films the great majority of cells have round, smooth contours and diameters within the comparatively narrow range of 6.0–8.5 µm. As a rough guide, normal red cell size appears to be about the same as that of the nucleus of a small lymphocyte on the dried film (Fig. 5.1). The red cells stain quite deeply with the eosin component of Romanowsky dyes, particularly at the periphery of the cell as a result of the cell's normal biconcavity. A small but variable proportion of cells in well-made films (usually <10%) are definitely oval rather than round, and a very small percentage may be contracted and have an irregular contour or appear to have lost part of their substance as the result of fragmentation (schistocytes). According to Marsh, the percentage of 'pyknocytes' (irregularly contracted cells) and schistocytes in blood from healthy adults does not exceed 0.1% and the proportion is usually considerably less than this, whereas in normal, full-term infants the proportion is higher, 0.3–1.9%, and in premature infants it is still higher, up to 5.6%.[1]

Normal and pathological red cells are subject to considerable distortion in the spreading of a film and, as already mentioned, it is imperative to scan films carefully to find an area where the red cells are least distorted before attempting to examine the cells in detail. Such an area can usually be found toward the tail of the film, although not actually at the tail. Rouleaux often form rapidly in blood after withdrawal from the body and may be conspicuous even in films made at a patient's bedside. They are particularly noticeable in the thicker parts of a film that have dried more slowly. Ideally, red cells should be examined in an area in which there are no rouleaux and the red cells are touching but with little overlap. The film in the chosen area must not be so thin as to cause red cell distortion; if the tail of the film is examined, a false impression of spherocytosis may be gained. The varying appearances of different areas of the same blood film are illustrated in Figures 5.2–5.4. The area illustrated in Figure 5.2 would clearly be the best for looking at red cells critically.

The advantages and disadvantages of examining red cells suspended in plasma have been referred to briefly in Chapter 4 (see p. 63). By this means, red cells can be seen in the absence of artefacts produced by drying, and abnormalities in size and shape can be better and more reliably appreciated than in films of blood dried on slides. However, the ease and rapidity with which dried films can be made, and their permanence, give them an overwhelming advantage in routine studies.

In disease, abnormality in the red cell picture stems from four main causes, which lead to characteristic cytological abnormalities (Table 5.1).

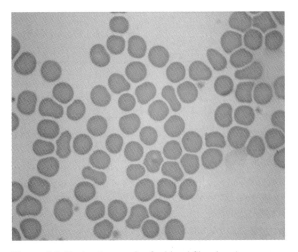

Figure 5.3 Photomicrograph of a blood film showing an area that is too thin for examination (same film as Fig. 5.2).

Figure 5.4 Photomicrograph of a blood film showing an area that is too thick for examination (same film as Fig. 5.2).

ABNORMAL ERYTHROPOIESIS

Anisocytosis ($\alpha\nu\iota\sigma o\zeta$, unequal) and Poikilocytosis ($\pi o\iota\kappa\iota\lambda o\zeta$, varied)

Anisocytosis and poikilocytosis are non-specific features of almost any blood disorder. The terms imply more variation in size or shape than is normally present (Figs 5.5, 5.6). Anisocytosis may be a result of the presence of cells larger than normal (macrocytosis), cells smaller than normal (microcytosis) or both; frequently both macrocytes and microcytes are present (Fig. 5.5).

Poikilocytes are produced in many types of abnormal erythropoiesis, for example, megaloblastic anaemia

Figure 5.2 Photomicrograph of a blood film. Ideal thickness for examination.

Table 5.1 Mechanisms of red cell abnormalities and resultant cytological features

CAUSE	RESULTANT ABNORMALITY
Attempts by the bone marrow to compensate for anaemia by increased erythropoiesis	Signs of less mature cells in the peripheral blood (polychromasia and erythroblastaemia)
Inadequate synthesis of haemoglobin	Reduced or unequal haemoglobin content and concentration (hypochromia, anisochromasia or dimorphism)
Abnormal erythropoiesis, which may be effective or ineffective	Increased variation in size (anisocytosis) and shape (poikilocytosis), basophilic stippling, sometimes dimorphism
Damage to, or changes affecting, the red cells after leaving the bone marrow, including the effects of reduced or absent splenic function	Spherocytosis, irregular contraction, elliptocytosis, ovalocytosis or fragmentation (schistocytosis); the presence of Pappenheimer bodies, Howell–Jolly bodies and variable numbers of certain specific poikilocytes (target cells, acanthocytes and spherocytes)

Figure 5.5 Photomicrograph of a blood film from a patient with a myelodysplastic/myeloproliferative neoplasm, unclassified. Shows moderate anisocytosis, anisochromasia and poikilocytosis. There is one neutrophil band form.

Figure 5.6 Photomicrograph of a blood film from a patient with compound heterozygosity for haemoglobin E and β° thalassaemia. Shows marked anisocytosis and poikilocytosis.

Figure 5.7 Photomicrograph of a blood film. Pernicious anaemia. Shows marked anisocytosis, moderate poikilocytosis (including oval macrocytes and teardrop cells) and a megaloblast.

(Fig. 5.7), iron deficiency anaemia, thalassaemia, myelofibrosis (both idiopathic and secondary) (Fig. 5.8), congenital dyserythropoietic anaemia (Fig. 5.9) and the myelodysplastic syndromes. Elliptocytes and ovalocytes are among the poikilocytes that may be present when there is dyserythropoiesis; they are often present in megaloblastic anaemia (macro-ovalocytes) and in iron deficiency anaemia ('pencil cells'), but they may also be seen in myelodysplastic syndromes and in primary myelofibrosis (Fig. 5.8). The number of elliptocytes and teardrop poikilocytes has been observed to correlate with the severity of iron deficiency anaemia.[2] Poikilocytes are not only characteristic of disordered erythropoiesis but are also seen in various congenital haemolytic anaemias caused by membrane defects and in acquired conditions such as microangiopathic haemolytic anaemia and oxidant damage; in these disorders, the abnormality of shape results from damage to cells after formation and is described later in this chapter.

Figure 5.8 Photomicrograph of a blood film. Idiopathic myelofibrosis. Many of the erythrocytes are elliptical or oval.

Figure 5.10 Photomicrograph of a blood film. Megaloblastic anaemia. Shows macrocytes, oval macrocytes and a hypersegmented neutrophil.

Figure 5.9 Photomicrograph of a blood film. Congenital dyserythropoietic anaemia type II. Shows marked anisocytosis, marked poikilocytosis, one unusually large macrocyte and one severely hypochromic cell.

Figure 5.11 Photomicrograph of a blood film. Liver disease. Shows macrocytosis and stomatocytosis.

Macrocytes

Classically found in megaloblastic anaemias (Fig. 5.10), but macrocytes are also present in some cases of aplastic anaemia, myelodysplastic syndromes and other dyserythropoietic states. In patients being treated with hydroxycarbamide (previously known as hydroxyurea) the red cells are often macrocytic. A common cause of macrocytosis is excess alcohol intake, and it occurs in alcoholic and other types of chronic liver disease. In these conditions, the red cells tend to be fairly uniform in size and shape and there may also be stomatocytes (Fig. 5.11). In the rare type III form of congenital dyserythropoietic anaemia, some of the macrocytes are exceptionally large. Another rare cause of macrocytosis is benign familial macrocytosis.[3] Macrocytosis also occurs whenever there is an increased rate of erythropoiesis, because of the presence of reticulocytes.

Their presence is suspected in routinely stained films because of the slight basophilia, giving rise to polychromasia (see p. 86) and is easily confirmed by special stains (e.g. New methylene blue, see p. 33). These polychromatic macrocytes should be distinguished from other macrocytes because the diagnostic significance is quite different.

Microcytes

The presence of microcytes usually results from a defect in haemoglobin formation. Microcytosis is characteristic of iron deficiency anaemia (Fig. 5.12), various types of thalassaemia (Fig. 5.13), and severe cases of anaemia of chronic disease. Causes that are rarer include congenital and acquired sideroblastic anaemias. Microcytosis related to a defect in haemoglobin synthesis should be distinguished from red cell fragmentation or schistocytosis (see p. 80).

Figure 5.12 Photomicrograph of a blood film. Iron deficiency anaemia. Shows hypochromia, microcytosis and poikilocytosis.

Figure 5.13 Photomicrograph of a blood film. Compound heterozygosity for Hb D-Punjab/β thalassaemia. Shows anisocytosis, poikilocytosis, hypochromia, microcytosis and basophilic stippling.

Figure 5.14 Photomicrographs of blood films. (A) β thalassaemia trait shows hypochromia, microcytosis and basophilic stippling. (B) Erythropoietic porphyria. Shows prominent basophilic stippling.

Both abnormalities can lead to a reduction of the mean cell volume (MCV). However, it should be noted that a low MCV is common in association with a defect in haemoglobin synthesis, whereas it is uncommon in fragmentation syndromes because the fragments usually comprise only a small percentage of erythrocytes.

Basophilic Stippling

Basophilic stippling or punctate basophilia means the presence of numerous basophilic granules distributed throughout the cell (Fig. 5.14); in contrast to Pappenheimer bodies (see below), they do not give a positive Perls' reaction for ionized iron. Punctate basophilia has quite a different significance from diffuse cytoplasmic basophilia. It is indicative of disturbed rather than increased erythropoiesis. It occurs in many blood diseases: thalassaemia, megaloblastic anaemias, infections, liver disease,

poisoning by lead and other heavy metals, unstable haemoglobins and pyrimidine-5'-nucleotidase deficiency.[4]

INADEQUATE HAEMOGLOBIN FORMATION

Hypochromia (Hypochromasia) (υπο, under)

The term *hypochromasia*, or now, more often, *hypochromia*, refers to the presence of red cells that stain unusually palely. (In doubtful cases, it is wise to compare the staining of the suspect film with that of a normal film stained at the same time.) There are two possible causes: a lowered haemoglobin concentration and abnormal thinness of the red cells. A lowered haemoglobin concentration results from impaired haemoglobin synthesis. This may stem from failure of haem synthesis – iron deficiency is a very common cause (Fig. 5.15) and sideroblastic anaemia (Fig. 5.16) is a rare cause – or failure of globin synthesis as in the thalassaemias (Fig. 5.17). Haemoglobin synthesis may also be impaired in chronic infections and other inflammatory conditions. Abnormally thin red cells (leptocytes) (see p. 82) can be the result of a defect in haemoglobin synthesis (e.g. in thalassaemias and iron deficiency) but they also occur in liver disease. It cannot be too strongly stressed that a hypochromic blood picture does not necessarily mean iron deficiency, although this is the most common cause. In iron deficiency, the red cells are characteristically hypochromic and microcytic, but the extent of these abnormalities depends on the severity;

hypochromia may be minor and may be overlooked if the haemoglobin concentration (Hb) exceeds 100 g/l. In heterozygous or homozygous α+ thalassaemia, heterozygous α° thalassaemia or heterozygous β thalassaemia, hypochromia is often less marked, in relation to the degree of microcytosis, than in iron deficiency. The presence of target cells or basophilic stippling also favours a diagnosis of thalassaemia trait rather than iron deficiency. In homozygous β thalassaemia, the abnormalities are greater than in iron deficiency at the same Hb and nucleated red cells are usually present, whereas they are not a feature of iron deficiency. If the patient is being transfused regularly, normal donor cells will also be present, producing a dimorphic blood film (Fig. 5.18).

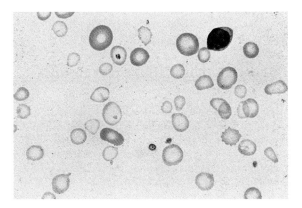

Figure 5.15 Photomicrograph of a blood film. Iron deficiency anaemia. Shows a marked degree of hypochromia, microcytosis, marked anisocytosis and mild poikilocytosis; there are some normally haemoglobinized cells.

Figure 5.17 Photomicrograph of a blood film. Haemoglobin H disease. Shows microcytosis, moderate hypochromia, moderate anisocytosis and some poikilocytes (including teardrop poikilocytes and red cell fragments).

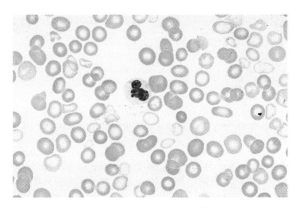

Figure 5.16 Photomicrograph of a blood film. Acquired sideroblastic anaemia (refractory anaemia with ring sideroblasts). Shows a dimorphic blood film with a mixture of normochromic normocytic cells and hypochromic microcytes; there are also several polychromatic macrocytes.

Figure 5.18 Photomicrograph of a blood film. β thalassaemia major. Shows a dimorphic blood film. The normal cells are transfused cells. The patient's own cells show severe hypochromia. There are two nucleated red blood cells.

Anisochromasia (ανισοζ, unequal) and Dimorphic Red Cell Population

A distinction should be made between anisochromasia, in which there is abnormal variability in staining of red cells, and a dimorphic picture, in which there are two distinct populations. Anisochromasia, in which some but not all of the red cells stain palely, is characteristic of a changing situation. It can occur during the development or resolution of iron deficiency anaemia (Fig. 5.19) or the anaemia of chronic disease. In thalassaemia trait, in contrast, anisochromasia is much less common. A dimorphic blood film can be seen in several circumstances. It can occur when an iron deficiency anaemia responds to iron therapy, after the transfusion of normal blood to a patient with a hypochromic anaemia (Fig. 5.19), and in sideroblastic anaemia (Fig. 5.20). In acquired sideroblastic anaemia as a feature of a myelodysplastic syndrome, the two populations of cells are usually hypochromic microcytic and normochromic macrocytic, respectively.

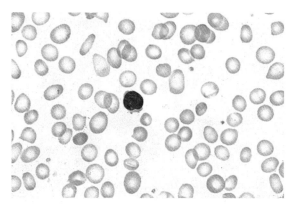

Figure 5.19 Photomicrograph of a blood film. Iron deficiency anaemia. Shows a constant gradation of haemoglobinization of cells (i.e. anisochromasia). There is one elliptocyte.

Figure 5.20 Photomicrograph of a blood film. Acquired sideroblastic anaemia. Shows two distinct populations of cells: hypochromic cells, which also tend to be microcytic, and normocytic normochromic cells.

DAMAGE TO RED CELLS AFTER FORMATION

Poikilocytosis can result not only from abnormal erythropoiesis but also from damage to red cells after their formation. The damage may be consequent on an intrinsic abnormality of the red cell such as a haemoglobinopathy, a membrane defect or an enzyme defect that renders the cell prone to shape alteration. Poikilocytosis can also result from extrinsic causes, as when a red cell is damaged by drugs, chemicals or toxins; by heat; or by abnormal mechanical forces. Poikilocytes of specific shapes suggest different aetiological factors.

Hyperchromasia (Hyperchromia) (υπερ, over)

Unusually deep staining of the red cells with a lack of central pallor may be seen in two circumstances: first, in the presence of macrocytes and second, when cells are abnormally rounded. In macrocytosis, as in neonatal blood and megaloblastic anaemias, it is the increased red cell thickness that causes the hyperchromia, and the mean cell haemoglobin concentration is normal. When hyperchromia results from cells being of abnormal shape, the red cell thickness is greater than normal and the MCHC is increased. Abnormally rounded cells may be either spherocytes or irregularly contracted cells. The distinction between these two cell types is of diagnostic importance.

Spherocytosis (σφαιρα, a sphere)

Spherocytes are cells that are more spheroidal (i.e. less disc-like) than normal red cells but maintain a regular outline. Their diameter is less and their thickness is greater than normal. Only in extreme instances are they almost spherical in shape. It is useful to draw a distinction between spherocytes of normal size and microspherocytes; the latter result from red cell fragmentation or from removal of a considerable proportion of the red cell membrane by splenic or other macrophages. Spherocytes may result from genetic defects of the red cell membrane as in hereditary spherocytosis (Fig. 5.21); from the interaction between immunoglobulin- or complement-coated red cells and phagocytic cells, as in delayed transfusion reactions, ABO haemolytic disease of the newborn (Fig. 5.22) and autoimmune haemolytic anaemia (Fig. 5.23); and from the action of bacterial toxins (e.g. *Clostridium perfringens* lecithinase; Fig. 5.24).

Figure 5.21 Photomicrograph of a blood film. Hereditary spherocytosis. Shows a moderate degree of spherocytosis and anisocytosis. Note the round contour of the spherocytes.

Figure 5.24 Photomicrograph of a blood film. *Clostridium perfringens* septicaemia. Shows an extreme degree of spherocytosis; note the round contour of the spherocytes. A markedly dimorphic picture.

Figure 5.22 Photomicrograph of a blood film. ABO haemolytic disease of the newborn. Spherocytosis is intense, and there are several polychromatic macrocytes.

Figure 5.25 Photomicrograph of a blood film. Sodium chlorate poisoning. Shows sphero-echinocytes, one keratocyte and one nucleated red cell.

Spherocytes usually appear perfectly round in contour in stained films; they have to be carefully distinguished from both irregularly contracted cells and 'crenated spheres' or sphero-echinocytes (Fig. 5.25), which are the end result of crenation (see p. 82). Sphero-echinocytes develop as artefacts, especially in blood that has been allowed to stand before films are spread (Fig. 5.26). The blood film of a patient who has been transfused with stored blood may show a proportion of sphero-echinocytes (Fig. 5.27).

Irregularly Contracted Red Cells

There are a number of causes of irregularly contracted cells. In drug- or chemical-induced haemolytic anaemias, a proportion of the red cells are smaller than normal and unusually densely stained (i.e. they appear contracted) and their margins are slightly or moderately irregular and may be partly concave (Fig. 5.28). These may be

Figure 5.23 Photomicrograph of a blood film. Autoimmune haemolytic anaemia. Shows marked spherocytosis and anisocytosis. There are numerous polychromatic macrocytes.

Figure 5.26 Photomicrograph of a blood film. Normal blood after 24 h at 20°C. Shows a marked degree of crenation; also degenerative changes in white cells.

cells from which Heinz bodies have been extracted by the spleen. Similar cells may be seen in films of some unstable haemoglobinopathies before splenectomy (e.g. that caused by the presence of Hb Köln or Hb St Mary's; Fig. 5.29) and in haemoglobin E homozygosity (Fig. 5.30) and, to a lesser extent, haemoglobin E heterozygosity. Heinz bodies are not normally visible in Romanowsky-stained blood films, but they may be seen in such films as pale pink–staining bodies at the cell margin or even protruding from the erythrocytes in severe unstable haemoglobin haemolytic anaemias after splenectomy and in acute oxidant-induced haemolytic anaemia, including that occurring in deficiency of glucose-6-phosphate dehydrogenase. An extreme degree of irregular contraction is characteristic of severe favism or any other

Figure 5.27 Photomicrograph of a blood film. Post-transfusion, showing one sphero-echinocyte.

Figure 5.29 Photomicrograph of a blood film. An unstable haemoglobin haemolytic anaemia (haemoglobin St Mary's). Shows several irregularly contracted cells.

Figure 5.28 Photomicrograph of a blood film. Haemolytic anaemia caused by an overdose of phenacetin. Shows four irregularly contracted cells and crenation.

Figure 5.30 Photomicrograph of a blood film. Haemoglobin E homozygosity showing four irregularly contracted cells and target cells.

very acute haemolytic episode in individuals who are glucose-6-phosphate dehydrogenase deficient. It is typical to see cells in which the haemoglobin appears to have contracted away from the cell membrane, an appearance sometimes referred to as a hemi-ghost (Fig. 5.31); there may also be ghost cells – cells with almost empty membranes containing negligible haemoglobin. Irregularly contracted cells can be seen in small numbers in β thalassaemia trait and in heterozygosity for haemoglobin C. There may be a considerable number in haemoglobin C homozygosity and in this condition haemoglobin C crystals may also be seen (Fig. 5.32).

A type of irregular contraction of unknown origin has been described by the term 'pyknocytosis'.[5] The pyknocytes closely resemble chemically damaged red cells. As already mentioned (see p. 70), a small number of pyknocytes may be found in the blood of infants in the first few weeks of life, especially in premature infants. The term 'infantile pyknocytosis' refers to a transient haemolytic anaemia, related to glutathione peroxidase and selenium deficiency, affecting infants in whom many pyknocytes are present (Fig. 5.33).[5,6]

Elliptocytosis and Ovalocytosis

Elliptocytes are often present in large numbers in hereditary elliptocytosis (Fig. 5.34). In hereditary pyropoikilocytosis, elliptocytes are only one of the many types of

Figure 5.31 Photomicrograph of a blood film. Acute drug-induced haemolysis in a patient with glucose-6-phosphate dehydrogenase deficiency. There are irregularly contracted cells, ghost cells (black arrows) and hemi-ghosts. Heinz bodies can be seen (blue arrows).

Figure 5.33 Photomicrograph of a blood film. Infantile pyknocytosis. Shows irregularly contracted cells similar to those seen in chemical- or drug-induced haemolytic anaemias.

Figure 5.32 Photomicrograph of a blood film. Haemoglobin C disease (homozygosity for haemoglobin C). Shows many target cells, irregularly contracted cells and a crystal of haemoglobin C. Sometimes it is apparent that haemoglobin C crystals are within otherwise empty red cell membranes.

Figure 5.34 Photomicrograph of a blood film. Hereditary elliptocytosis. Many of the cells are elliptical, and others are oval.

poikilocyte present (Fig. 5.35). South-east Asian ovalo-cytosis is characterized by the presence of a variable number of elliptocytes, macro-ovalocytes and stomatocytes (Fig. 5.36). In all these conditions, the reticulocytes are round in contour (i.e. the cell assumes an abnormal shape only in the late stages of maturation). Although the causative condition is inherited, the abnormalities of red cell shape only become apparent as the cells reach maturity.

SPICULATED CELLS AND RED CELL FRAGMENTATION

The terminology applied to spiculated cells has been confusing because the same terms have been used to designate different types of cells. For this reason the term 'burr cell' should be discarded and the terms recommended by Bessis[7] should be adopted. On the basis of

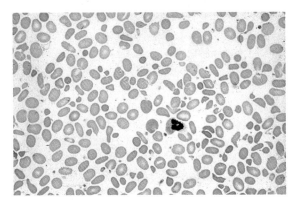

Figure 5.35 Photomicrograph of blood film from a child with hereditary pyropoikilocytosis. Shows spherocytes, elliptocytes, red cell fragments and polychromatic macrocytes.

scanning electron microscopy (discussed later), he distinguished four types of spiculated cell – schistocyte, keratocyte, acanthocyte and echinocyte. The term *echinocyte* is used for the crenated cell. It is differentiated from the acanthocyte on the basis of the number, shape and disposition of the spicules.

Schistocytosis (Fragmentation) ($\sigma\chi\iota\sigma\tau o\zeta$, cleft)

Schistocytes or erythrocyte fragments are found in many blood diseases. They are smaller than normal red cells and of varying shape. Sometimes they have sharp angles or spines (spurs), and sometimes they are round in contour, usually staining deeply but occasionally palely as the result of loss of haemoglobin at the time of fragmentation. If they are both round and densely staining, they may be referred to as microspherocytes. They occur in the following situations:

1. In certain genetically determined disorders (e.g. thalassaemias, congenital dyserythropoietic anaemia and hereditary pyropoikilocytosis)
2. In acquired disorders of red cell formation when erythropoiesis is megaloblastic or dyserythropoietic
3. As the consequence of mechanical stresses (e.g. in the microangiopathic haemolytic anaemias; Figs 5.37–5.39) and in cardiac haemolytic anaemias that are usually caused by a perivalvular leak accompanied by turbulence of left ventricular flow (Fig. 5.40)
4. As the result of direct thermal injury, as in severe burns (Fig. 5.41).

In burns, schistocytes are often rounded, being either microspherocytes or very small disc-shaped fragments. In addition, erythrocytes may be seen to be budding off small rounded blebs of cytoplasm. Not infrequently, as, for instance in the haemolytic-uraemic syndrome in children, the blood picture is made more bizarre by the

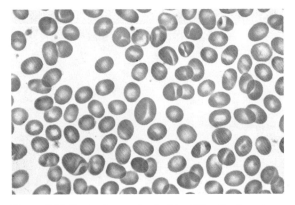

Figure 5.36 Photomicrograph of a blood film. South-east Asian ovalocytosis. Shows stomatocytes, macrostomatocytes and macro-ovalocytes.

Figure 5.37 Photomicrograph of a blood film. Microangiopathic haemolytic anaemia. Shows angular red cell fragments.

Figure 5.38 Photomicrograph of a blood film. Microangiopathic haemolytic anaemia in systemic lupus erythematosus. Shows one very dense microspherocyte and other red cell fragments.

Figure 5.39 Photomicrograph of a blood film. Microangiopathic haemolytic anaemia. Shows numerous bizarrely shaped red cell fragments.

Figure 5.40 Photomicrograph of a blood film. Postcardiac surgery haemolytic anaemia. Shows numerous irregularly shaped cell fragments.

superimposition of varying degrees of echinocytic change. Schistocytes are also a feature of thrombotic thrombocytopenia purpura.[8]

Keratocytes ($\kappa \epsilon \rho \alpha \zeta$, horn)

Keratocytes have pairs of spicules, usually either one pair or two pairs. They may be formed either by removal of a Heinz body by the pitting action of the spleen (Fig. 5.42) or by mechanical damage (Figs 5.43, 5.44). The terms 'helmet cell' and 'bite cell' have sometimes been used to describe keratocytes.

Acanthocytosis ($\alpha \kappa \alpha \nu \theta \alpha$, spine)

The term *acanthocytosis* was introduced to describe an abnormality of the red cell in which there are a small number of spicules of inconstant length, thickness and

Figure 5.41 Photomicrograph of a blood film. Severe burns. Shows many very small, rounded red cell fragments (microspherocytes) and one crenated cell.

Figure 5.42 Photomicrograph of a blood film. Keratocytes and irregularly contracted cells in a patient with haemolysis caused by glucose-6-phosphate dehydrogenase deficiency.

Figure 5.43 Photomicrograph of a blood film. Haemolytic anaemia caused by dapsone. Shows many irregularly contracted cells, three cells with haemoglobin retracted from the red cell membrane and one keratocyte.

Figure 5.44 Photomicrograph of a blood film. Two keratocytes in a patient with microangiopathic haemolytic anaemia.

shape, irregularly disposed over the surface of the cell (Fig. 5.45). They are often associated with abnormal phospholipid metabolism[9–11] or with inherited abnormalities of red cell membrane proteins, as in the McLeod phenotype, caused by lack of the Kell precursor (Kx).[12] They are present in varying numbers following splenectomy and in hyposplenism. A similar cell occurs in severe liver disease ('spur cell' anaemia).[13]

Echinocytosis (εχινοζ, sea-urchin or hedgehog)

Echinocytosis or crenation describes the process by which red cells develop numerous short, regular projections from their surface (Figs 5.25, 5.26). First described by Ponder[14] as disc-sphere transformation, crenation has many causes. A few crenated cells may be seen in many blood films, even in those from healthy subjects. Crenation regularly develops if blood is allowed to stand overnight at 20°C

Figure 5.45 Photomicrograph of a blood film. Liver failure. Acanthocytes are conspicuous.

before films are made (Fig. 5.26). It may be a marked feature, for obscure and probably diverse reasons, in freshly made blood films of patients suffering from a variety of illnesses, especially uraemia. Marked echinocytosis has been reported in premature infants after exchange transfusion or transfusion of normal red cells.[15] When crenation is superimposed on an underlying abnormality, the red cells may appear bizarre in the extreme.

Crenation also occurs as an artefact if red cells are washed free from plasma and suspended in 9 g/l NaCl between glass surfaces, particularly at a raised pH; it also occurs in the presence of traces of fatty substances on the slides on which films are made and in the presence of traces of chemicals that at higher concentrations cause lysis.

The end stages of crenation are the 'finely crenated sphere' and the 'spherical form', which closely resemble spherocytes. The disc-sphere transformation may be reversible (e.g. that produced by washing cells free from plasma), and in this respect the contracted 'spherical form' (which has not lost surface) is quite distinct from the 'spherocyte' (which has lost surface), although they may closely resemble one another in stained films.

If echinocytosis is observed in a film, it usually represents a storage artefact caused by delay in making the film. It is a warning that morphologic features in the blood film cannot be assessed reliably. If present in films made from fresh blood, it is a clinically significant observation.

MISCELLANEOUS ERYTHROCYTE ABNORMALITIES

Leptocytosis (λεπτοζ, thin)

The term *leptocytosis* has been used to describe unusually thin red cells, as in severe iron deficiency or thalassaemia in which the cells may stain as rings of membrane with a little attached haemoglobin with large, almost unstained, central areas (Fig. 5.46). They can also occur when there

Figure 5.46 Photomicrograph of a blood film. β thalassaemia major, after splenectomy. Shows one target cell and cells grossly deficient in haemoglobin, which are leptocytes. There are some transfused cells.

Figure 5.47 Photomicrograph of a blood film. Alcoholic liver disease. Shows many target cells.

Figure 5.48 Photomicrograph of a blood film. Haemoglobin C/β° thalassaemia compound heterozygosity showing target cells, irregularly contracted cells and one spherocyte.

Figure 5.49 Photomicrograph of a blood film. Haemoglobin C homozygosity. Shows numerous target cells and irregularly contracted cells.

is an excess of membrane in relation to cytoplasm, as can occur in liver disease.

Target Cells

The term *target cell* refers to a cell in which there is a central round stained area and a peripheral rim of haemoglobinized cytoplasm separated by non-staining or more lightly staining cytoplasm. Target cells result from cells having a surface that is disproportionately large compared with their volume. They may be normal in size, microcytic or macrocytic. They are seen in films in chronic liver diseases in which the cell membrane may be loaded with cholesterol (Fig. 5.47), in hereditary hypo-betalipoproteinaemia,[16] and in varying numbers in iron deficiency anaemia and in thalassaemia (Fig. 5.46). They are often conspicuous in certain haemoglobinopathies (e.g. haemoglobin C/β° thalassaemia; Fig. 5.48), haemoglobin C disease (Fig. 5.49), haemoglobin H disease (Fig. 5.50), sickle cell anaemia, sickle cell/haemoglobin C disease (Fig. 5.51), sickle cell/β thalassaemia, and haemoglobin E disease. Smaller numbers are usual in haemoglobin C trait, haemoglobin E trait and postsplenectomy. Splenectomy in thalassaemia may result in an extreme degree of leptocytosis and target cell formation.

Stomatocytosis (στομα, mouth)

Stomatocytes are red cells in which the central biconcave area appears slit-like in dried films. In 'wet' preparations, the stomatocyte is a cup-shaped red cell. The slit-like appearance of the cell's concavity, as seen in dried films, is thus to some extent an artefact. The term was first used to describe the appearance of some of the cells in a rare type of haemolytic anaemia, hereditary stomatocytosis.[17] They are

Figure 5.50 Photomicrograph of a blood film. Haemoglobin H disease. Shows target cells, hypochromic cells and poikilocytes.

Figure 5.52 Photomicrograph of a blood film. Patient with chronic myelogenous leukaemia taking hydroxycarbamide. Shows stomatocytosis. Many of the cells have a slit-like central unstained area.

Figure 5.51 Photomicrograph of a blood film. Sickle cell/haemoglobin C disease. Shows a sickle cell, target cells and two SC poikilocytes.

Figure 5.53 Photomicrograph of a blood film. Sickle cell anaemia (homozygosity for haemoglobin S). Shows a sickled cell, boat-shaped cells and a nucleated red cell and target cells.

also a feature of south-east Asian ovalocytosis. They have been described as being particularly frequent in films of Australians of Mediterranean origin.[18,19] Subsequently, stomatocytes were recognized in acquired conditions and occasionally they are prominent (Fig. 5.52). They are observed in liver disease, in alcoholism,[20] and occasionally in the myelodysplastic syndromes. There is a suspicion that in some films the occurrence of stomatocytosis is an *in vitro* artefact because it is known that the change can be produced by decreased pH and as the result of exposure to cationic detergent-like compounds and non-penetrating anions.[21]

Sickle Cells

The varied film appearances in sickle cell anaemia are illustrated in Figures 5.53–5.55. Sickle cells are almost always present in films of freshly withdrawn blood of adults with homozygosity for haemoglobin S. However, sickle cells are

Figure 5.54 Photomicrograph of a blood film. Sickle cell anaemia (homozygosity for haemoglobin S). Shows boat-shaped cells and a nucleated red blood cell.

Figure 5.55 Photomicrograph of a blood film. Sickle cell anaemia (homozygosity for haemoglobin S). Shows elliptical sickle cells, target cells and Pappenheimer bodies.

Figure 5.56 Photomicrograph of a blood film. Sickle cell/haemoglobin C disease showing SC poikilocytes and target cells.

usually absent in neonates and are rare in adult patients with a high haemoglobin F percentage. Sometimes many irreversibly sickled cells are present, and in all cases massive sickling takes place when the blood is subjected to anoxia (see p. 315). In films of fresh blood, the sickled cells vary in shape between boat-shaped forms and sickles. Target cells are also often a feature of blood films from patients with sickle cell anaemia, and Howell–Jolly bodies are found when there is splenic atrophy.

Haemoglobin C Crystals and SC Poikilocytes

In patients with homozygosity for haemoglobin C, target cells and irregularly contracted cells are usually numerous and there may be occasional straight-edged haemoglobin C crystals, either apparently extracellularly (Fig. 5.32) or within the ghost of a red cell. In patients who are compound heterozygotes for both haemoglobin S and haemoglobin C, the film sometimes resembles that of haemoglobin C disease (Fig. 5.32). In other patients, there are elliptical cells, rare sickle cells and sometimes distinctive SC poikilocytes (Fig. 5.56).

Erythrocyte Inclusions

The possibility of sometimes suspecting the presence of Heinz bodies on a routinely stained film and the detection of haemoglobin crystals within red cells has already been mentioned. Alpha chain inclusions can also sometimes be seen, e.g. in β thalassaemia major following splenectomy. Other red cell inclusions include Howell–Jolly bodies and Pappenheimer bodies.

Howell–Jolly Bodies

Howell–Jolly bodies are nuclear remnants. They are small, round cytoplasmic inclusions that stain purple on a Romanowsky stain. They are regularly present after splenectomy and when there is splenic atrophy (Fig. 5.57). They may be seen in a small percentage of red cells in pernicious anaemia. Usually only a few such inclusions are present, but they may be numerous in cases of coeliac disease and in other conditions in which there is splenic atrophy and megaloblastosis.

Pappenheimer Bodies

Pappenheimer bodies are small peripherally sited basophilic (almost black) erythrocyte inclusions. They are smaller than Howell–Jolly bodies. Usually only a small number are present in a cell. They are composed of haemosiderin and their presence is related to sideroblastic erythropoiesis and hyposplenism (Figs 5.58, 5.59). Sometimes they are found in the majority of circulating red cells. Their nature can be confirmed by means of a Perls' stain. They correspond to the siderotic granules of siderocytes and are never distributed in large numbers throughout the cells as in classical punctate basophilia. However,

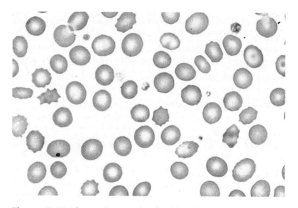

Figure 5.57 Photomicrograph of a blood film. Postsplenectomy. Shows acanthocytes, a target cell and a Howell–Jolly body.

Figure 5.60 Photomicrograph of a blood film. Increased rouleaux formation in a patient with bacterial infection.

Figure 5.58 Photomicrograph of a blood film. β thalassaemia major, patient of regular blood transfusions, showing Pappenheimer bodies in several poorly haemoglobinized cells.

Figure 5.59 Photomicrograph of a blood film. Autoimmune thrombocytopenic purpura, postsplenectomy, showing a Pappenheimer body and a Howell–Jolly body.

Figure 5.61 Photomicrograph of a blood film. Shows massive autoagglutination in a patient with chronic cold haemagglutinin disease (compare with Fig. 5.60).

a single cell may show both punctate basophilia and Pappenheimer bodies. With Perls' stain, the former granules are pink, whereas the latter are blue.

Rouleaux and Autoagglutination

Rouleaux occur to some extent in all films but increased rouleaux formation is significant. The differences between rouleaux and autoagglutination are described on p. 63, and there is usually no difficulty in determining which is which in stained films (Figs 5.60, 5.61). However, in myelomatosis and in other conditions in which there is intense rouleaux formation, the rouleaux may simulate autoagglutination. Even so, if the film, apparently showing autoagglutination, is carefully scanned, an area

in which rouleaux can be clearly seen will almost certainly be found, emphasizing the importance of careful selection of the area of film to be examined.

CHANGES ASSOCIATED WITH A COMPENSATORY INCREASE IN ERYTHROPOIESIS

Polychromasia (πολθζ, many)

The term *polychromasia* suggests that the red cells are being stained many colours. In practice, it means that some of the red cells stain shades of bluish grey (Fig. 5.62) – these

Figure 5.62 Photomicrograph of a blood film. Polychromasia. Some red cells stain shades of bluish grey.

Figure 5.63 Photomicrograph of a blood film. Primary myelofibrosis. Shows a leucoerythroblastic blood film, teardrop poikilocytes and ovalocytes.

are the reticulocytes. Cells staining shades of blue, 'blue polychromasia', are unusually young reticulocytes. 'Blue polychromasia' is most often seen when there is either an intense erythropoietic drive or when there is extramedullary erythropoiesis, as, for instance, in myelofibrosis or carcinomatosis. It should be noted that in certain circumstances the *absence* of polychromasia is significant; in a patient with severe anaemia it indicates that the bone marrow response is inadequate, e.g. in aplastic anaemia and pure red cell aplasia.

Erythroblastaemia

Erythroblasts may be found in the blood films of almost any patient with a severe anaemia; they are, however, very unusual in aplastic anaemia, and their presence should lead to this diagnosis being doubted. They are more common in children than in adults, and large numbers are a very characteristic finding in haemolytic disease of the newborn. Small numbers can be found in the cord blood of normal infants, whereas quite large numbers are found in that of premature infants.

When large numbers of erythroblasts are present, many of them may be derived from extramedullary foci of erythropoiesis (e.g. in the liver and spleen). This is likely, for instance, in haemolytic disease of the newborn and primary myelofibrosis. In myelofibrosis and carcinomatosis, the number of erythroblasts is often disproportionately high for the degree of anaemia, and a few immature granulocytes are usually also present (designated leucoerythroblastic anaemia) (Fig. 5.63).

Erythroblasts can usually be found in the peripheral blood after splenectomy, and many may be present in severe anaemia and in the presence of extramedullary erythropoiesis (Fig. 5.64). Large numbers are frequently seen in the blood films of patients with sickle cell anaemia in painful crises. Small numbers of erythroblasts are not uncommon in blood from patients suffering from cyanotic heart failure or septicaemia.

Figure 5.64 Photomicrograph of a blood film. β thalassaemia major with inadequate blood transfusion support. There are numerous erythroblasts; there are also hypochromic cells, target cells and a cell containing a Howell–Jolly body.

It should be noted that when the term *normoblast* is used, it implies that erythroid maturation is normoblastic. *Erythroblast* is a more general term that also includes megaloblasts.

EFFECTS OF SPLENECTOMY AND HYPOSPLENISM

Some of the effects of splenectomy and hyposplenism have already been mentioned – namely, the occurrence of target cells, acanthocytes, Howell–Jolly bodies and Pappenheimer bodies (Fig. 5.57). In addition, there may be neutrophilia (early after splenectomy), lymphocytosis, thrombocytosis and giant platelets. In people who are haematologically normal, the blood film features of hyposplenism are variable – sometimes striking and sometimes very minor.

SCANNING ELECTRON MICROSCOPY

The morphology of red cells, as illustrated in this chapter, may be distorted by spreading and drying films in the traditional way. A more authentic portrayal of red cell shape *in vivo* can be seen by scanning electron microscopy. This provided the means for a critical re-examination of red cell morphology. Bessis and his co-workers published excellent photographs of pathological red cells and, from their appearances, proposed a terminology[7,21,22] that has generally been adopted in this chapter. They also discussed the difficult question of the *in vivo* significance of crenation (echinocytic change) observed *in vitro*. It seems that neither echinocytosis nor acanthocytosis is necessarily associated with increased haemolysis. It cannot be concluded, either, that crenation is occurring *in vivo*, when the phenomenon is markedly evident in films made on glass slides. To ensure that cells are crenated in any blood sample as it is withdrawn, Brecher and Bessis recommended that the blood be examined immediately between plastic, instead of glass coverslips or slides, to avoid the known 'echinocytogenic' effect of glass surfaces, probably caused by alkalinity.[22] Nevertheless, for practical purposes, if a blood film of a freshly drawn blood specimen shows echinocytosis and films from other patients prepared using the same glass slides do not, the abnormality can be accepted as genuine.

The specialized procedure of scanning electron microscopy is not practical as a routine but helps in understanding the nature of cells observed in stained blood films. Morphological changes in red cells may be very complex. Echinocytic and stomatocytic change can be superimposed on other pathological forms, giving rise to 'sickle-stomatocytes' and 'stomato-acanthocytes'. Acanthocytes can undergo crenation, the product being termed an

Figure 5.65 Scanning electron microscope photograph. Normal red cells.

'acantho-echinocyte'. Following splenectomy in patients with hereditary spherocytosis, sphero-acanthocytes may be observed.

The appearance of various cells by scanning electron microscopy is illustrated in Figures 5.65–5.72.

MORPHOLOGY OF LEUCOCYTES

This section will include a description of the normal leucocytes, some congenital anomalies and reactive changes that are commonly encountered. To describe adequately the various changes found in malignant conditions would require a lengthy text and many illustrations that are beyond the scope of this book. They will be referred to briefly here, but for detailed reference readers should consult a specialist test[23] or an atlas on blood cells. For classification of the acute leukaemias, see the original description by the FAB (French-American-British) group[24] and the subsequent revision.[25] There is also a World Health Organization classification,[26] which supercedes the FAB classifications when facilities are available for fully characterizing leukaemia and is now in widespread use. However, the FAB classification remains useful as a widely accepted scheme for the initial morphologic description of leukaemias.

Figure 5.66 Scanning electron microscope photograph. Hereditary spherocytosis. Note the round shape of spherocytes but also that there are cells intermediate in form between spherocytes and normal discocytes. (Compare with Fig. 5.65; also see blood film appearances as shown in Fig. 5.21.)

Figure 5.67 Scanning electron microscope photograph. Normal blood after standing overnight. Note crenation.

POLYMORPHONUCLEAR NEUTROPHILS

In normal adults, neutrophils account for more than half the circulating leucocytes. They are the main defence of the body against pyogenic bacterial infections. Normal neutrophils are uniform in size, with an apparent diameter of *about* 13 μm on a film. They have a segmented nucleus and, when stained, pink/orange cytoplasm with fine granulation (Fig. 5.73). The majority of neutrophils have three nuclear segments (lobes) connected by tapering chromatin strands. The chromatin shows clumping and is usually condensed at the nuclear periphery. A small percentage have four lobes, and occasionally five lobes may be seen. Up to 8% of circulating neutrophils are unsegmented or partly segmented ('band' forms) (discussed later).

In women, 2–3% of the neutrophils show an appendage at a terminal nuclear segment. This 'drumstick' is about 1.5 μm in diameter and is connected to the nucleus by a short stalk. It represents the inactive X chromosome and corresponds to the Barr body of buccal cells.

Occasionally, red cells will adhere to neutrophils, forming rosettes. The mechanism is unknown, but it is likely

Figure 5.68 Scanning electron microscope photograph. Acanthocytosis. Some cells also show crenation and contraction. (Compare with Fig. 5.67; see also blood film appearances as shown in Fig. 5.45.)

89

Figure 5.69 Scanning electron microscope photograph. Oxidant drug-induced haemolysis; see blood film appearances shown in Figure 5.43.

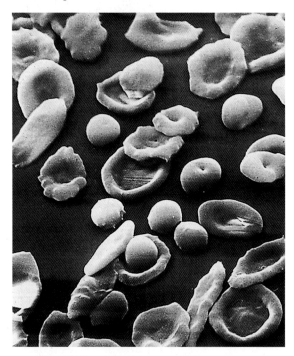

Figure 5.70 Scanning electron microscope photograph. Iron deficiency anaemia. (Compare with Fig. 5.71, and see also Fig. 5.12.)

to be immune; usually it appears to be of no clinical significance but occasionally it is seen in an immune haemolytic anaemia. Leucoagglutination also occurs as an *in vitro* artefact.[27] Occasionally neutrophils (and/or monocytes) have phagocytosed erythrocytes (Fig. 5.74).

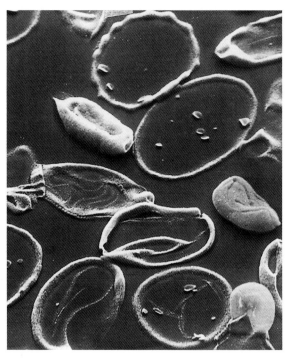

Figure 5.71 Scanning electron microscope photograph. β thalassaemia major, postsplenectomy. Shows cells grossly deficient in haemoglobin; there are also contracted cells and poikilocytes. In the hypochromic cells, inclusions are seen, corresponding to Pappenheimer bodies.

This is particularly common in paroxysmal cold haemoglobinuria.

It is extremely important to ensure the consistency of staining of the blood films using a standardized Romanowsky method (see Chapter 4) because changes in the staining density, colour and appearance of cytoplasmic granulation, if not artefact, may have diagnostic significance. Common neutrophil abnormalities are described later in this chapter.

Granules

Toxic granulation is the term used to describe an increase in staining density and possibly number of granules that occurs regularly with bacterial infection and often with other causes of inflammation (Fig. 5.75). It can also be a feature of administration of granulocyte colony-stimulating factor (G-CSF) and of aplastic anaemia. Poorly staining (hypogranular) and agranular neutrophils occur in the myelodysplastic syndromes (Fig. 5.76) and in some forms of myeloid leukaemia.

There are rare inherited disorders that are manifest by abnormal neutrophils. In the Alder–Reilly anomaly, the granules are very large, are discrete, stain deep red and may obscure the nucleus (Fig. 5.77). Other leucocytes, including some lymphocytes, also show the abnormal

Figure 5.72 Scanning electron microscope photograph. Sickle cell anaemia (homozygosity for haemoglobin S). Shows sickled cells.

Figure 5.74 Photomicrograph of a blood film. Erythrophagocytosis in a patient with a positive direct antiglobulin test.

Figure 5.75 Photomicrograph of a blood film. Severe infection. Neutrophils show toxic granulation.

Figure 5.73 Photomicrograph of a blood film. Normal polymorphonuclear neutrophil and normal eosinophil.

Figure 5.76 Photomicrograph of a blood film. Myelodysplastic syndrome. Shows a hypogranular neutrophil and a normally granulated neutrophil.

granules. In the Chédiak–Higashi syndrome there are giant but scanty azurophilic granules (Fig. 5.78), and the other leucocyte types may also be affected. Alder–Reilly neutrophils function normally, but in Chédiak–Higashi syndrome there is a functional defect that is manifested by susceptibility to severe infection.

Figure 5.77 Photomicrograph of a blood film. Alder–Reilly anomaly. The nucleus is obscured by the cytoplasmic granules.

Figure 5.78 Photomicrograph of a blood film. Chédiak–Higashi syndrome. Neutrophils show abnormal granules.

Figure 5.79 Photomicrograph of a blood film. Blood collected from infected site, showing bacteria (A) in scattered clumps and in a neutrophil (B).

Vacuoles

In blood films spread without delay, the presence of vacuoles in the neutrophils is usually indicative of severe sepsis, when toxic granulation is usually also present. Vacuoles will develop as an artefact with prolonged standing of the blood before films are made (see Chapter 1, Fig. 1.3, see p. 8).

Bacteria

Very rarely, in the presence of overwhelming septicaemia (e.g. meningococcal or pneumococcal), bacteria may be seen within vacuoles or apparently lying free in the cytoplasm of neutrophils. When blood is taken from an infected central line, clumps of bacteria or fungi may be seen scattered in the film as well as in neutrophils in phagocytic vacuoles (Fig. 5.79). In premature infants with staphylococcal septicaemia, the detection of bacteria in neutrophils helps in early diagnosis.[28] In endemic areas, detection of bacteria within neutrophils is important in the diagnosis of ehrlichiosis and anaplasmosis.

Döhle Bodies

Döhle bodies are small, round or oval, pale blue-grey structures usually found at the periphery of the neutrophil. They consist of ribosomes and endoplasmic reticulum. They are seen in bacterial infections but also following tissue damage, in inflammation, following administration of G-CSF and during pregnancy. There is also a benign inherited condition known as May–Hegglin anomaly with a similar but not identical morphologic structure; in this condition, the inclusions occur in all types of leucocytes except lymphocytes.

Nuclei

Segmentation of the nucleus of the neutrophil is a normal event as the cell matures from the myelocyte. With the three-lobed neutrophil as a marker, a shift to the left (less mature) or to the right (hypermature) can be recognized (Table 5.2). A left shift with band forms, metamyelocytes and perhaps occasional myelocytes is common in sepsis (Fig. 5.80), when it is usually accompanied by toxic granulation. If promyelocytes and myeloblasts are also present, it is likely to be a feature of a leucoerythroblastic anaemia or leukaemia (Fig. 5.81); occasionally this extreme picture may be seen in very severe infections, when it is called 'leukaemoid reaction'. A left shift, with a significant number of band forms, occurs normally in pregnancy.

Figure 5.80 Photomicrograph of a blood film. Infection. Shows left shift of the neutrophils with toxic granulation.

Figure 5.81 Photomicrograph of a blood film. Chronic myelogenous leukaemia. There is a left shift with band forms, metamyelocytes, myelocytes and one myeloblast.

Hypersegmentation

The presence of hypersegmented neutrophils is an important diagnostic feature of megaloblastic anaemias. Neutrophil hypersegmentation can be defined as the presence of neutrophils with six or more lobes or the presence of more than 3% of neutrophils with at least five lobes. In florid megaloblastic states, neutrophils are often enlarged and their nuclei may have six or more segments connected by particularly fine chromatin bridges (Fig. 5.10). A right shift with moderately hypersegmented neutrophils may also be seen in uraemia and not infrequently in iron deficiency.[29] Hypersegmentation can be seen after cytotoxic treatment, especially with methotrexate. Patients undergoing treatment with hydroxycarbamide or other drugs that induce megaloblastosis sometimes develop hypersegmented neutrophils (Table 5.2).[30]

Pelger–Huët Cells

The Pelger–Huët anomaly is a benign inherited condition in which neutrophil nuclei fail to segment properly. The majority of circulating neutrophils have only two discrete

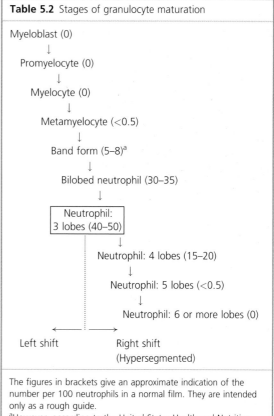

Table 5.2 Stages of granulocyte maturation

Myeloblast (0)
↓
Promyelocyte (0)
↓
Myelocyte (0)
↓
Metamyelocyte (<0.5)
↓
Band form (5–8)[a]
↓
Bilobed neutrophil (30–35)
↓
Neutrophil: 3 lobes (40–50)
↓
Neutrophil: 4 lobes (15–20)
↓
Neutrophil: 5 lobes (<0.5)
↓
Neutrophil: 6 or more lobes (0)

← Left shift | Right shift (Hypersegmented) →

The figures in brackets give an approximate indication of the number per 100 neutrophils in a normal film. They are intended only as a rough guide.
[a]However, according to the United States Health and Nutrition Examination surveys, the normal band count is lower – about 0.5% of the neutrophils.[30]

equal-sized lobes connected by a thin chromatin bridge (Fig. 5.82). The chromatin is coarsely clumped, and granule content is normal.

A similar acquired morphologic anomaly, known as pseudo-Pelger cells or the acquired Pelger–Huët anomaly, may be seen in myelodysplastic syndromes, acute myeloid leukaemia with dysplastic maturation, and occasionally in chronic myelogenous leukaemia (during the accelerated phase) (Fig. 5.83). In these conditions, the neutrophils are often hypogranular and they tend to have a markedly irregular nuclear pattern.

Pyknotic Neutrophils (Apoptosis)

Small numbers of dead or dying cells may normally be found in the blood, especially when there is an infection. They may also develop in normal blood *in vitro* after standing for 12–18 h, even if kept at 4°C. These cells have round, dense, featureless nuclei and their cytoplasm tends to be dark pink (see p. 8 and Fig. 1.4). It is important not to confuse these cells with erythroblasts.

EOSINOPHILS

Eosinophils are a little larger than neutrophils, 12–17 μm in diameter. They usually have two nuclear lobes or segments, and the cytoplasm is packed with distinctive spherical gold/orange (eosinophilic) granules (Figs 5.73, 5.84). The underlying cytoplasm, which is usually obscured by the granules, is pale blue. Prolonged steroid administration causes eosinopenia. Moderate eosinophilia occurs in allergic conditions; more severe eosinophilia (20–50 × 10⁹/l) may be seen in parasitic infections and even

Figure 5.83 Photomicrograph of a blood film. Chronic myelogenous leukaemia. There are five 'pseudo-Pelger' cells; this abnormality is not seen in the chronic phase of this disease.

Figure 5.84 Photomicrograph of a blood film. Normal adult. Shows a basophil, an eosinophil and a neutrophil.

greater numbers may be seen in other reactive eosinophilias, eosinophilic leukaemia and the idiopathic hypereosinophilic syndrome. Reactive eosinophilia with very high counts may be seen in T-cell lymphoma, B-cell lymphoma and acute lymphoblastic leukaemia. Eosinophils are part of the leukaemic population in chronic myelogenous leukaemia, and this is occasionally so in acute myeloid leukaemia. Cytological abnormalities in eosinophils are not very useful in distinguishing between leukaemic and reactive eosinophils.

BASOPHILS

Basophils are the rarest (<1%) of the circulating leucocytes. Their nuclear segments tend to fold up on each other, resulting in a compact irregular dense nucleus resembling a closed lotus flower. The distinctive, large,

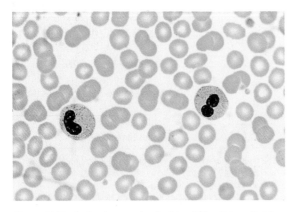

Figure 5.82 Photomicrograph of a blood film. Pelger–Huët anomaly. Shows hypolobated neutrophils.

variably sized, dark blue or purple granules of the cyto-plasm (Fig. 5.84) often obscure the nucleus; they are rich in histamine, serotonin and heparin. Basophils tend to degranulate, leaving cytoplasmic vacuoles.

Basophils are present in increased numbers in myelo-proliferative neoplasms and are especially prominent in chronic myelogenous leukaemia; in the latter condition, when basophils are more than 10% of the differential leu-cocyte count, this is a sign of impending accelerated phase or blast crisis.

MONOCYTES

Monocytes are the largest of the circulating leucocytes, 15–18 µm in diameter. They have bluish-grey cytoplasm that contains variable numbers of fine reddish granules. The nucleus is large and curved, often in the shape of a horseshoe, but it may be folded or curled (Figs 5.85, 5.86). It does not undergo segmentation. The chromatin is finer and more evenly distributed than in neutrophil nuclei. An increased number of monocytes occur in some chronic infections and inflammatory conditions such as tuberculosis and Crohn's disease, in chronic myeloid leu-kaemias (particularly atypical chronic myeloid leukaemia and chronic myelomonocytic leukaemia) and in acute leukaemias with a monocytic component. In chronic myelomonocytic leukaemia, the mature monocyte count may reach as high as $100 \times 10^9/l$. It is occasionally

Figure 5.86 Photomicrograph of a blood film. Healthy adult. Shows a monocyte and a lymphocyte.

difficult to distinguish abnormal monocytes from the large activated T lymphocytes produced in infectious mononucleosis or from circulating high-grade lymphoma cells.

LYMPHOCYTES

The majority of circulating lymphocytes are small cells with a thin rim of cytoplasm, occasionally containing scanty azurophilic granules (Figs 5.1, 5.87). Nuclei are remarkably uniform in size (about 9 µm in diameter).

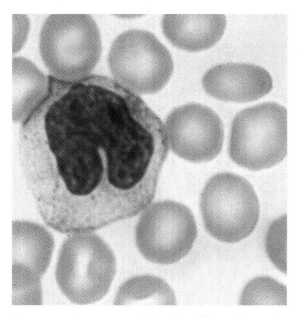

Figure 5.85 Photomicrograph of a blood film. Healthy adult. Monocyte.

Figure 5.87 Photomicrograph of a blood film. Shows a small lymphocyte and two large granular lymphocytes with azurophilic granules.

This provides a useful guide for estimating red cell size (normally about 7–8 µm) on the blood film. Some 10% of circulating lymphocytes are larger, with more abundant pale blue cytoplasm containing azurophilic granules (Fig. 5.87). The nuclei of lymphocytes have homogeneous chromatin with some clumping at the nuclear periphery. About 85% of the circulating lymphocytes are T cells or natural killer (NK) cells.

In infections, both bacterial and viral, transformed lymphocytes may be present. These immunoblasts or 'Türk' cells are 10–15 µm in diameter, with a round nucleus, often with a large nucleolus, and abundant, deeply basophilic cytoplasm (Fig. 5.88). They may develop into plasmacytoid lymphocytes and plasma cells, and these are occasionally seen in the blood in severe infections. In the absence of infection, multiple myeloma must be excluded. In viral infection, 'reactive lymphocytes' appear in the blood. These have slightly larger nuclei with more open chromatin and abundant cytoplasm that may be irregular. The most extreme examples of these cells are usually found in infectious mononucleosis (Fig. 5.89). These 'glandular fever' cells have irregular nuclei and abundant cytoplasm that is basophilic at the periphery; they have a tendency to appear, on a blood film, to have flowed around adjacent erythrocytes.

Malignant lymphoid cells vary enormously in their morphology. The commonest malignancy is chronic lymphocytic leukaemia, the leukaemic population being composed almost exclusively of small lymphocytes (Fig. 5.90), sometimes with a few larger nucleolated cells. In prolymphocytic leukaemia, the majority of cells are a little larger than small lymphocytes with more cytoplasm and usually one distinct nucleolus (Fig. 5.91). Lymphoblasts of acute lymphoblastic leukaemia (Figs 5.92, 5.93) vary in size from only slightly larger than lymphocytes to cells of 15–17 µm diameter. The nuclei generally have diffuse chromatin, but there may be some chromatin

Figure 5.89 Photomicrograph of a blood film. Infectious mononucleosis. There are two activated lymphocytes ('atypical mononuclear cells').

condensation in the smaller blasts. The cytoplasm varies from weakly to strongly basophilic.

Circulating lymphoma cells vary markedly in size, depending on the type of lymphoma. When there is a lymphocytosis, the lymphocytes are usually far less uniform than in chronic lymphocytic leukaemia, and the lymphoma cells frequently have irregular lobed, indented or cleaved nuclei and relatively scanty agranular cytoplasm that varies in its degree of basophilia. Lobulated lymphocytes are a

Figure 5.88 Photomicrograph of a blood film. Viral infection. Shows a Türk cell, another reactive lymphocyte and a small lymphocyte.

Figure 5.90 Photomicrograph of a blood film. Chronic lymphocytic leukaemia. The cells are small lymphocytes; note that rouleaux formation is increased.

Figure 5.93 Photomicrograph of a blood film. Acute lymphoblastic leukaemia (FAB L1 type). Shows lymphoblasts.

Figure 5.91 Photomicrograph of a blood film. Prolymphocytic leukaemia. There is a uniform population of prolymphocytes.

feature of HTLV-I (human T-lymphotropic virus type I) infection and of adult T-cell leukaemia/lymphoma. However, lymphocytes with definite lobulation are also a common storage artefact in blood kept for 18–24 h at room temperature (see p. 7).

Lymphocytes predominate in the blood films of infants and young children. In this age range, large lymphocytes and reactive lymphocytes tend to be conspicuous, and a small number of lymphoblasts may also be present.

There is no uniform approach to the terminology used to refer to cytologically abnormal lymphocytes, a problem compounded by the fact that sometimes it is difficult to distinguish reactive lymphocytes from neoplastic. The term 'variant lymphocyte' is sometimes used but it is not

a term that is known to many clinicians. It is not prudent to describe lymphocytes as 'reactive'; it is better to refer to 'atypical lymphocytes, appear reactive' or, in other circumstances, 'abnormal lymphocytes, suspect lymphoma'. In this way an opinion, which may be wrong, is differentiated from a factual morphologic description.

PLATELET MORPHOLOGY

Normal platelets are 1–3 μm in diameter. They are irregular in outline with fine red granules that may be scattered or centralized. A small number of larger platelets, up to 5 μm in diameter, may be seen in normal films. Larger platelets are seen in the blood when platelet production is increased (Fig. 5.94) and in hyposplenism (Fig. 5.95). Thus, for example, in severe immune thrombocytopenia,

Figure 5.92 Photomicrograph of a blood film. Philadelphia-positive acute lymphoblastic leukaemia (FAB L1 category). Shows three lymphoblasts.

Figure 5.94 Photomicrograph of a blood film. Essential thrombocythaemia. Shows platelet anisocytosis and increased numbers of platelets.

Figure 5.95 Photomicrograph of a blood film. Hyposplenism in coeliac disease. Shows giant platelet.

Figure 5.97 Photomicrograph of a blood film. Grey platelet syndrome. Shows severely hypogranular platelets.

some large platelets will be seen on the film. Very high platelet counts as a feature of a myeloproliferative neoplasm may be associated with extreme platelet anisocytosis, with some platelets being as large as red cells and often with some agranular or hypogranular platelets (Fig. 5.96). The platelet count frequently increases with acute inflammatory stress or bleeding but seldom to more than $1000 \times 10^9/l$. More than this, unless the patient is critically ill or hyposplenic, makes a myeloproliferative neoplasm a definite possibility.

Characteristic morphologic features are seen in various uncommon inherited platelet disorders associated with bleeding. These include the Bernard–Soulier syndrome, in which there are giant platelets with a defective ristocetin response, and the grey platelet syndrome, in which the platelets have decreased granules and have a ghost-like appearance on the stained blood film (Fig. 5.97). Thrombocytopenia with large platelets is also a feature of the May–Hegglin anomaly (see p. 92).

In about 1% of individuals, ethylenediaminetetra-acetic acid (EDTA) anticoagulant causes platelet clumping,

resulting in pseudothrombocytopenia.[31] It is much less likely to occur when the blood is collected into any other anticoagulant.[32] This phenomenon may be detected when it gives rise to a 'flag' on an automated blood cell counter; it is identifiable on the blood film. It is not associated with any coagulation disturbance and platelet function is normal. When this abnormality is detected it is important that the erroneous platelet count is deleted from the report. If the blood film shows that the platelet count is clearly normal, the statement 'Platelet count normal' is sufficient, rather than a repeat sample in an alternative anticoagulant being requested. Occasionally, EDTA inhibits the staining of platelets.[33]

Occasionally, platelets may be seen adhering to neutrophils (Fig. 5.98).[34–37] This has been reported in patients who have demonstrable antiplatelet autoantibodies,[38] but

Figure 5.96 Photomicrograph of a blood film. Myeloproliferative neoplasm. Shows platelet anisocytosis with some giant platelets.

Figure 5.98 Photomicrograph of a blood film. Shows adhesion of platelets to a neutrophil (platelet satellism).

it is more commonly seen in apparently healthy individuals. It is not seen in films made directly from blood that has not been anticoagulated. Sometimes the platelets are ingested by neutrophils.[39] If a blood film in a patient with platelet satellitism or phagocytosis shows that the automated count is erroneous and the platelet count is in fact normal, the erroneous count should be deleted from the report and an explanation given.

REFERENCES

1. Marsh GW. *Abnormal contraction, distortion and fragmentation in human red cells*. MD thesis: London University; 1966.
2. Rodgers MS, Chang C-C, Kass L. Elliptocytosis and tailed poikilocytes correlate with severity of iron deficiency anemia. *Am J Clin Pathol*. 1999;111:672–675.
3. Sechi LA, De Carll S, Catena C, et al. Benign familial macrocytosis. *Clin Lab Haematol*. 1996;18:41–43.
4. Rees DC, Dudley JA, Marinaki A. Review: pyrimidine 5'nucleotidase deficiency. *Br J Haematol*. 2003;120: 375–383.
5. Tuffy P, Brown AK, Zuelzer WW. Infantile pyknocytosis: a common erythrocyte abnormality of the first trimester. *Am J Dis Child*. 1959;98:227–241.
6. Keimowitz R, Desforges JF. Infantile pyknocytosis. *N Engl J Med*. 1965;273: 1152–1154.
7. Bessis M. Red cell shapes: an illustrated classification and its rationale. *Nouv Rev Fr Hematol*. 1972;12:721–745.
8. Burns ER, Lou Y, Pathak A. Morphological diagnosis of thrombotic thrombocytopenic purpura. *Am J Hematol*. 2004;75: 18–21.
9. Estes JW, Morley TJ, Levine IM, et al. A new hereditary acanthocytosis syndrome. *Am J Med*. 1967;42: 868–881.
10. Mier M, Schwartz SO, Boshes B. Acanthrocytosis [sic], pigmented degeneration of the retina and ataxic neuropathy: a genetically determined syndrome with associated metabolic disorder. *Blood*. 1960;16:1586–1608.
11. Salt HB, Wolfe OH, Lloyd JK, et al. On having no beta-lipoprotein: a syndrome comprising a-beta-lipoprotinaemia, acanthocytosis, and steatorrhoea. *Lancet*. 1960; ii:325–329.

12. Wimer BM, Marsh WL, Taswel HF, et al. Haematological changes associated with the McLeod phenotype of the Kell blood group system. *Br J Haematol*. 1977;36:219–224.
13. Silber R, Amorosi EL, Howe J, et al. Spur-shaped erythrocytes in Laennec's cirrhosis. *N Engl J Med*. 1966;275:639–643.
14. Ponder E. *Hemolysis and Related Phenomena*. New York: Grune & Stratton; 1948.
15. Feo CJ, Tchernia G, Subtu E, et al. Observation of echinocytosis in eight patients: a phase contrast and SEM study. *Br J Haematol*. 1978;40: 519–526.
16. Crook M, Williams W, Schey S. Target cells and stomatocytes in heterozygous familial hypobetalipoproteinaemia. *Eur J Haematol*. 1998;60:68–69.
17. Lock SP, Sephton Smith R, Hardisty RM. Stomatocytosis: a hereditary red cell anomaly associated with haemolytic anaemia. *Br J Haematol*. 1961;7:303–314.
18. Ducrou W, Kimber RJ. Stomatocytes, haemolytic anaemia and abdominal pain in Mediterranean migrants: some examples of a new syndrome? *Med J Aust*. 1969;ii:1087–1091.
19. Norman JG. Stomatocytosis in migrants of Mediterranean origin. *Med J Aust*. 1969;i:315.
20. Douglass C, Twomey J. Transient stomatocytosis with hemolysis: a previously unrecognized complication of alcoholism. *Ann Intern Med*. 1970;72:159–164.
21. Weed RI, Bessis M. The discocyte-stomatocyte equilibrium of normal and pathologic red cells. *Blood*. 1973;41:471–475.
22. Brecher G, Bessis M. Present status of spiculated red cells and their relationship to the discocyte-echinocyte transformation: a critical review. *Blood*. 1972;40: 333–344.

23. Bain BJ. *Leukaemia Diagnosis*. 4th ed. Oxford: Wiley-Blackwell; 2010.
24. Bennett JM, Catovsky D, Daniel MT, et al. Proposals for the classification of the acute leukaemias (FAB cooperative group). *Br J Haematol*. 1976;33:451–458.
25. Bennett JM, Catovsky D, Daniel MT, et al. Proposed revised criteria for the classification of acute myeloid leukemia. *Ann Intern Med*. 1985; 103:620–625.
26. Swerdlow SH, Campo E, Harris NL, et al. *World Health Classification of Tumours of Haematopoietic and Lymphoid Tissues*. Lyon: IARC; 2008.
27. Deal J, Hernandez AM, Pierre RV. Ethylenediamine tetraacetic acid-associated leukoagglutination. *Am J Clin Pathol*. 1995;103:338–340.
28. Howard MR, Smith RA. Early diagnosis of septicaemia in preterm infants from examination of the peripheral blood films. *Clin Lab Haematol*. 1999;21:365–368.
29. Van Assendelft OW, McGrath C, Murphy RS, et al. The differential distribution of leukocytes. In: Koepke JA, ed. *CAP Aspen Conference: Differential Leukocyte Counting*. Northfield, IL: College of American Pathologists; 1977.
30. Westerman DA, Evans D, Metz J. Neutrophil hypersegmentation in iron deficiency anaemia: a case control study. *Br J Haematol*. 1999;107:512–515.
31. Gowland E, Kay HEM, Spillman JC, et al. Agglutination of platelets by a serum factor in the presence of EDTA. *J Clin Pathol*. 1969;22: 460–1454.
32. Criswell KA, Breider MA, Bleavins MR. EDTA-dependent platelet phagocytosis. A cytochemical, ultrastructural and functional characterization. *Am J Clin Pathol*. 2001;115:376–384.
33. Stavem P, Berg K. A macromolecular serum component acting on

platelets in the presence of EDTA–'platelet stain preventing factor? *Scand J Haematol* 1973;10: 202–208.

34. Crome PE, Barkhan P. Platelet adherence to polymorphs. *Br Med J.* 1963;ii:871.

35. Field EJ, Macleod I. Platelet adherence to polymorphs. *Br Med J.* 1963;ii:388.

36. Greipp PR, Gralnick HR. Platelet to leucocyte adherence phenomena associated with thrombocytopenia. *Blood.* 1976;47:513–521.

37. Skinnider LF, Musclow CE, Kahn W. Platelet satellitism: an ultrastructural study. *Am J Hematol.* 1978;4: 179–185.

38. White LA Jr, Brubaker LH, Aster RH, et al. Platelet satellitism and phagocytosis by neutrophils: association with antiplatelet antibodies and lymphoma. *Am J Hematol.* 1978;4:313–323.

39. Campbell V, Fosbury E, Bain BJ. Platelet phagocytosis as a cause of pseudothrombocytopenia. *Am J Hematol.* 2009;84:362.

Chapter | 6 |

Supplementary techniques including blood parasite diagnosis

Andrew Osei-Bimpong, John Burthem

TESTS FOR THE ACUTE-PHASE RESPONSE

Inflammatory response to tissue injury includes alteration in serum protein concentration, especially increases in fibrinogen, haptoglobin, caeruloplasmin, immunoglobulins (Ig) and C-reactive protein (CRP), and decrease in albumin. The changes occur in acute infection, during active phases of chronic inflammation, with malignancy, in acute tissue damage (e.g. following acute myocardial infarction) with physical injury. Measurement of the acute-phase response is a helpful indicator of the presence and extent of inflammation or tissue damage and response to treatment. The usual tests are estimation of CRP and measurement of the erythrocyte sedimentation rate (ESR); some studies have suggested that plasma viscosity is also a useful indicator, but there is debate on the relative value of theses tests.[1,2]

Kits that are sensitive and precise are available for CRP assay; small increases in serum levels of CRP can often be detected before any clinical features become apparent, whereas as a tissue-damaging process resolves, the serum level rapidly decreases to within the normal range (<5 mg/l). The ESR is slower to respond to acute disease activity and it is insensitive to small changes in disease activity. It is less specific than CRP because it is also influenced by immunoglobulins (which are not acute-phase reactants) and by anaemia. Moreover, because the rate of change of ESR is slower than that of CRP, it rarely reflects the current disease activity and clinical state of the patient as closely as the CRP. The ESR is a useful screening test, and the conventional manual ESR method is simple, cheap and not dependent on power supply, thus making it suitable for point-of-care (near-patient) testing. It is recommended that, in clinical practice, both tests should be carried out in tandem.[3] Because CRP assay is a biochemical test usually performed in the clinical chemistry laboratory, it will not be discussed further here.

Erythrocyte Sedimentation Rate

The method for measuring the ESR recommended by the International Council for Standardization in Haematology (ICSH)[4] and also by various national authorities[5] is based on that of Westergren, who developed the test in 1921 for studying patients with pulmonary tuberculosis. ESR is the measurement of the sedimentation of red cells in diluted blood after standing for 1 h in an open-ended glass tube of 30 cm length mounted vertically on a stand.

Conventional Westergren Method

The recommended tube is a straight glass or rigid transparent plastic tube 30 cm in length and not less than 2.55 mm in diameter. The bore must be uniform to within 5% throughout. A scale graduated in mm extends over the lower 20 cm. The tube must be clean and dry and kept free from dust. If reusable, before being reused it should be thoroughly washed in tap water, then rinsed with deionized or distilled water and allowed to dry. Specially made racks with adjustable levelling screws are available for holding the sedimentation tubes firmly in an exactly vertical position. The rack must be constructed so that there will be no leakage of the blood from the tube. It is conventional to set up sedimentation-rate tests at room temperature (18–25°C). Sedimentation is normally accelerated as the temperature increases, and if the test is to be carried out at a higher ambient temperature, a normal range should be established for that temperature. Exceptionally, when high thermal amplitude cold agglutinins are present, sedimentation becomes noticeably less rapid as the temperature is increased toward 37°C.

For the diluent, prepare a solution of 109 mmol/l trisodium citrate (32 g/l $Na_3C_6H_5O_7.2H_2O$). Filter through a micropore filter (0.22 mm) into a sterile bottle. It can be stored for several months at 4°C but must be discarded if it becomes turbid through the growth of moulds.

Method

The method described below, originally described by the International Council for Standardization in Haematology (ICSH)[4] and now adopted by the Clinical and Laboratory Standards Institute (CLSI) as its approved method,[5] is intended to provide a reference method for verifying the reliability of any modification of the test.

Either collect venous blood in ethylenediaminetetraacetic acid (EDTA) and dilute a sample accurately in the proportion of 1 volume of citrate to 4 volumes of blood, or collect the blood directly into the citrate solution. The test should then be carried out on the diluted sample within 4 h of collecting the blood, although a delay of up to 6 h is permissible provided that the blood is kept at 4°C. EDTA blood can be used within 24 h if the specimen is kept at 4°C, provided that 1 volume of 109 mmol/l (32 g/l) trisodium citrate is added to 4 volumes of blood immediately before the test is performed.

Mix the blood sample thoroughly and then draw it up into the Westergren tube to the 200 mm mark by means of a teat or a mechanical device; mouth suction should never be used. Place the tube exactly vertical and leave undisturbed for exactly 60 min, free from vibrations and draughts and not exposed to direct sunlight. Then read to the nearest 1 mm the height of the clear plasma above the upper limit of the column of sedimenting cells. The result is expressed as ESR = X mm in 1 h. A poor delineation of the upper layer of red cells may sometimes occur, especially when there is a high reticulocyte count.

Range in health

The mean values and the upper limit for 95% of normal adults are given in Table 6.1. There is a progressive increase with age, but it is difficult to define a strictly healthy population for determining normal values in individuals older than 70 years.[6] In the newborn, the ESR is usually low. In childhood and adolescence, it is the same as for normal men with no differences between boys and girls. It is increased in pregnancy, especially in the later stages, and independent of anaemia;[7] this is due to the physiological effect of haemodilution (an increase in the plasma volume)

In the newborn, the ESR has been reported to be 0–2 mm in 1 h, increasing to 4 mm in 1 h at 1 week, up to 17 mm in 1 h by day 14, and then 10–20 mm in 1 h for both girls and boys, until puberty.[8] However, as the studies in infants were obtained by the capillary method, they are not strictly comparable to the Westergren method.

Table 6.1 Erythrocyte sedimentation rate ranges in health

AGE RANGE (YEARS)	ESR MEAN MM IN 1 H
10–19	8
20–29	10.8
30–39	10.4
40–49	13.6
50–59	14.2
60–69	16
70–79	16.5
80–91	15.8
Pregnancy	
Early gestation	48 (62 if anaemic)
Later gestation	70 (95 if anaemic)

Modified methods

Length of tube

The overall length of the tube is not a critical dimension for the test provided that it fits firmly in an appropriate holding device. The tube must, however, be long enough to ensure that packing of the cells does not start before the test has been completed.

Plastic glass tubes

A number of plastic materials (e.g. polypropylene and polycarbonate) are recommended as substitutes for glass in Westergren tubes. Nevertheless, not all plastics have similar properties, and it must be demonstrated that the ESR with the chosen tubes is reproducible and not affected by the plastic.

Disposable glass tubes

Disposable glass tubes should be supplied clean and dry and ready for use. It is necessary to show that neither the tube material nor the manufacturer's cleaning process affect the ESR.

Capillary method

Short tubes of narrower bore than in the standard tube are available mainly for tests on infants. These are, however, no longer in general use, and it is necessary to establish normal ranges or a correction factor to convert results to an approximation of ESR by the Westergren method.

Time

Sedimentation is measured after aggregation has occurred and before the cells start to pack, usually at 18–24 min.

From the rate during this time period the sedimentation that would have occurred at 60 min is derived and converted to the conventional ESR equivalent by an algorithm.[9]

Sloping tube

Red cells sediment more quickly when streaming down the wall of a sloped tube. This phenomenon has been incorporated into automated systems in which the end-point is read after 20 min with the tube held at an angle of 18° from the vertical.[10] Incorporating a low-speed centrifugation step (approx. 800 rpm) in this automated method reduces the end-point time further.[11] These have been shown to give results comparable to the conventional method.

Anticoagulant

EDTA blood can be used without citrate dilution, at least if packed cell volume (PCV) is below 0.36 (haemoglobin <110 g/l); less precise results are obtained when the PCV is higher. Because of the biohazard risk of blood contamination inherent in using open-ended tubes, it is now recommended that, where possible, a closed system be used in routine practice. Manual methods are available that avoid transfer of the blood into the sedimentation tube. Automated closed systems use either blood collected in special evacuated tubes containing blood anticoagulated with citrate or EDTA. A sample is taken up through a pierceable cap and then automatically diluted in the system if this is required.

Whenever a different method or tube is planned, a preliminary test should be carried out to check precision and to compare results with those obtained by the CLSI standardized method described earlier.

Evaluation of a new routine method

For the evaluation of a new ESR method the test should be carried out on at least 60 samples. These samples could be collected separately from the same subjects in accordance with specified requirements (e.g. directly into tubes containing citrate or undiluted EDTA samples). The samples should come from patients with a wide variety of diseases (as well as from normal subjects) to cover the range of ESR from 15 to 105 mm, with approximately the same number of samples in each quartile. If any test fails to give a clear-cut plasma erythrocyte interface in either the test system or the standardized test, the pair of values should be eliminated from the data.

Any new method may be considered to be satisfactory if 95% of results differ consistently by no more than 5%. However, because the ESR may be affected by several uncontrolled variables, the reference method cannot be used to adjust the measurements that are obtained. Thus if the new method gives disparate readings, it will be necessary to establish a normal range specifically for the method.

Quality Control

The standardized method can be used as a quality-control procedure for routine tests or alternatively stabilized whole blood preparations which are now available are suitable as a daily control for use with automated systems (e.g. ESR-Chex).[12] Three or four specimens of EDTA blood kept at 4°C will also serve as a control on the following day.

Another control procedure is to calculate the daily cumulative mean, which is relatively stable when at least 100 specimens are tested each day in a consistent setting (see Chapter 25). A coefficient of variation of <15% between daily sets appears to be a satisfactory index for monitoring instrument performance.[13]

Semiquantitative Slide Method

Enhanced red cell adhesion/aggregation can be demonstrated by allowing a drop of citrated blood to dry on a slide. An estimate of the amount of cell aggregation on the film by image analysis provides a semiquantitative measure of the acute-phase response that appears to correlate with the ESR.[14] Based on this principle, serial microscopic images of red cells aggregating on a glass slide taken every 30 s for 5 min can distinguish a normal ESR from a high value (Figs 6.1, 6.2). The images demonstrate greater spacing of cells in blood with higher ESR values compared with blood with lower ESR values.

Mechanism of Erythrocyte Sedimentation

The rate of fall of the red cells is influenced by a number of interacting factors. It depends on the difference in specific gravity between red cells and plasma, but it is influenced very greatly by the extent to which the red cells form rouleaux, which sediment more rapidly than single cells. Other factors that affect sedimentation include the ratio

Figure 6.1 ESR of 9 mm in 1 h after 2 min.

Figure 6.2 ESR of 69 mm in 1 h after 2 min.

of red cells to plasma (i.e. the PCV), the plasma viscosity, the verticality or otherwise of the sedimentation tube, the bore of the tube and the dilution (if any) of the blood.

The all-important rouleaux formation and the red cell clumping that are associated with the increased ESR are mainly controlled by the concentrations of fibrinogen and other acute-phase proteins (e.g. haptoglobin, ceruloplasmin, α_1-acid-glycoprotein, α_1-antitrypsin, and CRP). Rouleaux formation is also enhanced by the immunoglobins and is retarded by albumin. Defibrinated blood normally sediments extremely slowly (i.e. not more than 1 mm in 1 h) unless the serum globulin concentration is increased or there is an unusually high globulin:albumin ratio.

Anaemia, by altering the ratio of red cells to plasma, encourages rouleaux formation and accelerates sedimentation. In anaemia, cellular factors may also affect sedimentation. Thus, in iron deficiency anaemia, a reduction in the intrinsic ability of red cells to sediment may compensate for the accelerating effect of an increased proportion of plasma.

Sedimentation can be observed to take place in three stages: a preliminary stage of at least a few minutes during which time rouleaux occur and aggregates form; then a period in which the sinking of the aggregates takes place at a constant speed; and finally, a phase during which the rate of sedimentation slows as the aggregated cells pack at the bottom of the tube. It is obvious that the longer the tube used, the longer the second period can last and the greater the sedimentation rate may appear to be.

Although ESR is a non-specific phenomenon, its measurement is clinically useful in disorders associated with an increased production of acute-phase proteins. In rheumatoid arthritis or tuberculosis it provides an index of progress of the disease, and it is of considerable value in diagnosis of temporal arteritis and polymyalgia rheumatica. It is often used if multiple myeloma is suspected, but when the myeloma is non-secretory or light chain, a normal ESR does not exclude this diagnosis.

An elevated ESR occurs as an early feature in myocardial infarction.[15] Although a normal ESR cannot be taken to exclude the presence of organic disease, the vast majority of acute or chronic infections and most neoplastic and degenerative diseases are associated with changes in the plasma proteins that lead to an acceleration of sedimentation. An increased ESR in subjects who are HIV seropositive seems to be an early predictive marker of progression toward acquired immune deficiency syndrome (AIDS).[16] The ESR is less helpful in countries where chronic diseases are rife; however, one study has shown that very high ESRs (higher than 100 mm/h) have a specificity of 0.99 and a positive predictive value of 0.9 for an acute or chronic infection.[17] The ESR is influenced by age, stage of the menstrual cycle and medications taken (corticosteroids, contraceptive pills). It is especially low (0–1 mm) in polycythaemia, hypofibrinogenaemia and congestive cardiac failure and when there are abnormalities of the red cells such as poikilocytosis, spherocytosis, or sickle cells. In cases of performance-enhancing drug intake by athletes (discussed below) the ESR values are generally lower than the usual value for the individual and as a result of the increase in haemoglobin (i.e. the effect of secondary polycythaemia).

Plasma Viscosity

The ESR and plasma viscosity generally increase in parallel with each other.[1] Plasma viscosity is, however, primarily dependent on the concentration of plasma proteins, especially fibrinogen, and it is not affected by anaemia. Changes in the ESR may lag behind changes in plasma viscosity by 24–48 h, and viscosity seems to reflect the clinical severity of disease more closely than does the ESR.[18]

There are several types of viscometers, including rotational and capillary types that are suitable for routine use[1] and, as for ESR methods, automated closed-tube methods are available.[19] The main use of plasma viscosity is in the investigation of individuals with suspected hyperviscosity, myeloma and macroglobulinaemia. In conjunction with the ESR and CRP, the plasma viscosity can be used as a marker for inflammation. The viscosity test should be carried out as described in the instruction manual for the particular instrument used.

Reference Values

Each laboratory should establish its own reference values for plasma viscosity. As a general guide, ICSH has recorded that with the Harkness capillary viscometer normal plasma has a viscosity of 1.16–1.33 mPa/s (if expressed in poise (P), 1 cP = 1 mPa/s) at 37°C and 1.50–1.72 mPa/s at 25°C.[20] Plasma viscosity is lower in the newborn (0.98–1.25 mPa/s at 37°C), increasing to adult values by the 3rd year; it is slightly higher in old age. There are no significant differences in plasma viscosity between men and women or in pregnancy. It is remarkably constant in health, with little or no diurnal variation, and it is not affected by exercise. A change of only 0.03–0.05 mPa/s is thus likely to be clinically significant.

WHOLE BLOOD VISCOSITY

The viscosity of whole blood reflects its rheological properties; it is influenced by PCV, plasma viscosity, red cell aggregation and red cell deformability. It is especially sensitive to PCV, with which it is closely correlated. The clinical interpretation of its measurement must also take into account the interaction of the red cells with blood vessels, which greatly influences blood flow *in vivo*.

Guidelines for measuring blood viscosity and red cell deformability by standardized methods have been published.[21] Rotational and capillary viscometers are suitable for measuring blood viscosity; deformability can be measured by recording the rate at which red cells in suspension pass through a filter with pores 3–5 mm in diameter.

HETEROPHILE ANTIBODIES IN SERUM: DIAGNOSIS OF INFECTIOUS MONONUCLEOSIS

Infectious mononucleosis (IM) is caused by Epstein–Barr virus.[22] The immune response that develops in response to virus-infected cells includes not only antibodies to viral antigens but also characteristic heterophile antibodies. Before the nature of this reaction was understood, Paul and Bunnell[23] demonstrated the antibodies as agglutinins directed against sheep red cells. They are, in fact, not specific for sheep red cells but also react with horse and ox, but not human, red cells. They are IgM globulins, which are immunologically related to, but distinct from, antibodies that occur in response to the Forssman antigens. The latter are widely spread in animal tissue; they occur at low titre in healthy individuals and at high titre in serum sickness and in some leukaemias and lymphomas.[24,25] In these non-IM conditions, the antibody can be absorbed out by guinea pig cells. Thus, for the diagnosis of IM, it is necessary to demonstrate that the antibody present has the characters of the Paul–Bunnell antibody (i.e. it is absorbed by ox red cells but not by guinea pig kidney). This is the basis of the absorption tests for IM ('monospot' test). Immunofluorescent antibody tests have been developed to distinguish the IgM antibody, which occurs at high titre in the early phase of IM and diminishes during convalescence, from the IgG antibody, which persists at high titre for years after infection[26,27] and which also occurs in the non-IM infections.[22,28]

Screening Tests for Infectious Mononucleosis

The reagents for IM screening are available commercially in diagnostic kits from several manufacturers. Guinea pig cells can be also be manufactured locally as described in previous editions. Some kits are based on agglutination of stabilized horse red cells or antigen-coated latex particles to which IM antibody binds. An extensive evaluation of 14 slide tests for the UK Medical Devices Agency (MDA), showed them to have a sensitivity between 0.87 and 1.00 and specificity of 0.97 to 1.00, with an overall accuracy (positive and negative) in the order of 91–100%.[25] False-positive reactions have been reported in malaria, toxoplasmosis, and cytomegalovirus infection; autoimmune diseases; and even occasionally without any apparent underlying disease.[29,30] False-negative reactions occur if the test is carried out before the level of heterophile antibody has increased or conversely when it has decreased. False-negative reactions may also occur in the very young and the very old. In the UK MDA study the best performance was obtained with the Clearview test (*Unipath*), which uses latex-labelled bovine erythrocyte glycoprotein. IM heterophile antibody binds to this to form a complex that presents as a band in the result window (Fig. 6.3). The test can be performed with diluted whole blood as well as with plasma or serum.

Screening tests are also available based on enzyme-linked immunosorbent assay (ELISA) and immunochromatographic assay. These tests are more elaborate than the slide screening test described earlier, but they are less likely to give a false result.

Clinical Value

Tests for the heterophile antibody are useful for diagnosis. Antibodies are often present as early as the 4th to 6th day of the disease and are almost always found by the 21st day. They disappear as a rule within 4–5 months. There is no unanimity as to how frequently negative reactions are found in 'true' IM. Occasionally, the characteristic antibodies develop very late in the course of the disease, perhaps weeks or even months after the patient becomes ill. It is also known that a positive reaction may be transient and that the antibodies may be present at such low titres that they may be missed or may produce anomalous agglutination reactions when associated with the naturally occurring antibody at similar titres. For all of these reasons, it is difficult to state categorically that any particular patient has not or will not produce antibodies. Antibodies specific for Epstein–Barr virus have been demonstrated in

Figure 6.3 Screening for infectious mononucleosis with *Clearview* slide test. The sample is added to the bottom window, where, if positive, antibodies combine with bovine erythrocyte glycoprotein attached to blue microspheres; migration to the test window (centre) then occurs and here the complexes are bound to immobilized bovine erythrocytic glycoprotein, producing a blue line. The blue line in the upper window is a positive control.

the serum of 86% of patients with clinical and/or haematological features of IM.[31]

There is no substantial evidence that sera containing agglutinins in high concentration giving the typical reactions of IM are ever found in other diseases uncomplicated by IM. In particular, the heterophile antibody titres in the lymphomas are similar to those found in unselected patients not suffering from IM.[32]

DEMONSTRATION OF LUPUS ERYTHEMATOSUS CELLS

Antinuclear antibodies, or antinuclear factors (ANF), occur in the serum in a wide range of autoimmune disorders, including systemic lupus erythematosus (SLE). Descriptions of the LE cell test, which has now been superseded by immunological tests, can be found in the 8th and earlier editions of this book.

ERYTHROPOIETIN

Erythropoietin regulates red cell production. It is a heat-stable glycoprotein with a molecular weight of about 34 kDa. It is produced mainly in the kidney. Only a small quantity is demonstrable in normal plasma or urine.

A pure form of human erythropoietin from recombinant DNA (r-HuEpo) is available for diagnostic assay methods by ELISA, enzyme immunoassay and radioimmune assay. Commercial kits are available that are reliable and sensitive,[33] although there is some inter-method variability.[34] Results are expressed in international units by reference to an international (WHO) standard. This was originally a urinary extract, and a preparation is available with a potency of 10 iu per ampoule.[35] The present standard has been established for r-HuEpo with a potency of 86 iu per ampoule.[36]

Reference Range

The normal reference range in plasma or serum varies considerably according to the method of assay.[33] For the ELISA method used by the UK supraregional service, the normal range is 9.1–30.8 iu/l. With test kits, in the steady state without anaemia, it is usually given as 5–25 iu/l or slightly higher. In normal children, the levels are the same as in adults, except for infants younger than 2 months when the levels are low.[37]

There is a diurnal variation, with the highest values at night.[38] In pregnancy, erythropoietin concentration increases with gestation.[39]

Significance

Increased levels of erythropoietin are found in the plasma (or serum) in various anaemias,[40] and there is normally an inverse relationship between haemoglobin and erythropoietin. In thalassaemia, erythropoietin is lower than in iron deficiency with the same degree of anaemia, but there is a close inverse correlation with the red cell count.[41] In renal disease, there is a progressive decline in the erythropoietin response to anaemia, and in end-stage renal failure the concentration is normal or even lower than normal despite increasing anaemia. In renal patients receiving dialysis, erythropoietin treatment may cause functional iron deficiency.[42]

Some impairment of production of erythropoietin may occur in association with neoplasias and chronic inflammatory diseases. Increased concentrations of erythropoietin occur in secondary polycythaemia as a result of respiratory and cardiac disease; in the presence of abnormal haemoglobins with high oxygen affinity; and in association with carcinoma of the kidney and other erythropoietin-secreting tumours such as hepatoma, uterine fibroma and ovarian carcinoma.[40]

In primary polycythaemia ('polycythaemia vera'), the plasma erythropoietin level is usually lower than normal even when the haemoglobin has been reduced by venesection.[43,44] In secondary polycythaemia, the level of erythropoietin is never below normal. An assay is particularly useful in patients with erythrocytosis of undetermined cause; low erythropoietin has a specificity of 0.92 with moderate sensitivity for diagnosing primary polycythaemia.[43] However, in such cases there may be an intermittent increase in erythropoietin secretion. Thus, determining its level in a single sample of plasma may be misleading. Low levels have been found in one-third of cases of primary (essential) thrombocythaemia, especially when haemoglobin is at a high normal level.[43]

AUTONOMOUS *IN VITRO* ERYTHROPOIESIS

When mononuclear cells from blood or bone marrow are cultured, erythroid colonies (CFU-E) will normally develop only when erythropoietin is present in the culture medium. However, growth will occur in erythropoietin-free medium in primary polycythaemia. This provides a method for distinguishing primary from secondary polycythaemia.[45–47]

Mononuclear cells are collected from a blood sample by density separation (see p. 65) and added to an appropriate serum-free liquid culture medium[46,47] or collagen gel medium,[48] which is then divided into two portions. To one portion is added 1 iu/ml of erythropoietin. Both portions are plated and incubated for 7 days at 37°C. They are then stained with benzidine and examined directly under an inverted microscope or after spreading onto slides. The numbers of benzidine-positive cell clusters in the erythropoietin-free and erythropoietin-containing samples are counted and compared. A diagnosis of primary polycythaemia is indicated if there is an approximately equal growth in both samples. A method has been described in which flow cytometry with immunofluorescence is used to detect growth of the erythroid cells after only 2–5 days of culture.[49]

THROMBOPOIETIN

Thrombopoietin regulates megakaryocyte development and platelet production. It is a protein produced by the liver and has been purified from serum.[50] It is considerably larger than erythropoietin, with a molecular weight of about 335 kDa. A recombinant human thrombopoietin (rhTPO) has been produced and used to prepare a monoclonal antibody and develop a sensitive and specific ELISA. This has been used to measure thrombopoietin in normal serum and serum from patients with various blood disorders.[51] The normal range (mean and 2SD) is 0.79 ± 0.35 fmol/ml for men and 0.70 ± 0.26 fmol/ml for women. It is increased in thrombocytopenias and is especially high (18.5 ± 12.4 fmol/ml) in aplastic anaemia with severe thrombocytopenia. In essential thrombocythaemia, thrombopoietin is in the range of $1.01–4.82$ fmol/ml.[51]

HAEMATOLOGICAL TESTS IN SPORTS MEDICINE

Assays to detect the illicit use of hormones such as erythropoietin in endurance sports are becoming increasingly important.[52,53] Some of the current test methods for detecting erythropoietin used in this manner are described below.

Blood doping, often called induced erythrocythemia, is the practice of increasing the number of red blood cells through an intravenous infusion of blood, thereby enhancing performance in sports through the increase in red blood cell mass with an increased oxygen-carrying capacity.[52] Alternatively, recombinant hormones such as erythropoietin can be used to induce erythropoiesis. Blood doping is an illegal practice as it provides an unfair advantage of endurance and performance over other athletes;[52,54] It is also potentially dangerous due to the abnormal increase in red cell mass and the risk of acquiring infection from contaminated blood.[54] The International Doping Test and Management[55] collaborates with the World Anti-Doping Agency and other international and national sports authorities to coordinate the collection of blood and urine samples to be analysed in accredited laboratories.[56]

The full blood count, which includes the reticulocyte count, haemoglobin and packed cell volume, is the cheapest and most effective way to screen for suspected use of erythropoietin[55] as abnormal blood counts may suggest doping. The sports administrative bodies collect blood profiles on individual athletes and these are monitored over time so changes in blood parameters due to doping can be detected. Compared to population-derived upper limits of the reference range such as the 0.5 Hct limit or the 2.5% reticulocyte limit, the fluctuations allowed are smaller when using individual-based cut-offs.[52,54] Blood samples need to be analysed within 24 h of venesection[52] and the security and confidentiality of blood samples obtained should be maintained at all times. The abnormalities in the blood profile which may suggest doping are outlined in the following section.

Reticulocytes

The administration of recombinant erythropoietin can be suspected from a raised reticulocyte count.[57] Erythropoietin causes increased production of erythroblasts and immature reticulocytes, and accelerates their release from the bone marrow into peripheral blood. The mean haemoglobin content of the reticulocyte fraction is also raised.

Haemoglobin and Hct

Exogenous erythropoietin and intravenous infusion of blood both increase the haemoglobin and haematocrit.[57]

Whole Blood Viscosity and ESR

A large infusion of red blood cells can increase whole blood viscosity and reduce the ESR due to the change in red cell count:plasma ratio.

Erythropoietin

Changes in one or more of the full blood count parameters are only suggestive of the possible use of erythropoietin so they should be followed by tests to directly detect recombinant erythropoietin in the plasma.[53,58] The structural differences between the endogenous and the recombinant erythropoietin isoforms[59] make it possible to separate the two isoforms of erythropoietin, providing the samples are collected within 24 h of erythropoietin administration.[60] Alternatively, isoelectric focusing can detect exogenous (recombinant) erythropoietin in urine specimens[61,62]

PRINCIPLES OF PARASITE DETECTION

The essential method for a definitive diagnosis of malaria remains the finding of parasites in a blood film, followed by the identification of the particular species by morphology. Microscopic diagnosis can be a satisfying process in which parasites are identified then are assigned to their species based on fine morphological detail. Examination of thick or thin blood films remains the most sensitive routinely applied technique where microscopic expertise is available. Only brief outlines of how microscopic diagnoses may be reached are given in this chapter, and for more detailed accounts, readers are referred to a parasitology textbook. Where microscopic expertise is not available, antibody-based 'rapid diagnostic tests' (RDTs) are increasingly applied. RDTs have widespread application in developing countries, but increasingly are gaining use in all laboratories to screen potentially infected samples and to supplement microscopic diagnosis. It is important, however, that users appreciate the strengths and limitations that govern selection and interpretation of RDTs. Molecular approaches to malaria diagnosis and in particular to species identification, employ PCR-based assays and have the capability to be highly sensitive and specific.[63]

Cost and time constraints, however, mean that at present molecular techniques are employed principally in reference or research laboratories. Molecular techniques in parasite diagnosis are not discussed in this text.

In addition to the *Plasmodia* that give rise to malaria, the other important parasites to be found in the blood are leishmaniae, *Babesia*, trypanosomes, microfilaria, and ehrlichiae. Thick blood films are also useful for the detection of microfilaria. When they are used for this purpose, it is important to scan the entire film using a low-power objective, or parasites may be missed. Examination of wet preparations of blood can also be used for diagnosis of microfilariae and has the advantage that the parasites are easily detected because they are moving. A stained film is necessary for confirmation of species. Wet preparations are also useful for the detection of trypanosomes and the spirochaetes of relapsing fever. The presence of small numbers of trypanosomes or spirochaetes is revealed by occasional slight agitation of groups of red cells. Examination of a stained film confirms their nature.

EXAMINATION OF BLOOD FILMS FOR PARASITES

General Principles

Thick films are extremely useful when parasites are scanty, and these should be prepared and examined as a routine where malaria is suspected. Identification of the species is less easy than in thin films, and mixed infections may be missed, but if 5 min are spent examining a thick film, this is equivalent to about 1 h spent in traversing a thin film. Once the presence of parasites has been confirmed, a thin film should be used for determining the species and, in the case of *Plasmodium falciparum*, for assessing the severity of the infection by counting the percentage of positive cells. Low levels of parasitaemia may be missed by microscopy, and proficiency testing studies have demonstrated the need for all laboratories, and especially those lacking expertise, to take part in external quality control programmes and to refer problematic cases to more experienced centres.[64,65]

Staining Thin Films

Thin films should be stained with Giemsa's stain or Leishman's stain at pH 7.2, not with a standard May–Grünwald–Giemsa stain. The pH is important to maximize the visibility of cytological features important for diagnosis (Fig. 6.4).

MICROSCOPIC DIAGNOSIS OF MALARIA

Morphological criteria for differentiation of malaria parasites are given in Table 6.2 and illustrated in Figures 6.5–6.8. Mixed species infections are well recognized,

Figure 6.4 Effects of staining pH on parasite staining characteristics (*P. vivax*). At pH 7.2 (A) the parasite is readily distinguished from the adjacent blue/grey erythrocytes, chromatin staining is prominent and Schüffner's dots are readily distinguished. At pH 6.9 (B) the parasite remains visible, but there is less contrast from surrounding erythrocyte cytoplasm, relatively weak chromatin staining, and poor resolution of Schüffner's dots (which may not be visible at this pH).

Table 6.2 Morphological differentiation of malaria parasites

	P. falciparum	P. vivax	P. ovale	P. malariae
Infected red cells	Normal size;[a] Maurer's clefts[b]	Enlarged; Schüffner's dots[c]	Enlarged; oval and fimbriated; Schüffner's dots[c]	Normal or microcytic; stippling not usually seen
Ring forms (early trophozoites)	Delicate; frequently 2 or more; accolé forms;[d] small chromatin dot	Large, thick; usually single (occasionally 2) in cell; large chromatin dot	Thick, compact rings	Very small, compact rings
Later trophozoites	Compact, vacuolated; sometimes 2 chromatin dots	Amoeboid; central vacuole; light blue cytoplasm	Smaller than P. vivax; slightly amoeboid	Band across cell; deep blue cytoplasm
Schizonts	18–24 merozoites filling 2/3 of cell	12–24 merozoites, irregularly arranged	8–12 merozoites filling 3/4 of cell	6–12 merozoites in daisy-head around central mass of pigment
Pigment	Dark to black clumped mass	Fine granular; yellow-brown	Coarse light brown	Dark, prominent at all stages
Gametocytes	Crescent of sausage-shaped; diffuse chromatin; single nucleus	Spherical, compact, almost fills cell; single nucleus	Oval; fills 3/4 of cell; similar to but smaller than P. vivax	Round; fills 1/2 to 2/3 of cell; similar to P. vivax but smaller, with no Schüffner's dots

[a]In P. falciparum, it is important to report the percentage of red cells that are infected.
[b]Large, irregularly shaped, red-staining dots.
[c]Fine stippling.
[d]That is, marginalized to edge of cell ('appliqué').

and microscopists should be alert to morphological features that cannot be reconciled to a single disease type (Fig. 6.9). Films for malaria must be made no longer than 3–4 h after blood collection. Films prepared later may still reveal parasites, but the parasite morphology will differ from fresh samples making species identification more difficult and in some cases causing the appearances of parasite stages not normally occurring in blood (Fig. 6.10).

Two other morphology-based screening methods can be used for malaria diagnosis.

Fluorescence Microscopy

Red cells containing malaria parasites fluoresce when examined by fluorescence microscopy after staining with acridine orange. This has a sensitivity of about 90% in acute infections but only 50% at lower levels of parasitaemia, and false-positive readings may occur with Howell–Jolly bodies and reticulocytes. When positive, it is necessary to examine a conventionally stained blood film to identify the species.[66]

Quantitative Buffy Coat Method

The quantitative buffy coat (QBC) method (BD Diagnostic Systems) is another procedure for detection of parasites by fluorescent microscopy. The blood is centrifuged in capillary tubes that are coated with acridine orange. It is fairly sensitive but requires expensive equipment and has the disadvantage of false-positive results in the presence of Howell–Jolly bodies and reticulocytes. When positive, identification of species requires examination of a stained blood film, but it is useful as an initial screening test.[67]

RAPID DIAGNOSTIC TESTS FOR MALARIA

Rapid diagnostic tests (RDTs) for malaria employ specific antibodies that detect malaria antigens in the blood of infected individuals. RDTs use small blood samples obtained by finger prick or by venepuncture and employ a 'lateral diffusion' system similar to a pregnancy test to

Figure 6.5 Morphology of *P. falciparum*. Note that erythrocytes throughout this series are not enlarged or distorted. Early trophozoites (A) show high parasitaemia, with accolé (appliqué edge) forms, multiply infected erythrocytes and double chromatin dot forms. The late trophozoite (B) shows two thickened ring forms with characteristic Maurer's dots (clefts) in the erythrocyte cytoplasm. A typical crescent ('banana-shaped') gametocyte is shown (C). Schizonts are not shown since they rarely circulate in *P. falciparum* infection.

generate results. RDTs therefore display results in the form of visible 'bands' that can be interpreted by non-expert users with limited facilities. In general, a blood specimen to be tested (2–50 µl) is lysed in buffer solution containing one or more malaria-specific 'detection antibodies'. The detection antibody is coupled to a visually observable label. Where specific antigen is present, a complex is formed between that antigen and its cognate labelled antibody. The labelled antigen–antibody complex generated is then bound by a second 'capture-antibody' that recognizes the same antigen, and which is immobilized as a line on the test strip. A positive result therefore generates a visible line of antigen–antibody complex. A separate immobilized capture antibody recognizes the labelled detection antibody alone; this control band will produce a line in the absence of malaria antigen and confirms that

the test has been performed correctly and the result can be interpreted (Fig. 6.11).[72]

The antigen targets detected by RDTs fall into two groups. The first group of antigens are expressed in all malarial species. Antigens from this group therefore confirm malarial infection is present, but do not allow the parasite species to be determined. Antigens from this group are *Plasmodium* aldolase (PMA) or parasite lactate dehydrogenase (pLDH). The second group of antigens are specific for *P. falciparum*. Antigens from this group are histidine-rich protein-2 of *P. falciparum* (pfHRP2) or a *P. falciparum*-specific form of LDH (pfLDH). Antibodies from the two groups are used individually, or in combination, to produce two different test formats. A 'two line' test uses an anti-pfHRP2 band together with the positive control band to recognize *P. falciparum* only.

Figure 6.6 Morphology of *P. malariae*. Early trophozoites (A) are small but less fine than those of *P. falciparum*; in this case the ring is irregular and chromatin dot is within the main parasite cytoplasm. A late trophozoite (B) spans the erythrocyte as a thick 'band form'. A characteristic 'daisy head' schizont (C) has eight merozoites arrayed around the central pigment. Finally, the gametocyte (D) is typically small and does not fill the normally sized erythrocyte.

A 'three line' test uses a *P. falciparum* specific antibody band, together with PMA or pLDH, together with the positive control antibody. The three line test can therefore indicate the presence of *P. falciparum*, or if *P. falciparum* is not present the test will indicate the presence of other malarial species. Since the second antibody is pan-malarial, the three line test does not distinguish between infection by *P. vivax*, *P. ovale*, or *P. malariae*, and will not detect mixed infection. For field diagnosis in malaria-endemic areas the selection of a two line (*P. falciparum* only) test, or three line (pan-malarial) test, will depend on local species prevalence. It is considered that if >90% of malaria cases in an area are caused by *P. falciparum* an RDT that detects only that species is appropriate for use.

Figure 6.7 Morphology of *P. vivax*. The red cells are enlarged, distorted and contain visible Schüffner's dots in all these images. Note that the parasites are larger than in the other malarial forms. The early trophozoite (A) in this figure has the form of a thick ring with a large chromatin dot, but the later trophozoite (B) has a distorted 'amoeboid' form. Note that the large macrogametocyte (C) fills the enlarged erythrocyte.

The introduction of such tests in malaria endemic areas also requires careful consideration of ease of use; cost; and limitations imposed by transport, distribution and storage.[68]

In terms of diagnostic sensitivity, WHO requires RDTs to reliably detect infections of 100 parasites per microlitre of blood (95% sensitivity).[69] This is equivalent to the diagnostic sensitivity reasonably expected of a field microscopist diagnosing malaria in endemic regions.[70] Sensitivity becomes less reliable below 100 parasites per microlitre, and this contrasts with the 'gold standard' sensitivity achieved by an expert microscopist in good conditions, who should detect 5–10 parasites per microlitre.[70] Sensitivity does depend on species. For *P. falciparum* parasites, RDT sensitivity frequently exceeds 100 parasites per microlitre, although genetic variation

Figure 6.8 Morphology of *P. ovale*. Distinguishing *P. ovale* from *P. vivax* is perhaps the most difficult morphological distinction in malaria diagnosis. For both species, the red cells are enlarged, distorted, and contain visible Schüffner's dots. The features that help distinguish these forms are given in Table 6.2. In this figure, note that the parasites and erythrocytes are smaller than for *P. vivax*, and that in some cases the cytoplasm is fimbriated. Both early (A) and late trophozoites (B) have coarse 'ring' forms. The schizont (C) contains fewer than 16 developing merozoites. A microgametocyte (D) does not fill the erythrocyte and numerous dots can be seen in the erythrocyte cytoplasm.

of *P. falciparum* antigens may reduce sensitivity in some instances.[69] For other malarial species, sensitivity of detection is recognized to be less good, particularly for *P. ovale* and *P. malariae* where RDTs may not detect infections that are clinically significant. There is also a recognized incidence of false-positive reactions caused by cross-reaction with autoantibodies (particularly with rheumatoid factor) that varies between detection systems. In all instances, malaria antigens are recognized to persist for a number of weeks following successful treatment, and in these circumstances a positive result may not indicate current infection.

Figure 6.9 Mixed infection of *P. falciparum* and *P. ovale*. Diagnosis depends on recognition of features that cannot be reconciled with a single malarial species. (A) A typical fine double dot ring form of *P. falciparum* coexists with an enlarged ovoid erythrocyte containing a thickened parasite and numerous Schüffner's dots (*P. ovale*). (B) Gametocytes from the same two species with contrasting appearances and causing different effects on the host erythrocyte.

Figure 6.10 Delayed film preparation. These gametocytes of *P. falciparum* have very atypical morphology: showing rounding up and clumping (A) or exflagellation of microgametocytes (B). Biologically, such changes occur within the mosquito stomach during sexual reproduction of the parasite; when present on a blood film they indicate a delay in preparation.

The lower sensitivity of RDTs when compared with expert microscopic diagnosis means that all positive and negative results should be confirmed using microscopy. Symptomatic parasitaemia in non-immune subjects may occur with fewer than 100 parasites per microlitre of blood, and repeat testing of negative samples may be required to confirm a diagnosis. Users should also be aware that the positive line on the test only indicates a correctly performed test, and does not confirm effectiveness of parasite detection or accuracy of the test. Awareness of diagnostic performance for the selected test in the user's laboratory is therefore mandatory.[69]

Figure 6.11 Rapid diagnostic tests for malaria. An RDT of the 'three line' format, the image shows the output window. (A) The results of a negative test in which the positive control line shows a positive band to indicate the technical validity of the result. (B) The positive lines in all three positions, i.e. a technically interpretable result (control line positive), with *P. falciparum*-specific antigen detected (line 1), and pan-malarial antigen detected (line 2). This patient had a single-species infection (*P. falciparum*), although the test does not allow a mixed infection to be excluded.

LEISHMANIASIS

Leishmania species are transmitted by the bite of an infected female sandfly and are associated with a variety of clinical conditions including visceral and mucocutaneous leishmaniasis. Visceral leishmaniasis may present to the haematologist as splenomegaly, hepatomegaly, fever, lymphadenopathy or pancytopenia, and it is being increasingly reported in patients with HIV infection. Serological studies are recommended as the initial diagnostic tests in suspected leishmaniasis. In advanced stages of the disease, parasites can be found in phagocytic cells in spleen, lymph nodes, bone marrow and peripheral blood. Culture of aspirated bone marrow is, however, a more sensitive diagnostic technique than microscopy.

Diagnosis of Leishmaniasis in the Haematology Laboratory

Leishmaniasis is diagnosed in the haematology laboratory by direct visualization of the amastigotes (often referred to as Leishman–Donovan bodies). Buffy coat preparations of peripheral blood or aspirates (see p. 64 for preparation of buffy coats) from marrow, spleen, lymph nodes or skin lesions should be spread on a slide to make a thin smear and stained with Leishman's or Giemsa's stain (pH 7.2) for 20 min (see p. 66). Amastigotes are seen within monocytes or, less commonly, in neutrophils in peripheral blood and in macrophages in bone marrow aspirates. They are small, round bodies 2–4 mm in diameter with indistinct cytoplasm, a nucleus, and a small rod-shaped kinetoplast (Fig. 6.12A). Occasionally, amastigotes may be seen lying free between cells.

TRYPANOSOMIASIS

African Trypanosomiasis

African trypanosomiasis (sleeping sickness) is caused by *Trypanosoma brucei gambiense* (West Africa and western Central Africa) and Trypanosoma brucei rhodesiense (East, Central and Southern Africa); it is transmitted by a few species of tsetse fly. The trypomastigotes can be found in blood, lymph node aspirates, and cerebrospinal fluid, but repeated examinations and concentration techniques may be needed before they are detected. Serological investigations may also be helpful in diagnosis.

American Trypanosomiasis

American trypanosomiasis (Chagas' disease) is caused by *Trypanosoma cruzi*, which is transmitted by the Reduviidae bug, subfamily Triatominae. Chagas' disease is only found in tropical and subtropical South and Central American countries. Trypomastigotes can only be found circulating in the blood in the acute form of Chagas' disease. Because the trypomastigotes are more fragile than those causing African trypanosomiasis, serology rather than morphology is recommended for initial screening. In the haematology laboratory, tests that detect motile organisms are more sensitive than those that require fixed, stained preparations.

Diagnosis of Trypanosomiasis in the Haematology Laboratory

Care should be taken when handling samples suspected of being infected with trypomastigotes because infection can occur if the organisms penetrate the skin. Several techniques are available for examining specimens for the presence of trypomastigotes.

Figure 6.12 Bone marrow and blood parasites. (A) Leishmaniasis (Leishman–Donovan bodies); (B) African trypanosomiasis; (C) American trypanosomiasis (*T. cruzi*); and (D) microfilaria.

Wet Preparations

If present in high concentrations, trypomastigotes can be seen thrashing among the cells on a fresh, unstained wet preparation of blood or lymph node fluid. Preparations should be examined within 4 h of sampling (this time can be extended if a few milligrams of glucose are added to the specimen) using a ×40 objective and a partially closed condenser iris or dark-field or phase contrast microscopy.

Thick Blood Films or Chancre Aspirates

Examination of a thick film allows more of the sample to be examined rapidly, but *T. cruzi* are easily damaged by the spreading of specimens for thick films. Thick films are prepared by spreading a drop of blood on a slide to cover a 15–20-mm diameter area and staining with Giemsa staining technique or Field's rapid technique (see p. 62) as for malaria smears. Microscopically, *T. b. gambiense* and *T. b. rhodesiense* cannot be distinguished from each other; they are 13–42 mm long with a single flagellum, a centrally placed nucleus, and a small dot-like kinetoplast.

T. cruzi measures 12–30 mm and has a larger kinetoplast than *T. b. gambiense* and *T. b. rhodesiense* (Fig. 6.12B,C).

Concentration Techniques

Quantitative buffy coat method

The QBC method[71] is referred to on p. 110. After centrifugation, the tube should be left to stand upright for 5 min, and the plasma interface area is then examined for motile trypomastigotes. This has been suggested as the 'gold standard' for diagnosis.

Capillary tube method

Fill one or two micro-haematocrit capillary tubes with EDTA or citrated blood. Seal the ends and centrifuge for about 5 min as for microhaematocrit. Then lay the capillary tubes adjacent to each other on a microscope slide, and secure both ends onto the slide with adhesive tape (Fig. 6.13). Examine the plasma just below the red cell and buffy layer immediately for motile trypomastigotes using a ×20 or ×10 objective with the condenser iris partially closed or by dark-field microscopy.

Figure 6.13 Capillary tube concentration method. Method used for detecting trypomastigotes or microfilariae in blood.

FILARIASIS AND LOIASIS

Filariasis involving the lymphatics is the cause of elephantiasis. It is caused by the filarial worms *Brugia malayi*, *Wuchereria bancrofti* and *Brugia timori*, whereas filarial infection of the subcutaneous tissues is caused by *Loa loa*. The larvae of these worms, microfilariae, are transmitted by mosquito to humans, where they can be found in the blood and where they show periodicity with fluctuating levels at different times of the day (Fig. 6.12D).

Diagnosis of Filariasis in the Haematology Laboratory

Blood concentrations of microfilariae are often higher in capillary blood than venous blood. However, even when blood has been collected at the appropriate time, microfilariae can be scanty, so that serological or rapid immunochromatographic tests and concentration techniques may be required.

Wet Preparation

A thick blood film is prepared from 20 μl blood and stained as for malaria smears (see p. 66).

Concentration Techniques

Filtration method

The filtration method is the most sensitive concentration method for microfilariae, but samples must be handled gently to preserve the organisms. Anticoagulated blood (10 ml), followed by 10 ml of methylene blue or azure B saline solution, is passed through a transparent polycarbonate membrane filter of 3-mm porosity attached to a syringe. The filter is placed face upwards on a slide, a drop of saline is added, and a coverslip is placed on top. The entire membrane is examined microscopically for motile microfilariae using a ×10 objective and a partially closed condenser iris or dark-field microscopy.

Quantitative buffy coat and microhaematocrit methods

Microfilariae can be detected using the same methods as for detection of trypomastigotes (see above).

Lysed capillary blood

Blood (1 ml) is mixed with 9 ml of 2% formalin and centrifuged at 1000 *g* for 5 min. All the deposit is placed on a slide and 1 drop of Field's stain A or 1% methylene blue is added to facilitate species identification. Motile microfilariae can be seen using a ×10 objective with a partially closed condenser iris or dark-field microscopy.

BABESIOSIS

Babesiosis results from a tick-borne intraerythrocytic protozoan, *Babesia*. Humans are infected by chance in the natural cycle of transmission between the tick and its domestic or wild animal host. It is especially prevalent in subtropical and tropical countries. The infection results in high fever accompanied by jaundice and severe haemolytic anaemia with haemoglobinuria; there is a leucocytosis with neutrophilia.

The parasites can be seen in the erythrocytes in Giemsa-stained blood films. Morphologically they are variable round or oval bodies that may be mistaken for the ring form of plasmodium. However, in babesiosis the dividing cells characteristically consist of two daughter cells held together by a thin strand of cytoplasm; also, no pigment occurs in erythrocytes infected with older stages of *Babesia*.

EHRLICHIOSIS

Ehrlichiosis is a tick-borne fever in which clusters of small organisms may be seen in Giemsa-stained blood smears. The detection of organisms within neutrophils or monocytes is important for its diagnosis.

REFERENCES

1. International Committee for Standardization in Haematology. Guidelines on the selection of laboratory tests for monitoring the acute-phase response. *J Clin Pathol.* 1988;41:1203–1212.

2. Lowe GDO. Annotation: Should plasma viscosity replace the ESR? *Br J Haematol.* 1994;86:6–11.

3. Osei-Bimpong A, Meek JH, Lewis SM. ESR or CRP? A comparison of their clinical utility. *Haematology.* 2007;12: 353–357.

4. International Council for Standardization in Haematology. ICSH recommendations for measurement of erythrocyte sedimentation rate. *J Clin Pathol.* 1993;46:198–203.

5. National Committee for Clinical Laboratory Standards. *Reference and selected procedures for the erythrocyte sedimentation rate (ESR) test (H2-A4).* Wayne, PA: NCCLS; 2000.

6. Sharland DE. Erythrocyte sedimentation rate. The normal range in the elderly. *J Am Geriatr Soc.* 1980;28:346–348.

7. van den Broek NR, Letsky EA. Pregnancy and the erythrocyte sedimentation rate. *Br J Obstet Gynaecol.* 2001;108:1164–1169.

8. Adler SM, Denton RL. The erythrocyte sedimentation rate in the newborn period. *J Pediatr.* 1975;86:942–948.

9. Kallner A, Engervall P, Björkholm M. Kinetic measurement of the erythrocyte sedimentation rate. *Ups J Med Sci.* 1994;99:179–186.

10. Happe MR, Buttafarono DF, Dooley DP, et al. Validation of the Diesse Mini-Ves erythrocyte sedimentation rate (ESR) analyzer using the Westergren method in patients with systemic inflammatory conditions. *Am J Clin Pathol.* 2002;118:14–17.

11. Menarini A. *Features of the Vesmatic 30 analyser.* Available at: www. menarini.com/diagnostic_uk/uk/ diagnostic/products/hematology/ erythrocyte_sedimentation_rate/ ves_matic_30_plus/ Accessed 05.01.10.

12. Garvey BJ, Mahon A, Parker-Williams J, et al. *An evaluation of ESR-Chex control material for erythrocyte sedimentation rate determination (MDA 99/28).* Norwich: Medical Devices Agency, Stationery Office; 1999.

13. Plebani M, Piva E. Erythrocyte sedimentation rate: use of fresh blood for quality control. *Am J Clin Pathol.* 2002;117:621–626.

14. Rotstein R, Fusman R, Berliner S, et al. The feasibility of estimating the erythrocyte sedimentation rate within a few minutes by using a simple slide test. *Clin Lab Haematol.* 2001;23:21–25.

15. Froom P, Margaliot S, Caine Y, et al. Significance of erythrocyte sedimentation rate in young adults. *Am J Clin Pathol.* 1984;82: 198–200.

16. Lefrère JJ, Salmon D, Doinel C, et al. Sedimentation rate as a predictive marker in HIV infection. *AIDS.* 1988;2:63–64.

17. Fincher RF, Page MI. Clinical significance of extreme elevation of the erythrocyte sedimentation rate. *Arch Intern Med.* 1986;146:1581–1583.

18. Harkness J. The viscosity of human plasma: its measurement in health and disease. *Biorheology.* 1971;8:171–193.

19. Benson B. *BV 200 Viscometer features.* Available at: www. bensonviscometers.com/BV200. html; 2008.

20. International Committee for Standardization in Haematology. Recommendation for selected method for the measurement of plasma viscosity. *J Clin Pathol.* 1984;37:1147–1152.

21. International Committee for Standardization in Haematology. Guidelines for measurement of blood viscosity and erythrocyte deformability. *Clin Hemorheol.* 1986;6:439–453.

22. Henle W, Henle GE, Horwitz CA. Epstein-Barr virus specific diagnostic tests in infectious mononucleosis. *Hum Pathol.* 1974;5:551–565.

23. Paul JR, Bunnell WW. The presence of heterophile antibodies in infectious mononucleosis. *Am J Med Sci.* 1932;183:90.

24. Huh J, Cho K, Heo DS, et al. Detection of Epstein-Barr virus in Korean peripheral T-cell lymphoma. *Am J Hematol.* 1999;60:205–214.

25. Klein G. Epstein-Barr virus strategy in normal and neoplastic B cells. *Cell.* 1994;77:791–793.

26. Strand BC, Schuster TC, Hopkins RF, et al. Identification of an Epstein-Barr virus nuclear antigen by fluoro-immuno-electrophoresis and radioimmuno-electrophoresis. *J Virol.* 1981;38:996–1004.

27. Edwards JMB, McSwiggen DA. Studies on the diagnostic value of an immunofluorescence test for EB virus-specific IgM. *J Clin Pathol.* 1974;27:647–651.

28. Rea TD, Ashley RL, Russo JE, et al. A systematic study of Epstein-Barr virus serological assays following acute infection. *Am J Clin Pathol.* 2002;117:156–161.

29. Reed RE. False-positive monospot tests in malaria. *Am J Clin Pathol.* 1974;61:173–174.

30. Horwitz CA, Henle W, Henle G, et al. Persistent falsely positive rapid tests for infectious mononucleosis. Report of five cases with four-six year follow-up data. *Am J Clin Pathol.* 1979;72:807–811.

31. Evans AS, Niederman JC. EBV-IgA and new heterophile antibody tests in diagnosis of infectious mononucleosis. *Am J Clin Pathol.* 1982;77:555–560.

32. Goldman R, Fishkin BG, Peterson E. The value of the heterophile antibody reaction in the lymphomatous diseases. *J Lab Clin Med.* 1950;35:681–687.

33. Marsden JT, Sherwood RA, Peters TJ. *Evaluation of six erythropoietin kits.* Norwich: (MDA 95/57) Medical Devices Agency, Stationery Office; 1995.

34. Bechensteen AG, Lappin TRJ, Marsden J, et al. Unreliability in immunoassays of erythropoietin: anomalous estimates with an assay kit. *Br J Haematol.* 1993;83:663–664.

35. Annable L, Cotes PM, Mussett MV. The second international

preparation of erythropoietin. *Bull World Health Org.* 1972;47:99–112.

36. Storring PL, Gaines Das RE. The international standard for recombinant DNA-derived erythropoietin: collaborative study of four recombinant DNA-derived erythropoietins and two highly purified human erythropoietins. *J Endocrinol.* 1992;134:459–484.

37. Hellebostad M, Haga P, Cotes MP. Serum immunoreactive erythropoietin in healthy normal children. *Br J Haematol.* 1988;70: 247–250.

38. Wide L, Bengtsson C, Birgegard G. Circadian rhythm of erythropoietin in human serum. *Br J Haematol.* 1988;72:85–90.

39. Cotes PM, Canning CE, Lind T. Changes in serum immunoreactive erythropoietin during the menstrual cycle and normal pregnancy. *Br J Obstet Gynaecol.* 1983;90:304–311.

40. Kendall RG. Erythropoietin. *Clin Lab Haematol.* 2001;23:71–80.

41. Tassiopoulos T, Konstantopoulos K, Tassiopoulos S, et al. Erythropoietin levels and microcytosis in heterozygous beta-thalassaemia. *Acta Haematol.* 1997;98:147–149.

42. MacDougall IC, Cahill I, Hulme B, et al. Detection of functional iron deficiency during erythropoietin treatment: a new approach. *Br Med J.* 1992;304:225–226.

43. Messinezy M, Westwood NB, El-Hemaidi I, et al. Serum erythropoietin values in erythrocytoses and in primary thrombocythaemia. *Br J Haematol.* 2002;117:47–53.

44. Carneskog J, Safai-Kutti S, Wadenvik H, et al. The red cell mass, plasma erythropoietin and spleen size in apparent polycythaemia. *Eur J Haematol.* 1999;62:43–48.

45. Weinberg RS. In vitro erythropoiesis in polycythemia vera and other myeloproliferative disorders. *Semin Hematol.* 1997;34:64–69.

46. Lemoine F, Najman A, Baillou C, et al. A prospective study of the value of bone marrow erythroid progenitor cultures in polycythemia. *Blood.* 1986;68:996–1002.

47. Beckman BS, Anderson WF, Beltran GS, et al. Diagnostic use of CFU-E formation from peripheral blood in polycythemia vera. *Am J Clin Pathol.* 1983;79:496–499.

48. Dobo I, Mossuz P, Campos L, et al. Comparison of four serum-free, cytokine-free media for analysis of endogenous erythroid colony growth in polycythemia vera and essential thrombocythemia. *Hematol J.* 2001;2:396–403.

49. Manor D, Rachmilewitz EA, Fibach E. Improved method for diagnosis of polycythemia vera based on flow cytometric analysis of autonomous growth of erythroid precursors in liquid culture. *Am J Hematol.* 1997;54:47–52.

50. Kaushansky K. Thrombopoietin: the primary regulator of platelet production. *Blood.* 1995;86: 419–431.

51. Tahara T, Usuki K, Sato H, et al. A sensitive sandwich ELISA for measuring thrombopoietin in human serum: serum thrombopoietin levels in healthy volunteers and in patients with haemopoietic disorders. *Br J Haematol.* 1996;93:783–788.

52. Morkeberg JS, Belhage B, Damsgaard R. Strategies to combat doping in cycling. *International Sports Medical Journal.* 2008;9:155–161.

53. Robinson N, Giraud S, Saudan C, et al. Erythropoietin and blood doping. *Br J Sports Med.* 2006;40:30–34.

54. Catlin DH, Fitch KD, Ljungqvist A. Medicine and science in the fight against doping in sport. *J Intern Med.* 2008;264(2):99–114.

55. International Doping Test Management. *Diagnostic testing for drug abuse detection.* Available at: www.idtm.com; 2004. Accessed 30.12.09.

56. World Anti-doping Agency. *About WADA.* Available at: www.wada-ama.org/en/; 2010 Accessed 16.02.10.

57. Erslev AJ. Production of erythrocytes. In: Williams WJ, ed. *Hematology.* New York: McGraw-Hill; 1990:389–407.

58. World Anti-doping Agency. *The 2009 prohibition list world anti-doping code.* Available at: www.wada-ama.org/en/World-Anti-Doping-Program/Sports-and-Anti-Doping-Organizations/The-Code/; 2009. Accessed 30.12.09.

59. Rush RS, Derby PL, Smith DM, et al. Microheterogeneity of erythropoietin carbohydrate structure. *Anal Chem.* 1995;67:1442–1452.

60. Wide L, Bengtsson C, Berglund B, et al. Detection in blood and urine of recombinant erythropoietin administered to healthy men. *Med Sci Sports Exerc.* 1995;27: 1569–1576.

61. Lasne F, de Ceaurriz J. Recombinant erythropoietin in urine. *Nature.* 2000;405:635–636.

62. Lasne F, Martin L, Crepin N, et al. Detection of isoelectric profiles of erythropoietin in urine: differentiation of natural and administered recombinant hormones. *Anal Biochem.* 2002;311:119–126.

63. Johnston SP, Pieniazek NJ. PCR as a confirmatory technique for laboratory diagnosis of malaria. *J Clin Microbiol.* 2006;44:1087–1089.

64. Thomson ST, Lohmann RC, Crawford L, et al. External quality assessment in the examination of blood films for malaria parasites within Ontario, Canada. *Arch Pathol Lab Med.* 2000;124:57–60.

65. Bell D, GO R, Miguel C, et al. Diagnosis of malaria in a remote area of the Philippines: comparison of techniques and their acceptance by health workers and the community. *Bull World Health Org.* 2001;79:933–941.

66. Lowe BS, Jeffa NF, New L. Acridine orange fluorescence techniques as alternatives to traditional Giemsa staining for the diagnosis of malaria in developing countries. *Trans R Soc Trop Med Hyg.* 1996;90:30–34.

67. Bailey W, Smith D. The quantitative buffy coat for the diagnosis of trypanosomes. *Trop Doct.* 1994;24: 54–56.

68. World Health Organization. *The Use of Malaria Rapid Diagnosis Tests.* Geneva: WHO; 2004:1–20.

69. World Health Organization. *Towards Quality Testing of Malaria*

Rapid Diagnostic Tests: Evidence and Methods. Geneva: WHO; 2006:1–22.

70. *New Perspectives Malaria Diagnosis Report of a joint WHO/USAID informal consultation 25–27 October 1999. 4.2: Approaches to the diagnosis of malaria: microscopic diagnosis*. Geneva: WHO/SAID; 11.

71. Ali FM. *Separation of Human Blood and Bone Marrow Cells*. Bristol: Wright; 1986.

Chapter | 7 |

Bone marrow biopsy

Imelda Bates, John Burthem

Biopsy of the bone marrow is an indispensable adjunct to the study of diseases of the blood and may be the only way in which a correct diagnosis can be made. Marrow can be obtained by needle aspiration, percutaneous trephine biopsy or surgical biopsy. When performed correctly, bone marrow aspiration and trephine biopsy are simple and safe procedures that can be repeated many times and can be performed on outpatients.

The morphological assessment of aspirated or core biopsy specimens of bone marrow is based on two principles. First, that bone marrow has an organized structure such that in normal health, bone marrow cells display distinct numerical and spatial relationships to each other. Second, that individual bone marrow cells have distinctive cytological appearances that reflect the lineage and stage of maturation. Each or all of these features may specifically be disordered in disease. The specimens obtained by bone marrow aspiration or by bone marrow trephine biopsy are very different samples (Fig. 7.1) and contribute differently to diagnosis. Trephine biopsies provide excellent appreciation of spatial relationships between cells and of overall

Figure 7.1 Low-power appearances of spread bone marrow aspirate (A) and part section of bone marrow trephine biopsy (B).

bone marrow structure; aspirated material provides information about the numerical and cytological features of marrow cells. It is clear therefore that bone marrow aspirate and bone marrow biopsy specimens have important and complementary roles in clinical investigation and may have different relative merits in the assessment of marrow disease. Furthermore, in almost all cases marrow assessment is only one part of the overall diagnostic work-up.[1-3]

ASPIRATION OF THE BONE MARROW

Satisfactory samples of bone marrow can usually be aspirated from the sternum, iliac crest or anterior or posterior iliac spines. In the majority of patients, the procedure can be performed with local and oral analgesia without recourse to intravenous sedation.[4] in most circumstances the posterior iliac spines are the preferred biopsy site and selection of this site has the advantage that, if no material is aspirated, a trephine biopsy can be performed immediately. Biopsy from the posterior iliac spine may, however,

be technically difficult in subjects who are obese or immobile and puncture of the sternum is occasionally necessary.

Consent and Safety

Consent for the procedure of aspiration or trephine biopsy should take place according to local standard operating procedures, but should always include a discussion of the risks and benefits of the procedure. The risks associated with bone marrow aspiration and biopsy have been assessed using voluntary register data. Results show that risks are not dependent on operator experience and have a low incidence (around 0.1%). However, adverse events continue to be reported and may be severe. The most frequent adverse events relate to haemorrhage and are most frequently seen in the context of myeloproliferative neoplasms and thrombocytopenia or other bleeding disorders (including the use of antiplatelet agents).[5,6] Particular risks are associated with aspiration from the sternum. The operator should be aware of the additional risks and contraindications associated with aspiration from that site. The sternum should not be used as a site of biopsy in children or be used in adults if there is a disorder associated with increased bone resorption, such as myeloma. Operators should also be aware that unless the needle is correctly inserted in the sternum with an appropriate guard, there is a danger of perforating the inner cortical layer and damaging the underlying large blood vessels and right atrium, with serious consequences.[7]

Performing a Bone Marrow Aspiration

Only needles designed for the purpose should be used for marrow aspiration (discussed later). The operator should always wear surgical gloves to obtain a biopsy of bone marrow and should take great care to avoid needlestick injuries. A marrow aspiration or trephine biopsy should be performed in accordance with local guidelines for sterile procedures. Skin around the area should be cleaned, e.g. with 70% alcohol or 0.5% chlorhexidine (5% diluted 1 in 10 in ethanol). Infiltrate the skin, subcutaneous tissue and periosteum overlying the selected site with a local anaesthetic such as 2–5 ml 2% lidocaine. Wait until anaesthesia has been achieved. With a boring movement, pass the needle perpendicularly into the cavity of the ilium at the centre of the oval posterior superior iliac spine or 2 cm posterior and 2 cm inferior to the anterior superior iliac spine. When the bone has been penetrated, remove the stilette, attach a 1 or 2 ml syringe and suck up marrow contents for making films. If a larger sample is needed (e.g. for cytogenetic or immunophenotypic analysis), attach a second 5 or 10 ml syringe and aspirate a second sample. As a rule, material can be sucked into the syringe without difficulty; occasionally it may be necessary to reinsert the stilette, push the needle in a little further and suck again. Failure to aspirate marrow – a 'dry tap' – suggests bone marrow fibrosis or infiltration. Computed tomography-guided marrow sampling may be helpful in patients who are obese, in whom it is difficult to locate the iliac spine.[8]

Because bone marrow clots faster than peripheral blood, films should be made from the aspirated material without delay at the bedside. The remainder of the material may then be delivered into a bottle containing an appropriate amount of ethylenediaminetetra-acetic acid (EDTA) anticoagulant and used later to make more films. Preservative-free heparin should be used rather than EDTA if immunophenotyping or cytogenetic studies are needed. Some material can be preserved in fixative rather than anticoagulant for preparation of histological sections (see p. 133). Fix some of the films in absolute methanol as soon as they are thoroughly dry for subsequent staining by a Romanowsky method or Perls' stain for iron. Appropriately fixed films are also suitable for cytochemical staining (Chapter 15). If there has been a 'dry tap', insert the stilette into the needle and push any material in the lumen of the needle onto a slide and spread it; in lymphomas and carcinomas, especially, sufficient material may be obtained using this approach to allow a diagnosis.[9] Squash preparations of marrow fragments can be a useful supplement to bone marrow films. A drop of aspirated marrow is placed in the centre of a slide and, unless the aspirate is very cellular, the fragments are concentrated by removing the more dilute part of the aspirate with a plastic pipette. A second slide is then placed on top of the first and the fragments are crushed by rotating one slide on the other. Both squashes are then fixed and stained. Bone marrow aspirates in adults can be performed from the ilium, the sternum or the spinous processes; the latter site is rarely used and the procedure is described in the 10th edition of this book.

Puncture of the Ilium

The usual sites for puncture in adults are the posterior and, less commonly, the anterior iliac spine. If serial punctures are being performed, a different site should be selected for each to avoid aspirating marrow that has been diluted by intramedullary haemorrhage resulting from previous punctures. The posterior iliac spine overlies a large marrow-containing area and relatively large volumes of marrow can be aspirated from this site. Posterior iliac puncture can be carried out with the patient lying sideways, as for a lumbar puncture, or prone. The anterior superior iliac spine may be easier to locate in individuals who are very obese and the bone overlying it is said to be thinner than that of the iliac crest.

Puncture of the Sternum

The specific risks of sternal marrow aspiration were discussed earlier (see p. 124). Puncture of the sternum must be performed with care to avoid pushing the aspiration needle through the bone. The usual site for puncture is the manubrium or the first or second parts of the body of the sternum. The manubrium is formed of rather denser bone than the body of the sternum and, in elderly subjects at least, it tends to contain more fatty marrow than is found elsewhere in the sternum. The thickness of the cortex here varies from 0.2 mm to 5.0 mm, so it may be difficult to be certain that the needle point has reached the cavity of the bone.

The site for puncture of the manubrium should be about 1 cm above the sterno-manubrial angle and slightly to one side of the midline; if the body of the bone is to be punctured, this should be done opposite the second intercostal space slightly to one side of the midline. It is essential to use a needle with a guard that cannot slip, such as a Klima type. After piercing the skin and subcutaneous tissues, when the needle point reaches the periosteum, adjust the guard on the needle to allow it to penetrate about 5 mm further. If the guard cannot be advanced to this extent, it is not safe to proceed. Push the needle with a boring motion into the cavity of the bone. It is usually easy to appreciate when the cavity of the bone has been entered. Aspiration is then carried out as described earlier.

Comparison of Different Sites for Marrow Puncture

There is considerable variation in the composition of cellular marrow withdrawn from adjacent or different sites. Aspiration from only one site may give misleading information; this is particularly true in aplastic anaemia since the marrow may be affected patchily.[10] In general, however, the overall cellularity, the haemopoietic maturation pathways and the balance between erythropoiesis and leucopoiesis are similar at all sites. In practice, it is an advantage to have a choice of several sites for puncture, particularly when puncture at one site results in a 'dry tap' or when only peripheral blood is withdrawn. Aspiration at a different site may yield cellular marrow or strengthen suspicion of a widespread change affecting the bone marrow, such as fibrosis or hypoplasia. In aplastic anaemia, several punctures or, much to be preferred, a trephine biopsy may be necessary to arrive at the diagnosis.

ASPIRATION OF THE BONE MARROW IN CHILDREN

Iliac puncture, particularly in the region of the posterior spine, is usually the method of choice in children. Occasionally, in an older child who is obese, the posterior iliac spine cannot be felt. In this case, a satisfactory sample usually can be obtained from the anterior ilium. In small babies, marrow can be withdrawn from the medial aspect of the upper end of the tibia just below the level of the tibial tubercle. This site should be used with caution because it is vulnerable to fractures and laceration of the adjacent major blood vessels. In older children, the tibial cortical bone is usually too dense and the marrow within is normally less active. It must be remembered that sternal puncture in children should be avoided because the bone is thin and the marrow cavities are small.

MARROW PUNCTURE NEEDLES

Needles should be stout and made of hard stainless steel, about 7–8 cm in length, with a well-fitting stilette and they must be provided with an adjustable guard. With reusable needles, the point of the needle and the edge of the bevel must be kept well sharpened. The most common reusable needles are the Salah and Klima needles (Fig. 7.2). A slightly larger needle with a T-bar handle at the proximal end was developed by Islam (Fig. 7.3); it provides a better grip, is more manoeuvrable and is more successful for biopsies of excessively hard (e.g. osteosclerotic) or soft (e.g. profoundly osteoporotic) bone.[11] A modified version

Figure 7.2 Marrow puncture needles. Salah (A) and Klima (B).

Figure 7.3 Islam's bone marrow aspiration needle. The dome-shaped handle and T-bar are intended to provide stability and control during operation.

of the Islam needle has multiple holes in the distal portion of the shaft in addition to the opening at the tip to overcome sampling error when the marrow is not uniformly involved in a pathological lesion. Several types of disposable bone marrow aspiration and trephine biopsy needles are now available; their design is similar to the traditional reusable needles (Fig. 7.4). The increasing use of disposable needles by haematologists is based on considerations of safety for patient and operator.

PROCESSING OF ASPIRATED BONE MARROW

There is little advantage in aspirating more than 0.3 ml of marrow fluid from a single site for morphological examination because this increases peripheral blood dilution. If large amounts of marrow are needed for several tests, such as immunophenotyping, cytogenetic analysis and molecular studies, the syringe can be detached from the aspiration needle and the stilette can be replaced, leaving the aspiration needle in the bone. After the marrow smears have been prepared, the same or another syringe can be attached to the needle and another 5–10 ml of marrow can be aspirated.

It is good practice to obtain a sample of peripheral blood from the patient at the same time as the bone marrow so that films from both specimens can be examined and stored together. This can be done simply by preparing some films from blood obtained from a finger prick after completing the bone marrow sampling or by venepuncture so that a full blood count can be obtained. The blood film should be permanently stored with the bone marrow films.

Preparing Films from Bone Marrow Aspirates

Make films, 3–5 cm in length, of the aspirated marrow using a smooth-edged glass spreader of not more than 2 cm in width (Fig. 7.5). The marrow fragments are dragged behind the spreader and leave a trail of cells behind them. Spreading should be towards the area to which the label is to be applied to avoid having particles dragged to the tip of the slide, where it is difficult to examine them. If there are insufficient fragments, they can be concentrated. This is not usually necessary for marrows that are very cellular such as in acute and chronic myelogenous leukaemia and megaloblastic anaemia. Concentration of marrow can be achieved by delivering single drops of aspirate onto slides about 1 cm from one end. Most of the blood is quickly sucked off from the edge of the drop with the marrow syringe or a fine plastic pipette. The irregularly shaped marrow fragments tend to be left behind on the slide and can be lifted off with the spreader; films can then be prepared as explained earlier.

Figure 7.5 Film of aspirated bone marrow. The marrow particles are easily visible, mostly at the tail of the film (×1.5). Note that the bone marrow has been spread towards the label. This ensures that the area that is optimal for examination is easily positioned beneath the objective when the slide is placed on the stage.

After thorough drying, fix the films of bone marrow and stain them with Romanowsky dyes, as for peripheral blood films. However, a longer fixation time (at least 20 min in methanol) is essential for high-quality staining. If a film needs to be stained urgently, fix and stain one film only and permit the others to dry thoroughly. This avoids having all films showing artefacts caused by fixation of slides before thorough drying has been achieved. Films can also be stained by Perls' method (see p. 334) to demonstrate the presence or absence of iron.

The preparation can be considered satisfactory only when marrow particles and free marrow cells can be seen in stained films. It is in the cellular trails that differential counts should be made, commencing from the marrow fragment and working back toward the head of the film; in this way, smaller numbers of cells from the peripheral blood are included in a differential count.

Figure 7.4 Disposable bone marrow needles. For trephine biopsy (A) and aspiration (B).

When the aspirated marrow is put into an anticoagulant in a tube (e.g. EDTA) care should be taken that appropriate amounts are used for the volume of marrow to be anticoagulated. When films of marrow containing a gross excess of anticoagulant are spread (as when a few drops of marrow are added to a tube containing sufficient EDTA to prevent the clotting of 5 ml of blood), masses of pink-staining amorphous material may be seen and some of the erythroblasts and reticulocytes may clump together.

Concentration of Bone Marrow by Centrifugation

Centrifugation can be used to concentrate the marrow cells and to assess the relative proportions of marrow cells, peripheral blood and fat in aspirated material. While concentration of poorly cellular samples is useful, especially when an abnormal cell is present in small numbers,[12] it is unnecessary when the aspirated material is of average or increased cellularity. Volumetric data, too, are of little value in individual patients because of the wide range of values encountered even in health. Methods for separation of marrow cells are described on p. 65.

Preparation of Films of Post-mortem Bone Marrow

Films made of bone marrow obtained at post mortem are seldom satisfactory. If satisfactory results are to be achieved, the procedure must be carried out as soon after death as possible. When the marrow is spread in the ordinary way, the majority of the cells tend to break up and appear as smears.

The rate and pattern of cellular autolysis during the first 15 h after death has been studied and the differences between the changes of post-mortem autolysis and those that occur in life as a result of blood diseases have been defined.[13] Blood cells are much better preserved if a small piece of marrow is suspended in 1–2 ml of 5% bovine albumin (1 volume 30% albumin, 5 volumes 9 g/l NaCl). The suspension is then centrifuged and the deposited marrow cells are resuspended in a volume of supernatant approximately equal to, or slightly less than, that of the deposit. Films are made of this suspension in the usual way.

EXAMINATION OF ASPIRATED BONE MARROW

Principles of Marrow Aspirate Examination

Aspirated bone marrow material spread on glass slides yields individual separate bone marrow cells that have not been subject to prior processing or been cut to form sections. The specimen may therefore be examined using an oil-immersion lens to allow excellent assessment of cytological detail. Marrow aspiration therefore has particular value where recognition of individual cells or abnormal cytological features is paramount or where individual cells need to be recognized, classified and counted. Examples where bone marrow aspiration is of major value include the cytological assessment of abnormal cell maturation of bone marrow cells or the cytological classification and numerical assessment of acute leukaemia (Fig. 7.6).

Figure 7.6 (A) Aspirated cells from a case of megaloblastic anaemia. (B) Marrow aspirate spread of acute myeloid leukaemia arising from myelodysplastic syndrome. The films each illustrate very abnormal cells (megaloblastic or dysplastic, respectively) within the mature or maturing compartments. These cells are best recognized by their characteristic abnormal cytology.

Aspirated bone marrow cells are also well suited to further examination by cytogenetic, molecular or flow cytometric methods. However, the aspiration process generally disrupts structural elements within the marrow, preventing assessment of the structural relationships of normal or abnormal elements within marrow, and loose structural features such as lymphoid aggregates or granulomata are often not detected. The bone marrow aspirate may also be misleading if the cells of interest do not 'spill' from marrow particles and therefore do not appear on the slides. This problem is most readily apparent when marrow is subject to fibrotic processes; for example, the reticulin fibrosis of hairy cell leukaemia or the collagenous fibrosis of established myelofibrosis. An aspirate is also frequently insufficient when infiltrating cells form cohesive structures. Clumps of cells from carcinoma may on occasion be seen in aspirates, but are usually better revealed by biopsy.

Quantitative Cell Counts on Aspirated Bone Marrow

A number of values for the cell content of aspirated normal bone marrow have been given in the literature.[14,15] The percentage of marrow in the sternum of healthy adults that is cellular rather than fatty is 48–79%. However, quantification of the cell content of aspirated marrow is not reliable in view of the tendency of the marrow to be aspirated in the form of particles of varying size as well as free cells and the uncontrollable factor of dilution with peripheral blood, which according to some authors may amount to 40–100% in 0.25–0.5 ml bone marrow samples.

Quantitative cell counts on aspirated marrow are therefore difficult to interpret. For practical purposes, the degree of marrow cellularity can be assessed within broad limits as increased, normal or reduced by inspection of a stained film containing marrow particles. As a rough guide, if less than 25% of the particle is occupied by haemopoietic cells, it is hypocellular and if more than 75–80% is occupied, it is hypercellular. Less subjective quantitative measurement can be obtained by 'point counting' of sections; a normal range of 30–80% has been reported in the anterior iliac spine.

Physiological variation in the cell content has to be taken into account. The cellularity of the marrow is affected by age. In adults, a smaller proportion of the marrow cavity is occupied by haemopoietic marrow than in children and the proportion of fat cells to cellular marrow is increased. In one study, by means of point counting of sections from the iliac crest, the range of cellularity in children younger than 10 years was reported as 59–95% with a mean of 79%; at 30 years, the mean was 50% and at 70 years it was 30% with a range of 11–47%. The decrease in cellularity in elderly subjects is even more marked in the manubrium sterni. The marrow undergoes slight to moderate hyperplasia in pregnancy.

Differential Cell Counts on Aspirated Bone Marrow

For general purposes, it is not usually necessary to document the proportion of every stage of each cell type on the marrow slide. A 200–500-cell differential using the categories erythroid, myeloid, lymphoid and plasma cells is generally adequate providing that a systematic scheme for examining the morphology of these, and all other, cells is also used. In some conditions, such as acute and chronic myelogenous leukaemia and myelodysplastic syndrome, detailed differential counts are important because precise counts are essential for diagnosis and the results may indicate prognosis and affect treatment. Occasionally, it may be important to specifically count one cell type (e.g. blasts in acute leukaemia for assessing response to chemotherapy). Follow-up bone marrows should always be compared with previous bone marrow films to assess the course of a disease or the effect of treatment.

Sources of Error and Physiological Variations

Because of the naturally variegated pattern of the bone marrow, the irregular distribution of the marrow cells when spread in films and the variable amount of dilution with blood, differential cell counts on marrow aspirated from normal subjects vary widely. Aspirating only a small volume and counting cells in the trails left behind marrow particles as they are spread on the slide minimizes the dilutional effect of blood. When there is an increase in associated reticulin, some cell types may resist aspiration or remain embedded in marrow fragments and will therefore be under-represented in the differential count. Megakaryocytes in particular are irregularly distributed and tend to be carried to the tail of the film. The chance aspiration of a lymphoid follicle would result in an abnormally high percentage of lymphocytes.[16]

Ideally, differential counts should be performed on sectioned material, but difficulties in identification make this impractical. Methacrylate embedding offers a better opportunity for correctly identifying cells. The incidence of the various cell types is usually expressed as percentages. The normal values for cell differentials in bone marrow (Table 7.1) can only be taken as an approximate guide.[14,15] The cellular composition of the bone marrow varies between normal infants, children and young adults. Variation is marked in the first year, particularly in the first month. The percentage of erythroblasts decreases from birth and at 2–3 weeks they constitute only about 10% of the nucleated cells. Myeloid cells (granulocyte precursors) increase during the first 2 weeks of life, following which a sharp decrease occurs at about the 3rd week; however, by the end of the 1st month about 60% of the cells are myeloid. Lymphocytes constitute up to 40% of the nucleated

Table 7.1 Normal ranges for differential counts on aspirated bone marrow

	95% RANGE	MEAN[a]	MEAN[b]
Myeloblasts	0–3	0.4	1.4
Promyelocytes	3–12	13.7[c]	7.8
Myelocytes (neutrophil)	2–13	–	7.6
Metamyelocytes	2–6	–	4.1
Neutrophils	22–46	35.5	32.1[M]; 37.4[F]
Myelocytes (eosinophil)	0–3	1.6	1.3
Eosinophils	0.3–4	1.7	2.2
Basophils	0–0.5	0.2	0.1
Lymphocytes	5–20	16.1	13.1
Monocytes	0–3	2.5	1.3
Plasma cells	0–3.5	1.9	0.6
Erythroblasts[d]	5–35	23.5	28.1[M]; 22.5[F]
Megakaryocytes	0–2		0.5
Macrophages	0–2	2.0	0.4

[a]Den Ottolander (1996).[14]
[b]Bain (1996).[15]
[c]Includes all 'immature neutrophils'.
[d]Hammersmith Hospital data: proerythroblasts, 0.5–5; early erythroblasts, 2–20; late erythroblasts, 2–10.
[M]Males.
[F]Females.

cells in the marrow of small infants; the mean value at 2 years is approximately 20%, falling to about 15% during the rest of childhood. The percentage of plasma cells is especially low from infancy up to the age of 5 years.

The hyperplasia that occurs in pregnancy affects both erythropoiesis and granulopoiesis, the latter proportionately less, although with some increase in the relative proportion of immature cells. The hyperplasia is maximal in the 3rd trimester; a return to normal begins in the puerperium but is not completed until at least 6 weeks' postpartum.

Cellular Ratios

Ratios based on a count of 200–500 cells can provide useful qualitative information. The myeloid:erythroid ratio has been widely used and is the ratio of neutrophil and neutrophil precursor cells to erythroid precursors. The inclusion of monocytes, eosinophils and basophils is

controversial but in practice makes little difference to the overall ratio, which varies from 2:1 to 4:1. As an alternative, the leuco-erythrogenetic ratio can be calculated. For this, mature cells are excluded; the normal ratio has been reported as 0.56–2.67:1. The myeloid:lymphoid ratio varies widely, 1–17:1 and the lymphoid:erythroid ratio has a similarly wide variation, 0.2–4.0:1.

REPORTING BONE MARROW ASPIRATE FILMS

A systematic examination of the marrow aspirate, combined with knowledge of the clinical context, provides the best chance of arriving at a diagnosis.[3] Choose several of the best-spread stained films that contain easily visible marrow particles. Several particles should then be examined with a low-power ($\times10$) objective to estimate whether the marrow is hypocellular, normocellular or hypercellular. Megakaryocytes and clumps of non-haemopoietic cells (e.g. metastatic carcinoma cells) should be looked for at this stage of the examination; they are most often found toward the tail of the film.

Select for detailed examination – still using the $\times10$ objective – a highly cellular area of the film where the nucleated cells are well stained and well spread. Areas such as these can usually be found toward the tails of films behind marrow particles. The cells in these cellular areas should then be examined with a higher-power (e.g. $\times40$) objective and, subsequently, if necessary, with the $\times100$ oil-immersion objective. It is important always to examine marrows in a systematic fashion because it is easy to overlook subtle abnormalities. A suggested scheme for this is outlined below.

Systematic Scheme for Examining Bone Marrow Aspirate Films

Low Power ($\times10$)

Determine cellularity by examining several particles.

Identify megakaryocytes and note morphology and maturation sequence (higher power may be needed for smaller immature megakaryocytes and micromegakaryocytes).

Look for clumps of abnormal cells that could indicate infiltration by metastatic tumour (higher power may be needed to examine content and morphology of clumps).

Identify macrophages and examine at higher power for evidence of haemophagocytosis, malaria pigment and bacterial or fungal organisms that may be present in the cytoplasm.

Higher Power ($\times40$, $\times100$ Oil-Immersion)

Identify all stages of maturation of myeloid and erythroid cells. This is usually easiest to achieve by starting with mature red cells and working backward to the most immature cells.

Repeat the process for the myeloid series starting with mature neutrophils. Maturation abnormalities, such as giant proerythroblasts or evidence of dysfunctional maturation, including nuclear–cytoplasmic asynchrony, will suggest specific diagnoses such as parvovirus B19 infection, myelodysplastic syndrome or megaloblastic anaemia, respectively. Changes in the proportion of primitive to mature myeloid cells may reflect response to treatment in leukaemia or recovery from agranulocytosis. The actual percentage of blast cells is of significance in the differentiation of myelodysplastic syndromes from acute leukaemia, in determining prognosis in myelodysplastic syndrome and in assessing whether chronic myelogenous leukaemia is in chronic, accelerated or acute phase.

Determine the myeloid:erythroid ratio. Whereas a lack of myeloid cells may be obvious without performing a formal differential count, it is easy to overlook an increase in erythroid cells, which might suggest blood loss or peripheral destruction.

Perform a differential count using the categories erythroid, myeloid, lymphoid, plasma cell and 'others', simultaneously noting any morphological abnormalities. The normal lymphocyte percentage in the marrow is 5–20%; moderate increases to 30–40%, which may indicate a significant disorder such as lymphoma, are not likely to be identified simply by rapidly surveying the slide. Plasma cells should be less than 2%; in plasma cell dyscrasias, they may be increased, occur in clumps or have an abnormal morphological appearance.

Look for areas of bone marrow necrosis.[17] In necrotic areas, the cells stain irregularly, with blurred outlines, cytoplasmic shrinkage and nuclear pyknosis. Bone marrow necrosis may occur in sickle cell disease; it also occurs occasionally in lymphomas, acute lymphoblastic and chronic lymphocytic leukaemia, myeloproliferative neoplasms and metastatic carcinoma, as well as in septicaemia, tuberculosis and anorexia nervosa.[18] In patients with anorexia nervosa or cachexia, there may be gelatinous transformation of the ground substance of the marrow.[18]

Assess the iron content of macrophages and look for iron granules in erythroid cells on a slide stained with a Perls' stain. At least seven particles should be examined to optimally assess a bone marrow aspirate for iron stores.[19] If fewer particles are available, a diagnosis of iron deficiency can only be tentative. In sideroblastic anaemia, the granules incompletely encircle the nucleus. Abnormal patterns of iron staining may also be seen in dyserythropoietic anaemias such as the thalassaemias.

Reporting Results

It is helpful to report bone marrow films on a printed form on which the report and conclusion can be set out in an ordered fashion (Fig. 7.7).[3] Where a computerized reporting system is in use, it is useful to have a template with headings to ensure that the marrow reports are systematic and consistent. A list of the various descriptive comments that may be used can be provided in coded form to facilitate data entry. Report summaries should be intelligible to clinicians who are not haematology specialists.

PREPARATION OF SECTIONS OF ASPIRATED BONE MARROW FRAGMENTS

If it is not possible to obtain a trephine biopsy (see below), the small fragments obtained by marrow aspiration can be fixed, stained and examined to contribute to diagnosis. Such samples are useful for assessing cellularity and for detecting granulomas and tumour cells. If sections are required, it is convenient to let residual aspirated marrow clot within a plastic syringe and tease the sample out into the fixative once it has clotted.

PERCUTANEOUS TREPHINE BIOPSY OF THE BONE MARROW

Like marrow aspirations, trephine biopsy may be carried out in the inpatient ward or in outpatient departments. The posterior iliac spine is the usual site, although the anterior iliac spine can also be used. The posterior iliac spine is said to provide samples that are longer and larger and the aspiration is less uncomfortable for the patient.[20]

The trephine specimen is obtained by inserting the biopsy needle into the bone, using a to-and-fro rotation and then rocking the needle gently from side to side to detach a core of tissue that can be extracted within the needle. The main problems with this method are that the specimen may be crushed, thereby distorting the architecture, and it can be difficult to detach the core of bone from inside the marrow space. Trephine biopsy needles, both reusable and disposable, have been specifically designed to overcome these problems. The Jamshidi needle has a tapering end to reduce crush artefact (Fig. 7.8) and the Islam trephine has a core-securing device (Fig. 7.9). If larger specimens are needed, trephine needles that have bores of 4–5 mm may be used. Other needles occasionally used for trephine biopsy specimens are a 2 mm bore 'microtrephine' needle and a Vim-Silverman needle. However, compared with other needles, these yield smaller specimens of marrow that are prone to fracturing.

For the investigation of thrombocytopenia and neutropenia in neonates, sections of aspirated bone marrow can be obtained that allow assessment of marrow cellularity and architecture.[21] A 19G, half-inch Osgood needle (Cadence Inc, New York) is introduced 2 cm below the tibial tuberosity. The trocar is removed and the hollow needle is advanced by twisting 2–3 mm into the marrow space. A syringe is used to apply suction to the needle

| Surname: | First Name: | Sex: | Date of birth: |

Consultant:

| Date taken: | Hospital No: | Lab No: |

Clinical details:

WBC   Hb   MCV   Platelet count

Blood film:

Performed by: Aspiration Site: Ease of aspiration:

Particles:

Cellularity: M:E Ratio

Erythropoiesis:

Granulopoiesis:

Megakaryocytes:

Lymphocytes:

Plasma Cells:

Macrophages:

Other Cells:

Blast cells	Promyelocytes	Myelocytes and metamyelocytes	Neutrophils	Eosinophils
Basophils	Monocytes	Lymphocytes	Plasma cells	Erythroid

Storage iron: Siderotic granules:

Other tests to follow:

Conclusion:

Authorized by: Date:

Figure 7.7 Example of report form for bone marrow films.

Figure 7.8 Jamshidi trephine needle for bone marrow biopsy.

Figure 7.9 Islam trephine needle for bone marrow biopsy. The distal cutting edge is shaped to hold the core secure during extraction of the material.

until marrow appears; then the needle and syringe are withdrawn. The marrow clot is gently dislodged with the tip of a needle and placed into fixative. The specimen is processed as if it were an adult biopsy except that decalcification is not required.

Principles Behind Marrow Trephine Biopsy Examination

Bone marrow trephine biopsy provides a core of tissue, which is fixed and embedded to yield a histological specimen in which the structural relationships between cells, bone and bone marrow stroma are preserved. The nature of the specimen allows cellular distributions to be

recognized: for example, the tendency for precursor myeloid cells to mature close to bony trabeculae or the normal development of erythroid cells in the form of small islands (Fig. 7.10). Bone marrow biopsy also delineates the abnormal distribution of cells that is characteristic of particular pathological conditions. For example, the paratrabecular collection of abnormal cells that is typical of follicular lymphoma or the clustered megakaryocytes seen in certain myeloproliferative neoplasms (Fig. 7.11). In addition, since a trephinebiopsy specimen is a core of tissue, all cells present within the specimen will be represented irrespective of fibrosis or cohesion. Cell types within a bone marrow biopsy may be recognized by cytological characteristics, but that identification is reinforced by their distribution within the biopsy. Cellular recognition on trephine biopsy sections is frequently supplemented by immunostaining in which monoclonal or polyclonal antibodies are used (with cytochemical reactions) to detect a range of lineage, maturational or cell-type restricted markers. Such markers allow confirmation of cell lineage or of maturation stage within a particular lineage (Fig. 7.12). Markers may also highlight abnormal distribution of cells: for example, markers of B-cell lineage may highlight infrequent paratrabecular aggregates of cells in cases of follicular lymphoma. Specific cell markers may highlight infrequent abnormal cells that represent residual or recurrent disease (e.g. CD72 (DBA.44) can be used to highlight neoplastic cells in hairy cell leukaemia). Finally, since trephine biopsy tissue is fixed and preserved, additional tests may be performed some time after the specimen was obtained.

Imprints from Bone Marrow Trephine Biopsy Specimens

Whenever a trephine biopsy is obtained, imprints can be taken before the specimen is transferred into fixative. This is particularly useful if the bone marrow aspirate is inadequate. The bony core is gently dabbed or rolled across the slide, which is then fixed and stained as for bone marrow smears (see p. 61). This allows immediate examination of cells that fall out of the specimen onto the slide and may provide a diagnosis several days before the trephine biopsy specimen has been processed.

Processing of Bone Marrow Trephine Biopsy Specimens

The specimen should be fixed in 10% formal saline, buffered to pH 7.0, for 12–48 h prior to decalcifying, dehydrating and embedding in paraffin wax by the usual histological procedures. Cell shrinkage and distortion from the decalcification process may obscure cellular detail. These disadvantages can be overcome by methyl methacrylate ('plastic') embedding (Fig. 7.13). Details of the preparation of sections of bone marrow biopsies can be found in Bain et al.[22]

Figure 7.10 Areas of bone marrow trephine biopsy stained with H&E showing an erythroid island (upper left), maturing myeloid lineage cells (lower left) and paratrabecular area with early precursor cells (right).

Figure 7.11 Bone marrow trephine biopsy showing increased and abnormally clustered megakaryocytes.

Figure 7.12 Immunostaining of marrow infiltrated by plasma cells highlighting the abnormal cells.

Figure 7.13 Photomicrograph of section of normal bone marrow. Iliac crest biopsy. Methacrylate embedding. Stained by May–Grünwald–Giemsa.

Staining of Sections of Bone Marrow Trephine Biopsy Specimens

Bone marrow sections should be routinely stained with haematoxylin and eosin (H&E) and a silver impregnation method for reticulin. Sections can also be stained for iron by Perls' reaction. H&E staining is excellent for demonstrating the cellularity (Fig. 7.14) and pattern of the marrow and for revealing pathological changes such as fibrosis or the presence of granulomata or carcinoma cells. Haemopoietic cells may be more easily identified in a Romanowsky-stained preparation. Both paraffin- and plastic-embedded specimens are suitable for immunohistochemistry.

Silver impregnation stains the glycoprotein matrix, which is associated with connective tissue. The bone marrow always contains a small amount of this material, which is referred to as 'reticulin' and is an early form of collagen. The normal reticulin content of iliac bone marrow is shown in Figure 7.15A. An increase in marrow reticulin appears as an increase in the number, thickness and length of fibres (Fig. 7.15B). Increased reticulin deposition can occur in myeloproliferative neoplasms, particularly those associated with proliferation of megakaryocytes and in lymphoproliferative disorders, secondary carcinoma with marrow infiltration, osseous disorders such as hyperparathyroidism and Paget's disease and inflammatory reactions.[23] In primary myelofibrosis, a more 'mature' form of collagen is present, which, unlike reticulin, is visible on H&E staining (Fig. 7.16).

Figure 7.14 Photomicrographs of sections of bone marrow. Iliac crest bone marrow illustrating the range of cellularity. (A) hypocellular; (B,C) normal cellularity; (D) hypercellular.

Continued

Figure 7.14—cont'd

Figure 7.15 Photomicrographs of sections of bone marrow. Iliac crest biopsy. Stained for reticulin by silver impregnation method. (A) normal; (B) primary myelofibrosis.

Figure 7.16 Photomicrograph of a section of bone marrow. Iliac crest biopsy; fibroblast proliferation and collagen in primary myelofibrosis. Haematoxylin and eosin (H&E) stain.

REFERENCES

1. Bain BJ. Bone marrow aspiration. *J Clin Pathol*. 2001;54:657–663.

2. Bain BJ. Bone marrow trephine biopsy. *J Clin Pathol*. 2001;54: 737–742.

3. Lee S-H, Erber WN, Porwit A, et al. ICSH guidelines for the standardization of bone marrow specimens and reports. *International Journal of Laboratory Hematology*. 2008;30:349–364.

4. Hall R. Results of bone marrow biopsy patient satisfaction survey at the Royal Bournemouth Hospital. Abstract 200. *Br J Haematol*. 2004;125(supp 1):62.

5. Bain BJ. Bone marrow biopsy morbidity and mortality: 2002 data. *Clin Lab Haematol*. 2004;26: 315–318.

6. Bain BJ. Morbidity associated with bone marrow aspiration and trephine biopsy – a review of UK data for 2004. *Haematologica*. 2006;91:1293–1294.

7. Marti J, Anton E, Valenti C. Complications of bone marrow biopsy. *Br J Haematol*. 2004;124:555–563.

8. Devaliaf V, Tudor G. Bone marrow examination in obese patients. *Br J Haematol*. 2004;125:537–539.

9. Engeset A, Nesheim A, Sokolowski J. Incidence of 'dry tap' on bone marrow aspirations in lymphomas and carcinomas: diagnostic value of the small material in the needle. *Scand J Haematol*. 1979;22:417–422.

10. Ferrant A. Selective hypoplasia of pelvic bone marrow. *Scand J Haematol*. 1980;25:12–18.

11. Jacobs P. Choice of needle for bone marrow trephine biopsies. *Hematology Reviews*. 1995;9: 163–168.

12. Fillola GM, Laharrague PF, Corberand JX. Bone marrow enrichment technique for detection and characterization of scarce abnormal cells. *Nouv Rev Fr Hématol*. 1992;34:337–341.

13. Hoffman SB, Morrow Jr GW, Pease GL, et al. Rate of cellular autolysis in postmortem bone marrow. *Am J Clin Pathol*. 1964;41:281–286.

14. Den Ottolander GJ. The bone marrow aspirate of healthy subjects. *Br J Haematol*. 1996;95:574–575.

15. Bain B. The bone marrow aspirate of healthy subjects. *Br J Haematol*. 1996;94:206–209.

16. Maeda K, Hyun BH, Rebuck JW. Lymphoid follicles in bone marrow aspirates. *Am J Clin Pathol*. 1977;67:41–48.

17. Kiraly JF, Wheby MS. Bone marrow necrosis. *Am J Med*. 1976;60: 361–368.

18. Smith RRL, Spivak JL. Marrow cell necrosis in anorexia nervosa and involuntary starvation. *Br J Haematol*. 1985;60: 525–530.

19. Hughes DA, Stuart-Smith SE, Bain BJ. How should stainable iron in bone marrow films be assessed? *J Clin Pathol*. 2004;57:1038–1040.

20. Hernándes-Garciá MT, Hernández-Nieto L, Pérez-González E, et al. Bone marrow trephine biopsy: anterior superior iliac spine versus posterior superior iliac spine. *Clin Lab Haematol*. 1993;15: 15–19.

21. Sola M, Rimsza L, Christensen R. A bone marrow biopsy technique suitable for use in neonates. *Br J Haematol*. 1999;107:458–460.

22. Bain B, Clark DC, Wilkins BS. *Bone Marrow Pathology*. 4th ed. Oxford: Wiley-Blackwell; 2010.

23. McCarthy DM. Fibrosis of the bone marrow: content and causes. *Br J Haematol*. 1985;59:1–7.

Chapter | **8** |

Molecular and cytogenetic analysis

Tom Vulliamy, Jaspal Kaeda, Letizia Foroni, with contributions from Barbara J. Bain

INTRODUCTION TO THE ANALYSIS OF DNA

Our understanding of the molecular basis of both inherited and acquired haematological disorders is now considerable and there are several ways in which this knowledge is being applied in diagnostic haematology. These include the identification of genetic defects in haemoglobinopathies allowing the provision of early prenatal diagnosis, the assessment of genetic risk factors in thrombophilia, the diagnosis and characterization of leukaemias, the monitoring of minimal residual disease and the study of host–donor chimerism following bone marrow transplantation. In this chapter, we shall describe some of the methods that can be applied in these conditions, although this cannot be exhaustive and will reflect the specific interests of our laboratories.

The ability to manipulate DNA as recombinant molecules followed from the discovery of bacterial DNA-modifying enzymes that allowed genes to be isolated as cloned recombinant DNA molecules and their DNA to be sequenced. The sequence of the human genome is now complete (see: www.ornl.gov/sci/techresources/Human_Genome/project/timeline.shtml).[1,2] It has become extensively annotated and is accessible through a number of genome browsers. The ability to amplify specific DNA fragments from small amounts of starting material using the polymerase chain reaction (PCR)[3] is now the cornerstone of most routine DNA analysis. Because this technique is relatively simple, rapid, inexpensive and requires only some basic pieces of laboratory equipment, it has made molecular genetic analysis readily accessible in many laboratories.

Guidelines from the American Association for Molecular Pathology address the choice and development of appropriate diagnostic assays, quality control and validation and implementation of molecular diagnostic tests.[4] In the UK, a national external quality assessment scheme has been approved for the molecular genetics of thrombophilia and pilot studies are currently in progress for the molecular diagnosis of haematological malignancies and for haemophilia A. It is true, however, that the development and implementation of quality control methods and assurance standards still lag behind the rapid rate of expansion of molecular techniques.[5,6] To overcome this, both at national and international level, several groups are attempting to reach a standardization of molecular methodologies applied to fusion gene quantification (BCR–ABL1, PML–RARA, etc.) in myeloid malignancies as well as the molecular monitoring of residual disease using antigen receptor targets in acute and chronic lymphoid malignancies.

In this chapter, some of the applications of the PCR in a diagnostic haematology laboratory are described. For the reasons just mentioned, the analysis of PCR products has largely superseded other techniques, including Southern blot analysis, and capillary electrophoresis has replaced polyacrylamide gel electrophoresis. For situations in which these are still appropriate, the reader is referred to previous editions of this book.

EXTRACTION OF DNA

DNA can be extracted from blood, bone marrow or tissue samples. The quality and quantity of the DNA obtained will vary depending on the size, age and cell count of the sample. As a rule, 5–10 ml of blood in ethylenediaminetetra-acetic acid (EDTA) will suffice. The DNA is extracted from all nucleated cells and is called genomic DNA.

In the nucleus, the DNA is tightly associated with many different proteins as chromatin. It is important to remove these as well as other cellular proteins to extract the DNA. This is achieved through the use of organic solvents, salt precipitation or DNA-affinity columns. An aqueous solution of DNA is obtained, from which the DNA is further purified by precipitation. A number of DNA extraction kits have been developed. They are commercially available and cost-effective. In addition, equipment that can achieve simultaneous extraction from a large number of samples is available and will be discussed below. These can significantly reduce the amount of time required for DNA extraction, bypass the use of organic solvents and provide good quality control of the reagents used.

DNA Extraction Kits

We are currently using two different types of DNA extraction kit, depending essentially on the quantity of DNA required. The first (The *QIAamp* system, Qiagen, Crawley, West Sussex) is a robust method for obtaining ≈5 μg of DNA from 200 μl of whole blood. This method revolves around a high-affinity DNA binding matrix in a spin column, which can be used in a microcentrifuge or in an automated set-up. The DNA obtained is usually of high quality and sufficient for most routine analysis.

When larger amounts of DNA are required, perhaps for storage and more extensive analysis of important samples, we use from 3 to 10 ml blood in the *Gentra Puregene Blood kit* (Qiagen), which can yield upwards of 100 μg of DNA. This method depends on salting-out of proteins after sequential red cell and then white cell lysis, followed by isopropanol precipitation of the DNA.

Protocols are of course supplied with any kit method and will therefore not be given in detail here. For preparation of reagents, and a protocol for the manual extraction of DNA from blood using organic solvents, the reader is referred to previous editions of this book.

POLYMERASE CHAIN REACTION

Development of the PCR[3] has had a dramatic impact on the study and analysis of nucleic acids. Through the use of a thermostable DNA polymerase, Taq polymerase (available from various suppliers, including Applied Biosystems, Warrington and Thermo-Fisher, Runcorn) extracted from the bacterium *Thermus aquaticus*, the PCR results in the amplification of a specific DNA fragment such that it can be visualized using intercalating SYBR Safe (Invitrogen, Paisley) added to agarose gels. Ethidium bromide, a carcinogenic product, is no longer in use for safety reasons. The procedure takes only a few hours and requires only a very small amount of starting material.

Principle

A DNA polymerase will synthesize the complementary strand of a DNA template *in vitro*. A stretch of double-stranded DNA is required for the synthesis to be initiated. This double-stranded sequence can be generated by annealing an oligonucleotide (oligo), which is a short, single-stranded DNA molecule usually between 17 and 22 bases in length, to a single-stranded DNA template. These oligos, which are synthesized *in vitro*, will prime the DNA synthesis and are therefore referred to as primers.

In the PCR, at least two oligos are used. One primes the synthesis of DNA in the forward direction or along the coding strand of the DNA, whereas the other primes DNA synthesis in the reverse direction or along the non-coding strand. The other components of the reaction are the DNA template from which the DNA fragment will be amplified, the four deoxynucleotide triphosphates (dATP, dTTP, dCTP and dGTP) required as the building blocks of the newly synthesized DNA, a salt buffer containing $MgCl_2$ and the thermostable DNA polymerase (Taq polymerase).

The first step of the reaction is to denature the DNA, generating single-stranded templates, by heating the reaction mixture to 95°C. The reaction is then cooled to a temperature, usually between 50°C and 68°C, that permits the annealing of the primers to the DNA template but only at their specific complementary sequences. The temperature is then raised to 72°C, at which temperature the Taq polymerase efficiently synthesizes DNA, extending from the primers in a 5′ to 3′ direction. Cyclical repetition of the denaturing, annealing and extension steps, by simply changing the temperature of the reaction in an automated heating block, results in exponential amplification of the DNA that lies between the two primers (Fig. 8.1).

The specificity of the DNA fragment that is amplified is therefore determined by the sequences of the primers used. A sequence of 17–22 base pairs (bp) is statistically likely to be unique in the human genome and so primers of this length and longer will anneal at only one specific place on a template of genomic DNA. One general requirement of the PCR therefore is some knowledge of the DNA sequence of the gene that is to be amplified. The relative positioning of the two primers is another important consideration. They must anneal to complementary strands and must prime DNA synthesis in opposite directions pointing towards one another. There is also an upper limit to the distance apart that the oligos can be placed; fragments of several kilobase pairs (kb) in length can be amplified, but the process is most efficient for fragments of several hundred bp.

Reagents

Taq polymerase and oligonucleotide primers. These can be purchased from a variety of different companies, such as Applied Biosystems (Warrington), Thermo-Fisher (Runcorn) and Sigma-Genosys (Poole). The oligos are usually 17–22 bases in length.

PCR buffers. These are usually supplied with the Taq polymerase. Three different buffers can be prepared as follows:

> *×10 PCR buffer I:* 100 mmol/l Tris-HCl, pH 8.3, 500 mmol/l KCl, 15 mmol/l $MgCl_2$, 0.1% (w/v) gelatin, 0.5% (v/v) NP40 and 0.5% (v/v) Tween 20
>
> *×10 PCR buffer II:* 670 mmol/l Tris, pH 8.8, 166 mmol/l $(NH_4)_2SO_4$, 25 mmol/l $MgCl_2$, 670 μmol/l Na_2EDTA, 1.6 mg/ml bovine serum albumin (BSA) and 100 mmol/l β-mercaptoethanol. This buffer is used in conjunction with 10% dimethyl sulphoxide (DMSO) in the final reaction mixture

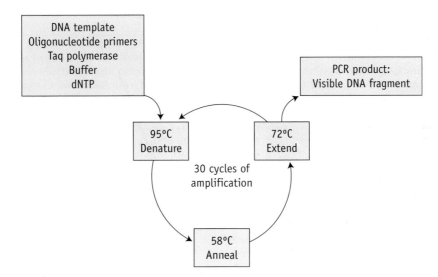

Figure 8.1 The polymerase chain reaction. Cyclical repetition of three temperatures for denaturing, annealing and extending DNA, respectively, gives rise to an exponential amplification of a DNA fragment between two primer sequences directing DNA synthesis on opposite strands of the DNA template.

×10 *PCR buffer III*: 750 mmol/l Tris, pH 8.8, 200 mmol/l $(NH_4)_2SO_4$, 0.1% (v/v) Tween 20. A solution of 25 mmol/l $MgCl_2$ is also prepared and added separately to the PCR reaction.

dNTP, 10 mmol/l. Take 10 μl of 100 mmol/l dATP, 10 μl of 100 mmol/l dTTP, 10 μl of 100 mmol/l dCTP, 10 μl of 100 mmol/l dGTP and 60 μl of water to make a 100 μl of 10 mmol/l dNTP.

DMSO

Agarose, Type II medium electroendosmosis.

×10 *Tris-borate-EDTA (TBE) buffer.* Add 216 g of Trizma base, 18.6 g of EDTA and 110 g of orthoboric acid to 1600 ml water. Dissolve and top up to 2l; dilute 1 in 20 for use as ×0.5 TBE buffer.

SYBR Safe DNA Stain, Invitrogen, Cat no S33102 (×10 000 *concentrated*). Add 5 μl every 50 ml of agarose gel preparation.

Tracking dye. Weigh 15 g of Ficoll (type 400), 0.25 g of bromophenol blue and 0.25 g of xylene cyanol. Make up to 100 ml with water, cover and mix by inversion; it will take a considerable amount of mixing to get the solution homogeneous. Dispense into aliquots.

Method

Optimal conditions for the reaction have to be derived empirically, with the magnesium concentration and annealing temperature being the most important parameters.[7] The choice of buffer depends on the enzyme being used and the company will usually supply the most appropriate one. For genes with a high GC content, buffer II in combination with 10% DMSO may give better amplification. In most cases, a 25 μl reaction volume suffices. A blank control should always be included (i.e. a reaction without any template) to control for contamination. If the blank control yields a product, the analysis is invalid. A DNA sample that is known to amplify can also be included and this sample may then be used as a normal or positive control.

The risk of contamination cannot be overemphasized. It can be minimized by using plugged tips and having dedicated micropipettes and areas for each step of the analysis. The optimum cycling conditions need to be determined for each thermocycler. Specificity is often improved by 'hot start' PCR. This is achieved by setting up all the PCR tests on wet ice and transferring the tubes to the thermocycler once it reaches 95°C or by using an enzyme that only becomes activated when heated at 95°C for several minutes. In preparing a group of reactions, a premix solution is prepared that can be dispensed into microcentrifuge tubes, tube strips or PCR reaction 96-well plates to which the template DNA is added. When a particular PCR is to be performed repetitively over a period of time, it is helpful to prepare a large volume (e.g. 10 ml) of the reaction mixture (without DNA or Taq polymerase), aliquot it and store it at –20°C.

1. Prepare a PCR mixture for 20 reactions (with a final volume of 25 μl for each DNA sample) as follows:

STOCK SOLUTION	VOLUME (μl)	FINAL CONCENTRATION
×10 PCR buffer III	50	×1
25 mmol/l $MgCl_2$	40	2.0 mmol/l
10 mmol/l dNTP	10	0.02 mmol/l
10 μmol/l Primer (1)	20	0.04 μmol/l
10 μmol/l Primer (2)	20	0.04 μmol/l
5 u/μl Taq polymerase	2	0.02 μ/ml
Water	358	
Final volume	500	

Add the Taq polymerase last, mix well and pulse-spin in a microcentrifuge to bring down the contents of the tube.

2. Aliquot 24 μl of the PCR reaction mix into each tube. Add 1 μl of template DNA at approximately 0.05 mg/ml into all except one of the reaction tubes.

3. Place the tubes in a PCR machine, using a heated lid, programmed for the following conditions: an initial step of 5 min at 95°C and then 30 cycles of 95°C for 45 s, 58°C for 45 s and 72°C for 1 min in sequence, followed by a final extension step at 72°C for 10 min. These conditions are suitable for many primer pairs, although some will require different annealing temperatures or longer extension times.

4. While the PCR program is running, a 1.5% agarose mini-gel is prepared: add 0.75 g of agarose to 50 ml of ×0.5 TBE buffer and heat until completely dissolved. Add 2 μl of SYBR Safe, allow the agarose to cool slightly and pour with the appropriate comb in position.

5. To check if the amplification has been successful, add 1 μl of tracking dye to a 10 μl aliquot of the PCR reaction mixture, being careful not to pipette the mineral oil overlaying the PCR reaction.

6. Load the gel and run at a constant voltage of 100 V for 1 h in ×0.5 TBE buffer. A molecular size marker should be included to establish the size of the amplified fragment; these are commercially available (e.g. *HyperLadder* from Bioline, London). The marker used in this chapter is the plasmid pEMBL 8 digested with Taq I and Pvu II to yield fragments of 1443, 1008, 613, 357, 278, 193 and 108 bp.

7. Visualize the DNA on an ultraviolet (UV) transilluminator and take a photograph.

Modifications and Developments

The procedure described earlier is a guideline for setting up and checking a standard PCR amplification. As the test dictates, modifications can be used, such as the following:

Radiolabelling. A PCR can be labelled with ^{32}P by adding 0.1 µl of [α^{32}P]dCTP per tube to the reaction mixture.

Multiplex. More than one fragment can be amplified in the same tube simply by adding further primer pairs. It is important that the different pairs all work equally well under the same conditions.

Nested PCR. This involves successive rounds of amplification using two pairs of primers; the second pair, located within the sequence amplified by the first, allows products to be generated from as little as a single cell.

Long-range amplification. Fragments upward of 10 kb can now be generated by PCR using modified polymerases.

Automation. High-throughput PCR amplification is being achieved through the use of robots and 96-well plate technology.

Automated fragment analysis. The method of gel electrophoresis is modified for the detection of fluorescentlylabelled PCR products on DNA fragment analysers (e.g. the ABI 3700 DNA analyser).

Problems and Interpretation

If the amplification has been successful, a discrete fragment of the expected size is seen in an SYBR Safe-stained agarose gel in all samples, except where a blank control (in which the DNA template is replaced by water) is loaded. If a product is seen in the blank control, then one of the solutions has been contaminated. In this case, the experiment and all the working solutions must be discarded and the micropipettes must be cleaned. Cleaning micropipettes prior to the start of each experiment is highly recommended. To avoid contamination, setting up a master mix of all reagents is recommended before DNA samples are added to each tube.

Conversely, the absence of a fragment in all tracks indicates that the PCR has failed. This could occur for a number of reasons, the most obvious being the poor quality or omission of one of the essential reagents. The reaction may also fail if the magnesium concentration is too low (standard concentration 1.5 mM) or if the annealing temperature is too high. DNA quality is often one of the major reasons for failure. If one particular DNA sample repeatedly fails to amplify, then the sample should be re-extracted using Proteinase K (Sigma, Poole) and phenol and chloroform and reprecipitated in one-tenth volume of 5 mol/l ammonium acetate or 3M sodium acetate pH 4.8 and 2.5 volumes of ethanol. We have also found that for samples prepared using the Gentra method, passing the DNA through a Qiagen column substantially improves DNA quality and PCR efficiency. Another problem is the presence of non-specific fragments or just a smear of amplified product. This can occur if the magnesium concentration is too high or if the annealing temperature is too low.

ANALYSIS OF POLYMERASE CHAIN REACTION PRODUCTS

Presence or Absence of a Polymerase Chain Reaction Product

Initially, PCR products are commonly and conveniently visualized by agarose gel electrophoresis. However, it has also become commonplace to visualize PCR products directly on DNA analysers – in particular the *Applied Biosystems 3130xl* (Warrington) – through the use of a fluorescent label on one of the primers. If appropriate primers and controls are included in an experiment, the actual presence of a product can be highly informative.

Amplification Refractory Mutation System
Principle

Point mutations and small insertions or deletions can be identified directly by the presence or absence of a PCR product using allele-specific primers.[8,9] Two different oligos are used that differ only at the site of the mutation (the amplification refractory mutation system or ARMS, primers) with the mismatch distinguishing the normal and mutant base located at the 3′ end of the oligo. In a PCR, an oligo with a mismatch at its 3′ end will fail to prime the extension step of the reaction. Each test sample is amplified in two separate reactions containing either a mutant ARMS primer or a normal ARMS primer. The mutant primer will prime amplification together with one common primer from DNA with this mutation but not from a normal DNA. A normal primer will do the opposite. To increase the instability of the 3′ end mismatch and so ensure the failure of the amplification, it is sometimes necessary to introduce a second nucleotide mismatch three or four bases from the 3′ end of both oligos. A second pair of unrelated primers at a distance from the ARMS primers is included in each reaction as an internal control to demonstrate that efficient amplification has occurred. This is essential because a failure of the ARMS primer to amplify is interpreted as a significant result and must not be the result of suboptimal reaction conditions.

Interpretation

In all the samples, apart from the blank control, the fragment produced by amplification with the internal control primers must be seen. If this is the case, then the presence or absence of a mutation is simply determined by the presence or absence of the expected fragment produced by amplification with the mutant ARMS primer and the common primer. The presence or absence of the normal allele is determined in the same way in the reaction that includes the normal ARMS primer. In this way, heterozygous, homozygous normal and homozygous mutant genes can be distinguished.

Gap-PCR

Large deletions can be detected by Gap-PCR. Primers located 5′ and 3′ to the breakpoints of a deletion will anneal too far apart on the normal chromosome to generate a fragment in a standard PCR. When the deletion is present, the sites at which these primers anneal will be brought together, enabling them to give rise to a product. An example of this is given for the detection of deletions in $\alpha°$ thalassaemia in Figure 8.4 on p. 149.

By the same principle, the sites at which primers anneal can be brought together by chromosomal translocation, giving rise to a diagnostic product. Breakpoints may be clustered over too large a region for genomic DNA to be used in these instances. However, leukaemic translocations can also give rise to transcribed fusion genes. Primer annealing sites in different genes are then juxtaposed in a hybrid messenger RNA (mRNA) molecule and can give rise to a reverse transcription-PCR (RT-PCR) product. Examples of this are given for the analysis of minimal residual disease in chronic myelogenous leukaemia (CML) in Figure 8.8 on p. 155.

Size of the PCR Product

Principle

Deletions and insertions can be identified using agarose gel electrophoresis, when the size of the PCR product significantly differs from the size of a normal control. A higher resolution of fragment sizes is obtained by capillary electrophoresis. This is particularly appropriate in the analysis of short tandem repeat (STR) sequences that can be highly variable in length and, therefore, useful as genetic markers of different individuals. High resolution of DNA fragments is now often performed on the capillaries of the *Applied Biosystems (ABI) 3700 or 3130xl DNA analysers* (Warrington). These read fluorescently labelled DNA fragments as they exit from the gel and enable single base resolution from around 50–800 bp. Several examples of these applications are given in this chapter.

Restriction Enzyme Digestion

Principle

Restriction enzymes (RE) cleave DNA at short specific sequences. Because many RE are available, it is not uncommon for a single point mutation to coincidentally create or

destroy an RE recognition sequence. If this is the case, digestion of the appropriate PCR product prior to agarose gel electrophoresis enables the mutation to be identified. A difference in the size of the restriction fragments seen in normal and mutant samples can be predicted from a restriction map of the amplified fragment and the site of the mutation that changes a restriction site. The observed fragments should be consistent with either the mutant or the normal pattern. An example is shown in Figure 8.2 on p. 147 in the diagnosis of the sickle cell mutation.

Reagents

A number of companies supply a comprehensive list of restriction enzymes (RE), including New England Biolabs (Hitchin) and Fermentas (York). Those that are in regular use are generally quite inexpensive compared with the more specialized enzymes that are used only occasionally, which may be 10–100 times more expensive. RE buffers are now almost always supplied with each RE. Buffer compositions are always given and will vary from enzyme to enzyme. Many commonly used REs cut perfectly well in a single 'universal' buffer. This is prepared using the following stock solutions:

Tris-acetate, 2 mol/l, pH 7.5. Dissolve 24.2 g of Trizma base in 60 ml of water, adjust the pH to 7.5 with glacial acetic acid and make up to 100 ml.
Potassium acetate, 2 mol/l. Weigh out 19.62 g, make up to 100 ml with water and dissolve.
Magnesium acetate, 2 mol/l. Weigh out 42.89 g, make up to 100 ml with water and dissolve.
BSA fraction V (molecular biology grade), 20 mg/ml.
Dithiothreitol (DTI), 0.5 mol/l. Weigh out 0.771 g, make up to 10 ml with water, dissolve and store at –20°C.
Spermidine (N-(3-aminopropyl)-1, 4-butane-diamine), 1 mol/l. Weigh out 1.273 g, make up to 10 ml with water, dissolve and store at –20°C.
×10 RE buffer. For a ×10 concentrated buffer, prepare a solution that is 300 mmol/l Tris-acetate, pH 7.5, 660 mmol/l potassium acetate, 100 mmol/l magnesium acetate, 1 mg/ml BSA, 10 mmol/l DTT and 30 mmol/l spermidine; aliquot into microcentrifuge tubes and store at –20°C.

Method

1. To 20 µl of a PCR product add 2.5 µl of ×10 restriction enzyme buffer, 2 µl of double-distilled water and 2–5 units of the appropriate restriction enzyme (usually 0.5 µl), giving a final volume of 25 µl. When preparing more than one digestion with the same restriction enzyme, sufficient buffer, enzyme and water can be premixed and dispensed into the PCR products.
2. Incubate at 37°C (or other temperature as specified by the manufacturer) for a minimum of 4 h.

3. Pour a 2.5% agarose mini-gel in a taped casting tray with the appropriate comb. The gel is made up as a 1:1 mixture of type II medium electroendosmosis agarose and NuSieve agarose (Cambrex Bioscience, Wokingham) – that is, 0.675 g of agarose and 0.675 g of NuSieve agarose in 50 ml of half-strength ($\times$0.5) TBE buffer.

4. After the incubation period, add 2 µl of tracking dye to the digests and load the samples on to the gel. The electrophoresis is continued until a clear separation of all the expected fragments is achieved, which may be checked at intervals by placing the gel on a UV transilluminator.

Allele-Specific Oligonucleotide Hybridization

Principle

Under appropriate conditions, short oligonucleotide probes will hybridize to their exact complementary sequence but not to a sequence in which there is even a single base mismatch.[10] A pair of oligos is therefore used to test for the presence of a point mutation: a mutant oligo complementary to the mutant sequence and a normal oligo complementary to the normal sequence, with the sequence difference placed near the centre of each oligo.

The stability of the duplex formed between the oligo and the target DNA being tested (the product of a PCR reaction) depends on the temperature, the base composition and length of the oligo and the ionic strength of the washing solution. For allele-specific oligonucleotide hybridization (ASOH) studies, an empirical formula has been derived for the dissociation temperature (Td), the temperature at which half of the duplexes are dissociated: for hybridization of oligonucleotides of 14–20 bases in length. The Td can be estimated as $2°C$ for each dA:dT pair plus $4°C$ for each dG:dC base pair. This value is used as a guideline; the exact temperature at which only perfect base pairing is maintained is usually determined by trial and error.

This methodology has been widely applied for the detection of point mutations using fluorescently labelled *TaqMan* probes that distinguish the two alleles. Two short allele-specific probes are used, one of which will hybridize only to the wild-type allele and one of which will hybridize only to the mutant allele. Each probe is labelled with a different fluorescent colour, which is quenched while the probe remains intact, but is released if and when the probe hybridizes to its perfectly complementary sequence during the PCR reaction, as it will then be broken up by the exonuclease activity of the Taq polymerase. An example of this analysis is the detection of the factor V Leiden mutation in Figure 8.5 on p. 150.

Interpretation

The oligos will hybridize to their perfectly complementary DNA sequence, such that the mutant oligo gives a signal only when the mutant allele is present, with the same happening for the wild-type allele. When this is the case, the interpretation of the result is straightforward; a positive signal from a particular oligo indicates the presence of that allele in the test sample. Heterozygotes and homozygotes are distinguished by using the mutant and normal oligos in tandem. With the two fluorescent colours of the Taqman probes, the heterozygote is identified as the sum of the two fluorochromes.

Other non-radioactive probes, with detection systems involving horseradish peroxidase, have also been quite widely used in this procedure.[11] The technique has also been modified such that the allele-specific oligonucleotides are immobilized onto nylon membranes and the patient-specific PCR product is used as the probe–the reverse dot blot procedure.[12] This allows for several different mutations to be analysed simultaneously and has proved particularly useful in the diagnosis of β thalassaemia mutations.[13]

DNA Sequencing

Principle

The Sanger chain termination method for direct DNA sequencing has become a standard diagnostic tool. In many laboratories, this procedure has superseded targeted mutation detection as it provides a robust and relatively rapid method to identify all sequence changes that may be present in a particular DNA fragment. This approach is particularly relevant where multiple different mutations may underlie a particular disorder. This is the case for β thalassaemia, glucose-6-phosphate dehydrogenase (G6PD) deficiency and the red cell membrane disorders among others and so it is not surprising that DNA sequencing has often become the method of choice for the molecular diagnosis of these diseases.

In outline, the method revolves around the *de novo* synthesis of DNA strands in one direction from a PCR-derived template DNA fragment. The chain is lengthened by a thermostable DNA polymerase using deoxynucleotide triphosphates in the normal way; however, included in the reaction mixture is a small proportion of labelled dideoxynucleotide triphosphates (ddNTPs), which when incorporated will prevent any further extension of the chain. This process happens millions of times along a relatively short piece of DNA (usually up to 1000 bases), which means that chaintermination will occur many times at each position along the fragment. In the *Applied Biosystems BigDye system* (Warrington), each of the ddNTPs is labelled with a different fluorochrome and so the products of the sequencing reaction will consist of single-stranded DNA fragments, each differing in size by one base pair and each labelled with a different colour. These fragments can then be separated by capillary electrophoresis and the order with which the different colours exit the capillary will correspond to the sequence of the DNA template.

Reagents

ExoSapIt, a mixture of exonuclease and shrimp alkaline phosphatase (GE Healthcare, Little Chalfont).
BigDye Terminator v3.1 cycle sequencing kit (Applied Biosystems Inc., Warrington).
125mM ethylenediaminetetra-acetic acid (EDTA).
MicroAmp optical plates (Applied Biosystems Inc, Warrington).
100% and 70% ethanol.
HiDi formamide (Applied Biosystems Inc, Warrington).

Method

1. Mix 5 μl of the PCR product with 2 μl of ExoSapIt (GE Healthcare, Little Chalfont) and incubate at 37°C for 45 min and then 80°C for 15 min. Cool to 4°C until ready for use.
2. Prepare 10 μl sequencing reactions by mixing 1–4 μl of the ExoSapIt-treated PCR reaction (see Note 7), 2 μl of the relevant oligonucleotide primer (diluted to 0.8 pmol/μl), 1 μl of the 5 times concentrated (5×) reaction buffer and 2 μl of the BigDye ddNTP terminator mix (both supplied with the kit), made up to 10 μl with water.
3. Run the sequencing reaction, incubating at 96°C for 10 s, 50°C for 5 s and 60°C for 4 min for 25 cycles.
4. Cool samples to 4°C. Add 2.5 μl 125 mM EDTA to each sample and mix well and then add 30 μl ice-cold ethanol and mix again (see Note 8). Incubate on ice for 10 min in a sealed MicroAmp plate.
5. Centrifuge 2000 *g* for 20 min to pellet the DNA. Carefully remove the seal, invert the plate onto some tissue and centrifuge the plate upside down for ≈10 s to remove all residual liquid.
6. Add 125 μl 70% ethanol and centrifuge at 2000 *g* for 5 min. Invert and briefly spin the plate upside down again. Place on a pre-heated 95°C block for 10 s to remove any residual ethanol.
7. Resuspend in 10 μl HiDi formamide, cover with the grey septa, heat to 95°C for 5 min, snap cool on ice and place in the DNA sequence analysis platform and run using the appropriate DNA fragment analysis protocol.

Interpretation

Reading the DNA sequence from a good trace – known as an electrophoretogram – is completely straightforward: As are called as green peaks; Ts as red; Cs as blue; and Gs as black. Free software packages, such as Chromas (at: http://chromas-lite-version.fyxm.net/), are available for viewing these traces and will call the DNA sequence in the file. Simple alignment of this sequence to the GenBank reference sequence can be performed at the National Center for Bioinformatics (NCBI) using the Blast program (at: http://blast.ncbi.nlm.nih.gov/Blast.cgi?CMD=Web&PAGE_TYPE=BlastHome) and will identify any sequence changes. Heterozygous point mutations will be seen as double peaks, with two colours overlaid. Small heterozygous insertions or deletions (indels) are harder to decipher, as the sequence 3′ of the mutation will be a double sequence, with the normal and indel allele superimposed on one another: the extent of the indel can be defined by subtracting from the expected normal sequence.

INVESTIGATION OF HAEMOGLOBINOPATHIES

Sickle Cell Disease

The presence of a sickle cell gene can be determined by haemoglobin cellulose acetate electrophoresis or a sickling test. However, there are occasions when it is beneficial to make this diagnosis by DNA analysis (e.g. in prenatal diagnosis, which can be performed at 10 weeks of pregnancy, in distinguishing HbS/S from HbS/β° thalassaemia or in confirming the diagnosis of sickle cell anaemia in a neonate). For the type of specimens collected for prenatal diagnosis, refer to p. 330.

The sickle cell mutation in codon 6 of the β globin gene (GAG → GTG) results in the loss of a Bsu36 I (or Mst II, Sau I, OxaN I or Dde I) restriction enzyme site that is present in the normal gene. It is therefore possible to detect the mutation directly by restriction enzyme analysis of a DNA fragment generated by the PCR. A pair of primers are used to amplify exons 1 and 2 of the β globin gene and the products of the PCR are digested with Bsu36 I. The loss of a Bsu36 I site in the sickle cell gene gives rise to an abnormally large restriction fragment that is not seen in normal individuals (Fig. 8.2).

β Thalassaemia

The ethnic groups with the highest incidence of β thalassaemia are the Mediterranean populations, Asian Indians, Chinese and Africans. Although more than 100 β thalassaemia mutations are known, each of these groups has its own subset of mutations, so that as few as five different mutations may account for more than 90% of the affected individuals in a population. This makes the direct detection of β thalassaemia mutations a reasonable possibility and it has become the method of choice where it is most important: in prenatal diagnosis.[13,14]

The majority of mutations causing β thalassaemia are point mutations affecting the coding sequence, splice sites

Figure 8.2 Detection of the sickle cell mutation. (A) A sketch of the β globin gene shows the position of the primers used to amplify a 768 bp fragment in a polymerase chain reaction (PCR). The sequence of β I-5' is 5'TAAGCCAGTGCCAGAAAGAGCC3' and that of β II-3' is 5'CATTCGTCTGTTTCCCATTCTA3'. Maps of the Bsu36 I restriction sites and the fragment sizes from β^A and β^S genes are shown below. (B) An ethidium-bromide-stained mini-gel illustrates the fragment sizes generated by Bsu36 I digestion of the PCR product from normal (A/A), sickle cell trait (A/S) and sickle cell anaemia (S/S) individuals, along with the undigested amplified fragment (U) and the molecular size marker (M).

or promoter of the β globin gene. Methods for their detection include either ARMS or reverse dot blot analysis, although more commonly now, they are detected by direct DNA sequence analysis. Unstable and other unusual haemoglobins may also cause disease and can also be identified by direct DNA sequence analysis. An example of such a case is shown in Figure 8.3, where a picture of moderate anaemia is seen in the heterozygote due to the highly unstable and electrophoretically silent variant, haemoglobin, Durham, NC.

α Thalassaemia

In contrast to the β thalassaemias, the most common α thalassaemia mutations are deletions. Two categories exist:

Figure 8.3 Sequencing of the β globin gene reveals Hb Durham-N.C. The sequencing electrophoretogram clearly shows the heterozygous mutation (arrowed), where a C peak and a T peak are superimposed and called as N. This mutation is c344T>C causing a p.Leu115Pro substitution (traditionally named as codon 114). (Courtesy of A. Tibepu.)

those that remove only one of the two alpha globin genes on any one chromosome (α^+ thalassaemia) and those that remove both of the alpha genes from one chromosome (α° thalassaemia). Although PCR amplification around the alpha globin locus has proved to be rather difficult, the common deletions can now be identified by a reasonably robust Gap-PCR.[15] In these reactions dimethylsulphoxide (DMSO) and betaine are added. Two different multiplex PCR reactions are set up, one for the common α^+ thalassaemias ($-\alpha^{3.7}$ and $-\alpha^{4.2}$) and one for the common α° thalassaemias ($-{}^{SEA}$, $-{}^{MED}$, $-{}^{FIL}$ and $-\alpha^{20.5}$). The fragment generated by these primers across the deletion breakpoint is different in size to a control fragment that is generated from the normal chromosome as a part of the multiplex reaction. The primers that flank the deletion breakpoint are too far apart to generate a fragment from the normal chromosome in the PCR. Only when these are brought closer together as a result of the deletion can a fragment be produced. Primer sequences used in this analysis are given in Table 8.1 and an example of their application in the detection of α thalassaemias is shown in Figure 8.4. More than 30 non-deletional forms of α thalassaemia have been described. Of these, Hb Constant Spring and the $\alpha^{Hph1}\alpha$ mutation are relatively common in South-east Asian and Mediterranean populations, respectively. These can be detected by ASOH, ARMS, restriction enzyme digestion or direct sequencing of the appropriate PCR product. Unlike the β thalassaemias, α thalassaemias are not easily diagnosed using routine haematological techniques. The diagnosis of α thalassaemias is often made following exclusion of β thalassaemia and iron deficiency. Because the vast majority of cases of α thalassaemia are of the clinically benign type (i.e. α^+ thalassaemia), it is debatable whether molecular analysis is justified to reach a diagnosis in these individuals. However, it is important that individuals with α° thalassaemia are identified and

Table 8.1 Primers used in Gap-PCR analysis of α-thalassaemia

PRIMER NAME	SEQUENCE, 5′→3′	CONCENTRATION (μmol/l)
α°	**Multiplex PCR**	**Clark and Thein (2004)[14]**
20.5(F)	GGGCAAGCTGGTGGTGTTACACAGCAACTC	0.1
20.5(R)	CCACGCCCATGCCTGGCACGTTTGCTGAGG	0.1
α/SEA(F)	CTCTGTGTTCTCAGTATTGGAGGGAAGGAG	0.3
α(R)	TGAAGAGCCTGCAGGACCAGGTCAGTGACCG	0.15
MED(F)	CGATGAGAACATAGTGAGCAGAATTGCAGG	0.15
MED(R)	ACGCCGACGTTGCTGCCCAGCTTCTTCCAC	0.15
SEA(R)	ATATATGGGTCTGGAAGTGTATCCCTCCCA	0.15
FIL(F)	AAGAGAATAAACCACCCAATTTTTAAATGGGCA	1.6
FIL(R)	GAGATAATAACCTTTATCTGCCACATGTAGCAA	1.6
α⁺	**Multiplex PCR**	**From JM Old (pers. comm.)**
3.7F	CCCCTCGCCAAGTCCACCC	0.4
3.7/20.5R	AAAGCACTCTAGGGTCCAGCG	0.4
4.2F	GGTTTACCCATGTGGTGCCTC	0.6
4.2R	CCCGTTGGATCTTCTCATTTCCC	0.8
α2R	AGACCAGGAAGGGCCGGTG	0.1
PCR, polymerase chain reaction.		

the only definitive diagnostic test is DNA analysis. The α° thalassaemias are almost entirely restricted to at-risk ethnic groups, particularly those of South-east Asian or Mediterranean origin and so it is most efficient to target these groups specifically. The diagnosis of α° thalassaemia is particularly relevant if prenatal diagnosis is to be offered to a couple who are at risk of having a fetus with hydrops, where there is an increased risk of maternal death at delivery. Guidelines derived from the UK experience as to how and when DNA analysis should be implemented have recently been updated.[16]

DISORDERS OF COAGULATION

Thrombophilia

Considerable advances have been made in our understanding of the genetic risk factors found in patients with venous thromboembolism (VTE).[17] Among these are the diverse mutations causing protein C, protein S and antithrombin deficiency. An increased factor VIII level is also a risk factor for VTE, but the genetic determinants of this are unclear. Homozygosity for the common C677T mutation of the methylenetetrahydrofolate reductase gene, which gives rise to a thermolabile variant of this protein, has been reported to be a risk factor for VTE, although other studies have not supported this claim. A point mutation in the 3′ UTR of the prothrombin gene associated with elevated protein levels has been identified as a genetic risk factor for VTE.[18] The most common of the known genetic risk factors for VTE is a resistance to the anticoagulant effect of activated protein C caused by the Arg506Gln substitution in factor V (factor V Leiden, FVL);[19] around 20% of subjects of north European origin presenting for the first time with thromboembolism are heterozygous for this mutation. Because of their prevalence and because the tests have become relatively simple, there is a tendency toward indiscriminate testing for these genetic risk factors in thrombophilia, but without careful and informed counselling this may often be inappropriate (see also Chapter 19).[20]

Figure 8.4 Detection of α° thalassaemia by multiplex Gap-PCR. The sequences of the primers used are shown in Table 8.1. A normal fragment of 1010 bp is generated by the primers α/SEA(F) and α/(R) in all lanes (although this is very faint in lane 11). In addition, a fragment of 660 bp is generated by the primer pair α/SEA(F) and SEA(R) in lanes 1, 4 and 8 in individuals who are heterozygous for the $-\,-^{SEA}$ deletion; a fragment of 550 bp is generated by the primer pair FIL(F) and FIL(R) in lane 9 in an individual who is heterozygous for the $-\,-^{FIL}$ deletion; a fragment of 875 bp is generated by the primer pair MED(F) and MED(R) in lane 10 in an individual who is heterozygous for the $-\,-^{MED}$ deletion; and a fragment of 1187 bp is generated by the primer pair 20.5(F) and 20.5(R) in lane 10 in an individual who is heterozygous for the $-\alpha^{20.5}$ deletion.

Method

A variety of different methods have been used to detect these mutations and we have recently adopted a Taq-Man-based assay. The reagents are provided by Applied Biosystems and the protocol provided has been adapted as described here. Differentially labelled, but quenched, TaqMan probes hybridize specifically to the normal and mutant alleles in a given patient's sample. Detection of the light that is emitted as the probes are released during the PCR amplification is used to discriminate between the presence of normal and mutant alleles in the sample.

Reagents

All are obtained from Applied Biosystems (Warrington): 96-well optical PCR plate, optical adhesive lid, pipettes and tips, TaqMan Genotyping master mix, FVL genotyping assay (C_11975250_10), PTM genotyping assay (C_8726802_20), ddH2O, Applied Biosystems 7900HT Fast or 7500 Real-Time PCR apparatus.

Method

Defrost the genotyping assay mixes on ice.

In each experiment, include a normal, heterozygous and homozygous control for both the factor V Leiden and the prothrombin mutations; also include three blanks to which no template DNA is added. In the remaining wells, aliquot 2 μl of test DNA into the bottom of the appropriate well.

Prepare a PCR mix for each test using 0.5 μl of the relevant genotyping assay, 10 μl of water and 12.5 μl of the TaqMan Genotyping master mix per sample to be analysed.

Aliquot 23 μl of this PCR mix to each well, seal the plate with the optical adhesive lid and spin briefly.

Use the 'Allele Discrepancy Assay' on the computer associated with the Applied Biosystems 7900HT Fast or 7500 Real-Time PCR System. Thermocycling conditions are a denaturation at 95°C, for 10 min for 1 cycle followed by denaturation at 92°C for 15 s and annealing/extension at 60°C for 60 s, repeated for 40 cycles.

Interpretation

The results can be evaluated using the allelic discrimination plots for the individual genotyping assays. Each data point represents one sample and they can be seen to fall into four clusters according to the genotype of the sample or the absence of the signal in the non-template control (NTC): see Figure 8.5. If the assay has worked, these clusters should be clearly distinct. An automatic genotype annotation is then based on this clustering. Some points will not be automatically called by the software: these data points can be annotated manually by assigning them to the appropriate cluster.

Haemostatic Disorders

Diverse mutations underlie haemophilia A and haemophilia B and these are usually identified in specialized laboratories by screening exons for mutation by single-stranded conformational polymorphism analysis (SSCP), denaturing high-performance liquid chromatography or direct DNA sequence analysis.[21] It may still be relevant to determine carrier status and offer prenatal diagnosis through genetic linkage analysis. Problems with this include the number of sporadic cases, lack of informative markers, unavailable family members and the possibility of recombination.

Of particular diagnostic significance is the fact that from between one-third and one-half of all patients with severe haemophilia A have a large genomic inversion mutation involving recombination between a region in intron 22 of the factor VIII gene and telomeric homologous sequences.[22] These inversions are readily detected by Southern blot analysis using the p482.6 probe[23] to Bcl I digests of genomic DNA. A method has also recently been described using long-distance PCR, enabling identification of these inversion mutations in a single tube reaction (see Chapter 18 for more information on bleeding disorders).[24]

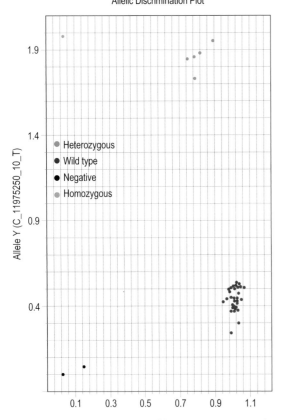

FVL allelic discrimination
Allelic Discrimination Plot

Allele Y (C_11975250_10_T)

- Heterozygous
- Wild type
- Negative
- Homozygous

Figure 8.5 Allelic discrimination of factor V Leiden using the TaqMan assay system. Each spot on the graph represents one well of the plate in which one DNA template is under test. In each well we either see no signal (bottom left) – NTC; only 'red' signals, coming from the wild-type probe (bottom right) – homozygous wild-type; only blue signals coming from the FVL probe (top left) – homozygous FVL; or a mixture of signals to give green spots coming from both the wild-type and FVL probes (top right) – heterozygous for FVL.

LEUKAEMIA AND LYMPHOMA

Cytogenetic Principles and Terminology

Cytogenetic analysis is usually carried out by specially trained cytogeneticists in a separate laboratory that often has no specific relationship to the haematology laboratory. For this reason, no details of techniques will be given. However, cytogenetic analysis is so crucial to the diagnosis and management of haematological neoplasms that it is necessary for haematologists to understand the principles and be able to understand the reports that are received. In addition, haematologists are often involved in collection of appropriate samples.

Classical cytogenetic analysis is carried out on cells that have entered mitosis and have been arrested in metaphase so that individual chromosomes can be recognized by their size and their banding pattern following staining (e.g. Giemsa staining [G-banding] or staining with a fluorescent dye). Alternating dark and light bands are numbered from the centromere toward the telomere to facilitate description of any abnormalities detected. An example showing the balanced translocation t(9;22) (q34;q11) in chronic myelogenous leukaemia (CML) is shown in Figure 8.6. The standard terminology applied to chromosomes is shown in Table 8.2.

The results of cytogenetic analysis may be displayed visually (a karyogram) or written according to standard conventions (a karyotype). Thus, 46,XY,t(3;3)(q21;q26) [20] indicates a pseudodiploid karyotype in a male; a reciprocal translocation has occurred between the paired chromosomes 3, following a break at 3q21 on one chromosome (i.e. involving the long arm of chromosome 3, band 2, sub-band 1) and at 3q26 on the other. The abnormality has been detected in 20 metaphases. 46,XY,inv(3) (q21q26) indicates a pseudodiploid karyotype with a paracentric inversion of the long arm of a single chromosome 3; the breakpoints are the same as in the first example but are on a single chromosome. Note the use of semicolons in describing a translocation, whereas these are absent from the notation of an inversion. Numbers shown within square brackets in a karyotype indicate the number of cells showing the specified normal or abnormal finding. Cytogenetic analysis can be carried out on the following:

1. Skin fibroblasts or phytohaemagglutinin (PHA)-stimulated lymphocytes (to study constitutional abnormalities)
2. Bone marrow cells
3. Blood cells
4. Cells isolated from lymph nodes or other organs suspected of being infiltrated by a lymphoid or other neoplasm
5. Cells isolated from serous effusions
6. Amniocytes, isolated from the amniotic fluid.

In studying suspected haematological neoplasms, there are two reasons for seeking to detect constitutional abnormalities. First, there may be a constitutional abnormality underlying a haematological neoplasm as when megakaryoblastic leukaemia occurs in Down syndrome. Second, there may be an irrelevant and previously undetected constitutional chromosomal abnormality that has to be recognized so that it can be distinguished from an acquired chromosomal abnormality associated with a neoplastic process.

The indications for cytogenetic analysis in a definite or suspected haematological neoplasm are as follows:

Figure 8.6 G-Banded karyotype. Female karyotype with a balanced reciprocal translocation between chromosomes 9 and 22 (arrowed) giving rise to the Philadelphia chromosome (Ph). *(Courtesy of J. Howard.)*

- To provide evidence of clonality and permit a diagnosis of a neoplastic condition when this is not otherwise demonstrated (e.g. in some patients with eosinophilia or an increase in natural killer lymphocytes)
- To confirm a specific diagnosis (e.g. acute promyelocytic leukaemia, Burkitt lymphoma)
- To permit classification (e.g. to apply the World Health Organization classification of acute myeloid leukaemia, acute lymphoblastic leukaemia [ALL], the myelodysplastic syndromes [MDS], non-Hodgkin lymphoma and neoplasms associated with rearrangement of *PDGFRB* or *FGFR1*)
- To give prognostic information (e.g. the detection of hyperdiploidy [prognostically good] in ALL)

- To indicate which fusion genes are likely to be present and thus give information permitting detection of minimal residual disease by molecular analysis
- To distinguish a phenotypic switch occurring within a single clone from a therapy-related leukaemia
- To distinguish therapy-related acute leukaemia following alkylating agents from that following topoisomerase II-interactive drugs.

For investigation of haematological neoplasms, a bone marrow aspirate is usually the preferred tissue. It is also possible to disaggregate bone marrow cells from a trephine biopsy specimen into tissue culture medium. Peripheral blood may yield metaphases when large numbers of immature cells are present, but it is generally less reliable than the bone marrow in yielding dividing cells. In theory, any infiltrated tissue can provide cells that can be

Table 8.2 Terminology and abbreviations used in classical cytogenetic analysis

TERM	ABBREVIATION	EXPLANATION
Centromere	cen	The junction of the short and long arms of a chromosome
Telomere	ter	The termination of the short or long arm of a chromosome, pter or qter
Long arm	q	The longer of the two arms of the chromosome that are joined at the centromere
Short arm	p	The shorter of the two arms of the chromosome that are joined at the centromere
Diploid		Having the full complement of 46 chromosomes, 44 paired autosomes and two sex chromosomes in a cell or clone
Haploid		Having 23 chromosomes, a single copy of each autosome and either an X or a Y chromosome in a cell or clone
Tetraploid		Having a total of 92 chromosomes, four of each autosome and four sex chromosomes in a cell or clone
Aneuploid		Having a chromosome number that is neither diploid nor a fraction or a multiple of the diploid number, in a cell or clone
Pseudodiploid		Having 46 chromosomes in a cell or clone but with either structural abnormalities or with loss and gain of different chromosomes so that not all chromosomes are paired
Hyperdiploid		The presence of more than 46 chromosomes in a cell or clone
Hypodiploid		The presence of fewer than 46 chromosomes in a cell or clone
Monosomy	− (a minus sign before the chromosome number, e.g. −7)	Loss of one of a pair of chromosomes
Trisomy	+ (a plus sign before the chromosome number, e.g. +13)	Gain of a chromosome so that there are three rather than two copies
Deletion	del or a minus sign after the number and the designation of the arm of a chromosome, e.g. del(20q) or 20q−	Loss of part of the long or the short arm of a chromosome
Translocation	t	Movement of a chromosomal segment or segments between two or more chromosomes; a translocation can be reciprocal or non-reciprocal
Reciprocal translocation		Exchange of segments between two or more chromosomes
Non-reciprocal translocation		Movement of a segment of a chromosome from one chromosome to another but without reciprocity
Balanced translocation		A translocation that occurs without loss of chromosomal material or at least without loss of sufficient chromosomal material to be detectable by microscopic examination of chromosomes
Unbalanced translocation		A translocation that is associated with gain or loss of part of a chromosome

Table 8.2 Terminology and abbreviations used in classical cytogenetic analysis – cont'd

TERM	ABBREVIATION	EXPLANATION
Inversion	inv	The inversion of a part of a chromosome, either pericentric or paracentric
Pericentric inversion		An inversion that follows breaking of both the long and short arms so that the part of the chromosome that is inverted includes the centromere
Paracentric inversion		An inversion that follows the occurrence of two breaks in either the long or the short arm of a chromosome so that the part of the chromosome that is inverted does not include the centromere
Insertion	ins	The insertion of a segment of one chromosome into another chromosome or into a different position on the same chromosomes. Can be direct or inverted
Isochromosome	i	A chromosome with two long arms or two short arms joined at the centromere, e.g. i(17q)
Derivative	der	A chromosome that is derived from another; a derivative chromosome derived from two or more chromosomes carries the number of the chromosome that contributed the centromere
Duplication	dup	The duplication of part of a chromosome
Clone		A population of cells derived from a single cell; in cytogenetic analysis a clone is considered to be present if two cells share the same structural abnormality or extra chromosome or if three cells have lost the same chromosome
Marker	mar	An abnormal chromosome of uncertain origin that 'marks' a clone
Constitutional	c	A chromosomal abnormality that is part of the constitution of an individual rather than being acquired, e.g. +21c in Down syndrome

disaggregated and analysed. In haematological practice it is mainly lymph node cells that are studied, but clinically relevant information is sometimes obtained from other infiltrated tissues.

A bone marrow aspirate for cytogenetic analysis should be anticoagulated by the addition of preservative-free heparin or tissue culture medium containing heparin. It can be stored at room temperature for some hours or at 4°C if delay in analysis is expected. If it is being sent to a central laboratory, detailed clinical and haematological information must accompany the sample so that the central laboratory is aware if there is clinical urgency in obtaining results and so that appropriate techniques are used.

Fluorescence *in situ* Hybridization

Fluorescence *in situ* hybridization (FISH) bridges classical cytogenetic analysis and molecular diagnostic techniques. Chromosomes can be stained and visualized but the technique is also dependent on the recognition of specific DNA sequences by means of a fluorescent probe that can anneal to a specific DNA sequence. FISH can be carried out on metaphase preparations or on cells in interphase. FISH probes may identify the following:

- Centromeres of a specific chromosome (useful for detecting trisomy or monosomy and chimerism following sex-mismatched bone marrow transplantation; Fig. 8.7A)
- Specific oncogenes (locus-specific probe, useful for detecting translocations; Fig. 8.7B,C)
- Specific tumour-suppressor genes (locus-specific probe, loss is relevant to tumour progression)
- Other diagnostically useful genes (locus-specific probe, for example, for the *CHIC2* gene, which is lost when an interstitial deletion leads to formation of a *FIP1L1–PDGFRA* fusion gene)
- Whole chromosomes (whole chromosome painting, useful in identifying complex chromosomal rearrangements).

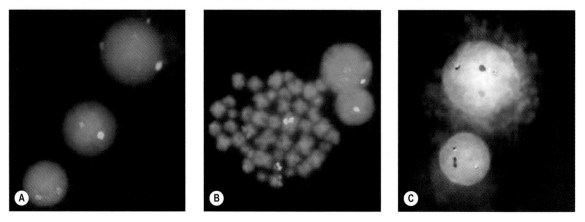

Figure 8.7 Fluorescence *in situ* hybridization (FISH). (A) Use of the X/Y dual-label probe (Abbott Diagnostics, Vysis) in a sex-mismatched bone marrow transplant patient. Two interphases show 1 red signal (X chromosome) and 1 green signal (Y chromosome) indicating male cells, whereas one interphase shows 2 red signals (X chromosomes) indicating a female cell. (B) Use of the *BCR/ABL* dual-colour, dual-fusion translocation probe (Abbott Diagnostics, Vysis). One metaphase and one interphase cell show 2 red signals (from the *ABL1* gene on chromosome 9) and 2 green signals (from the *BCR* gene on chromosome 22). These cells are therefore negative for the *BCR–ABL1* gene fusion at the molecular cytogenetic level. (C) Use of the *BCR–ABL* dual-colour, dual-fusion translocation probe (Abbott Diagnostics, Vysis). Interphase cells show 2 red/green fusion signals (from the *BCR–ABL1* fusion on chromosome 22 and the *ABL1-BCR* fusion on chromosome 9), 1 red signal (*ABL1* gene on chromosome 9) and 1 green signal (*BCR* gene on chromosome 22). This sample is therefore positive for the *BCR–ABL1* gene fusion at the molecular cytogenetic level. *(Courtesy of J. Howard.)*

- Advantages of FISH analysis in comparison with conventional chromosomal analysis include the following:
  - Many more cells can be examined (useful for detecting residual disease)
  - Metaphases are not essential, so abnormalities can be detected in non-dividing cells (useful in chronic lymphocytic leukaemia)
  - FISH can be performed in a shorter period of time (may be critical in confirming a diagnosis of acute promyelocytic leukaemia)
- Abnormalities that cannot be detected by conventional cytogenetic analysis may be detected [e.g. *SIL–TAL* fusion in T-lineage ALL or t(12;21)(p12;q22) in B-lineage ALL].

The main disadvantage is that only those abnormalities that are specifically sought will be found, whereas conventional cytogenetic analysis permits all chromosom'ses to be evaluated.

Translocations, Molecular Analysis and Minimal Residual Disease

The accurate characterization of haematological malignancies at the chromosomal and molecular level has advanced greatly in recent years and now makes an important contribution to initial treatment decisions. For example, many patients with acute leukaemia, CML and non-Hodgkin lymphoma have specific chromosomal lesions known to be associated with particularly favourable or unfavourable prognoses and the proportion of such patients with defined chromosomal lesions is increasing. The presence of a specific molecular abnormality may indicate the need for specific treatment (e.g. all-*trans*-retinoic acid [ATRA] or As$_2$O$_3$ when *PML–RARA* is detected or the use of a tyrosine kinase inhibitor when *BCR–ABL1* is detected). Usually cytogenetic abnormalities indicate the molecular lesion that is present, but in some cases molecular techniques are more informative.

The Philadelphia (Ph) chromosome (22q–) present in 95% of cases of CML may be identified by routine cytogenetic studies; its presence can be confirmed by demonstrating the presence of the *BCR–ABL1* fusion gene by RT-PCR. The Ph chromosome may also be found in 25% and 5% of adult and childhood ALL, respectively,[25] where it is associated with relatively poorer prognosis and indicates the need for specific therapy including a tyrosine kinase inhibitor. Patients suspected of having CML should be tested for *BCR–ABL1* for definitive diagnosis. Patients with apparent essential thrombocythaemia who do not have a *JAK2* mutation should also be tested for *BCR–ABL1*. To optimize clinical management, patients with ALL should likewise be tested for *BCR–ABL1*; in adult patients this should be regarded as an essential investigation.

Small cleaved lymphoid cells are observed in a number of conditions with different treatments and prognoses. In such cases, detection of t(11;14) involving *CCND1* indicates mantle cell lymphoma, whereas identification of t(14;18) involving *BCL2* implies a follicular lymphoma.[26] The former is much more aggressive with poor prognosis, thus requiring a more intensive treatment. Translocations associated with lymphomas often lead to the dysregulation of a normal gene: for example t(14;18) places the *BCL2* gene adjacent to the *IGH* locus, leading to dysregulation of *BCL2*. In contrast, the acute leukaemia-associated translocations often give rise to a chimeric gene that is transcribed: for example t(15;17), which yields a novel *PML–RARA* fusion gene.[27]

Frequently, the breakpoints within the translocation are too far apart to allow direct amplification of DNA by PCR. In such cases, the mRNA from the fusion gene can be reverse transcribed using RT to yield cDNA, which can then be amplified by PCR. In addition, RT-PCR is an exquisitely sensitive tool that has been exploited in the detection of residual disease.[28] We will illustrate this in the analysis of the *BCR–ABL1* fusion gene and describe the analysis of other translocations on p. 168.

BCR–ABL1 Reverse Transcriptase-Polymerase Chain Reaction

Principle and Interpretation

The *BCR–ABL1* analysis is performed by two-stage RT-PCR. The RNA extracted from nucleated cells is reverse transcribed by RT to generate coding or cDNA using random primers

6 bp long (hexamers). Following the RT step, the samples are subjected to multiplex PCR, to test for the presence or absence of *BCR–ABL1*.[29] Multiplex PCR is similar to conventional PCR but includes more than one pair of primers in a single PCR test. This strategy enables the detection of the vast majority of the *BCR–ABL1* transcripts. The most commonly observed transcripts are b3a2 (e14a2), b2a2 (e13a2) and e1a2, giving rise to 385, 310 and 481 bp amplicons, respectively (Fig. 8.8). However, the identification of fragments of different sizes may be indicative of the presence of a 'variant fusion gene' such as e6a2 (1125 bp), e6a3 (951 bp), e8a2 (1319 bp), e8a3 (1145 bp) or e19a2 (908 bp).

In addition to *BCR–ABL1*, the normal *BCR* gene is co-amplified, yielding an 808 bp amplicon. The co-amplification of *BCR* is an indication of the quality of RNA and the efficiency of cDNA synthesis. Absence of any fragments indicates failure of the procedure. The latter is often the result of an aged sample (i.e. more than 72 h old). For RT-PCR analysis, the sample should be processed to lysate stage (see Nuclear lysate preparation, below) within 48 h of collection. In addition, the *BCR* fragment is often not observed in diagnostic samples where the *BCR–ABL1* is preferentially amplified.

If *BCR–ABL1* is undetectable by multiplex PCR in follow-up samples from patients undergoing therapy, the

Figure 8.8 Detection of minimal residual disease in chronic myelogenous leukaemia (CML) by reverse transcriptase-polymerase chain reaction (RT-PCR). (A) Diagrammatic representation of the processed exons of the *BCR* and *ABL1* genes together with the relative position of the B2B and C5e-primers used to co-amplify *BCR* in the multiplex PCR. (B) Commonly observed *BCR–ABL1* derivatives, b2a2 and b3a2 which give rise to p210 *BCR–ABL1* and e1a2, which gives rise to p190 *BCR–ABL1*. The relative positions of the primers used to amplify the chimeric transcripts by multiplex PCR are shown. (C) A 2.0% agarose gel containing SYBR Safe dye through which amplicons generated by multiplex PCR using complementary DNA (cDNA) from five patients (lanes 1 to 5) were electrophoresed. The co-amplified normal *BCR* fragment, 808 bp in length, is seen in all samples except for the lanes containing the blank controls (B). The diagnostic sample from a patient with suspected CML, in lane 2, revealed a fragment corresponding to the b3a2 *BCR–ABL1* transcript, 385 bp in length, in addition to the *BCR* amplicon. *BCR–ABL1* is not detectable in lanes 1, 3, 4 and 5 containing follow-up samples from patients following stem cell transplantation (SCT). (D) The cDNA of these individuals was subjected to nested PCR to exclude residual disease. This reveals *BCR–ABL1* transcripts, b3a2 (385 bp) and b2a2 (310 bp) in lanes 1 and 4, previously undetectable by the less sensitive multiplex PCR. However, *BCR–ABL1* is not detectable in lanes 3 and 5, implying these samples are from patients in molecular remission post-SCT. B, blank controls; K (K562-b3a2) and BV (BV173-b2a2), positive controls; M, molecular size marker.

cDNA is tested at higher level of sensitivity by nested PCR.[30] Nested PCR enables the detection of one leukaemic cell in a background of 10^5 to 10^6 normal cells. The choice of primers for nested PCR is dependent on the type of transcript detected by multiplex PCR at presentation. The primers for e14a2 and e13a2 are the same; however, for e1a2 transcript a different set of primers is used. The nested PCR yields fragments of 385 bp (e14a2), 310 bp (e13a2) or 481 bp (e1a2) in length. Nested PCR is not indicated for testing cDNA from a patient suspected of having CML. Diagnosis is made by expression of *BCR–ABL1* by multiplex PCR. Furthermore, in post-therapy samples this will indicate molecular relapse.

Reagents

×10 concentrated red cell lysis buffer (RCLB). For 3 l, weigh 248.7 g of NH_4Cl (1.55 mol/l), 30.03 g of $KHCO_3$ (0.1 mol/l). Add 6 ml of 0.5 mol/l EDTA (0.1 mmol/l), pH 7.4, make up to 3 l with sterile water and store at 4°C
RCLB. Make 500 ml of ×10 RCLB up to 5 l with sterile water and cool to 4°C. Adjust the working solution pH to 7.4 with HCl and store at 4°C
1 mol/l citrate, pH 7.0. Neutralize 1 mol/l trisodium citrate with 1 mol/l citric acid
Sodium acetate. 3 mol/l sodium acetate is adjusted to pH 5.2 with glacial acetic acid
Guanidinium thiocyanate (GTC). Because GTC is highly toxic, it is advisable to use the entire amount as purchased from the manufacturer, rather than weighing a required amount. Thus, with 1 kg of GTC add 21.15 ml of 0.5 mol/l EDTA (5.0 mmol/l), pH 8.0, 52.87 ml of 1 mol/l citrate, pH 7.0, 35.25 ml of 30% Sarkosyl (0.5%) and make up to 2.115 l with sterile water. Store this solution in 50 ml aliquots. Add 7.1 µl of β-mercaptoethanol per ml of GTC immediately before use.

Solutions for the Complementary DNA Mix

5 mg/ml random hexamer primers: reconstitute 50 U pdN_6 (Pharmacia) with 539 µl of sterile water and add 21 µl of 0.5 mol/l KCl
5′ RT-buffer (usually supplied) with M-MLV reverse transcriptase (RT): 0.25 mol/l Tris-HCl, pH 8.3, 0.375 mmol/l KCl, 15 mmol/l $MgCl_2$
25 mM dNTP stock: Mix an equal volume of ultrapure 100 mmol/l dATP, dCTP, dGTP and dTTP 0.1 M dithiothreitol (DTT), which is usually supplied with M-MLV RT
cDNA mix: To 428 µl of 5′ RT-buffer, add 21.5 µl of DTT, 85.5 µl of 25 mmol/l dNTPs and 45 µl of 5 mg/ml random hexamers; make up to 1000 µl with sterile water.

The compositions for the multiplex and nested PCR mixes are given in Table 8.3, including the optimum $MgCl_2$ concentration for each mix as well as the primers used in the different PCR reactions.

Methods

Nuclear lysate preparation

1. Either blood or bone marrow aspirate can be analysed for MRD in CML, although bone marrow aspirates are preferred for ALL MRD studies. Centrifuge the anticoagulated peripheral blood sample at 700 *g* for 15 min. Bone marrow aspirates can be dealt with in the same way as buffy coats by proceeding directly to Step 4.
2. Carefully remove and discard the plasma, taking care not to disturb the buffy coat.
3. Using a sterile plastic Pasteur pipette, collect the buffy coat and transfer it to a 50 ml polypropylene tube. It is not necessary to collect all of the buffy coat layer if the white cell count is >50 × 10^9/l.
4. To lyse the contaminating red cells, resuspend the buffy coat in ice-cold RCLB to a final volume of 50 ml and vortex for a few seconds. The suspension is then incubated on wet ice for 10 min, inverting the tube occasionally.
5. Centrifuge again at 700 *g* for 10 min and discard the supernatant by inverting the tube, taking care not to lose the nuclear pellet.
6. Repeat steps 4 and 5 until the nuclear pellet is void of pink-red colour. Usually two washes with RCLB are sufficient.
7. Wash the nuclear pellet once with 20–30 ml of phosphate buffered saline (PBS) by centrifuging at 700 *g* for 10 min.
8. Resuspend the nuclear pellet in 1–2 ml GTC containing β-mercaptoethanol. Homogenize the suspension by passing it through a 2 ml syringe and 21G needle repeatedly until it loses its viscosity (i.e. the DNA is degraded). In some cases, it may be necessary to add more GTC.
9. The lysate can now be stored at −20°C or −70°C for several years.

RNA extraction

There are several protocols, including commercially available kits, yielding RNA of varying qualities. Qiagen extraction columns are used in our laboratory. The protocol described in the following, originally described by Chomczynski and Sacchi,[31] can easily be applied in a clinical laboratory.

1. Add 50 µl of 2 M NaOAc, pH 4.0, to 500 µl of GTC lysate in a 1.5 ml microcentrifuge tube and vortex briefly.
2. Add 500 µl of un-neutralized water saturated phenol and 100 µl of chloroform. Vortex the mixture for 10 s and transfer to wet ice for 20 min.
3. Centrifuge at 12 000 *g* for 30 min at 4°C.
4. After centrifugation, two distinct layers should be clearly discernible; if not, add a further 50 ml of chloroform. Vortex for 10 s and centrifuge again for

Table 8.3 Composition of PCR mixes used in the amplification of *BCR–ABL1* to create restriction enzyme recognition sites

| | MULTIPLEX PCR | NESTED PCR | | | |
| | | P210 | | P190 | |
		1ST STEP	2ND STEP	1ST STEP	2ND STEP
PCR buffer (×10)	1.2×	1.25×	1.0×	1.25×	1.0×
MgCl$_2$ (mmol/l)	1.8	3.125	1.75	2.25	1.75
dNTP (µmol/l)	240	250	200	250	200
Primer 1 (µmol/l)	C5e– (0.6)	NB1+ (0.625)	CA3– (0.5)	BCR 1+ (0.625)	CA3– (0.5)
Primer 2 (µmol/l)	CA3– (0.6)	Abl3– (0.625)	B2A (0.5)	Ab13– (0.625)	E1N+ (0.5)
Primer 3 (µmol/l)	B2B (0.6)				
Primer 4 (µmol/l)	BCR-C (0.6)				

Primer sequences are as follows:

BCR1+: 5′ GAA CTC GCA ACA GTC CTT CGA C 3′

BCR-C: 5′ ACC GCA TGT TCC GGG ACA AAA G 3′

C5e–: 5′ ata ggaTCC TTT GCA ACC GGG TCT GAA 3′[a]

NB1+: 5′ GAG CGT GCA GAG TGG AGG GAG AAC A 3′

Ab13–: 5′ GGT ACC AGG AGT GTT TCT CCA GAC TG 3′

B2A: 5′ TTC AGA AGC TTC TCC CTG ACA T 3′

CA3–: 5′ TGT TCA CTG GCG TGA TGT AGT TGC TTG G 3′

E1N+: 5′ AGA TCT GGC CCA ACG ATG ACG A 3′

PCR, polymerase chain reaction.
[a]Lower case letters represent changes introduced to create restriction enzyme site (underlined).

---

30 min at 4°C. Transfer the upper aqueous layer to another 1.5 ml microcentrifuge tube, taking care not to disturb the interface.

5. Add an equal volume of propan-2-ol (isopropanol), cap the tube, mix by inverting and incubate at –20°C for 2 h or overnight.

6. Microcentrifuge for 30 min at 4°C and discard the supernatant, taking care not to lose the pellet, which may be hard to see.

7. Wash the pellet in 1 ml of 80% ethanol. Do not mix. Centrifuge directly for 30 min at 4°C and discard the supernatant. Re-centrifuge briefly to collect the residual ethanol and discard using a micropipette.

8. Air dry the pellet for 10 min and reconstitute in 20–40 µl of sterile water. The RNA must be stored at –70°C. However, immediate reverse transcription is the preferred option.

cDNA synthesis

1. Incubate 19 µl of RNA in a 1.5 ml microcentrifuge tube (approx. 20 µg) at 65°C for 10 min. This is to denature the RNA, which readily forms secondary structures, reducing the efficiency of the reverse transcriptase. Centrifuge at 12 000 *g* briefly to collect the condensation to the bottom of the tube. Transfer the tube to wet ice.

2. On the wet ice, add 21 µl of cDNA mix containing 300 u M-MLV RT and 30 u of RNAsin.

3. Incubate the mixture at 37°C for 2 h. When using gene-specific primers in this reaction, the temperature should be increased to 42°C.

4. Terminate the reaction by incubating the mixture at 65°C for 10 min. cDNA can be stored at –20°C.

Multiplex PCR

Add 2 μl of cDNA to 20 μl of multiplex PCR mix (Table 8.3); add 0.5 u of Taq polymerase. Overlay with 1 drop of mineral oil and amplify using conditions as described in Appendix A. Carry out electrophoresis on the PCR products through 2.0% agarose gel containing SYBR Safe dye.

Nested PCR

Transfer 1 μl of the PCR products from the first-step to 19 μl of the second-step PCR mix (Table 8.3). Overlay with 1 drop of mineral oil and amplify using an annealing temperature of 64°C for 50 s. Then electrophorese the PCR products through 2.0% agarose gel containing SYBR Safe dye. The procedure for nested PCR is the same for both p210 (b3a2 and b2a2) and p190 (e1a2).

Monitoring Minimal Residual Disease

Effective clinical management of haematological malignancies depends on accurate and precise measurement of a patient's response to therapeutic agents. This includes examination of cellular morphology in peripheral blood and marrow specimens. Although these studies are essential, they lack sensitivity; therefore, the malignant clone has frequently expanded considerably before relapse is recognized. The last three decades have seen a remarkable advance in the development of technology to monitor patients' response to therapy to a sensitivity of 1 in 10^5 (i.e. the detection of one malignant cell in a background of 100 000 normal cells). To enable this, a disease-specific marker is essential, as illustrated by targeting the novel fusion gene BCR–ABL1, which maps to the Philadelphia chromosome associated with CML. The principal aim is to detect and measure MRD using the most sensitive techniques available to a clinical laboratory with accuracy and precision and thus recognize early signs of relapse. The clinical utility of such studies has been amply confirmed by close and regular measurement of MRD in patients with CML. This is increasingly being shown to apply to other adult and childhood leukaemias using disease-specific markers.

For purposes of clarity and because of space limitation, we will focus on CML to describe the principle and aims of MRD studies. Although qualitative PCR (i.e. multiplex and nested PCR; see above) is very useful, it provides no information about the kinetics of the disease. The latter can only be obtained by measuring the tumour load; this is achieved by quantification of BCR–ABL1 mRNA molecules.

Because the amount of total RNA added to each reverse transcription reaction and its quality (i.e. the degree of degradation) are variable, the transcripts of a housekeeping gene are quantified as an endogenous control. Furthermore, amplification of an endogenous control gene also allows for the inter-sample PCR dynamics variation. There are a number of control genes that can be used as endogenous control genes (e.g. GAPDH, B2M (β₂-microglobulin) and ABL1). An endogenous control gene should not be too highly expressed and should show no inter-sample variation in levels of expression; also, there should be no related pseudogenes or alternative splicing.[32] The introduction of real-time quantitative reverse transcriptase PCR (qRT-PCR) at the end of the last millennium made quantification of MRD more widely accessible.

Principle

qRT-PCR permits quantification of number of transcripts of gene of interest at high levels of sensitivity. This is achieved by developing a technology that permits the detection of PCR products as they accumulate. Furthermore, the rate of accumulation is proportional to the number of mRNA molecules of the target gene in the starting material during the exponential phase of the PCR. The accumulation of amplicons is detected by including a sequence-specific probe labelled with fluorochromes in addition to the primers as in a conventional PCR (Fig. 8.9). Since the advent of qRT-PCR several types of probes have been developed, although all are dependent on the fluorescence resonance energy transfer (FRET) principle. The two commonly used systems involve hybridization or hydrolysis of the probe. A widely used methodology is TaqMan, which involves hydrolysis of the probe.[33] This technology is based on the 5′ exonuclease assay, which exploits the inherent 5′ to 3′ exonuclease activity of the Taq DNA polymerase.[34] The Taq DNA polymerase cleaves a dual-labelled probe annealed to the target sequence during PCR amplification (Fig. 8.10A). Briefly, the cDNA synthesized from total RNA is added to the PCR reaction containing standard PCR components plus a probe that anneals to the template between the two primers as per conventional PCR. The probe has a fluorescent reporter dye, FAM, at the 5′-end (6′carboxyfluorescein; emission $\lambda_{max} = 518$ nm) and quencher dye, TAMRA, at the 3′-end (6-carboxy-tetramethyl-rhodamine; emission $\lambda_{max} = 582$ nm). While the probe is intact, the proximity of the quencher greatly reduces the fluorescence emitted by the reporter dye by Förster resonance energy transfer (FRET).[35] Adequate quenching is observed for probes with the reporter dye at the 5′ end and the quencher at the 3′ end.

Thus, while TAMRA and FAM are closely attached to the probe, fluorescence from the reporter dye is quenched by TAMRA. During PCR, as the Taq DNA polymerase replicates the DNA strand to which the TaqMan probe is annealed, the probe is degraded by the intrinsic 5′–3′ exonuclease activity of the polymerase. The effect is to dissociate FAM from TAMRA; therefore FRET is no longer applicable and fluorescence from FAM can be detected by a laser integrated in the sequence detector (TaqMan ABI 7500 Real-Time PCR system, Applied Biosystems, Warrington). Fluorescence increases in each cycle, proportional to the rate of probe degradation. The number of cycles taken for the fluorescence to cross a threshold value

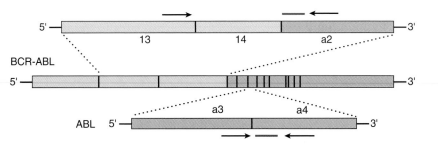

Figure 8.9 Probes and primers. The position of probes and primers used for quantification of *BCR–ABL1* and *ABL1* transcripts are shown. The *BCR–ABL1* fusion gene is shown in yellow- and purple-filled boxes, with the yellow representing the exons derived from the *BCR* gene and purple those originating from the *ABL1* gene. The dual-labelled probes are shown as red lines and primers are shown as arrows. Probes and primers were designed using the Primer Express software to detect e13a2 and e14a2 junctions in a single reaction by qRT-PCR. The *BCR–ABL1* (FAM-cccttcagcggccagtagcatctga-TAMRA) and *ABL1* (FAM-tgcttctgatggcaagctctacgtctcct-TAMRA) probes are dual labelled with 6-carboxyfluorescein (FAM) and 6-carboxy-tetramethyl-rhodamine (TAMRA). *BCR–ABL1* forward primer: 5′-tccgctgaccatcaayaagga-3′; *BCR–ABL1* reverse primer: 5′-cactcagaccctgaggctcaa-3′; *ABL1* forward primer: 5′-gatacgaagggagggtgtacca-3′; *ABL1* reverse primer: 5′-ctcggccagggtgttgaa-3′. The *BCR–ABL* probe and primer set was designed in association with Europe Against Cancer Collaborative study.

of 10× the standard deviation of baseline emission is used for quantitative measurement. The threshold is set significantly above the baseline and can be adjusted manually. The upper baseline limit can be altered by the operator. The fluorescence is plotted as ΔRN against number of cycles (Fig. 8.10B), where $\Delta RN = (Rn^+) - (Rn^-)$. The Passive reference, ROX (6-carboxy-X-rhodamine), is included in the qRT-PCR Universal master mix. The formulae used to calculate the Rn^+ and Rn^- follow:

From PCR with template :

$$Rn^+ = \frac{\text{Emission intensity of reporter}}{\text{Emission intensity of passive reference (ROX)}}$$

and from PCR without template or early cycles of PCR:

$$Rn^- = \frac{\text{Emission intensity of reporter}}{\text{Emission intensity of passive reference (ROX)}}$$

The number of cycles taken to pass the defined threshold is called the cycle threshold (Ct) and it is inversely proportional to the quantity of target starting material. The number of transcripts of the target is read off a standard curve. The quantity of target gene and endogenous control gene transcripts are measured off their respective standard curves, generated from dilutions of the appropriate plasmids and run on each plate. The level of expression of the target gene is then reported as a percentage ratio of the target gene to the control gene to obtain a normalized value for the gene of interest independent of the integrity of the RNA and efficiency of the reverse transcription reaction.

Interpretation

Patients who achieve complete cytogenetic remission may still harbour up to 1×10^{10} leukaemic cells. The kinetics of the leukaemic load in these patients and their response to therapeutic agents can only be monitored by measuring MRD.[36] However, it should be noted that patients in whom qRT-PCR fails to detect *BCR–ABL1* may still harbour up to 1×10^6 leukaemic cells. Of those who are in complete cytogenetic remission $(BCR–ABL1/ABL1) \times 100$ is invariably <2.0%. Investigators previously reported that patients who achieve $(BCR–ABL1/ABL1) \times 100$ <0.045% while receiving α-interferon therapy have a considerably reduced risk of cytogenetic relapse.[37] More recently, qRT-PCR has been used to monitor patients being treated with imatinib. An international multicentre study showed that a 3 log reduction in *BCR–ABL1* copies was consistent with a good prognosis.[38] Quantification of *BCR–ABL1* also helps to identify patients at risk of relapse and therefore provides a window for early clinical intervention with the aim of reversing disease progression. For patients who have undergone stem cell transplantation (SCT) this generally means infusion of lymphocytes isolated from the original donor (i.e. adoptive immunotherapy). Although there is some debate as to the precise criteria for molecular relapse, there is little doubt that a confirmed 1 log increase in *BCR–ABL1* transcripts is clinically significant (i.e. from 0.002% to 0.02%). Patients who achieve a 0.02% *BCR–ABL1/ABL1* ratio on three consecutive occasions are said to be in molecular relapse.

Advantages of qRT-PCR

The major advantage of qRT-PCR is the ability to detect accumulation of amplicons during the exponential phase of PCR. This permits quantification of the DNA of interest in the starting material. This is not possible with conventional PCR because samples are analysed at the end of the PCR run and therefore any differences in the copy number between samples in the starting material are generally not discernible. This is illustrated by the amplification plot shown in Figure 8.10B, where all the samples at the end

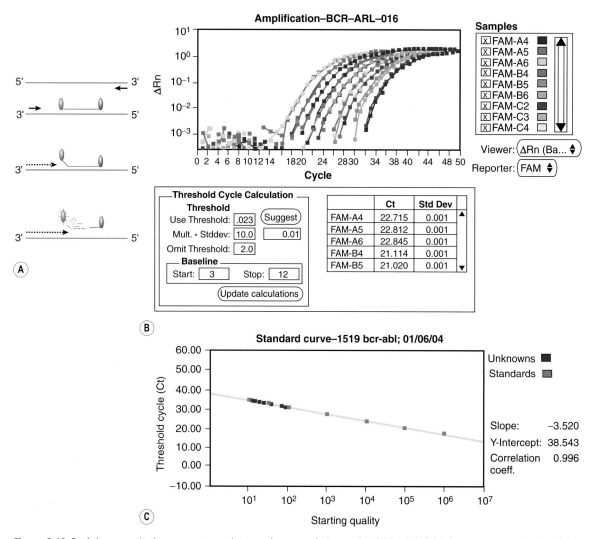

Figure 8.10 Real-time quantitative reverse-transcriptase polymerase chain reaction (qRT-PCR). (A) Schematic representation of the principle of real-time PCR. The forward and reverse primers (*blue lines*) are extended by the *Taq* DNA polymerase as per conventional PCR. The quencher (*red symbol*) suppresses the fluorescence from the reporter (*green symbol*) dye while the two are attached to the probe. As the forward primer is extended, the probe is displaced and is cleaved by the *Taq* DNA polymerase 5′–3′ exonuclease activity. Fluorescence is detected once the reporter dissociates from the quencher on probe being degraded and the synthesis of the new DNA continues to completion. Therefore the fluorescence increases with increment in number of amplicons. (B) Amplification plot. The real-time PCR amplification plot of the standards in log increments is shown. A 0.5 log standard between 10 and 100 *BCR–ABL1* copies is included. The number of cycles for the fluorescence to cross the threshold is reported as Ct (cycle threshold). The greater the number of copies, the lower the Ct value (i.e. it is inversely proportional). (C) A standard curve. A standard curve drawn from qPCR data from serial dilutions of plasmid containing *BCR–ABL1* (*black symbols*) is shown. The *BCR–ABL1* transcripts for the unknown samples (*red symbols*) are read off the standard curve.

of 50 cycles have the same level of fluorescence, despite having varying target copy numbers in the starting material as seen in the exponential phase of the PCR. Post-PCR handling is eliminated. On completion of an assay, the sealed microtitre plate is discarded, thereby minimizing risk of contamination. This also eliminates the need to handle stained gels on completion of the qRT-PCR assay.

The qRT-PCR offers a higher level of specificity because, in addition to primers annealing to DNA sequence of interest, a third oligonucleotide (the probe) anneals to the region between the primers at a higher temperature. To achieve a level of sensitivity that is similar to qRT-PCR, nested conventional PCR is required, but this is associated with a greater risk of contamination. Conventional PCR is also less amenable to automation. More importantly, because qRT-PCR can be automated, inter-laboratory standardization becomes feasible when measuring patients' responses to therapy. This permits rapid evaluation of new therapeutic modalities because methodology and protocols can be standardized, permitting international inter-laboratory studies.

With the aim of administrating an optimum dose it is critical to ensure negligible inter-laboratory variation as patients move from one place to another. This would also assist in simplifying multicentre therapeutic agent clinical trials as best illustrated by International Normalized Ratio (INR) for prothrombin time, used to monitor patients whose coagulation status is controlled with the anticoagulant warfarin. There have been efforts to establish a single internationally recognized scale for monitoring CML patients and this may be soon achieved by the establishment of a calibrated and accredited primary reference reagent for *BCR–ABL1* q-PCR assays.[39]

Reagents

×2 Universal master mix. The ×2 Universal master mix contains dATP, dCTP, dGTP and dTTP at 200 µmol/l each, 5.5 mmol/l $MgCl_2$ and 0.025 µmol/l AmpliTaq-Gold. It also contains the passive background reference dye, ROX. The Universal master mix can be purchased with or without uracil DNA glycosylase, which degrades any PCR contaminating products prior to starting the PCR by heating the plate to 95°C for 10 min (see later). It is possible to assemble master mixes by purchasing various components, such as dNTP, buffer, $MgCl_2$ and hot start *Taq* DNA polymerase. However, in-house preparation of master mixes is not recommended to minimize intra-assay and inter-assay variation and contamination, essential for monitoring patient response to therapy.

Probe–Primer mix. For convenience and to minimize inter-assay variation a bulk preparation of the qRT-PCR assay mix, containing the probes and primers at required concentration, minus the master mix, is recommended. The mixture is stored at –20°C or –70°C. This also avoids repeated freezing and thawing of probes and primers because this may affect the probe–primer integrity. Furthermore, the probe should not be left exposed for prolonged periods to direct sunlight because this leads to degradation. In general 300 nmol/l of each primer and 200 nmol/l of probe permits optimum qRT-PCR sensitivity; however, this should be determined for each assay by titrating one primer against the other. The optimum concentration of the primers is one that gives the lowest Ct. Similarly; the optimum probe concentration is determined by varying the quantity of the probe. The quantity yielding the lowest Ct is the optimum probe concentration. The probe–primer mixture is then prepared using the determined optimum concentrations. The mixture can then be aliquoted into microcentrifuge tubes for a required number of samples, allowing for standards and positive and negative controls. Furthermore, for MRD studies it is advisable to measure the target gene in replicates of three to minimize sampling error at low copy number values. Because the endogenous control gene copy number is expected, assays in duplicate will suffice. However, standards for the endogenous control should be performed in triplicate.

Designing probe and primers. The probe and primers are designed using Primer Express Software (Applied Biosystems, Foster City, CA). Optimum design of probes and primers is critical to the sensitivity of qRT-PCR. The probe is designed such that it has higher T_m than the primers and works optimally at default PCR conditions settings using the universal master mix. The probe should not have a guanine base at the 3′ end and the number of guanine bases should be fewer than the number of cytosine bases. Furthermore, there should not be more than four guanine bases in tandem. Similar rules apply to design of primers. The annealing temperature of the probe should be 10°C greater than that of the primers. It is essential to design probes and primers such that the assay is RNA specific. This is achieved by positioning the forward and reverse primers in separate exons or by placing either of the primers or the probe across a splice site.

Standard curve. It is acceptable to report data as Ct, with an increase of 3.3 being clinically significant, because this represents 1 log increase in *BCR–ABL1* copies; it takes 3.3 cycles for every log increase in amplicons. For clinical samples, however, it is essential to generate a standard curve from which the unknown test samples can be calculated. The standard curve can be generated using serially diluted cDNA derived from a cell line expressing the target gene at high levels (e.g. K562 for *BCR–ABL1*). As an alternative to using cDNA, a plasmid can be used to create this curve, which provides stability over time. The method of preparation of the plasmid is beyond the scope of this book. Serially diluted plasmids for commonly occurring fusion genes and endogenous control genes are commercially available. In the absence of a standard curve the MRD values are reported as a delta-delta Ct ($\Delta\Delta Ct$). This is calculated by first normalizing the fusion gene Ct (CtFG) to the control gene (CtCG) to obtain a ΔCt for the follow-up samples – that is, the ΔCt(follow-up) = $Ct_{FG} - Ct_{CG}$. The same calculation is performed for the Ct value for the sample taken at diagnosis to obtain a ΔCt(diagnosis). The ΔCt(diagnosis) is then subtracted from the ΔCt(follow-up) to obtain a $\Delta\Delta Ct$. From this the MRD value is calculated as $10^{\Delta\Delta Ct/3.3}$. To apply the $\Delta\Delta Ct$ method of reporting the slope and intercept values for the control and fusion genes must be similar. More precisely it is recommended that the slope values for the fusion and control gene should not differ by more than 0.01 (i.e. the PCR efficiency for CG and FG are similar). The major advantage of using $\Delta\Delta Ct$ is it obviates the need for a standard curve. Therefore, eliminating the need for a plasmid- or RNA-based standard curve reduces the risk of contamination further and frees microtitre plate wells for patient samples.

PCR cycling conditions. It is convenient to design the probes and primers so that they are able to work efficiently using standard qRT-PCR conditions to amplify the cDNA, which are 2 min at 50°C (to allow uracil DNA glycosylase-mediated elimination of exogenous PCR product contamination), an enzyme heat-activation step of 10 min at 95°C, followed by 50 cycles of 15 s at 95°C for denaturation and 1 min at 60°C for annealing and extension.

Method

The qRT-PCR assay is normally performed in 96-well microtitre plates in a 25 μl final reaction volume containing universal master mix. The composition of a 25 μl qRT-PCR reaction is shown in Table 8.4.

1. Dispense 20 μl or qRT-PCR mixture into the required number of microtitre wells. To minimize inter-sample differences, an eight-channel automatic pipette is recommended to dispense the qRT-PCR assay mix. Note the location of each sample, including the standards and controls, on a grid map in which each of the 96 wells is represented.
2. Using the grid map, add 5 μl of the appropriate cDNA or standard to each well.
3. To the No Template Control wells, genomic DNA is included in mRNA-based studies. Add HL60 cell line derived cDNA to the No Amplification Control wells for *BCR–ABL1* qRT-PCR assays because this cell line does not express this fusion gene.
4. Also included are cDNA derived from K562 and BV173 cell lines diluted to give a known number of copies.

5. On dispensing all the samples, secure the wells with optical caps or a film adhesive.
6. Centrifuge the plate for 2–3 s at 1000 rpm to collect all the contents to the bottom of the wells and expel any trapped bubbles prior to placing it in the instrument.
7. Initiate the run as per manufacturer's instructions, adjusting the sample volume and number of cycles accordingly. The plate is normally subjected to between 40 and 50 cycles.

The instrument sets the threshold at ×10 the standard deviation of baseline emission; however, this can be reset manually within the exponential phase of the PCR to avoid any background fluorescent interference. Alternatively, the threshold can be set at the same value for each assay, for instance, at 0.05, assuming this is within the exponential phase of PCR, thus avoiding operator variation. The data for any samples with a Ct >38 are considered unreliable.

The baseline limits are set by the instrument; however, this should be adjusted so that the upper limit of the baseline is 4 cycles less than the lowest Ct value for a sample. For example, if the lowest Ct is 20, then the upper baseline limit is set at 16, thus giving a clear margin between the baseline and the samples. The lower limit set by instrument rarely requires adjusting.

The standard curve is generated and accepted if the slope value is between –3.3 and –3.6. A slope value of –3.3 represents 100% PCR efficiency because it takes 3.3 cycles for every log increase in PCR products. Ideally the curve correlation coefficient should not be <0.98. If the standard curve is acceptable, then the copy number for the samples can be recorded. The qRT-PCR for the endogenous control gene is performed similarly using

Table 8.4 25 μl qRT-PCR assay

STOCK SOLUTION	CONCENTRATION	VOLUME (μl)	VOLUME (μl, 110 REACTIONS)	WORKING CONCENTRATION
Universal master mix	×2	12.5	1375	×1
Forward primer	80 μmol/l	0.094	10.31	300 nmol/l
Reverse primer	80 μmol/l	0.094	10.31	300 nmol/l
Dual-labelled probe	50 μmol/l	0.050	5.5	100 nmol/l
Complementary DNA	–	3.0	–	–
Sterile water	–	9.26	1018.88	–

qRT-PCR, quantitative reverse transcriptase polymerase chain reaction.
The volumes for bulk preparation of probe–primer mix are indicated; these are sufficient for 96 samples (i.e. 96-well microtitre plate) and allow for pipetting. The universal master mix is added just prior to setting up the qRT-PCR.

the target-specific probes and primers. On completion of qRT-PCR for target and endogenous control, the data are reported as a percentage (i.e. $(BCR–ABL1/ABL1) \times 100$).

Notes

To minimize sampling error, the target gene and the standards are assayed in triplicate. It is essential to include positive controls with a known number of transcripts. To minimize risk of contamination the patients' samples and standards should be handled in geographically separate locations. Because qRT-PCR assays are BCR–ABL1 transcript-type specific it is essential to perform a multiplex PCR on a presentation sample to assign the transcript type expressed by the patient. This ensures that correct qRT-PCR assay is used. A qRT-PCR assay designed for b2a2 or b3a2, now referred to as e13a2 and e14a2, respectively, would give rise to false-negative data in patients expressing e13a3 and/or e14a3. A single qRT-PCR for e13a2 and e14a2 is recommended rather than two separate assays for e13a2 and e14a2. This is achieved by designing the assay such that the probe and reverse primer map to the second exon (i.e. a2) of the ABL1 gene and the forward primer maps to the e13 exon (i.e. b2) of the BCR gene (Fig. 8.9). Apart from being cost-effective and efficient, it increases the accuracy of the assay because a significant minority of patients with a single nucleotide polymorphism in exon 13 of the BCR gene have the potential to express both e13a2 and e14a2.

The Lymphoproliferative Disorders

The majority of lymphoproliferative disorders can be readily diagnosed using cytological, histological and immunological techniques. However, in MRD and in certain cases in which the diagnosis is ambiguous, genetic techniques may be useful.[28,40] Examples include cases of controversial lineage, lymphomas in which the histology is ambiguous and occult lymphomas. DNA analysis may also help in determining whether a lymphocytosis is monoclonal, oligoclonal or polyclonal. Translocations do occur in these disorders and may be used in monitoring disease, as described for CML earlier. However, the most commonly used markers, because they are more universally applicable, are the rearranged immunoglobulin (IG) and T-cell receptor (TCR) genes.

Principle

This analysis is possible because the IGH@ and TCR genes undergo a rearrangement during the normal differentiation of B and T lymphocytes, respectively, but not during differentiation of other cells. This rearrangement results in a unique fusion of variable, diversity and joining (VDJ) segments, interdigitated by random nucleotide (N region) insertion or deletion. The sequence and length of the

DNA at these sites of recombination are therefore characteristic of any particular lymphocyte clone.

For many years, Southern blot analysis was the gold standard for the detection of rearranged IGH@ and TCR genes. For details on how these were performed and interpreted, we refer the reader to previous editions of this book. More recently, because of its simplicity, the small amount of DNA required and potential sensitivity, PCR has been used to detect rearrangement of the IGH@ and TCR genes. Because of the N region diversity, a polyclonal population of cells will give rise to a ladder of various fragment sizes. However, if one clone becomes abnormally large, a discrete fragment size will begin to dominate the products of the PCR – the basis of the so-called 'fingerprinting' method for the diagnosis of lymphoproliferative disorders.[41] This analysis can be refined using heteroduplex analysis or SSCP gels in which the sequence as well as the size of the amplified product determines its mobility. To gain further sensitivity in following disease, the product of a 'clonal' amplification can be sequenced to derive a clone-specific sequence at the site of rearrangement. This sequence can then be used for the design of clone-specific oligonucleotide probes or primers that can be used in ASOH, ARMS or qRT-PCR. This methodology has been used to monitor MRD in lymphoproliferative disorders.[42,43]

A comprehensive report has been published on the design and standardization of PCR primers and protocols for the detection of IGH@ and TCR gene rearrangements.[40] The detection rate of clonal rearrangements is very high, but the comprehensive nature of the test requires 107 primer pairs in 18 multiplex PCR tubes, which are now commercially available. The methods described here are more restricted but more widely applicable.

Method: Immunoglobulin Heavy Chain Gene Rearrangement

To study immunoglobulin gene rearrangement, the locus of choice is the heavy chain gene. A single primer can be used, which will anneal to a consensus sequence shared by all joining (JH) segments. The choice of variable (VH) segment primers is more difficult and for the more comprehensive analysis, primers from all three framework regions for each of the six or seven VH families are used.[39] A reasonable starting point, however, is to use the JH primer in conjunction with a different primer derived from a consensus sequence of the framework 1 region for each VH family. These primers are as follows:

JH 5′ CTT ACC TGA GGA GAC GGT GAC CAG 3′
VH1 5′ FAM-CCT CAG TGA AGG TCT CCT GCA AGG 3′
VH2 5′ HEX-TCCT GC GC TG GT GAA AGC CAC 3′
VH3 5′ FAM-GGT CCC TGA GAC TCT CCT GTG CA 3′
VH4 5′ HEX- TCG GAG ACC CTG TCC CTC ACC T 3′
VH5 5′ VIC- GAA AAA GCC CGG GGA GTC TCT GAA 3′
VH6 5′ VIC- CCT GTG CCA TCT CCG GGG ACA GTG 3′

PCR buffer I (see above) is used in these reactions, with an annealing temperature of 60°C. The products of the reactions are in the order of 310–350 bp and can be visualized as either a smear or discrete band in high-percentage agarose gels (1.5–2%). However, a better resolution is obtained when the products are resolved by capillary electrophoresis on an automated fragment analyser (e.g. the ABI 3130xl DNA Analyser). Fragments are visualized by attaching a fluorescent label (HEX or FAM or VIC) to the VH primers and reading the peaks of fluorescence as an electrophoretogram or 'genescan' Alternatively, the PCR products can be subjected to heteroduplex analysis, denaturing them at 95°C for 5 min and annealing at 50°C for 1 h, prior to electrophoresis in a non-denaturing 6% polyacrylamide gel.

Interpretation

Because of the variable number of nucleotides either removed or added at the point of joining of VDJ segments of the immunoglobulin heavy-chain gene, the distance between V segment and J segment primers will alter accordingly. For the gene to be functional, the reading frame must be maintained and therefore variations in length must be in multiples of 3 bp, although this may not always be the case in acute leukaemias where non-productive rearrangements may occur. The polyclonal population of B cells therefore gives rise to a characteristic 'ladder' or Gaussian size distribution, with maximal intensity observed at the median length at its centre. However, if one B-cell clone is abnormally large, it will give rise to a disproportionately intense peak at the size (and using a V primer from the appropriate family) corresponding to the length of VDJ fragment derived from that clone. At presentation of a B-cell malignancy, this band may be the only one visible, confirming the presence of a dominant abnormal B-cell clone. Subsequently, an abnormal intensity of this fragment size in the background of a ladder can be used to monitor the disease.

In heteroduplex analysis, the polyclonal population of B cells will give rise to fragments with many different sequences, which, on denaturing and reannealing, will generate heteroduplexes that will appear as a smear spreading across the gel. If one large B-cell clone is present, however, homoduplexes will form and these will migrate as a discrete fragment with a migration consistent with its size alone.

There are two main problems that can be encountered in this analysis. The first is that the consensus V primers may not amplify all V segments because of mutations in sequence of the region recognized by the primers (either J, V or both). To overcome this problem, primers for the leader region of the V gene and for the constant region of the heavy chain identified by immunofluorescence on the surface of the B-cell clones may be used on cDNA. The distance between the leader primers and the constant regions may be too large for DNA amplification. It is therefore important that in patients with chronic lymphocytic leukaemia (CLL), B-cell lymphomas and myeloma, RNA is also stored from diagnostic samples in case this approach is required. However, it is also important that appropriate diagnostic material is referred for analysis. For instance, lymph nodes in case of lymphomas, bone marrow (BM) in case of myeloma and peripheral blood (PB) in CLL. A BM or PB sample in a case of lymphoma may be totally 'empty' of disease and therefore not suitable for this type of investigation.

Another problem encountered, especially in ALL, is the emergence of a subclone or clones during the course of the disease, which may result in a change in the fragment size and family.

Method: T-Cell Receptor Gene Rearrangement

The first choice of locus for PCR analysis of the *TCR* gene rearrangement is the TCR gamma locus as it is rearranged in the vast majority of T-cell clones and does not have the complexity of the TCR beta locus, which has 24 different V segment families. Amplification of DNA around the joining region of the TCR gamma gene is performed in a similar way to that described earlier for the *IGH@* locus, using a consensus primer for the joining segment (JγC) and one for each of the four variable segment families (Vγ I–IV). The primer sequences are as follows:

JγC: 5′ FAM-CAA CAA GTG TTG TTC CAC 3′
VγI: 5′ TGC AGC CAG TCA GAA ATC TTC C 3′
VγII: 5′ TGC AGG TCA CCT AGA GCA ACC T 3′
VγIII: 5′ AGC AGT TCC AGC TAT CCA TTT CC 3′
VγIV: 5′ TGC AAT TGC ACT TGG GCA GTT G 3′

Standard PCR amplification conditions can be employed using these primer combinations and analysis is again performed on acrylamide gels or an automated fluorescence analyser.

Interpretation

As in the analysis of the *IGH@* gene, discrete bands of amplified product are obtained from clonal T-cell populations, whereas ladders are obtained from polyclonal populations by gene scanning or heteroduplex analysis. The main problem with the interpretation of this kind of data is that it does not distinguish reactive T-cell clones from malignant T-cell clones. Three different patterns are clearly distinguished: a large malignant clonal population, an oligoclonal population and a polyclonal population. However, because of the sensitivity of this method, problems can arise in trying to detect a small malignant clone against a polyclonal population compared to a clonal population stimulated by antigen, particularly when a patient is lymphopenic.

Immunoglobulin Heavy Chain and *TCR* Gene Rearrangements as Targets for Minimal Residual Disease Analysis

The value of detecting residual disease with greater sensitivity than light microscopy, using molecular or immunological techniques, has been extensively evaluated in childhood and adult ALL. Minimal residual disease is defined as the 'lowest level of disease detectable in patients in CR (i.e. complete remission) by the methods available' and the newly developed real-time quantitative PCR techniques have revolutionized MRD investigation and patient management. The methodology makes use of the information derived from the cloning and sequencing of the rearranged clonal leukemic clone and the generation of an allele-specific primer able to identify the unique rearrangement belonging to the leukaemic cell with a sensitivity of 1 in 100 000 normal cells. Guidelines for the interpretation of real-time quantitative PCR data in the analysis of minimal residual disease by *IGH@/TCR* gene rearrangement have been generated by a European study group. These are currently being followed and applied in a large study at international level and we refer the reader to such extensive publications[43] for further information.

In brief, these studies in children have concluded that conversion to MRD negativity shortly after induction therapy and maintenance of MRD negativity are prerequisites for long-term disease-free survival and that MRD positivity often precedes clinical relapse.[44] In adults also, MRD analysis carried out during induction therapy provides a strong predictor of outcome and should also be applied to harvested BM to exclude patients with detectable leukaemia burden of more than $1:10^3$ normal cells. Finally, predictions of outcome based on MRD analysis in children and adults are more accurate than predictions based on other prognostic indicators, such as age, gender, immunophenotype, presenting white cell count, karyotype and time taken to achieve first CR.[45–47]

The Myeloproliferative Neoplasms

JAK2 Mutation Analysis

In 2005 several groups independently identified a unique mutation in the JAK homology 2 (JH2) pseudokinase domain of the Janus kinase 2 (*JAK2*) gene in patients with a variety of myeloproliferative neoplasms (MPNs), including polycythemia vera (PV), essential thrombocythemia (ET) and primary myelofibrosis (PMF).[48,49] The mutation was reported in up to 90%, 40% and 25% of patients in the three diseases, respectively, but not in chronic myelogenous leukaemia or in 700 normal controls. It consisted of a G to T substitution at nucleotide 1849 of exon 14, leading to a valine to phenylalanine substitution at codon 617 (V617F). This mutation caused loss of JAK2 autoinhibition and constitutive activation of the cytoplasmic

JAK2 kinase and has become recognized for definitive molecular diagnosis of PV. Until this mutation was identified the distinction between primary and secondary polycythemia was sometimes difficult to establish.

A variety of molecular methods have been employed to establish the presence of this mutation, including direct DNA sequencing, allele-specific PCR, amplification refractory mutation system, real-time quantitative PCR and melting curve analysis as a semi-quantitative method, restriction fragment length polymorphism (RFLP) analysis and pyrosequencing. There are other methods which could be applicable to this type of mutation analysis, including SSCP or denaturing high-performance liquid chromatography (DH-PLC), both of which are technically challenging and labour intensive.

More recently, some relatively rare mutations in the exon 12 of the *JAK2* gene have been identified in V617F-negative patients with polycythaemia vera or unexplained erythrocytosis (thus redefined as polycythaemia vera) using PCR and direct DNA sequencing as well as allele-specific PCR. We are currently screening for these mutations by denaturing HPLC analysis, but a full description of this test lies beyond the scope of this chapter and readers are referred to reference 52 for information. For these investigations, granulocytes represent the preferred source for DNA or RNA preparation, but total white blood cells are also commonly used. DNA and RNA are prepared according to the protocols described in other sections of this chapter.

Principle: *JAK2* Exon 14 Mutation Analysis

Mutation of exon 14 of the *JAK2* gene in MPNs is characterized by a single nucleotide mutation which is identical in all patients carrying this defect. PCR amplification can be designed to exploit the specific annealing of a primer at the 3′ end in single or multiplex conditions. By designing a primer that matches the codon 617 wild-type (G) sequence, the primer will bind and amplify only the wild-type DNA. Conversely, the primer designed to match the mutant sequence (T) will amplify the mutant allele and not the wild type. After the PCR has been carried out, the products can be visualized in several ways. One can simply run the product on a 2% agarose gel and visualize the products by incorporating SYBR Safe dye in the gel and using a UV transilluminator. This methodology is marred by problems, such as possible lack of specificity and false-positive results.

A more successful approach in our hands is the use of primers designed to include a fluorescent label that differs between the wild-type and the mutant primer. The PCR product can then be run on a fragment analyser (the ABI 3130 for instance, Applied Biosystems, Warrington) with the wild-type and mutant allele appearing as two distinct fragments of the expected size in separate channels (Fig. 8.11).

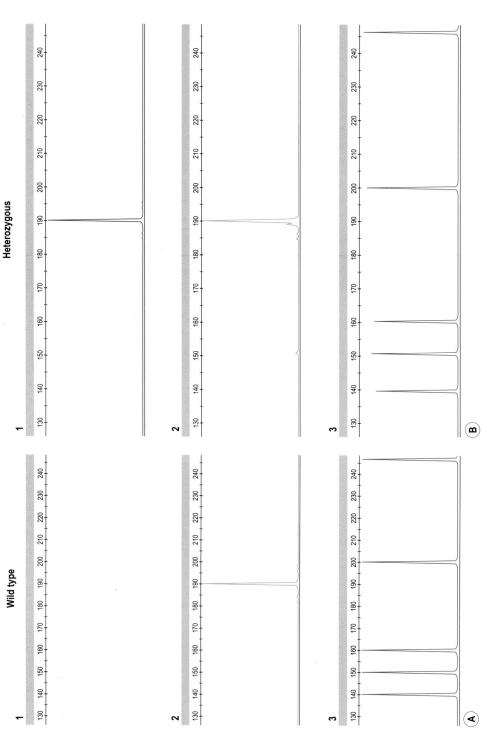

Figure 8.11 *JAK2* genotype analysis by genescanning. Primers specific for the wild-type *JAK2* sequence (*green fluorescent signal*) and for the mutant allele (*blue fluorescent signal*) have been applied to two samples and run on a gene-scanning ABI apparatus. (A) The presence of a single signal in the wild-type amplification indicates that this sample is wild type for the G>T mutation. (B) The presence of a signal on both PCR amplifications indicates that this sample is heterozygous for the mutation.

This represents a rapid and cost-effective method for the analysis of large cohort of patients: 100–200 ng of total DNA or 1/20th of a cDNA reaction (normally containing 2 µg of total RNA in a 50 µl final volume reaction) is sufficient for this test, which is described in more detail below.

A different approach, pyrosequencing, is also extensively used in our laboratory for detecting *JAK2* mutations. This approach involves the amplification of a fragment containing the nucleotide mutation by PCR using a biotinylated primer. The amplified product is captured on streptavidin-coated beads and is then used as a substrate for sequencing by synthesis at the mutated nucleotide/s. The four nucleotides are added stepwise and – when they are incorporated – a pyrophosphate (PPi) molecule is released. This is subsequently converted to ATP by ATP sulphurylase, which in turn enables a luciferin molecule to become oxidized in a luciferase reaction, producing light in amounts that are proportional to the amount of ATP. Unincorporated nucleotides and ATP are degraded by the apyrase and the reaction can restart with another nucleotide. Therefore the incorporation of the mutant and/or wild-type nucleotide will be captured and converted into a light emission signal, which can be measured and quantified. By comparing the relative intensity of the signal obtained after incorporation of the mutant and wild-type nucleotides, their relative abundance in the target sequence can be established. In this respect, pyrosequencing is a quantitative method and therefore offers a great advantage compared to other methodologies.

Method A: Using a DNA fragment analyser

In this protocol a reverse common primer (5′ CCT ACA GTG TTT TCA GTT TCA AAA ATA 3′) is used in combination with two different forward primers in two separate reactions. The two forward primers differ by one nucleotide at their 3′ end with a G in the wild-type (exon14 Forward wild-type: 5′ AGC ATT TGG TTT TAA ATT ATG GAG TAT GT**G** 3′) and a T in the mutated PCR reaction (exon 14 Forward mutated 5′ AGC ATT TCC TTT TAA ATT ATG GAG TAT GT**T** 3′) and by being labelled with a different fluorochrome.

1. Set up a PCR reaction, with 100–200 ng of genomic DNA in the presence of 100 ng of each nucleotide and 1.5 mM final concentration of $MgCl_2$. PCR cycling conditions are as follows: 94°C for 5 min; then 30 repeated cycles of 94°C for 30 s, 61°C for 30 s and 72°C for 1 min; followed by 72°C for 10 min.
2. Check the amplicons by agarose gel electrophoresis to verify amplification of the correct-size fragment.
3. Run these fragments on the ABI 3130 genetic analyser to determine the presence or absence of the mutant allele. DNA from HEL cell line (a human erythroleukaemia cell line: AML-M6 that carries a homozygous mutant for *JAK2*, V617F) is used as a positive control in each experiment.

Method B: Using pyrosequencing

Primer sequences are as follows. Pyro-JAK2Ex14 Forward: 5′ GAA GCA GCA AGT ATG ATG AGC A 3′; Pyro-JAK2 Ex14Reverse-Biotinylated: 5′-[Btn]TAT AGT TTA CAC TGA CAC CTA GCT-3′; JAK2 SNP (for sequencing): 5′ TTT TAA ATT ATG GAG TAT GT 3′.

1. Prepare 1 ml of the *JAK2* exon 14 master mix as follows: ten times concentrated (10×) PCR buffer: 100 µl; 50 mM $MgCl_2$: 36 µl; primers Pyro-JAK2Ex14 Forward and Pyro-JAK2 Ex14Reverse-BIO, both to 500 nM; 15 mM dNTP: 17 µl; ddH_2O: 815 µl.
2. 0.1 µl Taq polymerase enzyme per sample is added to the master mix before distributing 28 µl of the mastermix into each PCR tube; 2 µl of DNA from each patient's sample is added to each tube, except for the blank in which water is added.
3. Cycling condition are as follows: initial denaturation at 94°C for 5 min. Then 94°C for 30 s, 57°C for 1 min and 72°C for 2 min with repeated cycling for 28 cycles. Then a final extension of 72°C for 7 min.
4. Check for PCR amplification on a 2% agarose gel running at 100 V for approximately 1 h.
5. Prepare the (SQA)/SNP pyrosequencing kit, which includes the lyophilized enzymes, substrate mix and reconstituted nucleotides (including the alpha thio form of dATP), 70% ethanol; 0.2 M NaOH, wash buffer (10 time concentrated – 10× – stock, working solution 1×), ddH_2O; 96 well microtitre plate/caps, pyrosequencing, binding buffer and annealing buffer; streptavidin-coated Sepharose beads (Amersham) and vacuum pump. Primer sequence is: JAK2 SNP: 5′ TTT TAA ATT ATG GAG TAT GT 3′.
6. Prepare the pyrosequencing binding mixture for double number of the samples as follows: for each well, use 38 µl binding buffer, 30 µl water and 2 µl Sepharose beads.
7. Add 70 µl of this mix is to each well. Then add 10 µl of the PCR product to the relevant well. Shake the plate for 10–15 min on a shaker with mixing rate of 1200 rpm at room temperature.
8. Meanwhile, prepare the annealing mixture consisting of 11.5 µl annealing buffer and 0.5 µl 10 µM JAK2 SNP primer for each well; 12 µl of this mixture is added to each well in the pyro-plate.
9. Remove the caps from the microtitre plate after the end of shaking. The biotinylated strand is separated from the unlabelled complementary strand by sequentially washing with 70% ethanol, 0.2 M NaOH and washing buffer using a vacuum pump. The biotinylated strand is then transferred to the related well in the pyro-plate.
10. Put the pyro-plate in a thermocycler, heat to 80°C for 2 min and then slowly cool to room temperature to allow annealing of JAK2 SNP primer to the biotinylated DNA strand.

167

11. Put the plate in the pyrosequencing machine. Instructions for the operation of equipment may vary from model to model.

This analysis will produce a measurement of the amplification of each product as a percentage of the wild-type and mutated allele. Normally any amplification of the mutated allele above 5% is considered a positive. Between 1 and 5% is borderline and a repeat sample is recommended. Below 1% is reported as negative.

Interpretation

All tests are carried out including a positive control (DNA from HEL cell line, grown *in vitro* or any other DNA from cell lines or patients carrying a homozygous mutant allele), a negative control (normal individual DNA) and a non-template control, containing all reagents and water in place of DNA. Samples are tested in duplicate for the pyrosequencing and evaluated for the presence of a peak in the amplification well containing primers for the mutant allele. The amplitude of the luminescence signal provides quantification of wild-type and mutant allele amplicons as percentages of total. If using agarose gels, the presence of a band in the wild-type combination but not in the mutant will identify a wild-type patient; the presence of a band only in the mutant reaction will identify a homozygous patient, while the heterozygous cases will show amplification in both wild-type and mutant wells. The same principle applies when using a fragment analyser (Fig. 8.11). Fragment analysis can be semi-quantitative if the PCR cycle number is kept low, with the peak height reflecting the amount of target sequence present in the starting material. Several quantitative PCR tests have recently being developed and we refer to the wider literature for information on such tests.[50]

Acute Myeloid Leukaemia

Testing for Other Common Fusion Gene Products

In addition to the *BCR–ABL1* fusion gene, a variety of fusion genes have been identified and characterized at the molecular level in acute and chronic leukaemias, all suitable for PCR amplification and use as markers at diagnosis and for application for minimal residual disease detection. The identification of these at the time of diagnosis may carry prognostic significance and subsequently influence treatment modalities. There are a great number of potential fusion genes, but the *PML–RARA*, *ETV6–RUNX1* and *MLL–MLLT2* are among the most frequent targets of investigation in acute myeloid leukaemia (AML) and acute lymphoblastic leukaemia (ALL). They are the result of the t(15;17), t(12;21) and t(4;11) translocations, respectively. The former two chromosomal aberrations are commonly associated with good response to therapy and patients rarely require transplantation.

However, the t(4;11) is associated with a less favourable response to therapy. For this group even the option of transplant offers limited advantages for long-term survival and this is especially in adults. Each of these translocations will be briefly discussed in the following sections.

t(15;17)(q22;q21); *PML-RARA* Fusion Gene

The t(15;17)(q22;q21) translocation, associated with acute promyelocytic leukaemia (APL)(French–American–British – FAB – M3), fuses the *PML* gene, on 15q22, to the *RARA* gene on 17q21. The breakpoint cluster region on chromosome 17 localizes within *RARA* intron 2. Within *PML* there are three breakpoint cluster regions: breakpoint cluster region 3 (bcr3) in intron 3, bcr2 in exon 6 (rarely in intron 5) and bcr1 in intron 6. At the messenger RNA level, bcr1, bcr2 and bcr3 are also known as the long (L), variant (V) and short (S) isoforms, respectively. Alternative splicing within *PML* transcripts and the alternative use of two *RARA* polyadenylation sites are responsible for the production of additional *PML–RARA* transcripts of different sizes.

There are at least four variant translocations involving the *RARA* gene, with the same breakpoint, associated with the APL or similar phenotype. The fusion partners are *NPM1* at 5q35, *ZNF145* (previously *PLZF*) at 11q23, *NUMA1* at 11q13 and *STAT5B* at 11q11.

As a consequence of the t(15;17)(q22;q21) translocation, both *PML–RARA* and *RARA–PML* fusions can be transcribed. While *PML–RARA* is consistently found in APL patients, *RARA–PML* is detectable in only 70% of cases. Thus, *PML–RARA* is most widely used for diagnosis and MRD monitoring in APL. This transcript can be detected by RT-PCR with a sensitivity of $1:10^4$.

The *PML–RARA* transcript can be detected with increased sensitivity by qRT-PCR compared to semi-quantitative nested/two-round PCR techniques. Accurate quantification can identify patients with an increasing number of transcripts preceding haematological relapse. Patients treated at the time of molecular relapse have 2-year event-free survival (EFS) rates superior to those treated at the time of haematological relapse.

11q23 Abnormalities

Rearrangements involving the *MLL* (mixed leukaemia lymphoma) gene (previously also called *ALL1*, *HRX* or *Htrx1*) on chromosome 11q23 and multiple partner genes are found in precursor B-ALL, T-ALL, AML, MDS and therapy-related leukaemia. The presence of *MLL* rearrangements is usually associated with a poor prognosis.

In ALL, the most common translocation partner of *MLL* is the *MLLT2* gene on chromosome 4q21. Between 50% and 70% of infant ALL cases and approximately 5% of paediatric and adult ALL cases are *MLL–MLLT2* positive and are associated with a pro-B-ALL ('null') phenotype (CD19+, CD34+, terminal deoxynucleotidyl transferase+, cytoplasmic CD79a+, CD10−). There is also frequent expression of myeloid antigens (CD15 and/or CD65).

The *MLL* and *MLLT2* genes are composed of 37 and 20 exons, respectively, and at least 10 different fusion transcripts have been identified due to translocation breakpoints occurring in different introns of both genes. Breakpoints downstream of the *MLL* exon 9 in adult and paediatric ALL, but downstream of exon 11 in infant ALL and upstream of exon 4 of the *MLLT2* gene, are commonly detected by PCR. Differential splicing is a common finding, leading to more than one fusion transcript in some patients. All t(4;11)-positive cases transcribe the *MLL–MLLT2* fusion gene, while only 70% of cases transcribe the reciprocal, *MLLT2–MLL*, product. Interestingly, low levels of the *MLL–MLLT2* transcript have been detected in some ALL cases without cytogenetically detectable t(4;11) and in haemopoietic tissues of healthy individuals.

Using a nested PCR strategy, the various *MLLT2–MLL* transcripts can be identified with a detection limit of $1:10^4–10^5$. MRD studies have shown that early conversion and persisting MRD negativity is consistently associated with complete cytogenetic remission.

t(12;21)(p13;q22); *ETV6-RUNX1* Fusion Gene

The t(12;21)(p13;q22) is a cryptic translocation not readily observed by conventional cytogenetics and the ETV6 (TEL)–RUNX1 (AML1 or CBFA2) fusion transcript can be detected in patients with and without a cytogenetically visible chromosome 12 and/or 21 abnormality. FISH and PCR are therefore important techniques employed for its detection.

The t(12;21) is usually associated with a common ALL (cALL) and more rarely pre-B ALL. It is rarely seen in adult ALL, although it is the commonest translocation in childhood ALL, with a peak incidence in the 2–5-year age group. The breakpoint region usually lies between exons 5 and 6 of the *ETV6* gene and between exon 1 and 3 of *RUNX1*. Fusion transcripts resulting from splicing of *ETV6* exon 5 to other *RUNX1* exons can also be formed. The majority of positive patients have the *ETV6* gene deleted on the non-translocated allele and it has been suggested that the translocation occurs during fetal development. The *ETV6–RUNX1* fusion transcript can be identified with a sensitivity of $1:10^4–10^5$ using a nested RT-PCR approach. Accurate quantification of *ETV6–RUNX1* has shown that MRD measurements are a good prognostic indicator.

Method and Interpretation

The above three translocations are determined and monitored by amplification of the mRNA, resulting from the fusion gene, as this is leukaemia-specific in the same way as the *BCR–ABL1* testing for the t(9;22) (see p. 155 for the preparation of cDNA and conditions of PCR

amplification). However, for primers specific for amplification at diagnosis and for qRT-PCR for follow-up samples we follow the protocols and guidelines for interpretation of results provided by the Europe Against Cancer Consortium.[51,52]

It is worth noting that due to the multiplicity of the MLL–MLLT2 fusion products and the limitations of hydrolysis probe amplicon size, a genomic DNA-based assay may be employed for following affected patients as previously described.[53] This involves the characterization of the individual breakpoint by direct sequencing and designing an ASO in a manner similar to that for Ig/TCR-based MRD.[54] As controls for amplification we use the Ipsogen plasmids (www.ipsogen.com). For interpretation of data, we refer to the Europe Against Cancer guidelines.[50,51]

FLT3 PCR-based Mutation Analysis

In the past 10 years, genetic changes identified in the leukaemic cells at the time of diagnosis have greatly influenced treatment and management of AML. In addition to chromosomal abnormalities, mutations in specific genes have also emerged as important prognostic indicators. Among the most common are mutations in tyrosine kinase genes such as *FLT3* and *NPM1*.[55–57]

Principle

The *fms-like* tyrosine kinase gene 3, *FLT3*, shows an internal tandem duplication (ITD) in approximately 15–30% of patients with AML. The mutations are restricted to the leukaemic cells and patients with *FLT3*-ITD have a poorer outcome and may require transplant or more aggressive chemotherapy. Therefore, the rapid identification of these leukaemic-specific changes is important and analysis should be carried out in pre-treatment samples of all AML patients.

FLT3-ITD occurs with higher frequency in older adults than younger patients. Mutations map to the negative regulatory juxta-membrane (JM) domain and change the amino acid sequence, which subsequently interrupts inhibition and constitutively activates the protein.

Between 8% and 12% of AML patients have other types of *FLT3* mutation that map to the activation loop, most frequently involving aspartic acid 835 or the immediately adjacent isoleucine 836. Neither mutation appears to carry prognostic significance and therefore they are less often tested for than *FLT3*-ITD.

Methods

To investigate the presence of an ITD in the *FLT3* gene, the method of choice is PCR amplification using primers flanking the region containing the mutation and this can be carried out on DNA or cDNA.

For DNA amplification:

G11F 5′ GCA ATT TAG GTA TGA AAG CCA GC 3′
G12R 5′ VIC-CTT TCA GCA TTT TGA CGG CAA CC 3′.

For cDNA amplification:

R5F: 5′ TGT CGA GCA GTA CTC TAA ACA TG 3′,
R6R: 5′ VIC-GAG TTT GGG AA GG TA CTA GGG AT 3′.

See Figure 8.12 for PCR strategy and amplicon size.

PCR cycling conditions are: 95°C for 5 min initial denaturation and then 30 cycles using 95°C for 30 s denaturation step, 56°C for 45 s annealing step and 72°C for 30 s extension with a final 72°C for 7 min extension step. Analysis of amplicon size is carried out using Genescanning on a fragment analyser (Applied Biosystems, Warrington).

Interpretation

A 328 bp amplicon using cDNA (R5F–R6R primers; Fig. 8.12) and a 365 bp amplicon when using DNA (and G11F and G12R primers; Fig. 8.12) are detected in the presence of a wild-type allele. The mutant allele gives rise to a larger amplicon of variable size depending on the size of the internal tandem repeat, different in each individual patient. Because the wild-type and mutant amplicons are very similar in size the PCR product is better visualized using a fragment analyser. This offers a more accurate separation of similar-size products but requires one of the primers used in the reaction to be fluorescently labelled. The samples can be reported as 'wild-type' or 'mutated' depending on the results obtained and the size of the mutant allele should be noted in the report (in bp).

The other common FLT3 mutation (D835) results in the introduction of an EcoRV restriction site absent in the wild-type allele. This facilitates the identification of this mutation by digestion of the PCR product containing this site.

Figure 8.12 *FLT3*-ITD mutation analysis. Primers specific for the DNA amplification (G11–G12) and RNA amplification (R5 and R6) can be used on DNA and RNA, respectively. The amplicon size in an unmutated/wild-type allele is given in bp. In the presence of an internal tandem duplication (ITD), the size will increase according to the size of the insertion and, consequently, this may vary from individual to individual and will be restricted to the leukaemic cell population.

NPM1 PCR-based Mutation Analysis

The nucleophosmin-1 (*NPM1*) gene maps to chromosome 5q35. The cDNA has a coding sequence equivalent to a protein of 294 amino acids. Nucleophosmin is an abundant nucleolar phosphoprotein constantly shuffling between the nucleus/nucleolus and cytoplasm. *NPM1* mutations represent the most frequent gene alteration in AML. More than 26 different *NPM1* mutations have been identified, at breakpoint positions from 956 to 971, characterized by simple 1- or 2-tetranucleotide insertions, a 4-base pair (bp) or 5-bp deletion combined with a 9-bp insertion or a 9-bp deletion combined with a 14-bp insertion. *NPM1*-mutated AML occurs in all FAB categories except French–American–British (FAB) M3. However, the frequency among the FAB subgroups varies: it is lower in M2 (about 20%) and higher in M4 (acute myelomonocytic leukemia, 40–50%), M5a (acute monoblastic leukaemia, 40–50%) and especially M5b (acute monocytic leukemia, up to 90%). In the World Health Organization 2008 classification, *NPM1*-mutated AML comprises a specific provisional category. The most common *NPM1* mutation type, accounting for 75–80% of cases, is referred to as mutation A (*NPM1*-mutA). *NPM1* gene mutations are common in AML with a normal karyotype, occurring in 50–60% of cases. There is a high frequency of *FLT3* gene mutations in *NPM1*-mutated AML, mostly of the internal tandem duplication type. However, no association between *NPM1* gene mutations and *TP53*, *NRAS*, *CEBPA* (*CCAAT/enhancer binding protein-α*) and *MLL* gene mutations or recurrent genetic abnormalities has been found. These *NPM1* alterations have been shown to possess prognostic significance because they appear to identify patients who will respond well to chemotherapy and may not require transplantation.

Reagents and Methods

It is important to note that since analysis for *NPM1* mutations is carried out on cDNA samples, every effort to reduce DNA contamination should be made to avoid cross-amplification of DNA regions which contain pseudogenes. These may amplify using the primers commonly used for this test. To this end, samples are treated with DNAse prior to RNA extraction using Qiagen DNAse Free RNA extraction kit (Cat. No. 79294).

Primer sequences for the test and PCR amplification strategy on cDNA are as follows:

Forward: NPM1-F2 5′ ATC AAT TAT GTG AAG AAT TGC TTC C 3′
Reverse: NPM1-Rev6: 5′ FAM-ACC ATT TCC ATG TCT GAC CAC C 3′.

PCR amplification conditions are standard using a 20 µl final volume and 1.5 mM MgCl$_2$ concentration. Amplification is carried out using the following cycling conditions: initial extended denaturation at 95°C for 5 min; then 30 cycles using a denaturation at 95°C for 30 s, annealing at 56°C for 45 s; extension at 72°C for 30 s; and a final 72°C for 7 min extension.

Interpretation

The *NPM1* amplification should result in the production of one peak corresponding to 348 bp wild-type amplicon and another 352 bp mutant amplicon, when the mutant version with an insertion of 4 bp is present. The samples can be reported as 'wild-type' or 'mutated' and the size of the mutant allele should be noted in the report (in bp).

The test is analysed on a gene-scanning apparatus and frequently run as a duplex test in combination with *FLT3*. This is possible because *NPM1 and FLT3* primer pairs have been designed to yield fragments of different sizes.

HOST–DONOR CHIMERISM STUDIES

Following allogeneic stem cell transplantation it is important to monitor the engraftment of donor cells in the host. This can be achieved in a number of ways, one of which is the use of DNA markers. The method of choice is the PCR amplification of short tandem repeat (STR) loci, which, because of their highly polymorphic nature, are likely to give informative differences between any host–donor pair.[58]

Principle

Provided the amplification cycle number is kept reasonably low (25 cycles), the PCR reaction is semi-quantitative and the amount of product will reflect the amount of starting material. Therefore, once an informative difference is established, the amount of PCR product of the different host and donor alleles will reflect the proportions of host and donor DNA in a sample. Fluorescent-labelled primers are used in multiplex PCR reactions that are run on a capillary-based genetic analyser.

Method

This method has been modified from Mann et al.[59] by Griffiths and Mason (pers. comm.). Five primer pairs are used, as listed in Table 8.5. PCR reactions are carried out using buffer III with 1.5 mM MgCl$_2$. Amplification conditions are 94°C for 5 min, then 25 cycles of 94°C for 30 s, 57°C for 1 min and 72°C for 2 min followed by an extension at 72°C for 5 min. Products are then analysed by genotyping as follows. One μl of the PCR product, which may need to be diluted from 1:4 to 1:10 in water, is added to 10 μl of formamide containing the size marker Rox 500 (Applied Biosystems, Warrington) diluted 7.5 μl per 500 μl of formamide, aliquoted into an optical 96-well reaction plate and run on the ABI 3700 DNA analyser (or equivalent). Peaks representing the DNA fragments are visualized with the Genotyper software (Applied Biosystems, Warrington).

Interpretation

Comparing the host (pre-transplant) and donor DNA samples, an informative difference is sought at one or

Table 8.5 PCR primers used for multiplex STR amplification

MARKER	LABEL	PRIMER SEQUENCE (5′–3′)	CONCENTRATION (μmol/l)
D13S634F	6-FAM	GGCAGATTCAATCGGATAAATAGA	0.12
D13S634R	–	GTAACCCCTCAGGTTCTCAAGTCT	0.12
D18S386F	HEX	TGAGTCAGGAGAATCACTTGGAAC	0.2
D18S386R	–	CTCTTCCATGAAGTAGCTAAGCAG	0.2
D18S391F	HEX	TAGACTTCACTATTCCCATCTGAG	0.12
D18S391R	–	TAGACTTCACTATTCCCATCTGAG	0.12
FGAF	6FAM	CCATAGGTTTTGAACTCACAG	0.2
FGAR	–	CTTCTCAGATCCTCTGACAC	0.2
MBPF	6FAM	GGACCTCGTGAATTACAATC	0.6
MBPR	–	ATTTACCTACCTGTTCATCC	0.6

PCR, polymerase chain reaction; STR, short tandem repeat.

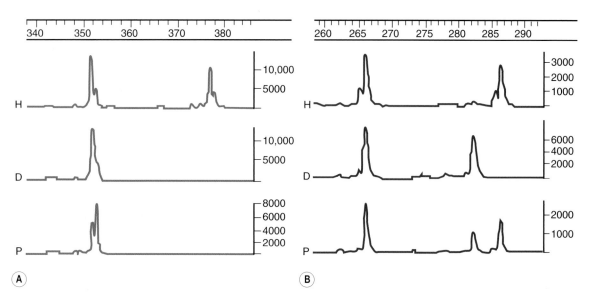

Figure 8.13 Short tandem repeat (STR) analysis of bone marrow engraftment. Capillary electrophoresis of the polymerase chain reaction (PCR) products of STR amplification as viewed by the Genotype software. H, host DNA; D, donor DNA; P, post-transplant DNA. (A) The host and donor share an allele at 352 bp, whereas a host-specific allele is seen at 376 bp with the marker D18S386; the latter is not detected in the post-transplant sample. (B) The host and donor share an allele at 266 bp but have specific alleles at 286 and 282 bp, respectively. All three alleles are seen in the post-transplant DNA, indicating that the sample is chimeric. From the relative area under the host- and donor-specific peaks, the proportion of donor DNA is estimated at 39%.

more of the STR loci such that host- and/or donor-specific alleles are identified. Correction factors are established by comparing the relative peak heights of the two host or donor alleles at these STRs. Post-transplant, the area under each informative peak is recorded and used to assess the relative proportion of host and donor DNA. Examples of full-engraftment and mixed chimerism are given in Figure 8.13.

REFERENCES

1. International Human Genome Sequencing Consortium. Initial sequencing and analysis of the human genome. *Nature.* 2001;409:860–921.

2. Venter JC, Adams MD, Myers EW, et al. The sequence of the human genome. *Science.* 2001;291:1304–1351.

3. Saiki RK, Gelfand DH, Stoffel S, et al. Primer-directed enzymatic amplification of DNA with a thermostable DNA polymerase. *Science.* 1988;239:487–491.

4. Association for Molecular Pathology. Recommendations for in-house development and operation of molecular diagnostic tests. *Am J Clin Pathol.* 1999;111:449–463.

5. Schwartz MK. Genetic testing and the clinical laboratory improvement amendments of 1988: present and future. *Clin Chem.* 1999;45:739–745.

6. Williams LO, Cole EC, Lubin IM, et al. Quality assurance in human molecular genetics testing: status and recommendations. *Arch Pathol Lab Med.* 2003;127:1353–1358.

7. Harris S, Jones DB. Optimization of the polymerase chain reaction. *Br J Biomed Sci.* 1997;54:166–173.

8. Newton CR, Graham A, Heptinstall LE, et al. Analysis of any point mutation in DNA. The amplification refractory mutation system (ARMS). *Nucleic Acids Res.* 1989;17:2503–2516.

9. Old JM, Varawalla NY, Weatherall DJ. Rapid detection and prenatal diagnosis of β-thalassaemia: studies in Indian and Cypriot populations in the UK. *Lancet.* 1990;336:834–837.

10. Wallace RB, Shaffer J, Murphy RF, et al. Hybridization of synthetic oligodeoxyribonucleotides to PhiX174 DNA: the effect of single base pair mismatch. *Nucleic Acids Res.* 1979;6:3543–3547.

11. Saiki RK, Chang CA, Levenson CH, et al. Diagnosis of sickle cell anemia and beta-thalassemia with enzymatically amplified DNA and non-radioactive allele specific oligonucleotide probes. *N Engl J Med.* 1988;319:537–541.

12. Kawasaki E, Saiki R, Erlich H. Genetic analysis using polymerase chain reaction-amplified DNA and immobilized oligonucleotide probes: reverse dot-blot typing. *Methods Enzymol.* 1993;218:369–381.

13. Old J. Haemoglobinopathies. *Prenat Diagn.* 1996;16:1181–1186.

14. Clark BE, Thein SL. Molecular diagnosis of haemoglobin disorders. *Clin Lab Haematol.* 2004;26:159–176.

15. Liu YT, Old JM, Miles K, et al. Rapid detection of alpha-thalassaemia deletions and alpha-globin triplication by multiplex polymerase chain reactions. *Br J Haematol.* 2000;108:295–299.

16. Ryan K, Bain BJ, Worthington D, et al. On behalf of the British Committee for Standards in Haematology. Significant haemoglobinopathies: guidelines for screening and diagnosis. *Br J Haematol.* 2010;149:35–49.

17. Cumming AM, Shiach CR. The investigation and management of inherited thrombophilia. *Clin Lab Haematol.* 1999;21:77–92.

18. Poort SR, Rosendaal FR, Reitsma PH, et al. A common genetic variation in the 3′-untranslated region of the prothrombin gene is associated with elevated plasma prothrombin levels and an increase in venous thrombosis. *Blood.* 1996;88: 3698–3703.

19. Bertina RM, Koeleman BP, Koster T, et al. Mutation in blood coagulation factor V associated with resistance to activated protein C. *Nature.* 1994;369:64–67.

20. Baglin T, Gray E, Greaves M, et al. British Committee for Standards in Haematology. Clinical guidelines for testing for heritable thrombophilia. *Br J Haematol.* 2010;149:209–220.

21. Vidal F, Farssac E, Altisent C, et al. Rapid hemophilia A molecular diagnosis by a simple DNA sequencing procedure: identification of 14 novel mutations. *Thromb Haemost.* 2001;85:580–583.

22. Lakich D, Kazazian Jr HH, Antonarakis SE, et al. Inversions disrupting the factor VIII gene are a common cause of severe haemophilia A. *Nat Genet.* 1993;5:236–241.

23. Wion KL, Tuddenham EGD, Lawn R. A new polymorphism in the factor VIII gene for prenatal diagnosis of haemophilia A. *Nucleic Acids Res.* 1986;14:4535–4542.

24. Liu Q, Nozari G, Sommer SS. Single-tube polymerase chain reaction for rapid diagnosis of the inversion hotspot of mutation in hemophilia A. *Blood.* 1998;92:1458–1459.

25. Secker-Walker LM, Craig JM, Hawkins JM, et al. Philadelphia-positive acute lymphoblastic leukaemia in adults: age distribution. BCR-breakpoint and prognostic significance. *Leukaemia.* 1991;5:196–199.

26. Macintyre EA, Delabesse E. Molecular approaches to the diagnosis and evaluation of lymphoid malignancies. *Semin Hematol.* 1999;36:373–389.

27. Biondi A, Rambaldi A, Pandolfi PP, et al. Molecular monitoring of the myl/retinoic acid receptor-α fusion gene in acute promyelocytic leukaemia by polymerase chain reaction. *Blood.* 1992;80:492–497.

28. Delabesse E, Asnafi V, Macintyre E. Application of molecular biology techniques to malignant haematology. *Transfus Clin Biol.* 2003;10:335–352.

29. Cross NCP, Melo JV, Lin F, et al. An optimised multiplex polymerase chain reaction for detection of BCR-ABL fusion mRNAs in haematological disorders. *Leukaemia.* 1994;8:186–189.

30. Lin F, Goldman JM, Cross NCP. A comparison of the sensitivity of blood and bone marrow for the detection of minimal residual disease in chronic myeloid leukaemia. *Br J Haematol.* 1994;86:683–685.

31. Chomczynski P, Sacchi N. Single step method of RNA isolation by acid guanidinium thiocyanate-phenol-chloroform extraction. *Annals of Biochemistry.* 1987;162:156–159.

32. Gabert J, Beillard E, van der Velden, et al. Standardization and quality control studies of 'real-time' quantitative reverse transcriptase polymerase chain reaction of fusion gene transcripts for residual disease detection in leukemia – a Europe Against Cancer program. *Leukaemia.* 2003;17:2318–2357.

33. Menisk E, van de Locht A, Schattenberg A. Quantification of minimal residual disease in Philadelphia chromosome positive chronic myeloid leukaemia patients using real-time quantitative RT-PCR. *Br J Haematol.* 1998;102:768–774.

34. Holland PM, Abramson RD, Watson R, et al. Detection of specific polymerase chain reaction product by utilizing the 5′–3′ exonuclease activity of *Thermus aquaticus* DNA polymerase. *Proc Natl Acad Sci U S A.* 1991;88: 7276–7280.

35. Livak KJ, Flood SJ, Marmaro J, et al. Oligonucleotides with fluorescent dyes at opposite ends provide a quenched probe system useful for detecting PCR product and nucleic acid hybridization. *PCR Methods Appl.* 1995;4:357–362.

36. Kaeda J, Chase A, Goldman JM. Cytogenetic and molecular monitoring of residual disease in chronic myeloid leukaemia. *Acta Haematol.* 2002;107:64–75.

37. Hochhaus A, Lin F, Reiter A, et al. Quantification of residual disease in chronic myeloid leukaemia on interferon-alpha therapy by competitive polymerase chain reaction. *Blood.* 1996;87:1549–1555.

38. Hughes T, Kaeda J, Branford S, et al. For the International Randomized Study of Interferon Versus STI571 (IRIS) Study Group. Frequency of major molecular responses to imatinib or interferon alfa plus cytarabine in newly diagnosed chronic myeloid leukemia. *N Engl J Med.* 2003;349:1397–1431.

39. White HE, Matejtschuk P, Rigsby P, et al. Establishment of the 1st World Health Organization International Genetic Reference Panel for quantitation of BCR-ABL mRNA. *Blood.* 2010; 10.1182/blood-2010-1182/b06-1182/blood-2010-11291641 [Epub ahead of print].

40. van Dongen JJ, Langerak AW, Bruggemann M, et al. Design and standardization of PCR primers and protocols for detection of clonal immunoglobulin and T-cell receptor gene recombinations in suspect lymphoproliferations: report of the BIOMED-2 Concerted Action BMH4-CT98–BMH4-3936. *Leukaemia.* 2003;17:2257–2317.

41. Deane M, Norton JD. Detection of immunoglobulin gene rearrangement in B lymphoid

malignancies by polymerase chain reaction gene amplification. *Br J Haematol.* 1990;74:251–256.

42. Cave H, van der Werff ten Bosch J, Suciu S, et al. Clinical significance of minimal residual disease in childhood acute lymphoblastic leukemia. *N Engl J Med.* 1998;339:591–598.

43. van der Velden VH, Hochhaus A, Cazzaniga G, et al. Detection of minimal residual disease in hematologic malignancies by real-time quantitative PCR: principles, approaches and laboratory aspects. *Leukemia.* 2003;17:1013–1034.

44. Goulden N, Bader P, van der Velden V, et al. Minimal residual disease prior to stem cell transplant for childhood acute lymphoblastic leukaemia. *Br J Haematol.* 2003;122:24–29.

45. Patel B, Rai L, Buck G, et al. Minimal residual disease is a significant predictor of treatment failure in non T-lineage adult acute lymphoblastic leukaemia: final results of the international trial UKALL XII/ ECOG2993. *Br J Haematol.* 2010;148:80–89.

46. Giebel S, Stella-Holowiecka B, Krawczyk-Kulis M, et al. Status of minimal residual disease determines outcome of autologous hematopoietic SCT in adult ALL. *Bone Marrow Transplant.* 2009;45:1095–1101.

47. Gökbuget N, Raff R, Brügge-Mann M, et al. Risk/MRD adapted GMALL trials in adult ALL. *Ann Hematol.* 2004;83(suppl 1): S129–S131.

48. Baxter EJ, Scott LM, Campbell PJ, et al. Cancer Genome Project.

Acquired mutation of the tyrosine kinase JAK2 in human myeloproliferative disorders. *Lancet.* 2005;365:1054–1061.

49. Steensma DP, Dewald GW, Lasho TL, et al. The JAK2 V617F activating tyrosine kinase mutation is an infrequent event in both 'atypical' myeloproliferative disorders and myelodysplastic syndromes. *Blood.* 2005;106:1207–1209.

50. Denys B, El Housni H, Nollet F, et al. A real-time polymerase chain reaction assay for rapid, sensitive and specific quantification of the JAK2V617F mutation using a locked nucleic acid-modified oligonucleotide. *J Mol Diagn.* 2010;12:512–519.

51. Gabert J, Beillard E, van der Velden VH, et al. Standardization and quality control studies of 'real-time' quantitative reverse transcriptase polymerase chain reaction of fusion gene transcripts for residual disease detection in leukemia – a Europe Against Cancer program. *Leukemia.* 2003;17: 2318–2357.

52. Beillard E, Pallisgaard N, van der Velden VH, et al. Evaluation of candidate control genes for diagnosis and residual disease detection in leukemic patients using 'real-time' quantitative reverse-transcriptase polymerase chain reaction (RQ-PCR) – a Europe against cancer program. *Leukemia.* 2003;17:2474–2486.

53. Reichel M, Gillert E, Breitenlohner I, et al. Rapid isolation of chromosomal breakpoints from patients with t(4;11). Acute

lymphoblastic leukemia. *Cancer Res.* 1999;59:3357–3362.

54. Szczepański T, Willemse MJ, Brinkhof B, et al. Comparative analysis of Ig and TCR gene rearrangements at diagnosis and at relapse of childhood precursor-B-ALL provides improved strategies for selection of stable PCR targets for monitoring of minimal residual disease. *Blood.* 2002;99: 2315–2323.

55. Horiike S, Yokota S, Nakao M, et al. Tandem duplications of the FLT3 receptor gene are associated with leukemic transformation of myelodysplasia. *Leukemia.* 1997;11: 1442–1446.

56. Cazzaniga G, Dell'Oro MG, Mecucci C, et al. Nucleophosmin mutations in childhood acute myelogenous leukemia with normal karyotype. *Blood.* 2005;106: 1419–1422.

57. Bacher U, Schnittger S, Haferlach T. Molecular genetics in acute myeloid leukemia. *Curr Opin Oncol.* 2010; 22(6):646–655.

58. Van Deerlin VM, Leonard DG. Bone marrow engraftment analysis after allogeneic bone marrow transplantation. *Clinical and Laboratory Medicine.* 2000;20: 197–225.

59. Mann K, Fox SP, Abbs SJ, et al. Development and implementation of a new rapid aneuploidy diagnostic service within the UK National Health Service and implications for the future of prenatal diagnosis. *Lancet.* 2001;358:1057–1061.

Chapter | 9 |

Iron deficiency anaemia and iron overload

Mark Worwood, Alison May

CHAPTER CONTENTS

IRON METABOLISM

The iron content of the body and its distribution among the various proteins is summarized in Table 9.1. Most of the iron is present in the oxygen-carrying protein of the red blood cell, haemoglobin, the synthesis and breakdown of which dominates iron turnover. Haem of haemoglobin is synthesized in nucleated red cells in the bone marrow by a pathway ending with the incorporation of iron into protoporphyrin IX by ferrochelatase. Haem breakdown from haemoglobin takes place mainly in phagocytic cells, largely those in the spleen, liver and bone marrow. Iron is released from haem by haem oxygenase and is largely reused for haem synthesis. Every day about 30 mg iron is used to make new haemoglobin and most of this is obtained from the breakdown of old red cells.

Relatively little iron is lost from the body (about 1 mg/d in men) and these losses are not influenced by body iron content or the requirement of the body for iron. The body iron content is maintained by variation in the amount of iron absorbed. In women, menstruation

and childbirth increase iron losses to about 1.5 mg/d. Iron absorption may not increase sufficiently to compensate for these iron losses and this may eventually lead to the development of iron deficiency anaemia. In most men and postmenopausal women there is some 'storage' iron. This is iron in ferritin or its insoluble derivative haemosiderin, which is available for haem synthesis if necessary. Many young women and children have little or no storage iron.

The iron-binding protein transferrin is responsible for extracellular transport. Each molecule of transferrin can bind up to two molecules of ferric iron. Most cells obtain iron from diferric transferrin which binds to transferrin receptors (TfR) on the cell surface. This is followed by internalization into vesicles, release of iron, transport of iron into the cytoplasm and recycling of the apotransferrin (the protein without iron) into the plasma (Fig. 9.1).

Dietary Iron Absorption

Iron absorption[1] depends on the amount of iron in the diet, its bioavailability and the body's need for iron. A normal Western diet provides approximately 15 mg iron daily. Of that iron, digestion within the gut lumen releases about half in a soluble form, from which only

Table 9.1 Distribution of iron in the body in a 70 kg man[a]		
PROTEIN	**LOCATION**	**IRON CONTENT (mg)**
Haemoglobin	Red blood cells	3000
Myoglobin	Muscle	400
Cytochromes and iron sulphur proteins	All tissues	50
Transferrin	Plasma and extravascular fluid	5
Ferritin and haemosiderin	Liver, spleen and bone marrow	100–1000

[a]The numbers are different for women.

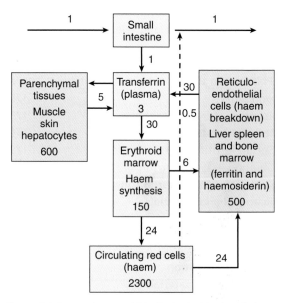

Figure 9.1 Iron exchange within the body. Numbers in boxes refer to amount of iron (mg) in the various compartments and the numbers alongside arrows indicate transfer in mg/d. The iron in parenchymal tissues is largely haem in muscle and ferritin/haemosiderin in hepatic parenchymal cells. The dotted line indicates the small daily loss of iron (0.5 mg) into the gut from red cells; the remaining iron loss is mostly in exfoliated gut cells and bile.

about 1 mg (5–10% of dietary iron) is transferred to the portal blood in a healthy adult male.

Dietary and Luminal Factors

Most of the dietary iron is non-haem iron derived from cereals (often fortified with additional iron), with a lesser, but well-absorbed, component of haem iron from meat and fish. With iron deficiency, the maximum iron absorption from a mixed Western diet is no more than 3–4 mg daily. This amount is much less in the more vegetarian, cereal-based diets of many populations.

Non-haem iron is released from protein complexes by acid and proteolytic enzymes in the stomach and small intestine. It is maximally absorbed from the duodenum and less well from the jejunum, probably because the increasingly alkaline environment leads to the formation of insoluble ferric hydroxide complexes. Many luminal factors enhance (e.g. meat and vitamin C) or inhibit (e.g. phytates and tannins) non-haem iron absorption. Therapeutic ferrous iron salts are well absorbed (approximately 10–20%) on an empty stomach, but when taken with meals, absorption is reduced by the same dietary interactions that affect non-haem food iron.

Iron Absorption at the Molecular Level

Several membrane transport proteins, regulatory proteins and associated oxidoreductases involved in iron transport through the intestinal cell have been identified. Non-haem iron is released from food as Fe^{3+} (ferric iron) and reduced to Fe^{2+} (ferrous iron) by a membrane-bound, ferrireductase, duodenal cytochrome b (DCYTB). Iron is then transported across the brush-border membrane by the divalent metal transporter, DMT1. Some iron is incorporated into ferritin and lost when the cells are exfoliated. Iron destined for retention by the body is transported across the serosal membrane by ferroportin-1. Before uptake by transferrin, Fe^{2+} is oxidized to Fe^{3+} by hephaestin (a membrane protein homologous to the plasma copper-containing protein caeruloplasmin) or by plasma caeruloplasmin.

Haemoglobin and myoglobin are digested in the stomach and small intestine. Haem is initially bound by haem receptors at the brush border membrane and the iron is released intracellularly by haem oxygenase before entering the labile iron pool and following a common pathway with iron of non-haem origin.

Regulation of Iron Absorption

Iron absorption may be regulated both at the stage of mucosal uptake and at the stage of transfer to the blood. Recent studies show that in mice HIF-2α, a mediator of cellular adaptation to hypoxia, regulates DMT1 transcription and thus mucosal uptake of iron.[2] As the epithelial cells develop in the crypts of Lieberkuhn, their iron status reflects that of the plasma (transferrin saturation) and this programmes the cells to absorb iron appropriately as they differentiate along the villus. Transfer to the plasma depends on the requirements of the erythron for iron and the level of iron stores. This regulation is mediated directly by hepcidin, a peptide synthesized in the liver in response to iron and inflammation.[3]

Cellular Iron Uptake and Release

Diferric transferrin binds with high affinity to the transferrin receptor (TfR1) on the membrane of the cell to form a complex which initiates clathrin-dependent endocytosis of the local membrane. The resulting endosome contains the holotransferrin–transferrin receptor complex.[4] The pH of the endosome is reduced by a proton pump and a conformational change in holotransferrin is induced causing iron release. Iron is then reduced by a membrane-bound ferrireductase (six transmembrane epithelial antigen of the prostate 3, STEAP3 in erythroid cells[5]) and transported into the cytoplasm by DMT1. This iron is then either stored as ferritin or used within the cell. Iron destined for haem and mitochondrial iron sulphur (Fe-S) clusters is transported into mitochondria by mitoferrin for incorporation into protoporphyrin by ferrochelatase[6] and for Fe-S cluster assembly on the scaffold protein ISCU.[7] Export by ABCB7 of an as-yet unknown component to the cytoplasm stimulates Fe-S cluster protein assembly there, essential for cellular iron homeostasis.[7] Apotransferrin and the transferrin receptor of the endosome return rapidly to the cell surface where they dissociate at neutral pH so that the cycle can start again.[7a]

The reticuloendothelial macrophages play a major role in recycling iron resulting from the degradation of haemoglobin from senescent erythrocytes. They engulf red blood cells and release the iron within using haem oxygenase. The iron is rapidly released to plasma transferrin or stored as ferritin. The protein transporting iron to plasma is ferroportin or SLC40A1. Ferroportin activity is regulated in a negative manner by the mainly liver-derived peptide, hepcidin that binds to ferroportin externally, inducing endocytosis and degradation.

Hepcidin synthesis in the hepatocyte is controlled at the transcriptional level through the alteration of levels within the nucleus of different transcription factors able to bind to the gene. Interaction of diferric transferrin, bone morphogenetic proteins (BMPs), interleukin (IL)-6 and other inflammatory cytokines with cell surface receptors TfR1, TfR2, hemojuvelin (HJV) and IL-6 receptor lead to upregulation of the hepcidin gene through different and sometimes interacting signalling pathways. TMPRSS6, a plasma membrane serine protease, inhibits the HJV-BMP-SMAD signaling pathway by cleaving HJV from the surface of the cell, thus preventing overproduction of hepcidin and maintaining iron homeostasis.[8,9] A soluble form of HJV (sHJV) produced within the cell by the enzyme furin and released into the plasma antagonizes and also inhibits this pathway.[10]

The mechanism of action of the HFE protein is less clear. HFE binds to both TfR1 and TfR2, decreasing the affinity of each for transferrin. Stabilization and endocytosis of TfR2 stimulates hepcidin production and there is evidence that diferric transferrin displaces the protein HFE from TfR1, leaving it free to interact with TfR2, thus stimulating hepcidin production in response to plasma iron levels.[11-13]

Increased erythropoiesis causes decreased hepcidin, increased iron absorption and increased iron availability for haemoglobin production. So far, two plasma antagonists of the BMP-HJV-SMAD pathway, GDF15 and TWSG1, produced by erythroid cells and associated with expanded ineffective erythropoiesis, have been found.[14,15] Alteration of the function of key regulators leads to body iron overload or iron deficiency (see later). The extent and the manner in which these regulatory pathways vary between different tissues await further investigation.

Iron Storage

All cells require iron for the synthesis of proteins but have the ability also to store excess iron. There are two forms of storage iron: a soluble form, known as ferritin and insoluble haemosiderin.[16] Ferritin consists of a spherical protein (molecular mass 480 000) enclosing a core of ferric-hydroxy-phosphate, which may contain up to 4000 atoms of iron. Haemosiderin is a denatured form of ferritin in which the protein shells have partly degraded, allowing the iron cores to aggregate. Haemosiderin deposits are readily visualized with the aid of the light microscope as areas of Prussian-blue positivity after staining of tissue sections with potassium ferrocyanide in acid (see Chapter 4). Ferritin is found in all cells and in the highest concentration in liver, spleen and bone marrow.

Regulation of Iron Metabolism

The expression of a number of iron proteins involved in both transport and storage is largely controlled posttranscriptionally by iron regulatory proteins (IRP1 and 2).[4] The conformation of IRP1 required for binding to mRNA iron-responsive elements (IREs) and the turnover of IRP2 are directly affected by the amount of iron within a cell. Depending on where the target IRE elements are found these proteins may inhibit or enhance translation of many proteins involved in iron metabolism.

IREs are regions of mRNA that form hairpin-like stem-loop structures. These consist of a base-paired stem of variable length interrupted by an asymmetrical region including a 5′ unpaired cytosine, followed by an upper stem of five paired bases and a six-membered loop. When the labile iron pool is deficient of iron, IRP1 has an available binding site for IRE. When the labile iron pool is saturated with iron, the iron binds to IRP1 to produce a 4Fe-4S cluster which blocks the IRE binding site and prevents IRP1 binding to the IRE. Fe-saturated IRP1 is then able to function as the enzyme aconitase. In the presence of iron, IRP2 (which is not an Fe-S protein) is degraded. The turnover of IRP1 is also affected by iron levels.

Different iron proteins are regulated by IRP in different ways, depending on where the IRE is located. If the IRE is at the 3′ UTR of the mRNA, IRP binding will stabilize translation by protecting the translation product from endonucleolytic cleavage (e.g. TfR1 and DMT1). If the IRE is at the 5′ UTR of the mRNA, IRP binding will inhibit the translation of mRNA. Both L and H ferritin subunits have 5′ UTR IRE. When iron is abundant, the IRP does not bind to the 5′ IRE so ferritin expression is not inhibited and excess iron can be stored adequately. When iron is scarce, the IRP binds to the IRE and inhibits ferritin synthesis.

Plasma Iron Transport

Almost all the iron in plasma is tightly bound to transferrin, which is usually less than 50% saturated with iron. Transferrin, when incompletely saturated with iron, exists in four forms: apo, monoferric (iron bound at the 'A' site), monoferric (B) and diferric. The distribution may be determined by urea-polyacrylamide electrophoresis.[17] Delivery to cells requires specific binding to transferrin receptors. The plasma iron pool (transferrin-bound iron) is about 3 mg, although the daily turnover is more than 10 times his amount. In addition, smaller amounts of iron are carried in the plasma by other proteins.

Haptoglobin is a serum glycoprotein that avidly binds haemoglobin αβ dimers released into the bloodstream by haemolysis. The haemoglobin–haptoglobin complex is rapidly removed from the plasma by a specific receptor, CD163, highly expressed on tissue macrophages.[18]

Hemopexin[19] is a plasma glycoprotein of molecular mass approximately 60 kDa that binds haem and transports the haem to cells by a process that involves receptor-mediated endocytosis and recycling of the intact protein.

Low concentrations of *ferritin* are found in the plasma and ferritin concentrations in healthy subjects reflect body iron stores. Much of this ferritin appears to be glycosylated and has a relatively low iron content.[20] Such ferritin has a half life ($T_{1/2}$) of approximately 30 h. Ferritin is also released into the circulation as a result of tissue damage (most strikingly after necrosis of the liver). Tissue ferritin is cleared rapidly from the circulation ($T_{1/2}$ in approximately 10 min) by the liver.

Non-transferrin-bound iron describes a form of iron that is not bound to transferrin, is of low molecular mass and can be bound by specific iron chelators.[21] Several assays have been described that have demonstrated such a fraction in plasma from patients with iron overload. The chemical form of this iron is unknown, but it is probably rapidly removed from the circulation by the liver. Recent studies implicate the involvement of the zinc transporter ZIP14 in this process.[22]

IRON STATUS

Normal iron status implies a level of erythropoiesis that is not limited by the supply of iron and the presence of a small reserve of 'storage iron' to cope with normal physiological needs. The ability to survive the acute loss of blood (iron) that may result from injury is also an advantage. The limits of normality are difficult to define and some argue that physiological normality is the presence of only a minimal amount of storage iron[23] but the extremes (i.e. iron deficiency anaemia and haemochromatosis) are well understood.[23a]

Apart from too little or too much iron in the body, there is also the possibility of a maldistribution (Fig. 9.2). An example is anaemia associated with inflammation or infection where there is a partial failure of erythropoiesis and of iron release from the phagocytic cells in liver, spleen and bone marrow, which results in accumulation of iron as ferritin and haemosiderin in these cells. Determination of iron status requires an estimate of the amount of haemoglobin iron (usually by measuring the haemoglobin concentration (Hb) in the blood; see Chapter 3) and the level of storage iron (measuring serum ferritin concentration). Iron deficiency should be suspected in hypochromic, microcytic anaemia, but in the early stages of iron deficiency red cells may be normocytic and normochromic. Another feature of iron deficiency is an increased concentration of protoporphyrin in the red cells; normally, there is a small amount present, but defective haem synthesis caused by lack of iron results in the accumulation of zinc protoporphyrin and occasionally free protoporphyrin may be increased as well.[24]

DISORDERS OF IRON METABOLISM

Clinical aspects of iron metabolism have been reviewed[25–27] and are summarized in Table 9.2. A guideline on the management of genetic haemochromatosis is available.[28]

METHODS FOR ASSESSING IRON STATUS

The methods used to assess iron status are summarized in Table 9.3. Some are not generally applicable but have value in the standardization of indirect methods. The determinations of Hb and red cell indices are described in Chapter 3.

Serum Ferritin Assay

With the recognition that the small quantity of ferritin in human serum (15–300 µg/l in healthy men) reflects body iron stores, measurement of serum ferritin has been widely adopted as a test for iron deficiency and iron overload. The first reliable method to be introduced was an immunoradiometric assay in which excess radiolabelled antibody was reacted with ferritin and antibody not bound to ferritin was removed with an immunoadsorbent.[31] This assay was supplanted by the two-site immunoradiometric assay, which is sensitive and convenient. Since then the principle of this assay has been extended to non-radioactive labelling, including enzymes (enzyme-linked immunosorbent assay or ELISA). Most current laboratory immunoassay systems for clinical

Figure 9.2 Body iron content and distribution in different conditions. Additional assays are sometimes required. In genetic haemochromatosis, early iron accumulation is indicated by increased transferrin saturation alone. The serum ferritin concentration increases only later as the level of stored iron increases. In the anaemia of chronic disease, patients often have normal serum ferritin concentrations even when storage iron in the bone marrow is absent (see p. 336). In this situation, the assay of serum transferrin receptor may help detect tissue iron deficiency.

Table 9.2 Disorders of iron metabolism

Iron deficiency

Deficient iron intake

Diet of low bioavailability

Increased physiological requirements due to rapid growth in early childhood and in adolescence

Blood loss: physiological (e.g. menstruation) or pathological (e.g. gastrointestinal)

Malabsorption of iron intake

Reduced gastric acid secretion (e.g. after partial gastrectomy)

Reduced duodenal absorptive area (e.g. in coeliac disease)

Rare, inherited iron-refractory iron deficiency anaemia

TMPRSS6 deficiency

Redistribution of iron

Macrophage iron accumulation

Inflammatory, infectious or malignant diseases ('anaemia of chronic disease')

Iron overload

Due to increased iron absorption

e.g. Hereditary haemochromatosis – commonly homozygosity for *HFE* C282Y but sometimes involving other genes (*HAMP, HJV, TFR2, SLC40A1*)

Substantial ineffective erythropoiesis (e.g. β thalassaemia syndromes of intermediate and major severity, some types of sideroblastic anaemia, congenital dyserythropoietic anaemia)

Sub-Saharan iron overload ('Bantu siderosis') – only in combination with increased dietary iron

Other rare inherited disorders (e.g. congenital atransferrinaemia, DMT1 deficiency)

Inappropriate iron therapy (rare)

Due to multiple blood transfusions in refractory anaemias

e.g. Thalassaemia major

Aplastic anaemia

Myelodysplastic syndromes

---

laboratories include ferritin in the assay repertoire. Factors to be considered when selecting an immunoassay system are discussed later. The method described in the next section is an ELISA. The most sophisticated equipment required is a microtitre plate reader.

Immunoassay for Ferritin

Preparation and Storage of Ferritin

Ferritin may be prepared from iron-loaded human liver or spleen obtained at operation (spleen) or postmortem. The informed consent of the patient or the patient's relatives should be obtained for use in preparation of ferritin. Tissue should be obtained as soon as possible after death and may be stored at $-20°C$ for 1 year. The usual precautions must be taken to avoid the risk of infection when handling tissues and extracts. Ferritin is purified by methods that exploit its stability at $75°C$. Further purification is obtained by precipitation from cadmium sulphate solution and gel-filtration chromatography.[32] Purity should be assessed by polyacrylamide gel electrophoresis,[33] and the protein content determined by the method of Lowry and colleagues, as described by Worwood.[33] Buffered solutions of human ferritin may be stored at $4°C$, at concentrations of 1–4 mg protein/ml, in the presence of sodium azide as a preservative, for up to 3 years. Such solutions should not be frozen. Ferritin, from human liver or spleen, may be obtained from several suppliers of laboratory reagents. This should be used as an assay standard only after calibration against the international standard (see p. 183).

Antibodies to Human Ferritin

High-affinity antibodies to human liver or spleen ferritin are suitable. Polyclonal antibodies may be raised in rabbits or sheep by conventional methods,[34] and the titre checked by precipitation with human ferritin.[33] An immunoglobulin G (IgG)-enriched fraction of antiserum is required for labelling with enzyme in the assay. The simplest method is to precipitate IgG with ammonium sulphate.[35] Monoclonal antibodies that are specific for 'L' subunit-rich ferritin (liver or spleen ferritin) are also suitable. A mouse monoclonal antibody and a horseradish peroxidase (HRP)-labelled antibody are available from NIBSC (www.nibsc.ac.uk; codes 87/654 and 87/662). Suitable antibodies are available from commercial suppliers.

Reagents and Materials

Before handling any of the reagents and materials described below a risk assessment should be carried out. If there is significant risk of harm, the word 'caution' has been added.

Conjugation of Antiferritin IgG Preparation to Horseradish Peroxidase[36]

1. Dissolve 4 mg horseradish peroxidase (Sigma Type VI P-8375) in 1 ml water and add 200 μl of freshly prepared 0.1 mol/l sodium periodate solution (caution). The solution should turn greenish-brown. Mix gently by inverting and leave for 20 min at room temperature, mixing gently every 5 min. Dialyse overnight against 1 mmol/l sodium acetate buffer, pH 4.4.

2. Add 20 μl of 0.2 mol/l sodium carbonate buffer, pH 9.5, to a solution of antiferritin IgG fraction (8 mg in 1 ml). Add 20 μl of 0.2 mol/l sodium carbonate buffer, pH 9.5, to the horseradish peroxidase solution to increase the pH to 9.0–9.5 and immediately mix the two solutions. Leave at room temperature for 2 h and mix by inversion every 30 min.

3. Add 100 μl freshly prepared sodium borohydride solution (caution) (4 mg/ml in water) and let it stand at $4°C$ for 2 h. Dialyse overnight against 0.1 mol/l borate buffer, pH 7.4.

4. Add an equal volume of 60% v/v glycerol in 0.1 mol/l borate buffer to the conjugate solution and store at $4°C$.

Table 9.3 Assessment of body iron status and confounding factors

MEASUREMENT	REFERENCE RANGE (ADULTS)	DIAGNOSTIC USE	CONFOUNDING FACTORS
Haemoglobin concentration	Male: 13–17 g/dl Female: 12–15 g/dl	Defining anaemia and assessing its severity; response to a therapeutic trial of iron confirms iron deficiency anaemia (IDA)	Other causes of anaemia besides iron deficiency
Red cell indices 　Mean cell volume 　Mean cell haemoglobin	83–101 fl 27–32 pg	Low values indicate iron deficient erythropoiesis	May be reduced in disorders of haemoglobin synthesis, other than iron deficiency (thalassaemia, sideroblastic anaemias, anaemia of chronic disease)
Tissue iron supply 　Serum iron	10–30 μmol/l	Low values in iron deficiency, high values in iron overload	Reduced in acute and chronic disease; labile, use of fasting morning sample reduces variability
Total iron binding capacity (TIBC)	47–70 μmol/l	High values characteristic of tissue iron deficiency. Low values in iron overload. May also be calculated from transferrin concentration (Tf g/l × 25)	Rarely used on its own. Reliable reference ranges not available
Unsaturated iron binding capacity (UIBC)	See text		
Transferrin saturation (TS) (iron/TIBC × 100)	16–50%	Low values in iron deficiency, high values in iron overload. Raised TS is an early indicator of iron accumulation in genetic haemochromatosis	See serum iron (above)
Iron supply to the bone marrow 　Serum transferrin receptor (sTfR) 　Red cell zinc protoporphyrin (ZPP) 　Red cell ferritin ('L' type) 　% hypochromic red cells	2.8–8.5 mg/l[a] <80 μmol/mol Hb 3–40 ag/cell <6%	Reduced red cell ferritin or increased ZPP, sTfR and % hypochromic red cells indicate impaired iron supply to the bone marrow. Useful for identifying early iron deficiency and, with a measure of iron stores, distinguishing this from anaemia of chronic disease (ACD). In ACD, sTfR only increases in the presence of tissue iron deficiency	sTfR concentration is related to extent of erythroid activity as well as iron supply to cells; ZPP, red cell ferritin and % hypochromic cells are stable measures determined at time of red cell formation. ZPP may be increased by other causes of impaired iron incorporation into haem (sideroblastic anaemias, lead poisoning, inflammation). % hypochromic cells will be affected by change in red cell volume on sample storage

Continued

Table 9.3 Assessment of body iron status and confounding factors – cont'd

MEASUREMENT	REFERENCE RANGE (ADULTS)	DIAGNOSTIC USE	CONFOUNDING FACTORS
Iron stores Serum ferritin	Male 15–300 µg/l Female 15–200 µg/l	Correlated with body iron stores from deficiency to overload	Increased: as acute-phase protein and by release of tissue ferritin after organ damage (particularly liver disease). Increased in rare inherited disorders of ferritin overproduction. Decreased: vitamin C deficiency

Tissue biopsy iron
Chemical assay
    Liver
Perls' stain
    Liver
	3–33 µmol/g dry weight
	(Grade)
		Confirmation of iron overload
		
		Confirmation of iron overload, also to distinguish between parenchymal and macrophage iron accumulation
			Adequate sample required

Bone marrow	(Grade)	Graded as absent, present or increased. Most commonly used to differentiate ACD from IDA	Adequate sample required
Quantitative phlebotomy	<2 g Fe	Treatment of genetic haemochromatosis including measurement of initial amount of storage iron	Also treatment of secondary iron overload of non-transfused iron-loading anaemias
Urine chelatable Fe (after intramuscular injection of deferoxamine)	<2 mg/24 h	Rarely used but may provide confirmation of iron overload	
Imaging MRI (magnetic resonance imaging)		Available both for hepatic and cardiac iron deposition	Machines widely available but special analysis and software required
SQID (superconducting quantum interface device)[29]		Quantitation of liver iron overload using magnetic properties of iron	Not available in UK

Modified from Pippard (2003).[30]

[a]Units and reference ranges are specific to method.

Buffer A

Phosphate-buffered saline, pH 7.2, containing 0.05% v/v Tween 20. Prepare a ×10 concentrated (1.5 mol/l) stock solution by dissolving 80 g sodium chloride, 2 g potassium chloride, 11.5 g anhydrous disodium phosphate and 2 g anhydrous potassium phosphate (KH_2PO_4) in 1 litre of water. Store at room temperature. Prepare Buffer A by diluting 100 ml stock solution to 1 litre with water and adding 0.5 ml Tween 20. Store at 4°C for up to 2 weeks.

Buffer B

Prepare by dissolving 5 g bovine serum albumin (BSA; Sigma A-7030) in 1 litre of Buffer A. Store at 4°C for up to 2 weeks.

Buffer C

Carbonate buffer, 0.05 mol/l, pH 9.6. Dissolve 1.59 g sodium carbonate and 2.93 g sodium bicarbonate in 1 litre of water and store at room temperature.

Buffer D

Citrate phosphate buffer, 0.15 mol/l, pH 5.0. Dissolve 21 g of citric acid monohydrate in 1 litre of water and store at 4°C. Dissolve 28.4 g of anhydrous disodium phosphate in 1 litre of water and store at room temperature. Prepare fresh buffer on the day of assay by mixing 49 ml citric acid solution with 51 ml phosphate solution.

Substrate Solution

Prepare immediately before use by adding 33 µl 30% w/v hydrogen peroxide (CAUTION: causes burns) to 100 ml Buffer D and mixing well. Add 1 tablet containing 30 mg of *o*-phenylenediamine dihydrochloride (Sigma P 8412) and mix (caution).

Sulphuric Acid

Purchase as a 4 M solution (CAUTION: poison, corrosive). Consider using a commercial ELISA 'Stop' solution.

Preparation and Storage of a Standard Ferritin Solution

Dilute a solution of human ferritin to approximately 200 µg/ml in water. Measure the protein concentration by the method of Lowry after diluting further to 20–50 µg/ml. Then dilute the ferritin solution (approx. 200 µg/ml) accurately to a concentration of 10 µg/ml in 0.05 mol/l sodium barbitone solution containing 0.1 mol/l NaCl, 0.02% NaN_3 and BSA (5 g/l) and adjusted to pH 8.0 with HCl. Deliver 200 µl into 200 small polypropylene tubes, cap tightly and store at 4°C for up to 1 year. For use, dilute in Buffer B to 1000 ng/ml, then prepare a range of standard solutions between 0.2 and 25 ng/ml. Calibrate this working standard against the World Health Organization (WHO) standard for the assay of serum ferritin 94/572, recombinant human L type ferritin. (Information available at: www.nibsc.ac.uk.)

Coating of Plates

Microtitre plates (96-well) for immunoassay are required. Do not use the outer wells until you have established the assay procedure and can check that all wells give consistent results. Coat the plates by adding to each well 200 µl antiferritin IgG preparation diluted to 2 µg/ml in Buffer C. Cover the plate with a lid and leave overnight at 4°C. On the day of the assay, empty the wells by sharply inverting the plate and dry them by tapping briefly on paper towels. Block uncoated sites by adding 200 µl 0.5% (w/v) BSA in Buffer C. After 30 min at room temperature, wash each plate three times by filling each well with Buffer A (using a syringe and blunt needle and emptying and draining as described earlier). Plates may be stored dry at 4°C for up to 1 week.

Preparation of Test Sera

Collect clotted venous blood and separate the serum. Serum samples may be stored for 1 week at 4°C or for 2 years at −20°C. Plasma obtained from either ethylenediaminetetra-acetic acid (EDTA) or heparinized blood is also suitable. For assay, dilute 50 µl of serum to 1 ml with Buffer B. Further dilutions may be made in the same buffer if required.

Assay Procedure

The use of a multichannel pipette for rapid addition of solutions is recommended. For each plate standards and sera, in duplicate, should be added within 15 min.

Add 200 µl standard solution or diluted serum to each well of a pre-coated plate. Cover the plate and leave for 2 h at room temperature on a draught-free bench away from direct sunlight. Empty the wells by sharply inverting the plate and drain by standing them on paper towels with occasional tapping for 1 min. Wash three times by filling each well with Buffer A, leaving for 2 min at room temperature and draining as described earlier. Dilute the anti ferritin IgG-horseradish peroxidase conjugate in 1% BSA in Buffer A. The optimal dilution (of the order of 10^3–10^4 times) must be ascertained by experiment. Add 200 µl of diluted conjugate to each well and leave the covered plate for a further 2 h at room temperature. Wash three times with Buffer A. Add 200 µl of peroxidase substrate solution to each well. Incubate the plate for 30 min in the dark. Stop the reaction by adding 50 µl of 4 M sulphuric acid to each well (alternative 'stop' reagents are available) and within 30 min read the absorbance at 492 nm using a microtitre plate reader. Alternatively, after stopping the reaction, transfer 200 µl from each well to a tube containing 800 µl of water and read the absorbance in a spectrophotometer.

Calculation of Results

Calculate the mean absorbance for each point on the standard curve and plot against ferritin concentration using semilogarithmic paper. Read concentrations for the sera from this curve. If results are captured on a file and calculated with a computer program, the log-logit plot provides a linear dose response. For serum ferritin concentrations >200 µg/l, re-assay at a dilution of ≥100 times. Control sera should be included in each assay.

Selecting an Assay Method

The following notes may be of use for those considering introducing a ferritin assay into a clinical laboratory using an immunoassay system. The major manufacturers of immunoassay analysers include ferritin in the test menu and allow for either batch or random access operation. Most use chemiluminescent signal detection with microparticle separation of free and ferritin-bound labelled antibody.

1. *Limit of detection.* Most current assays have a lower limit of <1 μg/l. This is adequate for all clinical purposes.
2. *The 'high-dose hook'.* This is a problem peculiar to labelled-antibody assays when sera with very high ferritin concentrations give anomalous readings in the lower part of the standard curve. Most current commercial assays are not affected. Because of the wide range of serum ferritin concentrations that may be encountered in hospital patients (0–40 000 μg/l), it is good practice to dilute and re-assay any samples giving readings higher than the working range of the assay. This may be done automatically in some systems but might require manual dilution.
3. *Interference by non-ferritin proteins in serum.* This may occur with any method but particularly with labelled antibody assays. Serum proteins may inhibit the binding of ferritin to the solid phase when compared with binding in buffer solution alone. Such an effect may be avoided by diluting the standards in a buffer containing a suitable serum or by diluting serum samples as much as possible. For example, in the assay described earlier, the sample is diluted 20 times with buffer. Another cause of error, difficult to detect, is interference by antibodies to animal immunoglobulins.[37] These antibodies bind to the animal immunoglobulins used to detect the antigen and form artefactual 'sandwiches', thereby falsely elevating the reading. Such antibodies are found in up to 10% of patients and normal subjects. Interference may be reduced by adding the appropriate species of animal immunoglobulins to block the cross-reaction, but this is not always successful.[38] One solution is to use antibodies from different species as solid-phase and labelled antibodies. Thus one may use a polyclonal, rabbit antiferritin to coat plates in the ELISA with a polyclonal sheep antiferritin labelled with horseradish peroxidase as the second antibody. Rabbit serum (0.5%) replaces BSA in Buffer B.
4. *Reproducibility.* Most assays are satisfactory. With microtitre plate assays there may be 'edge' effects (differences between readings for inner and outer wells).
5. *Dilution of serum samples.* It should be established that both standard and serum samples dilute in parallel over a 100-fold range.
6. *Accuracy.* The use of the WHO standard ferritin preparation is recommended (see earlier discussion).

Interpretation

The use of serum ferritin for the assessment of iron stores has become well-established.[31] In most normal adults, serum ferritin concentrations lie within the range of 15–300 μg/l. During the first months of life, mean serum ferritin concentrations change considerably, reflecting changes in storage iron concentration. Concentrations are lower in children (<15 years) than in adults and from puberty to middle life are higher in men than in women. In adults, concentrations <15 μg/l indicate an absence of storage iron. Reference ranges quoted by kit manufacturers vary and this is partly a result of the selection of 'normal' subjects. Sometimes subjects with iron deficiency are included and sometimes they are excluded. The interpretation of serum concentration in many pathological conditions is less straightforward, but concentrations <15 μg/l indicate depletion of storage iron. In children, mean levels of storage iron are lower and a 12 μg/l threshold has been found to be appropriate for detecting iron deficiency.[39]

Iron overload causes high concentrations of serum ferritin, but these may also be found in patients with liver disease, infection, inflammation or malignant disease.[31] In addition some rare inherited causes of increased ferritin production unlinked to iron stores occur. Careful consideration of the clinical evidence is required before concluding that a high serum ferritin concentration is primarily the result of iron overload and not a result of tissue damage or enhanced synthesis of ferritin. A normal ferritin concentration provides good evidence against iron overload but does not exclude genetic haemochromatosis. This is because haemochromatosis is a late-onset condition and iron stores may remain within the normal range for many years.

Serum ferritin concentrations are high in patients with advanced haemochromatosis, but the serum ferritin estimation should not be used alone to screen the relatives of patients or to assess re-accumulation of storage iron after phlebotomy. The early stages of iron accumulation are detectable by an increased serum iron concentration, a decreased unsaturated iron-binding capacity and increased transferrin saturation; the serum ferritin concentration may be within the normal range. In this situation, the measurement of serum iron and total iron-binding capacity provides useful clinical information not given by the ferritin assay.

In patients with acute or chronic disease, interpretation of serum ferritin concentrations is less straightforward and patients may have serum ferritin concentrations up to 100 μg/l despite an absence of stainable iron in the bone marrow. Ferritin synthesis is enhanced by interleukin-1 – the primary mediator of the acute-phase response.[40] In patients with chronic disease, the following approach should be adopted: low serum ferritin concentrations indicate absent iron stores, values within the normal range indicate either low or normal levels and high values indicate either normal or high levels. In terms of adequacy of iron stores for replenishing haemoglobin in patients with anaemia, the degree of anaemia must also be considered. Thus a patient with Hb 10 g/dl may benefit from iron therapy if the serum ferritin concentration is <100 μg/l because below this level there is unlikely to be sufficient iron available for full regeneration. Here, measurement of serum transferrin receptor concentration may be of value (see p. 190).

Immunologically, plasma ferritin resembles the 'L-rich' ferritins of liver and spleen and only low concentrations are detected with antibodies to heart or HeLa cell ferritin, ferritins rich in 'H' subunits. The heterogeneity of serum ferritin on isoelectric focusing is largely the result of glycosylation and the presence of variable numbers of sialic acid residues and not variation in the ratio of H to L subunits.[41] Attempts to assay for 'acidic' (or 'H'-rich) isoferritins in serum as tumour markers have not been successful.[41] The iron content of serum ferritin is low[41] and measurement of this iron has no diagnostic use.[42]

ESTIMATION OF SERUM IRON CONCENTRATION

Iron is carried in the plasma bound to the protein transferrin (molecular mass 78 000). This molecule binds two atoms of iron as Fe^{3+} and delivers iron to cells by interaction with membrane transferrin receptors. The following method is a modification of that recommended by the International Council for Standardization in Haematology (ICSH) and is based on the development of a coloured complex when ferrous iron released by serum protein denaturation in the presence of reducing agent is treated with a chromogen solution.[43]

Reagents and Materials

Reagents must be at least of analytical grade with the lowest obtainable iron content. Before handling any of the reagents and materials described below a risk assessment should be carried out. If there is significant risk of harm, the word 'caution' has been added.

Preparation of Glassware

It is essential to avoid contamination by iron. If possible, use disposable plastic tubes and bottles. If glassware is to be used, wash in a detergent solution, soak in 2 mol/l HCl (caution) for 12 h and finally rinse in iron-free water.

Protein Precipitant

100 g/l trichloroacetic acid (0.61 M) and 22.7 mmol/l ascorbic acid in 0.9 mol/l HCl. The original reducing agent was thioglycolic acid.[43] Ascorbic acid is an alternative reducing agent, although there may be more interference from copper. However, any benefit from reduced copper interference is usually outweighed by the associated health and safety problems of working with thioglycolic acid. To 45 ml 1 mol/l HCl in a 50 ml screwcap polypropylene tube add 5 ml 6.1 mol/l trichloroacetic acid solution (Sigma 490–10; caution). Add 200 mg ascorbic acid and mix. Make a fresh solution when required and discard after 4 h.

Chromogen Solution (Ferrozine)

In 100 ml 1.5 mol/l sodium acetate dissolve 25 mg ferrozine [Sigma-Aldrich 82950, monosodium 3-(2-pyridyl)-5, 6-bis(4-phenylsulphonic acid)-1, 2, 4-triazine] (caution). Store in the dark for up to 4 weeks.

Iron-free Water

Use deionized water for the preparation of all solutions.

Iron Standard 80 μmol/l

Add 22.1 ml deionized water to a universal container (the easiest way is by weight). Add 200 μl 2 mol/l HCl and mix. Add 100 μl iron standard solution (1000 μg Fe/ml in 1% v/v HCl, Aldrich No. 30, 595–2) and mix. Store for up to 2 months at room temperature.

Method

Place 0.5 ml serum (free of haemolysis), 0.5 ml working iron standard and 0.5 ml iron-free water (as a blank), respectively, in each of three 1.5 ml polypropylene microcentrifuge tubes with lids. Add 0.5 ml protein precipitant to each and replace the lid. Mix the contents vigorously (e.g. with a vortex mixer) and allow to stand for 5 min. Centrifuge the tube containing the serum at 13 000 g for 4 min (in a microfuge) to obtain an optically clear supernatant. To 0.5 ml of this supernatant and to 0.5 ml of each of the other mixtures, add 0.5 ml chromogen solution with thorough mixing. After standing for 10 min, measure the absorbance in a spectrophotometer against water at 562 nm. If a microcentrifuge is not available, use double the volume of serum and reagents in a 3 ml plastic tube with lid and centrifuge at 1500 g for 15 min in a bench centrifuge.

If EDTA-plasma is used, the colour develops more slowly and the preparation should be allowed to stand for at least 15 min before measuring the absorbance. The use of EDTA-plasma is not recommended. Iron chelators (e.g. deferoxamine) also delay colour development.[44]

Calculation

$$\text{Serum iron(μmol/l)} = \frac{(A_{562}\text{test} - A_{562}\text{blank})}{(A_{562}\text{standard} - A_{562}\text{blank})} \times 80$$

ALTERNATIVE PROCEDURE: SERUM IRON WITHOUT PROTEIN PRECIPITATION

This is a microtitre plate method developed from the assay of Persijn et al.[45]

Reagents and Materials

Iron Standards 80 μmol/l and 40 μmol/l

Dilute with an equal volume of water to make the 40 μmol/l standard.

Phosphate–Ascorbate Buffer (Stock)

Add approximately 200 ml deionized water to an acid-washed plastic beaker. Add 17.5 g sodium dihydrogen orthophosphate ($NaH_2PO_42H_2O$) to the water and dissolve fully by stirring (plastic stirrer). Adjust the pH to 4.9 using 2 M NaOH solution (2 g NaOH in 25 ml water; caution). Make the volume up to 250 ml and add 25 ml of the buffer to 10 universal containers. Store for up to 1 month at room temperature. Prior to use, add 50 mg of ascorbic acid to each universal container required and shake to dissolve. Discard after 4 h.

Chromogen Solution

Add 50 mg ferrozine (see p. 185) to 25 ml deionized water and shake to dissolve. Store for up to 1 month in the dark at room temperature.

Microtitre Trays

Microtitre trays should be optical grade, with flat-bottomed wells.

Control Serum

Suitable control sera are Lyphochek Assayed Chemistry Control (Bio-Rad).

Method

Add 80 μl deionized water ('O'), standard solution (40, 80 μmol/l), controls (C1, C2) and samples (S1, S2, etc.) to the microtitre plate (see plate map, Table 9.4).

Add 80 μl phosphate–ascorbate buffer to each well, using a multichannel pipette. Tap the tray to mix. Leave for 20 min at room temperature. During this time, take an initial absorbance reading of the tray at 560–570 nm on a microtitre plate reader. Add 40 μl of chromogen solution to each well, then tap the tray to mix. Cover with a film or lid. Incubate for 40 min at 37°C. Take a second absorbance reading. Calculate the net absorbance increment values.

Calculations

Calculate the difference in absorbance (δA) between the final and initial readings for the water blank (δA_0), each standard (δA_{40}, δA_{80}) and serum sample (δA_{sample}).

The approximate values are 0.015–0.03 for the water blank (zero standard) and 0.25–0.28 for the 40 μmol Fe/l standard. Subtract the mean net value of the zero standard (δA_0) from each standard or sample (δA_{sample}).

Table 9.4 Plate map for serum iron determination

	1	2	3	4	5	6	7	8	9	10	11	12
A	0	80	C1	S1	S5	S9	S13	S17	S21	S25	S29	S33
B	0	80	C1	S1	S5	S9	S13	S17	S21	S25	S29	S33
C	0	80	C1	S2	S6	S10	S14	S18	S22	S26	S30	S34
D	0	80	C1	S2	S6	S10	S14	S18	S22	S26	S30	S34
E	40	0	C2	S3	S7	S11	S15	S19	S23	S27	S31	S35
F	40	0	C2	S3	S7	S11	S15	S19	S23	S27	S31	S35
G	40	0	C2	S4	S8	S12	S16	S20	S24	S28	S32	S36
H	40	0	C2	S4	S8	S12	S16	S20	S24	S28	S32	S36

The net value of the 80 μmol/l standard δA_{80} should be 2× that of the 40 μmol/l standard δA_{40}.

Serum iron concentrations are:

$$\frac{\delta A_{sample} - \delta A_0 \times 40\ \mu mol/l}{\delta A_{40} - \delta A_0}$$

The data may be downloaded from the plate reader and imported into a suitable spreadsheet or statistical program (e.g. Excel or Minitab) for these calculations.

Automated Methods for Serum Iron

Procedures for measuring serum iron are available for most clinical chemistry analysers. A non-precipitation method similar to that described above is available from Randox Ltd (www.randox.com). The performance of several methods was reviewed by Tietz et al.[46] who found differences between the various methods, particularly at low values of serum iron concentration. More recently, Blanck et al.[47] carried out an interlaboratory comparison and found no significant differences in results generated by methods currently in use. Variability across laboratories and across methods was low. Serum iron concentrations may be measured by atomic absorption spectroscopy, but this has the disadvantage of measuring any haem iron present as a result of haemolysis and is not used for diagnostic purposes.

SERUM IRON CONCENTRATIONS IN HEALTH AND DISEASE

Jacobs et al.[48] measured serum iron concentrations in a random sample of 517 women and 499 men in the general population of Wales. Serum iron concentrations[44] approximated to a normal distribution. The mean (±SD) of 16.1 ± 7.4 μmol/l in women was slightly lower than for men (18.0 ± 6.3 μmol/l). These figures do not refer to 'iron replete' subjects because subjects with absent iron stores or with frank anaemia were included. Using the microtitre plate method described earlier, Jackson and co-workers[49] determined serum iron concentrations in 10 500 blood donors from South Wales. For 1502 'first time' donors, mean age of 28 years, the mean (±SD) was 16.7 ± 6.0 μmol/l for men and 14.4 ± 6.7 μmol/l for women. Again subjects included potential donors who failed the screening test for anaemia and were not permitted to give blood on that occasion. In the first month of life mean concentration of serum iron is higher (22 μmol/l) than in adults, falls to about 12 μmol/l by the age of 1 year and remains at that level throughout childhood.[50,51]

Measurement of the serum iron concentration alone provides little useful clinical information because, although methodological variation is low, there is considerable variation from hour to hour and day to day in normal individuals (see p. 193). Low concentrations are found in patients with iron deficiency anaemia; in chronic disease (including inflammation, infection and cancer); and during the acute-phase response, including after surgery. Therefore, low serum iron concentrations do not necessarily indicate an absence of storage iron. High concentrations are found in liver disease, hypoplastic anaemias, ineffective erythropoiesis and iron overload.

IRON-BINDING CAPACITY, SERUM TRANSFERRIN AND TRANSFERRIN SATURATION

Estimation of Total Iron-Binding Capacity

In the plasma, iron is bound to transferrin and the total iron-binding capacity (TIBC) is a measure of this protein. The additional iron-binding capacity of transferrin is known as the unsaturated iron-binding capacity (UIBC). The serum iron concentration plus the UIBC together give TIBC.

Iron-binding capacity is usually measured by adding an excess of iron and measuring the iron retained in solution after the addition of a suitable reagent such as 'light' magnesium carbonate or an ion-exchange resin that removes excess iron. All methods are empiric and none is completely satisfactory. The method described as follows was developed by the ICSH.[52]

Principle

Excess iron as ferric chloride is added to serum. Any iron that does not bind to transferrin is removed with excess magnesium carbonate. The iron concentration of the iron-saturated serum is then measured.

Reagents

Basic magnesium carbonate, $MgCO_3$, 'light grade'.
Saturating solution (100 μmol Fe/l).
Add 17.7 ml deionized water to a universal container (by weight is most convenient). Add 100 μl of 1 mol/l HCl. Add 100 μl commercial iron standard solution (see p. 185. Mix and store for up to 2 months at room temperature. The 'saturating iron solution' contains 5.6 μg Fe/ml (100 μmol Fe/l).

Method

Place 0.5 ml serum (EDTA-plasma should not be used) in a 1.5 ml polypropylene microcentrifuge tube and add 0.5 ml saturating iron solution. Mix carefully by hand

and leave at room temperature for 15 min. Use a plastic scoop or tube to add 100 mg ($\pm$ 15 mg) light magnesium carbonate and cap the tube. Shake vigorously and allow to stand for 30 min with occasional mixing. Centrifuge at 13 000 g for 4 min in a microcentrifuge. If the supernatant contains traces of magnesium carbonate, remove the supernatant and re-centrifuge. Carefully remove 0.5 ml supernatant and treat as serum for the iron estimation described earlier (p. 185). Multiply the final result by 2.

DETERMINATION OF UNSATURATED IRON-BINDING CAPACITY

The UIBC may be determined by methods that detect iron remaining and able to bind to chromogen, after adding a standard and excess amount of iron to the serum.[45] The UIBC is the difference between the amount added and the amount binding to the chromogen.

Reagents and Materials

Saturating Solution

2000 μmol iron/l. Add 7.95 ml deionized water to a universal container (by weight is most convenient). Add 1.0 ml Commercial Iron Standard Solution (1000 μg Fe/ml; see p. 185). Mix. Store for up to 2 months at room temperature.

Tris Buffer (Stock)

0.22 M, pH 7.8. Add approximately 200 ml of deionized water to a weighed acid-washed plastic beaker. Add 6.8 g Tris to the water and fully dissolve by stirring with a magnetic stirrer. Adjust the pH to 7.8 using 2 M HCl. Adjust the volume to 250 ml with water (by weight), mix and dispense 24.5 ml (24.5 g) into universal containers. Store for up to 1 month at room temperature.

Tris–Ascorbate–Iron Buffer

Immediately prior to use, add 50 mg ascorbic acid to each universal container of Tris buffer required and dissolve by mixing. Add 0.5 ml saturating solution (2000 μmol Fe/l) and mix. Discard after 4 h.

Chromogen Solution

See p. 185.

Microtitre Trays

See p. 186.

Control Serum

See p. 186.

Method

Add 80 μl deionized water ('O'), control (C1, C2) and sample (S1, S2, etc.) to the microtitre plate (Table 9.5). Add 160 μl Tris–ascorbate–iron buffer to each well, using a multichannel pipette. Tap the tray to mix. Leave the tray for 20 min. During this time, take an initial reading ($A_{initial}$) of the $A_{560-570\,nm}$. Add 40 μl of chromogen solution to each sample and tap the tray to mix; cover with a film or lid. Incubate for 40 min at 37°C. Take a final absorbance reading (A_{final}).

Calculations

The saturating solution added to each well (160 μl) contains 6.4 nmol Fe. Calculate the absorbance reading corresponding to 6.4 nmol Fe from the mean value of

Table 9.5 Plate map for UIBC determination

	1	2	3	4	5	6	7	8	9	10	11	12
A	0	C1	S1	S5	S9	S13	S17	S21	S25	S29	S33	S37
B	0	C1	S1	S5	S9	S13	S17	S21	S25	S29	S33	S37
C	0	C1	S2	S6	S10	S14	S18	S22	S26	S30	S34	S38
D	0	C1	S2	S6	S10	S14	S18	S22	S26	S30	S34	S38
E	0	C2	S3	S7	S11	S15	S19	S23	S27	S31	S35	S39
F	0	C2	S3	S7	S11	S15	S19	S23	S27	S31	S35	S39
G	0	C2	S4	S8	S12	S16	S20	S24	S28	S32	S36	S40
H	0	C2	S4	S8	S12	S16	S20	S24	S28	S32	S36	S40

the readings in column 1 as $A_{final} - A_{initial}$ (A_s). (Note: this absorbance reading should be within 5% of the 80 μmol/l value for the iron determination.)

Once A_s has been calculated, it is used in the following equation:

For controls 1 and 2 and samples:

$$UIBC = [1 - (A_{final} - A_{initial})]/A_s \times 80 \ \mu mol/l$$

Data may be imported into a spreadsheet for calculation. As with the serum iron determination, protocols for clinical chemistry analysers sometimes include a method for UIBC.

Determination of total iron-binding capacity from UIBC:

$$TIBC = serum \ iron + UIBC \ (\mu mol/1)$$

Fully Automated Methods

A number of methods to determine the TIBC using clinical chemistry analysers require a pretreatment step. Direct (fully automated procedures) have been developed.[53] A non-precipitation method (UIBC) similar to that described above is available from Randox Ltd (Cat. No. S1250; www.randox.com).

SERUM TRANSFERRIN

An alternative approach is to measure transferrin directly by an immunological assay. This avoids some of the spuriously high values of TIBC found when the transferrin is saturated and non-transferrin iron is measured.[43] Rate immunonephelometric methods are rapid and precise. There is generally a good correlation between the chemical and immunological TIBC,[54,55] although when TIBC was calculated as the sFe + UIBC, values were lower than the direct TIBC.[53] Transferrin concentrations (g/l) may be converted to TIBC (μmol/l) by multiplying by 25.

Normal Ranges of Transferrin and Total Iron-Binding Capacity

In health, the serum transferrin is 2.0–3.0 g/l and 1 mg of transferrin binds 1.4 μg of iron. The normal serum TIBC (mean ± SD) was 68.0 ± 12.6 μmol/l in a random sample of 517 women and 63.2 ± 9.1 μmol/l for 499 men.[48] For 890 first-time, female blood donors of mean age 27 years the mean TIBC (determined by the UIBC method described earlier) was 56.7 ± 12.1 μmol/l. In 612 first-time, male blood donors of mean age 28 years the mean was 54.2 ± 10 μmol/l (mean ± SD).[49] In both surveys, the sample included some individuals with iron deficiency. Note the comment earlier about lower values given by the colorimetric UIBC method. The TIBC is increased in iron deficiency anaemia and in pregnancy;

it is lower than normal in infections, malignant disease and renal disease. In pathological iron overload, the TIBC of the serum is reduced.

Diagnostically, although a raised TIBC is characteristic of iron deficiency anaemia, the TIBC is usually used to calculate the transferrin saturation. The UIBC has attracted little diagnostic use, but is being evaluated as a screening test for iron overload in genetic haemochromatosis. In genetic haemochromatosis (subjects homozygous for *HFE* C282Y), a UIBC (determined as described earlier) of <20 μmol Fe/l was found in most men and in about 50% of women.[49] UIBC and transferrin saturation were equally sensitive and specific. For UIBC methods, optimum thresholds for detecting subjects with genetic haemochromatosis have varied. Murtagh and co-workers[56] determined the optimum threshold to be 25.6 μmol/l (sensitivity 0.91 and specificity 0.95). In this case, fasting blood samples were taken. UIBC was as reliable as transferrin saturation in detecting HFE haemochromatosis in both reports.

TRANSFERRIN SATURATION

The transferrin saturation is the ratio of the serum iron concentration and the TIBC expressed as a percentage. If transferrin is measured immunologically, then the corresponding TIBC (μmol/l) may be calculated by multiplying the transferrin concentration (g/l) by 25. In a sample of the Welsh population, the mean transferrin saturation in 499 men was 29.1 ± 11.0%; in 517 women it was 24.6 ± 11.8%.[48] For first-time blood donors from South Wales the mean transferrin saturation was 31.1 ± 10.9% for 612 men and 25.5 ± 12.9% for 890 women.[49] A transferrin saturation of <16% is usually considered to indicate an inadequate iron supply for erythropoiesis.[57] The most valuable use of transferrin saturation is for the detection of genetic haemochromatosis. Even in the early stages of the development of iron overload,[49,58] an elevated transferrin saturation is indicative of the disorder (suggested thresholds vary but >55% for men and >50% for women are an appropriate compromise),[28] although a more recent guideline suggests >50% for men and >45% for women.[23a]

Transferrin Index

Beilby and co-workers[59] have recommended that the transferrin saturation is replaced by the 'transferrin index'. This is the serum iron concentration (μmol/l) divided by the transferrin concentration (determined immunologically and expressed as μmol/l). They claimed that the transferrin index had better precision that the transferrin saturation and showed greater specificity for detecting iron overload than the transferrin saturation. However, the transferrin index has attracted little use.

SERUM TRANSFERRIN RECEPTOR

Almost all cells in the body obtain iron from the plasma protein transferrin, but transferrin has a very high affinity for iron at neutral pH and iron release takes place through a specific membrane receptor. There are two types of transferrin receptors – TfR1 and TfR2 – encoded by different genes. TfR1 is essential for tissue iron delivery and is a homodimer consisting of two identical protein subunits of molecular mass 95 kDa. Transferrin binds to TfR1, the complex is internalized and iron is released when the pH of the internal vesicles is reduced to about 5.5. After iron release, apotransferrin remains bound to the receptor until exposed to an alkaline pH at the cell surface, returns to the circulation and can undertake further cycles of iron uptake and delivery.[60] The cells that require most iron are the nucleated red cells in the bone marrow which synthesize haemoglobin and have the greatest number of transferrin receptors. TfR1 synthesis is also controlled by iron supply. The mechanism involves five IREs (see p. 178) at the 3′ untranslated region of the receptor mRNA. In the absence of iron, an IRP binds to each RNA IRE, thus stabilizing it and permitting synthesis of the protein chain. In the presence of adequate iron concentrations, binding of iron by the IRP changes the conformation of the protein and prevents its binding to the mRNA. The mRNA is rapidly broken down and synthesis of transferrin receptors is reduced. The second receptor, TFR2, also binds transferrin, but it is not required for iron delivery to cells and its synthesis is not regulated by IRPs.[61]

In 1986, Kohgo and co-workers[62] reported that transferrin receptors were detectable in the plasma by immunoassay. Since then, there has been much investigation of the physiological and diagnostic significance of circulating transferrin receptors.[63] The protein is derived by proteolysis at the cell membrane and circulates bound to transferrin. Plasma concentrations reflect the number of cellular receptors and, in patients with adequate iron stores, the number of nucleated red cells in the bone marrow. Because the number of cellular transferrin receptors per cell increases in iron deficiency, concentrations also increase when erythropoiesis becomes iron limited. Table 9.6 summarizes the conditions associated with reduced or elevated levels of circulating transferrin receptor.

Assays for the Serum Transferrin Receptor

There has been no agreement about the source of transferrin receptor as standard or as an antigen for the raising of antibodies. Transferrin receptors have been purified from placenta and from serum. The receptor may or may not

Table 9.6 Serum transferrin receptor (sTfR) concentrations in human disease

sTfR CONCENTRATION	CONDITION
Increased	Increased erythroid proliferation: Autoimmune haemolytic anaemia Hereditary spherocytosis β Thalassaemia intermedia or major β Thalassaemia/HbE Haemoglobin H disease Sickle cell anaemia Polycythaemia vera Decreased tissue iron stores: Iron deficiency anaemia
Normal to increased	Idiopathic myelofibrosis Myelodysplastic syndrome Chronic lymphocytic leukaemia
Normal	Haemochromatosis (but see text) Acute and chronic myeloid leukaemia Most lymphoid malignancies Solid tumours Anaemia of chronic disease
Decreased	Chronic renal failure Aplastic anaemia After bone marrow transplantation

Modified from Feelders et al (1999).[60]

be bound to transferrin as a standard or to raise antibodies. No 'reference' method is therefore described here. Three enzyme immunoassay kits (Orion; Ramco; R&D) for the determination of serum transferrin receptor concentrations have been evaluated for the Medical Devices Agency.[64] All have been approved for diagnostic purposes in the USA by the Food and Drug Administration. Assays for fully automated, diagnostic, immunoassay systems are now being introduced and offer improved sensitivity, reproducibility and speed.

The different reference ranges in the available commercial assays reflect the differences in preparations of transferrin receptor used to raise antibodies and as a standard in the various assays. For the Orion, Ramco and R&D kits Akesson et al.[65] and Worwood et al.[64] noted some assay drift but found acceptable intra-assay coefficient of variance (CV) values. The determined sensitivity was adequate for clinical purposes for the three assay systems. Four different units (nmol/l, μg/ml, mg/l and ku/l) and different normal ranges are in use.[66] At the present time, serum transferrin receptor (sTfR) is not included in the national external quality control schemes for the UK (NEQAS) and the Welsh External Quality Assessment Scheme (WEQAS). A WHO reference reagent for the serum transferrin receptor has now been established and an international collaborative study showed that using this reagent as a standard markedly improved agreement between methods. Currently available commercial assays are listed in this report.[67]

Reference Ranges

sTfR concentrations are high in neonates and decline until adult concentrations are reached at 17 years. Concentrations are similar in normal men and non-pregnant women. During pregnancy sTfR levels increase, returning to non-pregnant values 12 weeks after delivery.[68] sTfR concentrations obtained with different assay systems cannot be directly compared because reference ranges differ.

Samples

The information provided by the manufacturers shows good recovery of standard and linearity but some problems with interference.[64] Although serum is the preferred matrix, the R&D and Ramco assays give the same results with EDTA, heparin and citrate plasma. Orion states that EDTA-plasma is not acceptable. It is recommended that sera are stored for no more than 2 days at room temperature, 7 days at 2–8°C, 6 months at –20°C and 1 year at –70°C. Repeated freezing and thawing are not advisable. Moderate haemolysis is not a problem.

Transferrin Receptor Concentrations in Diagnosis

Erythropoiesis

The function of the TfR1 in delivering iron to the immature red cell immediately suggested an application in the clinical laboratory for the assay of circulating TfR. The use of the assay to monitor changes in the rate of erythropoiesis has been explored by several authors.[69] When iron supply is not limiting, the assay can provide a replacement for ferrokinetic investigations that required the injection of radioactive iron.

Iron Deficiency

The major application of the serum transferrin receptor assay has been to detect patients with an absence of stored iron (ferritin and haemosiderin in cells). In infants (age 8–15 months) sTfR concentration increases with increased severity of iron deficiency.[70] When normal subjects undergo quantitative phlebotomy, serum ferritin concentrations decrease steadily as iron stores are depleted, but there is little change in sTfR concentration. As iron stores become exhausted (serum ferritin <15 µg/l), sTfR levels

increase and continue increasing as haemoglobin concentrations decrease.[71] In this study the increased rate of erythropoiesis during phlebotomy had little effect on sTfR levels as long as iron stores were adequate so that most of the increase in sTfR level was the result of iron deficiency rather than increased erythropoiesis. However, the rate of phlebotomy was only 250 ml per week (about 500 ml per week is usually removed during treatment of haemochromatosis) and higher rates might cause an immediate increase in sTfR levels during phlebotomy. The log[sTfR/serum ferritin] gives a linear relationship with storage iron that has considerable potential for assessing iron stores in epidemiological studies.[72]

Circulating transferrin receptor levels increase, not only in patients with simple iron deficiency but also in patients with the anaemia of chronic disease who lack stainable iron in the bone marrow.[73] Identifying a lack of storage iron in patients with the anaemia of chronic disease is difficult without this measurement because serum iron concentrations are low regardless of iron stores and serum ferritin concentrations are higher than in patients not suffering from chronic disease who have similar levels of stainable iron in the bone marrow (see p. 336). Unfortunately, the sTFR has not proved to be superior to serum ferritin for detecting iron deficiency in all studies (Table 9.7).

In both iron deficiency anaemia and the anaemia of chronic disease, sTfR levels are also influenced by changes in the rate of erythropoiesis. Ineffective erythropoiesis – an increase in the proportion of immature red cells destroyed within the bone marrow – increases in iron deficiency anaemia.[86] In the anaemia of chronic disease, erythropoiesis is normal or depressed[87]; nevertheless, iron deficiency increases the number of receptors.

Although it has been claimed that sTfR measurements provide a sensitive indicator of iron deficiency in pregnancy,[88] questions remain about the decreased erythropoiesis in early pregnancy because this may mask iron deficiency at this time[89] and increases in sTfR in later pregnancy appear to relate to increased erythropoiesis rather than iron depletion.[68] Measurement of sTfR did not enhance the sensitivity and specificity for the detection of iron deficiency anaemia in pregnant women from Malawi, where anaemia and chronic disease are both common.[90]

Iron Overload

Normal concentrations of sTfR have been reported for patients with genetic haemochromatosis (although some had been venesected) and also for patients with African iron overload.[91] In contrast, lower mean values of sTfR were found in subjects with a raised transferrin saturation.[92,93] However, there is considerable overlap with the normal range of sTfR concentration and measurement of sTfR in iron overload is unlikely to be of diagnostic value.

Table 9.7 Overall variability (%) of assays for iron status (within subject, day-to-day coefficient of variation for healthy subjects)

Hb	SERUM FERRITIN	SERUM IRON	TIBC	ZPP	sTfR	REFERENCE
	15 (M; F)					74
1.6 (F)	15 (M; F)					75
		29 (F)				76
		27 (M)				77
3 (M; F)						78
	15 (M; F)	29 (M; F)				79
	13 (M; F)[a]	33 (M; F)[a]	11 (M; F)[a]			80
4 (M; F)	14 (M)	27 (M)				81
	26 (F)	28 (F)				81
	27 (M; F)	29 (M; F)	7 (M; F)		14 (M; F)	82
	26 (F)[V]				14 (F)	83
	15 (M)[V]				12 (M)	83
	28 (F)[C]				11 (F)	83
	12 (M)[C]				10 (M)	83
				5 (M; F)		84
3 (F)[b]	11 (F)[b]	26 (F)[b]	4 (F)[b]		13 (F)[b]	85

F, female; M, male; sTfR, serum transferrin receptor; TIBC, total iron-binding capacity; ZPP, zinc protoporphyrin;
[C], capillary blood; [V], venous blood.
[a]Patients with anaemia.
[b]70–79-year-old healthy women.

ERYTHROCYTE PROTOPORPHYRIN

Protoporphyrin IX is the immediate precursor to haem. The enzyme ferrochelatase is able to insert ferrous iron to produce haem or zinc cation to form zinc protoporphyrin (ZPP). When iron supply to ferrochelatase is limiting, ZPP increases. When ferrochelatase is limiting, free protoporphyrin accumulates. Different assays differ in the extent to which they measure and/or discriminate between these two forms of erythrocyte protoporphyrin (EP). Assay of EP[94] has been performed for many years as a screening test for lead poisoning. More recently, there has been considerable interest in its use in evaluating the iron supply to the bone marrow. The protoporphyrin concentration of red blood cells increases in iron deficiency. Usually, more than 95% is present as ZPP. The original method converts zinc to free protoporphyrin, requires a chemical extraction and use of a fluorescence spectrometer.[94] This has now been largely replaced for detection of iron deficiency by the direct measurement of the fluorescence of ZPP (μmol/mol haem) in an instrument called a haematofluorometer.[24]

Analysers

Two dedicated analysers are available: the Proto Fluor Z from Helena Laboratories, Beaumont, Texas (www. helena.com) and the ZPP 206D from Aviv Biomedical, Inc (www.avivbiomedical.com). These should be operated exactly as described by the manufacturer. The small sample size (about 20 μl of venous or skin-puncture blood), simplicity, rapidity and reproducibility within a laboratory are advantages. Furthermore, the test has an interesting retrospective application. Because it takes weeks for a significant proportion of the circulating red blood cells to be replaced with new cells, it is possible to make a diagnosis of iron deficiency anaemia some time after iron therapy has commenced. Chronic diseases that reduce serum iron concentration, but do not reduce iron stores, also increase protoporphyrin levels.[95]

Diagnostic Applications

The measurement of EP levels as an indicator of iron deficiency has particular advantages in paediatric haematology and in large-scale surveys in which the small sample size and simplicity of the test are important. The normal range in adults is less than 70 μmol/mol haem. Mean values in normal women are slightly higher than in men.[96] One potential confounder is the contribution of other fluorescent compounds (including drugs) in the plasma and concentrations are lower if washed red cells are assayed.[84] However, washing is a tedious process and is rarely undertaken. Paediatric reference ranges have been determined in 6478 subjects (ages 0–17 years).[97] Mean ZPP values were higher in females than males and declined slightly with age. A diurnal variation was noted, with ZPP concentrations being higher between 18.00 h and midnight. No explanation was offered.

The WHO[39] has recommended levels for the detection of iron deficiency. For children younger than age 5 years, levels should be >61 μmol/mol haem; for all other subjects, levels should be >70 μmol/mol haem. These are higher than the 97.5 percentile established from surveys of healthy children[97] and are based on the sensitivity and specificity for detecting the absence of storage iron.

Units

To convert between the various units used to express protoporphyrin levels, the following calculations apply:

μg EP/dl red cell = (μg EP/dl whole blood)/haematocrit
From μg EP/dl red cell to μg EP/g Hb multiply by 0.037
From μg EP/dl red cell to μmol EP/mol haem multiply by 0.87.

These factors are based on an assumed normal mean cell haemoglobin concentration, although this may be measured in individual samples and an appropriate factor calculated.

Infection and inflammation, lead poisoning and haemolytic anaemia all cause significant elevation of ZPP. Measurement of ZPP is most useful when iron deficiency is common and the other conditions are rare. In the general clinical laboratory, therefore, ZPP provides less information about iron storage levels in patients with anaemia than does the serum ferritin assay.[98]

Although blood samples may be taken at any time of day, fresh blood is required (samples must not be frozen) and the method has not been automated.

HEPCIDIN

Reliable assays for serum hepcidin have now been developed but their role in the differential diagnosis of both iron deficiency and iron overload is not yet clear although a number of useful diagnostic applications are being investigated.[99] An international survey of urinary and plasma hepcidin assays demonstrated that absolute concentrations vary widely. However, analytical variation was generally low and similar for the six methods included in the study.[100]

METHODOLOGICAL AND BIOLOGICAL VARIABILITY OF ASSAYS

The blood assays vary greatly in both methodological and biological stability. Haemoglobin concentrations are stable and a simple and well-standardized method ensures relatively low day-to-day variation in individuals (Table 9.7). Automated cell counters analyse at least 10 000 cells and thus increase precision. ZPP values also appear to be relatively stable. The more complicated procedures involved in immunoassays result in higher methodological variation for serum ferritin assays (CV of about 5%) and this, coupled with some physiological variation, gives an overall CV for serum ferritin for an individual over a period of weeks of the order of 15%. There is, however, little evidence of any significant diurnal variation in serum ferritin concentration.[74] On the other hand, the serum iron determination has a reasonably low methodological variation coupled with extreme physiological variability, giving an overall 'within subject' CV of approximately 30% when venous samples are taken at the same time of day. A diurnal rhythm has been reported with higher values in the morning than in late afternoon, when the concentration may fall to 50% of the morning value.[44] However, variations are not consistently diurnal.[101] The circadian fluctuation is largely the result of variation in the release of iron from the reticuloendothelial system to the plasma. It should be noted that for the studies summarized in Table 9.7 the type of blood sample, length of study period and statistical analysis vary. The somewhat higher variability for Hb and ferritin reported by Borel et al.[81] may be a result of their use of capillary blood and plasma. Pootrakul et al.[102] have demonstrated that mean plasma ferritin concentration is slightly higher in capillary specimens than venous specimens and that within- and between-sample variation was approximately three-fold greater. Variability was less for capillary serum than plasma but still greater than for venous serum. However, the increased variability of capillary samples may be related to sampling technique, because Cooper and Zlotkin[83] found little difference in variability between venous and capillary samples.

The effect of menstruation on iron-status indicators was examined in 1712 women aged 18–44 years after adjusting for potential confounders.[103] Adjusted mean values of Hb, transferrin saturation and serum ferritin were lowest for women whose blood was drawn during menses and highest for women examined in luteal or late luteal phase of the menstrual cycle (Hb, 13.0 versus 13.3 g/dl; transferrin saturation, 21.2% versus 24.8%, $p<0.01$ for both; serum ferritin, 17.2 versus 24.0 µg/l, $p<0.05$). The prevalence estimate of impaired iron status was significantly higher for women whose blood was drawn during the menstrual phase than for women whose blood was drawn during the luteal and late luteal phases. The authors concluded that cyclic variations in indicators of iron status are a potential source of error when iron status is assessed in large population surveys that include women of reproductive age.[103]

Starvation, or even fasting for a short period, can cause elevation of the serum ferritin concentration,[104] and vitamin C deficiency can reduce ferritin concentration.[105] Moderate exercise has little effect on serum ferritin concentration,[106] although exhausting exercise leads to increases in serum ferritin concentration as a result of muscle damage and inflammatory reactions.[107,108] Seasonal changes in red cell parameters have been reported[109] and Maes et al.[82] found statistically significant seasonal patterns for serum iron, transferrin, serum ferritin and sTfR. The peak–trough difference in the yearly variation, expressed as a percentage of the mean, was greatest for serum ferritin (39%) and least for sTfR and transferrin (12%).

These results have clear implications for the use of these assays in population studies. For accurate diagnosis, either a multiparameter analysis is required or several samples should be assayed. For haemoglobin, one sample was required for 95% confidence and 20% accuracy;[110] for sTfR, one sample was required,[83,111] but for ferritin one to three samples were required.[83,110]

PREDICTIVE VALUE OF BLOOD TESTS FOR IRON DEFICIENCY

The major diagnostic use of the various measures of iron status is in the differential diagnosis of hypochromic anaemia. The large amount of iron present as haemoglobin means that the degree of any anaemia must always be considered in assessing iron status. There is an overall reduction in body iron in iron deficiency anaemia. No single measurement of iron status is ideal for all clinical circumstances because all are affected by confounding factors (Table 9.3). The anaemia of chronic disorders is associated with normal or increased iron stores (normal or increased serum ferritin), accompanied by a reduced

tissue iron supply (low serum iron and low to normal TIBC). Although the serum ferritin is an acute-phase reactant, values below 50 µg/l are usually associated with absent iron stores in rheumatoid arthritis, renal disease and inflammatory bowel disease. Serum transferrin receptor levels may also provide valuable diagnostic information on iron deficiency in chronic disease.

Despite years of investigations, there is little definitive evidence of how different measurements compare in their ability to diagnose iron deficiency. The main reason for this is the difficulty of distinguishing between the presence and absence of storage iron. Most investigators have used the grade of storage iron in the bone marrow as a 'gold standard'. This is an invasive procedure and therefore limits drastically the number of patients investigated. It is often difficult to justify bone marrow aspiration to determine a patient's iron status and even more difficult in the case of normal volunteers. Furthermore, bone marrow aspiration followed by staining for iron is not a reproducible procedure. Observer error,[112] inadequate specimens and lack of correlation with response to iron therapy[113] have been described. Demonstrating a response in Hb to oral iron therapy has been the method of choice to diagnose iron deficiency retrospectively in paediatric practice.

Iron Deficiency Anaemia in Adults

Almost all measures show a high sensitivity and specificity for distinguishing between subjects with iron deficiency and those with iron stores and normal haemoglobin levels in the absence of any other disease process. Guyatt et al.[114] conducted a systematic review of the diagnostic value of the various laboratory tests for iron deficiency. They concluded that serum ferritin was the most powerful test for simple iron deficiency and also for iron deficiency in hospital patients. However, this analysis did not include measurements of sTfR.

Detection of Iron Deficiency in Acute or Chronic Disease

Table 9.8 summarizes a number of studies in which bone marrow iron was assessed and the sensitivity and specificity of various assays was compared. Despite very different results between studies, some general points may be made.

Conventional red cell parameters, mean cell volume (MCV) and mean cell haemoglobin (MCH), do not distinguish between the presence or absence of bone marrow iron in patients with chronic disease. The serum iron concentration is almost invariably low in chronic disease and, although the TIBC (or transferrin concentration) is higher for patients with no storage iron, neither this measurement, nor the transferrin saturation derived from the serum iron and TIBC, provides useful discrimination.

Table 9.8 Sensitivity/specificity of methods for diagnosis of iron deficiency in the presence of chronic disease

In adults, iron stores were determined by staining for iron in bone marrow. Optimum diagnostic thresholds selected vary. The various studies are described in the references at the top of the table.

	REFERENCE							
	115	116[a]	73[a]	117	118	119	120	121
MCV	–	–	0.86	–	–	0.42/0.83	–	–
% Hypo	–	–	–	0.77/0.90	–	–	–	–
Serum iron	–	–	0.68	L	–	–	NS	–
TIBC	–	–	0.84[b]	L	–	–	–	–
% Saturation	–	–	0.79[c]	L	–	0.38/0.89	–	–
Serum ferritin	0.79/0.97	0.870	0.89	0.86/0.90	1.00/0.81	0.25/0.99	0.94/0.95	0.92/0.98
ZPP	0.74/0.94		–	L	–	–	–	–
sTfR	0.63/0/81	0.704	0.98	L	1.00/0.84	0.71/0.74	0.61/0.68	0.92/0.84
sTfR/log ferritin	0.74/0.97	0.865	1.00	–	1.00/0.97	0.67/0.93	–	–

L, Lower sensitivity/specificity than serum ferritin, individually or in combination. The combination of ferritin and erythrocyte sedimentation rate or C-reactive protein did not improve efficiency. MCV, mean cell volume; TIBC, total iron-binding capacity; ZPP, zinc protoporphyrin; sTfR, serum transferrin receptor.
[a]Area under receiver operating characteristics (ROC) curve.
[b]Transferrin concentration (equivalent to TIBC; see text).
[c]Transferrin index (equivalent to % saturation; see text).

In chronic disease serum ferritin concentrations reflect storage iron levels but are higher than in normal subjects with the same amount of storage iron. It is necessary to set a threshold of 30–50 μg/l to distinguish between the presence and absence of storage iron. Even with this limit sensitivity is low.

Combinations of serum ferritin, erythrocyte sedimentation rate (ESR) or C-reactive protein (CRP) either in a discriminant analysis[111] or logistic regression[122] provide only marginal improvement in the ability to detect a lack of storage iron.

The serum transferrin receptor level discriminates between the presence and absence of storage iron, although there is disagreement as to whether the assay is superior to serum ferritin. Several studies show that the sTfR/log$_{10}$ ferritin ratio provides superior discrimination to either test on its own. The use of log ferritin decreases the influence of serum ferritin (and thus the acute-phase response) on the overall ratio. Although the log[sTfR/ferritin] is an excellent measure of iron stores in healthy subjects,[72] this transformation (i.e. after calculating the ratio of sTfR/ferritin) may not provide the best discrimination for clinical applications. When the assay of sTfR is readily available on high-throughput immunoanalysers the sTfR/log ferritin ratio may provide the best discriminator for identifying the coexistence of iron deficiency in chronic disease. However, this will also require standardization of units and ranges for the various sTfR assays if the use of the ratio is to gain wide acceptance.

Functional Iron Deficiency

Functional iron deficiency is the situation in which iron stores are apparently adequate but iron supply for erythropoiesis remains inadequate. This often occurs during the treatment of patients with anaemia and renal failure with erythropoietin. The diagnostic question is to identify those patients with a functional iron deficiency who will require parenteral iron therapy to respond to erythropoietin with an acceptable increase in Hb. The percentage hypochromic erythrocytes is a good predictor of response.[123] Fishbane and colleagues[124] concluded that reticulocyte haemoglobin content (CHr) was a markedly more stable analyte than serum ferritin or transferrin saturation and it predicted functional iron deficiency more efficiently. They did not include percentage hypochromic cells in their analysis. Fernandez-Rodriguez and colleagues[125] assessed the sensitivity and specificity of ferritin, TIBC, transferrin saturation index, red blood cell ferritin and sTfR in 63 patients with anaemia and chronic renal failure undergoing dialysis, who were not being treated with erythropoietin. Storage iron was assessed by bone marrow iron staining. For serum ferritin, a cut-off value of 121 µg/l gave a sensitivity and specificity of 75%. Efficiency was lower for sTfR and RBC ferritin. MCV, transferrin saturation index and TIBC showed the lowest values for sensitivity and specificity.

Iron Deficiency in Infancy and Childhood

In infants, thresholds for the diagnosis of iron deficiency and iron deficiency anaemia are not universally agreed. There are rapid changes in iron status in the first year of life as fetal haemoglobin is replaced by adult haemoglobin. The serum ferritin concentration is a less useful guide to iron deficiency than in adults partly because of the rapid decline in concentration in the first 6 months and the low concentrations generally found in children older than 6 months of age. Domellof et al.[126] have suggested revised cut-offs for iron deficiency, including serum ferritin and sTfR, for infants up to age 1 year.

In children, the reason for detecting iron deficiency is to identify those who will respond to iron therapy. Margolis et al.[127] found that the best predictor of response was the initial Hb, although sensitivity was only 66% and specificity was 60%. Serum ferritin, transferrin saturation and erythrocyte protoporphyrin (EP) had even lower efficiencies and combination of the various measures made little improvement. Hershko et al.[128] studied children in villages from the Golan Heights (Israel) and concluded that EP was a more reliable index of iron deficiency than serum ferritin. They suggested that a significant incidence of chronic disease affected both ferritin and iron values. ZPP provides a useful indicator of iron-deficient erythropoiesis, although high values may indicate lead poisoning rather than iron deficiency. The small sample volume for ZPP determination is also an advantage in paediatric practice.

A report published in 2003 confirms the effect of low-level infection on measures of iron status. Abraham et al.[129] studied 101 healthy, 11-month-old infants. On the morning of blood sampling, slight clinical signs of airway infection were observed for 42 infants. Extensive blood analyses were done, including a high sensitivity one for C-reactive protein (CRP). CRP measured by the routine methods gave values of <6 mg/l for all infants, but with the high sensitivity assay values were higher for many infants with symptoms of airway infection. Serum iron concentration was depressed in these children and correlated significantly with CRP level. When a further blood sample was taken, serum ferritin concentration was higher for the children with the higher CRP level, serum iron was reduced, but sTfR and transferrin levels were unaffected.

Pregnancy

In early pregnancy serum ferritin concentrations usually provide a reliable indication of iron deficiency. Haemodilution in the 2nd and 3rd trimesters of pregnancy reduces the concentrations of all measures of iron status and this means that the threshold values for iron deficiency established in non-pregnant women are not appropriate. In principle, determination of values as ratios (ZPP µmol/mol haem, transferrin saturation and sTfR/ferritin) should be more reliable. In healthy women who were not anaemic and who were supplemented with iron,[68] serum iron, transferrin saturation and serum ferritin fell from the 1st to the 3rd trimester and increased after delivery; TIBC increased during pregnancy and fell after delivery. sTfR concentrations showed a substantial increase (approximately two-fold) during pregnancy and this probably reflects increased erythropoiesis.[68] In contrast, Carriaga et al.[88] had reported that the mean sTfR concentration of pregnant women in the 3rd trimester did not differ from that in non-pregnant women and that sTfR concentration was not influenced by pregnancy *per se*. Choi et al.[68] suggest that different assays and different ages in the control groups may explain this discrepancy.

CONCLUSION

Body iron status can usually be assessed by considering the Hb, red cell indices and serum ferritin concentration, along with evidence of inflammation, infection and liver disease. The sTfR may provide useful discrimination between the presence and absence of iron stores in the anaemia of chronic disease, but its use is hindered by the lack of agreement about units and reference ranges. Measurement of transferrin saturation is essential for evaluating iron accumulation in genetic haemochromatosis.

REFERENCES

1. Miret S, Simpson RJ, McKie AT. Physiology and molecular biology of dietary iron absorption. *Annu Rev Nutr*. 2003;23:283–301.

2. Mastrogiannaki M, Matak P, Keith B, et al. HIF-2 alpha, but not HIF-1 alpha, promotes iron absorption in mice. *J Clin Invest*. 2009;119:1159–1166.

3. Ganz T. Hepcidin: a key regulator of iron metabolism and mediator of anemia of inflammation. *Blood*. 2003;102:783–788.

4. Hentze MW, Muckenthaler MU, Andrews NC. Balancing acts: molecular control of mammalian iron metabolism. *Cell*. 2004;117:285–297.

5. Ohgami RS, Camagna DR, Greer EL, et al. Identification of a ferrireductase required for efficient transferrin-dependent iron uptake in erythroid cells. *Nat Genet.* 2005;37:1264–1269.

6. Paradkar PN, Zumbrennen KB, Paw BH, et al. Regulation of mitochondrial iron import through differential turnover of mitoferrin 1 and mitoferrin 2. *Mol Cell Biol.* 2009;29:1007–1016.

7. Lill R. Function and biogenesis of iron-sulphur proteins. *Nature.* 2009;460:831–838.

7a. Anderson GJ, Vulpe CD. Mammalian iron transport. *Cell Mol Life Sci.* 2009;66:3241–3261.

8. Silvestri L, Pagani A, Nai I, et al. The serine protease matriptase-2 (TMPRSS6) inhibits hepcidin activation by cleaving membrane hemojuvelin. *Cell Metab.* 2008;8:502–511.

9. Finberg KE, Whittlesey RL, Fleming MD, et al. 2010; Downregulation of Bmp/Smad signaling by Tmprss6 is required for maintenance of systemic iron homeostasis. *Blood.* Epub Mar 03.

10. Lin L, Goldberg YP, Ganz T. Competitive regulation of hepcidin mRNA by soluble and cell-associated hemojuvelin. *Blood.* 2005;106:2884–2889.

11. Andriopoulos Jr B, Corradini E, Xia Y, et al. BMP6 is a key endogenous regulator of hepcidin expression and iron metabolism. *Nat Genet.* 2009;41:482–487.

12. Johnson B, Chen J, Murchison N, et al. Transferrin receptor 2: evidence for ligand-induced stabilization and redirection to a recycling pathway. *Mol Biol Cell.* 2007;18:743–754.

13. Ramey G, Deschemin J-C, Vaulont S. Cross-talk between the mitogen activated protein kinase and bone morphogenetic/hemojuvelin pathways is required for the induction of hepcidin by holotransferrin in primary mouse hepatocytes. *Haematologica.* 2009;94:765–772.

14. Tanno T, Bhanu NV, Oneal PA, et al. High levels of GDF15 in thalassaemia suppress expression of the iron regulatory protein hepcidin. *Nat Med.* 2007;13:1096–1101.

15. Tanno T, Parayette P, Sripichai O, et al. Identification of TWSG1 as a second novel erythroid regulator of hepcidin expression in murine and human cells. *Blood.* 2009;114: 181–186.

16. Harrison PM, Arosio P. The ferritins: molecular properties, iron storage function and cellular regulation. *Biochim Biophys Acta.* 1996;1275: 161–203.

17. Leibman A, Aisen P. Distribution of iron between the binding sites of transferrin in serum: methods and results in normal human subjects. *Blood.* 1979;53:1058–1065.

18. Kristiansen M, Graversen JH, Jacobsen C, et al. Identification of the haemoglobin scavenger receptor. *Nature.* 2001;409:198–201.

19. Tolosano E, Altruda F. Hemopexin: structure, function and regulation. *DNA Cell Biol.* 2002;21:297–306.

20. Worwood M. Ferritin. *Blood Rev.* 1990;4:259–269.

21. Hider RC. Nature of nontransferrin-bound iron. *Eur J Clin Invest.* 2002;32:50–54.

22. Liuzzi JP, Aydemir F, Nam H, et al. Zip14 (Slc39a14) mediates non-transferrin-bound iron uptake into cells. *Proc Natl Acad Sci U S A.* 2006;103:13612–13617.

23. Sullivan JL. Iron and the sex difference in heart disease risk. *Lancet.* 1981;1:1293–1294.

23a. EASL clinical practice guidelines for HFE hemochromatosis . *J Hepatol.* 2010;53:3–22.

24. Labbe RF, Vreman HJ, Stevenson DK. Zinc protoporphyrin: a metabolite with a mission. *Clin Chem.* 1999;45:2060–2072.

25. Hoffbrand AV, Worwood M. Iron overload. In: Hoffband AV, Tuddenham E, Catovsky D, eds. *Postgraduate Haematology.* Oxford: Blackwell; 2005.

26. Worwood M, Hoffband AV. Iron metabolism and iron deficiency. In: Hoffband AV, Tuddenham E, Catovsky D, eds. *Postgraduate Haematology.* Oxford: Blackwell; 2005.

27. Finberg KE. Iron-refractory iron deficiency anemia. *Semin Hematol.* 2009;46:378–386.

28. Dooley J, Worwood M. *Guidelines on diagnosis and therapy: genetic haemochromatosis.* British Committee for Standards in Haematology; 2000. Available at: www. bcshguidelines.com.

29. Brittenham GM. Noninvasive methods for the early detection of hereditary hemochromatosis. [Review]. *Ann N Y Acad Sci.* 1988;526:199–208.

30. Pippard MJ. Iron-deficiency anemia, anemia of chronic disorders and iron overload. In: Wickramasinghe SL, McCullough J, eds. *Blood and Bone Marrow Pathology.* London: Churchill Livingstone; 2003:203–228.

31. Worwood M. Ferritin in human tissues and serum. *Clin Haematol.* 1982;11:275–307.

32. ICSH (Expert Panel on Iron). Proposed international standard of human ferritin for the serum ferritin assay. *Br J Haematol.* 1985;61:61–63.

33. Worwood M. Serum ferritin. In: Cook JD, ed. *Iron.* New York: Churchill Livingstone; 1980:59–89.

34. Dresser DW. Immunization of experimental animals. In: Weir DM, ed. *Handbook of Experimental Immunology.* Oxford: Blackwell Science; 1986:8.1–8.21.

35. Johnson GD, Holborow EJ. Preparation and use of fluorochrome conjugates. In: Weir DM, ed. *Handbook of Experimental Immunology.* Oxford: Blackwell Science; 1986:28.1–28.21.

36. Wilson MB, Nakane PK. Recent developments in the periodate method of conjugating horseradish peroxidase (HRPO) to antibodies. In: Knapp W, Houlbar K, eds. *Immunofluorescence and Related Staining Techniques.* Amsterdam: Elsevier/North-Holland; 1978: 215–224.

37. Boscato LM, Stuart MC. Heterophilic antibodies: a problem for all immunoassays. *Clin Chem.* 1988;34: 27–33.

38. Zweig MH, Csako G, Benson CC, et al. Interference by anti-immunoglobulin G antibodies in immunoradiometric assays of thyrotropin involving mouse monoclonal antibodies. *Clin Chem.* 1987;33:840–844.

39. World Health Organization. *Iron deficiency anemia. Assessment, prevention and control. A guide for*

programme managers. 2001. Available at: www.who.int/nut/documents/ida_assessment_prevention_control.

40. Rogers JT, Bridges KR, Durmowicz GP, et al. Translational control during the acute phase response. Ferritin synthesis in response to interleukin-1. *J Biol Chem.* 1990;265:14572–14578.

41. Worwood M. Serum ferritin. *Clin Sci.* 1986;70:215–220.

42. Nielsen P, Gunther U, Durken M, et al. Serum ferritin iron in iron overload and liver damage: correlation to body iron stores and diagnostic relevance. *J Lab Clin Med.* 2000;135:413–418.

43. ICSH. Revised recommendations for the measurement of serum iron in human blood. *Br J Haematol.* 1990;75:615–616.

44. Bothwell TH, Charlton RW, Cook JD, et al. *Iron Metabolism in Man.* Oxford: Blackwell Scientific; 1979.

45. Persijn J-P, van der Slik W, Riethorst A. Determination of serum iron and latent iron-binding capacity (LIBC). *Clinica Chimica Acta.* 1971;35:91–98.

46. Tietz NW, Rinker AD, Morrison SR. When is a serum iron really a serum iron? A follow-up study on the status of iron measurements in serum. *Clin Chem.* 1996;42:109–111.

47. Blanck HM, Pfeiffer CM, Caudill SP, et al. Serum iron and iron-binding capacity: a round-robin interlaboratory comparison study. *Clin Chem.* 2003;49: 1672–1675.

48. Jacobs A, Waters WE, Campbell H, et al. A random sample from Wales III. Serum iron, iron binding capacity and transferrin saturation. *Br J Haematol.* 1969;17:581–587.

49. Jackson HA, Carter K, Darke C, et al. HFE mutations, iron deficiency and overload in 10 500 blood donors. *Br J Haematol.* 2001;114:474–484.

50. Koerper MA, Dallman PR. Serum iron concentration and transferrin saturation in the diagnosis of iron deficiency in children: normal developmental changes. *J Pediatr.* 1977;91:870–874.

51. Saarinen UM, Siimes MA. Developmental changes in serum iron, total iron binding capacity

and transferrin saturation in infancy. *J Pediatr.* 1977;91:877.

52. International Committee for Standardization in Haematology. The measurement of total and unsaturated iron binding capacity in serum. *Br J Haematol.* 1978;38:281–290.

53. Siek G, Lawlor J, Pelczar D, et al. Direct serum total iron-binding capacity assay suitable for automated analyzers. *Clin Chem.* 2002;48:161–166.

54. Yamanishi H, Iyama S, Yamaguchi Y, et al. Total iron-binding capacity calculated from serum transferrin concentration or serum iron concentration and unsaturated iron-binding capacity. *Clin Chem.* 2003;49: 175–178.

55. Gambino R, Desvarieux E, Orth M, et al. The relation between chemically measured total iron-binding capacity concentrations and immunologically measured transferrin concentrations in human serum. *Clin Chem.* 1997;43:2408–2412.

56. Murtagh LJ, Whiley M, Wilson S, et al. Unsaturated iron binding capacity and transferrin saturation are equally reliable in detection of HFE hemochromatosis. *Am J Gastroenterol.* 2002;97: 2093–2099.

57. Bainton DF, Finch CA. The diagnosis of iron deficiency anemia. *Am J Med.* 1964;37:62–70.

58. Edwards CQ, Kushner JP. Screening for hemochromatosis. *N Engl J Med.* 1993;328:1616–1620.

59. Beilby J, Olynyk J, Ching S, et al. Transferrin index: an alternative method for calculating the iron saturation of transferrin. *Clin Chem.* 1992;38:2078–2081.

60. Feelders RA, Kuiperkramer EPA, Vaneijk HG. Structure, function and clinical significance of transferrin receptors. *Clin Chem Lab Med.* 1999;37:1–10.

61. Trinder D, Baker E. Transferrin receptor 2: a new molecule in iron metabolism. *Int J Biochem Cell Biol.* 2003;35:292–296.

62. Kohgo Y, Nishisato T, Kondo H, et al. Circulating transferrin receptor in human serum. *Br J Haematol.* 1986;64:277–281.

63. Cook JD. The measurement of serum transferrin receptor. *Am J Med Sci.* 1999;318:269–276.

64. Worwood M, Ellis RD, Bain BJ. *Three Serum Transferrin Receptor ELISAs.* MDA/2000/09. Norwich: HMSO; 2000.

65. Akesson A, Bjellerup P, Vahter M. Evaluation of kits for measurement of the soluble transferrin receptor. *Scand J Clin Lab Invest.* 1999;59:77–81.

66. Kuiperkramer EPA, Huisman CMS, Vanraan J, et al. Analytical and clinical implications of soluble transferrin receptors in serum. *Eur J Clin Chem Clin Biochem.* 1996;34: 645–649.

67. Thorpe SJ, Heath A, Sharp G, et al. A WHO Reference reagent for the Serum Transferrin Receptor (sTfR): international collaborative study to evaluate a recombinant soluble transferrin receptor preparation. *Clin Chem Lab Med.* 2010;48:815–820.

68. Choi JW, Im MW, Pai SH. Serum transferrin receptor concentrations during normal pregnancy. *Clin Chem.* 2000;46:725–727.

69. Beguin Y, Clemons GK, Pootrakul P, et al. Quantitative assessment of erythropoiesis and functional classification of anemia based on measurements of serum transferrin receptor and erythropoietin. *Blood.* 1993;81:1067–1076.

70. Olivares M, Walter T, Cook JD, et al. Usefulness of serum transferrin receptor and serum ferritin in diagnosis of iron deficiency in infancy. *Am J Clin Nutr.* 2000;72: 1191–1195.

71. Skikne B, Flowers CH, Cook JD. Serum transferrin receptor: a quantitative measure of tissue iron deficiency. *Blood.* 1990;75: 1870–1876.

72. Cook JD, Flowers CH, Skikne BS. The quantitative assessment of body iron. *Blood.* 2003;101:3359–3364.

73. Punnonen K, Irjala K, Rajamaki A. Serum transferrin receptor and its ratio to serum ferritin in the diagnosis of iron deficiency. *Blood.* 1997;89:1052–1057.

74. Dawkins S, Cavill I, Ricketts C, et al. Variability of serum ferritin concentration in normal subjects. *Clin Lab Haematol.* 1979;1:41–46.

75. Gallagher SK, Johnson LK, Milne DB. Short-term and long-term variability of indexes related to nutritional-status. I. Ca, Cu, Fe, Mg and Zn. *Clin Chem.* 1989;35: 369–373.

76. Statland BE, Winkel P. Relationship of day-to-day variation of serum iron concentration to iron-binding capacity in healthy young women. *Am J Clin Pathol.* 1977;67:84–90.

77. Statland BE, Winkel P, Bokieland H. Variation of serum iron concentration in healthy young men: within day and day-to-day changes. *Clin Biochem.* 1976;9:26–29.

78. Statland BE, Winn RK, Harris SC. Evaluation of biologic sources of variation of leucocyte counts and other hematologic quantities using very precise automated analysers. *Am J Clin Pathol.* 1977;69:48–54.

79. Pilon VA, Howantitz PJ, Howanitz JH, et al. Day-to-day variation in serum ferritin concentration in healthy subjects. *Clin Chem.* 1981;27:78–82.

80. Romslo I, Talstad I. Day-to-day variations in serum iron, serum iron binding capacity, serum ferritin and erythrocyte protoporphyrin concentrations in anaemic subjects. *Eur J Haematol.* 1988;40:79–82.

81. Borel MJ, Smith SM, Derr J, et al. Day-to-day variation in iron-status indices in healthy men and women. *Am J Clin Nutr.* 1991;54:729–735.

82. Maes M, Bosmans E, Scharpe S, et al. Components of biological variation in serum soluble transferrin receptor: relationships to serum iron, transferrin and ferritin concentrations and immune and haematological variables. *Scand J Clin Lab Invest.* 1997;57:31–41.

83. Cooper MJ, Zlotkin SH. Day-to-day variation of transferrin receptor and ferritin in healthy men and women. *Am J Clin Nutr.* 1996;64:738–742.

84. Hastka J, Lasserre JJ, Schwarzbeck A, et al. Washing erythrocytes to remove interferents in measurements of zinc protoporphyrin by front-face hematofluorometry. *Clin Chem.* 1992;38:2184–2189.

85. Ahluwalia N. Diagnostic utility of serum transferrin receptors measurement in assessing iron status. *Nutr Rev.* 1998;56:133–141.

86. Kuiperkramer PA, Huisman CMS, Vandermolensinke J, et al. The expression of transferrin receptors on erythroblasts in anaemia of chronic disease, myelodysplastic syndromes and iron deficiency. *Acta Haematol.* 1997;97:127–131.

87. Fitzsimons EJ, Houston T, Munro R, et al. Erythroblast iron metabolism and serum soluble transferrin receptor values in the anemia of rheumatoid arthritis. *Arthritis Rheum.* 2002;47:166–171.

88. Carriaga MT, Skikne BS, Finley B, et al. Serum transferrin receptor for the detection of iron deficiency in pregnancy. *Am J Clin Nutr.* 1991;54:1077–1081.

89. Akesson A, Bjellerup P, Berglund M, et al. Serum transferrin receptor: a specific marker of iron deficiency in pregnancy. *Am J Clin Nutr.* 1998;68:1241–1246.

90. Van den Broek NR, Letsky EA, White SA, et al. Iron status in pregnant women: which measurements are valid? *Br J Haematol.* 1998;103: 817–824.

91. Baynes RD, Cook JD, Bothwell TH, et al. Serum transferrin receptor in hereditary hemochromatosis and African siderosis. *Am J Hematol.* 1994;45:288–292.

92. Khumalo H, Gomo ZAR, Moyo VM, et al. Serum transferrin receptors are decreased in the presence of iron overload. *Clin Chem.* 1998;44: 40–44.

93. Looker AC, Loyevsky M, Gordeuk VR. Increased serum transferrin saturation is associated with lower serum transferrin receptor concentration. *Clin Chem.* 1999;45:2191–2199.

94. Piomelli S. The diagnostic utility of measurements of erythrocyte porphyrins. *Hematol Oncol Clin North Am.* 1987;1:419–430.

95. Hastka J, Lasserre JJ, Schwarzbeck A, et al. Zinc protoporphyrin in anemia of chronic disorders. *Blood.* 1993;81:1200–1204.

96. Yip R. Changes in iron metabolism with age. In: Brock JH, Halliday JW, Pippard MJ, et al. *Iron Metabolism in Health and Disease.* London: WB Saunders; 1994:427–448.

97. Soldin OP, Miller M, Soldin SJ. Pediatric reference ranges for zinc protoporphyrin. *Clin Biochem.* 2003;36:21–25.

98. Zanella A, Gridelli L, Berzuini A, et al. Sensitivity and predictive value of serum ferritin and free erythrocyte protoporphyrin for iron deficiency. *J Lab Clin Med.* 1989;113:73–78.

99. Bergamaschi G, Villani L. Serum hepcidin: a novel diagnostic tool in disorders of iron metabolism. *Haematologica.* 2009;94:1631–1633.

100. Kroot JJC, Hendriks JCM, Laarakkers CMM, et al. (Pre) analytical imprecision, between-subject variability and daily variations in serum and urine hepcidin: Implications for clinical studies. *Anal Biochem.* 2009;389:124–129.

101. Dale JC, Burritt MF, Zinsmeister AR. Diurnal variation of serum iron, iron-binding capacity, transferrin saturation and ferritin levels. *Am J Clin Pathol.* 2002;117:802–808.

102. Pootrakul P, Skikne BS, Cook JD. The use of capillary blood for measurements of circulating ferritin. *Am J Clin Nutr.* 1983;37:307–310.

103. Kim I, Yetley EA, Calvo MS. Variations in iron-status measures during the menstrual cycle. *Am J Clin Nutr.* 1993;58: 705–709.

104. Lundberg PA, Lindstedt G, Andersson T, et al. Increase in serum ferritin concentration induced by fasting. *Clin Chem.* 1984;30:161–163.

105. Chapman RW, Gorman A, Laulicht M, et al. Binding of serum ferritin to concanavalin A in patients with iron overload and with chronic liver disease. *J Clin Pathol.* 1982;35:481–486.

106. Nikolaidis MG, Michailidis Y, Mougios V. Variation of soluble transferrin receptor and ferritin concentrations in human serum during recovery from exercise. *Eur J Appl Physiol.* 2003;89:500–502.

107. Fallon KE. The acute phase response and exercise: the ultramarathon as prototype exercise. *Clin J Sport Med.* 2001;11:38–43.

108. Stupnicki R, Malczewska J, Milde K, et al. Day to day variability in the transferrin receptor/ferritin index in female athletes. *Br J Sports Med.* 2003;37:267–269.

109. Kristalboneh E, Froom P, Harari G, et al. Seasonal changes in red-blood-cell parameters. *Br J Haematol.* 1993;85:603–607.

110. Lammikeefe CJ, Lickteig ES, Ahluwalia N, et al. Day-to-day variation in iron status indexes is similar for most measures in elderly women with and without rheumatoid arthritis. *J Am Diet Assoc.* 1996;96:247–251.

111. Ahluwalia N, Lammikeefe CJ, Bendel RB, et al. Iron-deficiency and anemia of chronic disease in elderly women: a discriminant–analysis approach for differentiation. *Am J Clin Nutr.* 1995;61:590–596.

112. Bentley DP, Williams P. Serum ferritin concentration as an index of storage iron in rheumatoid arthritis. *J Clin Pathol.* 1974;27:786–1738.

113. Tessitore N, Solero GP, Lippi G, et al. The role of iron status markers in predicting response to intravenous iron in haemodialysis patients on maintenance erythropoietin. *Nephrol Dial Transplant.* 2001;16:1416–1423.

114. Guyatt G, Oxman AD, Ali M, et al. Laboratory diagnosis of iron-deficiency anemia – an overview. *J Gen Intern Med.* 1992;7:145–153.

115. van Tellingen A, Kuenen JC, de Kieviet W, et al. Iron deficiency anaemia in hospitalized patients: value of various laboratory parameters. Differentiation between IDA and ACD. *Neth J Med.* 2001;59:270–279.

116. Lee EJ, Oh EJ, Park YJ, et al. Soluble transferrin receptor (sTfR), ferritin and sTfR/log ferritin index in anemic patients with nonhematologic malignancy and chronic inflammation. *Clin Chem.* 2002;48:1118–1121.

117. Kurer SB, Seifert B, Michel B, et al. Prediction of iron deficiency in chronic inflammatory rheumatic disease anaemia. *Br J Haematol.* 1995;91:820–826.

118. Bultink IEM, Lems WF, de Stadt RJV, et al. Ferritin and serum transferrin receptor predict iron deficiency in anemic patients with rheumatoid arthritis. *Arthritis Rheum.* 2001;44:979–981.

119. Means RT, Allen J, Sears DA, et al. Serum soluble transferrin receptor and the prediction of marrow iron results in a heterogeneous group of patients. *Clin Lab Haematol.* 1999;21:161–167.

120. Joosten E, Van Loon R, Billen J, et al. Serum transferrin receptor in the evaluation of the iron status in elderly hospitalized patients with anemia. *Am J Hematol.* 2002;69:1–6.

121. Mast AE, Blinder MA, Gronowski AM, et al. Clinical utility of the soluble transferrin receptor and comparison with serum ferritin in several populations. *Clin Chem.* 1998;44:45–51.

122. Kotru M, Rusia U, Sikka M, et al. Evaluation of serum ferritin in screening for iron deficiency in tuberculosis. *Ann Hematol.* 2004;83:95–100.

123. Macdougall IC, Cavill I, Hulme B, et al. Detection of functional iron-deficiency during erythropoietin treatment: a new approach. *Br Med J.* 1992;304:225–226.

124. Fishbane S, Shapiro W, Dutka P, et al. A randomized trial of iron deficiency testing strategies in hemodialysis patients. *Kidney Int.* 2001;60:2406–2411.

125. Fernandez-Rodriguez AM, Guindeo-Casasus MC, Molero-Labarta T, et al. Diagnosis of iron deficiency in chronic renal failure. *Am J Kidney Dis.* 1999;34:508–513.

126. Domellof M, Dewey KG, Lonnerdal B, et al. The diagnostic criteria for iron deficiency in infants should be reevaluated. *J Nutr.* 2002;132:3680–3686.

127. Margolis HS, Huntley HH, Bender TR, et al. Iron deficiency in children: the relationship between pretreatment laboratory tests and subsequent hemoglobin response to iron therapy. *Am J Clin Nutr.* 1981;34:2158–2168.

128. Hershko C, Baror D, Gaziel Y, et al. Diagnosis of iron-deficiency anemia in a rural-population of children: relative usefulness of serum ferritin, red-cell protoporphyrin, red-cell indexes and transferrin saturation determinations. *Am J Clin Nutr.* 1981;34:1600–1610.

129. Abraham K, Muller C, Gruters A, et al. Minimal inflammation, acute phase response and avoidance of misclassification of vitamin A and iron status in infants: importance of a high-sensitivity C-reactive protein (CRP) assay. *Int J Vitam Nutr Res.* 2003;73:423–430.

Chapter | **10** |

Investigation of megaloblastic anaemia: cobalamin, folate and metabolite status

Malcolm S. Hamilton, Sheena Blackmore

proteins by pepsin and acid and bound initially by transcobalamin I or haptocorrin (R binder). This binder also binds other cobinamides in the diet which are metabolically inert. Pancreatic enzymes release the cobalamin from transcobalamin I and permit binding by intrinsic factor. The intrinsic factor–cobalamin complex is attached to cubam, a multiligand receptor, which is a combination of cubilin[2] and amnionless and is taken up by endocytosis, into the ileal cell. The cobalamin is then released from the endosome and bound to transcobalamin II (holotranscobalamin) in the ileal cell and exported into the portal circulation. Cobalamin undergoes enterohepatic circulation via the liver and bile ducts with 1.4 µg/day excreted in the bile, of which 1 µg/day is reabsorbed in the ileum. Holotranscobalamin is the active form of cobalamin and is taken up by holotranscobalamin receptors (TCII receptors) on cells throughout the body, particularly liver, kidney and bone marrow cells. At the cellular level in the target tissue the holotranscobalamin undergoes endocytosis via the transmembrane TCII receptor. Holotranscobalamin then undergoes lysosomal degradation, releasing cobalamin for metabolic reactions.

Cobalamin is a cofactor in two important biochemical reactions. In the first, methylcobalamin acts as a cofactor for methionine synthase in the production of methionine from homocysteine. The remethylation of cobalamin requires the donation of the methyl group from methyltetrahydrofolate as it is converted to tetrahydrofolate, thus linking cobalamin to folate and 1-carbon metabolism. The second cobalamin reaction occurs in the mitochondrion. Cobalamin is converted to adenosylcobalamin, a cofactor for the enzyme methylmalonyl-CoA mutase, which converts methylmalonyl-CoA (the product of propionate metabolism) to succinyl-CoA. Methionine produced in the first reaction is converted to adenosylmethionine and is a vital source of methyl groups critical for a series of methylation reactions involving proteins, phospholipids, neurotransmitters, RNA and DNA. In cobalamin deficiency, methylmalonic acid and homocysteine levels are therefore elevated. Reduced methionine synthesis is thought to result in a decrease in methylation of myelin basic protein, resulting in the neuropathies associated with cobalamin deficiency which are irreversible once subacute combined degeneration[3] of the cord has occurred.

COBALAMIN ABSORPTION AND METABOLISM

Cobalamin in the human diet is a bacterial product ingested and stored by animals and strict vegans are therefore liable to deficiency. The prevalence of cobalamin deficiency, as defined by serum vitamin B$_{12}$ <200 ng/l and methylmalonic acid >0.27 µmol/l, is 1.6% of subjects over 51 years of age in the 2001–2004 National Health and Nutrition Examination Survey[1] in the USA. Of this age group, 3.2% have a low serum B$_{12}$ <200 ng/l. Ingested cobalamin is released from food

FOLATE ABSORPTION AND METABOLISM

Dietary folate polyglutamates are thermolabile, water-soluble vitamins found in leafy green vegetables. Folate deficiency arises from dietary deficiency, impaired absorption or increased requirements. Folate polyglutamates in the diet must be hydrolysed to monoglutamates by hydrolases, operating maximally at pH 5.5 in the presence of zinc and further converted to pteroylglutamate, before absorption can take place. Folate carriers transport pteroylpolyglutamate rapidly into the luminal cells where it is methylated using methyl cobalamin as cofactor and reduced to 5-methyltetrahydrofolate (5-methyl THF) in the enterocyte before entering the portal venous system. Unconverted pteroylglutamate remains in the luminal cells.

Just like cobalamin, there is significant enterohepatic recirculation of folate, amounting to 90 μg/day, and biliary drainage results in rapid fall in serum folate levels, whereas deprivation of dietary folate takes up to 3 weeks to cause serum levels to fall. Two-thirds of plasma folate is non-specifically bound to plasma folate binding proteins including albumen and one-third circulates as free folate.

There is sufficient retention of folate by the renal tubules to prevent urinary vitamin loss; this is achieved by megalin uptake of filtered folate-binding protein[4] and bound folate. Cubam,[2] which binds intrinsic factor-cobalamin complex, is also important in the uptake of albumen from the renal tubules, which may also contribute to folate retention.

Folate transport into cells is dependent upon two mechanisms, reduced folate carrier (58 kDa), which is a low-affinity high-capacity system, and folate receptors (44 kDa), of which there are three isoforms – alpha and beta are attached to the cell surface through a glycosylphosphatidylinositol anchor and gamma is secreted by enteric mucosal cells. Methyltetrahydrofolate bound to the folate receptor undergoes endocytosis by clathrin-coated pits or caveolae. Antimetabolites such as methotrexate also bind to the reduced folate carrier and folate receptor. Passive diffusion is an alternative mechanism by which folate can enter cells. The relative contributions of the different mechanisms are not known. Folate receptors may be expressed on malignant cells and have become potential targets for delivery of cytotoxic agents linked to folate.

Folates participate in 1-C metabolism and thereby facilitate the essential cellular metabolism of methionine, serine, glycine, choline and histidine in the biosynthesis of purine and deoxythymidine monophosphate (dTMP) in the synthesis of pyrimidines and thus DNA (Fig. 10.1).

Intracellular folates are compartmentalized between the cytosol and mitochondria and the major forms are tetrahydrofolate (THF), 5-methyl THF and 10-formyltetrahydrofolate (10-formyl THF). Homocysteine is converted to methionine by methionine synthetase using cobalamin as a cofactor and methyl THF as the methyl group donor. Cobalamin deficiency therefore results in inactivation of methionine synthase, resulting in accumulation of 5-methyl THF, which cannot be converted back to 5,10-methylene THF. Folate is then unavailable for pyrimidine and purine synthesis – the methyl-trap hypothesis, which was advanced to explain why cobalamin deficiency often results in a functional folate deficiency. Furthermore, methyl THF is a very poor substrate for the enzyme responsible for folate polyglutamation, folylpoly-γ-glutamate synthetase, which prefers THF and 10-formyl THF. Folate deficiency is thought to cause megaloblastic anaemia by inhibiting the production of 5,10-methylene THF polyglutamate form, which acts as a cofactor in the rate-limiting step in the production of DNA, the synthesis of deoxythymidine

Figure 10.1 Metabolic diagram. *Note:* Cobalamin bound to transcobalamin II is in its most oxidized 3+ state and enters the cell by TCII receptor, it undergoes one reductase step to cobalamin (I) in the cytoplasm and a second reductase step to cobalamin (II) in the mitochondria. The methionine cycle takes place in the cytoplasm and the succinyl-CoA synthesis in the mitochondria.

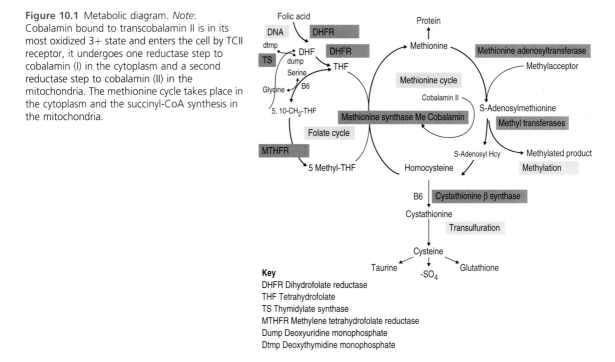

Key
DHFR Dihydrofolate reductase
THF Tetrahydrofolate
TS Thymidylate synthase
MTHFR Methylene tetrahydrofolate reductase
Dump Deoxyuridine monophosphate
Dtmp Deoxythymidine monophosphate

monophosphate (dTMP). Thus, in the absence of cobalamin, polyglutamate synthesis ceases and monoglutamate forms are not retained by cells. This explains why in cobalamin deficiency serum folate levels may be found to be elevated and red cell folate levels normal or low. These metabolic pathways explain the interrelationship of serum B_{12}, serum folate and red cell folate results seen in the clinical laboratory.

Folate deficiency is therefore associated with elevation of homocysteine levels, reduced methionine synthesis and defective purine and pyrimidine synthesis, the latter resulting in morphologically visible megaloblastic change in bone marrow cells. Cobalamin deficiency also results in a functional folate deficiency with indistinguishable megaloblastic change and/or the more insidious and dangerous potential for neurological damage.

RATIONALE FOR INVESTIGATION OF COBALAMIN OR FOLATE STATUS

Investigation of the vitamin B_{12} and folate status of individuals is not restricted to investigation of individuals with classical features of megaloblastic anaemia alone because neuropathy and neuro-psychiatric changes may occur in B_{12} deficiency in the absence of macrocytosis or anaemia.[5-9] The finding that folate supplementation reduced the incidence of neural tube defects[10] by 25–46% in the USA and Canada highlights the importance of defining optimum population folate levels. Increased plasma homocysteine and serum methylmalonic acid (MMA) levels have been advocated[11-14] as sensitive indicators of folate and cobalamin deficiency that may be subclinical. Introduction of metabolite testing to routine laboratory practice was limited in the past as a result of technical difficulty in measurement but is now becoming more available, though the clinical benefit of this approach has been questioned by some authors.[15,16] Elevated homocysteine levels are an independent vascular disease risk factor[17] and are also associated with risk of idiopathic venous thrombosis.[18] In the USA, dietary supplementation with folate was introduced in 1998 to reduce neural tube defects and by lowering homocysteine levels may achieve a further health gain in reduced myocardial infarction and stroke. Food supplementation with folate remains a controversial step in European countries because of a possible increased risk of cancers[19,20] (see Scientific Advisory Committee on Nutrition, at: www. sacn.gov.uk, for update). Increased plasma homocysteine levels occur in both B_{12} and folate deficiency as a result of reduction in methionine synthesis (Fig. 10.1). Some laboratories have utilized homocysteine as an initial screening test for abnormalities of cobalamin and folate metabolism which may be particularly appropriate for investigation of suspected inherited cobalamin or folate disorders in children.[21,22] MMA measurement though not widely available in the UK, requiring gas chromatography-

mass spectrometry (GC-MS), is available at a limited number of university departments. In contrast, plasma homocysteine measurement by high-performance liquid chromatography (HPLC) and commercial enzyme immunoassays is widely available. The limitations of total serum B_{12} measurement have been highlighted by studies that showed poor positive predictive value (i.e. healthy persons with a low level or low cobalamin levels with no evidence of deficiency) and <100% negative predictive value of 95% (i.e. 5% clinically deficient with normal level).[15,23] In addition, some publications have highlighted the presence of severe cobalamin deficiency concurrent with a normal cobalamin level using some of the current commercial assays.[24,25] The introduction of holotranscobalamin assays,[26-28] now available on an Abbott automated immunoassay platform, provides a readily accessible method of assessing the physiologically active form of cobalamin rather than the less relevant total B_{12}. The advent of a commercial holotranscobalamin assay occurred over 20 years after depletion of serum holotranscobalamin II was identified as an early sign of cobalamin deficiency.[29] Adoption of new methodology in laboratory medicine in the UK requires careful evaluation in a clinical setting and this research appears inhibited by lack of training in research methodology and financial constraints in service laboratories. Serum methylmalonic acid is increased in renal impairment and 7.9% of subjects over 51 have levels in excess of 0.27 μmol/l.[1] MMA must therefore be used in conjunction with serum cobalamin and holotranscobalamin and must be interpreted in the light of renal function. Urinary MMA measurement can be used to compensate for the impact of renal impairment.

HAEMATOLOGICAL FEATURES OF MEGALOBLASTIC ANAEMIA

Megaloblastic anaemia resulting from impaired DNA synthesis is characterized by the presence of megaloblastic red cell precursors in the bone marrow and occasionally also in the blood. Megaloblasts have a characteristic chromatin pattern (Fig. 10.2) and increased cytoplasm as a result of asynchrony of nuclear and cytoplasmic maturation with a relatively immature nucleus for the degree of cytoplasmic haemoglobinization. The delay in nuclear maturation caused by delay in DNA synthesis resulting from lack of vitamin B_{12} or folate is also seen in all lineages, particularly granulocytic marrow precursors with giant metamyelocytes (Fig. 10.3) and hyperlobated neutrophils with increased lobe size as well as number of nuclear segments (see Chapter 5, Fig. 5.10). In severe pernicious anaemia, a progressive increase in mean red cell volume (MCV) up to 130 fl occurs, with oval macrocytes, poikilocytes and hypersegmentation of neutrophils (>5% with more than five nuclear lobes).[31] The neutrophil hypersegmentation index is an equivalent automated

A

B

Figure 10.2 Photomicrographs of bone marrow films stained by May–Grünwald–Giemsa. (A) Megaloblasts. (B) Normoblasts for comparison.

Figure 10.3 Photomicrograph of bone marrow film stained by May–Grünwald–Giemsa showing giant metamyelocytes.

parameter on some cell counters, although hypersegmentation does not always respond to a therapeutic trial. The mean platelet volume is decreased and there is increased platelet anisocytosis, as detected by the platelet distribution width (PDW). The MCV falls to 110–120 fl as megaloblastic change advances. Howell–Jolly bodies and basophilic stippling are seen in the red cells.

Differential Diagnosis of Macrocytic Anaemia

Macrocytic red cells are also seen in myelodysplastic syndromes, which can be suspected from the presence of hypogranular neutrophils (see Chapter 5, Fig. 5.76) or monocytosis. Excess alcohol consumption results in an increased MCV as a result of round macrocytes, although rarely does it go higher than 110 fl unless coexisting folate deficiency is present. Hypothyroidism, liver disease, aplastic anaemia, rare inherited orotic aciduria or Lesch–Nyhan syndrome also have a high MCV. Automated reticulocyte counts facilitate detection of increased red cell turnover and high MCV as a result of haemolysis or bleeding. Coexisting iron deficiency or thalassaemia trait may mask macrocytic changes, although a high red cell distribution width indicates anisocytosis and the need for blood film review. Congenital dyserythropoietic anaemias types I and III and erythroleukaemia exhibit some features of megaloblastic erythropoiesis that are unrelated to B_{12} and folate. Drugs interfering with DNA synthesis (e.g. azathioprine, zidovudine or hydroxycarbamide) result in macrocytosis and megaloblastic erythropoiesis. Anticonvulsant therapy interferes with folate metabolism,[32] whereas the impact of oral contraceptives on folate absorption and metabolism is controversial.[33] Prolonged nitrous oxide anaesthesia destroys methylcobalamin and causes acute megaloblastic change.[34] Methotrexate inhibits dihydrofolate reductase and toxicity can be reversed with folinic acid, which is already in the tetrahydrofolate form and effectively reverses the metabolic block, which is not achieved solely with folic acid.

TESTING STRATEGY FOR SUSPECTED COBALAMIN OR FOLATE DEFICIENCY

Microbiological cobalamin and folate assays and competitive radiodilution binding assays for measurement of cobalamin and folate, which were often performed together, have largely been replaced by separate analysis by automated binding assays. The application of a suitable testing strategy for patients suspected of having cobalamin or folate deficiency is shown in Tables 10.1–10.3.

Table 10.1 Significance of clinical details

SYMPTOMS OR SIGNS	POSSIBLE SIGNIFICANCE
Tiredness, palpitations, pallor	Anaemia
Slight jaundice	Ineffective erythropoiesis
Neurological Cognitive impairment, optic atrophy, loss of vibration sense, joint position sense; plantar responses normal or abnormal; tendon reflexes depressed or increased	Cobalamin deficiency, subacute combined degeneration of the spinal cord and sensori/motor peripheral neuropathies
Dietary and gastrointestinal history Vegetarian or vegan; poor nutrition (e.g. tea and toast diet in elderly or students); dietary fads	Low iron stores and iron deficiency Cobalamin deficiency in babies born to mothers who are vegans Folate deficiency (often with iron deficiency)
Weight loss, bloating and steatorrhoea, particularly nocturnal bowel movements	Features of malabsorption and folate deficiency, e.g. due to coeliac disease, tropical sprue
Mouth ulcers, abdominal pain, perianal ulcers, fistulae	Terminal ileal Crohn's disease – cobalamin deficiency
Glossitis, angular cheilosis and koilonychia	Cobalamin and combined iron deficiency
Alcohol history	Poor diet and interference with folate metabolism
History of autoimmune disease in patient or family Hypothyroidism, pernicious anaemia or coeliac disease	Increased likelihood of pernicious anaemia or coeliac disease
Surgery Gastrectomy/bowel resection	Cobalamin deficiency usually 2 years post-gastrectomy Ileal disease resulting in cobalamin deficiency Blind loop syndromes
Physical appearance Grey hair, blue eyes, vitiligo	Association with pernicious anaemia
Pregnancy	Increased iron and folate requirements. Cobalamin levels fall by 30% in the 3rd trimester Holotranscobalamin levels are unaltered in late pregnancy
Malabsorptive syndrome Tropical sprue, bacterial overgrowth, fish tape worm in Scandinavian countries	Combined folate and iron deficiency Cobalamin deficiency
Drug history	See text
Other haematological disorders Myeloproliferative neoplasms, haemolytic anaemias, leukaemias	Increased folate utilization may result in folate deficiency
Myeloma	Paraprotein interference with cobalamin assays resulting in falsely low cobalamin levels, which normalize on treatment of myeloma

Table 10.1 highlights the important clinical details that should be elicited by the clinician and submitted with the request to assist the laboratory in interpretation of the numeric results of cobalamin and folate assays. Ideally, test requests should not be accepted without this information, which could be incorporated into electronic order communication from user to laboratory.

Table 10.2 lists the important laboratory investigations that should be performed – results must not be reported in isolation from other laboratory results and clinical

Table 10.2 Laboratory tests in suspected cobalamin or folate deficiency

DIAGNOSTIC TESTS	DIAGNOSTIC FEATURES SUGGESTIVE OF COBALAMIN OR FOLATE ABNORMALITY	WILL HELP TO EXCLUDE	PITFALLS
Full blood count	Macrocytosis	–	Macrocytosis and anaemia may be absent despite neuropathy
Blood film	Oval macrocytes, hypersegmented neutrophils (>5% with >5 lobes) Howell–Jolly bodies suggests hyposplenism and therefore coeliac disease as a cause of the deficiency	Myelodysplastic syndrome (hypogranular or hypolobulated neutrophils, dimorphic red cells) alcohol excess/liver disease (round macrocytes, target cells, stomatocytes), haemolytic anaemia (see Chapter 5)	Hypersegmented neutrophils are not invariably present; they may occur during cytotoxic therapy
Reticulocyte count	Absolute count low pre-treatment	Reticulocyte response at day 6 post-therapy confirms response to B_{12} or folate therapy provided only low dose is given	Reticulocyte response may be blunted if inadequate iron stores
Bone marrow aspirate (including Perls' stain) before treatment or within 24 h of cobalamin or folate therapy – indicated if severe, unexplained macrocytic anaemia	Megaloblastic erythropoiesis, giant metamyelocytes, hypersegmented neutrophils, ring sideroblasts infrequent	Myelodysplastic syndromes, aplastic anaemia	Megaloblastic change is not necessarily a result of deficiency; can be drug induced or a feature of a myelodysplastic syndrome
Serum B_{12}	B_{12} <180 ng/l suggestive of cobalamin deficiency, may be a result of pernicious anaemia, veganism, or gastrectomy; in the absence of these causes, may result from malabsorption of protein-bound B_{12} (e.g. as a result of achlorhydria). B_{12} <150 ng/l highly suggestive of cobalamin deficiency	B_{12} <180 ng/l with no clinical signs or symptoms and normal MMA and homocysteine reflects poor sensitivity of total B_{12} assay. B_{12} levels may be borderline low due to severe folate deficiency; give folic acid and monitor B_{12} level unless neurological abnormalities present	B_{12} >180 ng/l but presence of neuropathy or strong clinical suspicion of B_{12} deficiency requires a therapeutic trial or additional tests, such as MMA, holotranscobalamin and homocysteine: if holotranscobalamin is low then treat with B_{12} and monitor response by repeat metabolite levels at day 6; B_{12} deficiency is confirmed by high MMA and homocysteine which fall on treatment
Serum folate	Low level, particularly if red cell folate also low confirms deficient state		Subject to diurnal variation. Low levels may result from recent deterioration in diet. Conversely low serum folate levels are rapidly corrected by improved diet

Continued

Table 10.2 Laboratory tests in suspected cobalamin or folate deficiency – cont'd

DIAGNOSTIC TESTS	DIAGNOSTIC FEATURES SUGGESTIVE OF COBALAMIN OR FOLATE ABNORMALITY	WILL HELP TO EXCLUDE	PITFALLS
Red cell folate	Low level, particularly if B_{12} deficiency is excluded		Low red cell folate and high serum folate occur in cobalamin deficiency – treat with B_{12}
Serum holotranscobalamin	Early marker of B_{12} deficiency. Low levels <23 μmol/l often as low as 5 μmol/l in pernicious anaemia		Subject to recent dietary change, within 24 h. Particularly useful in pregnancy, where levels unaffected by trimester
Elevation of serum holotranscobalamin levels at 24 h from baseline in response to oral 10 μg cyanocobalamin 6 hourly ×3 doses	Subjects with dietary deficiency show rapid elevation of HoloTC by >15 pmol/l. Pernicious anaemia show enhanced HoloTC levels after addition of oral recombinant intrinsic factor		Non-isotopic B_{12} absorption tests utilizing HoloTC levels at 24–48 h and recombinant intrinsic factor are in development
Intrinsic factor antibody test (test if serum B_{12} is <150 ng/l)	Positive in 50–60% of cases of pernicious anaemia and, when positive, obviates Schilling test		False positive (rare) Negative in 40–50% of cases of pernicious anaemia; if negative, proceed to Schilling test (if available)
Schilling test (Part I, basic test; Part II, with intrinsic factor; Part III, following course of antibiotics)	Part I <5% and part II normal or near normal confirms malabsorption as a result of lack of intrinsic factor (e.g. pernicious anaemia); Parts I and II abnormal, suggests malabsorption not resulting from intrinsic factor deficiency[a]		Reagents not currently available. Awaiting recombinant intrinsic factor supplier. Invalid in renal failure; Part II may not correct in pernicious anaemia if intrinsic factor antibodies are present at high concentration in gastric juice
Upper gastrointestinal endoscopy and duodenal biopsy[b]	Villous atrophy in coeliac disease		
Serum gastrin or gastric juice pH	Raised serum gastrin or gastric juice pH of >6 confirms achlorhydria: if not present, diagnosis of pernicious anaemia is suspect		

Table 10.2 Laboratory tests in suspected cobalamin or folate deficiency – cont'd

DIAGNOSTIC TESTS	DIAGNOSTIC FEATURES SUGGESTIVE OF COBALAMIN OR FOLATE ABNORMALITY	WILL HELP TO EXCLUDE	PITFALLS
Serum MMA and plasma or serum homocysteine, before treatment or before and 6 days after treatment[c]	Raised homocysteine in folate and B_{12} deficiency; raised MMA in B_{12} deficiency, which is helpful to confirm deficiency if B_{12} is low and IF antibodies are absent. Correction of elevated metabolite levels after cobalamin therapy provides evidence of biochemical response	Lack of significance of low B_{12} is indicated by normal MMA and homocysteine and no clinical signs. Note serum homocysteine requires sample taken on ice and separated before any haemolysis	Both MMA and homocysteine are elevated in renal impairment. MMA cannot be used in isolation without either B_{12} or HoloTC measurement. Homocysteine is not specific for cobalamin deficiency, being elevated in folate deficiency, smokers and hyperhomocystinaemia.

HoloTC, holotranscobalamin; IF, intrinsic factor; MMA, methylmalonic acid; MTHF, methyltetrahydrofolate.
[a]If Part II fails to correct, proceed to barium follow through or small bowel enema to diagnose ileal disease (e.g. Crohn's disease); Parts I and II abnormal, Part III normal indicates malabsorption resulting from bacterial overgrowth (e.g. blind loop syndrome).
[b]Upper gastrointestinal tract endoscopy also useful if dyspepsia develops in known pernicious anaemia so as to exclude gastric carcinoma.
[c]Plasma homocysteine assay is now widely available; in suspected B_{12} deficiency it provides a useful test of biochemical cobalamin deficiency. Correction of elevated levels after treatment provides confirmation of deficiency.

Table 10.3 Clinical and laboratory checklist for diagnosis of pernicious anaemia

	LABORATORY CRITERIA	CLINICAL CRITERIA
Minor criteria	Macrocytosis	Parasthesiae, numbness or ataxia
	Anaemia	Hypothyroidism
	Raised plasma homocysteine	Vitiligo
	Gastric pH above 6	Family history of pernicious anaemia or hypothyroidism
	Raised serum gastrin	
	Positive gastric parietal cell antibody	
Major criteria	Low serum B_{12} (<180 ng/l) or raised serum methylmalonic acid (>0.75 µmol/l) in presence of normal renal function. Megaloblastic anaemia not resulting from folate deficiency. Positive intrinsic factor antibodies using high-specificity test. Holotranscobalamin level <23 µmol/l	
Reference standard criteria	Schilling test[a] shows malabsorption of oral cyanocobalamin corrected by coadministration of intrinsic factor	

[a]Reagents for Schilling tests currently unavailable. A non-isotopic B_{12} absorption test utilizing recombinant intrinsic factor and holotranscobalamin measurement is under development.

details. If investigations are performed in different laboratories, authorization and release of results requires access to all laboratory data on the individual patient. Laboratory information systems should facilitate this cross-disciplinary access. For example, intrinsic factor antibody results should be available to haematology or clinical chemistry laboratories undertaking cobalamin, MMA or homocysteine assays.

Table 10.3 provides a list of clinical and laboratory features for diagnosis of pernicious anaemia. These criteria

Table 10.4 The calculation to derive specificity and sensitivity for the *Siemens Centaur B$_{12}$* assay

Community study of 1621 subjects with normal renal function in Banbury, UK	True cobalamin deficiency defined by methylmalonic acid of >0.75 µmol/l with normal renal function	Absence of cobalamin deficiency defined by methylmalonic acid of <0.75 µmol/l	
Siemens Centaur B$_{12}$ assay <270 ng/l	53 true positives (TP)	437 false positives (FP) (27% of subjects studied)	Positive predictive value = TP/(TP+FP) = 53/490 = 13.2%
Siemens Centaur B$_{12}$ >270 ng/l	17 false negatives (FN)	1114 true negatives (TN)	Negative predictive value = TN/(TN+FN) = 1114/1131 = 98.4%
	70 cobalamin-deficient individuals (4.3% of subjects studied). Sensitivity = TP/(TP+FN) = 53/70 = 75.7%	1551 non-deficient. Specificity = TN/(TN+FP) = 1114/1551 = 71.8%	

False-positive rate (α) = FP/(FP+TN) = 437/1551 = 28.2% = 1 − specificity. False-negative rate (β) = FN/(TP+FN) = 17/70 = 24.3% = 1 − sensitivity.

avoid undue reliance on a single B$_{12}$ assay and should help clinicians to make a diagnosis even when some critical tests, e.g. Schilling tests, are not available.

In view of the lack of specificity and sensitivity of serum cobalamin assays and frequent lack of availability of other diagnostic tests, basing the diagnosis of pernicious anaemia, which requires lifelong parenteral B$_{12}$ therapy, solely on laboratory results, is not straightforward. A checklist of laboratory and clinical diagnostic criteria, as shown in Table 10.2, helps to achieve a greater degree of diagnostic certainty than any single diagnostic test and permits the diagnosis to be made even when a single diagnostic test is anomalous or unavailable. Clinical and other laboratory criteria thus provide additional supportive evidence of an autoimmune aetiology, even if the more demanding diagnostic laboratory criteria are not met.

Limitations of Cobalamin Assays

Sensitivity and Specificity of Cobalamin and Holotranscobalamin Assays

Utility of receiver operator characteristic curves

There has been little data on sensitivity and specificity of current B$_{12}$ assays, due to the difficulty in defining a truly deficient study population. Some authors have suggested B$_{12}$ assays and measurement of methylmalonic acid are no better than tossing a coin, to determine the presence or absence of deficiency. The study by Clarke et al.[28] provides data which permits calculation of the specificity and sensitivity of a current B$_{12}$ immunoassay in the detection of cobalamin deficiency in a community study of 1621 subjects over age 65 with normal renal function. Subjects were defined as cobalamin deficient if the

methylmalonic acid was elevated above 0.75 µmol/l. Deficiency was found in 4.3% of subjects over 65 years of age with normal renal function. The mean B$_{12}$ level of these subjects was 151 pmol/l (202 ng/l) by Siemens Centaur assay (range 110–199 pmol/l). Table 10.4 illustrates the calculation to derive specificity and sensitivity for the Siemens Centaur B$_{12}$ assay using a cut-off point of 200 pmol/l (270 ng/l).

This study demonstrates that, while values over 270 ng/l have a high (98.4%) negative predictive value for the presence of disease, values below 270 ng/l include a high percentage (28.2%) of individuals with normal methylmalonic acid levels and presumably no evidence of cobalamin deficiency, resulting in a large grey area. This is reflected in the poor specificity (71.8%) of the assay using this cut-off point. The choice of the appropriateness of the cut-off point can be explored further using receiver operator characteristic (ROC) curves. Laboratories able to construct ROC curves will be able to select an appropriate cut-off point to identify those patients with possible or definite disease.

Selection of a cut-off point for cobalamin of below 150 ng/l, will identify subjects with higher probability of presence of cobalamin deficiency. Some authors[13] have advocated choosing a cut-off point 25% below the reference range lower limit for any particular assay.

If, for example, a cut-off point of 125 pmol/l (168 ng/l) is chosen, the specificity of a value below this level, i.e. the number of normal individuals who fall below the cut-off point, will be markedly reduced (FP) and therefore the specificity of the test (TN/TN+FP) improves to 95%, although the detection of individuals with true deficiency who lie above the cut-off point, i.e. false negatives will be markedly increased, resulting in a sensitivity (TP/TP+FN) of 35%. The ROC curve therefore allows a laboratory to select a cut-off point that meets the objective of the laboratory – to have either a highly specific but low sensitivity test or to have a test of poor specificity but high sensitivity. Clearly cobalamin assays do not meet the criteria for an ideal test of high sensitivity and high specificity which would lie on the coordinates 0.1 to the left of the graph. The Axis-Shield/Abbott holotranscobalamin assay in this pivotal study is seen to have slightly superior ROC curves (see Fig. 10.4).

Utility of holotranscobalamin, methylmalonic acid and homocysteine assays

Holotranscobalamin assays gave a greater area under the curve, 0.85 versus 0.76 in the above study, and superior sensitivity and specificity. Holotranscobalamin is the physiologically active fraction of total cobalamin.[27–29] An isolated abnormal result of serum B_{12} should not be the sole criterion on which treatment decisions are based and a repeat assay and other confirmatory and clinical evaluation are necessary prior to a diagnostic conclusion. Additional secondary testing with metabolite levels, or holotranscobalamin and monitoring of treatment response is recommended. High B_{12} levels have been described in subjects with no myeloproliferative neoplasm and who are not on cobalamin therapy or vitamin supplementation.[35] This is thought to be due to immunoglobulin-complexed B_{12} resulting in assay interference. False normal B_{12} levels[24,25] have been described in subjects with high titre intrinsic factor antibody[25] and may also occur due to presence of heterophile antibody interference.

Holotranscobalamin assays[27,28] may challenge total B_{12} assays as a first-line test in cobalamin assessment. Holotranscobalamin has been shown to be unaffected by assay interference from high-titre intrinsic factor antibody levels.[36] In addition, holotranscobalamin is not subject to the 30% fall in total B_{12} levels seen in normal pregnancy, which makes low total B_{12} levels uninterpretable during pregnancy (Fig. 10.5).[30]

Access to homocysteine, methylmalonic acid and holotranscobalamin assays facilitates more precise definition of cobalamin and folate status in patients in whom

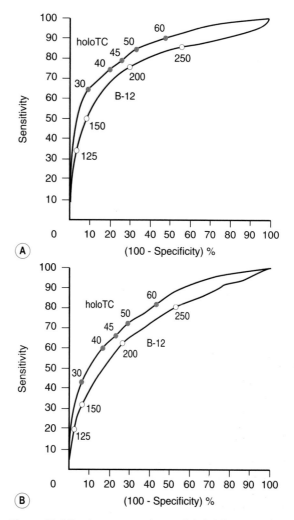

Figure 10.4 Receiver operator characteristic (ROC) curves (showing holotranscobalamin levels in µmol/l (abnormal <44 µmol/l) and B_{12} levels in pmol/l (1 pmol/l = 1.344 ng/l). (A) The ROC curve for methylmalonic acid levels >0.75 µmol/l (definite metabolic B_{12} deficiency). (B) Methylmalonic acid levels of >0.45 µmol/l (probable B_{12} deficiency). *(Redrawn from Clarke et al. 2007).[28]*

Figure 10.5 Comparison of HoloTC, cobalamins and HoloHC in pregnant women at 18th, 32nd, 39th gestational week (gw) and at 8 weeks' postpartum (8 pp) (n = 141). Means and 95% CI (calculated from the normal distributed log transformed data) for HoloTC (white), cobalamins (white + grey shaded) and measured HoloHC (grey + black shaded) are shown. The grey shaded area indicates HoloHC saturated with true cobalamins (cobalamins – HoloTC) and the black shaded area indicates HoloHC saturated with analogues (measured HoloHC + HoloTC – cobalamins). CI, confidence interval.
(Redrawn from Morkbak et al. (2007), Figure 1.[30])

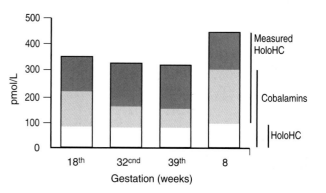

prolonged B_{12} therapy may have been initiated inappropriately and continued unnecessarily or, conversely, discontinued inappropriately because of lack of confidence in the original assessment. The study by Gorringe et al.[16] showed that only 27/49 patients were anaemic or macrocytic with a low total B_{12} of <170 ng/l and elevated MMA. All of these patients treated with B_{12} therapy corrected elevated MMA levels, suggesting the presence of a metabolic deficiency. However, only 15/27 showed a haematological response.

Homocysteine levels also fell by >25% in 47/49 patients after B_{12} treatment. Many of these patients had no clinical evidence or symptoms of cobalamin deficiency and may reflect subjects with subclinical deficiency, which could have subtle cognitive impairment, or may just represent a compensated metabolic state of no clinical consequence. Elevation of homocysteine levels is seen in folate deficiency and is therefore less specific than MMA measurement. The causes of cobalamin deficiency are shown in Table 10.5.

Table 10.5 The causes of cobalamin deficiency

	SUPPORTIVE INFORMATION/DIAGNOSTIC TESTS
Reduced intake	
Strict vegetarian/vegan	Dietary history
Dietary fad that excludes dairy products and meat	Ethnic origin/culture
Breastfed babies of mothers who are vegetarian or cobalamin deficient	
Poor dietary intake in elderly	
Malabsorption as a result of loss or inactivity of intrinsic factor	
Addisonian pernicious anaemia	Diagnostic criteria for pernicious anaemia (see Table 10.3)
Gastrectomy (partial or total)	History of gastric surgery
Bacterial overgrowth or parasitic infestation of small bowel	Radiolabelled lactose breath tests for bacterial overgrowth; Repeat Schilling test post-antibiotic therapy
Pancreatic dysfunction: failure of trypsin release of B_{12} from R binding proteins	Pancreatic function tests; exocrine pancreatic dysfunction results in abnormal Schilling test but clinical deficiency is rare
Malabsorption as a result of failure of B_{12}-intrinsic factor complex uptake in ileum – ileal resection	Radiological, enteroscopic or capsule camera study of small bowel for Crohn's disease of terminal ileum or tuberculous ileitis
Congenital Imerslund–Gräsbeck syndrome	Subjects of Scandinavian origin
Tropical sprue	Small bowel biopsy
Zollinger–Ellison syndrome	Multiple gastric and duodenal ulcers; Pancreatic adenoma on imaging
Food cobalamin malabsorption	
Atrophic gastritis with achlorhydria	Endoscopic and gastric biopsy findings
Gastric surgery	
Abnormal transport proteins	
Transcobalamin II deficiency	Megaloblastic anaemia in presence of normal cobalamin levels; transcobalamin II and holotranscobalamin levels reduced
Transcobalamin I deficiency	No evidence of clinical deficiency but low serum cobalamin levels; Possible fall in holotranscobalamin levels in elderly
Inborn errors of cobalamin metabolism (see reviews[21,22])	Serum and urinary methylmalonic acid and metabolite measurement
Acquired drug effects	
Nitrous oxide: chronic repeated exposure	Drug history
Colchicine: chronic usage impairs B_{12} uptake resulting from diarrhoea	
Metformin reduces B_{12} levels in diabetics.	

Clinical and Diagnostic Pitfalls of Folate Assays

Serum folate is altered by acute dietary change and interruption of enterohepatic recycling; it can therefore be low without significant tissue deficiency. This may be a particular problem in hospital inpatients. Red cell folate was originally advocated as correlating better with megaloblastic change[37,38] reflecting the folate status over the lifespan of the red cells (2–3 months), but a subsequent study suggested that little was to be gained by the addition of red cell folate analysis because only 14% of patients with low serum folate also have low red cell folate levels.[39] Minor haemolysis *in vitro* may cause spurious elevation of serum folate levels because the red cell folate may be 10–20 times the serum value. More than half of the patients with severe cobalamin deficiency have a low red cell folate because impaired methionine synthesis results in accumulation of methyltetrahydrofolate (MTHF) monoglutamate, which diffuses out of cells resulting in a high serum folate.[40,41] Treatment with cobalamin alone will correct the low red cell folate and high serum folate levels. Concern over the inter-method variability of red cell folate assays, and questions about the additional benefits[39] of measurement of both serum and red cell folate, have reduced the use of red cell folate assays. However, satisfactory results are possible if appropriate care is taken with preanalytical sample preparation and analysis. 5-methyl THF is a very labile substance and the addition of sodium ascorbate has reduced the coefficient of variation by half in serum folate assays in external quality assurance surveys.[42] The interplay between serum B_{12}, serum folate and red cell folate and plasma homocysteine and MMA is shown in Table 10.7. In view of the limitations of both serum and red cell folate assays, it is prudent to measure both. An international reference method[43,44] for serum folate has been recognized by the Joint Committee on Traceability in Laboratory Medicine (JCTLM) and is now used to verify the target values in UK National External Quality Assessment Scheme (NEQAS) Haematinics surveys (www.ukneqas-haematinics.org.uk). This should improve the accuracy of serum folate assays, which have been bedevilled by inter-method differences and variation in recommended reference ranges between manufacturers. Red cell folate assays still suffer from a lack of a standardized method for haemolysate preparation and matrix effects, which result in large inter-method differences.

Clinicians and patients using different laboratories require information about derivation of reference ranges, which will now be included in the standards for laboratory accreditation in the UK. Definition of population reference ranges for both serum and red cell folate have been difficult to achieve due to changing diet and food supplementation and assay variability. Elevated levels of homocysteine have been found in elderly subjects,[45,46] indicating possible subclinical folate deficiency in the elderly. Folate reference ranges provided by kit manufacturers also show large inter-method differences. In the USA, some authors have advocated cessation of folate testing since, following dietary supplementation of flour, folate deficiency is very unusual. The causes of clinical deficiency and supportive information or diagnostic tests are shown in Table 10.6 and the interactions between cobalamin and folate are shown in Table 10.7.

Standards, Accuracy and Precision of Cobalamin and Folate Assays

There are currently no internationally recognized reference methods for serum cobalamin measurement, but isotope dilution liquid chromatography tandem mass spectrometric methods have recently been accepted as international reference methods for the quantification of folate species in serum.[43,44] As a result, international reference materials have been developed (by the World Health Organization, WHO 03/178, and by the National Institute of Standards and Technology, NIST SRM), with values assigned for folate species by the tandem mass spectrometric methods.[47] Although reference methods have not been verified for the whole blood matrix as yet, there is a WHO whole blood international standard (95/528) with consensus values for total folate.[48]

Evaluation of commercial automated binding assays by recovery experiments has shown under-recovery of added 5-methyl THF and over-recovery of pteroylglutamic acid (PGA),[49] whereas a suitably calibrated microbiological assay recovers closer to 100%.[50] Differential sensitivity of assays to pteroylglutamic acid and genetic variability in the proportion of *in vivo* formyl folates may be a factor in inter-method variability.

A microbiological assay was the method used to assign a potency value to the British Standard for human serum B_{12},[51] and this was later re-classified as the 1st WHO International Standard (IS) (81/563). The 2nd WHO IS for serum B_{12}, 03/178, was ratified in 2007,[47] the values adopted being a consensus of the contemporary B_{12} protein-binding assays.

External quality assessment schemes have shown serum B_{12} intra-method coefficients of variation (CV) of 6–10% and as much as 20% at clinically relevant levels; there is thus a substantial 'grey' indeterminate range between normal and low values. Serum folate intra-method CVs are between 6% and 12% and higher CVs of up to 20% are seen for red cell folate assays. Overall between-method CVs may be as high as 35% for the serum methods and can reach 50% for the whole blood assays, suggesting considerable method differences. The causes of this variability include patient factors as well as pre-analytical, analytical and post-analytical factors, as discussed later.

Table 10.6 The causes of folate deficiency

	SUPPORTIVE INFORMATION/ DIAGNOSTIC TESTS
Reduced intake 　Poor diet particularly alcoholics (wine and spirits because beer contains folate) 　Elderly or students 'tea and toast diet' 　Dietary fads 　Premature babies 　Unsupplemented parenteral nutrition	Dietary and alcohol history
Malabsorption 　Coeliac disease (often with coexisting iron deficiency) 　Tropical sprue 　Small bowel resection, malabsorption syndromes	Antiendomysial, antigliadin tests, antitissue transglutaminase Small bowel biopsy
Drug effects 　Sulphasalazine, methotrexate, trimethoprim-sulphamethoxazole, pyrimethamine, phenytoin, sodium valproate, oral contraceptives	Drug history Bone marrow aspiration
Hereditary hyperhomocysteinaemia 　Homozygotes for C677T MTHFR have lower folate levels	
Increased folate turnover 　Pregnancy: progressive fall in 3rd trimester 　Increased requirements for breastfeeding 　Skin disease – severe psoriasis or exfoliation 　Haemodialysis 　Haemolysis: haemoglobinopathy, paroxysmal nocturnal haemoglobinuria, autoimmune haemolytic anaemia (see Chapters 11–13)	

Genetic Factors

A number of methylenetetrahydrofolate reductase polymorphisms that alter the proportion of formylfolate in serum have been described[52] and this could be a potential source of disparity in the response of some sera to different assays. Individuals homozygous for C677T genetic polymorphism have 25% higher plasma homocysteine levels than controls.[53] A genetic–nutrient interactive effect is noted in that the polymorphism confers a greater effect on homocysteine levels in those individuals with low folate levels. Cigarette smoking, age, renal disease, drugs including levodopa and folate supplements all affect homocysteine levels.

Pre-analytical Sample Preparation

Serum B_{12} is stable at room temperature and is not affected by sample handling, unless the sample is haemolysed. Holotranscobalamin is a sensitive marker of recent cobalamin intake and day-to-day variation is 10%. A change in value of twice the day-to-day variation may be taken as a significant change. Folate is affected by recent dietary intake and ideally fasting samples should be taken. However, this is difficult in practice and assumes that the reference range was also based on fasting samples. Marked loss of folate activity is observed as a result of light and temperature instability. Because red cells contain 30–50 times more folic acid than serum, even slight haemolysis will affect serum folate analysis. Thus, rapid transportation and separation prior to analysis, avoidance of storage at room temperature and the storage of samples at 2–8°C for a maximum of 48 h, or at −20°C for no longer than 28 days are all critical factors in the accuracy and precision of serum folate assays. Presence of haemoglobin as a result of lysis in a plasma or serum sample can be readily determined and may be quantified by haemoglobinometry.

The addition of sodium ascorbate 5 mg/ml will stabilize folate in serum, extending sample storage times. Stabilization of serum folate with sodium ascorbate added to the primary blood collection tube would improve the reproducibility of routine serum folate assays as shown in external quality control surveys,[42] but would necessitate introduction of separate B_{12} and folate sample tubes since

Table 10.7 Interaction between serum cobalamin, serum folate, red cell folate, plasma homocysteine, serum methylmalonic acid, urinary methylmalonic acid and holotranscobalamin

CLINICAL STATUS	NORMAL B$_{12}$ AND FOLATE STATUS	B$_{12}$ DEFICIENT	FOLATE DEFICIENT
Serum B$_{12}$[a]	Usually normal, but may be high in liver disease, myeloproliferative neoplasms, acute inflammation, recovery from autoimmune neutropenia. High levels may be due to immunoglobulin-complexed B$_{12}$. Low total B$_{12}$ in 25% of elderly subjects	Usually low, but up to 5% of patients with megaloblastic anaemia may have results within reference range	Usually normal, but low B$_{12}$ may be seen in severe folate deficiency, which corrects when monotherapy with folic acid is given
Serum folate[a]	Usually normal	Usually normal; high serum folate may occur in B$_{12}$ deficiency	Usually low, but normal levels are found with recent dietary improvement
Red cell folate[a,b]	Usually normal	Low	Usually low, but normal in very acute deficiency state
Plasma homocysteine	Usually normal; but may be high in renal failure or in *MTHFR* C677T mutation. Levels may fall with folate supplements	High in B$_{12}$ deficiency and in 50% of samples from patients with low B$_{12}$ consistent with metabolic B$_{12}$-deficient state	High in folate deficiency – corrected with folic acid therapy
Serum methylmalonic acid	Usually normal; high in 10% of normals or with high intake of methionine or renal failure	High in B$_{12}$ deficiency and in 50% of samples from patients with low B$_{12}$ consistent with metabolic B$_{12}$-deficient state	Usually normal, but high in 5% of patients who are folate deficient
Urinary methylmalonic acid	Normal even in renal failure	High	Normal
Holotranscobalamin	Normal although lower levels in elderly	Low (<23 μmol/l) in B$_{12}$ deficiency	Normal

[a]For normal reference values, see Chapter 2. Folic acid, pteroylglutamic acid; MTHF, methyltetrahydrofolate; *MTHFR*, gene encoding methyl-tetrahydrofolate reductase.
[b]Folate assays may exhibit different responses to folic acid compared to MTHF. Assays may not be optimized for haemolysate matrix. Definition of reference range requires reference method and population studies.

ascorbate interferes with cobalamin analysis. EDTA plasma is unsuitable and heparinized plasma may result in higher values. Samples must be fibrin free and without bubbles.

Analytical Factors

Analytical sensitivity or limit of detection (LOD) varies between methods. It is defined as the concentration of analyte at 2SD of 20 replicates above the zero standard and for B$_{12}$ assays is normally in the region of 22 pmol/l (30 ng/l) and for folate is 0.68 nmol/l (0.3 μg/l). This is sometimes confused with the functional sensitivity of an assay, a term that defines the analyte concentration at

which the CV of the assay is 20%. It is preferable that the functional sensitivity limit of serum B$_{12}$ assays is closer to 37 pmol/l (50 ng/l) than the 111 pmol/l (150 ng/l) quoted by some kits because this provides increased sensitivity at the clinically important lower end of the reference range.

For many folate assays, functional sensitivity is in the region of 2.26 nmol/l (1.0 μg/l) or less, although the Roche Elecsys assay quotes 4.5 nmol/l (2.0 μg/l).

Limitations and Interference

Ascorbic acid destroys vitamin B$_{12}$; therefore ascorbate-treated serum cannot be used for B$_{12}$ assays.

Methotrexate and folinic acid interfere with folate measurement because these drugs cross-react with folate-binding proteins. Minor degrees of haemolysis significantly increase serum folate values as a result of high red cell folate levels. Lipaemia with >2.25 mmol/l (2 g/l) of triglycerides and bilirubin >340 µmol/l (200 mg/l) may affect assays.

High cobalamin levels were thought to be due to B_{12} therapy, vitamin supplementation, myeloproliferative neoplasms or liver disease. In the absence of these factors, assay interference may result from immunoglobulin–B_{12}–transcobalamin complexes.[35]

Post-analytical Factors

The clinical interpretation of laboratory data should take account of the positive or negative predictive value of a result. The report should include a reference range, the derivation of which should be indicated. Food supplementation with folate or voluntary additional vitamin intake has resulted in bimodal distributions of vitamin levels in some populations, further complicating the definition of normality.

METHODS FOR COBALAMIN AND FOLATE ANALYSIS

Microbiological bioassays and radiodilution assays for serum B_{12} and folate[54] are still used, albeit by a decreasing minority of laboratories and continue to play an important role in the evaluation of new automated methods. They are also used in population studies where they are useful in providing information on the long-term comparability of results. (They are detailed in the 9th edition of this book.)

Modern methods are highly automated, heterogeneous, competitive protein-binding assays with chemiluminescence or fluorescence detection systems.

GENERAL PRINCIPLES OF COMPETITIVE PROTEIN BINDING ASSAYS

The majority of automated single-platform, multianalyte, random-access analysers offer assays for serum B_{12}, folate and homocysteine by non-isotopic competitive protein binding or immunoassays. Second antibodies may be utilized as part of the separation procedures. These assays have been designed for serum assays and the assay platforms may not be optimized for analysis of haemolysates.

SERUM B_{12} ASSAYS

Release from Endogenous Binders and Conversion of Analyte to Appropriate Form

Nearly 99% of serum B_{12} is bound to endogenous binding proteins (transcobalamin I, II and III) and must be released from these before measurement. The release step utilizes alkaline hydrolysis (NaOH at pH 12–13) in the presence of potassium cyanide (KCN), which converts cobalamin to the more stable cyanocobalamin and dithiothreitol (DTT) to prevent rebinding of released B_{12}. Alkaline hydrolysis requires subsequent adjustment of pH to be optimal for the binding agent.

Binding of B_{12} to Kit Binder

The binding of B_{12} to kit binder is the competitive step of the assay. Serum-derived cyanocobalamin competes with labelled cobalamin, which is usually complexed to a chemiluminescent or fluorescent substrate or enzyme, for limited binding sites on porcine intrinsic factor. Specificity for cobalamin is ensured by purification of the intrinsic factor (IF) or by blocking contaminating corrinoid binders (R binders) by addition of excess blocking cobinamide. Specificity of pure and blocked IF can be demonstrated by the addition of cobinamide to sera. There should be no increase in assay value. Some assays use only the alkaline denaturation step to inactivate the endogenous binders. It is important that assays are not be affected by the presence of high-titre anti-intrinsic factor antibody in patient sera. The Siemens Centaur, Beckman Access, Siemens Immulite 2000/2500 and Tosoh assays have all been vulnerable to this false normal B_{12} effect and carry product literature warnings to this effect. Roche and Abbott assays have not demonstrated this problem with such sera and the holotranscobalamin assay by Axis-Shield is also unaffected.[25,26,36]

Separation of Bound and Unbound B_{12}

Following competitive binding, the separation of bound and unbound B_{12} is achieved by a number of electro- or physico-chemical and immunological methods. The *Roche Elecsys* utilizes an electrochemiluminescence measuring cell in which the bound B_{12}–ruthenium–IF complex, attached to paramagnetic particles by biotin–streptavidin, is magnetically captured onto the surface of an electrode. The *Abbott Axsym* uses polymer microparticles (beads) coated with porcine IF to bind B_{12} and the bound B_{12} is then immobilized by irreversible binding to a glass fibre matrix. These methods are designed to improve separation of bound and unbound B_{12}; they may utilize murine anti-intrinsic factor antibody–enzyme conjugates as part of the signal generation.

Signal Generation

The bound fraction is then detected by addition of a chemiluminescent, fluorescent or colorimetric enzyme substrate, which results in generation of fluorescence or light emission. There are two types of signal: flash, which is pH or electrically induced, and plateau, which is sustained. The initial rate of reaction or the area under the curve is used to calculate the result.

Electrochemiluminescence Immunoassay

In the *Roche Elecsys* platforms a voltage is applied to the electrode on which the bound B_{12}–ruthenium–IF complexes have been immobilized by magnetic attraction. This generates electrochemical luminescence that is measured by the photomultiplier, the relative light units being inversely proportional to the sample B_{12} concentration. The signal that is produced is timed and integrated by the instrument's software.

Enzyme-linked Fluorescence Generation

In the *Abbott Axsym* substrates such as 4-methyl-umbelliferyl phosphate are cleaved by an enzyme (i.e. alkaline phosphatase–ligand complex) and the resulting reaction generates fluorescence, the intensity of which is inversely proportional to the B_{12} concentration in the sample.

The *Siemens Centaur* and the *Abbott Architect* use acridinium esters bound to B_{12}–IF complex coupled to paramagnetic particles; photons are emitted in response to pH change. The Siemens *Immulite 2000/2500* (formerly *DPC*) uses adamantyl dioxatane phosphate as an alternative substrate, which is cleaved by alkaline phosphatase-labelled B_{12}–IF complex, resulting in generation of a plateau chemiluminescent signal. Alkaline phosphatase/4 methyl-umbelliferyl phosphate is utilized by the *Tosoh Eurogenetics* method and *Beckman Coulter Access* employs alkaline phosphatase/dioxatane phosphate (Lumi-Phos) for signal generation. Precise descriptions of the assay methods are given in the product literature.

HOLOTRANSCOBALAMIN ASSAYS

Principle

About 6–20% of B_{12} is bound to TC II forming the physiologically active complex HoloTC and in this form is taken up by cells. Levels of holotranscobalamin (HoloTC) B_{12} are 30–160 pmol/l. The remainder of the serum B_{12} is bound to transcobalamin I (haptocorrin), which is involved in the transport of B_{12} to the liver and enterohepatic circulation thereof. Haptocorrin also binds B_{12} in the gastric contents and B_{12} is released from haptocorrin by pancreatic proteases prior to capture by IF. HoloTC is thought to be the first metabolite to decrease following reduced intake or absorption of B_{12}.[28,29] A commercial assay is available from Axis-Shield and Abbott.[27] The clinical utility of this assay is being confirmed particularly in pregnancy sera where changes in transcobalamin I make total B_{12} levels uninterpretable. The relative merits of HoloTC compared with metabolite measurement remain to be clarified. As a sensitive marker of cobalamin malabsorption, holotranscobalamin levels that correct with small oral doses of B_{12} and the use of recombinant intrinsic factor[55–58] could provide the basis for a non-isotopic B_{12} absorption test to replace the Schilling test, currently unavailable in the UK.

Holotranscobalamin 'Active B_{12}' Immunoassay

Measurement of the 'active form of B_{12}'[27] is based on a monoclonal antibody to cobalamin bound to TCII known as HoloTC. This 'active' form of B_{12} amounts to 20% of the total serum B_{12}. Reference range values are 19–134 pmol/l; pernicious anaemia values are <5 pmol/l. HoloTC is thought to be more sensitive to early deficiency than the measurement of total B_{12} and may be a better indicator of vulnerability to impaired cognitive function.[28] Levels are elevated by renal failure, but are unaffected by pregnancy.[30]

HoloTC levels below 23 pmol/l show an increase in macrocytosis and red cell distribution width. The HoloTC assay appears to be unaffected by assay interference due to high intrinsic factor antibody levels which has caused false normal B_{12} levels in severely deficient patients, as reported to the Medicines and Healthcare products Regulatory Agency (MHRA) by UK NEQAS for three of five major manufacturers of serum B_{12} assays. As expected, HoloTC levels do not correlate with total serum B_{12} and there is an indeterminate zone with borderline levels which may represent early or subclinical deficiency. HoloTC levels below 20 pmol/l occur in approximately 10% of laboratory requests for B_{12}.

HoloTC Radioimmunoassay

The HoloTC radioimmunoassay[59] uses magnetic microspheres coated with monoclonal antibody to holotranscobalamin and achieves separation from haptocorrin by magnetic separator. A [57]Co B_{12} tracer together with a reducing and a denaturing agent are then added to destroy the HoloTC linkage. When the B_{12} binder containing IF is added, the free B_{12} and tracer compete for binding. The unbound tracer is removed by centrifugation and the bound fraction is measured using a gamma counter. The measured radioactivity reflects the competition between tracer and vitamin B_{12} bound to transcobalamin (i.e. HoloTC). The concentration of vitamin B_{12} in the sample is calculated from a calibration curve using recombinant human HoloTC. The assay only requires a 0.4 ml sample volume, the coefficient of variation is <10%, the limit of detection is 10 pmol/l and the assay time is 4 h.

Quantitation of Transcobalamin Saturation

Nexo and colleagues[60,61] described a method permitting measurement of total TC and HoloTC. The method uses B_{12} modified by acid treatment and bound to magnetic beads, which can then be used to remove unsaturated TC or apoTC from serum. The remaining HoloTC is then measured by an enzyme-lined immunosorbent assay (ELISA). Thus the total and HoloTC can be measured and the TC saturation (HoloTC/Total TC) can be quantitated.

In a study of 137 healthy blood donors the reference range for HoloTC was 40–150 pmol/l. Some 10% of circulating TC is saturated with a reference range of 5–20%; 15–50% of B_{12} is bound to TC. In subjects who were B_{12} deficient, HoloTC was 2–34 pmol/l and the TC saturation was 0.4–3%, well below the reference interval, providing a clear cut-off from normal sera. Nexo's method combines a sensitive ELISA[60] for HoloTC with a simple procedure for removal of the unsaturated TC or apoTC.

SERUM FOLATE METHODS

The first methods used for measurement of serum folate were microbiological assays. Radioisotope dilution (RID) assays were subsequently developed and the newer commercial, automated, competitive-binding assays are based on similar principles. As with B_{12}, the use of the original microbiological and RID procedures for serum and red cell folate measurements has diminished. Definition of assay response to different forms of folate is crucial for inter-assay comparisons, particularly in view of the effect of dietary supplementation with folate.

Release from Endogenous Binders

Serum folate present as 5-methyl THF is released from endogenous binders (two-thirds weakly bound to serum proteins and a minority to membrane-derived soluble folate receptors) by alkaline denaturation. DTT or mono-thioglycerol (MTG) is used in most folate assays to prevent reattachment of folate to the endogenous binders and to keep the folate in its reduced form.

Binding of Folate to Folate-Binding Protein

β-Lactoglobulin, isolated from cow's milk, is commonly used as a binding agent in folate assays, i.e. as the folate-binding protein (FBP). Unfortunately, these lactoglobulins are not specific for the attachment of 5-methyl THF and will bind many forms of folate, dependent on pH. These properties have been utilized for the standardization of folate assay. The physiologically active form (5-methyl THF) is very unstable. Pteroylglutamic acid (PGA), present in vitamin supplements, is more stable, binds to FBP and has been used as an alternative standard for the folate assays. Its use as a standard depends on the observation that the binding affinities for 5-methyl THF and PGA are equivalent[62] at pH 9.3 ± 0.1. It is therefore essential that the pH is strictly maintained at the binding stage of the procedure. In most of these assays, serum-derived folate competes with chemiluminescent or enzyme-labelled folate for limited sites on FBP. In the *Roche Elecsys* methods the FBP is labelled with ruthenium and competition exists between endogenous and biotin-labelled folate.

Separation of Bound and Unbound Folate

Following competitive binding the separation of bound and unbound folate is achieved by a number of electro- or physico-chemical and immunological methods.

In the *Abbott Axsym* ion capture assay, murine anti-FBP immunoglobulin G (IgG) results in negatively charged polyanion–folate complexes. These are captured electrostatically using a positively charged glass fibre matrix (charge imparted by high molecular-weight quaternary ammonium compound) that removes the bound fraction. The *Beckman Access* uses murine anti-FBP goat antimouse IgG coated on paramagnetic particles. The *Siemens Immulite* platforms use murine anti-FBP coated on polystyrene beads with separation by centrifugation.

Signal Generation

Generation of electro-chemiluminescence, chemiluminescent, fluorescent or light emission is similar to that for B_{12} methods. In assays where the bound B_{12} complex is labelled with chemiluminescent esters, signal is generated in response to pH change or is electrically induced.

RED CELL FOLATE METHODS

Whereas *Lactobacillus casei* responds equally to both triglutamates and monoglutamates, the affinity of the FBP varies with the number of glutamate residues. Reproducible protein-binding assays for red cell folate can only be achieved by release and conversion of the protein-bound folate polyglutamates, mainly 5-methyl THF with four or five additional glutamate moieties, to a monoglutamate form. There must be adequate dilution of the red cells in hypotonic solution, a pH between 3.0 and 6.0 (ideally pH 4.5–5.2) for optimal conditions for plasma folate deconjugase (polyglutamate hydrolase) and ascorbic acid to stabilize the reduced forms.[63,64]

Haemolysate preparations for the newer assay platforms vary widely. The concentration of ascorbic acid varies from 0.09% to 1%, dilution factors from 1:5 to 1:31 and the duration of haemolysate preparation from 40 to 180 min. Some assays require the addition of protein to lysates before analysis and use bovine serum or human serum albumin, whereas others need only aqueous solutions. The pH of lysing diluent varies from 3.0 to 4.0 and that of the deconjugase step from 4.0 to 6.8 (the final pH of the lysate after protein addition varies from 4.4 to 7.5). These various factors may help to explain the large inter-method differences detected in external quality assessment surveys. Inadequate lysis and deconjugation will give falsely low results.[65,66]

If advice is not given by the manufacturer a suitable haemolysate method described below may be used. However, when the haemolysate is analysed using the serum folate methodology, this preparation method may not be suitable for all instruments.

Haemolysate Preparation

Red cell folate samples are usually collected in EDTA tubes and may be stored at 4°C for up to 48 h prior to lysate preparation. The lysate is prepared by adding 0.1 ml of whole blood of known haematocrit (Hct) to 1.9 ml of 1 g/dl freshly prepared aqueous ascorbic acid, incubated at room temperature for 60 min, in the dark. The ascorbic acid stabilizes the folate and the pH of 4.6 allows plasma folate deconjugase to convert the polyglutamate forms to the monoglutamate form. Folate activity should be assayed straight away although the lysate may be stored at 4°C for no more than 24 h prior to analysis. Storage at −20°C for longer periods is permissible, but approximately 10% decrease in activity is noted following a single freeze/thaw cycle. Whole blood in heparin, EDTA, or citrate–phosphate–dextrose (CPD) can be used in some, but not all, assays.

Calculation of Red Blood Cell Folate from Haemolysate Folate Result

1. Multiply the haemolysate folate value by the dilution factor (e.g. 21 if a 1:21 dilution) to obtain the folate concentration of whole blood in µg/l.

2. For an uncorrected red cell folate value in µg/l, divide the whole blood folate result in (1) by the Hct (l/l).

3. The result obtained in (2) should, if possible, be corrected for the serum folate value, which for patient populations taking supplemented dietary folate may now be quite significant, as is illustrated in the following worked example:

Corrected red cell folate (µg/l) =
Red cell folate in µg/l − [serum folate in µg/l × (1 − Hct)/Hct]
e.g. when Hct is 0.45, red cell folate is 180 µg/l and serum folate is 28 µg/l, then
Corrected red cell folate (µg/l) = 180 − [28 × (1 − 0.45)/0.45] = 145.8.

Many serum assays have an upper limit of 22–28 µg/l and the serum sample must therefore also be diluted and retested to obtain accurate results. Serum folate is traditionally quoted as µg/l or ng/ml; to convert to SI units (Système International d'unités); µg/l × 2.265 = nmol/l and nmol/l × 0.44 = µg/l.

Serum B$_{12}$ and Folate and Red Cell Folate Assay Calibration

Cobalamin in serum is protein bound and therefore standards for total B$_{12}$ assays should be gravimetrically prepared cyanocobalamin in either a lyophilized serum or protein adjusted matrix. A WHO lyophilized serum standard with consensus values for serum B$_{12}$ is available from the National Institute for Biological Standards and Control (NIBSC) (www.nibsc.ac.uk);[47] however, the protein binding B$_{12}$ assays are not usually calibrated with this material.

For serum folate analysis, 5-methyl THF is the physiologically active folate form and therefore should be used as the standard. However, 5-methyl THF is highly unstable and historically PGA has been used as the primary calibrator either gravimetrically added to aqueous standards or used to assign values to secondary serum matrix standards. The principle underlying the use of PGA is dependent on the equimolar binding of 5-methyl THF or PGA at pH 9.3.[62] More recent work suggests the pH of equimolar binding may be nearer 8.9 than 9.3.

The recent development of isotope dilution, liquid chromatography, tandem mass spectrometry (ID-LC/MS/MS) reference methods for folate derivatives in serum[43,44] has permitted the introduction of higher-order serum and plasma reference materials with accurate values for folates. A lyophilized serum standard (WHO 03/178)[47] is available from NIBSC and three frozen plasma preparations (FPP) with assigned values for 5-methyl THF and folic acid (FA) are available from the NIST in the USA (www.nist.gov/index.html).

Whole Blood Folate Standards

An international reference preparation for whole blood folates[48] is available from NIBSC although the haemolysate preparations are generally analysed using the serum method protocols and calibration curves.

Primary Instrument Calibration

The majority of manufacturers still use gravimetric PGA calibrators or PGA values assigned to serum matrix calibrators referenced to older RID methods as their primary instrument calibration. Siemens now utilizes 5-methyl THF as its instrument calibrator, although this is referenced to aqueous gravimetric factory standards. Methods calibrated in this way should be optimized for the detection of 5-methyl THF and should not require the adjustment of the binding pH to 9.3. Currently only one major manufacturer has opted to harmonize the calibration of its serum folate assay with the WHO 1st International Standard for Total Folate in Serum. Results from recent surveys of the UK NEQAS External Quality Assessment (EQA) Haematinics Scheme suggest that this method (Abbott) is now accurate when compared to values obtained by the ID-LC/MS/MS reference method (UKNEQAS Haematinics steering committee report October 2009).

Internal Adjustment Calibration

Most automated assay systems use calibration curves that are stored on barcode systems with each reagent lot. The barcode also contains the mathematical formulae for shifting or adjusting the observed responses to the master curve when the instrument requires routine calibration. The calibration interval within reagent lots usually varies from 7 to 28 days. Most instruments will also require at least a 2-point calibration when changing lot numbers of reagent packs, when replacing system components and when internal quality control results are out of range. Reagents should be discarded at the end of the stability intervals and should not be used beyond the expiry dates. Particular care should be taken to ensure that calibrators and reagents are correctly mixed and homogeneous, especially those containing particulates. Aliquots of reagents may be stored at 2–8°C or at –20°C if permitted by the manufacturer.

Internal Quality Control

As a minimum requirement, two levels of quality control material should be assayed daily when samples are being analysed. A choice of batch analysis, or true random access, may be preferred by the operator, although in view of folate instability prolonged on-board times are to be avoided by consideration of the test repertoire for a given set of samples. Suitable controls are available commercially (Bio-Rad Laboratories).

METHYLMALONIC ACID MEASUREMENT

Principle

Methylmalonic acid (MMA) is one of several dicarboxylic acids present in urine and plasma. Before separating MMA from other interfering substances it is necessary to obtain derivatives of these compounds. Urine concentration of MMA is higher than plasma concentration and needs to be normalized for urine creatinine concentration and corrected for the effects of renal impairment or dehydration.

Serum measurement offers added convenience, is unaffected by diet and can use the same sample as that obtained for B_{12}.

Methods

Plasma or serum MMA is extracted, purified and, using *tert*-butyldimethylsilyl derivatives of MMA, measured by GC-MS. A deuterated stable isotope of MMA is used as an internal standard. The use of dicyclohexyl, another derivative of MMA, is described by Rasmussen.[67]

A method for screening for inborn errors of metabolism using *O*-(2,3,4,5,6-pentafluorobenzyl) hydroxylamine HCl to derive oxoacids, followed by liquid partition chromatography, was described by Hoffman et al.[68] In more recent HPLC or capillary electrophoresis methods,[69,70] MMA can be derivatized using the fluorescent compound 1-pyrenyldiazomethane to yield a fluorescent monoester adduct. After separation by HPLC or capillary electrophoresis, short-chain dicarboxylic acids are quantified following laser-induced fluorescence activation.

Reference ranges for serum MMA measured by GC-MS and using mean $\pm$ 3SD of log transformed data are 53–376 nmol/l[71] and 50–440 nmol/l (Rasmussen et al.[72]).

HOMOCYSTEINE MEASUREMENT

Principle

Homocysteine is a disulphide amino acid present at low concentrations in cells (<1 µmol/l) and in plasma at 5–15 µmol/l.[73] Homocysteine has a reactive sulphydryl group that forms disulphide bonds with homocysteine or cysteine or protein sulphydryl groups to form the oxidized form of homocysteine: homocystine, homocysteine-cysteine mixed disulphide and protein-bound homocysteine. The free homocysteine is <2% of plasma homocysteine and 80% is as protein-bound homocysteine; the remainder is homocystine or mixed disulphides. Reducing conditions convert all these species to homocysteine by reduction of disulphides; therefore total homocysteine is measured.

For quantification, plasma homocysteine requires protein precipitation and reduction of disulphide bonds. The S-H group of homocysteine is derivatized using a thiol-specific reagent and the resulting adduct is detected. A variety of methods have evolved[73] from ion-exchange amino acid analysers,[74] radioenzymatic determination, capillary gas chromatography[75] stable isotope dilution combined with capillary GC-MS,[76] liquid chromatography electrospray tandem mass spectrometry[77] and HPLC methods using fluorochromophore detection.

HPLC methods that use fluorochromophore detection systems are still available but are not as widely used in clinical laboratories as previously. These methods first reduce the disulphide bonds followed by the removal of protein and the derivatization of the thiol groups. Separation requires reverse-phase HPLC and high organic mobile phase such as heptane sulphonic acid/methanol mobile phase at pH 1.9–2.0 for example. In the method from *Drew Scientific*, detection is by fluorescence of the fluorophore at λ_{ex} 385 nm and λ_{em} 515 nm.

Development of enzymatic and immunoassays for homocysteine has dramatically changed the availability of its measurement in routine laboratories. These are discussed further in the following section.

Immunoassay for Homocysteine Measurement

Automated enzyme immunoassays[78] for homocysteine have now been developed by a number of manufacturers and have reduced the dependence of clinical laboratories on highly specialized instrumentation such as gas chromatography, mass spectrometry and HPLC. The general principle of these methods is the release of protein-bound homocysteine by buffered DTT and the reduction of homocystine and mixed disulphides to homocysteine. The enzymatic conversion of free homocysteine to s-adenosyl-L-homocysteine (sAH) is then achieved with s-adenosyl homocysteine hydrolase in the presence of excess adenosine. Competitive reactions are used to quantify total homocysteine and methods are further sub-classified based on differences in the separation and detection of sAH. These include fluorescence polarization immunoassay (FPIA), chemiluminescent immunoassay (CIA), enzyme-linked immunosorbent assay (ELISA) and other enzyme immunoassays (EIA). More recently latex enhanced agglutination immunoassays have also been developed for homocysteine quantitation.

In the *Axis-Shield, Siemens Centaur* and *Siemens Immulite 2000/2500* (formerly *Diagnostic Products*) methods, synthetically derived sAH is bound to the separator system (coated wells, paramagnetic particles, or polystyrene beads). Labelled murine anti-sAH is added and in the presence of sample-derived sAH competes for binding to immobilized sAH. The concentration of labelled anti-sAH bound to the separation phase sAH is inversely proportional to the concentration of sAH derived from the original sample. An appropriate substrate and suitable conditions for colour, chemiluminescence, or fluorescence generation permit analyte quantitation.

The enzyme immunoassays methods utilize enzyme systems in the detection phase of the assay. For example, in the *Axis-Shield EIA* method a second rabbit anti-mouse antibody labelled with enzyme horseradish peroxidase is added to the bound fraction. Colour is generated by the addition of the substrate, tetramethylbenzidine and read at 450 nm.

Immunoturbidimetric assays, suitable for use on a coagulation analyser, have also been developed. One such method has been produced by *Instrumentation Laboratory* (IL). This assay converts all homocysteine forms enzymatically to sAH in the same way as described above. Plasma-derived sAH and a homocysteine conjugate with multiple binding sites compete for limited binding sites on microlatex particles coated with anti-SAH antibodies. The resultant agglutination is measured at 405 nm.

Other Enzyme Assays for Homocysteine

One of the more novel methods for homocysteine measurement is described by its manufacturer (*Diazyme Europe GmbH*) as an enzyme cycling system with amplification of the detection signal. The sample total homocysteine is converted to methionine and sAH by homocysteine-s-methyltransferase in the presence of s-adenosylmethionine (sAM). sAH is hydrolysed to adenosine and homocysteine which is cycled back into the conversion reaction. The adenosine formed is hydrolysed to inosine and ammonia that reacts with glutamate dehydrogenase in the presence of NADH. The conversion to NAD^+ is detected spectrophotometrically at 340 nm. The kit is transferable to a number of platforms, including the *Roche Diagnostics Hitachi, Siemens* (formerly Dade) *Vista Dimension* and the *Beckman Synchron CX, LX* and *DXC*.

Standardization of Homocysteine Methods

Although the exact process differs between techniques, the chromatographic methods are calibrated, using gravimetrically prepared standards of homocysteine and other closely related thiol compounds, as a ratio to a stable internal standard such as 2-mercaptoethylamine. The ratio of the sample signal to internal standard is used to quantify the unknown concentration. Where this is described in any detail, most immunoassays are standardized with synthetically derived sAH that may be dispersed in buffered aqueous solution or added in modified human serum. This means that the standard material is not subject to the release, reduction and enzymatic conversion of the endogenous homocysteine but has the advantage of stability. Some enzymatic methods employ gravimetrically prepared homocysteine.

Reference Methods for Homocysteine

There are three procedures quoted on the Joint Committee for Traceability in Laboratory Medicine (JCTLM) database as high-order reference procedures for homocysteine in human serum.[79,80] Methods include isotope dilution, gas chromatography, mass spectrometry (ID/GC/MS) and two methods based on isotope dilution, liquid chromatography, tandem mass spectrometry (ID/LC/MS/MS). These methods are used to assign homocysteine (and folate) values to frozen serum reference material (SRM 1955) produced by NIST in the USA. Lyophilized materials with values assigned by the reference procedures are not available yet.

Relative Performance of Homocysteine Methods

Proficiency testing shows that there are small but significant differences in the values produced by the enzymatic methods when compared with HPLC and immunoassays.[81-85] While the within-run precision is acceptable for all three types of technology the between-laboratory data reveals a greater imprecision in the HPLC method group.[85] When evaluated in the light of intra-individual variability in homocysteine levels, FPIA meets the performance goal suggested by Fraser and Petersen.[86]

Pre-analytical Variables in Homocysteine Testing

Plasma homocysteine is elevated in both B_{12} and folate deficiency and is elevated in individuals with a common genetic polymorphism of methylenetetrahydrofolate reductase, C677T polymorphism, the homozygous form of which is present in 10% of Western populations and results in homocysteine levels 25% above the normal upper limit. A raised homocysteine level is an independent risk factor for vascular disease, including myocardial infarction and stroke.[18] Homocysteine levels are affected by age, renal function, smoking, excessive coffee consumption and drugs, including levodopa. Correction of elevated homocysteine levels in patients with cobalamin or folate deficiency by administration of one or both vitamins provides proof of a deficiency state, which may be subclinical.

Factors affecting albumin levels will alter homocysteine because it is protein bound and venepuncture should not be performed after venous stasis or following the subject resting in supine position. Plasma is preferred because cells leak homocysteine, resulting in an increase of 10% during clot formation from uncoagulated samples. Even plasma will show an increase of 10% per hour at room temperature as a result of leakage from red cells.[87] Samples should be kept on ice and centrifuged as soon as possible, at least within 1 h.

DYNAMIC TESTING OF COBALAMIN FOLATE METABOLISM

Measurement of metabolite response at 1 week following cobalamin or folate treatment provides the opportunity to perform an *in vivo* dynamic function test of the cobalamin–folate metabolic pathways and confirm a diagnosis of tissue deficiency of one vitamin or the other.

Another dynamic functional test of cobalamin–folate metabolism, utilized primarily in research laboratories, is the deoxyuridine suppression test,[88] in which failure of suppression by deoxyuridine of tritiated thymidine ^{3}H-TdR incorporation into DNA in cobalamin or folate deficient is corrected by treatment with the appropriate haematinic. (The method was described in the 9th edition of this book.)

INVESTIGATION OF THE CAUSE OF COBALAMIN DEFICIENCY

Once cobalamin deficiency has been confirmed by the finding of an unequivocally low serum B_{12} result (with or without confirmatory raised metabolite levels and response to therapy), the aetiology of the low cobalamin should be elucidated as in Table 10.5. Gastric parietal cell antibodies are present in 90% of patients with pernicious anaemia, but this is of low specificity, being found in 15% of elderly subjects, and is therefore of little discriminatory use. Achlorhydria as a cause of cobalamin malabsorption may be suspected by the presence of raised gastrin levels.[89]

INTRINSIC FACTOR ANTIBODY MEASUREMENT

Principle

Two types of antibody to IF have been detected in the sera of patients with pernicious anaemia. Type I blocks the binding of B_{12} to IF, whereas type II prevents the attachment of IF or the IF–B_{12} complex to ileal receptors. Type II antibodies (precipitating antibodies) may be precipitated by IF–B_{12} complex and sodium sulphate at pH 8.3 in barbitone buffer. More than 60% of patients with pernicious anaemia are reported to have type I or type II antibodies.[90,91] Automated competitive binding assays are now available and have largely superseded radiodilution assays. A number of manufacturers are developing IF antibody assays for their multianalyte immunoassay platforms.

Assay methods have been reviewed[90] and one method for detection of types I and II IF antibody based on radiodilution competitive binding was described in the 9th edition of this book.

Intrinsic Factor Antibody Kits

Radioisotopic competitive binding assay kits that only detect blocking (type I) antibodies are being superseded by automated competitive binding assays for inclusion in the test repertoire of these multianalyte platforms. ELISA (enzyme-linked immunosorbent assay) kits that detect both type I and type II antibodies are available from a number of companies.

Principle of Binding Assay for Type I Intrinsic Factor Antibodies

Current methods for serum type I intrinsic factor antibodies (IFAb) are adaptations of the B_{12} competitive binding assays. Patient serum is incubated with an intrinsic factor alkaline phosphatase conjugate and intrinsic factor antibody in the patient sample binds to the intrinsic factor conjugate. Paramagnetic particles coated with murine monoclonal antibody specific for the vitamin B_{12} binding site on intrinsic factor are added to the reaction vessel and intrinsic factor conjugate that has not been blocked by sample intrinsic factor antibody binds to the mouse monoclonal antibody on the solid phase (paramagnetic particles). Separation is achieved by the application of a magnetic field to hold the particles and the excess unbound material (IF conjugate) is washed away. The chemiluminescent substrate is added to the reaction vessel and the light generated read at 530 nm in a luminometer.

This type of method is potentially subject to interference from free B_{12} in the patient's serum because it binds to the IF conjugate, which is then removed in the washing step. Under normal circumstances 99% of B_{12} in serum is bound but patients with high levels of circulating free B_{12} (>444 ng/l), as might be the case following treatment with intramuscular B_{12}, may record disproportionately elevated levels of intrinsic factor antibody.

ELISA Methods for Type I and Type II Intrinsic Factor Antibodies

Serum is incubated in the presence of IF bound to a solid phase in such a way that both the type I and type II binding sites are available for binding IFAb.[91] Excess unbound serum is removed and the solid phase is further incubated with conjugate-labelled (e.g. horseradish peroxidase) antihuman IgG. Unbound conjugate is removed and substrate is added to develop the signal, which is proportional to the amount of IFAb in the original serum. The specificity of the IF antibody assay will depend on the purity of the solid-phase IF. Purified porcine intrinsic factor or recombinant intrinsic factor are used in different ELISAs and the UK NEQAS intrinsic factor antibody quality control surveys have shown variable positive rates for different types of ELISA,[92] perhaps reflecting different sensitivities and specificity of patient sera.

Interpretation

International reference and calibration material for IFAb is not available and results of both types of method are expressed in arbitrary units or as a ratio of a cut-off deemed as positive by each manufacturer. As a consequence of the use of arbitrary units and the requirement to detect both antibodies concurrently, independent quality control material is not available.

INVESTIGATION OF ABSORPTION OF B_{12}

In patients who are B_{12} deficient and who are IFAb negative, it is important to establish whether the capacity to absorb the vitamin is normal. Absorption tests should be reserved for those individuals in whom low B_{12} levels result in genuine tissue deficiency, confirmed by supportive laboratory or clinical findings (e.g. macrocytosis, hypersegmented neutrophils, megaloblastic anaemia, neuropathy, neuropsychiatric features or elevation of cobalamin dependent metabolites) to avoid excessive investigation of 'falsely low or indeterminate' serum B_{12} levels.

The withdrawal of reagents for the traditional radiolabelled Schilling tests has hampered the full investigation of patients with cobalamin deficiency.

Development of Non-Isotopic B_{12} Absorption Tests Using Holotranscobalamin Levels and Recombinant Intrinsic Factor

Holotranscobalamin levels increase 3–4 h after oral cobalamin intake and, after 3 doses of 9 µg cyanocobalamin given 6-hourly on day 1, peak serum HoloTC was detected at 24 h in healthy adults maintained on a normal diet and given bread and juice to aid absorption of each cobalamin dose. Cellular uptake of HoloTC will be greater in deficient individuals and therefore the time course of a rise in HoloTC and the dose of cyanocobalamin may vary. Further work to optimize this approach to develop a standardized B_{12} absorption test is ongoing.[55-57] Bhat et al.[58] gave 10 μg of cyanocobalamin at 6-hourly intervals ×3 and defined a normal response as a rise in plasma HoloTC of >15% and >15 pmol above baseline measurement; the majority of Asian women studied corrected low holotranscobalamin levels, suggesting dietary deficiency as the cause.

Non-Isotopic B_{12} Absorption Test Utilizing Recombinant Intrinsic Factor in Combination with Holotranscobalamin Levels

Native (human) or bovine intrinsic factor is no longer commercially available. Hvas et al.[57] have therefore utilized recombinant intrinsic factor from 1 g of the plant leaves of transgenic *Arabidopsis thaliana* (Pharma Skan, Skanderborg, Denmark) to show enhanced cobalamin absorption and holotranscobalamin levels in subjects with B_{12} deficiency. Three patterns were observed: one group showed a large increase in HoloTC (mean rise 13 pmol/l) from baseline levels with cyanocobalamin, indicating dietary deficiency; clinically deficient individuals showed only a small rise (mean 5 pmol/l) in HoloTC after cyanocobalamin, which could be enhanced (>10 pmol by day 3) by addition of intrinsic factor, indicating a lack of intrinsic factor (e.g. gastrectomy or autoimmune pernicious anaemia); and a third group with no increase in HoloTC, with or without intrinsic factor, a finding consistent with malabsorption.

Urinary Excretion of Radiolabelled B_{12} With and Without Intrinsic Factor (Schilling Test)

Radiolabelled cyanocobalamin and bovine intrinsic factor reagents are no longer available. (Details of the principles of the Schilling tests can be found from the references[93,94] and in the 10th edition of this book.)

B_{12} BINDING CAPACITY OF SERUM OR PLASMA: TRANSCOBALAMIN MEASUREMENT

Principle

Transcobalamin I (TCI) binds 80% or more of the total serum B_{12} and the B_{12}-TCI complex is known as holohaptocorrin. TCII is the minor but important transport protein that delivers B_{12} to the tissues. The B_{12}-TCII complex is known as holotranscobalamin (HoloTC) and

6–25% of total serum B_{12} is carried in this complex. HoloTC is believed to be the first B_{12} metabolite that decreases on inadequate B_{12} absorption. TCII and III are normally virtually unsaturated unless an individual is undergoing B_{12} treatment. TCII and III should therefore be measured prior to B_{12} treatment. TCI and III (R binders) are glycosylated proteins differing in their sugar moiety. Chronic myeloid leukaemia, myelofibrosis and other myeloproliferative neoplasms are characterized by increased levels of TCI and therefore total serum B_{12}. Primary liver cancer (fibrolamellar hepatoma) is also associated with synthesis of large quantities of an abnormal form of TCI. It has been suggested that some low B_{12} levels without evidence of B_{12} deficiency may result from a decrease in R binder concentration.[95] Congenital absence of R binders TCI and III results in very low serum B_{12} but no evidence of B_{12} deficiency.[96] In congenital absence of TCII,[21,22] which results in fulminating pancytopenia and megaloblastosis within 2 months of birth, the serum B_{12} is normal, unsaturated B_{12} binding capacity is decreased as a result of absent TCII and B_{12} absorption is reduced; the deoxyuridine suppression test is abnormal and corrected by B_{12}.

UNSATURATED B_{12} BINDING CAPACITY AND TRANSCOBALAMIN IDENTIFICATION AND QUANTITATION

Measurement of unsaturated B_{12} binding capacity is rarely undertaken and is only available in reference laboratories. (Details of the method were given in the 9th edition of this book.) It is mainly of use for detection of transcobalamin I deficiency as a cause for very low serum B_{12} with no clinical features of cobalamin deficiency. It is also required for diagnosing the rare TCII deficiency. In addition, the assay has been used as a tumour marker for primary liver cancer.

Reference Ranges for Transcobalamins

The normal range[97] for serum unsaturated B_{12} binding capacity is 670–1200 ng/l; for plasma collected into EDTA-sodium fluoride it is 505–1208 ng/l,[98] for TCI, 49–132 ng/l, TCII, 402–930 ng/l and for TCIII, 80–280 ng/l.

ACKNOWLEDGEMENTS

The description of metabolic pathways for cobalamin, folate and homocysteine were assisted by *Hematology Basic Principles and Practice*[99] and *Homocysteine in Health and*

Disease.[100] We wish to thank Annie Lee, Julie Bonser, staff at UK NEQAS Haematinics Department of Haematology and Good Hope NHS Trust for collaboration on production of international reference standards and experimental work on folate and B[12] assays, Dr Christine Pfeiffer at Centers for Disease Control and Prevention (CDC) Atlanta for collaborative work on the international reference method for serum folate and inter-method comparisons and Dr Susan Thorpe at NIBSC for collaborative work on international reference standards. Thanks also to family, friends and colleagues for ever-present support and encouragement.

REFERENCES

1. Centers for Disease Control and Prevention. Available at: www.cdc.gov/ncbddd/B[12]/table4.html.

2. Fyle JC, Madsen M, Hojrup P, et al. The functional cobalamin (vitamin B[12])-intrinsic factor receptor is a novel complex of cubilin and amnionless. *Blood.* 2004;103:1573–1579.

3. Pearce J. Subacute combined degeneration of the cord. *Putnam–Dana Syndrome European Neurology.* 2008;60:53–56.

4. Birn H. The kidney in vitamin B[12] and folate homeostasis: characterization of receptors for tubular uptake of vitamins and carrier proteins. *Am J Physiol Renal Physiol.* 2006;291:F22–F36.

5. Waters AH, Mollin DL. Observations on the metabolism of folic acid in pernicious anaemia. *Br J Haematol.* 1963;9:319–327.

6. Jewsbury EC. Subacute combined degeneration of the cord and achlorhydric peripheral neuropathies without anaemia. *Lancet.* 1954;3:307–312.

7. Healton EH, Savage DG, Brust JCM, et al. Neurologic aspects of cobalamin deficiency. *Medicine.* 1991;70:229–245.

8. Lindenbaum J, Healton EB, Savage DG, et al. Neuropsychiatric disorders caused by cobalamin deficiency in the absence of anaemia or macrocytosis. *N Engl J Med.* 1988;318:1720–1728.

9. Smith D, Refsum H. Vitamin B[12] and cognition in the elderly. *Am J Clin Nutr.* 2009;89:707S–711S.

10. Rush D. Folate supplements prevent recurrence of neural tube defects. FDA Dietary Supplement Task Force. *Nutr Rev.* 1992;50:22–28.

11. Savage DG, Lindenbaum J, Stabler SP, et al. Sensitivity of serum methylmalonic acid and total homocysteine for diagnosing cobalamin and folate deficiencies. *Am J Med.* 1994;96:239–246.

12. Holleland G, Schneede J, Ueland PM, et al. Cobalamin deficiency in general practice. Assessment of the diagnostic utility and cost benefit analysis of methylmalonic acid determination in relation to current diagnostic strategies. *Clin Chem.* 1999;45:189–198.

13. Hvas AM, Nexo E. Diagnosis and treatment of vitamin B[12] deficiency – an update. *Haematologica.* 2006;91:1506–1512.

14. Klee G. Cobalamin and folate evaluation: Measurement of methylmalonic acid and homocysteine vs vitamin B[12] and folate. *Clin Chem.* 2000;46:1277–1283.

15. Solomon LR. Cobalamin responsive disorders in the ambulatory care setting: unreliability of cobalamin, methylmalonic acid and homocysteine testing. *Blood.* 2005;105:978–985.

16. Gorringe A, Ellis R, McDowell I, et al. The limited value of methylmalonic acid, homocysteine and holotranscobalamin in the diagnosis of early B[12] deficiency. *Haematologica.* 2006;91:231–234.

17. Nygard O, Vollset SE, Refsum H, et al. Total homocysteine and cardiovascular disease. *J Intern Med.* 1999;246:425–454.

18. Ridker PM, Hennekens CH, Selhub J, et al. Interrelation of hyperhomocystinaemia, factor V Leiden and risk of future venous thromboembolism. *Circulation.* 1997;95:1777–1782.

19. Smith AD, Kim Y, Refsum H. Is folic acid good for everyone? *Am J Clin Nutr.* 2008;87:517–533.

20. Ebbing M, Bonaa KH, Nygard O, et al. Cancer incidence and mortality after treatment with folic acid and vitamin B[12]. *J Am Med Assoc.* 2009;302:2119–2126.

21. Briddon A. Homocysteine in the context of cobalamin metabolism and deficiency states. *Amino Acids.* 2003;24:1–12.

22. Whitehead VM. Acquired and inherited disorders of cobalamin and folate in children. *Br J Haematol.* 2006;134:125–136.

23. Stabler SP, Allen RH, Savage DG, et al. Clinical spectrum and diagnosis of cobalamin deficiency. *Blood.* 1990;76:871–881.

24. Devalia V. Diagnosing vitamin B-12 deficiency on the basis of serum B-12 assay. *Br Med J.* 2006;333:385–386.

25. Hamilton MS, Blackmore S, Lee A. Possible cause of false normal B-12 assays. *Br Med J.* 2006;333:654–655.

26. Ulleland M, Eilertsen I, Quadros EV, et al. Direct assay for cobalamin bound to Transcobalamin (holotranscobalamin) in serum. *Clin Chem.* 2002;48:526–532.

27. Brady J, Wilson L, McGregor L, et al. Active B[12]: a rapid automated assay for holotranscobalamin on the Abbott AxSYM analyser. *Clin Chem.* 2008;54:567–573.

28. Clarke R, Sherliker P, Hin H, et al. Detection of vitamin B[12] deficiency in older people by measuring vitamin B[12] or the active fraction of vitamin B[12] holotranscobalamin. *Clin Chem.* 2007;53:963–970.

29. Herzlich B, Herbert V. Depletion of serum holotranscobalamin. II. An early sign of negative vitamin B[12] balance. *Lab Invest.* 1988;58:332–337.

30. Morkbak AL, Hvas AM, Milman N, et al. Holotranscobalamin remains unchanged during pregnancy. Longitudinal changes of cobalamins and their binding proteins during pregnancy and post partum. *Haematologica.* 2007;92:1711–1712.

31. Lindenbaum J, Nath BJ. Megaloblastic anaemia and neutrophil hypersegmentation. *Br J Haematol.* 1980;44:511–513.

32. Rose M, Johnson I. Reinterpretation of the haematological effects of anti-convulsant treatment. *Lancet.* 1978;1:1349–1350.

33. Shojania AM, Hornady GJ. Oral contraceptives: effect of folate and B_{12} metabolism. *Can Med Assoc J.* 1982;126:244–247.

34. Lassen HC, Henriksen A, Neukirch F, et al. Treatment of tetanus: severe bone marrow depression after prolonged nitrous oxide anaesthesia. *Lancet.* 1956; 270:527–530.

35. Jeffery J, Millar H, MacKenzie P, et al. An IgG complexed form of vitamin B_{12} is a common cause of elevated serum concentrations. *Clin Biochem.* 2010;43:82–88.

36. Hamilton MS, Blackmore S, Lee A, et al. Ability of holotranscobalamin assay (active B_{12}) to detect severe cobalamin deficiency evidenced by high methylmalonic acid in the presence of high titre intrinsic factor antibody and false normal B_{12} results. *Br J Haematol.* 2010;149 (supp 1):26: Abs 54.

37. Hoffbrand AV, Newcombe BF, Mollin DL. Method of assay of red cell folate activity and the value of the assay as a test for folate deficiency. *J Clin Pathol.* 1966;19:17–28.

38. Jaffe JP, Schilling RE. Erythrocyte folate levels: a clinical study. *Am J Hematol.* 1991;36:116–121.

39. Phekoo K, Williams Y, Schey SA, et al. Folate assays serum or red cell? *J R Coll Physicians Lond.* 1994;31: 291–295.

40. Lavoie A, Tripp E, Hoffbrand AV. The effect of vitamin B_{12} deficiency on methylfolate metabolism and pteroylpolyglutamate synthesis in human cells. *Clin Sci Mol Med.* 1974;47:617–630.

41. Perry J, Lumb M, Laundy M, et al. Role of vitamin B_{12} in folate coenzyme synthesis. *Br J Haematol.* 1976;32:243–248.

42. Blackmore S, Lee A, Hamilton MS. The impact of sample stabilization with sodium ascorbate on the analysis of serum folate in the UKNEQAS Haematinics surveys.

Clinica Chimica Acta. 2005;355 UKNP 1.3:S459.

43. Pfeiffer CM, Fazili Z, McCoy L, et al. Determination of folate vitamers in human serum by stable-isotope-dilution tandem mass spectrophotometry and comparison with radioassay and microbiologic assay. *Clin Chem.* 2004;50:423–432.

44. Nelson B, Pfeiffer CM, Margolis S, et al. Solid phase extraction-electrospray ionization mass spectrometry for the quantification of folate in human plasma or serum. *Anal Biochem.* 2004;325:41–51.

45. Selhub J, Jacques PF, Wilson PW, et al. Vitamin status and input as primary determinants of homocystinaemia in an elderly population. *J Am Med Assoc.* 1993;270:2693–2698.

46. Selhub J, Jacques PF, Rosenbery IH, et al. Serum total homocysteine concentrations in the third National Health and Nutrition Survey 1991–1994. Population reference ranges and contribution of vitamin status to high serum concentrations. *Ann Intern Med.* 1999;131:331–339.

47. Thorpe SJ, Heath A, Blackmore S, et al. International standard for serum B_{12} and serum folate: international collaborative study to evaluate a batch of lyophilised serum for B_{12} and folate content. *Clin Chem Lab Med.* 2007;45: 380–386.

48. Thorpe S, Sands D, Heath AB, et al. An international standard for whole blood folate: evaluation of a lyophilised haemolysate in an international collaborative study. *Clin Chem Lab Med.* 2004;42: 533–539.

49. Blackmore S, Pfeiffer C, Hamilton MS, et al. Recoveries of folate species from serum pools sent to participants of the UKNEQAS Haematinics scheme in February and March 2004. *Clinica Chimica Acta.* 2005;355 UKNP 1.2:S459.

50. Fazili Z, Pfieffer CM, Zhang M. Comparison of serum folate species analysed by LC-MS/MS with total folate measured by microbiologic assay and Bio-Rad radioassay. *Clin Chem.* 2007;53:781–784.

51. Curtis AD, Mussett MV, Kennedy DA. British Standard for

human serum vitamin B_{12}. *Clin Lab Haematol.* 1986;8:135–147.

52. Bagley PJ, Selhub J. A common mutation in the methylenetetrahydrofolate reductase gene is associated with an accumulation of formylated tetrahydrofolates in red blood cells. *Proc Natl Acad Sci U S A.* 1998;95: 13217–13220.

53. Jacques PF, Bostom AG, Williams RR, et al. Relation between folate status, a common mutation in methylenetetrahydrofolate reductase and plasma homocysteine concentrations. *Circulation.* 1996; 93:7–9.

54. O'Broin SD, Kelleher BP. Microbiological assay on microtitre plates of folate in serum and red cells. *J Clin Pathol.* 1992;45: 344–347.

55. Castel-Roberts KM, Morkbak AL, Nexo E, et al. Holotranscobalamin is an indicator of vitamin B_{12} absorption in healthy adults with adequate vitamin B_{12} status. *American Journal of Nutrition.* 2007;85:1057–1061.

56. Hvas AM, Morkbak AL, Nexo E. Plasma holotranscobalamin compared with plasma cobalamins for assessment of vitamin B_{12} absorption: optimization of a non radioactive vitamin B_{12} absorption test. *Clin Chim Acta.* 2007;376: 150–154.

57. Hvas AM, Buhl T, Laursen NB, et al. The effect of recombinant human intrinsic factor on the uptake of vitamin B_{12} in patients with evident vitamin B_{12} deficiency. *Haematologica.* 2006;91:805–807.

58. Bhat DS, Thuse NV, Lubree H, et al. Increases in plasma holotranscobalamin can be used to assess vitamin B_{12} absorption in individuals with low plasma vitamin B_{12}. *J Nutr.* 2009;139:2119–2123.

59. Ulleland M, Eilertsen I, Quadros EV, et al. Direct assay for cobalamin bound to transcobalamin (holotranscobalamin) in serum. *Clin Chem.* 2002;48:526–532.

60. Nexo E, Christensen A, Petersen TE, et al. Measurement of transcobalamin by ELISA. *Clin Chem.* 2000;46:1643–1649.

61. Nexo E, Christensen A, Hvas A, et al. Quantification of

holotranscobalamin, a marker of vitamin B_{12} deficiency. *Clin Chem.* 2002;48:561–562.

62. Givas J, Gutcho S. pH dependence of the binding of folate to milk binder in radioassay of folates. *Clin Chem.* 1975;21:427–428.

63. Bain BJ, Wickramasinghe SN, Broom GW, et al. Assessment of the value of a competitive protein binding radioassay of folic acid in the detection of folic acid deficiency. *J Clin Pathol.* 1984;37:888–894.

64. Omer A. Factors influencing the release of assayable folate from erythrocytes. *J Clin Pathol.* 1969;22:217–221.

65. Netteland B, Bakke OM. Inadequate sample preparation as a source of error in determination of erythrocyte folate by competitive binding radioassay. *Clin Chem.* 1977;23:1505–1506.

66. Shane B, Tamura T, Stokstad ELR. Folate assay: a comparison of radioassay and microbiological methods. *Clin Chim Acta.* 1980;100:13–19.

67. Rasmussen K. Solid phase sample extraction for rapid determination of methylmalonic acid in serum and urine by a stable isotope dilution method. *Clin Chem.* 1989;35:260–264.

68. Hoffmann G, Aramaki S, Blum-Hoffmann E, et al. Quantitative analysis for organic acids in biological sample: batch isolation followed by gas chromatographic-mass spectrometric analysis. *Clin Chem.* 1989;35:587–595.

69. Schneede J, Ulleland PM. An automated assay for methylmalonic acid in serum and urine based on derivatization with 1-pyrenyldiazomethane, liquid chromatography and fluorescence detection. *Clin Chem.* 1993;39:392–393.

70. Schneede J, Ulleland PM. Application of capillary electrophoresis with laser-induced fluorescence detection for routine determination of methylmalonic acid in human serum. *Anal Chem.* 1995;67:812–819.

71. Allen RH, Stabler SP, Savage DG, et al. Diagnosis of cobalamin deficiency. I. Usefulness of serum methylmalonic acid and total homocysteine concentrations. *Am J Hematol.* 1990;34:90–98.

72. Rasmussen K, Moller J, Ostergaard K, et al. Methylmalonic acid concentrations in serum of normal subjects: biological variability and effect of oral l-isoleucine loads before and after intramuscular administration of cobalamin. *Clin Chem.* 1990;36:1295–1299.

73. Ulleland PM, Refsum H, Stabler SP, et al. Total homocysteine in plasma or serum: methods and clinical applications. *Clin Chem.* 1993;39:1764–1779.

74. Rasmussen K, Moller J. Methodologies of testing. In: Carmel R, Jacobsen DW, eds. *Homocysteine in Health and Disease.* Cambridge: Cambridge University Press; 2001:9–20.

75. Kataoka H, Takagi K, Makita M. Determination of total plasma homocysteine and related aminothiols by gas chromatography with flame photometric detection. *J Chromatogr B Biomed Appl.* 1995;664:421–425.

76. Stabler SP, Marcell PD, Podell ER, et al. Quantitation of total homocysteine, total cysteine and methionine in normal serum and urine using capillary gas chromatography-mass spectrometry. *Anal Biochem.* 1987;162:185–196.

77. Magera MJ, Lacey JM, Casetta B, et al. Method for the determination of total homocysteine in plasma and urine by stable isotope dilution and electron spray tandem mass spectrometry. *Clin Chem.* 1999;41:1517–1522.

78. Shipchandler MT, Moore EG. Rapid fully automated measurement of plasma homocysteine with the Abbott Imx analyser. *Clin Chem.* 1995;41:991–994.

79. Satterfield MB, Sniegoski LT, Welch M, et al. Comparison of isotope dilution mass spectrometry methods for the determination of total homocysteine in plasma and serum. *Anal Chem.* 2003;75:4631–4638.

80. Satterfield MB, Sniegoski LT, Welch M, et al. Comparison of isotope dilution mass spectrometry methods for the determination of total homocysteine in plasma and serum. [Comparability assessment studies.] *Anal Chem.* 2003;75:775–784.

81. Pfeiffer CM, Twite D, Shih J, et al. Method comparison for total plasma homocysteine between the Abbott Imx analyser and an HPLC assay with internal standardization. *Clin Chem.* 1999;45:152–153.

82. Pfeiffer CM, Huff DL, Smith SJ, et al. Comparison of plasma total homocysteine measurements in 14 laboratories: an international study. *Clin Chem.* 45:1261–1288.

83. Nexo E, Engbaek F, Ueland PM, et al. Evaluation of novel assays in clinical chemistry: quantification of plasma total homocysteine. *Clin Chem.* 2000;46:1150–1156.

84. Huijgen HJ, Tegelaers FP, Schoenmakers CHH, et al. Multicentre analytical evaluation of an enzymatic method for the measurement of plasma homocysteine and comparison with HPLC and immunochemistry. *Clin Chem.* 2004;50:937–940.

85. Hanson NQ, Eckfeldt JH, Schwichtenberg K, et al. Interlaboratory variation of plasma total homocysteine measurements: results of three successive homocysteine proficiency testing surveys. *Clin Chem.* 2002;48:1539–1545.

86. Fraser CG, Petersen PH. Analytical performance characteristic should be judged against objective quality specifications. *Clin Chem.* 1999;45:321–323.

87. Andersson A, Isaksson A, Hultberg B. Homocysteine export from erythrocytes and its implications for plasma sampling. *Clin Chem.* 1992;38:1311–1315.

88. Wickramasinghe SN, Matthews JH. Deoxyuridine suppression: biochemical basis and diagnostic applications. *Blood Rev.* 1988;2:168–177.

89. Slingerland DW, Cararelli JA, Burrows BA, et al. The utility of serum gastrin levels in assessing the significance of low serum B_{12} levels. *Arch Intern Med.* 1984;144:1167–1168.

90. Shackleton PJ, Fish DI, Dawson DW. Intrinsic factor antibody tests. *J Clin Pathol*. 1989;42:210–212.

91. Waters HM, Smith C, Howarth JE, et al. A new enzyme immunoassay for the detection of total type I and type II intrinsic factor antibody. *J Clin Pathol*. 1989;42:307–312.

92. Lee A, Blackmore S, Hamilton MS. A new external quality assessment (EQA) scheme for intrinsic factor antibody (IFAb) assays: a key diagnostic criterion for pernicious anaemia. *Clinica Chimica Acta*. 2005;355 UKTP 4.42:S297.

93. Schilling RF. Intrinsic factor studies. II. The effect of gastric juice on the urinary excretion of radioactivity after the oral administration of radioactive vitamin B_{12}. *J Lab Clin Med*. 1953;42:860–866.

94. International Committee for Standardization in Haematology. Recommended method for the measurement of vitamin B_{12} absorption. *J Nucl Med*. 1981;22:1091–1093.

95. Carmel R. R-binder deficiency: a clinically benign cause of cobalamin deficiency. *J Am Med Assoc*. 1988;250:1886–1890.

96. Jacob E, Herbert V. Measurement of unsaturated 'granulocyte-related' (TCI and TCIII) and 'liver-related' (TCII) binders by instant batch separation using a microfine precipitate of silica (QUSO G32). *J Lab Clin Med*. 1975;88:505–512.

97. Nexo E, Christensen A, Hvas AB, et al. Quantification of holotranscobalamin, a marker of vitamin B_{12} deficiency. *Clin Chem*. 2002;48:561–562.

98. Scott JM, Bloomfield FJ, Stebbins R, et al. Studies on derivation of transcobalamin III from granulocytes: enhancement by lithium and elimination by fluoride of in vitro increments in vitamin B_{12}-binding capacity. *J Clin Invest*. 1974;53:228–239.

99. Hoffman R, Furie B, McGlave P, et al. *Hematology Basic Principles and Practice*, Ch. 39, 5th ed. London: Churchill Livingstone Elsevier; 2009.

100. Carmel R, Jacobsen DW. *Homocysteine in Health and Disease*. Cambridge: Cambridge University Press; 2001.

Chapter | **11** |

Laboratory methods used in the investigation of the haemolytic anaemias

David Roper

Red cells are typically removed from the circulation at the end of their lifespan of about 120 days. A shortened lifespan due to premature destruction may lead to haemolytic anemia when bone marrow activity cannot compensate for the erythrocyte loss. The causes can be divided into three groups:

1. Defects within red cells from dysfunction of enzyme-controlled metabolism, abnormal haemoglobins and thalassaemias
2. Loss of structural integrity of red cell membrane and cytoskeleton in hereditary spherocytosis, hereditary elliptocytosis, paroxysmal nocturnal haemoglobinuria (PNH) and immune and drug-associated antibody damage
3. Damage by outside factors such as mechanical trauma, microangiopathic conditions (including thrombotic thrombocytopenic purpura) and chemical toxins.

At the end of a normal lifespan, red cells are destroyed within the reticuloendothelial system in the spleen, liver and bone marrow. In some haemolytic anaemias, the haemolysis occurs predominantly in the reticuloendothelial system (extravascular) and the plasma haemoglobin concentration (Hb) is barely increased. In other disorders, a major degree of haemolysis takes place within the bloodstream (intravascular haemolysis), the plasma Hb increases substantially and in some cases, the amount of Hb so liberated may be sufficient to lead to Hb being excreted in the urine (haemoglobinuria). However, there is often a combination of both mechanisms. The two pathways by which Hb derived from effete red cells is metabolized are illustrated in Figure 11.1.

INVESTIGATION OF HAEMOLYTIC ANAEMIA

The cardinal signs of haemolysis in adults – anaemia, jaundice and reticulocytosis – may be mimicked by non-haemolytic conditions unique to the newborn. Because of changes associated with Hb F and Hb A concentrations as a result of the shift from γ- to β-globin production, differences in glycolytic enzyme activities and reduction

or absence of haptoglobins during the first month or so of life, it is essential to compare results with age-matched sample(s) or age-adjusted reference values.

The clinical and laboratory associations of increased haemolysis reflect the nature of the haemolytic mechanism, where the haemolysis is taking place and the response of the bone marrow to the anaemia resulting from the haemolysis, namely, erythroid hyperplasia and reticulocytosis.

The investigation of patients suspected of suffering from a haemolytic anaemia comprises several distinct stages: recognizing the existence of increased haemolysis; determining the type of haemolytic mechanism; and making the precise diagnosis. In practice, the procedures are often telescoped because the diagnosis in some instances may be obvious to the experienced observer from a glance down the microscope at the patient's blood film.

The following practical scheme of investigation is recommended. In each group, tests are listed in order of importance and practicability.

Is There Evidence of Increased Haemolysis?

1. Hb estimation; reticulocyte count; inspection of a stained blood film for the presence of spherocytes, elliptocytes, irregularly contracted cells, schistocytes or agglutination (see Chapters 3 and 5)

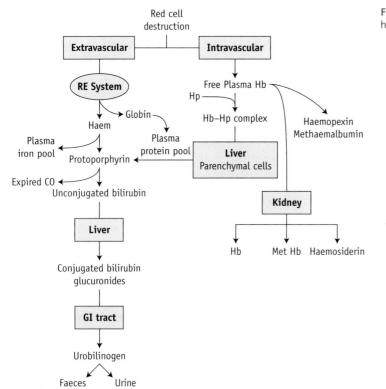

Figure 11.1 Catabolic pathway of haemoglobin.

2. Test for increased unconjugated serum bilirubin and urinary urobilinogen excretion; measurement of haptoglobin or haemopexin
3. Detection of urinary Hb or haemosiderin.

What is the Type of Haemolytic Mechanism?

1. Direct antiglobulin test (DAT) with broad-spectrum antiserum
2. Osmotic fragility and glycerol lysis test
3. Measurement of Hb in urine; plasma Hb; Schumm's test.

What is the Precise Diagnosis?

1. If a hereditary haemolytic anaemia is suspected:
   a. Osmotic-fragility determination after 24 h of incubation at 37°C or eosin-5-maleimide (EMA) dye binding test; screening test for red cell glucose-6-phosphate dehydrogenase (G6PD) deficiency (formal assay if reticulocytosis present); red cell pyruvate kinase assay; assay of other red cell enzymes involved in glycolysis; estimation of red cell glutathione (see Chapter 12).
   b. Estimation of % Hb A_2 and % Hb F; electrophoresis or high-performance liquid chromatography for abnormal Hb; tests for sickling; tests for unstable Hb; blood count parameters, especially mean cell volume (MCV) and mean cell Hb (MCH); gene analysis (see Chapter 8).
   c. Examination of the proteins of the red cell membrane and cytoskeleton (e.g. spectrin) by gel electrophoresis and by specific radioimmunoassay.
2. If an autoimmune acquired haemolytic anaemia is suspected:
   a. Direct antiglobulin test using anti-immunoglobulin and anti-complement sera; tests for autoantibodies in the patient's serum; titration of cold agglutinins; Donath–Landsteiner test; electrophoresis of serum proteins; demonstration of thermal range of autoantibodies; tests for agglutination and/or lysis of enzyme-treated cells by autoantibodies; tests for lysis of normal cells by autoantibodies.
3. If the haemolytic anaemia is suspected of being drug induced:
   a. Screening test for red cell G6PD; glutathione stability test; staining for Heinz bodies; identification of methaemoglobin (Hi) and sulphaemoglobin (SHb); tests for drug-dependent antibodies.
4. If mechanical stress is suspected:
   a. Red cell morphology; platelet count; renal function tests; coagulation screen; fibrinogen assay; test for fibrinogen/fibrin degradation products (see Chapters 5 and 18).
5. In obscure cases:
   a. Investigations for paroxysmal nocturnal haemoglobinuria (PNH) (e.g. acidified serum test [Ham's test], sucrose lysis test, flow cytometric immunophenotyping for erythrocyte and neutrophil antigens) (see Chapter 13).
   b. Measurement of lifespan of patient's red cells (see Chapter 17).
   c. If splenectomy is contemplated, determination of sites of haemolysis by radionuclide imaging (see Chapter 17).

PLASMA HAEMOGLOBIN

Methods for estimation of plasma Hb are based on (1) peroxidase reaction and (2) direct measurement of Hb by spectrometry. In the peroxidase method, the catalytic action of haem-containing proteins brings about the oxidation of tetramethylbenzidine* by hydrogen peroxide to give a green colour, which changes to blue and finally to reddish violet. The intensity of reaction may be compared using a spectrometer with that produced by solutions of known Hb. Hi and Hb are measured together.

A pink tinge to the plasma is detectable by eye when the Hb is higher than 200 mg/l. When the plasma Hb is >50 mg/l, it can be measured as haemiglobincyanide (HiCN) or oxyhaemoglobin by a spectrometer at 540 nm[1] (p. 26). Lower concentrations can also be measured reliably provided that the spectrometer plots of concentration/absorbance give a linear slope passing through the origin. This facility is provided by the Low Hb HemoCue (Hemocue Ltd, Dronfield, Derbyshire, UK), which can reliably measure plasma Hb at or higher than 100 mg/l.[2]

Sample Collection

Every effort must be made to prevent haemolysis during the collection and manipulation of the blood. For this, it may be preferable to use a syringe rather than an evacuated tube system. A clean venipuncture is essential; a plastic syringe and relatively wide-bore needle should be used. When the required amount of blood has been withdrawn, the needle should be detached with care and 9 volumes of blood should be added to 1 volume of 32 g/l sodium citrate.

---

*This is an analogue of benzidine that can be used with the standard safety precautions for handling any toxic chemicals; benzidine itself is a carcinogenic substance, the use of which is prohibited in many countries.

Peroxidase Method[3]

Reagents

Benzidine compound

Dissolve 1 g of 3,3',5,5'-tetramethylbenzidine in 90 ml of glacial acetic acid and make up to 100 ml with water. The solution will keep for several weeks in a dark bottle at 4°C.

Hydrogen peroxide

Dilute 1 volume of 3% ('10 vols') H_2O_2 with 2 volumes of water before use.

Acetic acid

Use 100 g/l glacial acetic acid.

Standard

A blood sample of known Hb content is diluted with water to a final concentration of 200 mg/l. It is convenient to use an HiCN standard solution as the source of Hb.

Method

Add 20 μl of plasma to 1 ml of the benzidine reagent in a large glass tube. At the same time, set up a control tube, in which 20 μl of water are substituted for the plasma and a standard tube, containing 20 μl of the Hb standard. Add 1 ml of the H_2O_2 solution to each tube and mix the contents well.

Allow the mixture to stand at about 20°C for 20 min and then add 10 ml of the acetic acid solution to each tube; after mixing, allow the tubes to stand for a further 10 min. Compare the coloured solutions at 600 nm, using the colour developed by the control tube as a blank. If the Hb of the plasma to be tested is unusually high, it can be measured by the method used with whole blood (described later).

Spectrophotometric Method

A normal EDTA anticoagulated blood sample should be washed three times in isotonic saline (0.15 mol/l). Lyse one volume of washed packed red cells in two volumes of water. Alternatively, lyse by freezing and thawing. Centrifuge the haemolysate at 3000 rpm (1200 g) for 30 min and transfer the clear solution to a clean tube. Adjust the haemoglobin concentration to 80 g/l.

Dilute 1:100 with phosphate buffer, pH 8, to obtain an Hb concentration of 800 mg/l. By six consecutive double dilutions with phosphate buffer, make a set of seven lysate standards with values from 800 to 12.5 mg/l.

Read the absorbance of each solution at 540 nm, with water as a blank. Prepare a calibration graph by plotting the readings of absorbance (on y axis) against Hb

concentration (on x axis) on arithmetic graph paper and draw the slope. Check that the slope is linear.

Read the absorbance of the plasma directly at 540 nm with a water blank and read the Hb concentration from the calibration graph. If absorbance is greater than the maximum value plotted on the graph, repeat the reading with a sample diluted with buffer.

When using the Low Hb HemoCue haemoglobinometer, fill the special cuvette with plasma and carry out the test in accordance with the instructions that are provided.

Normal Range

The normal range is 10–40 mg/l.

Significance of increased plasma haemoglobin

Hb liberated from the intravascular or extravascular breakdown of red cells interacts with the plasma haptoglobins to form an Hb–haptoglobin complex,[4] which, because of its size, does not undergo glomerular filtration, but it is removed from the circulation by and is degraded in, reticuloendothelial cells. Hb in excess of the capacity of the haptoglobins to bind it passes into the glomerular filtrate; it is then partly excreted in the urine in an uncomplexed form, resulting in haemoglobinuria, and partly reabsorbed by the proximal glomerular tubules where it is broken down into haem, iron and globin. The iron is retained in the cells and eventually excreted in the urine (as haemosiderin). The haem and globin are reabsorbed into the plasma.

The haem complexes with albumin forming methaemalbumin and with haemopexin (p. 235); the globin competes with Hb to form a complex with haptoglobin. In effect, the plasma Hb level is further increased in haemolytic anaemias when haemolysis is sufficiently severe for the available haptoglobin to be fully bound. The highest levels are found when haemolysis takes place predominantly in the bloodstream (intravascular haemolysis). Thus, marked haemoglobinaemia, with or without haemoglobinuria, may be found in PNH, paroxysmal cold haemoglobinuria, cold-haemagglutinin syndromes, blackwater fever, march haemoglobinuria and other mechanical haemolytic anaemias (e.g. that after cardiac surgery). In warm-type autoimmune haemolytic anaemias, sickle cell anaemia and severe β thalassaemia, the plasma Hb level may be slightly or moderately increased, but in hereditary spherocytosis, in which haemolysis occurs predominantly in the spleen, the levels are normal or only very slightly increased.

Haem within the proximal tubular epithelium undergoes further degradation to bilirubin with liberation of iron, some of which is retained intracellularly incorporated into ferritin and haemosiderin. When haemolysis is severe, the excess of Hb that occurs in the glomerular filtrate will lead to an accumulation of intracellular haemosiderin in the glomerular tubular cells; when these cells slough, haemosiderin will appear in the urine (p. 236).

The presence of excess Hb in the plasma is a reliable sign of intravascular haemolysis only if the observer can be sure that the lysis has not been caused during or after the withdrawal of the blood. It is also necessary to exclude colouring of the plasma from certain foods and food additives.

Increased levels may occur as a result of violent exercise, as well as occurring in runners and joggers as a result of mechanical trauma caused by continuous impact of the soles of the feet with hard ground.[4]

SERUM HAPTOGLOBIN

Haptoglobin is a glycoprotein that is synthesized in the liver. It consists of two pairs of α chains and two pairs of β chains. With haemolysis, free Hb readily dissociates into dimers of α and β chains; the α chains bind avidly with the β chains of haptoglobin in plasma or serum to form a complex that can be differentiated from free Hb by column chromatographic separation or by its altered rate of migration in the α_2 position on electrophoresis.

Direct measurement of haptoglobin is also possible by turbidimetry or nephelometry and by radial immunodiffusion.[5] The methods described below are cellulose acetate electrophoresis and radial immunodiffusion.

Electrophoresis Method[6,7]

Principle

Known amounts of Hb are added to serum. The Hb–haptoglobin complex is separated by electrophoresis on cellulose acetate; the presence of bound and free Hb is identified in each sample and the amount of haptoglobin is estimated by noting where free Hb appears.

Reagents

Buffer (pH 7.0, ionic strength 0.05)

$Na_2HPO_4.H_2O$ 7.1 g/l, 2 volumes; $NaH_2PO_4.H_2O$ 6.9 g/l, 1 volume. Store at 4°C.

Haemolysates

A normal EDTA anticoagulated blood sample should be washed three times in isotonic saline (0.15 mol/l). Lyse one volume of washed packed red cells in three volumes of water. Alternatively, lyse by freezing and thawing. Centrifuge the haemolysate at 3000 rpm (1200 g) for 30 min and transfer the clear solution to a clean tube. Adjust the Hb to 30 g/l with water and dilute this preparation further with water to obtain a batch of solutions with Hb concentrations of 2.5, 5, 10, 20 and 30 g/l. These solutions are stable at 4°C for several weeks.

Stain

Dissolve 0.5 g of *o*-dianisidine (3,3′-dimethoxybenzidine) in 70 ml of 95% ethanol; prior to use, add together 10 ml of acetate buffer, pH 4.7 (sodium acetate 2.92 g, glacial acetic acid 1 ml, water to 1 litre), 2.5 ml of 3% (10 volumes) H_2O_2 and water to 100 ml.

Clearing solution

Glacial acetic acid 25 ml, 95% ethanol 75 ml.

Acetic acid rinse

Glacial acetic acid 50 ml/l.

Method

Serum is obtained from blood allowed to clot undisturbed at 37°C. As soon as the clot starts to retract, remove the serum with a pipette and centrifuge it to rid it of suspended red cells. The serum may be stored at –20°C until used.

Mix well 1 volume of each of the diluted haemolysates with 9 volumes of serum. Allow to stand for 10 min at room temperature.

Impregnate cellulose acetate membrane filter strips (12 × 2.5 cm) in buffer solution and blot to remove all obvious surface fluid. Apply 0.75 ml samples of the serum–haemolysate mixtures across the strips as thin transverse lines. As controls, include strips with serum alone and Hb lysate alone. Electrophorese at 0.5 mA/cm width. Good separation patterns about 5–7 cm in length should be obtained in 30 min (see Fig. 11.2).

After electrophoresis is completed, immerse the membranes in freshly prepared *o*-dianisidine stain for 10 min. Then rinse with water and immerse in 50 ml/l acetic acid for 5 min. Remove the membranes and place in 95% ethanol for exactly 1 min. Transfer the membranes to a tray containing freshly prepared clearing solution and immerse for exactly 30 s. While they are still in the solution, position the membranes over a glass plate placed in the tray. Remove the glass plate with the membranes on it, drain the excess solution from the membranes, transfer the glass plate to a ventilated oven preheated to 100°C and allow the membranes to dry for 10 min.

Interpretation

The patterns of free Hb and Hb–haptoglobin complex migration are shown in Figure 11.2. Hb–haptoglobin complex appears in the α_2 globulin position. When there is more Hb than can be bound to the haptoglobin, the free Hb migrates in the β globulin position. The amount of haptoglobin present in the serum is determined semi-quantitatively as between the lowest concentration of Hb, which shows only a free Hb band, and the adjacent strip, which shows a band of Hb–haptoglobin complex. In the total absence of haptoglobin, an Hb band alone will be seen even at 2.5 g/l. In severe intravascular haemolysis

A α₁ α₂ β

Figure 11.2 Demonstration of serum haptoglobin. (A) Serum from case of haemolytic anaemia with no haptoglobin: the added haemoglobin is demonstrated as a band in the β-globulin position. (B) Normal serum with added haemoglobin: there are bands in the β-globulin (Hb) and α_2-globulin (Hb–haptoglobin complex) positions, respectively. The line of origin is indicated by the arrow. The pattern of serum electrophoresis is shown below (A, albumin; α_1, α_2 and β, components of globulin).

with depleted haptoglobin, some of the haem may bind in the β-globulin position to haemopexin (see below) and some to serum albumin to form methaemalbumin.

The concentration of haptoglobin can be determined quantitatively with a densitometer. The test is carried out as described earlier, but only one haemolysate is required with an Hb of 30–40 g/l. After the plate has cooled, the membranes are scanned by a densitometer at 450 nm with a 0.3-mm slit width. The density of the haptoglobin band is calculated as a fraction of the total Hb in the electrophoretic strip:

$$\text{Haptoglobin (g/l)} = \text{Haptoglobin fraction} \times \text{Hb (g/l)}$$

Radial Immunodiffusion (RID) Method

Principle

The test serum samples and reference samples of known haptoglobin concentration are dispensed into wells in a plate of agarose gel containing a monospecific antiserum to human haptoglobin. Precipitation rings form by the reaction of haptoglobin with the antibody; the diameter of each ring is proportional to the concentration of haptoglobin in the sample.

Reagents

Phosphate buffer, iso-osmotic, pH 7.4:

(A) $NaH_2PO_4.2H_2O$ (150 mmol/l) – 23.4 g/l
(B) NaH_2PO_4 (150 mmol/l) – 21.3 g/l.

Add 18 ml reagent A to 82 ml reagent B.

Single diffusion plates*

Dissolve agarose (20 g/l) in boiling phosphate buffered water, pH 7.4. Allow to cool to 50°C. Add 5% sheep or goat antihuman haptoglobin antiserum diluted in buffered water, pH 7.4. Mix well but without creating bubbles. Pour the gel onto thin plastic trays (plates) to a thickness of <1 mm. After the gel has set, cut out a series of wells about 2 mm in diameter, about 2 cm apart. Extract the core by using a pipette tip with a negative pressure pump. Cover the plates with fitted lids and store in sealed packets at 4°C until used.

Reference sera

Preparations of human serum with stated haptoglobin concentration are available commercially. They should be stored at 4°C.

Test serum

Test serum can be kept at 4°C for 2–3 days, but if it is not used within this time, store at –20°C. Thaw completely and mix well immediately before use.

Method

Allow the plate (in its sealed packet) and the sera to equilibrate at room temperature for 15 min. Remove the lid from the plate. Check for moisture; if present, allow to evaporate. Add 5 µl of each serum into one of the wells in the plate. Stand for about 10 min to ensure that the serum is completely absorbed into the gel. Then cover the plate, return it to its container and reseal the packet. Leave on a level surface at room temperature for 18 h. From measurements of the reference sera, construct a reference curve on log-linear graph paper by plotting haptoglobin concentration on the vertical axis (logarithmic scale) and the diameter of the rings on the horizontal scale (linear scale). Measure the diameter of the precipitation ring formed by the test serum and express concentration in g/l (Fig. 11.3).

Normal Ranges

By direct measurement[5] results are expressed as haptoglobin concentration; slightly different normal reference values have been reported for the different methods:

RID: 0.8–2.7 g/l
Nephelometry: 0.3–2.2 g/l
Turbidimetry: 0.5–1.6 g/l.

When measured as Hb-binding capacity, in normal sera haptoglobins will bind 0.3–2.0 g/l of Hb. With this wide range of values there are no obvious sex differences, but in both men and women levels increase after the age of 70 years.

---

*Gel plates containing the antiserum are available commercially (e.g. The Binding Site Group Ltd, PO Box 11712, Birmingham, B14 4ZB, UK).

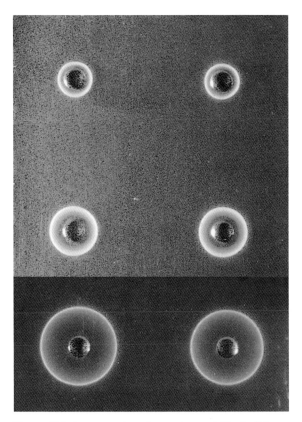

Figure 11.3 Demonstration of serum haptoglobin. Radial immunodiffusion: (top) low; (middle) normal; and (bottom) increased concentrations.

Significance

Haptoglobins begin to be depleted when the daily Hb turnover exceeds about twice the normal rate.[6] This occurs irrespective of whether the haemolysis is predominantly extravascular or intravascular; but rapid depletion, often with the formation of methaemalbumin, occurs as a result of small degrees of intravascular haemolysis, even when the daily total Hb turnover is not increased appreciably above normal. Low concentrations of haptoglobins, in the absence of increased haemolysis, may be found in hepatocellular disease and are characteristic of congenital anhaptoglobinaemia, which is uncommon except in populations of African origin.[8] Low concentrations may also be found in megaloblastic anaemias, probably because of increased haemolysis and following haemorrhage into tissues.

The haptoglobin–Hb complex is cleared by the reticuloendothelial system, mainly in the liver. The rate of removal is influenced by the concentration of free Hb in the plasma: at levels below 10 g/l, the clearance $T_{1/2}$ is 20 min; at higher concentrations, clearance is considerably slower.

Increased haptoglobin concentrations may be found in pregnancy, chronic infections, malignancy, tissue damage, Hodgkin's lymphoma, rheumatoid arthritis, systemic lupus erythematosus and biliary obstruction and as a consequence of steroid therapy or the use of oral contraceptives. Under these circumstances, a normal haptoglobin concentration does not exclude haemolysis.

SERUM HAEMOPEXIN

Haemopexin is a β_1 glycoprotein of molecular weight 70 000, synthesized in the liver. It has a transport function. Haem derived from Hb, which fails to bind to haptoglobin, complexes with either haemopexin or albumin. The former has a much higher affinity and only when all the haemopexin has been used up will the haem combine with albumin to form methaemalbumin. The haem–haemopexin complex is eliminated from the circulation (e.g. by the liver Kupffer cells) over a period of several hours, depleting the haemopexin.

Haem binds in a 1:1 molar ratio to haemopexin; 6 µg/ml of free haem is required to deplete the normal binding levels of haemopexin. In normal adults of both sexes, its concentration is 0.5–1.15 g/l (by nephelometry) or 0.5–1.5 g/l (by electrophoresis);[5] there is less in newborn infants, about 0.3 g/l, but adult levels are reached by the end of the first year of life. In severe intravascular haemolysis, when haptoglobin is depleted, haemopexin is low or absent and plasma methaemalbumin is elevated. With less severe haemolysis, although haptoglobin is likely to be reduced or absent, haemopexin may be normal or only slightly lowered. Haemopexin seems to be disproportionately low in thalassaemia major and low levels may be found in certain pathological conditions other than haemolytic disease: namely, renal and liver diseases. The concentration is increased in diabetes mellitus, infections and carcinoma.[9]

Haemopexin can be measured by the same methods as for haptoglobin with radial immunodiffusion or electrophoresis.[10]

EXAMINATION OF PLASMA (OR SERUM) FOR METHAEMALBUMIN

A simple but not very sensitive method is to examine the plasma using a hand spectroscope.

Free the plasma from suspended cells and platelets by centrifuging at 1200–1500 g for 15–30 min. Then view it in bright daylight with a hand spectroscope using the greatest possible depth of plasma consistent with visibility. Methaemalbumin gives a rather weak band in the red (at 624 nm) (Fig. 11.4). Because HbO_2 is usually present as well, its characteristic bands in the yellow–green may also be visible. The position of the methaemalbumin

Figure 11.4 Visible light spectrum showing wavelengths of the colours of the spectrum. This ranges from 380 to 780 nm. Fraunhofer lines should be seen at approximately 431 nm, 486 nm, 518 nm, 527 nm, 589 nm, 656 nm and 687 nm.

absorption band in the red can be readily differentiated from that of Hi by means of a reversion spectroscope.

Presumptive evidence of the presence of small quantities of methaemalbumin, giving an absorption band too weak to recognize, can be obtained by extracting the pigment by ether and then converting it to an ammonium haemochromogen, which gives a more intense band in the green (Schumm's test).

Schumm's Test

Method

Cover the plasma (or serum) with a layer of ether. Add a one-tenth volume of saturated yellow ammonium sulphide and mix it with the plasma. Then view it with a hand spectroscope. If methaemalbumin is present, a relatively intense narrow absorption band at 558 nm will be seen in the green.

Significance of Methaemalbuminaemia

Methaemalbumin is found in the plasma when haptoglobins are absent in haemolytic anaemias in which lysis is predominantly intravascular. It is a haem–albumin compound formed subsequent to the degradation of Hb liberated into plasma. It remains in the circulation for several days or until the haem is transferred from albumin to the more highly avid haemopexin.

Quantitative Estimation by Spectrometry

To 2 ml of plasma (or serum) add 1 ml of iso-osmotic phosphate buffer, pH 7.4. Centrifuge the mixture for 30 min at 1200–1500 g and measure its absorbance in a spectrophotometer at 569 nm. Add about 5 mg of solid sodium dithionite to the diluted plasma. Shake the tube gently to dissolve the dithionite and leave for 5 min to allow complete reduction of the methaemalbumin. Remeasure the absorbance. The difference between the two readings represents the absorbance due to methaemalbumin; its concentration can be read from a calibration graph.

Calibration Graph

Prepare solutions containing 10–100 mg/l methaemalbumin by dissolving appropriate amounts of haemin (bovine or equine) in a minimum volume of 40 g/l human serum albumin. Measure the absorbance of each solution in a spectrophotometer at 569 nm and draw a graph from the figures obtained.

DEMONSTRATION OF HAEMOSIDERIN IN URINE

Method

Centrifuge 10 ml of urine at 1200 g for 10–15 min. Transfer the deposit to a slide, spread out to occupy an area of 1–2 cm and allow to dry in the air. Fix by placing the slide in methanol for 10–20 min and then stain by the method used to stain bone marrow films for haemosiderin (p. 334). Haemosiderin, if present, appears in the form of isolated or grouped blue-staining granules, usually from 1 to 3 μm in size (Fig. 11.5); they may be both intracellular and extracellular. If haemosiderin is present in small amounts and especially if distributed irregularly on the slide or if the findings are difficult to interpret, the test should be repeated on a fresh sample of urine collected into an iron-free container and centrifuged in an iron-free tube. (For the preparation of iron-free glassware: wash thoroughly in a detergent solution, then soak in 3 mol/l HCl for 24 h; finally, rinse in deionized, double-distilled water.)

Significance of Haemosiderinuria

Haemosiderinuria is a sequel to the presence of Hb in the glomerular filtrate. It is a valuable sign of intravascular haemolysis because the urine will be found to contain iron-containing granules even if there is no haemoglobinuria

Figure 11.5 Photomicrograph of urine deposit stained by Perls' reaction.

at the time. However, haemosiderinuria is not found in the urine at the onset of a haemolytic attack even if this is accompanied by haemoglobinaemia and haemoglobinuria because the Hb has first to be absorbed by the cells of the renal tubules. The intracellular breakdown of Hb liberates iron, which is then re-excreted. Haemosiderinuria may persist for several weeks after a haemolytic episode.

CHEMICAL TESTS OF HAEMOGLOBIN CATABOLISM

Measurement of serum or plasma bilirubin, urinary urobilin and faecal urobilinogen can provide important information in the investigation of haemolytic anaemias. In this section, their interpretation and significance in haemolytic anaemias will be described, but because currently the tests are seldom performed in a haematology laboratory, for details of the techniques readers are referred to textbooks of clinical chemistry.[5]

Serum Bilirubin

Bilirubin is present in serum in two forms: as unconjugated prehepatic bilirubin and bilirubin conjugated to glucuronic acid. Normally, the serum bilirubin concentration is <17 µmol/l (10 mg/l) and mostly unconjugated. As illustrated in Figure 11.1, when there is increased red cell destruction, the protoporphyrin gives rise to an increased amount of unconjugated bilirubin and carbon monoxide. The bilirubin is then conjugated in the liver and this bilirubin glucuronide is excreted into the intestinal tract. Bacterial action converts bilirubin glucuronide to urobilin and urobilinogen. In haemolytic anaemias, the serum bilirubin usually lies between 17 and 50 µmol/l (10–30 mg/l) and most is unconjugated. Sometimes the level may be normal, despite a considerable increase in haemolysis. Levels >85 µmol/l (50 µg/l) and/or a large proportion of conjugated bilirubin suggest liver disease or post-hepatic obstruction. In haemolytic disease of the newborn (HDN), the bilirubin level is an important factor in determining whether an exchange transfusion should be carried out because high values of unconjugated bilirubin are toxic to the brain at this age and can lead to kernicterus. In normal newborn infants, the level often reaches 85 µmol/l, whereas in infants with HDN levels of 350 µmol/l are not uncommon and need to be urgently reduced by exchange transfusion. Moderately raised serum bilirubin levels are frequently found in dyshaemopoietic anaemias (e.g. pernicious anaemia), where there is ineffective erythropoiesis. Although part of the bilirubin comes from red cells that have circulated, a major proportion is derived from red cell precursors in the bone marrow that have failed to complete maturation.

Total bilirubin can be measured by direct reading spectrophotometry at 454 (or 461) and 540 nm; the former are the selected wavelengths for bilirubin, whereas the latter automatically corrects for any interference by free Hb. The instrument can be calibrated with bilirubin solutions of known concentration or with a coloured glass standard. Another direct reading method is by reflectance photometry on a drop of serum that is added to a reagent film.

An alternative 'wet chemistry' method is by the reaction with aqueous diazotized sulphanilic acid. A red colour is produced, which is compared in a photoelectric colorimeter with that of a freshly prepared standard or read in a spectrophotometer at 600 nm. Only conjugated bilirubin reacts directly with this aqueous reagent; unconjugated bilirubin, which is bound to albumin, requires either the addition of ethanol to free it from albumin or an accelerator such as methanol or caffeine to enable it to react. A positive urine spot test indicates a condition in which there is an elevated serum conjugated bilirubin. There is also a simple optical method, the Lovibond Comparator (Tintometer Ltd., Salisbury, UK), in which the colour produced by reaction with sulphanilic acid is matched against graded colour scales.

Bilirubin is destroyed by exposure to direct sunlight or any other source of ultraviolet (UV) light, including fluorescent lighting. Solutions are stable for 1–2 days if kept at 4°C in the dark.

Urobilin and Urobilinogen

Urobilin and its reduced form urobilinogen are formed by bacterial action on bile pigments in the intestine. The excretion of faecal urobilinogen in health is 50–500 µmol (30–300 mg) per day. It is increased in patients with a haemolytic anaemia. Quantitative measurement of faecal urobilinogen should, in theory, provide an estimate of the total rate of bilirubin production. This is, however, a crude method of assessing rates of haemolysis and minor degrees are more reliably demonstrated by red cell lifespan studies. Urobilinogen excretion is also increased in dyshaemopoietic anaemias such as pernicious anaemia because of ineffective erythropoiesis.

The amount of urobilinogen in the urine in health is up to 6.7 µmol (4 mg) per day. However, these measurements are method dependent and laboratories should establish their own normal reference values. This is not a reliable index of haemolysis, as excessive urobilinuria can be a consequence of liver dysfunction as well as of increased red cell destruction.

For estimation in the faeces, the bile-derived pigments (stercobilin) are reduced to urobilinogen, which is extracted with water. The solution is then treated with Ehrlich's dimethylaminobenzaldehyde reagent to produce a pink colour, which can be compared with either a natural or an artificial standard in a quantitative assay.

Qualitative Test for Urobilinogen and Urobilin in Urine

Schlesinger's Zinc Test

To 5 ml of urine, add 2 drops of 0.5 mol/l iodine to convert urobilinogen to urobilin. After mixing the sample and then leaving it standing on the bench for 1–2 min, add 5 ml of a 100 g/l suspension of zinc acetate in ethanol and centrifuge the mixture. A green fluorescence becomes apparent in the clear supernatant if urobilin or urobilinogen is present. If a spectroscope is available, the fluid may be examined for the broad absorption band (caused by urobilin) at the green–blue junction (Fig. 11.4). Urobilinogen can also be detected in freshly voided urine by commercially available reagent strip methods.

PORPHYRINS

Haem synthesis is initiated by succinyl coenzyme A and glycine, activated by the rate-limiting enzyme δ-aminolaevulinic (ALA)-synthase. ALA is the precursor of the porphyrins (Fig. 11.6). The porphyrins of clinical importance in man are protoporphyrin, uroporphyrin and coproporphyrin together with their precursor ALA. Protoporphyrin is widely distributed in the body and, in addition to its main role as a precursor of haem in Hb and myoglobin, it is a precursor of cytochromes and catalase. Uroporphyrin and coproporphyrin, which are precursors of protoporphyrin, are normally excreted in small amounts in urine and faeces. Red cells normally contain a small amount of coproporphyrin (5–35 nmol/l) and protoporphyrin (0.2–0.9 μmol/l). Deranged haem synthesis (e.g. in sideroblastic anaemias or lead toxicity) and iron deficiency anaemia result in an increased concentration of protoporphyrin in the red cells.

Appropriate tests are usually performed in clinical chemistry laboratories, including sophisticated methods for measuring red cell porphyrins, as described in an Association of Clinical Pathology Best Practice document.[11] Simple qualitative screening tests for urinary porphobilinogen and urinary porphyrin are described later. Urinary porphobilinogen will help to diagnose the acute forms of porphyria, particularly when the patient is symptomatic and this test can lead to a definite diagnosis in a critical clinical situation.

Demonstration of Porphobilinogen in Urine

Principle

Ehrlich's dimethylaminobenzaldehyde reagent reacts with porphobilinogen to produce a pink aldehyde compound, which can be differentiated from that produced by urobilinogen by the fact that the porphobilinogen compound is insoluble in chloroform.

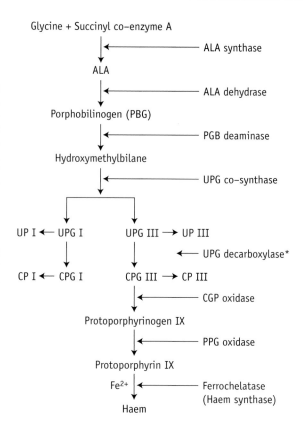

acts on both isomer I and isomer III

Figure 11.6 Biosynthesis of porphyrin. (See Table 11.1 for explanation of abbreviations.)

Ehrlich's Reagent

Dissolve 0.7 g of *p*-dimethylaminobenzaldehyde in a mixture of 150 ml of 10 mol/l HCl and 100 ml of water.

Method

Specimens must be protected from light and the test is best carried out on freshly passed urine. Mix a few ml of urine and an equal volume of Ehrlich's reagent in a large test tube. Add 2 volumes of a saturated solution of sodium acetate. The urine should then have a pH of about 5.0, giving a red reaction with Congo red indicator paper.

If a pink colour develops in the solution, add a few ml of chloroform and shake the mixture thoroughly to extract the pigment. The colour due to urobilinogen or indole will be extracted by the chloroform, whereas that owing to porphobilinogen will not and remains in the supernatant aqueous fraction. A kit is available for a semiquantitative test using anion-exchange resin (Microgenics, Thermo Fisher Scientific, UK). When present, the concentration of porphobilinogen in the urine may be measured quantitatively by a test kit method (Bio-Rad Laboratories UK Ltd, Hemel Hempstead, UK) or by spectrophotometry at 555 nm.

Aminolaevulinic Acid

When ALA is present in the urine, it can be concentrated with acetyl acetone. It then reacts with Ehrlich's reagent in the same way as porphobilinogen to give a red solution with an absorbance maximum at 553 nm. It can be separated from porphobilinogen by ion-exchange resins and estimated quantitatively by a spectrometric method.

Demonstration of Porphyrins in Urine

Principle

Porphyrins exhibit pink-red fluorescence when viewed by UV light (at 405 nm). Uroporphyrin can be distinguished from coproporphyrin by the different solubilities of the two substances in acid solution.

Method

Mix 25 ml of urine with 10 ml of glacial acetic acid in a separating funnel and extract twice with 50 ml volumes of ether. Set the aqueous fraction (Fraction 1) aside. Wash the ether extracts in a separating funnel with 10 ml of 1.6 mol/l HCl and collect the HCl fraction (Fraction 2). View both fractions in UV light (at 405 nm) for pink-red fluorescence. Its presence in Fraction 1 indicates uroporphyrin; its presence in Fraction 2 indicates coproporphyrin. The presence of the porphyrins should be confirmed spectroscopically (described later).

If uroporphyrin has been demonstrated, the reaction can be intensified by the following procedure. Adjust the pH of Fraction 1 to 3.0–3.2 with 0.1 mol/l HCl and extract the fraction twice with 50 ml volumes of ethyl acetate. Combine the extracts and extract three times with 2 ml volumes of 3 mol/l HCl. View the acid extracts for pink-red fluorescence in UV light and spectroscopically for acid porphyrin bands.

Spectroscopic Examination of Urine for Porphyrins

Spectroscopic examination of urine for porphyrins is carried out on extracts, made as described earlier, or on urine that is acidified with a few drops of 10 mol/l HCl. If porphyrins are present, a narrow band will appear in the orange at 596 nm and a broader band will appear in the green at 552 nm (see Fig. 11.4). Qualitative tests are adequate for screening purposes. Accurate determinations require spectrophotometry or chromatography. Porphyrins

are stable in ethylenediaminetetra-acetic acid (EDTA) blood for up to 8 days at room temperature if protected from light. Urine should be collected in a brown bottle or, if in a clear container, kept in a light-proof bag. If the urine is rendered alkaline to pH 7–7.5 with sodium bicarbonate, porphyrins will not be lost for several days at room temperature.

Significance of Porphyrins in Blood and Urine

Normal red cells contain <650 nmol/l of protoporphyrin and <64 nmol/l of coproporphyrin.[11] Increased amounts are present during the first few months of life. At all ages, there is an increase in red cell protoporphyrin in iron deficiency anaemia or latent iron deficiency, lead poisoning, thalassaemia, some cases of sideroblastic anaemia and the anaemia of chronic disease. Zinc protoporphyrin is also elevated in these conditions (p. 192).

Normally, a small amount of coproporphyrin is excreted in the urine (<430 nmol/day). This is demonstrable by the qualitative test described earlier, the intensity of pink-red fluorescence being proportional to the concentration of coproporphyrin. The excretion of coproporphyrin is increased when erythropoiesis is hyperactive (e.g. in haemolytic anaemias and polycythaemia), in pernicious anaemia and in sideroblastic anaemias. It is high in liver disease; renal impairment results in diminished excretion. In lead poisoning, there is an increase in red cell protoporphyrin and coproporphyrin, with excretion of exceptionally high levels of urinary ALA, coproporphyrin III and uroporphyrin I.

Normally, porphobilinogen cannot be demonstrated in urine and only traces of uroporphyrin (<50 nmol/day), not detectable by the qualitative test described earlier, are present.[11] ALA excretion is normally <40 mmol/day; it is increased in lead poisoning.

The increase in urinary coproporphyrin excretion occurring in the previously mentioned conditions is known as porphyrinuria. There is no increase in uroporphyrin excretion. The porphyrias, however, are a group of disorders associated with abnormal porphyrin metabolism.

There are several forms of porphyria, caused by specific enzyme defects, each with a different clinical effect and pattern of excretion of porphyrin and precursors[12] (Table 11.1). The most common type is acute intermittent porphyria, in which the defect in the enzyme porphobilinogen deaminase presents in one of three ways:

Type 1: Decreased enzyme activity together with reduced amount of the enzyme in the red cells
Type 2: Decreased enzyme activity in lymphocytes and liver cells but normal red cell activity
Type 3: Reduced red cell enzyme activity but normal amount of enzyme in the red cells.

The different mutations of the porphobilinogen deaminase in the three types can be identified by DNA hybridization

Table 11.1 Distribution of porphyrins in red cells, urine and faeces in different forms of porphyria

DISEASE	CLINICAL EFFECT	ENZYME DEFECT[a]	RED CELLS	URINE	FAECES
ALA dehydratase deficiency porphyria	(a)	ALA dehydratase (porphobilinogen synthase)	ZnP ALA	CPIII	–
Acute intermittent porphyria	(a)	PBG deaminase	–	PBG ALA	–
Congenital erythropoietic porphyria	(b)	UPG III cosynthase	UP I C PI ZnP	UP I CP I	UP I CP I
Acquired cutaneous hepatic porphyria (symptomatic)	(b)	UPG decarboxylase	–	UP I CP III	–
Hereditary coproporphyria	(a), (b)	CPG oxidase	–	CP III	CP III
Variegate porphyria (South African genetic)	(a), (b)	PPG oxidase	–	PBG[b] ALA[b]	CP III PP
Erythropoietic protoporphyria	(b)	Ferrochelatase	PP	–	PP

[a]See Figure 11.6.
[b]Mainly during acute attacks.
(a) Gastrointestinal and/or nervous system disorders.
(b) Photosensitive dermatitis.
ALA, α-aminolaevulinic acid; PBG, porphobilinogen; UP, uroporphyrin; CP, coproporphyrin; PP, protoporphyrin; UPG, uroporphyrinogen; CPG, coproporphyrinogen; PPG, protoporphyrinogen; ZnP, zinc protoporphyrin.

using specific oligonucleotides.[13] Other acute forms are variegate porphyria and coproporphyria.

The most common hepatic type is *porphyria cutanea tarda*, which results in photosensitivity, dermatitis and often hepatic siderosis; it is the result of a defect in uroporphyrinogen decarboxylase. In this and other porphyrias associated with photosensitive dermatitis (Table 11.1) plasma porphyrins are elevated. There are two erythropoietic types: *congenital erythropoietic porphyria*, caused by defective uroporphyrinogen cosynthase and *erythropoietic protoporphyria*, caused by defective ferrochelatase. In the former, uroporphyrin and coproporphyrin are present in red cells and urine in increased amounts; in the latter, increased protoporphyrin is found in the red cells, but the urine is normal. In erythropoietic porphyria, haemolytic anaemia may occur.

ABNORMAL HAEMOGLOBIN PIGMENTS

Methaemoglobin (Hi; also called MetHb), sulphaemoglobin (SHb) and carboxyhaemoglobin (HbCO) are of clinical importance and each has a characteristic absorption spectrum demonstrable by simple spectroscopy or, more definitely, by spectrometry. If the absorbance of a dilute solution of blood (e.g. 1 in 200) is measured at wavelengths between 400 and 700 nm, characteristic absorption spectra are obtained[14–16] (Fig. 11.7 and Table 11.2). In practice, the abnormal substance represents usually only a fraction of the total Hb (except in carbon monoxide poisoning) and its identification and accurate measurement may be difficult. Hi can be measured more accurately than SHb.

Absorption spectroscopy is a method by which a substance can be characterized by the wavelengths at which the colour spectrum is absorbed when light is passed through a solution of the substance. The specific absorption bands are identifiable by their positions (Fig. 11.4).

Spectroscopic Examination of Blood for Methaemoglobin and Sulphaemoglobin

Method

Dilute blood 1 in 5 or 1 in 10 with water and then centrifuge. Examine the clear solution, if possible in daylight, using a hand spectroscope. It is important that the greatest possible depth or concentration of solution consistent with visibility should be examined and that a careful search should be made (with varying depths or concentrations of solution)

Figure 11.7 Absorption spectra of various haemoglobin pigments. HbCO, carboxyhaemoglobin; HbO$_2$, oxyhaemoglobin; SHb, sulphaemoglobin; Hi, methaemoglobin.

Table 11.2 Positions in spectrum for optimal absorbance of haemoglobin derivatives in absorption spectrometry (in nm)

Oxyhaemoglobin	542, 577
Deoxygenated haemoglobin	431, 556
Carboxyhaemoglobin	538, 568
Methaemoglobin	500, 630
Sulphaemoglobin	620
Methaemalbumin	624
Haemochromogen (Schumm's test)	558

Some approximations where slightly different figures have been reported in different studies.

for absorption bands in the red part of the spectrum at 620–630 nm. If bands are seen in the red, add a drop of yellow ammonium sulphide to the solution. A band caused by Hi, but not that caused by SHb, will disappear. For comparison, lysed blood may be treated with a few drops of potassium ferricyanide (50 g/l) solution, which will cause the formation of Hi; SHb may be prepared by adding to 10 ml of a 1 in 100 dilution of blood, 0.1 ml of a 1 g/l solution of phenylhydrazine hydrochloride and a drop of water that has been previously saturated with hydrogen sulphide.

The spectra of the unknown and the known pigments may then be compared in a reversion spectroscope. The absorption band in the red caused by Hi is at 630 nm (compare with methaemalbumin at 624 nm) (Fig. 11.4).

Hi and SHb are formed intracellularly; they are not found in plasma except under very exceptional circumstances (e.g. when their formation is associated with intravascular haemolysis).

Measurement of Methaemoglobin

Principle

Hi has a maximum absorption at 630 nm. When cyanide is added, this absorption band disappears and the resulting change in absorbance is directly proportional to the concentration of Hi. Total Hb in the sample is then measured after complete conversion to HiCN by the addition of ferricyanide-cyanide reagent. The conversion will measure oxyhaemoglobin and Hi but not SHb. Thus, the presence of a large amount of SHb will result in an erroneously low measurement of total Hb. Turbidity of the haemolysate can be overcome by the addition of a non-ionic detergent.[14,15]

Reagents

Phosphate buffer: 0.1 mol/l, pH 6.8:
    (A) Weigh out 7.45 g of Na$_2$HPO$_4$, dissolve in distilled water and adjust final volume to 500 ml.
    (B) Weigh out 6.8 g of KH$_2$PO$_4$, dissolve in distilled water and adjust final volume to 500 ml.
    Add 2 volumes of solution (A) to 1 volume of solution (B).
Potassium cyanide: 50 g/l
Potassium ferricyanide: 50 g/l
Non-ionic detergent: 10 ml/l (Triton X-100* or Nonidet P40†)

Method

Lyse 0.2 ml of blood in a solution containing 4 ml of buffer and 6 ml of detergent solution. Divide the lysate into two equal volumes (A and B). Measure the absorbance of A in a spectrophotometer at 630 nm (D_1). Add 1 drop of potassium cyanide solution and measure the absorbance again, after mixing (D_2). Add 1 drop of potassium ferricyanide solution to B, and after 5 min, measure the absorbance at the same wavelength (D_3). Then add 1 drop of potassium cyanide solution to B and after mixing make a final reading (D_4). All the measurements are made against a blank containing buffer and detergent in the same proportion as present in the sample.

---

*Sigma-Aldrich.
†VWR International.

Calculation

$$\text{Hi}\,(\%) = \frac{D_1 - D_2}{D_3 - D_4} \times 100$$

The test should be carried out within 1 h of collecting the blood. After dilution, the buffered lysate can be stored for up to 24 h at 2–4°C without significant autooxidation of Hb to Hi.

Screening Method for Sulphaemoglobin

Principle

An absorbance reading at 620 nm measures the sum of the absorbance of oxyhaemoglobin and SHb in any blood sample. In contrast to oxyhaemoglobin, the absorption band caused by SHb is unchanged by the addition of cyanide. The residual absorbance, as read at 620 nm, is therefore proportional to the concentration of SHb. The absorbance of the oxyhaemoglobin alone at 620 nm can only be inferred from a reading at 578 nm and a conversion factor, A^{578}/A^{620}, has to be determined experimentally for each instrument on a series of normal blood samples.[16,17] The absorbance of SHb is obtained by subtracting the absorbance of the oxyhaemoglobin from that of the total Hb. This provides an approximation only, but it may be regarded as adequate for clinical purposes in the absence of a more reliable method.

Method

Mix 0.1 ml of blood with 10 ml of a 20 ml/l solution of a non-ionic detergent (Triton X-100 or Nonidet P40; see footnote p. 241). Record the absorbance (A) at 620 nm (total Hb). Add 1 drop of 50 g/l potassium cyanide, and after letting it stand for 5 min, record A at 620 nm and at 578 nm.

Calculation

$$\text{SHb}\,(\%) = \frac{2 \times A^{620}\text{SHb}}{A^{620}\text{HbO}_2}$$

$$\text{where } A^{620}\text{HbO}_2 = \frac{\text{Absorbance read at 578 nm}}{\text{Conversion factor}}$$

$$\text{and } A^{620}\text{SHb} = A^{620}\text{total Hb} - A^{620}\text{HbO}_2$$

Significance of methaemoglobin and sulphaemoglobin in blood

Hi is present in small amounts in normal blood and constitutes 1–2% of the total Hb. Its concentration is very slightly higher in infants, especially in premature infants, than in older children and adults. An excessive amount of Hi occurs as the result of oxidation of Hb by drugs and chemicals such as phenacetin, sulphonamides, aniline dyes, nitrates and nitrites.

The Hi produced by drugs is chemically normal and the pigment can be reconverted to oxyhaemoglobin by reducing agents such as methylene blue.

Other (rare) types of methaemoglobinaemia are caused by inherited deficiency of the enzyme NADH-Hi reductase and by inherited Hb abnormalities (types of Hb M). The absorption spectra of the Hb Ms differ from that of normal Hi and they react slowly and incompletely with cyanide; their concentration cannot be estimated by the method of Evelyn and Malloy.[14] Methaemoglobinaemia leads to cyanosis which becomes obvious with as little as 15 g/l of Hi: that is, about 10%.

SHb is usually formed at the same time as methaemoglobin; it represents a further and irreversible stage in Hb degradation. It is present as a rule at a much lower concentration than is Hi.

Demonstration of Carboxyhaemoglobin

Principle

Oxyhaemoglobin, but not HbCO, is reduced by sodium dithionite and the percentage of HbCO in a mixture can be determined by reference to a calibration graph.

Calibration Graph

Dilute 0.1 ml of normal blood in 20 ml of 0.4 ml/l ammonia and divide into two parts. To each add 20 mg of sodium dithionite. Then bubble pure carbon monoxide into one for 2 min, so as to provide a 100% solution of HbCO.

Add various volumes of the HbCO solution to the reduced Hb solution to provide a range of concentrations of HbCO. Within 10 min of adding the dithionite, measure the absorbance of each solution at 538 nm and 578 nm. Plot the quotient A^{538}/A^{578} on arithmetic graph paper against the % HbCO in each solution.

Method

Dilute 0.1 ml of blood in 20 ml of 0.4 ml/l ammonia and add 20 mg of sodium dithionite. Measure the absorbance in a spectrophotometer at 538 nm and 578 nm within 10 min. Calculate the quotient A^{538}/A^{578} and read the % HbCO in the blood from the calibration curve[16] or calculate it from the equation.[16,17]

$$\%\text{HbCO} = \frac{\{2.44 \times A^{538}\}}{A^{578}} - 2.68$$

Significance of carboxyhaemoglobin in circulating blood

Carbon monoxide has an affinity for Hb $c200$ times that of oxygen. This means that even low concentrations of carbon monoxide rapidly lead to the formation of HbCO. Less than 1% of HbCO is present in normal blood and up to 10% in smokers.[17,18] There is also an increased production and excretion in the lungs, in haemolytic anaemias. A high concentration in blood from inhalation of the gas causes tissue anoxia and may lead to death. However, recovery can take place because HbCO dissociates in time in the presence of high concentrations of oxygen.

Identification of Myoglobin in Urine

Myoglobin is the principal protein in muscle and it may be released into the circulation when there is cardiac or skeletal muscle damage. Some may be excreted in the urine where its concentration can be measured by a specific and relatively sensitive radioimmunoassay.[19] Because the absorption spectra of myoglobin and Hb are similar, although not identical, it is not possible to distinguish them readily by spectroscopy or spectrometry, but they can be separated by column chromatography.[20] Normally, men have <80 µg/l and women have <60 µg/l, increasing slightly in old age, whereas children have very low values.[5]

REFERENCES

1. Moore GL, Ledford ME, Merydith A. A micromodification of the Drabkin hemoglobin assay for measuring plasma hemoglobin in the range of 5 to 2000mg/dl. *Biochem Med.* 1981;26:167–173.

2. Morris LD, Pont A, Lewis SM. Use of a new HemoCue system for measuring haemoglobin at low concentrations. *Clin Lab Haematol.* 2001;23:91–96.

3. Standefer JC, Vanderjogt D. Use of tetramethyl benzidine in plasma hemoglobin assay. *Clin Chem.* 1977;23:749–751.

4. Davidson RJL. March or exertional haemoglobinuria. *Semin Hematol.* 1969;6:150–161.

5. Burtis CA, Ashwood ER. *NW Tietz's Fundamentals of Clinical Chemistry.* 5th ed. Philadelphia: Saunders; 2000.

6. Brus I, Lewis SM. The haptoglobin content of serum in haemolytic anaemia. *Br J Haematol.* 1959;5: 348–355.

7. Valeri CR, Bond JC, Flower K, et al. Quantitation of serum hemoglobin-binding capacity using cellulose acetate membrane electrophoresis. *Clin Chem.* 1965;11:581–588.

8. Teye K, Quaye IK, Koda Y, et al. A-61C and C-101G Hp gene promoter polymorphisms are, respectively, associated with ahaptoglobinaemia and hypohaptoglobinaemia in Ghana. *Clin Genet.* 2003;64: 439–443.

9. Hanstein A, Muller-Eberhard U. Concentration of serum hemopexin in healthy children and adults and in those with a variety of hematological disorders. *J Lab Clin Med.* 1968;71: 232–239.

10. Heide K, Haupt H, Störiko K, et al. On the heme-binding capacity of hemopexin. *Clin Chim Acta.* 1964;10: 460–469.

11. Deacon AC, Elder GH. Frontline tests for the investigation of suspected porphyria: ACP Best Practice No. 165. *J Clin Pathol.* 2001;54:500–507.

12. Bottomley SS, Muller-Eberhard U. Pathophysiology of heme synthesis. *Semin Hematol.* 1988;25:282–302.

13. Sassa S. Diagnosis and therapy of acute intermittent porphyria. *Blood Rev.* 1996;10:53–55.

14. Van Kampen EJ, Zijlstra WG. Determination of hemoglobin and its derivates. *Adv Clin Chem.* 1965;8: 141–187.

15. Zijlstra WG, Buursma A, van Assendelft OW. *Visible and near infrared absorption spectra of human and animal haemoglobin: determination and applications.* Zeist, Netherlands: VSP; 2003.

16. Zwart A, van Kampen EJ, Zijlstra WG. Results of routine determination of clinically significant hemoglobin derivatives by multicomponent analysis. *Clin Chem.* 1986;32: 972–978.

17. Shields CE. Elevated carbon monoxide level from smoking in blood donors. *Transfusion (Phil).* 1971;11:89–93.

18. Russell MAH, Wilson C, Cole PV, et al. Comparison of increases in carboxyhaemoglobin after smoking 'extra mild' and 'non mild' cigarettes. *Lancet.* 1973;ii:687–690.

19. Stone MJ, Willerson JT, Waterman MR. Radioimmunoassay of myoglobin. *Methods Enzymol.* 1982;84:172–177.

20. Cameron BF, Azzam SA, Kotite L, et al. Determination of myoglobin and hemoglobin. *J Lab Clin Med.* 1965;65:883–890.

Chapter | 12 |

Investigation of the hereditary haemolytic anaemias: membrane and enzyme abnormalities

David Roper, Mark Layton

The various initial steps to be taken in the investigation of a patient suspected of having a haemolytic anaemia are outlined in Chapter 11 and the changes in red cell morphology that may be found in haemolytic anaemias are illustrated in Chapter 5. This chapter describes procedures useful in investigating haemolytic anaemias suspected to result from defects within the red cell membrane or deficiency of enzymes important in red cell metabolism.

The precise identification of an enzyme defect is beyond the scope of most haematology laboratories; it may require the isolation and purification of the enzyme and the determination of its kinetic and structural properties. In a service laboratory, it is sufficient to identify the general nature of the defect, whether it be in the membrane or the metabolic pathways of the red cell. In the case of putative metabolic defects, an attempt should be made, where possible, to pinpoint the enzyme involved. The first part of this chapter describes screening tests for spherocytosis, including hereditary spherocytosis (HS) and for glucose-6-phosphate dehydrogenase (G6PD) deficiency. The later sections of the chapter describe specific enzyme assays and the measurement of 2,3-diphosphoglycerate (2,3-DPG) and reduced glutathione (GSH).

Most of the enzyme assays have been standardized by the International Council for Standardization in Haematology (ICSH). Commercial kits are also available for some quantitative assays and screening tests. These are noted in the relevant sections.

INVESTIGATION OF MEMBRANE DEFECTS

The osmotic fragility test gives an indication of the surface area/volume ratio of erythrocytes. Its greatest usefulness is in the diagnosis of hereditary spherocytosis. The test may also be used in screening for thalassaemia. Red cells that are spherocytic, for whatever cause, take up less water in a hypotonic solution before rupturing than do normal red cells.

Other tests that demonstrate red cell membrane defects include glycerol lysis time, cryohaemolysis, autohaemolysis and, more specifically, membrane protein analysis.

Procedures to assess red cell flexibility (rigidity) using polycarbonate membrane filtration,[1] and red cell deformability measurements on specialized equipment such as the Laser-assisted Optical Rotational Cell Analyser (LORCA)[2] have been described elsewhere.

OSMOTIC FRAGILITY AS MEASURED BY LYSIS IN HYPOTONIC SALINE

Principle

The method to be described is based on that of Parpart et al.[3] Small volumes of blood are mixed with a large excess of buffered saline solutions of varying concentration. The fraction of red cells lysed at each saline concentration is determined colorimetrically. The test is normally carried out at room temperature (15–25°C).

Reagents

Prepare a stock solution of buffered sodium chloride, osmotically equivalent to 100 g/l (1.71 mol/l) NaCl, as follows: dissolve NaCl, 90 g; Na_2HPO_4, 13.65 g (or $Na_2H-PO_42H_2O$, 17.115 g); and $NaH_2PO_4.2H_2O$, 2.34 g in water. Adjust the final volume to 1 litre. This solution will keep for months at 4°C in a well-stoppered bottle. Salt crystals may form on storage and must be thoroughly redissolved before use.

In preparing hypotonic solutions for use, it is convenient to make first a 10 g/l solution from the 100 g/l NaCl stock solution by dilution with water. Dilutions equivalent to 9.0, 7.5, 6.5, 6.0, 5.5, 5.0, 4.0, 3.5, 3.0, 2.0 and 1.0 g/l are convenient concentrations. Intermediate concentrations such as 4.75 and 5.25 g/l are useful in critical work and an additional 12.0 g/l dilution should be used for incubated samples.

It is convenient to make up 50 ml of each dilution. The solutions keep well at 4°C if sterile, but should be inspected for moulds before use and discarded if moulds develop.

Method

Heparinized venous blood or defibrinated blood may be used; oxalated or citrated blood is not suitable because of the additional salts added to it. The test should be carried out within 2 h of collection with blood stored at room temperature or within 6 h if the blood has been kept at 4°C.

1. Deliver 5.0 ml of each of the 11 saline solutions into 12 × 75 mm test tubes. Add 5.0 ml of water to the 12th tube.
2. Add to each tube 50 μl of well-mixed blood and mix immediately by inverting the tubes several times, avoiding foam.
3. Leave the suspensions for 30 min at room temperature. Mix again and then centrifuge for 5 min at 1200 *g*.
4. Remove the supernatants and estimate the amount of lysis in each using a spectrometer at a wavelength setting of 540 nm or a photoelectric colorimeter provided with a yellow-green (e.g. Ilford 625) filter. Use as a blank the supernatant from tube 1 (osmotically equivalent to 9 g/l NaCl).
5. Assign a value of 100% lysis to the reading with the supernatant of tube 12 (water) and express the readings from the other tubes as a percentage of the value of tube 12. Plot the results against the NaCl concentration (Fig. 12.1).

Notes

1. The measurement of osmotic fragility is a simple procedure that requires a minimum of equipment. It will yield gratifying results if carried out carefully.
2. The blood must be delivered into the 12 tubes with great care. The critical point is not that the amount be exactly 50 μl, but rather that the amount added to each tube must be the same. Two methods are recommended:
   a. Using an automatic pipette, after aspirating the blood gently, wipe the outside with tissue paper, taking care not to suck out any blood from the inside of the tip by capillary action. The blood is then delivered into the saline solution and the pipette is rinsed in and out several times until no blood is visible inside its tip.

Figure 12.1 Osmotic fragility curves. Osmotic fragility curves of patients suffering from the following: sickle cell anaemia, β thalassaemia major, hereditary spherocytosis and 'idiopathic' warm autoimmune haemolytic anaemia. The normal range is indicated by the unbroken lines.

The tip has to be changed before moving on to the next tube. This procedure takes time and may result in an increased exposure for the first few tubes. It is therefore advisable to start the timing only after the addition of the sample to the first tube.

b. Using a Pasteur pipette with a perfectly flat end, 1 mm in diameter, suck up about 1 ml of blood, avoiding any bubbles and wipe the outside of the pipette. With the pipette held vertically above tube 1, deliver a single drop (about 50 μl) without the blood touching the wall of the tube. Then deliver single drops into the remaining 11 tubes. Method b appears to be primitive, but with practice it is perfectly satisfactory; it is also more economical and much faster than Method a. With either method, the best way to test its accuracy is to do a preliminary test by delivering the blood into several tubes all containing the same saline solution (e.g. either 3.0 or 1.0 g/l). The readings with the supernatants should be all within 5% of each other.

3. If the amount of blood available is limited (e.g. from babies) and the spectrometer takes 1 ml cuvettes, the volumes can be scaled down to 1 ml of saline solution and 10 μl of blood. However, to deliver 10 μl of blood reproducibly is not easy. With Method b, a Pasteur pipette or capillary pipette with a much smaller diameter, calibrated to give 10 μl drops of blood, would have to be used. It is then more difficult to maintain accuracy. Method a may be preferable in this case.

4. With the method using 50 μl of blood and with non-anaemic blood, the reading for 100% lysis will be about 0.7. With a modern spectrometer, any figure between 0.5 and 1.5 is acceptable. If the value is lower than 0.5, the test should be repeated using more blood or less saline (the reverse if the reading is higher than 1.5). With photoelectric colorimeters, values higher than 0.5 are often not very accurate.

5. When transferring the supernatant from a tube to the spectrometer cuvette, care has to be taken not to disturb the pellet. If it is well packed, the supernatant can simply be poured from the tube into the cuvette; with a spectrometer provided with an automatic suction device, this is usually satisfactory. Alternatively, a plastic Pasteur pipette should be used.

6. Even when a normal range has been established, it is essential always to run a normal control sample along with that of the patients to be tested to check, for example, the saline solutions.

The sigmoid shape of the normal osmotic fragility curve indicates that normal red cells vary in their resistance to hypotonic solutions. Indeed, this resistance varies gradually (osmotically) as a function of red cell age, with the youngest cells being the most resistant and the oldest cells being the most fragile. The reason for this is that old cells have a higher sodium content and a decreased capacity to pump out sodium.

Osmotic Fragility after Incubating the Blood at 37°C for 24 Hours

Method

Defibrinated blood should be used, care being taken to ensure that sterility is maintained.

Incubate 1 ml or 2 ml volumes of blood in sterile 5 ml bottles. It is advisable to set up the samples in duplicate in case one has become infected, as indicated by gross lysis and change in colour.

After 24 h, if no infection is evident, pool the contents of the duplicate bottles after thoroughly mixing the sedimented red cells in the overlying serum and estimate the fragility as previously described.

0 Hours

Hereditary spherocytosis
Pyruvate-kinase deficiency
Hereditary non spherocytic
haemolytic anaemia of undiagnosed
type

24 Hours

Figure 12.2 Osmotic fragility curves before and after incubating blood at 37°C for 24 h. Results are from patients suffering from the following: hereditary spherocytosis, pyruvate kinase deficiency and hereditary non-spherocytic haemolytic anaemia of undiagnosed type. The normal range is indicated by the unbroken lines.

Because the fragility may be markedly increased (Fig. 12.2), set up additional hypotonic solutions containing 7.0 g/l and 8.0 g/l NaCl. In addition, use a solution equivalent to 12.0 g/l NaCl because sometimes, as in HS, lysis may take place in 9.0 g/l NaCl. In this case, use the supernatant of the tube containing 12.0 g/l NaCl as the blank in the colorimetric estimation.

The incubation fragility test is conveniently combined with the estimation of the amount of spontaneous auto-haemolysis (p. 252).

Factors Affecting Osmotic Fragility Tests

In carrying out osmotic fragility tests by any method, three variables capable of markedly affecting the results must be controlled, quite apart from the accuracy with which the saline solutions have been made up. These are as follows:

1. The relative volumes of blood and saline
2. The final pH of the blood in saline suspension
3. The temperature at which the tests are carried out.

A proportion of 1 volume of blood to 100 volumes of saline is chosen because the concentration of blood is so small that the effect of the plasma on the final tonicity of the suspension is negligible. When weak suspensions of blood in saline are used, it is necessary to control the pH of the hypotonic solutions and it is for this reason that phosphate buffer is added to the saline. Even so, small differences will be found between the fragility of venous blood and maximally aerated (i.e. oxygenated) blood. For the most accurate results, it is recommended that the blood should be mixed until bright red. Finally, it is ideal for tests to be carried out always at the same temperature, although for most purposes room temperature is sufficiently constant.

The extent of the effect of pH and temperature on osmotic fragility was well illustrated in the paper of Parpart et al.[3] The effect of pH is more important: a shift of 0.1 of a pH unit is equivalent to altering the saline concentration by 0.1 g/l, the fragility of the red cells being increased by a decrease in pH. An increase in temperature decreases the fragility, an increase of 5°C being equivalent to an increase in saline concentration of about 0.1 g/l.

Lysis is virtually complete at the end of 30 min at 20°C and the hypotonic solutions may be centrifuged at the end of this time.

Further details of the factors that affect and control haemolysis of red cells in hypotonic solutions were given by Murphy.[4]

Recording the Results of Osmotic Fragility Tests

In the past, osmotic fragility most often has been expressed in terms of the highest concentration of saline at which lysis is just detectable (initial lysis or minimum resistance) and the highest concentration of saline in which lysis appears to be complete (complete lysis or maximum resistance). It is, however, useful also to record the concentration of saline causing 50% lysis (i.e. the median corpuscular fragility, MCF) and to inspect the entire fragility curve (Fig. 12.1). The findings in health are summarized in Table 12.1.

Table 12.1 Osmotic fragility in health (at 20°C and pH 7.4)		
	FRESH BLOOD (g/l NaCl)	BLOOD INCUBATED 24 h, 37°C (g/l NaCl)
Initial lysis	5.0	7.0
Complete lysis	3.0	2.0
MCF (50% lysis)	4.0–4.45	4.65–5.9
MCF, median corpuscular fragility.		

Alternative methods of recording osmotic fragility

Two simple alternative methods of recording the results quantitatively are available: the data may be plotted on probability paper or increment-haemolysis curves can be drawn. Both methods emphasize heterogeneity of the cell population with respect to osmotic fragility. If the observed amounts of lysis of normal blood are plotted on the probability scale against concentrations of saline, an almost straight line can be drawn through the points; the line is only skewed where lysis is almost complete. This method enables the MCF to be read off with ease.

In disease, tailed curves also skew the line to varying degrees at the other end of the probability plot. To obtain increment-haemolysis curves, the differences in lysis between adjacent tubes are plotted against the corresponding saline concentrations. Definitely bimodal curves may be obtained during recovery from a haemolytic episode.[5]

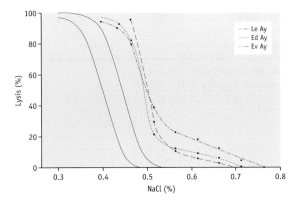

Figure 12.3 Osmotic fragility curves of three patients suffering from hereditary spherocytosis belonging to the same family (brother, sister and uncle [Le Ay]). The area between the unbroken lines represents the normal range.

Interpretation of Results

The osmotic fragility of freshly taken red cells reflects their ability to take up a certain amount of water before lysing. This is determined by their volume-to-surface area ratio. The ability of the normal red cell to withstand hypotonicity results from its biconcave shape, which allows the cell to increase its volume by about 70% before the surface membrane is stretched; once this limit is reached lysis occurs.[6] Spherocytes have an increased volume-to-surface area ratio; their ability to take in water before stretching the surface membrane is thus more limited than normal and they are therefore particularly susceptible to osmotic lysis. The increase in osmotic fragility is a property of the spheroidal shape of the cell and is independent of the cause of the spherocytosis. Characteristically, osmotic fragility curves from patients with HS who have not been splenectomized show a 'tail' of very fragile cells (Fig. 12.3). When plotted on probability paper, the graph indicates two populations of cells: the very fragile and the normal or slightly fragile. After splenectomy the red cells are more homogeneous, the osmotic fragility curve indicating a more continuous spectrum of cells, from fragile to normal.

Decreased osmotic fragility indicates the presence of unusually flattened red cells (leptocytes) in which the volume-to-surface area ratio is decreased. Such a change occurs in iron deficiency anaemia and thalassaemia in which the red cells with a low mean cell haemoglobin (MCH) and mean cell volume (MCV) are unusually resistant to osmotic lysis (Fig. 12.1). A simple one-tube osmotic fragility is a useful screening test for β thalassaemia and some haemoglobinopathies in countries with a high incidence of these abnormalities (p. 612). Reticulocytes and red cells from patients who have been splenectomized also tend to have a greater amount of membrane compared with normal cells and are osmotically resistant. In liver disease, target cells may be produced by passive accumulation of lipid and these cells, too, are resistant to osmotic lysis.[7]

The osmotic fragility of red cells after incubation for 24 h at 37°C is also a reflection of their volume-to-surface area ratio, but the factors that alter this ratio are more complicated than in fresh red cells. The increased osmotic fragility of normal red cells, which occurs after incubation (Fig. 12.2), is mainly caused by swelling of the cells associated with an accumulation of sodium that exceeds loss of potassium. Such cation exchange is determined by the membrane properties of the red cell, which control the passive flux of ions, and the metabolic competence of the cell, which determines the active pumping of cations against concentration gradients. During incubation for 24 h, the metabolism of the red cell becomes stressed and the pumping mechanisms tend to fail, one factor being a relative lack of glucose in the medium.

The osmotic fragility of red cells that have an abnormal membrane, such as those of HS and hereditary elliptocytosis (HE), increases abnormally after incubation (Fig. 12.2). Similar results occur in hereditary stomatocytosis.[8] The results with red cells with a glycolytic deficiency, such as those of pyruvate kinase (PK) deficiency, are variable. In severe deficiencies, osmotic fragility may increase substantially (Fig. 12.2), but, in other cases, the fragility may decrease owing to a greater loss of potassium than gain of sodium. In thalassaemia major and minor, osmotic fragility is frequently markedly reduced after incubation, again owing to a marked loss of potassium.[9] A similar, although usually less marked, change is seen in iron deficiency anaemia.

To summarize, measurement of red cell osmotic fragility provides a useful indication as to whether a patient's red cells are normal because an abnormal result invariably indicates abnormality. The reverse is, however, not

Table 12.2 Osmotic fragility in haemolytic anaemias: a summary

CONDITION	NOTES
A. Associated with increased osmotic fragility (OF)	
Hereditary spherocytosis (HS)	Entire curve may be 'shifted to the right', or most of it may be within the normal range but with a 'tail' of fragile cells. Curve within normal range in 10–20% of cases. After incubation for 24 h, abnormalities usually more marked, but still some false-negative results. Splenectomy does not affect MCF but reduces the tail of fragile cells
Hereditary elliptocytosis (HE)	As in HS, but in general changes less marked. Abnormal OF usually correlates with severity of haemolysis (i.e. OF is normal in non-haemolytic HE)
Hereditary stomatocytosis	As in HS with large osmotically fragile cells with low MCHC
Other inherited membrane abnormalities	Results variable; with milder disorders curve more likely to be abnormal after incubation for 24 h
Autoimmune haemolytic anaemia	Tail of fragile cells roughly proportional to number of spherocytes; rest of curve normal (or even left-shifted on account of reticulocytosis)
B. Associated with decreased OF	
Thalassaemia	MCF decreased in all forms of thalassaemia, except in some α thalassaemia heterozygotes; usually the entire curve is left-shifted
Enzyme abnormalities	OF usually normal (anaemia originally referred to as hereditary nonspherocytic), but tail of highly resistant cells may be seen on account of high reticulocyte court. After incubation for 24 h, there may be a tail of fragile cells
Hereditary xerocytosis	Increased resistance to osmotic lysis and increased MCHC
Iron deficiency	Curve shifted to left, wholly or partly, depending on proportion of hypochromic red cells

OF, osmotic fragility; HE, hereditary elliptocytosis; HS, hereditary spherocytosis; MCF, median corpuscular fragility; MCHC, mean cell haemoglobin concentration.

true (i.e. a result that is within the normal range does not mean that the red cells are normal). The findings in some important haemolytic anaemias are summarized in Table 12.2.

FLOW CYTOMETRIC (DYE-BINDING) TEST

Principle

The osmotic fragility test lacks specificity and sensitivity and fails to detect atypical or mild HS. Moreover, it can be affected by factors unrelated to red cell cytoskeletal defects; for example, positive results may be obtained for red cells from patients who are pregnant or who have immune or other haemolytic anaemias or renal failure. The flow cytometric (dye-binding) test of King and colleagues[10] measures the fluorescent intensity of intact red cells labelled with eosin-5-maleimide (EMA), which reacts covalently with Lys-430 on the first extracellular loop of Band 3 protein. The N-terminal cytoplasmic domain of Band 3 interacts with ankyrin and protein 4.2, which in turn crosslink with the spectrin-based cytoskeleton and stabilizes the membrane lipid bilayer.[11] Deficiency or abnormality of Band 3 may result in decreased fluorescence. This is seen in HS red cells but has also been observed in cases of South-east Asian ovalocytosis, congenital dyserythropoietic anaemia Type II and the stomatocytic variant, cryohydrocytosis. Blood samples in ethylenediaminetetra-acetic acid (EDTA) may be analysed for up to 48 h after collection provided they have been stored in the refrigerator.

Reagents

EMA

EMA is light sensitive and must be kept in the dark, preferably wrapped in aluminium foil and stored at 4°C. Prepare a stock solution by dissolving 1 mg in 1 ml of phosphate buffered saline (PBS). Mix well and store in 200 μl aliquots at −20°C.

Bovine serum albumin (30%) solution (BSA)

Available commercially. Dilute to 0.5% with PBS.

PBS

Tablets are available commercially for dissolving in water (e.g. Oxoid Dulbecco 'A' tablets). Alternatively, prepare by adding equal volumes of iso-osmotic phosphate buffer and 9 g/l NaCl:

Phosphate buffer, iso-osmotic, pH 7.2:
  (A) $NaH_2PO_4.2H_2O$ (150 mmol/l) – 23.4 g/l
  (B) NaH_2PO_4 (150 mmol/l) – 21.3 g/l.
  Add 24 ml reagent A to 76 ml reagent B.

Method

Thaw a tube of stock EMA solution in the dark at room temperature and dilute with an equal volume of PBS to obtain a working solution of 0.5 mg/ml. Mix 5 μl of washed packed red cells with 25 μl of EMA working solution in a plastic microfuge tube. Set up control tubes from blood of normal individuals and perform all tests in duplicate. Leave a rack with the tubes in a cupboard in the dark at room temperature for 30 min. Mix and return to the cupboard for a further 30 min.

Then, spin the tubes in a bench-top microfuge for 5–10 s and remove the supernatant dye carefully with a fine-tip pipette.

Wash the labelled red cells three times with 500 μl PBS containing 0.5% BSA. The third wash should be colourless. If it is still pink, suggesting that traces of dye particle remain in the tube, discard the sample and repeat the cell labelling procedure.

Resuspend the packed red cells in 500 μl of the PBS–BSA wash solution. Transfer 100 μl of the cell suspension into a plastic flow cytometer tube and add 1.4 ml of wash solution. Keep the cell suspensions in the dark by wrapping in aluminium foil until use. Set the analyser thresholds (gate) for red blood cells and count each sample for a minimum of 15 000 events. Select the FITC (fluorescein isothiocyanate) channel and record the mean fluorescence intensity (MFI). Compare the test with the mean value of several control samples.

Interpretation of Results

Results should be expressed as a ratio of mean value of the test to control sample. Each laboratory should set the reference range and cut-off values for its own instrument. In our laboratory, a ratio of 0.8 or more is regarded as normal.

GLYCEROL LYSIS-TIME TESTS

The osmotic fragility test is somewhat cumbersome and requires 2 ml or more of whole blood. It is thus not suitable for use in newborn babies or as a population screening test.

In 1974, Gottfried and Robertson[12] introduced a glycerol lysis-time (GLT) test, a one-tube test, to measure the time taken for 50% haemolysis of a blood sample in a buffered hypotonic saline–glycerol mixture. The original method had greater sensitivity in the osmotic-resistant range, but it also could identify most patients with HS by a shorter GLT_{50}. Better identification of HS blood from normal was obtained by 24-h incubation of samples and by modifying the glycerol reagent.[13] Zanella et al modified the original test further by decreasing the pH.[14] There is some loss of specificity for HS with the acidified glycerol lysis-time test (AGLT) compared with the original method, but in practice this loss is unimportant.

Acidified Glycerol Lysis-Time Test

Principle

Glycerol present in a hypotonic buffered saline solution slows the rate of entry of water molecules into the red cells so that the time taken for lysis may be more conveniently measured. Like the osmotic fragility test, differentiation can be made between spherocytes and normal red cells.

Reagents

Phosphate buffered saline

Add 9 volumes of 9.0 g/l (154 mmol/l) NaCl to 1 volume of 100 mmol/l phosphate buffer (2 volumes of 14.9 g/l Na_2HPO_4 added to 1 volume of 13.61 g/l KH_2PO_4). Adjust the pH to 6.85 ± 0.05 at room temperature (15–25°C). This adjustment must be accurate.

Glycerol reagent

300 mmol/l. Add 23 ml of glycerol (27.65 g AR grade) to 300 ml of PBS and bring the final volume to 1 litre with water.

Method

Add 20 μl of whole blood, anticoagulated with EDTA, to 5.0 ml of PBS, pH 6.85. Mix the suspension carefully.

Transfer 1.0 ml to a standard 4 ml cuvette of a spectrometer equipped with a linear-logarithmic recorder. Fix the wavelength at 625 nm and start the recorder. Add 2.0 ml of the glycerol reagent rapidly to the cuvette with a 2 ml syringe or automatic pipette and mix well.

The rate of haemolysis is measured by the rate of fall of turbidity of the reaction mixture. The results are expressed as the time required for the optical density to fall to half the initial value ($AGLT_{50}$). The test can also be carried out using a colorimeter and stopwatch.

Results

Normal blood takes more than 30 min (1800 s) to reach the $AGLT_{50}$. The time taken is similar for blood from normal adults, newborn infants and cord samples. In patients with HS, the range of the $AGLT_{50}$ is 25–150 s. A short $AGLT_{50}$ may also be found in chronic renal failure, chronic leukaemias and autoimmune haemolytic anaemia; it also may be found in some pregnant women.[14]

Significance of the AGLT

The same principles apply as with the osmotic fragility test. Cells with a high volume-to-surface area ratio resist swelling for a shorter time than normal cells. This applies to all spherocytes, whether the spherocytosis is caused by HS or other mechanisms. The test is particularly useful in screening family members of patients with HS where morphological changes are too small to indicate clearly whether the disorder is present.

CRYOHAEMOLYSIS TEST

Principle

Whereas osmotic fragility may be abnormal in any condition where spherocytes occur, it has been suggested that cryohaemolysis is specific for HS.[15] This appears to result from the fact that the latter is dependent on factors that are related to molecular defects of the red cell membrane rather than to changes in the surface area-to-volume ratio. The test can be carried out on EDTA blood up to 1 day old.

Reagent

Buffered 0.7 mol/l sucrose

23.96 g sucrose in 100 ml of 50 mmol/l phosphate buffer, pH 7.4. This can be stored frozen in 2 ml aliquots in tubes ready for use.

Method[15]

1. Centrifuge the blood and wash the red cells three times with cold (4°C) 9 g/l NaCl. Make a suspension of 50–70% cells in the saline and keep on ice until tested.
2. Prepare 2 ml volumes of reagent, thawing if frozen, and stand for 10 min in a 37°C waterbath to equilibrate.
3. Pipette 50 μl of the cell suspension into each of 2 tubes of the warmed reagent, vortex immediately for a few seconds and then incubate for exactly 10 min at 37°C.
4. Without delay, transfer the tubes to an icebath for another 10 min, vortex for a few seconds and then centrifuge to sediment the remaining cells. Transfer some of the supernatant to a clean tube.
5. Prepare a 100% haemolysate solution by pipetting 50 μl of the original sample into 2 ml of water. Centrifuge and dilute 200 μl of the supernatant in 4 ml of water.
6. Read absorbance at 540 nm of the test and the 100% lysis samples.

$$\% \text{ cryohaemolysis} = \left[\frac{A^{540}\text{test}}{\left[A^{540}\text{haemolysate} \times 21\right]} \right] \times 100$$

Interpretation

Streichman et al.[15] report the range of cryohaemolysis in normal subjects to be 3–15%, whereas in hereditary spherocytosis there is >20% lysis. However, it is recommended that individual laboratories establish their own reference values for the method. We have found that most normal samples give <3% lysis. Increased lysis is not exclusive to hereditary spherocytosis and may be observed in hereditary stomatocytosis.

AUTOHAEMOLYSIS: SPONTANEOUS HAEMOLYSIS DEVELOPING IN BLOOD INCUBATED AT 37°C FOR 48 HOURS

The autohaemolysis test is useful as an initial screen in suspected cases of haemolytic anaemia. It provides information about the metabolic competence of the red cells and helps to distinguish membrane and enzyme defects if the results of the tests are taken together with other observations such as morphology, inheritance and the presence or absence of associated clinical disorders.[16]

Principle

Aliquots of blood are incubated both with and without sterile glucose solution at 37°C for 48 h. After this period, the amount of spontaneous haemolysis is measured colorimetrically.

Method

It is essential to use aseptic techniques in setting up the autohaemolysis test to maintain sterility throughout the incubation period.

Defibrinating Blood

Defibrinate blood, as described on p. 5.

Use sterile defibrinated blood and deliver four 1 ml or 2 ml samples into sterile 5 ml capped bottles. Retain a portion of the original sample; separate and store this as the preincubation serum.

Add to two of the bottles 50 or 100 μl of sterile 100 g/l glucose solution, so as to provide a concentration of glucose in the blood of at least 30 mmol/l. Make sure that the caps of the bottles are tightly closed and place the series of bottles in the incubator at 37°C. A sample from a known normal individual should be run in parallel as a control.

After 24 h, thoroughly mix the content by gentle swirling. After incubating for 48 h, inspect the samples for signs of infection, thoroughly mix again, then from each bottle remove a sample for the estimation of the packed cell volume (PCV) (by the microhaematocrit method) and haemoglobin (Hb) concentration and centrifuge the remainder to obtain the supernatant serum.

Estimate the spontaneous lysis by means of a colorimeter or a spectrometer at 540 nm.

As a rule, it is convenient to make a 1 in 10 dilution of the incubated serum in cyanide-ferricyanide (Drabkin's) solution (p. 25), unless there is marked haemolysis, when a 1 in 25 or 1 in 50 dilution is more suitable. A corresponding dilution of the preincubation serum is used as a blank and a 1 in 100 or 1 in 200 dilution of the whole blood in Drabkin's solution indicates the total amount of Hb present and serves as a standard.

Calculate the percentage lysis, allowing for the change in PCV resulting from the incubation as follows:

$$\text{Lysis (\%)} = \frac{R_t - B}{R_0} \times \frac{D_0}{D_t} \times (1 - PCV_t) \times 100$$

where R_0 = reading of diluted whole blood; R_t = reading of diluted serum at 48 h; B = reading of blank; PCV_t = packed cell volume at time t; D_0 = dilution of whole blood (e.g. 1 in 200 = 0.005); and D_t = dilution of serum (e.g. 1 in 10 = 0.1).

The reading at time t is multiplied by $(1 - PCV_t)$ so as to give the concentration that would be found if the liberated Hb was dissolved in whole blood (i.e. in both plasma and red cell compartments), not in the plasma compartment alone.

Normal Range of Autohaemolysis

Lysis at 48 h: without added glucose, 0.2–2.0%; with added glucose, 0–0.9%.

The results obtained are sensitive to slight differences in technique and each laboratory should use a carefully standardized procedure and establish its own normal range. If the amount of liberated Hb is small, it is more accurate (although more time consuming) to measure lysis by a chemical method rather than by a direct spectrometric method (p. 231). It can also be measured directly by a simple and rapid procedure with a *HemoCue Plasma/Low Hb system*.[17]

Significance of Increased Autohaemolysis

Little or no lysis takes place when normal blood is incubated for 24 h under sterile conditions and the amount present after 48 h is small.[16] If glucose is added so that it is present throughout the incubation, the development of lysis is markedly slowed. The amount of autohaemolysis that occurs after 48 h with and without glucose is determined by the properties of the membrane and the metabolic competence of the red cell. In membrane disorders such as HS, the rate of glucose consumption is increased to compensate for an increased cation leak through the membrane.[8] During the 48-h incubation, glucose is therefore used up relatively rapidly so that energy production fails more quickly than normal unless glucose is added. This is one factor that contributes to the increased rate of autohaemolysis in HS. Usually, but not always, the addition of glucose to the blood decreases the rate of autohaemolysis in HS. This was referred to as Type 1 autohaemolysis.[16] When the utilization of glucose via the glycolytic pathway is impaired, as in PK deficiency, the rate of autohaemolysis at 48 h is usually increased but glucose fails to correct or may even aggravate lysis (Type 2 autohaemolysis).[8] Although a similar result may be seen in severe HS (Type B), in the absence of spherocytosis failure of glucose to diminish autohaemolysis is a strong indication of a glycolytic block. Blood from patients with G6PD deficiency or other disorders of the pentose phosphate pathway may undergo a slight increase in autohaemolysis (without additional glucose), which is corrected by the addition of glucose. Commonly, the result is normal, but examination of the incubated blood may show an increase in methaemoglobin (Hi) (discussed later). Not all glycolytic enzyme deficiencies give a Type 2 reaction so that a Type 1 result does not exclude the possibility of such a defect.

In the acquired haemolytic anaemias, the results of the autohaemolysis test are variable and generally not very helpful in diagnosis. In the autoimmune haemolytic anaemias, lysis may be increased in the absence of additional glucose but the effect of added glucose is unpredictable. In paroxysmal nocturnal haemoglobinuria (PNH), the autohaemolysis of aerated defibrinated blood is usually normal.

Autohaemolysis may be increased in haemolytic anaemias caused by oxidant drugs or when there are defects in the reducing power of the red cell. Heinz bodies, Hi or both will be detectable at the end of incubation. Normally, red cells produce <4% Hi after 48 h incubation and Heinz bodies are not seen. Red cells containing an unstable Hb also contain Heinz bodies at the end of the incubation period and increased amounts of Hi.

The nucleosides adenosine, guanosine and inosine, like glucose, diminish the rate of autohaemolysis when added to blood. Remarkably, adenosine triphosphate (ATP) strikingly retards haemolysis in PK deficiency, although glucose itself is ineffective.[18] ATP does not pass the red cell membrane.

The autohaemolysis test lacks specificity. This has drawn much criticism on the test, including the suggestion that it has no place in the screening of blood for inherited defects.[19] The best way to detect metabolic defects in red cells is undoubtedly to measure glucose consumption, lactate production and the contribution to metabolism of the pentose phosphate pathway. These measurements are, unfortunately, difficult and are likely to be undertaken only by specialized laboratories. The autohaemolysis test does provide some information about the metabolic competence of the red cells and helps to distinguish membrane defects from enzyme defects.

In summary, we feel that the autohaemolysis test is still useful in the investigation of patients who have or who may have chronic haemolytic anaemia for the following reasons:

1. If the result is entirely normal, an intrinsic red cell abnormality is unlikely.
2. If abnormal haemolysis is fully corrected by glucose, a metabolic abnormality is unlikely and a membrane abnormality is likely.
3. If abnormal haemolysis shows little or no correction by glucose, a metabolic abnormality is likely, provided that obvious features of spherocytosis are not present on the blood film.

Thus, in our experience, a combination of red cell morphology with the results of the autohaemolysis tests makes it possible to differentiate membrane abnormalities from enzyme deficiencies in the vast majority of cases.

MEMBRANE PROTEIN ANALYSIS

Defects of red cell membrane proteins that constitute the cytoskeleton are associated with congenital haemolytic anaemias accompanied by characteristic morphological features. Their analysis is generally only possible in the setting of a reference laboratory. Sodium dodecyl sulfate (SDS) – polyacrylamide gel electrophoresis of the membranes will identify qualitative and quantitative alterations in the specific proteins. Densitometry of protein bands on the gel gives an overall profile, showing spectrin, ankyrin, Band 3 (the anion transport protein) and protein 4.2. Spectrin variants may be detected after limited trypsin digestion of spectrin extracted from the red cell membranes; an increase in spectrin dimer is indicative of an unstable tetramer, leading to susceptibility to red cell fragmentation in hereditary elliptocytosis and hereditary pyropoikilocytosis.[20]

Membrane protein defects implicated in hereditary haemolytic anaemias are listed in Table 12.3.

DETECTION OF ENZYME DEFICIENCIES IN HEREDITARY HAEMOLYTIC ANAEMIAS

It is feasible for most haematology laboratories to identify the enzyme deficiencies of G6PD and PK and to indicate where the probable defect lies in less common disorders.

Table 12.3 Haemolytic anaemias associated with defects of red cell membrane proteins[20]

BAND	PROTEIN	HAEMOLYTIC ANAEMIA
1	α Spectrin	HE, HS, HPP
2	β Spectrin	HE, HS
2.1	Ankyrin	HS
3	Anion exchanger	HS, SAO, CDAII
4.1	Protein 4.1	HE
4.2	Pallidin	HS
7	Stomatin	HSt
PAS-1	Glycophorin A	CDAII
PAS-2	Glycophorin C	HE

CDAII, congenital dyserythropoietic anaemia Type II; HE, hereditary elliptocytosis; HPP, hereditary pyropoikilocytosis; HS, hereditary spherocytosis; HSt, hereditary stomatocytosis; SAO, South-east Asian ovalocytosis.

Detailed investigation of the aberrant enzymes and of the metabolism of the abnormal cells is probably best undertaken by specialized laboratories. Comprehensive accounts of methods available for studying red cell metabolism are to be found in Beutler's *Red Cell Metabolism, a Manual of Biochemical Methods*[21] and in the ICSH recommendations.[22]

There are two stages in the diagnosis of red cell enzyme defects: first, screening procedures; and second, specific enzyme assays. The simple nonspecific screening procedures such as the osmotic fragility and autohaemolysis tests, which have already been described, may indicate the presence of a metabolic disorder and simple biochemical tests are available to show whether the disorder is in the pentose phosphate or the Embden–Meyerhof pathways; these intermediate stages of glycolysis are illustrated in Figure 12.4.

These investigations may be augmented by quantitation of the major red cell metabolites 2,3-DPG, ATP and GSH, which are present at millimolar concentrations and which can be assayed conveniently by spectrometric techniques. Metabolic block in the Embden–Meyerhof pathway is most accurately pinpointed by measurement of the concentration of glycolytic intermediates with demonstration of accumulation of metabolites proximal and depletion of metabolites distal to the defective step (Fig. 12.4). These assays, which are generally confined to specialized laboratories, must be performed on deproteinized red cell extracts immediately after preparation.

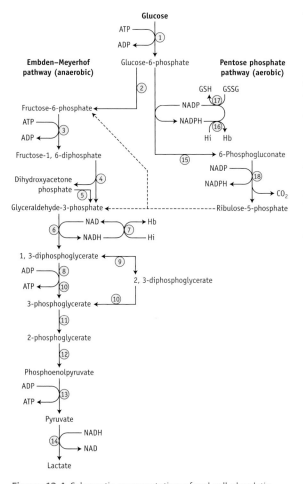

Glucose

Embden–Meyerhof pathway (anaerobic)

Pentose phosphate pathway (aerobic)

Figure 12.4 Schematic representation of red cell glycolytic pathways. The enzymes are indicated as follows: 1: hexokinase; 2: glucosephosphate isomerase; 3: phosphofructokinase; 4: aldolase; 5: triose phosphate isomerase; 6: glyceraldehyde-3-phosphate dehydrogenase; 7: NADH-methaemoglobin reductase; 8: phosphoglycerate kinase; 9: diphosphoglyceromutase; 10: diphosphoglycerate phosphatase; 11: phosphoglyceromutase; 12: enolase; 13: pyruvate kinase; 14: lactate dehydrogenase; 15: glucose-6-phosphate dehydrogenase; 16: NADPH-methaemoglobin reductase; 17: glutathione reductase; 18: 6-phosphogluconate dehydrogenase. NADH, reduced form of nicotinamide adenine dinucleotide; NADPH, reduced form of nicotinamide adenine dinucleotide phosphate.

Screening Tests for G6PD Deficiency and Other Defects of the Pentose Phosphate Pathway

Many variants of the red cell enzyme G6PD have been detected and the methods used to identify variants have been standardized.[23] Inheritance is sex-linked because

the enzyme is controlled by one gene locus in the X chromosome. Variants that have deficient activity produce one of several types of clinical disorders. The two most common variants are the Mediterranean type, which has very low activity and which may lead to favism (i.e. acute intravascular haemolysis following the ingestion of broad beans), and the A– type found in Black populations in West Africa, the USA, the UK and elsewhere, which leads to primaquine sensitivity. Both groups are susceptible to haemolysis produced by oxidant drugs and infections.

Much less frequently, a chronic non-spherocytic haemolytic anaemia is produced by rare variants of the enzyme. Severe neonatal jaundice with anaemia occurs in about 5% of patients who have major deficiencies of enzyme activity.

G6PD deficiency in hemizygous (male) or homozygous (female) individuals may be readily detected by screening tests, but it is more difficult to detect heterozygous (female) carriers. Other defects of the pentose phosphate pathway (left) also lead to deficiency in the reducing power of the red cell. The clinical syndromes associated with these defects include intravascular haemolysis, with or without methaemoglobinaemia, in response to oxidative drugs.

G6PD catalyses the oxidation of glucose-6-phosphate (G6P) to 6-phosphogluconate (6PG) with the simultaneous reduction of nicotinamide adenine dinucleotide phosphate (NADP) to reduced NADP (NADPH):

$$G6P + NADP \overset{G6PD}{\rightarrow} 6PG + NADPH$$

In a second, consecutive, oxidative reaction, 6PG is converted to 6-phosphogluconolactone, with reduction of a further molecule of NADP to NADPH. The lactone then undergoes decarboxylation to ribulose 5-phosphate through a reaction catalysed by a specific lactonase, but which can also take place spontaneously. Thus the overall reaction catalysed by 6PG dehydrogenase (6PGD) can be written as follows:

$$6PG + NADP \overset{6PGD}{\rightarrow} Ru5P + CO_2 + NADPH$$

The release of CO_2 drives the reaction to the right so that in practice the pathway is not reversible.

NADPH is an important reducing compound for the conversion of oxidized glutathione (GSSG) to GSH (Fig. 12.4) and, under conditions of stress, the reconversion of Hi to Hb. Screening tests for G6PD deficiency depend on the inability of cells from deficient subjects to convert an oxidized substrate to a reduced state. The substrates used may be the natural one of the enzyme, NADP or other naturally occurring substrates linked by secondary reactions to the enzyme, for example, GSSG or Hi or artificial dyes such as methylene blue. The reaction is demonstrated by fluorescence,[24] colour change when a dye is used,[25] or deposit of a dye (e.g. a blue ring of formazan from diphenyltetrazolium bromide in the presence of phenazine methosulphate).[26]

Which screening test is used in any particular laboratory will depend on a number of factors such as cost, time required, temperature and humidity and availability of reagents. Two tests that are commonly used and that are generally reliable are described here.

Fluorescence Screening Test for G6PD Deficiency

The method of fluorescent screening test for G6PD deficiency is that of Beutler and Mitchell[24] modified as recommended by ICSH.[22]

Principle

NADPH, generated by G6PD present in a lysate of blood cells, fluoresces under long-wave ultraviolet (UV) light. In G6PD deficiency, there is an inability to produce sufficient NADPH; this results in a lack of fluorescence.

Reagents

D-glucose-6-phosphate

10 mmol/l. Dissolve 305 mg of the disodium salt or an equivalent amount of the potassium salt, in 100 ml of water.

NADP+

7.5 mmol/l. Dissolve 60 mg of NADP+, disodium salt, in 10 ml of water.

Saponin (white, suitable for haemolysis)

1%.

Tris-HCl buffer

750 mmol/l, pH 7.8. Dissolve 9.1 g of Tris (hydroxymethyl) aminomethane in 80 ml of water. Adjust the pH to 7.8 with HCl and make up the volume to 100 ml with water.

Oxidized glutathione (GSSG)

8 mmol/l. Dissolve 49 mg of GSSG in 10 ml of water.

Mix the reagents in the following proportion: 2 volumes of G6P, 1 volume of NADP+, 2 volumes of saponin, 3 volumes of buffer, 1 volume of GSSG and 1 volume of water.

The combined reagent is stable at $-20°C$ for 2 or more years and for at least 2 months if kept at 4°C. Azide may be added to prevent growth of contaminants without loss of activity. Dispense 100 µl volumes into appropriate small tubes and keep at $-20°C$ ready for use.

Method

Thaw out sufficient tubes to set up test and controls. Allow reagents to reach room temperature before use.

Add 10 µl of whole blood (EDTA, heparin, ACD [acid–citrate–dextrose] or CPD [citrate–phosphate–dextrose]) to 100 µl volumes of the reagent mixture and keep at room temperature (15–25°C).

Place 10 µl of the reaction mixture on a Whatman No. 1 filter paper at the beginning of the reaction and again after 5–10 min. A shorter interval may be appropriate at a high ambient temperature (c 25–30°C). Allow to air dry thoroughly before examining the spots under UV light. Record whether fluorescence is present $(+)$ or absent $(-)$. Always set up samples of normal blood and known G6PD-deficiency blood in parallel.

If the samples are to be collected away from the laboratory or where delay is envisaged (e.g. during population screening) place about 10 µl of blood on Whatman No. 1 filter paper and allow it to dry. Cut out the disc of dried blood in the laboratory and add it to the reaction mixture. A sample of normal blood should always be tested as a positive fluorescence (i.e. normal) control.

The test can be carried out on blood stored in ACD (provided it is sterile) for up to 21 days at 4°C and for about 5 days at room temperature.

Interpretation

Fluorescence is produced by NADPH formed from NADP+ in the presence of G6PD. Some of the NADPH produced is oxidized by GSSG, but this reaction, catalysed by glutathione reductase, is normally slower than the rate of NADPH production. Red cells with <20% of normal G6PD activity do not cause detectable fluorescence.

Like all screening tests, this method is useful when large numbers of samples are to be tested, but the result must be interpreted with caution in an individual patient. The main causes of erroneous interpretations are as follows:

False-normal. If there is reticulocytosis, a vivid fluorescence may be seen with a genetically G6PD-deficient blood sample because young red cells have more G6PD activity. If the test is carried out during an acute haemolytic episode, the patient's blood should be retested when the reticulocyte count has returned to normal.

False-deficient. If the patient is anaemic, very little fluorescence may be seen despite the G6PD being genetically normal, simply because there are relatively few red cells in the 10 µl of blood used.

Although it is possible to correct for either or both of these contingencies, if in doubt, it is best to proceed directly to a quantitative enzyme assay (discussed later).

The test is meant to give only a + or − (normal or deficient) result by comparison with the controls and it does not make sense to grade by eye the intensity of fluorescence. If a control G6PD-deficient sample is not available, the appearance of the 'zero time' spot can be used for reference. The threshold for a 'deficient' result can be worked out by making dilutions of a normal blood sample in saline and is best set by regarding as deficient the fluorescence obtained when G6PD activity is 20% of normal or less (corresponding to a 1 in 5 dilution of normal blood). This means that very mildly deficient variants, and a substantial proportion of heterozygotes (see below), will be missed. However, clinically important haemolysis is unlikely to occur in subjects who have more than 20% G6PD activity and therefore this seems an appropriate (although arbitrary) threshold for a diagnostic laboratory. Because the test depends on visual inspection, it is best to select the time of incubation in relation to ambient temperature in preliminary trials. NADPH production is a cumulative process. Therefore, given enough time, a G6PD-deficient sample will fluoresce. The time allowed for the reaction should be one at which the contrast in fluorescence between a G6PD-normal and a G6PD-deficient sample is maximal.

Methaemoglobin Reduction Test

Principle

Sodium nitrite converts Hb to Hi. When no methylene blue is added, methaemoglobin persists, but incubation of the samples with methylene blue allows stimulation of the pentose phosphate pathway in subjects with normal G6PD levels. The Hi is reduced during the incubation period. In G6PD-deficient subjects, the block in the pentose phosphate pathway prevents this reduction.[25]

Reagents

Sodium nitrite

180 mmol/l.

Dextrose

280 mmol/l. Dissolve 5 g of dextrose (analytical grade) and 1.25 g of $NaNO_2$ in 100 ml of water.

Methylene blue

0.4 mmol/l. Dissolve 150 mg of methylthionine chloride (methylene blue chloride, Sigma) in 1 litre of water.

Nile blue sulphate

22 mg in 100 ml of water. This may be used as an alternative to methylene blue.

The reagents may be used in a variety of ways to suit the convenience of the laboratory. A batch of tubes may be prepared in advance of use by mixing equal volumes of the reagents (sodium nitrite with methylene blue or Nile blue sulphate) and pipetting 0.2 ml of the combined reagent into individual glass tubes. Glass tubes must be used because plastic may adsorb some reagents. The contents of the tubes are allowed to evaporate to dryness at room temperature (15–25°C) or in an oven at a temperature not exceeding 37°C. The tubes must then be tightly stoppered. The reagent will keep for 6 months at room temperature. The reagents may however be used fresh, without drying.

Method

Use anticoagulated blood (EDTA or ACD) and test the samples preferably within 1 h of collection if left on the bench or within 6 h if kept at 4°C. Blood in ACD can be stored for up to 1 week but will be unsatisfactory if there is any haemolysis. With blood from patients who are severely anaemic, adjust the PCV to 0.40 ± 0.05.

Add 2 ml of blood to the tube containing 0.2 ml of the combined reagent either freshly prepared or dried. Close the tube with a stopper and gently mix the contents by inverting it 15 times.

Prepare control tubes by adding 2 ml of blood to a similar tube without reagents (normal reference tube) and to a tube containing 0.1 ml of sodium nitrite–dextrose mixture without methylene blue ('deficient' reference tube).

Incubate the samples at 37°C for 90 min. If the blood has been heparinized, incubation should be continued for 3 h.

After the incubation, pipette 0.1 ml volumes from the test sample, the normal reference tube and the deficient reference tube into 10 ml of water in separate, clear glass test tubes of identical diameter. Mix the contents gently. Compare the colours in the different tubes (see below).

Interpretation

Normal blood yields a colour similar to that in the normal reference tube (i.e. a clear red). Blood from deficient subjects gives a brown colour similar to that in the deficient reference tube. Heterozygotes give intermediate reactions.

Although this method takes longer than the fluorescent test, its advantages include the fact that it is extremely inexpensive and that the only equipment required is a waterbath. In addition, the test can be complemented by cytochemical analysis that lends itself to detecting G6PD deficiency in patients with reticulocytosis and in heterozygotes.

Detection of Heterozygotes for G6PD Deficiency

Females heterozygous for G6PD deficiency have two populations of cells, one with normal G6PD activity and the other with deficient G6PD activity. This is the result of inactivation of one of the two X chromosomes in individual cells early in the development of the embryo. All progeny cells (i.e. somatic cells) in females will have the characteristics of only the active X chromosome.[27] The total G6PD activity of blood in the female will depend on the proportion of normal to deficient cells. In most cases, the activity will be between 20% and 80% of normal. However, a few heterozygotes (about 1%) may have almost only normal or almost only G6PD-deficient cells.

Screening tests for G6PD deficiency fail to demonstrate most heterozygotes. The deficient red cells may, however, be identified in blood films by a cytochemical elution procedure (see below).

Test Kits

Several commercial kits are available for detection of G6PD deficiency. A fluorescent spot test (Trinity Biotech 203-A) and a test based on reduction of the dye dichloroindophenol to a colourless state in the presence of phenazine methosulphate (Trinity Biotech 400) are available commercially.*

The Quantase kit[†] is a photometric method for use on whole blood or dried blood spots; NADPH produced by oxidation of G6P to 6PG is measured by an increase in absorption at 340 nm.

Each test or batch of tests should include a normal and a G6PD-deficient sample. Sheep blood is a useful source of naturally deficient blood. Where possible, participation in an external quality assessment (or proficiency testing) scheme is also recommended.

CYTOCHEMICAL TESTS FOR DEMONSTRATING DEFECTS OF RED CELL METABOLISM

Cytochemical methods have been developed by means of which some of these defects are demonstrable in individual cells. Thus tests have been described for demonstrating red cells deficient in G6PD.[28–30] The principle on which the methods are based is that red cells are treated with sodium nitrite to convert their oxyhaemoglobin (HbO$_2$) to methaemoglobin (Hi). In the presence of G6PD, Hi reconverts to HbO$_2$, but in G6PD deficiency, Hi persists. The blood is then incubated with a soluble tetrazolium compound (MTT), which will be reduced by HbO$_2$ (but not by Hi) to an insoluble formazan form.

Attempts have been made to improve the reliability of the test for detecting heterozygotes (e.g. by controlled slight fixation of the red cells and accelerating the reaction with an exogenous electron carrier, 1-methoxyphenazine methosulphate).[31] These cytochemical procedures are not more sensitive in the demonstration of G6PD deficiency than are the simple screening tests described above. They may, however, be useful in genetic studies and when assessing G6PD activity in women[32]; they may be the only way to detect deficiency in the heterozygous state.

Demonstration of G6PD-deficient Cells

Reagents

Sodium nitrite

0.18 mol/l (12.5 g/l). The solution must be stored in a dark bottle and made up monthly.

---

*Trinity Biotech, Bray, Co. Wicklow, Ireland; see their website for full product list.
†Quantase Ltd., Frierton, Perth, Scotland.

Incubation medium

9 g/l NaCl, 4 ml; 50 g/l glucose, 1.0 ml; 0.3 mol/l phosphate buffer, pH 7.0, 2.0 ml; 0.11 g/l Nile blue sulphate, 1.0 ml; water, 2.0 ml.

MTT tetrazolium

5 g/l of 3-(4,5-dimethyl-thiazolyl-1–2)-2,5 diphenyltetrazolium bromide in 9 g/l NaCl.

Hypotonic saline

6 g/l NaCl.

Method

Venous blood collected into ACD should be used. The test should be carried out within 8 h of collection and the blood should be kept at 4°C until it is tested. Centrifuge the blood at 4°C for 20 min at 1200–1500 g.[28]

Discard the supernatant and add 0.5 ml of the packed red cells to 9 ml of 9 g/l NaCl and 0.5 ml of sodium nitrite solution contained in a 15 ml glass centrifuge tube. Incubate at 37°C for 20 min. Centrifuge at 4°C for 15 min at approx. 500 g, then discard the supernatant fluid without disturbing the buffy coat and uppermost layer of red cells. Wash the cells three times in cold saline. After the last washing, remove the buffy coat, mix the packed cells well and transfer 50 μl to a glass tube containing 1 ml of the incubation medium. Incubate the suspension undisturbed at 37°C for 30 min. Then add 0.2 ml of MTT solution, shake gently and incubate at 37°C for 1 h. Resuspend the cells thoroughly. Place one drop adjacent to one drop of hypotonic saline on a glass slide, mix the drops thoroughly and cover with a coverglass.

Examine the red cells with an oil-immersion objective, noting the presence of formazan granules (Fig. 12.5).

Figure 12.5 Cytochemical demonstration of G6PD (glucose-6-phosphate dehydrogenase). Normal blood; positive reaction with formazan granules in the red cells.

Interpretation

When G6PD activity is normal, all the red cells are stained. In G6PD hemizygotes, the majority of the red cells are unstained. In heterozygotes, mosaicism is usually seen; usually 40–60% of the cells are unstained, but the proportion may be much less and in extreme cases only as few as 2–3% may be unstained.

PYRIMIDINE-5′-NUCLEOTIDASE SCREENING TEST

Pyrimidine-5′-nucleotidase (P5N) was first described by Valentine et al.[33] as a cytosolic enzyme in human red cells. Deficiency of P5N-1 (uridine monophosphate hydrolase-1), which shows autosomal recessive inheritance, is associated with congenital haemolytic anaemia. Heterozygotes are clinically and haematologically normal and typically have about half the normal red cell P5N activity. Homozygous P5N deficiency, in which enzyme activity is generally 5–15% of normal, results in a chronic non-spherocytic haemolytic anaemia. This is characterized by mild to moderate haemolysis, pronounced basophilic stippling visible in up to 5% of red cells and marked increase in both red cell glutathione and pyrimidine nucleotides. Osmotic fragility is normal. The rate of autohaemolysis is increased with little or no reduction in lysis by added glucose.[8]

P5N deficiency appears to be a comparatively rare cause of hereditary non-spherocytic haemolytic anaemia. Because lead is an inhibitor of P5N, an acquired deficiency occurs in lead toxicity and this may be important in the pathogenesis of the associated anaemia. The definitive diagnostic test is a quantitative assay of P5N activity; but the finding of supranormal levels of red cell nucleotides (mostly pyrimidines) is strongly suggestive and can be used for screening.

Activity of P5N may be measured by a colorimetric method[33] or by a radiometric method.[34] For the screening of P5N deficiency, the method recommended by ICSH is the determination of the UV spectra of a blood extract.[35]

Principle

The nucleotide pool of normal red cells consists largely (>96%) of purine (adenine and small amounts of guanine) derivatives. The levels of cytidine and uridine are normally extremely low. However, in P5N-deficient cells, more than 50% of this pool consists of pyrimidine nucleotides.

In acidic solutions, cytidine nucleotides have an absorbance maximum at approx. 280 nm, whereas adenine, guanine and uridine nucleotides absorb maximally at 260 nm. The ratio of absorbance at 260 nm to absorbance at 280 nm reflects the relative abundance of cytidine nucleotides; the absorbance ratio is lower when pyrimidine derivatives are increased.

Reagents

Sodium chloride solution

NaCl, 9 g/l.

Perchloric acid

4%. 28.6 ml of a 70% perchloric acid solution are diluted to a final volume of 500 ml with water.

Glycine buffer

1 mol/1, pH 3.0. 7.51 g of glycine are dissolved in about 80 ml of water, the pH is adjusted to 3.0 with concentrated hydrochloric acid (HCl) and the solution is made up to a final volume of 100 ml with water.

Method

For sample preparation, centrifuge blood freshly collected in EDTA at 1200 g for 5 min, remove the plasma and wash the cells three times with ice-cold 9 g/l NaCl solution. Add 1 ml of a 50% suspension of the washed red cells to 4 ml of ice-cold 4% perchloric acid (PCA) solution and then shake vigorously for 30 s. Transfer the clear supernatant obtained after centrifugation at 1200 g for 15 min to a small test tube. Prepare a sham extract by adding 1 ml of 9 g/l NaCl to 4 ml of 4% PCA solution.[35]

Add 500 μl of water and 300 μl of 1 mol/l glycine buffer to each of two cuvettes. To correct for optical differences between the cuvettes, read the sample cuvette against the blank at 260 and at 280 nm, giving readings B^{260} and B^{280}. Add 200 μl of the red cell extract to the sample cuvette and 200 μl of the sham extract to the blank cuvette. With the spectrometer zeroed at 260 nm on the blank cuvette, read the sample cuvette to obtain the value S^{260}. Repeat the process at 280 nm to obtain the reading S^{280}.

The A^{260}/A^{280} absorbance ratio (R) is calculated by subtracting the cuvette blank readings (positive or negative) at 260 and 280 nm from the readings obtained on the red cell extract when blanked against the sham extract:

$$R = \frac{S^{260} - B^{260}}{S^{280} - B^{280}}$$

Interpretation

The A^{260}/A^{280} absorbance ratio of freshly collected washed red cells has been reported to be 3.11 ± 0.41 (mean ± SD). Absorbance ratios of <2.29 imply that the concentration of cytidine nucleotide is increased and suggest a reduced level of P5N. Selective accumulation of pyrimidines owing to putative defect in CDP choline phosphotransferase has been reported in rare patients with a disorder that resembles P5N deficiency characterized by haemolytic anaemia and basophilic stippling.

Samples showing a significantly reduced absorbance ratio should have a specific assay for P5N carried out.[36] This is likely to require referral to a reference laboratory where a nucleotide profile may also be undertaken. Nucleotide extraction followed by radiolabelling and separation by high-performance liquid chromatography can be performed. The nucleotides have characteristic UV absorption spectra and retention times, which permit subsequent radiodetection and quantification.

RED CELL ENZYME ASSAYS

As is illustrated in Figure 12.4, a large number of enzymes play a part in the metabolism of glucose in the red cell and genetically determined variants of almost all the enzymes are known to occur. This means that in investigating a patient suspected of suffering from a hereditary enzyme-deficiency haemolytic anaemia, multiple enzyme assays may be needed to identify the defect. In practice, however, G6PD deficiency and PK deficiency should be excluded first because of the relative frequency (common in the case of G6PD, not rare in the case of PK) with which variants of these enzymes are associated with deficiency and increased haemolysis.

Many methods are available for assaying each enzyme and for this reason the ICSH has produced simplified methods suitable for diagnostic purposes.[37] These methods are not necessarily the most appropriate for detailed study of the kinetic properties of the variant enzymes, but they are relatively simple to set up and allow comparison of results between different laboratories.

General Points of Technique

Collection of Blood Samples

Blood samples may be anticoagulated with heparin (10 iu/ml blood), EDTA (1.5 mg/ml blood) or ACD (for formulae and volumes see below). In any of these anticoagulants, all normal enzymes are stable for 6 days (and most for 20 days) at 4°C and for 24 h at 25°C. However, enzyme variants in samples from patients may be less stable. Therefore, we recommend that ACD is used as anticoagulant and that the samples are tested promptly. Ideally, samples of blood should be transferred to central laboratories in tubes surrounded by wet ice at 4°C. Frozen samples are unsuitable because the cells are lysed by freezing. Further details of enzyme stability were given by Beutler.[21] Approx. 1 ml of blood is required for each enzyme assay.

Preparation of Acid–Citrate–Dextrose (ACD) Solution – NIH-A

Trisodium citrate, dihydrate (75 mmol/l) – 22 g
Citric acid, monohydrate (42 mmol/l) – 8 g
Dextrose (139 mmol/l) – 25 g
Water to 1 litre.

Sterilize the solution by autoclaving at 121°C for 15 min. Its pH is 5.4. For use, add 10 volumes of blood to 1.5 volumes of solution.

Separation of Red Cells from Blood Samples

Leucocytes and platelets generally have higher enzyme activities than red cells. Moreover, with many enzyme deficiencies, notably PK deficiency, the decrease in enzyme activity may be much less pronounced in leucocytes and platelets than in red cells or it even may be absent. It is therefore necessary to prepare red cells which are as free from contamination as possible. Various methods are suitable (see ICSH);[37] two are described in the following.

Washing the Red Cells

Centrifuge the anticoagulated blood at 1200–1500 g for 5 min and remove the plasma together with the buffy coat layer.

Resuspend the cells in 9 g/l NaCl (saline) and repeat the procedure three times. This will remove about 80–90% of the leucocytes.

This simple method is adequate in most instances when more complicated manoeuvres are impractical, but it has the disadvantage that some of the reticulocytes and young red cells are lost together with the buffy coat. In addition, the remaining leucocytes may still be sufficient to cause misleading results – for instance, in PK deficiency. Therefore, ideally the following method should be adopted.

Filtration through Microcrystalline Cellulose Mixtures

Pure red cell suspensions can be made from whole blood by filtering the blood through a mixed bed of microcrystalline cellulose (mean size 50 μm) and α-cellulose. Mix approx. 0.5 g of each type of cellulose with 20 ml of ice-cold saline; this gives sufficient slurry for 3–5 columns. The barrel of a 5 ml syringe is used as a column. The outlet of the syringe is blocked with absorbent cotton wool, equal in volume to the 1 ml mark on the barrel. Pour the well-shaken slurry into the column to give a bed volume of 1–2 ml after the saline has run through. Wash the bed with 5 ml of saline to remove any 'fines.' When the saline has run through, pipette 1–2 ml of whole blood onto the column, taking care not to disturb the bed. Collect the filtrate, and once the blood has completely run into the bed, wash the column through with 5–7 ml of saline. The column should be made freshly for each batch of enzyme assays and used promptly.

By this method, about 99% of the leucocytes and about 90% of the platelets are removed. About 97% of the red cells are recovered and reticulocytes are not removed selectively. The procedure should not alter the age or size of distribution of the recovered red cells compared to native blood. This should be checked with each new batch of cellulose by counting reticulocytes.

Wash the cells collected from the column twice in 10 volumes of ice-cold saline and finally resuspend them in the saline to give a 50% suspension.

Determine the Hb and/or red cell count in a sample of the suspension.

Preparation of Haemolysate

Mix 1 volume of the washed or filtered suspension with 9 volumes of lysing solution consisting of 2.7 mmol/l EDTA, pH 7.0, and 0.7 mmol/l 2-mercaptoethanol (100 mg of EDTA disodium salt and 5 μl of 2-mercaptoethanol in 100 ml of water); adjust the pH to 7.0 with HCl or NaOH.

Ensure complete lysis by freeze-thawing. Rapid freezing is achieved using a dry-ice acetone bath or methanol that has been cooled to −20°C. Thawing is achieved in a waterbath at 25°C or simply in water at room temperature. Usually the haemolysate is ready for use without further centrifugation, but a 1-min spin in a microfuge is recommended to remove any turbidity (this may be unsuitable for some red cell enzymes that are stroma-bound). Dilutions, when necessary, are carried out in the lysing solution. The haemolysate should be prepared freshly for each batch of enzyme assays. Most enzymes in haemolysates are stable for 8 h at 0°C, but it is best to carry out assays immediately. G6PD is one of the least stable enzymes in this haemolysate and its assay should be conducted within 1 or 2 h of the lysate being prepared. The storing of frozen cells or haemolysates is not recommended; it is preferable to store whole blood in ACD.

Control Samples

Control samples should always be assayed at the same time as the test samples even when a normal range for the various enzymes has been established.

Take the control samples of blood at the same time as the test samples and treat them in the same way. When receiving samples from outside sources, always ask for a normal 'shipment control' to be included.

Reaction Buffer

The ICSH recommendation is for a Tris-HCl/EDTA buffer that is appropriate for all the common enzyme assays. The buffer consists of 1 mol/l Tris-HCl and 5 mmol/l Na$_2$EDTA, the pH being adjusted to 8.0 with HCl.

Dissolve 12.11 g of Tris (hydroxymethyl) methylamine and 168 mg of Na$_2$EDTA in water; adjust the pH to 8.0 with 1 mol/l HCl and bring the volume to 100 ml at 25°C.

Only two assays will be described in detail – those for G6PD and PK. However, the principles of these assays apply

to all other enzyme assays. The assays are carried out in a spectrometer at a wavelength of 340 nm unless otherwise indicated. A final reaction mixture of 1.0 ml (or 3.0 ml) is suitable, the quantities given in the text being for 1.0 ml reaction mixtures unless otherwise stated. All dilutions of auxiliary enzymes are made in the lysing solution and all working materials should be kept in an icebath until ready for use. The assays are carried out at a controlled temperature, 30°C being the most appropriate. Cuvettes loaded with the assay reagents should be preincubated at this temperature for 10 min before starting the reaction. In most cases, the reaction is started by the addition of substrate. Many spectrometers have a built-in or attached recorder, by which the absorbance changes can be conveniently measured. If no recorder is available, visual readings should be made every 60 s. In any case, the reaction should be followed for 5–10 min and it is essential to ensure that during this time the change in absorbance is linear with time.

G6PD Assay

The reactions involving G6PD have already been described (p. 255). The activity of the enzyme is assayed by following the rate of production of NADPH, which, unlike NADP, has a peak of UV light absorption at 340 nm.

Method

The assays are carried out at 30°C; the cuvettes containing the first four reagents and water are incubated for 10 min before starting the reaction by adding the substrate, as shown in Table 12.4. Commercial kits are also available.*

The change in absorbance following the addition of the substrate is measured over the first 5 min of the reaction. The value of the blank is subtracted from the test reaction, either automatically or by calculation.

Calculation of Enzyme Activity

The activities of the enzymes in the haemolysate are calculated from the initial rate of change of NADPH accumulation:

$$\text{G6PD activity in the lysate (in mol/ml)} = \Delta A/\min \times \frac{10^3}{6.22}$$

where 6.22 is the mmol extinction coefficient of NADPH at 340 nm and 10^3 is the factor appropriate for the dilutions in the reaction mixture. Results are expressed per 10^{10} red cells, per ml red cells or per g Hb by reference to the respective values obtained with the washed red cell suspension. However, the ICSH recommendation is to

*Trinity Biotech, Bray, Co. Wicklow, Ireland.

Table 12.4 Glucose-6-phosphate dehydrogenase assay		
REAGENTS	ASSAY (μl)	BLANK (μl)
Tris-HCl EDTA buffer, pH 8.0	100	100
MgCl$_2$ 100 mmol/l	100	100
NADP 2 mmol/l	100	100
1:20 haemolysate	20	20
Water	580	680
Start reaction by adding: G6P 6 mmol/l	100	–

EDTA, ethylenediaminetetra-acetic acid; NADP, nicotinamide adenine dinucleotide phosphate; G6P, glucose-6-phosphate.

express values per g Hb and it is ideal to determine the Hb concentration of the haemolysate directly. When doing this, use a haemolysate to Drabkin's solution ratio of 1:25.

G6PD is very stable and, with most variants, venous blood may be stored in ACD for up to 3 weeks at 4°C without loss of activity.

Some enzyme-deficient variants lose activity more rapidly and this will cause deficiency to appear more severe than it is. Therefore, for diagnostic purposes, a delay in assaying well-conserved samples should not be a deterrent.

Normal Values

The normal range for G6PD activity should be determined in each laboratory. If the ICSH method is used, values should not differ widely from the given values. Results are expressed in enzyme units (eu), which are the μ moles (μmol) of substrate converted per min.

For adults, these values are 8.83 ± 1.59 eu/g Hb at 30°C. However, newborns and infants may have enzyme activity that deviates appreciably from the adult value.[37,38] In one study, the newborn mean activity was about 150% of the adult mean.[39]

Interpretation of Results

In assessing the clinical relevance of a G6PD assay result, three important facts must be kept in mind:

1. The gene for G6PD is on the X-chromosome and therefore males, having only one G6PD gene, can be only either normal or deficient hemizygotes. By contrast, females, who have two allelic genes, can be either normal homozygotes or heterozygotes

with 'intermediate' enzyme activity or deficient homozygotes.

2. Red cells are likely to haemolyse on account of G6PD deficiency only if they have less than about 20% of the normal enzyme activity.

3. G6PD activity falls off markedly as red cells age. Therefore, whenever a blood sample has a young red cell population, G6PD activity will be higher than normal, sometimes to the extent that a genetically deficient sample may yield a value within the normal range. This usually, but not always, will be associated with a marked reticulocytosis.

In practice, the following notes may be useful:

1. In males, diagnosis does not present difficulties in most cases because the demarcation between normal and deficient subjects is sharp. There are very few acquired situations in which G6PD activity is decreased (one is pure red cell aplasia where there is reticulocytopenia), whereas an increased G6PD activity is found in all acute and chronic haemolytic states with reticulocytosis. Therefore a G6PD value below a well-established normal range always indicates G6PD deficiency. A value in the low-normal range in the face of reticulocytosis should also raise the suspicion of G6PD deficiency because with reticulocytosis G6PD activity should be *higher* than normal. In such suspicious cases, G6PD deficiency can be confirmed by repeating the assay when the reticulocytosis has subsided or by assaying older red cells after density fractionation or by conducting family studies.

2. In females, all the same criteria apply, with the added consideration that heterozygosity can *never* be rigorously ruled out by a G6PD assay; for this purpose, the cytochemical test described on p. 258 is more useful than a spectrometric assay and a counsel of perfection is to use the two in conjunction with each other and with family studies. However, in most cases, a normal value in a female means that she is a normal homozygote, and a value of <10% of normal means that she is a deficient homozygote (Table 12.5); but a few heterozygotes may fall in either of these ranges because of the 'extreme phenotypes' that can be associated with an unbalanced ratio of the mosaicism consequent on X-chromosome inactivation. Any value between 10% and 90% of normal usually means a heterozygote, except for the complicating effect of reticulocytosis. As far as the clinical significance of heterozygosity for G6PD deficiency is concerned, it is important to remember that, because of mosaicism, a fraction of red cells in heterozygotes (on the average, 50%) is as enzyme-deficient as in a hemizygous male and therefore susceptible to haemolysis. The severity of potential clinical complications is roughly proportional to the fraction of deficient red cells.

Table 12.5 Glucose-6-phosphate dehydrogenase in various clinical situations (activity in enzyme units [eu] per g haemoglobin)

Male genotypes	Gd⁺	Gd⁻	
Female genotypes	Gd⁺/ Gd⁺	Gd⁻/ Gd⁻	Gd⁺/ Gd⁻
In health	7–10	<2	2–7
In increased haemolysis unrelated to G6PD deficiency	15	4	4–9
During recovery from G6PD-related anaemia	–	6.5	6–10

G6PD, glucose-6-phosphate dehydrogenase.
The values quoted are examples.
Gd⁺ designates an allele encoding normal G6PD; *Gd⁻* designates an allele encoding a variant associated with G6PD deficiency.

Therefore, within the heterozygote range, the actual value of the assay (or the proportion of deficient red cells estimated by the cytochemical test) correlates with the risk of haemolysis. During an acute episode, heterozygotes may be missed if their deficient red cells have undergone haemolysis, thus leaving only the normal population in circulation. This can occur before a reticulocyte response becomes apparent and may result in G6PD activity within the normal range.

Identification of G6PD Variants

There are many variants of G6PD in different populations with enzyme activities ranging from nearly 0 to 500% of normal activity.[40] Classification and provisional identification of variants are based on their physicochemical and enzymic characteristics.[41] Criteria were laid down by a World Health Organization scientific group[23] for the minimum requirements for identification of such variants and these recommendations have now been revised.[42] The tests are carried out on male hemizygotes and are as follows:

Red cell G6PD activity
Electrophoretic migration
Michaelis constant (K_m) for G6PD
Relative rate of utilization of 2-deoxyG6P (2dG6P)
Thermal stability.

The full amino acid sequence of G6PD has been established and definitive identification can be made by sequence analysis at the DNA level.[43,44] Diagnosis of G6PD deficiency by molecular analysis may be clinically useful when a patient has received a large volume of transfused blood or when a reticulocytosis results in a normal enzyme assay level; also,

females who are heterozygous deficient can readily be identified.

PYRUVATE KINASE ASSAY

Many variants of PK have deficient enzyme activity *in vivo*.[45,46] In most cases, deficient activity can be identified by simple enzyme assay. However, PK activity in red cells is subject to regulation by a number of effector molecules. With some PK variants, the maximum velocity (V_{max}) of the enzyme is normal or nearly so, but at the low-substrate concentrations found *in vivo* PK activity may be sufficiently low to cause haemolysis, either because affinity for the substrates, phosphoenolpyruvate (PEP) and ADP, is low or because binding of the important allosteric ligand, fructose-1,6-diphosphate, is altered. Some of these unusual variants can be identified by carrying out the enzyme assay not only understandard conditions but also at low-substrate concentrations. Functional PK deficiency can also be identified by finding high concentrations of the substrates immediately above the block in the glycolytic pathway, particularly 2,3-DPG.[47] (For measurement of 2,3-DPG, see p. 266).

PK deficiency is inherited as an autosomal recessive condition.

Method

The preparation of haemolysate, buffer and lysing solution is exactly the same as for the G6PD assay. In the PK assay it is particularly important to remove as many contaminating leucocytes and platelets as possible because these cells may be unaffected by a deficiency affecting the red cells and may have high activities of PK. The principle of the assay is as follows:

$$PEP + ADP \xrightarrow{PK} pyruvate + ATP$$

The pyruvate so formed is reduced to lactate in a reaction catalysed by lactate dehydrogenase (LDH) with the conversion of NADH (reduced form of nicotinamide adenine dinucleotide) to NAD:

$$pyruvate + NADH \xrightarrow{LDH} lactate + NAD$$

To ensure that this secondary reaction is not rate limiting, LDH is added in excess to the reaction mixture and the PK activity is measured by the rate of fall of absorbance at 340 nm.

The reaction conditions are established in a 1 ml cuvette at 30°C by adding all the reagents shown in Table 12.6, except the substrate PEP, to the cuvette and incubating them at 30°C for 10 min before starting the reaction by the addition of the PEP.

The amounts to be added for low-substrate conditions are also shown in Table 12.6.

Table 12.6 Reagents for pyruvate kinase assay

REAGENTS	ASSAY (μl)	BLANK (μl)	LOW-S (μl)
Tris-HCl EDTA buffer, pH 8.0	100	100	100
KCl 1 mol/l	100	100	100
MgCl$_2$ 100 mmol/l	100	100	100
NADH 2 mmol/l	100	100	100
ADP, neutralized 30 mmol/l	50	–	20
LDH 60 u/ml	100	100	100
1:20 haemolysate	20	20	20
Water	330	380	455
PEP 50 mmol/l	100	100	5

Low-S, low-substrate conditions; EDTA, ethylenediaminetetra-acetic acid; NADH, reduced form of nicotinamide adenine dinucleotide; ADP, adenosine diphosphate; LDH, lactate dehydrogenase; PEP, phosphoenolpyruvate:

The change in absorbance (A) is measured over the first 5 min and the activity of the enzyme in micromoles of NADH reduced/min/ml haemolysate is calculated as follows:

$$\frac{\Delta A/min}{6.22} \times 10$$

where 6.22 is the millimolar extinction coefficient of NADH at 340 nm.

Express results as for G6PD.

A blank assay should be carried out to be certain that the LDH is free of PK activity. Use the 2-mercapto-ethanol-EDTA stabilizing solution (p. 261) in place of haemolysate for both the blank and system mixtures. If no change in absorbance is observed, indicating that the LDH is free of contaminating PK, it is unnecessary to recheck on subsequent assays. Otherwise, the blank rate must be subtracted in computing the true enzyme activity each time.

Normal Values

As with all enzyme assays, a normal range should be determined for each laboratory. Values should however, not be widely different between laboratories if the ICSH methods are used. The normal range of PK activity at 30°C is 10.3 ± 2 eu/g Hb. At a low-substrate concentration, the normal activity is 15 ± 3% of that at the high-substrate concentration. Mean neonatal value is about 140% that of adults.[39]

Interpretation of Results

PK, like G6PD, is an age-dependent red cell enzyme. But unlike G6PD deficiency, PK deficiency is usually associated with *chronic* haemolysis. Therefore patients in whom PK deficiency is suspected almost invariably have a reticulocytosis and if their PK level is below the normal range, they can be considered to be PK deficient. Thus, once the technique and normal values are well established in a laboratory, and provided controls are always included, the main problem is of underdiagnosis rather than of overdiagnosis of PK deficiency. One additional way to pick up abnormal variants has been included in the method recommended (i.e. the use of low-substrate concentrations). Even so, PK deficiency may be missed because marked reticulocytosis may increase PK activity significantly. This means that a PK activity in the normal range in the presence of a marked reticulocytosis is highly suspicious of inherited PK deficiency (because with reticulocytosis the activity ought to be *higher* than normal). In such cases, the importance of family studies cannot be overemphasized. Heterozygotes have about 50% of the normal PK activity, sometimes less, but they do not suffer from haemolysis. Therefore, the heterozygous parents of a patient may have a red cell PK activity lower than that of their homozygous PK-deficient offspring; this finding may clinch the diagnosis. In this context, assay of an alternative red cell age-dependent enzyme (e.g. G6PD or hexokinase) may be a useful aid to interpretation.

ESTIMATION OF REDUCED GLUTATHIONE

The red cell has a high concentration of the sulphydryl containing tripeptide, GSH. An important function of GSH in the red cell is the detoxification of low levels of hydrogen peroxide, which may form spontaneously or as a result of drug administration. GSH may also function in maintaining the integrity of the red cell by reducing sulphydryl groups of Hb, membrane proteins and enzymes that may have become oxidized. Maintenance of normal levels of GSH is a major function of the hexose monophosphate shunt. Reduction of GSSG (oxidized glutathione) back to the functional GSH is linked to the rate of reduction of NADP$^+$ in the initial step of the shunt.[48]

Principle

The method described is based on the development of a yellow colour when 5,5'-dithiobis (2-nitrobenzoic acid) (Ellman's reagent, DTNB) is added to sulphydryl compounds. The colour that develops is fairly stable for about 10 min and the reaction is little affected by variation in temperature.

The reaction is read at 412 nm. GSH in red cells is relatively stable and venous blood samples anticoagulated with ACD maintain GSH levels for up to 3 weeks at 4°C. GSH is slowly oxidized in solution, so only fresh lysates should be used for the assay.

Reagents

Lysing solution

Disodium EDTA, 1 g/l.

Precipitating reagent

Metaphosphoric acid (sticks), 1.67 g; disodium EDTA, 0.2 g; NaCl, 30 g; water to 100 ml.

Solution is more rapid if the reagents are added to boiling water and the volume is made up after cooling. This solution is stable for at least 3 weeks at 4°C. If any EDTA remains undissolved, the clear supernatant should be used.

Disodium hydrogen phosphate

300 mmol/l. $Na_2HPO_4.12H_2O$, 107.4 g/l or Na_2HPO_4. $2H_2O$, 53.4 g/l or anhydrous Na_2HPO_4, 4.6 g/l.

Sodium citrate

34 mmol/l, pH 8.0. Dissolve 1 g of sodium citrate (trisodium salt) in 100 ml water.

DTNB reagent

Dissolve 20 mg of DTNB in 100 ml of 34 mmol/l sodium citrate solution.

The solution is stable for up to 3 months at 4°C.

Glutathione standards

When standard curves are constructed, suitable dilutions are made from a 1.62 mmol/l (50 mg/dl) stock solution of GSH.

The stock solution should be made freshly with degassed (boiled) water or saline for each run because GSH oxidizes slowly in solution.

Method

Add 0.2 ml of well-mixed, anticoagulated blood of which the PCV, red cell count and Hb have been determined, to 1.8 ml of lysing solution and allow to stand at room temperature for no more than 5 min for lysis to be completed, because glutathione oxidizes very rapidly when exposed to air.

Add 3 ml of precipitating solution, mix the solution well and allow to stand for a further 5 min.

After re-mixing, filter through a single-thickness Whatman No. 42 filter paper.

Add 1 ml of clear filtrate to 4 ml of freshly made Na_2HPO_4 solution. Record the absorbance at 412 nm (A_1). Then add 0.5 ml of the DTNB reagent and mix well by inversion.

The colour develops rapidly but begins to fade after about 10 min so the second reading should be within this period. Record the absorbance at 412 nm (A_2) and calculate the change in absorbance (ΔA^{412}).

A reagent blank is made using saline or plasma instead of whole blood.

If assays are carried out frequently, it is not necessary to construct standard curves for each batch. They are, however, essential initially to calibrate the apparatus used and should be done regularly to check the suitability of the reagents. Suitable dilutions of GSH are achieved by substituting 5, 10, 20 and 40 μl of the 1.62 mmol/l stock solution (make up to 0.2 ml with lysing solution) for the blood in the reaction.

Calculation

Determination of extinction coefficient (ε)

The molar extinction coefficient of the chromophore at 412 nm is 13 600. This only applies when a narrow band wavelength is available. When a broader waveband is used, the extinction coefficient is lower.

The system may be calibrated by comparing the extinction absorbance in the test system (D_2) with that obtained in a spectrometer with a narrow band at 412 nm (D_1). The derived correction factor, E_1, is given by D_1/D_2 and is constant for the test system.

Calculation of GSH Concentration

The amount of GSH in the cuvette sample (GSH_c) is given by the following:

$$\Delta A^{412} \times \frac{E_1}{\varepsilon} \times 5.5 \ \mu mol$$

The concentration of GSH in the whole blood sample is as follows:

$$\frac{GSH_c \times 5}{0.2} \mu mol/ml$$

The unit is often expressed in terms of mg/dl of red cells. The molecular weight of GSH is 307. Thus, GSH in mg/ dl packed red cells is given by the following:

$$\frac{GSH_c \times 5}{0.2} \times \frac{1}{PCV} \times 307 \times 100$$

Normal Range

The normal range may be expressed in a number of ways (e.g. 6.57 ± 1.04 μmol/g Hb or 223 ± 35 μmol (or 69 ± 11 mg)/dl packed red cells). Neonatal mean value is about 150% that of adults.[39]

Significance

Glutathione replenishment in mature red cells is accomplished through the consecutive action of two enzymes: γ-glutamylcysteine synthetase and glutathione synthetase. Although very rare, hereditary deficiency of either enzyme virtually abolishes the synthesis of GSH. The deficient cells are very prone to oxidative destruction and are short lived, resulting in a non-spherocytic haemolytic anaemia.

Increases in GSH have been described in various conditions such as dyserythropoiesis, primary myelofibrosis, pyrimidine 5′-nucleotidase deficiency and other rare congenital haemolytic anaemias of unknown aetiology.

Glutathione Stability Test

Principle

In normal subjects, incubation of red cells with the oxidizing drug acetylphenylhydrazine has little effect on the GSH content because its oxidation is reversed by glutathione reductase, which in turn relies on G6PD for a supply to NADPH. Therefore, in subjects who are G6PD deficient, the stability of GSH is significantly reduced.

Reagents

Acetylphenylhydrazine

670 mmol/l. Dissolve 100 mg in 1 ml of acetone.

Transfer 0.05 ml volumes (containing 5 mg of acetylphenylhydrazine) by pipette to the bottom of 12×75 mm glass tubes. Dry the contents of the tubes in an incubator at 37°C, stopper and store in the dark until used.

Method

Venous blood, anticoagulated with EDTA, heparin or ACD, may be used; it may be freshly collected or previously stored at 4°C for up to 1 week.

Add 1 ml to a tube containing acetylphenylhydrazine and place another 1 ml in a similar tube not containing the chemical. Invert the tubes several times and then incubate them at 37°C.

After 1 h, mix the contents of the tubes once more and incubate the tubes for a further 1 h. At the end of this time determine and compare the GSH concentration in the test sample and in the control sample.

Interpretation

In normal adult subjects, red cell GSH is lowered by not more than 20% by incubation with acetylphenylhydrazine. In subjects who are G6PD deficient, it is lowered by more than this: in heterozygotes (females), the fall may amount to about 50%, whereas in hemizygotes (males) the fall is often much greater and almost all may be lost.

The test is not specific for G6PD deficiency and other rare defects of the pentose phosphate pathway may give abnormal results.

Glutathione and Glutathione Stability in Infants

During the first few days after birth, the red cells have a normal or high content of GSH. On the addition of acetylphenylhydrazine, the GSH is unstable in both normal infants and infants who are G6PD deficient. In normal infants, however, the instability can be corrected by the addition of glucose and, by the time the normal infant is 3–4 days old, the cells behave like adult cells.[49,50]

2,3-DIPHOSPHOGLYCERATE

The importance of the high concentration of 2,3-DPG in the red cells of man was recognized at about the same time by Chanutin and Curnish[51] and Benesch and Benesch.[52] 2,3-DPG binds to a specific site in the β chain of Hb and it decreases its oxygen affinity by shifting the balance of the so-called T and R conformations of the molecule. The higher the concentration of 2,3-DPG, the greater the partial pressure of oxygen (pO_2) needed to produce the same oxygen saturation of Hb. This is reflected in a 2,3-DPG-dependent shift in the oxygen dissociation curve.

Measurement of the concentration of 2,3-DPG in red cells may also be useful in identifying the probable site of an enzyme deficiency in the metabolic pathway. In general, enzyme defects cause an increase in the concentration of metabolic intermediates above the level of the block and a decrease in concentration below the block. Thus 2,3-DPG is increased in PK deficiency and decreased in hexokinase deficiency. In most other disorders of the glycolytic pathway, however, the 2,3-DPG concentration is normal because increased activity through the pentose phosphate pathway allows a normal flux of metabolites through the triose part of the glycolytic pathway.

Measurement of Red Cell 2,3-Diphosphoglycerate

Various methods have been used to assay 2,3-DPG. Krimsky[53] used the catalytic properties of 2,3-DPG in the conversion of 3-phosphoglycerate (3PG) to 2-phosphoglycerate (2PG) by phosphoglycerate mutase (PGM). At very low concentrations of 2,3-DPG, the rate of conversion is proportional to the concentration of 2,3-DPG. This method is elegant and extremely sensitive but too cumbersome for routine use. A fluorometric method was described by Lowry et al.,[54] and this has been modified for spectrometry.

Rose and Liebowitz[55] found that glycolate-2-phosphate increased the 2,3-DPG phosphatase activity of PGM and a quantitative assay of the substrate, 2,3-DPG, was evolved on this basis.

Principle

2,3-DPG is hydrolysed to 3PG by the phosphatase activity of PGM stimulated by glycolate-2-phosphate. This reaction is linked to the conversion of NADH to NAD by glyceraldehyde-3-phosphate dehydrogenase (Ga3PD) and phosphoglycerate kinase (PGK):

$$2,3\text{-}DPG \xrightarrow[\text{(glycolate-2-phosphate)}]{\text{2,3-DPG phosphatase}} 3PG + Pi$$

$$3PG + ATP \xrightarrow{\text{PGK}} 1,2\text{-}DPG + ADP$$

$$1,3\text{-}DPG + NADH \xrightarrow{\text{Ga3PD}} Ga3P + Pi + NAD^+$$

The fail in absorbance at 340 nm, as NADH is oxidized, is measured.

Reagents

Triethanolamine buffer

0.2 mol/l, pH 8.0.

Dissolve 9.3 g of triethanolamine hydrochloride in $c200$ ml of water; then add 0.5 g of disodium EDTA and 0.25 g of $MgSO_4.7H_2O$. Adjust the pH to 8.0 with 2 mol/l KOH (approx. 15 ml) and make up the volume to 250 ml with water.

ATP, sodium salt

20 mg/ml. Dissolved in buffer, this is stable for several months when frozen.

NADH, sodium salt

10 mg/ml. When dissolved in buffer, this is relatively unstable and should be made freshly each day.

Glyceraldehyde-3-phosphate dehydrogenase/ phosphoglycerate kinase

Mixed crystalline suspension in ammonium sulphate.

phosphoglycerate mutase

Crystalline suspension from rabbit muscle in ammonium sulphate ($c2500$ u/ml).

Glycolate-2-phosphate

2-Phosphoglycolic acid, 10 mg/ml. After dissolving in water, this is stable for several months if kept frozen.

Method

Freshly drawn blood in EDTA or heparin may be used. If there is an unavoidable delay in starting the assay, blood (4 volumes) should be added to CPD anticoagulant (1 volume) and stored at 4°C. A control blood sample should be taken at the same time.

2,3-DPG levels are stable for 48 h if the blood is stored in this way. The Hb, red cell count and PCV should be measured on part of the sample. It is not necessary to remove leucocytes or platelets.

Deproteinization

Add 1 ml of blood to 3 ml of ice-cold 80 g/l trichloroacetic acid (TCA) in a 10 ml conical centrifuge tube.

Shake the tube vigorously, preferably on an automatic rotor mixer, and then allow to stand for 5–10 min for complete deproteinization. The shaking is important; otherwise some of the precipitated protein will remain on the surface of the mixture.

Centrifuge at about 1200 g for 5–10 min at 4°C to obtain a clear supernatant. The 2,3-DPG in the supernatant is stable for 2–3 weeks when stored at 4°C; it is stable indefinitely if frozen.

Reaction

Deliver the reagents into a silica or high-quality glass cuvette, with a 1 cm light path. The quantities in Table 12.7 are for a 4 ml cuvette:

Warm the mixtures at 30°C for 10 min and record the absorbance of both test and blank mixtures at 340 nm. Then start the reaction by the addition of 100 μl of glycolate-2-phosphate.

Remeasure the absorbance (at 35 min) of the test and blank mixtures on completion of the reaction.

Make further measurements after a further 5 min to make sure the reaction is complete.

Only one blank is required for each batch of test samples.

Table 12.7 Quantities for a 4 ml cuvette		
	TEST	**BLANK**
Triethanolamine buffer	2.50 ml	2.50 ml
ATP	100 μl	100 μl
NADH	100 μl	100 μl
Deproteinized extract	250 μl	–
Ga-3-PD/PGK mixture	30 μl	30 μl
PGM	20 μl	20 μl
Water	–	250 μl
	3.00 ml	3.00 ml

Calculation

2,3-DPG (μmol/ml blood)

$$= (\Delta A\ \text{test} - \Delta A\ \text{blank}) \times \frac{3.10}{6.22} \times 16$$

$$= (\Delta A\ \text{test} - \Delta A\ \text{blank}) \times 8 = D$$

where 3.10 = the volume of reaction mixture, 6.22 = mmolar extinction coefficient of NADH at 340 nm and 16 = dilution of original blood sample (1 ml in 3.0 ml of TCA, 0.25 ml added to cuvette).

The results of 2,3-DPG assays are best expressed in terms of Hb content or red cell volume. Thus, if the result of the previous calculation is represented by D, then:

$$\frac{D \times 1000}{(\text{Hb})} = 2,3\text{-DPG in } \mu\text{molg/ Hb}$$

or

$$\frac{D \times 1000}{(\text{Hb})} \times \frac{64}{1000} = 2,3\text{-DPG in } \mu\text{mol}/\mu\text{mol Hb}$$

and

$$D \times \frac{1}{\text{PCV}} = 2,3\text{-DPG in } \mu\text{mol/ml (packed) red cells}$$

where Hb = Hb in g/l of whole blood and 64 is the molecular weight of Hb $\times 10^{-3}$.

The molar ratio of 2,3-DPG to Hb in normal blood is about 0.75:1.

Normal Range

The normal range is 4.5–5.1 μmol/ml packed red cells or 10.5–16.2 μmol/g Hb. Neonatal values are about 20% lower than adult.[39]

Each laboratory should determine its own normal range.

Significance of 2,3-DPG Concentration

An increase in 2,3-DPG concentration is found in most conditions in which the arterial blood is undersaturated with oxygen, as in congenital heart and chronic lung diseases, in most acquired anaemias, at high altitudes, in alkalosis and in hyperphosphataemia. Decreased 2,3-DPG levels occur in hypophosphataemic states and in acidosis.

Acidosis, which shifts the oxygen dissociation curve to the right, causes a fall in 2,3-DPG, so that the oxygen dissociation curve of whole blood from patients with chronic acidosis (such as patients in diabetic coma or precoma) may have nearly normal dissociation curves. A rapid correction of the acidosis will lead to a major shift of the curve to the left (i.e. to a marked increase in the affinity of Hb for oxygen, which may lead to tissue hypoxia). Caution should

therefore be exercised in correcting acidosis. Measurement of oxygen dissociation is described below.

From the diagnostic point of view, the main importance of 2,3-DPG determination is (1) in haemolytic anaemias and (2) in the interpretation of changes in the oxygen affinity of blood.

1. As already mentioned, increased or decreased 2,3-DPG may be associated with glycolytic enzyme defects and increased 2,3-DPG (up to 2 to 3 times normal) is particularly characteristic of most patients with PK deficiency. Although this finding certainly cannot be regarded as diagnostic, a normal or low 2,3-DPG makes PK deficiency most unlikely.

2. Whenever a shift in the oxygen dissociation curve is observed and an abnormal Hb with altered oxygen affinity is suspected, determination of 2,3-DPG is essential. Indeed, there is a simple correlation between 2,3-DPG level and p_{50}, from which it is possible to work out whether any change in p_{50} is explained by an altered level of 2,3-DPG.[56]

2,3-DPG levels are generally slightly lower than normal in HS and this probably accounts for the slight erythrocytosis that is sometimes seen after splenectomy. Extremely low red cell 2,3-DPG concentration associated with erythrocytosis has been reported in a kindred with complete 2,3-diphosphoglycerate mutase deficiency.[57]

OXYGEN DISSOCIATION CURVE

The oxygen dissociation curve is the expression of the relationship between the partial pressure of oxygen and oxygen saturation of Hb. Details of this relationship and the physiological importance of changes in this relationship were worked out in detail at the beginning of this century by the great physiologists Hüfner, Bohr, Barcroft, Henderson and many others. Their work was summarized by Peters and Van Slyke in *Quantitative Clinical Chemistry*.[58] The relevant chapters of this book have been reprinted and it would be difficult to improve their description of the importance of the oxygen dissociation curve.

The physiological value of Hb as an oxygen carrier lies in the fact that its affinity for oxygen is so nicely balanced that in the lungs Hb becomes 95%–96% oxygenated, whereas in the tissues and capillaries it can give up as much of the gas as is demanded. If the affinity were much less, complete oxygenation in the lungs could not be approached; if it were greater, the tissues would have difficulty in removing from the blood the oxygen they need. Because the affinity is adjusted as it is, both oxyhaemoglobin and reduced Hb exist in all parts of the circulation but in greatly varied proportions.

Measuring the Oxygen Dissociation Curve

Determination of the oxygen dissociation curve depends on two measurements: pO_2 with which the blood is equilibrated and the proportion of Hb that is saturated with oxygen. Methods for determining the dissociation curve fall into three main groups:

1. The pO_2 is set by the experimental conditions and the percentage saturation of Hb is measured.
2. The percentage saturation is predetermined by mixing known proportions of oxygenated and deoxygenated blood and the pO_2 is measured.
3. The change in oxygen content of the blood is plotted continuously against pO_2 during oxygenation or deoxygenation and the percentage saturation is calculated.

The multiplicity of methods available for measuring the oxygen dissociation curve suggests that no method is ideal. The advantages and disadvantages of the various techniques have been reviewed.[59,60] The standard method with which new methods are compared is the gasometric method of Van Slyke and Neill.[61] This method is slow, demands considerable expertise and is not suitable for most haematology laboratories. Commercial instruments are now available for performing the test and drawing the complete oxygen dissociation curve.* Such analysers are extremely quick and accurate and are therefore ideal for laboratories performing multiple determinations. Approximate measurement of oxygen saturation of Hb can also be obtained at the bedside by non-invasive pulse oximetry.

Figure 12.6 Effect of pH on the oxygen dissociation curve.

Interpretation

Figure 12.6 shows the sigmoid nature of the oxygen dissociation curve of Hb A and the effect of hydrogen ions on the position of the curve. A shift of the curve to the right indicates decreased affinity of the Hb for oxygen and hence an increased tendency to give up oxygen to the tissues; a shift to the left indicates increased affinity and so an increased tendency for Hb to take up and retain oxygen. Hydrogen ions, 2,3-DPG and some other organic phosphates such as ATP shift the curve to the right. The amount by which the curve is shifted may be expressed by the $p_{50}O_2$ (i.e. the partial pressure of oxygen at which the Hb is 50% saturated).

The oxygen affinity, as represented by the $p_{50}O_2$, is related to compensation in haemolytic anaemias;[62] 1 g of Hb can carry about 1.34 ml of O_2. Figure 12.7 shows the O_2 dissociation curves of Hb A and Hb S plotted according to the volume of oxygen contained in 1 litre of blood when the Hb concentrations is 146 g/l and 80 g/l, respectively. The $p_{50}O_2$ of Hb A is given as 26.5 mmHg (3.5 kPa) and

---

*For example, Hemox-Analyzer, TCS Scientific Corporation, New Hope, Pennsylvania.

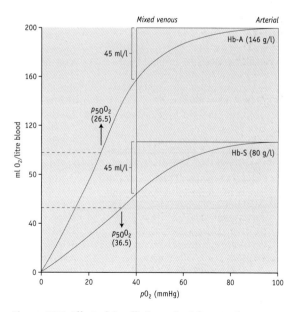

Figure 12.7 Effect of O_2 affinity on O_2 delivery to tissues.

Hb S as 36.5 mmHg (4.8 kPa). It will be seen that in the change from arterial to venous saturation, the same volume of oxygen is given up despite the difference in Hb concentration. Patients with a high $p_{50}O_2$ achieve a stable Hb at a lower level than normal and this should be taken into account when planning transfusion for these patients.

Bohr Effect

An increase in CO_2 concentration produces a shift to the right (i.e. a decrease in oxygen affinity). This effect originally described by C. Bohr,[63] is mainly a result of changes in pH, although CO_2 itself has some direct effect. The Bohr effect is given a numeric value, $\triangle \log p_{50}O_2/ \triangle pH$, where $\triangle \log p_{50}O_2$ is the change in $p_{50}O_2$ produced by a change in pH ($\triangle pH$). The normal value of the Bohr effect at physiological pH and temperature is about 0.45.

Hill's Constant ('n')

Hill's constant ('n') represents the number of molecules of oxygen that combine with one molecule of Hb.[64] Experiments showed that the value was 2.6 rather than the expected 4. The explanation for this lies in the effect of binding 1 molecule of oxygen by Hb on the affinity for binding further oxygen molecules by Hb, the so-called allosteric effect of haem–haem interaction: 'n' is a measure of this effect and the calculation of the 'n' value helps in identifying abnormal Hbs, the molecular abnormality of which leads to abnormal haem–haem interaction.[65]

REFERENCES

1. Johnsson R, Vuopio P. Studies on red cell flexibility in spherocytosis using a polycarbonate membrane filtration method. *Acta Haematol.* 1978;60: 329–340.

2. *LORCA.* Available at: www. mechatronics.nl/products/ download/lorrca.pdf.

3. Parpart AK, Lorenz PB, Parpart ER, et al. The osmotic resistance (fragility) of human red cells. *J Clin Invest.* 1947;26:636–640.

4. Murphy JR. The influence of pH and temperature on some physical properties of normal erythrocytes and erythrocytes from patients with hereditary spherocytosis. *J Lab Clin Med.* 1967;69:758–775.

5. Suess J, Limentani D, Dameshek W, et al. A quantitative method for the determination and charting of the erythrocyte hypotonic fragility. *Blood.* 1948;3:1290–1303.

6. Jacob HS, Jandl JH. Increased cell membrane permeability in the pathogenesis of hereditary spherocytosis. *J Clin Invest.* 1964;43: 1704–1720.

7. Cooper RA. Lipids of human red cell membrane normal composition and variability in disease. *Semin Hematol.* 1970;7:296–322.

8. John DS. *The Haemolytic Anaemias, Vol. 1. The Hereditary Haemolytic Anaemias, Part 1.* Edinburgh: Churchill Livingstone; 1985:292, 146, 352.

9. Gunn RB, Silvers DN, Rosse WF. Potassium permeability in β-thalassaemia minor red blood cells. *J Clin Invest.* 1972;51:1043–1050.

10. King M-J, Behrens J, Rogers C, et al. Rapid flow cytometric test for the diagnosis of membrane cytoskeleton-associated haemolytic anaemia. *Br J Haematol.* 2000;111: 924–933.

11. Golan DE, Corbett JD, Korsgren C, et al. Control of band 3 lateral and rotational mobility by band 4.2 in intact erythrocytes: release of band 3 oligomers from low affinity binding sites. *Biophys J.* 1996;70:1534–1542.

12. Gottfried EL, Robertson NA. Glycerol lysis time as a screening test for erythrocyte disorders. *J Lab Clin Med.* 1974;83:323–333.

13. Gottfried EL, Robertson NA. Glycerol lysis time of incubated erythrocytes in the diagnosis of hereditary spherocytosis. *J Lab Clin Med.* 1974;84:746–751.

14. Zanella A, Izzo C, Rebulla P, et al. Acidified glycerol lysis test: a screening test for spherocytosis. *Br J Haematol.* 1980;45:481–486.

15. Streichman S, Gescheidt Y. Cryohemolysis for the detection of hereditary spherocytosis: correlation studies with osmotic fragility and autohemolysis. *Am J Hematol.* 1998;58:206–210.

16. Selwyn JG, Dacie JV. Autohemolysis and other changes resulting from the incubation in vitro of red cells from patients with congenital hemolytic anemia. *Blood.* 1954;9: 414–438.

17. Morris LD, Pont A, Lewis SM. Use of the HemoCue for measuring haemoglobin at low concentrations. *Clin Lab Haematol.* 2001;23:91–96.

18. de Gruchy GC, Santamaria JN, Parsons IC, et al. Nonspherocytic congenital hemolytic anemia. *Blood.* 1960;16:1371–1397.

19. Beutler E. Why has the autohemolysis test not gone the way of the cephalin flocculation test? *Blood.* 1978;51:109–110.

20. Palek J, Jarolim P. Clinical expression and laboratory detection of red blood cell membrane protein mutations. *Semin Hematol.* 1993;30: 249–283.

21. Beutler E. *Red Cell Metabolism. A Manual of Biochemical Methods.* 2nd ed. Orlando: Grune & Stratton; 1984.

22. Beutler E, Blume KG, Kaplan JC, et al. International Committee for Standardization in Haematology. Recommended screening test for glucose-6-phosphate dehydrogenase (G-6-PD) deficiency. *Br J Haematol.* 1979;43:465–477.

23. World Health Organization Scientific Group. *Standardization of procedures for the study of glucose-6-phosphate dehydrogenase.* Technical Report Series, No. 366, Geneva: WHO; 1967.

24. Beutler E, Mitchell M. Special modification of the fluorescent screening method for glucose-6-phosphate dehydrogenase deficiency. *Blood.* 1968;32:816–818.

25. Brewer GJ, Tarlov AR, Alving AS. The methemoglobin reduction test for primaquine-type sensitivity of erythrocytes. A simplified procedure for detecting a specific hypersusceptibility to drug hemolysis. *JAMA*. 1962;180: 386–388.

26. Fujii H, Takahashi K, Miwa S. A new simple screening method for glucose-6-phosphate dehydrogenase deficiency. *Acta Haematologica Japonica*. 1984;47: 185–188.

27. Lyon MF. Gene action in the X-chromosomes of the mouse (*Mus musculus L.*). *Nature (London)*. 1961;190:372–373.

28. Fairbanks VF, Lampe LT. A tetrazolium-linked cytochemical method for estimation of glucose-6-phosphate dehydrogenase activity in individual erythrocytes: applications in the study of heterozygotes for glucose-6-phoshate dehydrogenase deficiency. *Blood*. 1968;31:589–603.

29. Gall JC, Brewer GJ, Dern RJ. Studies of glucose-6-phosphate dehydrogenase activity of individual erythrocytes: the methemoglobin-elution test for identification of females heterozygous for G6PD deficiency. *Am J Hum Genet*. 1965;17:350–363.

30. Tönz O, Rossi E. Morphological demonstration of two red cell populations in human females heterozygous for glucose-6-phosphate dehydrogenase deficiency. *Nature (London)*. 1964;202:606–607.

31. Kleihauer E, Betke K. Elution procedure for the demonstration of methaemoglobin in red cells of human blood smears. *Nature (London)*. 1963;199:1196–1197.

32. Vogels IMC, Van Noorden CJF, Wolf BHM, et al. Cytochemical determination of heterozygous glucose-6-phosphate dehydrogenase deficiency in erythrocytes. *Br J Haematol*. 1986;63:402–405.

33. Valentine WN, Fink K, Paglia DE, et al. Hereditary haemolytic anaemia with human erythrocyte pyrimidine 5′-nucleotidase deficiency. *J Clin Invest*. 1974;54:866–879.

34. Torrance J, West C, Beutler E. A simple radiometric assay for pyrimidine 5′-nucleotidase. *J Lab Clin Med*. 1977;90:563–568.

35. International Committee for Standardization in Haematology. Recommended screening test for pyrimidine 5′-nucleotidase deficiency. *Clin Lab Haematol*. 1989;11:55–56.

36. Fairbanks LD, Jacomelli G, Micheli V, et al. Severe pyridine nucleotide depletion in fibroblasts from Lesch-Nyhan patients. *Biochem J*. 2002;366: 265–272.

37. International Committee for Standardization in Haematology. Recommended methods for red-cell enzyme analysis. *Br J Haematol*. 1977;35:331–340.

38. Konrad PN, Valentine WN, Paglia DE. Enzymatic activities and glutathione content of erythrocytes in the newborn. Comparison with red cells of older normal subjects and those with comparable reticulocytosis. *Acta Haematol*. 1972;48:193–201.

39. Oski FA. Red cell metabolism in the newborn infant: V. Glycolytic intermediates and glycolytic enzymes. *Pediatrics*. 1969; 44:84–91.

40. Luzzatto L, Mehta A. Glucose-6-phosphate dehydrogenase deficiency. In: Scriver CR, Beaudet A, Sly WS, Valle D, eds. *The Metabolic Basis of Inherited Disease*. New York: McGraw-Hill; 1989:2237–2265.

41. Yoshida A, Beutler E, Motulsky AG. Human glucose-6-phosphate dehydrogenase variants. *Bull World Health Organ*. 1971;45: 243–253.

42. World Health Organization Scientific Group on Glucose-6-Phosphate Dehydrogenase. *Bull World Health Organ*. 1990;67:601.

43. Vulliamy TJ, D'urso M, Battistuzzi G, et al. Diverse point mutations in the human glucose-6-phosphate dehydrogenase gene cause enzyme deficiency and mild or severe hemolytic anemia. *Proc Natl Acad Sci U S A*. 1988;85:5171–5175.

44. Beutler E. Glucose-6-phosphate dehydrogenase: new perspectives. *Blood*. 1989;73:1397–1401.

45. Miwa S, Fujii H, Takegawa S, et al. Seven pyruvate kinase variants characterised by the ICSH recommended methods. *Br J Haematol*. 1980;45: 575–583.

46. Miwa S, Nakashima K, Ariyoshi K, et al. Four new pyruvate kinase (PK) variants and a classical PK deficiency. *Br J Haematol*. 1975;29:157–169.

47. International Committee for Standardization in Haematology. Recommended methods for the characterisation of red cell pyruvate kinase variants. *Br J Haematol*. 1979;43:275–286.

48. Beutler E, Duron O, Kelly B. Improved method for the determination of blood glutathione. *J Lab Clin Med*. 1963;61:882–888.

49. Lubin BH, Oski FA. An evaluation of screening procedures for red cell glucose-6-phosphate dehydrogenase deficiency in the newborn infant. *J Pediatr*. 1967;70:488–492.

50. Zinkham WH. An in-vitro abnormality of glutathione metabolism in erythrocytes from normal newborns: mechanism and clinical significance. *Pediatrics*. 1959;23:18–32.

51. Chanutin A, Curnish RR. Effect of organic and inorganic phosphates on the oxygen equilibrium of human erythrocytes. *Arch Biochem Biophys*. 1967;121:96–102.

52. Benesch R, Benesch RE. The effect of organic phosphates from the human erythrocyte on the allosteric properties of haemoglobin. *Biochem Biophys Res Commun*. 1967;26:162–167.

53. Krimsky I. D-2,3-diphosphoglycerate. In: Bergmeyer HU, ed. *Methods of Enzymatic Analysis*. New York: Academic Press; 1965.

54. Lowry OH, Passonneau JV, Hasselberger FX, et al. Effect of ischemia on known substrates and cofactors of the glycolytic pathway in brain. *J Biol Chem*. 1964;239:18–30.

55. Rose ZB, Liebowitz J. Direct determination of 2,3-diphosphoglycerate. *Ann Biochem Exp Med*. 1970;35:177–180.

56. Duhm J. Effects of 2,3-diphosphoglycerate and other organic phosphate compounds on oxygen affinity and intracellular pH of human erythrocytes. *Pflügers Arch Gesamte Physiol Menschen Tiere*. 1971;326:341–356.

57. Rosa R, Prehu MO, Beuzard Y, et al. The first case of a complete deficiency of diphosphoglycerate mutase in

human erythrocytes. *J Clin Invest.* 1978;62:907–915.

58. Peters JP, Van Slyke DD. Hemoglobin and oxygen. In: *Quantitative Clinical Chemistry, Vol. 1. Interpretations.* Baltimore: Williams & Wilkins; 1931:525.

59. Bellingham AJ, Lenfant C. Hb affinity for O_2 determined by O_2–Hb dissociation analyser and mixing technique. *J Appl Physiol.* 1971;30: 903–904.

60. Torrance JD, Lenfant C. Methods for determination of O_2 dissociation curves, including Bohr effect. *Respir Physiol.* 1969;8: 127–136.

61. Van Slyke DD, Neill JM. The determination of gases in blood and other solutions by vacuum extraction and manometric measurement. *J Biol Chem.* 1924;61: 523–573.

62. Bellingham AJ, Huehns ER. Compensation in haemolytic anaemias caused by abnormal haemoglobins. *Nature (London).* 1968;218:924–926.

63. Bohr C, Hasselbach K, Krogh A. Ueber einen in biologischer Beziehung wichtigen Einfluss, den die Kohlensäurespannung des Blutes auf dessen Sauerstoffbindungübt. *Skandinavisches Archiv für Physiologie.* 1904;16:402.

64. Hill AV. The possible effect of the aggregation of the molecules of haemoglobin on its dissociation curves. *J Physiol.* 1910;40:4.

65. Bellingham AJ. The physiological significance of the Hill parameter 'n'. *Scand J Haematol.* 1972;9:552–556.

Chapter | **13** |

Acquired haemolytic anaemias

Barbara J. Bain, Nay Win

ASSESSING THE LIKELIHOOD OF ACQUIRED HAEMOLYTIC ANAEMIA

Haemolytic anaemia may be suspected from either clinical or laboratory abnormalities. Suggestive clinical features include anaemia, jaundice and splenomegaly. Other relevant clinical features that should be sought are a history of autoimmune disease, recent blood transfusion, recent infection, exposure to drugs or toxins, the presence of a cardiac prosthesis and risk of malaria. Previous clinical history and laboratory results will help to establish that the disorder is acquired. The basic laboratory investigations when a haemolytic anaemia is suspected are listed in Chapter 11. In this chapter, tests are described that are more specific for the diagnosis of acquired haemolytic anaemia.

ASSESSMENT OF THE BLOOD FILM AND COUNT IN SUSPECTED ACQUIRED HAEMOLYTIC ANAEMIA

If haemolytic anaemia is suspected, a full blood count, reticulocyte count and blood film should always be performed. The blood count shows a reduced haemoglobin concentration (Hb) and, usually, an increased mean cell volume (MCV). The increased MCV is attributable to the fact that reticulocytes, which may constitute a significant proportion of total red cells, are larger than mature red cells. The abnormalities that may be detected in the blood film and their possible significance in acquired haemolytic anaemia are shown in Table 13.1. Abnormalities detected

Table 13.1 Abnormalities that may be detected on blood film examination and their possible significance

MORPHOLOGICAL ABNORMALITY OBSERVED ON BLOOD FILM EXAMINATION	TYPE OF ACQUIRED HAEMOLYTIC ANAEMIA SUGGESTED
Schistocytes	Fragmentation syndromes including microangiopathic haemolytic anaemia and mechanical haemolytic anaemia
Spherocytes	Autoimmune, alloimmune or drug-induced immune haemolytic anaemia, paroxysmal cold haemoglobinuria, burns, *Clostridium perfringens* sepsis
Microspherocytes	Burns, fragmentation syndromes
Irregularly contracted cells	Oxidant damage, Zieve's syndrome
Ghost cells, hemi-ghosts and suspicion of Heinz bodies	Acute oxidant damage
Marked red cell agglutination	Cold-antibody-induced haemolytic anaemia
Minor red cell agglutination	Warm autoimmune haemolytic anaemia, paroxysmal cold haemoglobinuria
Red cell agglutination plus erythrophagocytosis	Particularly characteristic of paroxysmal cold haemoglobinuria
Hypochromia, microcytosis and basophilic stippling	Lead poisoning
Erythrophagocytosis	Paroxysmal cold haemoglobinuria
Atypical lymphocytes	Cold-antibody-induced haemolytic anaemia associated with infectious mononucleosis or, less often, other infections
Lymphocytosis with mature small lymphocytes and smear cells	Autoimmune haemolytic anaemia associated with chronic lymphocytic leukaemia
Thrombocytopenia	Autoimmune haemolytic anaemia (Evans' syndrome), thrombotic thrombocytopenic purpura, microangiopathic haemolytic anaemia associated with disseminated intravascular coagulation, paroxysmal nocturnal haemoglobinuria
Neutropenia	Paroxysmal nocturnal haemoglobinuria
No specific red cell features	Paroxysmal nocturnal haemoglobinuria

in the blood film will direct further investigations. For example, a Heinz body preparation would be relevant if irregularly contracted cells were present, particularly if there appeared to be red cell inclusions. Similarly, a direct antiglobulin test (DAT) would be indicated if the blood film showed spherocytes. Various inherited forms of haemolytic anaemia enter into the differential diagnosis of suspected acquired haemolytic anaemia. Thus, spherocytes could be attributable to hereditary spherocytosis as well as to autoimmune or alloimmune haemolytic anaemia. Haemolysis with irregularly contracted cells could be attributable not only to oxidant exposure but also to an unstable haemoglobin, homozygosity for haemoglobin C or glucose-6-phosphate dehydrogenase (G6PD) deficiency.

IMMUNE HAEMOLYTIC ANAEMIAS

Acquired immune-mediated haemolytic anaemias are the result of autoantibodies to a patient's own red cell antigens or alloantibodies in a patient's circulation, either present in the plasma or completely bound to red cells (e.g. transfused or neonatal red cells). Alloantibodies may be present in a patient's plasma and react with antigens on transfused donor red cells to cause haemolysis. Alloantibodies may also occur in maternal plasma and cause haemolytic disease of the newborn. Autoimmune haemolytic anaemia (AIHA) may be 'idiopathic' or secondary, associated mainly with lymphoproliferative disorders and autoimmune diseases, particularly systemic lupus erythematosus. AIHA may also follow atypical (*Mycoplasma pneumoniae*) pneumonia or infectious mononucleosis and other viral infections. AIHA has also been reported following allogeneic bone marrow transplantation[1] and other hematopoietic stem cell transplantation in both adult[2] and paediatric patients.[3] Paroxysmal cold haemoglobinuria (PCH) also belongs to this group of disorders. Occasionally, drugs may give rise to a haemolytic anaemia of immunological origin that closely mimics idiopathic AIHA both clinically and serologically. This was a relatively common occurrence with α-methyldopa, a drug that is now used very infrequently, but it also occurs occasionally with other drugs. A larger range of drugs give rise to an antibody that is directed primarily against the drug and only secondarily involves the red cells. This is an uncommon occurrence. Such drugs include penicillin, phenacetin, quinidine, quinine, the sodium salt of *p*-aminosalicylic acid, salicylazosulphapyridine and cephalosporins.[4]

Types of Autoantibody

The diagnosis of an AIHA requires evidence of anaemia and haemolysis and demonstration of autoantibodies attached to the patient's red cells (i.e. a positive DAT, see p. 279). A positive DAT may also be caused by the presence of *allo*antibodies (e.g. owing to a delayed haemolytic transfusion reaction), so details of any transfusion in the past months must be sought.

Autoantibodies can often be demonstrated free in the serum of a patient suffering from an AIHA. The ease with which the antibodies can be detected depends on how much antibody is being produced, its affinity for the corresponding antigen on the red cell surface and the effect that temperature has on the adsorption of the antibody, as well as on the technique used to detect it. The autoantibodies associated with AIHA can be separated into two broad categories depending on how their interaction with antigen is affected by temperature: warm antibodies, which are able to combine with their corresponding red cell antigen readily at 37°C and cold antibodies, which cannot combine with antigen at 37°C but form an increasingly stable combination with antigen as the temperature falls from 30–32°C to 2–4°C.

Cases of AIHA can similarly be separated into two broad categories according to the temperature characteristics of the associated autoantibodies: warm-type AIHA and the less frequent cold-type AIHA. The relative frequency of the two categories is illustrated in Table 13.2.[5] In unusual instances, both warm autoantibody and cold autoantibody are detected in the patient's serum and those cases are referred to as mixed-typed AIHA. This can be further classified into idiopathic or secondary, the latter often associated with systemic lupus erythematosus or lymphoma.[6,7]

Table 13.2 Relative incidence of different types of autoimmune haemolytic anaemia[5]

	MALES	FEMALES	TOTAL
Warm antibodies			
'Idiopathic'	46	65	111
Associated with drugs (mostly α-methyldopa)	1	10	11[a]
Secondary, associated with			
Lymphomas	14	23	37
Systemic lupus erythematosus	1	15	16
Other possible or probable autoimmune disorders	8	13	21
Infections and miscellaneous	9	4	13
Ovarian teratoma	0	1	1
Totals	79	131	210
Cold antibodies			
'Idiopathic' (CHAD)[b]	16	22	38
Secondary, associated with			
Atypical or *Mycoplasma pneumoniae* infection	5	18	23
Infectious mononucleosis	1	1	2
Lymphoma	3	4	7
Paroxysmal cold haemoglobinuria			
Other secondary	4	3	7
'Idiopathic'	7	1	8
Totals	36	49	85

[a]It should be noted that since this study was done the use of α-methyldopa has declined and this is now a rare cause of haemolytic anaemia.
[b]CHAD, chronic cold haemagglutinin disease. Although is often regarded as 'idiopathic,' it is actually consequent on an occult lymphoproliferative disorder, which leads to production of a cold agglutinin by a clone of neoplastic cells.

Warm Autoantibodies

The most common type of warm autoantibody is an immunoglobulin (Ig) G, which behaves *in vitro* very similarly to an Rh alloantibody; indeed, many IgG autoantibodies have a mimicking Rh specificity. IgA and IgM warm autoantibodies are much less common and when present they are usually formed in addition to an IgG autoantibody (Table 13.3).[8]

Table 13.3 Direct antiglobulin test in warm-antibody autoimmune haemolytic anaemia: incidence of different reactions to specific antiglobulin sera[8]

ANTI-IgG	ANTI-IgA	ANTI-IgM	ANTI-C'	PATIENTS (N)	(%)
+	−	−	−	43	36
−	+	−	−	3	2
+	+	−	−	4	3
+	−	−	+	52	43
+	−	+	+	6	5
−	−	−	+	13	11
				121	100

Ig, immunoglobulin.

Frequently, patients with warm-type AIHA have complement adsorbed onto their red cells and the red cells are therefore agglutinated by antisera specific for complement or a complement component such as C3d (Table 13.3). In these cases, the complement is probably not being bound by an IgG antibody but is on the cell surface as the result of the action of small and otherwise undetected amounts of IgM autoantibody.

IgG can fix complement and sometimes patients with warm-type AIHA appear to have a positive DAT with complement components only on the red cell surface. Similar results (positive DAT with complement only) are seen in some patients with no evidence of increased red cell destruction, due to binding of circulating immune complexes to the red cells.

Warm autoantibodies free in the patient's serum are best detected by means of the indirect antiglobulin test (IAT) or by the use of enzyme-treated (e.g. trypsinized or papainized) red cells. (Antibodies that agglutinate unmodified cells directly *in vitro* are seldom present.) Not infrequently, antibodies that agglutinate enzyme-treated cells, sometimes at high titres, are present in the sera of patients in whom the IAT using unmodified cells is negative (Table 13.4). Occasionally, too, they are present in the sera of patients in whom the DAT is negative.

Antibodies in serum that can be shown to lyse (rather than simply agglutinate) unmodified red cells at 37°C in the presence of complement (warm haemolysins) are rarely demonstrable. If they are present, the patient is likely to suffer from extremely severe haemolysis. Antibodies in

Table 13.4 Results of testing for free autoantibodies in the sera of 210 patients with warm-antibody autoimmune haemolytic anaemia[5]

INDIRECT ANTIGLOBULIN TEST (IAT)	AGGLUTINATION OF ENZYME-TREATED RED CELLS AT 37°C	LYSIS OF ENZYME-TREATED RED CELLS AT 37°C	AGGLUTINATION OF NORMAL RED CELLS AT 20°C	NO. AND PERCENTAGE OF PATIENTS IN GROUP	
+	+	+	+	4	
+	+	+	−	16	
+	+	−	−	64	41%
+	−	−	−	2	
+	−	−	+	1	
−	+	+	+	16	
−	+	+	−	31	
−	+	−	−	29	40%
−	+	−	+	7	
−	−	−	−	39	19%

Notes
1. In 41% of the patients, the IAT was positive, and in 80% of the patients, the tests with enzyme-treated cells were positive (in half of these patients, the IAT was negative).
2. In 19% of the patients, all tests were negative.
3. In 13% of the patients, normal red cells were agglutinated at 20°C, probably by cold agglutinins.

serum that lyse as well as agglutinate enzyme-treated cells but do not affect unmodified cells are, however, quite common. Their specificity is uncertain – they are not anti-Rh – and their presence is not necessarily associated with increased haemolysis.

Cold Autoantibodies

Cold autoantibodies are nearly always IgM in type. *In vivo* the majority do not cause haemolysis, although a minority can cause chronic intravascular haemolysis, the intensity of which is characteristically influenced by the ambient temperature. The resultant clinical picture is generally referred to as the cold haemagglutinin syndrome or disease (CHAD). Haemolysis results from destruction of the red cells by complement that is bound to the red cell surface by the antigen–antibody reaction, which takes place in the blood vessels of the exposed skin where the temperature is 28–32°C or less. The cold autoantibody in CHAD is monoclonal because this syndrome is the result of a low-grade lymphoproliferative disorder.

The red cells of patients suffering from CHAD characteristically give positive antiglobulin reactions only with anticomplement (anti-C′) sera. (The C′ notation is used to distinguish anticomplement antibodies from anti-C antibodies of the Rh system.) This is because of the presence of red cells that have irreversibly adsorbed sublytic amounts of complement; it is an indication of an antigen–antibody reaction that has taken place at a temperature below 37°C. The complement component responsible for the reaction with anti-C′ sera is the C3dg derivative of C3 (see p. 494).

In vitro, a cold-type autoantibody will often lyse normal red cells at 20–30°C in the presence of fresh human complement, especially if the cell-serum mixture is acidified to pH 6.5–7.0; it will usually lyse enzyme-treated red cells readily in unacidified serum and agglutination and lysis of these cells may still occur at 37°C. Most of these cold-type autoantibodies have anti-I specificity (i.e. they react strongly with the vast majority of adult red cells and only weakly with cord-blood red cells). A minority are anti-i and react strongly with cord-blood cells and weakly with adult red cells. Rarely, the antibodies have anti-Pr or anti-M specificity and react with antigens on the red cell surface that are destroyed by enzyme treatment.

Combined Warm and Cold Autoantibodies

In approximately 7% of cases with AIHA, both warm IgG antibody and cold IgM autoantibody are simultaneously detected in the patient's serum.[6,7] These cases are referred to as 'combined warm and cold AIHA' or mixed-type AIHA. The serological characteristics in these patients are the presence of IgM cold autoantibody with a high thermal amplitude (reacting at or above 30°C) in association with a warm IgG autoantibody. In some cases, high-titre cold agglutinins (>1024 at 4°C) were reported[9,10] and in others the cold agglutinin titre were reported as >64 at 4°C.[11,12]

Another quite distinct, but rarely encountered, type of cold antibody is the Donath–Landsteiner (D–L) antibody. This is IgG and has anti-P specificity. The clinical syndrome the antibody produces is PCH.

PCH is caused by a biphasic IgG autoantibody, usually with anti-P specificity, and is commonly seen as an acute condition in children. This antibody binds to the red cells in the cold but activates complement and causes haemolysis on rewarming to 37°C. Cases may be idiopathic or can be secondary to acute viral infection in children. Other tests of value in the diagnosis of PCH are discussed on p. 287.

The DAT is positive for complement only. A negative antibody screen by the standard IAT at 37°C is a common finding in a suspected case of PCH because of the low thermal amplitude of the autoantibody. If the antibody investigation is carried out at a lower temperature in PCH cases, panreactive cold antibodies may be detected because the majority of autoantibodies show anti-P specificity with thermal amplitude range up to 15–24°C. Usually the antibody titre is low (<64), even when investigated at 4°C.

Some of the characteristics of IgG, IgM and IgA antibodies are listed in Table 13.5.

The clinical, haematological and serological aspects of the AIHAs have been summarized by Dacie[13] and others.[14–18]

Methods of Investigation

Many of the methods used in the investigation of a patient suspected of suffering from AIHA are described in Chapter 21. Detailed description is given here of precautions to be taken when collecting blood samples from patients and of methods of particular value in the investigations.

Collection of Samples of Blood and Serum

To determine the true thermal amplitude or titre of cold agglutinins requires that the blood sample is collected and maintained strictly at 37°C until serum and cells are separated. This can be achieved by collecting venous blood (clotted and ethylenediaminetetra-acetic acid [EDTA]-anticoagulated samples) and keeping it warmed at 37°C – ideally in an insulated thermos, but usually, in practice, by placing the sample tube in a beaker containing water at 37°C.

The red cells are available for antibody elution and the serum can be examined for free antibody or other abnormalities. The clotted sample should then be centrifuged to separate the serum at 37°C (e.g. in an ordinary

Table 13.5 Main characteristics of IgG, IgM and IgA autoantibodies

	IgG	IgM	IgA
Molecular weight (daltons)	146 000	970 000	160 000
Sedimentation constant (s)	7	19	7
Number of heavy-chain subclasses	4	1	2
Cross placenta	Yes	No	No
Cause activation of complement	Yes	Yes	No
Cause monocyte/macrophage attachment	Yes	No	No
Number of antigen-binding sites	2	5 or 10	2
Types of AIHA produced	Warm; PCH	Usually cold	Warm

Ig, immunoglobulin; AIHA, autoimmune haemolytic anaemia; PCH, paroxysmal cold haemoglobinuria.

centrifuge into the buckets of which has been placed water warmed to 37–40°C). The EDTA sample is used for the DAT and other tests involving the patient's red cells. If the autoantibody in a particular case is known to be warm in type, the blood may be separated at room temperature; otherwise, as already indicated, this should be carried out at 37°C. When samples are sent by post, it is best to send separately: (1) serum (separated at 37°C) and (2) whole blood added to acid–citrate–dextrose (ACD) or citrate–phosphate–dextrose (CPD) solution. Sterility must be maintained.

Storage of Samples

Samples of a patient's blood, while keeping quite well in ACD or CPD at 4°C, are more difficult to preserve than normal red cells. In particular, if marked spherocytosis is present, considerable lysis develops on storage. However, satisfactory eluates can be made from washed red cells that are frozen at –20°C for weeks or months.

The patient's serum should be stored at –20°C or below in small (1–2 ml) volumes. If complement is to be titrated and the titration is not performed immediately, the serum should be frozen as soon as practicable at −70°C or below.

Scheme for Serological Investigation of Haemolytic Anaemia Suspected to be of Immunological Origin

It is important to consider which are the most useful tests to carry out and the order in which they should be done. A suggested scheme has been set out in the form of answers to questions.[19] Whereas some information may be helpful in classifying the type of AIHA, the single most important practical consideration is to determine whether, in addition to an autoantibody, there is any underlying alloantibody present. This should be identified before transfusion is undertaken to avoid a delayed haemolytic transfusion reaction that would compound existing haemolysis.

1. **Are the patient's red cells 'coated' by immunoglobulins or complement (indicating an antigen–antibody reaction)?**
    Perform a DAT using a polyspecific 'broad-spectrum' reagent, which contains both anti-IgG and anti-C'. (If the DAT is negative, it is unlikely, although not impossible, that the diagnosis is AIHA. See DAT-negative AIHA, p. 281)

2. **If the DAT is positive, are immunoglobulins or complement adsorbed to the red cells?**
    Repeat the DAT using monospecific sera (see p. 500) (i.e. anti-IgG and anti-C3d).

3. **If immunoglobulins are present on the red cells, is there antibody specificity?**
    Prepare eluates from the patient's red cells. Test these later (see item 6).

4. **What is the patient's blood group?**
    Determine the patient's ABO and RhD and Kell type. The Rh phenotype is particularly important in warm-type AIHA; other antigens must be determined if alloantibodies are to be differentiated from autoantibodies (see p. 507).

5. **Is there free antibody in the serum? How does it react and at what temperatures and by what methods can it be demonstrated? Is there any underlying alloantibody present?**

Screen the serum with two or three red cell suspensions suitable for routine pretransfusion antibody screening (see p. 528) looking for agglutination and lysis at 37°C by the IAT (see p. 500). If positive, identify the antibody using an antibody identification panel.

a. If an alloantibody is identified, blood lacking the corresponding antigen must be selected for transfusion.

b. If no alloantibody is identified in the serum or plasma, it is safe to assume there is no alloantibody present, unless the patient has been transfused in the last month; in the latter case, a red cell eluate is required because an alloantibody may be bound to the recently transfused cells and there may not be free antibody detectable in the serum/plasma.

c. If the autoantibody is pan-reacting (i.e. is reacting against all panel cells), antibody adsorption tests are needed to remove the autoantibody so as to identify any underlying alloantibody. If the patient has not had a transfusion within the last 3 months, a ZZAP autoadsorption test is appropriate (see p. 283). If the patient has had a transfusion within the last 3 months, differential alloadsorption tests are needed. However, if the patient has had a transfusion within the last month, an eluate is required, irrespective of results of adsorption tests.

6. If there is a warm autoantibody, what is the specificity of the autoantibody?

Test the serum also at 20°C against antibody-screening cells to show whether cold or warm antibodies or a mixture of the two, are present in the serum.

Test the eluate against the antibody identification panel of red cells by IAT and by using enzyme-treated red cells (see p. 498). Titration of autoantibody may be useful in the presence of a strong alloantibody.

Titrate the serum/plasma by the methods that have given positive results in the screening test using the same panel of red cells (see item 5a).

7. If there is a cold antibody:

a. Has the antibody any specificity? Is it an autoantibody or an alloantibody? What is its titre?

b. What is the thermal range of the antibody?

Test the serum/plasma against a panel of O cells, O cord cells and patient's own cells at 20°C. If an autoantibody is found, titrate at 4°C with ABO-compatible adult (I) cells, cord blood (i) cells, the patient's cells and adult (i) cells (if possible):

i. Determine the highest temperature at which autoagglutination of the patient's whole blood takes place (see p. 287).

ii. Titrate the patient's serum/plasma at 20°C, 30°C and 37°C with pooled O adult cells, O cord cells, patient's own cells and the panel of cells described earlier. If there was any agglutination or lysis at 37°C in the screening test (item 5), titrate with the appropriate cells at this temperature.

iii. If PCH is suspected, carry out the direct and two-stage indirect Donath–Landsteiner tests (see p. 287).

8. Is there is a mixture of both warm autoantibody and cold autoantibody?

The diagnosis of mixed-type AIHA can only be made after appropriate characterization of the serum autoantibodies. The serological characteristic in these cases is the presence of a cold IgM antibody with a high thermal amplitude (reacting at or above 30°C) in association with a warm IgG autoantibody.[6,9]

9. Is a drug suspected as the cause of the haemolytic anaemia?

a. If a penicillin-induced haemolytic anaemia is suspected, test for antibodies using cells pre-incubated with penicillin (see p. 290).

b. If haemolysis induced by other drugs is suspected, add the drug in solution to a mixture of the patient's serum, normal cells and fresh normal serum (see p. 290). Look for agglutination of normal and enzyme-treated cells and use the IAT.

10. Are there any other serological abnormalities?

Consider carrying out the following tests: serum protein electrophoresis and quantitative estimation of immunoglobulins, estimation of complement, tests for antinuclear factor, a screening test for heterophile antibodies (infectious mononucleosis screening test) and a test for mycoplasma antibodies. The suggested scheme summarizes what may be done by way of serological investigation of a patient suspected of having AIHA. Close collaboration between clinician and laboratory helps in deciding what tests should be done in any particular case.

Detection of Incomplete Antibodies by Means of the Direct Antiglobulin (Coombs) Test

Principle

As already described, the DAT involves testing the patient's cells without prior exposure to antibody *in vitro*. For the investigation of cases of AIHA, antiglobulin reagents specific for IgG, IgM, IgA, C3c and C3d can be used.

Precautions

A blood sample in EDTA is preferred. (If a clotted sample is used, complement could be bound by normal incomplete cold antibody and give a false-positive result with anti-C3d.) Certain precautions are necessary when investigating a patient with possible AIHA. If a cold-reacting autoantibody is present, the patient's red cells should be washed four times in a large volume of saline (throughout this chapter, 'saline' refers to 9 g/l NaCl buffered to pH 7.0), warmed to 37°C to wash off cold antibodies and obtain a smooth suspension of cells; there is no risk of washing off adsorbed complement components. However, the washing process should be accomplished as quickly as possible and the test should be set up immediately afterward because bound warm antibody occasionally elutes from the cells when they are washed and false-negative results may be obtained. If for any reason the washing process has to be interrupted once it has begun, the cell suspension should be placed at 4°C to slow down the dissociation of the antibody.

Method

A spin tube technique, as described on p. 501, is recommended.

Make a 2–5% suspension of red cells that have been washed four times in saline. Add 1 volume (drop) of the cell suspension to 2 volumes (drops) of antiglobulin reagent. Centrifuge for 10–60 s. Refer to reagent manufacturer's instructions for specific details.

Examine for agglutination after gently resuspending the button of cells. A concave mirror and good light help in macroscopic readings. If the result appears to be negative, confirm this microscopically.

Each DAT or batch of tests should be carefully controlled as previously described.

Check negative results with the polyspecific antihuman globulin (AHG) or anti-IgG reagents by the addition of IgG-sensitized cells and anti-C′ by the addition of complement-coated cells.

DAT Using Column Agglutination Technology

A card of several microtubes enables multiple sample testing. The microtubes contain a solid-phase matrix and the antiglobulin reagent to which the patient's red cells are added. During centrifugation, unagglutinated cells pass to the tip of the tube, but agglutinates fail to pass through the gel, which acts as a sieve. As the antiglobulin reagent is already present in the microtubes, no washing or addition of IgG-coated cells to negative tests is required. Refer to individual manufacturer's instructions for details of methods for performing the tests.

Significance of Positive Direct Antiglobulin Test

A positive DAT plus anaemia does not necessarily mean that the patient has autoimmune haemolytic anaemia.[5,8,20] The causes of a positive test include the following:

1. An autoantibody on the red cell surface with or without haemolytic anaemia
2. An alloantibody on the red cell surface, as for example in haemolytic disease of the newborn or after an incompatible transfusion
3. Antibodies provoked by drugs adsorbed to the red cell (see p. 289)
4. Normal globulins adsorbed to the red cell surface as the result of damage by drugs (e.g. some cephalosporins)
5. Complement components alone:
    a. About 10–11% of patients with warm AIHA have red cells with a positive DAT as a result of C3 coating alone[6] (Table 13.3)
    b. Cold haemagglutinin disease/paroxysmal cold haemoglobinuria
    c. Drug-dependent immune haemolytic anemia (complement-induced lysis)
    d. Adsorption of immune complexes to the red cell surface. This may be the mechanism of the (usually weak) reactions that are found in approximately 8% of hospital patients suffering from a wide variety of disorders (see below)
6. Passive infusion of alloantibodies in donor plasma/derivatives that react with recipient's red cells
    a. Transfusion of group O platelets with high-titre anti-A,B to group A or B recipient
    b. Administration of intravenous immunoglobulin, which may contain ABO or anti-D antibodies.[21]

    In one study of patients treated with intravenous immunoglobulin after bone marrow transplantation, 49% of recipients developed a positive DAT and 25% had a positive antibody screen (passively transfused anti-A, -B, -D or -K) of short duration (2–5 days).
7. Administration of anti-D for the treatment of autoimmune thrombocytopenia purpura
8. Antibodies produced by passenger lymphocytes in solid organ transplant and bone marrow transplantation.[22,23]

    Non-specific binding of immunoglobulins to red cells in patients with hypergammaglobulinemia or multiple myeloma and in recipients of antilymphocyte globulin and antithymocyte globulin.[24]

    Szymanski et al.[25] used an AutoAnalyser and used Ficoll and polyvinylpyrrolidone (PVP) to enhance agglutination by an anti-IgG serum highly diluted (usually to 1 in 5000) in 0.5% bovine serum albumin. In this sensitive system, the strength of agglutination was positively correlated with the serum γ-globulin concentration, being subnormal in hypogammaglobulinaemia and supranormal in hypergammaglobulinaemia.[26]

Similar findings were observed in patients with multiple myeloma. Non-specific binding of IgG to red cells was related to the level of monoclonal protein in the patient's serum.[26]

Usually, in patients with hypergammaglobulinaemia in whom the DAT is positive, attempts to demonstrate antibodies in eluates fail (i.e. eluates are non-reactive).[27,28]

9. Cross-reacting antiphospholipid antibodies adsorbing non-specifically on to red cell membrane and binding to phospholipid-dependent epitopes. Positive DAT as a result of antiphospholipid antibodies has been documented in patients with primary antiphospholipid syndrome and antiphospholipid syndrome with systemic lupus erythematosus.[29] It has also been described in healthy blood donors.[30]

10. Incidental findings of positive DAT with no clear correlation between DAT and anaemia. A positive DAT is a common finding in patients with sickle cell disease because of abnormal amounts of IgG coating red cells. There was no correlation between the amount of IgG on the patient's red cells and the severity of anaemia.[31]

There was an association demonstrated between an elevated blood urea nitrogen and a positive DAT.[32] Urea may alter the red cell membrane and enhance non-specific IgG adsorption.[32]

11. Sensitization *in vitro* if a sample other than EDTA is used. If, for instance, clotted or defibrinated normal blood is allowed to stand in a refrigerator at 4°C or even at room temperature, and the antiglobulin test is subsequently carried out, the reaction may be positive because of the adsorption of incomplete cold antibodies and complement from normal sera. Samples of blood taken into EDTA or ACD and subsequently chilled do not give this type of false-positive result because the anticoagulant inhibits the complement reaction.

12. False-positive agglutination may occur with a silica gel derived from glass.[33] Also, albeit rarely, the DAT has been positive with the blood of apparently perfectly healthy individuals (e.g. blood donors). Such occurrences have not been satisfactorily explained (see below).

Positive DATs in Normal Subjects

The occurrence of a clearly positive DAT in an apparently healthy subject is a rare but well-known phenomenon. Worlledge[20] reported a prevalence in blood donors of approximately 1 in 9000. In a later report, Gorst et al.[34]

estimated that the prevalence was approximately 1 in 14 000 with an increasing likelihood of a positive test with increasing age. Their report and subsequent reports,[25,35] suggest that the finding of a positive DAT, using an anti-IgG serum, in an apparently healthy person is usually of little clinical significance and that, although overt AIHA may subsequently develop, this is infrequent. In some such individuals the DAT eventually becomes negative.

Positive DATs in Hospital Patients

In contrast to the rarity of positive DATs in healthy people, positive tests are much more frequent in hospital patients. Worlledge[20] reported that the red cells of 40 out of 489 blood samples (8.9%) submitted for routine tests were agglutinated by anti-C′ sera. Only one sample was agglutinated by an anti-IgG serum and this had been obtained from a patient being treated with α-methyldopa. Freedman[36] reported a similar incidence – 7.8% positive tests with anti-C′ sera. Lau et al.[37] used anti-IgG sera only. The tests were seldom positive (0.9% positive out of 4664 tests). The probable explanation for the relatively high incidence of positive tests with anti-C′ sera is that the reaction is between anti-C′ antibodies and immune complexes adsorbed to the red cells.

False-Negative Antiglobulin Test Results

There are several causes of false-negative test results:

1. Failure to wash the red cells properly: the antisera may then be neutralized by immunoglobulins or complement in the surrounding serum or plasma (see p. 501).
2. Excessive agitation at the reading stage: this may break up agglutinates, leading to a false-negative result.
3. The use of impotent antisera so that weakly sensitized cells are not detected.
4. The use of antisera lacking the antibody corresponding to the subclass of immunoglobulin responsible for the red cell sensitization.
5. The presence of an antibody that is readily dissociable and is eluted in the washing process.

These phenomena are largely negated by the use of column agglutination technology.

DAT-Negative Autoimmune Haemolytic Anaemia

Most hospital blood banks use polyspecific 'broad-spectrum' AHG reagents for screening for diagnosis of AIHA. These reagents contain antibody to human IgG and the C3d component of human complement and have little activity against IgA and IgM proteins. The incidence of IgA-only warm AIHA has been reported as 0.2% to 2.7%,[38] and the diagnosis may be missed if such polyspecific AHG is used for the DAT screen. In approximately

2–6% of patients who present with the clinical and haematological features of AIHA, the DAT is negative on repeated testing.[20,39,40]

Low-affinity IgG autoantibodies dissociate from the red cells during the washing phase if a tube technique is used, resulting in a negative DAT. Alternatively, there may be few IgG molecules coating the red cells and this number may fall below the threshold of detection, which is 300–4000 molecules per red blood cell if a tube technique is used. In such cases, a positive DAT may be demonstrated by a more sensitive technique, such as a column agglutination method, an enzyme-linked immunoabsorbant assay or flow cytometry.[41–43]

If polyspecific AHG is used and the DAT remains negative with clinical evidence of haemolysis, a more sensitive technique should be used for further investigation.[44]

The DiaMed DAT gel card, which contains a set of monospecific AHG reagents (i.e. anti-IgG, -IgA, -IgM, -C3c, -C3d and an inert control) can be used. Because there is no washing phase, this permits the detection of low-affinity IgG, IgA and IgM antibodies. A gel card can also pick up the rare IgA-only autoimmune haemolytic anaemia. In warm-type AIHA the DAT may be positive with anti-IgG or anti-IgG plus anti-C3d. In cold–type AIHA the DAT may be positive with anti-IgM or anti-IgM plus anti-C3d and in mixed-type AIHA the DAT may be positive with anti-IgG, anti-IgM and anti-C3d.

Preparing and Testing a Concentrated Eluate

The eluate technique concentrates low levels of immunoglobulin present on the red cell surface so that antibody may then be detected by screening the eluate with group O red cells by the IAT. Elution techniques reverse or neutralize the binding forces that exist between the red cell antigens and the antibody coating the cells. This may be achieved by several techniques (e.g. heat or alterations to the pH).

Manual Direct Polybrene Test

The following method[45] is modified from that of Lalezari and Jiang.[46] Polybrene is a polyvalent cationic molecule, hexadimethrine bromide, that can overcome the electrostatic repulsive forces between adjacent red cells, bringing the cells closer together. When low levels of IgG are present on the red cell surface, antibody linkage of adjacent red cells is enhanced. The Polybrene is then neutralized using a negatively charged molecule such as trisodium citrate. Sensitized red cells remain agglutinated after neutralization of the Polybrene. Unsensitized red cells will disaggregate after neutralization.

Reagents

Polybrene stock. 10% Polybrene in 9 g/l NaCl, pH 6.9 (saline).

Working Polybrene solution. Dilute the stock Polybrene solution 1 in 250 in saline.

Resuspending solution. 60 ml of 0.2 mol/l trisodium citrate added to 40 ml of 50 g/l dextrose.

Washing solution. 50 ml of 0.2 mol/l trisodium citrate in 950 ml of saline.

Low-ionic medium. 50 g/l dextrose containing 2 g/l disodium EDTA. Adjust the pH of half the batch to 6.4. Store the remainder at the original pH (approx. 4.9); use this to repeat tests that are negative using a low-ionic medium at pH 6.4.

Method

Ensure that all reagents are at room temperature.

Positive control

Dilute an IgG anti-D in normal group AB serum. Find a dilution that gives a positive result with papainized cells but is negative by the IAT on standard testing with group O, D-positive red cells (a dilution of 1 in 10 000 is often suitable).

Negative control

Normal group AB serum that fails to agglutinate papainized group O, D-positive red cells.

1. Wash the cells four times in saline and make 3–5% suspensions of test and normal group O RhD red cells in saline.
2. Set up three 75 × 10 mm tubes as shown in Table 13.6. Leave at room temperature for 1 min.
3. Add 1 drop of working Polybrene solution to each tube and mix gently. Leave for 15 s at room temperature.
4. Centrifuge for 10 s at 1000 g. Decant, taking care to remove all the supernatant.

Table 13.6 Setting up a direct manual Polybrene test

	TEST	POSITIVE CONTROL	NEGATIVE CONTROL
AB serum (drops)	2	0	2
Dilute anti-D in AB serum (drops)	0	2	0
3–5% test cells (drops)	1	0	0
3–5% normal O RhD cells (drops)	0	1	1
Low ionic medium	0.6 ml	0.6 ml	0.6 ml

5. Leave for 3–5 min at room temperature before adding 2 drops of resuspending solution and mixing gently. Within 10 s aggregates will dissociate, leaving true agglutination in the positive tubes.
6. Read macroscopically after 10–60 s. Check all negative results microscopically and compare with the negative control.
7. Repeat negative tests using low-ionic medium at the lower pH (about 4.9).

If the direct Polybrene test is negative, a supplementary antiglobulin test may be performed by washing the cells twice in the washing solution and testing with an anti-IgG antiglobulin reagent.

Determination of the Blood Group of a Patient with AIHA

ABO Grouping

No difficulty should be encountered in ABO grouping patients with warm-type AIHA using monoclonal reagents, but the presence of cold agglutinins may cause difficulties. The cells should in all cases be washed in warm (37°C) saline. They should then be groupable without any problem; the reactions must, however, be controlled with normal AB serum. Reverse grouping should be performed strictly at 37°C. Warm the known A_1, B and O cells to 37°C before adding them to the patient's serum at 37°C. Read the results macroscopically.

RhD Grouping

When the DAT is positive, monoclonal anti-D reagents should be used; if cold agglutinins are present, perform the test at 37°C. Appropriate controls should be included (see p. 524).

Demonstration of Free Antibodies in Serum

The sera of patients suffering from AIHA often contain free autoantibodies. However, free autoantibody is also found with no haemolysis. As a result of improved reagent sensitivity, any clinically significant IgG complement-binding antibodies will be detected by current antibody screening methods.

Identification by Adsorption Techniques of Coexisting Alloantibodies in the Presence of Warm Autoantibodies

Adsorption techniques for the detection of alloantibodies present in the sera or eluates of patients with suspected or proved AIHA can be helpful in the following situations:

1. In screening for coexisting alloantibodies in patients with AIHA who have been pregnant or previously transfused and are found to have a panreactive antibody in their serum

2. In differentiating between autoantibodies and alloantibodies in the eluate of recently transfused patients with AIHA
3. In investigating haemolytic transfusion reactions owing to red cell alloantibodies in patients with AIHA.

In some cases of AIHA, an underlying alloantibody may be detected by titrating the patient's serum and eluate against a panel of phenotyped reagent red cells. However, a high-titre autoantibody may mask the alloantibody; hence the need for adsorption techniques, especially in the situations outlined earlier.

Use of ZZAP Reagent in Autoadsorption Techniques

'ZZAP' reagent is a mixture of dithiothreitol and papain.[47] It dissociates an autoantibody already coating the patient's red cells and enzyme treats the cells, thus increasing the amount of autoantibody that can subsequently be adsorbed onto the patient's cells in vitro.

Reagents

Dithiothreitol (DTT). 0.2 mol/l.
Papain. 1%.
Phosphate-buffered saline (PBS). pH 6.8–7.2.
   Prepare a suitable volume of ZZAP by making up the reagents in the following ratio: 0.2 mol/l DTT 5 volumes; and 1% papain 1 volume.
   Check the pH and adjust to pH 6.0–6.5 using one drop at a time of 0.2 mol/l HCl or 0.2 mol/l NaOH.

Method

1. Add 2 volumes of ZZAP to 1 volume of packed red cells that have been washed four times. Incubate at 37°C for 30 min, mixing occasionally.
2. After incubation, wash the cells four times in saline, packing hard after the last wash.
3. Divide the cells into two equal volumes. To one volume, add an equal volume of the serum to be adsorbed. Incubate at 37°C for 1 h.
4. Centrifuge at 1000 g. Remove the serum and add to the remaining volume of cells.
5. Repeat the adsorption procedure.
6. Remove the adsorbed serum and store at −20°C or below for alloantibody screening or cross-matching, which may be performed by standard techniques.

Notes

The autoadsorption techniques should only be used in the following circumstances:

1. When the patient has not had a transfusion in the previous 3 months because the presence of transfused red cells may allow the adsorption of alloantibody as well as autoantibody

2. When at least 2–3 ml of packed red cells are available from the patient
3. When the autoantibodies present react well with enzyme-treated red cells. If they do not, heat elution should be substituted for ZZAP treatment. Heat elution may be performed by shaking the washed cells for 5 min in a 56°C waterbath and then washing the cells.

Alloadsorption Using Papainized R_1R_1, R_2R_2 and rr Cells

The method of alloadsorption using papainized R_1R_1, R_2R_2 and rr cells may be used when autoadsorption is not appropriate – for instance, when the patient has had a transfusion in the previous 3 months or when less than 2–3 ml of the patient's red cells are available.

1. Select three group O antibody screening cells, which individually lack some of the blood-group antigens that commonly stimulate the production of clinically significant antibodies (e.g. c, e, C, E, K, Fy^a, Fy^b, Jk^a, Jk^b, S, s) (Table 13.7).
2. Papainize 2 ml of packed cells from each sample after washing the cells in saline four times.
3. Add to 1 ml of each sample of washed, packed, papainized cells, 1 ml of the patient's serum. Incubate for 20 min at 37°C.
4. Centrifuge to pack the cells. Remove the supernatant serum and add it to the second 1 ml volume of papainized cells. Incubate for 1 h at 37°C.
5. Centrifuge again to pack the cells. Remove the supernatant and store at –20°C or below for further testing (e.g. alloantibody screening and cross-matching).

Method for Testing Alloadsorbed Sera

For alloantibody screening, each adsorbed serum is tested against a panel of phenotyped red cells by the IAT. For cross-matching, each adsorbed serum must be tested separately against the donor red cells by the IAT, using undiluted serum.

Example of alloantibody detection using the alloadsorption technique in a recently transfused patient with AIHA

The patient's serum when first tested against a panel of group O phenotyped red cells revealed only panreactive antibodies. In contrast, three absorbed sera, A, B and C, obtained by adsorbing the patient's serum with three selected phenotyped samples of group O cells, were shown to contain anti-E and anti-Jk^a when tested against a panel of phenotyped group O cells using the IAT. The results of testing the adsorbed sera, A, B and C, are shown in Table 13.7. The patient's red cell phenotype was R_1r Jk (a– b–).

Explanation of the results of testing alloadsorbed sera, A, B and C

1. Because the R_1R_1-adsorbing cells were negative for the E and Jk^a antigens, adsorbed serum A could contain anti-E and anti-Jk^a. Testing the adsorbed serum A against the panel of cells suggested that this was the case.
2. Because the R_2R_2-adsorbing cells were positive for the E antigen but negative for the Jk^a antigen, adsorbed serum B could contain anti-Jk^a but not anti-E. Testing adsorbed serum B against the panel of cells confirmed the presence of anti-Jk^a.
3. Because the rr-adsorbing cells were negative for the E antigen but positive for the Jk^a antigen, adsorbed serum C could contain anti-E but not anti-Jk^a. Testing adsorbed serum C against the panel of cells confirmed the presence of anti-E.
4. Because the phenotype of the patient's own red cells was R_1r, Jk (a– b–), the anti-E and anti-Jk^a detected in the alloadsorbed sera must be alloantibodies. Blood for transfusion should be E-negative, Jk^a-negative.

Additional notes on adsorption techniques

1. If the patient has had a transfusion in the past month, an eluate must also be tested because alloantibody may be present on red cells but not in serum/plasma.
2. If the patient's serum contains a haemolytic antibody, EDTA should be added to prevent the uptake of complement and subsequent lysis of the cells used for adsorption. Add 1 volume of neutral EDTA (potassium salt) (see p. 620) to 9 volumes of serum. More commonly, a plasma sample is used.
3. It is often useful to alloadsorb both serum and eluate to differentiate between autoantibodies and alloantibodies, particularly if the autoantibody is the mimicking type described by Issitt.[18]
4. If the autoantibody does not react with papainized cells, do *not* papainize the cells for adsorption.

Elution of Antibodies from Red Cells

The selection of any elution technique is often based on personal choice and the availability of the necessary reagents and equipment. However, heat elution techniques are best used for the elution of primary cold reactive (IgM) antibodies such as anti-A, anti-N, anti-M and anti-I and IgG anti-A and anti-B antibodies associated with ABO hemolytic disease of the newborn (HDN). The Lui freeze and thaw technique (see below) may also be used for investigation of ABO HDN. Commercially prepared kits that alter the pH of the red blood cells are equally effective and circumvent the hazards of using organic solvents. Refer to the manufacturer's instructions for details. Methods for heat elution and Lui's elution techniques are given below. Commercial kits are now widely available.

Table 13.7 Testing an alloabsorbed serum against a phenotyped panel of red cells

NO.	Rh	M	N	S	s	P_1	Lu^a	Le^a	Le^b	K	Kp^a	Fy^a	Fy^b	Jk^a	Jk^b	Serum A	Serum B	Serum C
						RED CELL PHENOTYPES										RESULTS OF IAT		
1.	R_1R_1	+	+	+	+	+	−	−	−	+	−	+	+	+	+	1+	1+	−
2.	R_1R_1	+	−	−	+	−	+	−	+	−	−	+	+	+	+	1+	3+	−
3.	R_2R_2	+	+	+	+	+	+	+	−	−	−	−	+	−	+	1+	−	3+
4.	R_1R_2	+	+	+	−	+	−	−	+	−	−	−	+	+	−	1+	4+	1+
5.	$r'r$	+	−	+	+	+	−	−	+	−	−	+	+	−	+	−	−	−
6.	$r''r$	+	+	+	−	+	−	−	+	−	−	+	−	+	+	2+	2+	2+
7.	rr	+	+	−	+	+	−	−	−	+	−	+	+	+	−	2+	2+	−
8.	rr	+	−	+	+	+	−	+	−	−	−	+	−	+	−	1+	2+	(+)
9.	rr	−	+	−	+	+	−	+	−	−	+	+	+	+	+	2+	2+	−
10.	R_1R_2	−	+	+	+	−	−	−	+	+	−	−	+	+	−	1+	3+	2+

PHENOTYPE OF CELLS SELECTED FOR ABSORPTION OF SERUM								ABSORBED SERUM
1.	R_1R_1,	C^w+,	K−,	Fy(a+ b−),	Jk(a− b+),	M+, N−, s−		Serum A
2.	R_2R_2,	C^w-,	K−,	Fy(a− b+),	Jk(a− b+),	M+, N+, s+		Serum B
3.	rr,	C^w	K+	Fy(a+ b−),	Jk(a+ b−),	M+, N−, s−		Serum C

IAT, indirect antiglobulin test.

Notes

1. A large volume of red blood cells is required to obtain enough eluate for testing.
2. The red blood cells must be washed at least six times and the last wash must be kept for testing to ensure removal of all free antibody.
3. Depending on the elution technique used, the prepared eluate may be frozen if testing is not possible immediately after preparation.

Heat Elution

Mix equal volumes of washed packed cells and saline or 6% bovine serum albumin (BSA). Incubate at 56°C for 5 min. Agitate periodically. Centrifuge to pack the red cells. Remove the supernatant (the eluate), which may be haemoglobin stained. Test the eluate[48] by appropriate techniques in parallel with the last wash from the red cells.

Freeze and Thaw Elution (Lui)

Mix 0.5 ml of washed packed red cells with 3 drops of PBS or AB serum. Stopper the tube and rotate to coat the glass surface with red cells. Place at –20°C for 10 min. Thaw the red cells rapidly in a 37°C waterbath. Remove the stopper and centrifuge to sediment red cell stroma. Remove the supernatant and test in parallel with the last wash from the red cells by appropriate techniques.[49]

Screening Eluates

The eluate and the saline of the last wash (control) are first screened against two or three samples of washed normal group O cells to see if they contain any antibodies using the IAT. If anti-A or anti-B is suspected, include A and B cells. To 4–6 drops of eluate and control, add 2 drops of a 2% suspension of *normal ionic strength saline* (NISS).

Incubate for 1–1.5 hours at 37°C. Wash four times and, using optimal dilutions of anti-IgG, carry out the IAT by the tube method.

If the control preparation (the supernatant saline from the last washing) gives positive reactions, the possibility that an eluate contains serum antibody has to be considered.

Determination of the Specificity of Warm Autoantibodies in Eluates and Sera

When tested against a phenotyped panel, about two-thirds of autoantibodies appear to have Rh specificity and in about half of these cases specificity against a particular antigen can be demonstrated.[5,15,18] Within the Rh system, anti-e-like is the most common specificity. D – – and Rh_{null} cells are an advantage.

The other one-third of autoantibodies may show specificity against other, very high incidence antigens (e.g. Wrb

and Ena) and rarely other blood-group specificities are involved. It is essential to differentiate between autoantibodies and alloantibodies, especially if transfusion is being considered. The presence of alloantibodies in addition to autoantibodies is suggested by any discrepancy between the serum and eluate results.

As already mentioned, the presence of alloantibodies in a serum complicates the determination of the specificity of an autoantibody and it can be argued that it would be better to test only the eluted autoantibody and to leave the serum strictly alone. However, only a small volume of an eluate may be available, especially in patients who are anaemic and it is generally wise to test both serum and eluate. The procedure is the same for both.

Titration of Warm Antibodies in Eluates or Sera

The methods used are those described in Chapter 21. The exact technique chosen, and the red cells used, should be those that have given the clearest results in the screening tests. Titration of the eluate can be useful in the presence of a panreacting autoantibody to exclude an underlying alloantibody.

In investigating cold autoantibodies, the following tests may sometimes provide clinically useful information.

Determination of the Specificity of Cold Autoantibodies

High-titre cold autoantibodies have a well-defined blood-group specificity, which is very often within the I/i system.[18,50,51] Because the I antigen is poorly developed in cord-blood red cells, whereas the i antigen is well developed, group O cord blood red cells should be included in the panel used to test for I/i specificity. Adult cells almost always have the I antigen well expressed, but the strength of the antigen varies and it is of considerable advantage to have available adult cells known to possess strong I antigen. (The rare adult i cells, if available, can also be used.)

Titration of Cold Antibodies

If the screening test is positive for cold auto-agglutinins, titrate as follows.

Prepare doubling dilutions of the serum in saline ranging from 1 in 1 to 1 in 512 and add 1 drop of each serum dilution into three series of (12 × 75 mm) tubes so that three replicate titrations can be made. Add 1 drop of a 2% suspension of pooled saline-washed adult group O (I) cells to the first row, 1 drop of cord-blood group O (i) cells to the second row and 1 drop of the patient's own cells to the third row. Mix and leave for several hours at 4°C. Before reading, place pipettes and a tray of slides at 4°C. Read macroscopically at room temperature using chilled slides.

Normal range

Using sera from normal White adults and normal adult I red cells, the cold-agglutinin titre at 4°C is 1 to 32; and with cord-blood (i) cells the titre is 0 to 8. In chronic CHAD, the end-point may not have been reached at a dilution of 1 in 512; if that is the case, further dilutions should be prepared and tested.

If a cold agglutinin is present at a raised titre, the presence of a cold alloantibody has to be excluded. In this case, the patient's own red cells will be found to react *much* less strongly than do normal adult I red cells. It should be noted that in CHAD the patient's cells commonly react less strongly than do normal adult I cells (Table 13.8).

Cold Agglutinin Titration Patterns

The presence of high-titre cold agglutinins in a patient's serum will be indicated by the screening procedure described earlier. To demonstrate that the agglutinins are autoantibodies, it is necessary to show that the patient's own cells are also agglutinated. The titre using the patient's cells is usually less than that of control normal adult red cells (one-half or one-quarter) (Table 13.8).

In CHAD, whether 'idiopathic' or secondary to mycoplasma pneumonia or lymphoma, the autoantibodies usually have anti-I specificity (Patient A.G. in Table 13.8).

In rare cases of haemolytic anaemia associated with infectious mononucleosis, an autoantibody of anti-i specificity has been demonstrated (Patient F.B. in Table 13.8) and this specificity, too, has been found in certain patients with lymphoma. Rarely, in CHAD, the antibody has been shown to have anti-Pr or anti-M specificity: if enzyme-treated red cells are used, then in either type of case the

Table 13.8 Agglutination titres using various types of cold autoantibodies and normal adult and normal cord red cells, the patient's red cells and enzyme-treated (papainized) normal adult red cells

PATIENT	AGGLUTINATION TITRE (4°C)			
	Adult (I) cells	Cord (i) cells	Patient's cells	Papainized adult (I) cells
A.G.	4000	512	2000	8000
F.B.	512	32 000	128	8000
A.R.	2000	2000	2000	16

A.G. This patient had chronic cold haemagglutinin disease. The antibody was of the common anti-I type.
F.B. This patient had haemolytic anaemia associated with a lymphoma. The antibody was of the anti-i type.
A.R. This patient had chronic cold haemagglutinin disease. The antibody was of the rare anti-Pr type.

antigen is destroyed by enzyme treatment (Patient A.R. in Table 13.8).

Determination of the Thermal Range of Cold Agglutinins

From a series of master doubling dilutions of serum in saline, place 1 drop of serum or serum dilution into three rows of (12 × 75 mm) tubes. Set them up at 30°C and at room temperature (20–25°C); to each tube add 1 drop of a 2% saline suspension of the following cells:

1. Pooled normal adult group O (I) red cells
2. Pooled cord-blood group O (i) red cells
3. Patient's red cells.

Titration should also be carried out at 37°C, if there had been agglutination at this temperature in the screening tests. After incubation at the appropriate temperature for 1 h, determine the presence or absence of agglutination macroscopically over a light.

Detection and Titration of the Donath–Landsteiner Antibody

The D–L antibody of PCH differs from the high-titre cold antibodies referred to previously in that it is an IgG antibody and has a quite different specificity. It is also far more lytic to normal cells in relation to its titre than are anti-I or anti-i. The lysis titre of a D–L antibody may be the same or greater than its agglutination titre. Almost maximal lysis develops in unacidified serum.

Direct Donath–Landsteiner Test

Collect two samples of venous blood into tubes containing no anticoagulant, previously warmed at 37°C. Incubate the first sample at 37°C for 1.5 h. Put the second sample in a beaker packed with ice and allow to stand for 1 h, then place this tube at 37°C for a further 20 min. Centrifuge both tubes at 37°C and examine the supernatant serum for lysis. A positive test is indicated by lysis in the sample that had been chilled. If positive, investigate the antibody specificity (as described later). If negative, proceed to an indirect Donath–Landsteiner test.

A false-negative direct Donath–Landsteiner test result is not uncommon for several reasons:

1. Low antibody level
2. Low complement level (complement is consumed during the haemolytic process)
3. Presence of C3dg on the patient's red cells (does not lead to complement-mediated haemolysis).

This can be overcome by performing an indirect Donath–Landsteiner test.

Indirect Donath–Landsteiner Test

Serum obtained from the patient's blood that has been allowed to clot at 37°C is used for this test. Add 1 volume of a 50% suspension of washed normal group O, P-positive red cells to 9 volumes of the patient's unacidified serum in a tube. Chill the suspension in crushed ice at 0°C for 1 h, then place the tube at 37°C for 30 min. Centrifuge at 37°C and examine for lysis. Three controls should be set up at the same time:

1. A duplicate of the test cell–serum suspension but kept strictly at 37°C for the duration of the test.
2. A duplicate of the test cell–serum suspension, except that an equal volume of ABO-compatible fresh normal serum is first added to the patient's serum as a source of complement. One volume of the 50% cell suspension is added and the suspension is chilled and subsequently warmed in the same way as the test suspension. (This control excludes false-negative results owing to the patient's serum being deficient in complement.)
3. A duplicate of the test cell–serum suspension, except that fresh normal serum is used in place of the patient's serum. This control also is chilled and subsequently warmed.

A positive test will be indicated by lysis in the test suspension and in control No. 2. If ABO-compatible *pp* cells are available, they should be used in a duplicate set of tubes. No lysis will develop, confirming the P specificity of the antibody.

A false-negative indirect Donath–Landsteiner test can occur. This is a result of the presence of globoside in the serum added as a source of complement. Globoside is the most abundant red cell membrane glycolipid and is present in the serum of all P+ individuals. Addition of ABO-compatible fresh serum as a source of complement could result in cross-reacting with anti-P and this can lead to a false-negative indirect Donath–Landsteiner test. Therefore the indirect Donath–Landsteiner[52] test can be modified into two stages.

Two-Stage Indirect Donath–Landsteiner Test

ABO-compatible fresh serum is only added to the red cell–serum suspension after the initial 1-h incubation at 0°C. This prevents antibody inhibition during the cold phase and allows maximum sensitization of the red cells.[9]

Another possible cause of a false-negative indirect Donath–Landsteiner test result is a low antibody level. Papain treatment of the red cells will expose P antigen and can enhance the sensitization.[52]

Titration of a Donath–Landsteiner Antibody

Prepare doubling or fourfold dilutions of the patient's serum in fresh normal human serum. To each tube, add a one-tenth volume of a 50% suspension of washed group O, P-positive red cells and immerse each of the tubes in crushed ice at 0°C. After 1 h, place in a 37°C incubator for a further 30 min. Then centrifuge and inspect for lysis.

Detection of a Donath–Landsteiner Antibody by the Indirect Antiglobulin Test

Because the D–L antibody is an IgG antibody, it can be detected by the IAT using an anti-IgG serum if the cells that have been exposed to the antibody in the cold are washed in cold (4°C) saline. At this temperature, the antibody will not be eluted during washing. It should be noted, however, that exposing normal red cells at 4°C to many fresh normal sera results in a positive IAT with broad-spectrum antiglobulin sera because of the adsorption of incomplete anti-H (a normally occurring cold antibody) on to the red cells. At a low temperature, complement is bound too, and it is its adsorption that gives rise to the positive tests with broad-spectrum sera. The adsorption of complement can be prevented by adding a chelating agent, such as EDTA, to the serum.

Method

Add a one-tenth volume of EDTA, buffered to pH 7.0 (see p. 620) to the patient's serum. Prepare doubling dilutions in saline from 1 in 1 to 1 in 28.

Add 1 volume (drop) of a 50% suspension of group O, P-positive red cells to 10 volumes (drops) of each dilution. Mix and chill at 4°C (preferably in a cold room).

After 1 h, wash the red cells four times in a large volume of cold (4°C) saline. Then carry out an antiglobulin test using an anti-IgG reagent, as described on p. 500, but keeping the red cell-antiglobulin serum suspension at 4°C.

As controls, set up a series of tests using a serum known to contain a D–L antibody (if available) and a normal serum, respectively.

This technique is the most sensitive way of detecting, especially in stored sera, the presence of a D–L antibody in an amount insufficient to bring about actual lysis.

Thermal range of Donath–Landsteiner antibody

The highest temperature at which D–L antibodies are usually adsorbed onto red cells is about 18°C. Hence little or no lysis can be expected unless the cell–serum suspension is cooled below this temperature. Chilling in crushed ice results in maximum adsorption of the antibody and leads to the binding of complement, which brings about lysis when the cell suspension is subsequently warmed at 37°C. Hence the 'cold-warm' biphasic procedure necessary for lysis to be demonstrated with a typical D–L antibody.

Specificity of the Donath–Landsteiner antibody

The D–L antibody appears to have a well-defined specificity within the GLOB blood-group system: namely, anti-P. However, in practice, almost all samples of red cells are acted upon because the cells that will not react (P[k] and pp) are extremely rare.[53] Cord blood cells are lysed to about the same extent as are adult P_1 and P_2 cells.

Treatment of Serum with 2-Mercaptoethanol or Dithiothreitol

Weak solutions of 2-mercaptoethanol (2-ME) or dithiothreitol (DTT) destroy the inter-chain sulphydryl bonds of gamma globulins. IgM antibodies treated in this way lose their ability to agglutinate red cells while IgG antibodies do not.[18] IgA antibodies may or may not be inhibited depending upon whether or not they are made up of polymers of IgA. Since almost all autoantibodies are either IgM or IgG, treatment of serum or an eluate with 2-ME or DTT gives a reliable indication of the Ig class of autoantibody under investigation.[18,54]

Method

2-Mercaptoethanol

To 1 volume of undiluted serum add 1 volume of 0.1 mol/l 2-ME in phosphate buffer, pH 7.2 (see p. 622).

As a control, add a volume of the serum to the phosphate buffer alone. Incubate both at 37°C for 2 h. Then titrate the treated serum and its control with the appropriate red cells.

If IgG antibody is present, the antibody titration in the control serum will be the same as that of the treated serum. However, if the antibody is IgM, the treated serum will fail to agglutinate the test cells or will agglutinate them to a much lower titre compared with the control untreated serum.

The control must remain active to show that the absence of agglutination is the result of reduction of IgM antibody and not dilution.

Dithiothreitol

0.01 mol/l DTT can be used in place of 0.1 mol/l 2-ME in the previous method.

Drug-Induced Haemolytic Anaemias of Immunological Origin

As already mentioned, acquired haemolytic anaemias may develop as the result of immunological reactions consequent on the administration of certain drugs.[15,55–57] Clinically, they often closely mimic AIHA of 'idiopathic' origin and for this reason a careful enquiry into the taking of drugs is a necessary part of the interrogation of any patient suspected of having an acquired haemolytic anaemia.

Two immunological mechanisms leading to a drug-induced haemolytic anaemia are recognized. These mechanisms can be referred to as 'drug-dependent immune' and 'drug-induced autoimmune'. Both types of antibody may be present in some patients.[58,59] In a unifying concept, the target orientation of these antibodies covers a spectrum in which the primary immune response is initiated by an interaction between the drug or its metabolites and a component of the blood cell membrane to create a neoantigen.[60] Drug-dependent antibodies bind to both the drug and the cell, membrane but not to either separately. If the drug is withdrawn, the immune reaction subsides. It has been postulated that in the case of the autoantibodies, the greater part of the neoantigen is sufficiently similar to the normal cell membrane to allow binding without the drug being present. Similar mechanisms have been described for drug-induced immune thrombocytopenia and neutropenia of immunological origin (see p. 508).

In drug-dependent immune haemolytic anaemia, the drug is required in the *in vitro* system for the antibodies to be detected. The red cells become damaged by one of two mechanisms:

1. *Complement lysis.* A typical history is for haemolysis, which may be severe and intravascular, to follow the readministration of a drug with which the patient has previously been treated and for the haemolysis to subside when the offending drug is withdrawn. The DAT is likely to become strongly positive during the haemolytic phase, the patient's red cells being agglutinated by anti-C′ and sometimes by anti-IgG. Drugs that have been shown to cause haemolysis by the previously explained mechanism include quinine, quinidine and rifampicin, chlorpropamide, hydrochlorothiazide, nomifensine, phenacetin, salicylazosulphapyridine, the sodium salt of *p*-aminosalicylic acid and stibophen. Petz and Branch listed 25 drugs reported to have brought about haemolysis by this mechanism.[56]

2. *Extravascular haemolysis.* This is brought about by IgG antibodies that usually do not activate complement or if they do, not beyond C3. The DAT will be positive with anti-IgG and sometimes also with anti-C′. The haemolytic anaemia associated with prolonged high-dose penicillin therapy is caused by the previously mentioned mechanism and other penicillin derivatives, as well as cephalosporins and tetracycline, may cause haemolysis in a similar fashion. Haemolysis ceases when the offending drug has been withdrawn.

Cephalosporins, in addition to causing the formation of specific antibodies, may alter the red cell surface so as to cause non-specific adherence of complement and immunoglobulins. This may lead to a positive DAT but is seldom associated with increased haemolysis, although where it occurs it can be very severe.

Drug-Induced Autoimmune Haemolytic Anaemias

In the case of drug-induced autoimmune haemolytic anaemias, the antibody reacts with the red cell in the absence of the drug (these are sometimes referred to as 'drug-independent antibodies'). The anti-red cell autoantibodies seem to

Table 13.9 Serological features of the different types of drug-induced haemolytic anaemia of immunological origin

MECHANISM	PROTOTYPE DRUG	DAT	IAT		
			No drug	**Serum + drug**	**Eluate + drug**
Drug-dependent antibody					
C′ activation	Quin(id)ine	C′ᵃ	Neg	C′ᵃ	Neg
No C′ activation	Penicillin	IgG	Neg	IgG	IgG
Autoantibody	α-Methyldopa	IgG	IgG		

ᵃOccasionally also IgG.

be serologically identical to those of 'idiopathic' warm-type AIHA. When the drug was widely used, the great majority of cases followed the use of the antihypertension drug α-methyldopa. The red cells are coated with IgG and the serum contains autoantibodies that characteristically have Rh specificity.

Other drugs that have been reported to act in a similar fashion to α-methyldopa include L-dopa, chlordiazepoxide, mefenamic acid, flufenamic acid and indometacin.[5]

Typical serological features of the different types of drug-induced haemolytic anaemia of immunological origin are summarized in Table 13.9.

Detection of Antipenicillin Antibodies

The characteristic features of penicillin-induced haemolytic anaemia are as follows:

1. Haemolysis occurs only in patients receiving large doses of a penicillin for long periods (e.g. weeks).
2. The DAT is strongly positive with anti-IgG reagents.
3. The patient's serum and antibody eluted from the patient's red cells react *only* with penicillin-treated red cells – they do not react with normal untreated red cells.

Reagents

Barbitone buffer. 0.14 mol/l, pH 9.5 (see p. 621).

Penicillin solution. 0.4 g of penicillin G dissolved in 6 ml of barbitone buffer.

Penicillin-Coated Normal Red Cells

Wash group O reagent red cells three times in saline and make an approximately 15% suspension in saline to which a one-tenth volume of barbitone buffer has been added. Add 2 ml of the red cell suspension to 6 ml of penicillin solution and incubate at 37°C for 1 h. Then wash four times in saline and make 2% red cell suspensions in saline (for tube tests).

Control normal red cells

Control normal red cells should be treated in exactly the same way as the penicillin-coated red cells except that the 6 ml of penicillin solution is replaced by 6 ml of barbitone buffer.

Method

Antipenicillin antibodies can be detected by the IAT in the usual way using the penicillin-coated red cells in place of normal unmodified cells. However, three extra controls are necessary.

1. Red cells that have not been exposed to penicillin should be added to the patient's serum.
2. Penicillin-treated red cells should be added to two normal sera known not to contain antipenicillin antibodies (*negative controls*).
3. Penicillin-treated red cells should be added to a serum (if one is available) known to contain antipenicillin antibodies (*positive control*).

Cephalosporin can be used in a similar way to sensitize red cells. Control (item 2) is particularly important when drugs such as cephalosporins are used because overexposure *in vitro* to these drugs can lead to positive results with normal sera.

Note

Some drugs do not dissolve easily; incubation at 37°C, crushing tablets with a pestle and mortar and vigorous shaking of the solution may help.

High-titre IgG antipenicillin antibodies often cause direct agglutination of penicillin-treated red cells in low dilutions of serum. The antibodies can be differentiated from IgM agglutinating antibodies by treatment with 2-ME or DTT (see p. 289).

Detection of Antibodies against Drugs Other than Penicillin

In a patient with an immune haemolytic anaemia whose serum and red cell eluate does *not* react with normal red

Table 13.10 Investigation of a suspected drug-induced immune haemolytic anaemia

	TUBE No.					
	1	2	3	4	5	6
Patient's serum (drops)	10	10	5	5	0	0
Fresh normal serum (drops)	0	0	5	5	10	10
Drug solution volumes (drops)	2	0	2	0	2	0
Saline volumes (drops)	0	2	0	2	0	2
50% normal group O cells volumes (drops)	1	1	1	1	1	1

cells and who is receiving a drug or drugs other than penicillin or a penicillin derivative, antibodies that react with red cells only in the presence of the suspect drugs or drugs should be looked for in the following way.

The patient's serum and red cell eluates should be tested with normal and enzyme-treated group O red cells, carrying out the tests with and without the drug that the patient is receiving. The approach is essentially empirical. A saturated solution of the drug or its metabolite should be prepared in saline and the pH should be adjusted to 6.5–7.0.

Set up six tubes containing the patient's serum and the drug solution in the proportions shown in Table 13.10 and add 1 drop of a 50% saline suspension of group O cells to each tube. Incubate at 37°C for 1 h, then examine for agglutination and lysis. Wash the red cells four times in saline, and carry out an IAT using anti-IgG and anti-C′ separately.

Interpretation

Tubes 1 and 2 test the patient's serum (? drug-dependent antibody) and normal red cells in the presence of the drug (Tube 1) and without the drug (Tube 2). Tubes 3 and 4 test the effect of added complement on the previous reactions. Tubes 5 and 6 without the patient's serum act as controls for tubes 3 and 4.

OXIDANT-INDUCED HAEMOLYTIC ANAEMIA

Oxidant-induced haemolytic anaemia should be suspected when the blood film of a patient exposed to an oxidant drug or chemical shows irregularly contracted cells. A Heinz-body test (see p. 336) is confirmatory. The oxidant

may also cause methaemoglobinaemia or sulphaemoglobinaemia, both of which can be confirmed by spectroscopy (see p. 240) or co-oximetry. The differential diagnosis of haemolysis induced by an exogenous oxidant includes other causes of haemolysis with irregularly contracted cells (e.g. Zieve's syndrome), G6PD deficiency and the presence of an unstable haemoglobin. In Zieve's syndrome (haemolysis associated with alcohol excess, fatty liver and hyperlipidaemia), the plasma may be visibly lipaemic; if this syndrome is suspected, further investigations should include liver function test and serum lipid measurements.

MICROANGIOPATHIC AND MECHANICAL HAEMOLYTIC ANAEMIAS

Microangiopathic or mechanical haemolytic anaemia should be suspected when a blood film shows schistocytes. Examination of the blood film is, in fact, the most important laboratory procedure in making this diagnosis, although some automated blood cell counters will also detect the presence of red cell fragments. Because haemolysis is intravascular, useful confirmatory tests include serum haptoglobin estimation (see p. 233) and, when the condition is chronic, a Perls' stain of urinary sediment to detect the presence of haemosiderin (see p. 236). Because a microangiopathic haemolytic anaemia is often part of a more generalized syndrome resulting from microvascular damage or fibrin deposition, other tests are also indicated in unexplained cases. They include tests of renal function, a platelet count and a coagulation screen including tests for D-dimer or fibrin degradation products (see p. 440). Tests for verotoxin-secreting *E. coli* are indicated in cases of microangiopathic haemolytic anaemia with renal failure. If available, quantification of von Willebrand factor-cleaving protease (ADAMTS13) is indicated in suspected thrombotic thrombocytopenic purpura.

PAROXYSMAL NOCTURNAL HAEMOGLOBINURIA

Paroxysmal nocturnal haemoglobinuria (PNH) is an acquired clonal disorder of haemopoiesis, in which the patient's red cells are abnormally sensitive to lysis by normal constituents of plasma. In its classical form, it is characterized by haemoglobinuria during sleep (nocturnal haemoglobinuria), jaundice and haemosiderinuria. Not uncommonly, however, PNH presents as an obscure anaemia without obvious evidence of intravascular haemolysis or it develops in a patient suffering from aplastic anaemia or more rarely from primary myelofibrosis or chronic myeloid leukaemia.[61,62]

PNH red cells are unusually susceptible to lysis by complement.[63,64] This can be demonstrated *in vitro* by a variety of tests (e.g. the acidified-serum [Ham],[65] sucrose,[66] thrombin,[67] cold-antibody lysis,[68] inulin[69] and cobravenom[70] tests). In the acidified serum, inulin and cobravenom tests, complement is activated via the alternative pathway, whereas in the cold-antibody test and probably in the thrombin test, complement is activated by the classical sequence initiated through antigen–antibody interaction. In the sucrose lysis test, a low ionic strength is thought to lead to the binding of IgG molecules non-specifically to the cell membrane and to the subsequent activation of complement via the classical sequence. In addition, the alternative pathway appears to be activated.[71] In each test, PNH cells undergo lysis because of their greatly increased sensitivity to lysis by complement.

Minor degrees of lysis may be observed in the cold-antibody lysis and sucrose tests with the red cells from a variety of dyserythropoietic anaemias (e.g. aplastic anaemia, megaloblastic anaemia and primary myelofibrosis).[72,73] Weak positive results in these tests thus have to be interpreted with care. PNH red cells, however, almost always undergo considerable lysis in these tests.

A characteristic feature of a positive test for PNH is that not all the patient's cells undergo lysis, even if the conditions of the test are made optimal for lysis (Fig. 13.1). This is because only a proportion of any PNH patient's red cell population is hypersensitive to lysis by complement. This population varies from patient to patient and there is a direct relationship between the proportion of

red cells that can be lysed (in any of the diagnostic tests) and the severity of *in vivo* haemolysis.

The phenomenon of some red cells being sensitive to complement lysis and some being insensitive was studied quantitatively by Rosse and Dacie, who obtained two-component complement sensitivity curves in a series of patients with PNH.[64] Later, Rosse reported that in some cases three populations of red cells could be demonstrated.[74,75]

1. Very sensitive (type III) cells, 10–15 times more sensitive than normal cells
2. Cells of medium sensitivity (type II), 3–5 times more sensitive than normal cells
3. Cells of normal sensitivity (type I).

In vivo the proportion of type III cells parallels the severity of the patient's haemolysis.

PNH is an acquired clonal disorder[76] resulting from a somatic mutation occurring in a haemopoietic stem cell. It has been demonstrated that a proportion of granulocytes, platelets and lymphocytes are also part of the PNH clone.[77,78] The characteristic feature of cells belonging to the PNH clone is that they are deficient in several cell-membrane–bound proteins including red cell acetylcholinesterase,[79–81] neutrophil alkaline phosphatase,[82–84] CD55 (decay accelerating factor or DAF),[85,86] homologous restriction factor (HRF),[63,87] and CD59 (membrane inhibitor of reactive lysis or MIRL),[88–90] among others. CD55, CD59 and HRF all have roles in the protection of the cell against complement-mediated attack. CD59 inhibits the formation of the terminal complex of complement and it has been established that the deficiency of CD59 is largely responsible for the complement sensitivity of PNH red cells. PNH type III red cells have a complete deficiency of CD59, whereas PNH type II red cells have only a partial deficiency and it is this difference that accounts for their variable sensitivities to complement.[91,92] The analysis of these deficient proteins on PNH cells by flow cytometry, particularly of the red cells and neutrophils, has become a useful research and diagnostic tool but is only applicable in centres with a significant number of patients requiring investigation for PNH. By comparing the proportion of cells with deficient CD59 to the percentage lysis in the Ham test, it has been possible to assess the sensitivity of the Ham test. The standard Ham test is reasonably good at estimating the proportion of PNH red cells as long as they are PNH type III cells and comprise <20% of the total. In cases in which the PNH cells are type II and >20% are present, the standard Ham test significantly underestimates the proportion of PNH red cells. The standard Ham test can be negative when there are <5% PNH type III cells or <20% PNH type II cells. When the Ham test is supplemented with magnesium, to optimize the activation of complement, the percentage lysis gives a more accurate estimation of the proportion of PNH cells (Fig. 13.2).[93]

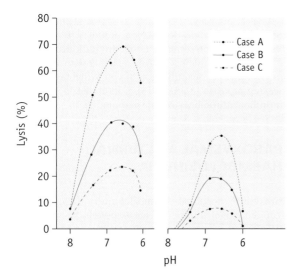

Figure 13.1 Effect of pH on lysis *in vitro* of paroxysmal nocturnal haemoglobinuria (PNH) red cells by human sera. The red cells of three patients with disease of different severity and two fresh normal sera, one serum being more potent than the other, were used.

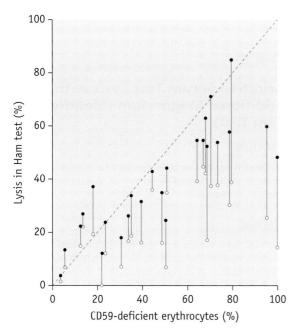

Figure 13.2 Comparison of the proportion of CD59-deficient red cells with the lysis in the Ham test. The percentage lysis in the Ham test with added magnesium (●) and without added magnesium (o) is plotted against the proportion of CD59-deficient red cells in the same samples from 25 patients with paroxysmal nocturnal haemoglobinuria (PNH). *(With thanks to P. Hillmen, M. Bessler, D. Roper and L. Luzzatto, unpublished observation.)*

Certain chemicals, in particular sulphydryl compounds, can act on normal red cells *in vitro* so as to increase their complement sensitivity. In this way, PNH-like red cells can be created in the laboratory and can be used as useful reagents.

Acidified-Serum Lysis Test (Ham test)

Principle

The patient's red cells are exposed at 37°C to the action of normal or the patient's own serum suitably acidified to the optimum pH for lysis (pH 6.5–7.0) (Table 13.11).

The patient's red cells can be obtained from defibrinated, heparinized, oxalated, citrated or EDTA blood and the test can be satisfactorily carried out even on cells that have been stored at 4°C for up to 2–3 weeks in ACD or Alsever's solution, if kept sterile. The patient's serum is best obtained by defibrination because in PNH if it is obtained from blood allowed to clot in the ordinary way at 37°C or at room temperature, it will almost certainly be markedly lysed. Normal serum should similarly be obtained by defibrination, although serum derived from blood allowed to clot spontaneously at room temperature or at 37°C can be used. Normal serum known to be strongly lytic to PNH red cells is to be preferred to patient's serum, the lytic potentiality of which is unknown. However, if the test is positive using normal serum, it is important, particularly if the patient appears not to be suffering from overt intravascular haemolysis, to obtain a positive result using the patient's serum to exclude hereditary erythroid multinuclearity associated with a positive acidified-serum test (HEMPAS) (see p. 294). The variability between the sera of individuals

Table 13.11 The acidified-serum lysis test with added magnesium

REAGENT	TEST (ml)			CONTROLS (ml)		
	1	2	3	4	5	6
Fresh normal serum	0.5	0.5	0	0.5	0.5	0
Heat-inactivated normal serum	0	0	0.5	0	0	0.5
0.2 mol/l HCl	0	0.05	0.05	0	0.05	0.05
50% patient's red cells	0.05	0.05	0.05	0	0	0
50% normal red cells	0	0	0	0.05	0.05	0.05
Magnesium chloride (250 mmol/l; 23.7 g/l)[a]	0.01	0.01	0.01	0.01	0.01	0.01
Lysis (in a positive modified test)	Trace (2%)	+++ (30%)	–	–	–	–

[a]Only for modified test.

in their capacity to lyse PNH red cells is shown in Figure 13.1. The activity of a single individual's serum also varies from time to time,[94] and it is always important to include in any test, as a positive control, a sample of known PNH cells or artificially created 'PNH-like' cells (see p. 296).

The sera should be used within a few hours of collection. Their lytic potency is retained for several months at –70°C, but at 4°C, and even at –20°C, this deteriorates within a few days.

Method

Deliver 0.5 ml samples of fresh normal serum, group AB or ABO-compatible with the patient's blood, into 3 pairs of 75 × 12 mm tubes. Place two tubes at 56°C for 10–30 min to inactivate complement. Keep the other 2 pairs of tubes at room temperature and add to the serum in two of the tubes one-tenth volumes (0.05 ml) of 0.2 mol/l HCl. Add similar volumes of acid to the inactivated serum samples. Then place all the tubes in a 37°C waterbath.

While the serum samples are being dealt with, wash samples of the patient's red cells and of control normal red cells (compatible with the normal serum) twice in saline and prepare 50% suspensions in the saline. Then add one-tenth volumes of each of these cell suspensions (0.05 ml) to one of the tubes containing unacidified fresh serum, acidified fresh serum and acidified inactivated serum, respectively. Mix the contents carefully and leave the tubes at 37°C. Centrifuge them after about 1 h.

Add 0.05 ml of each cell suspension to 0.55 ml of water so as to prepare a standard for subsequent quantitative measurement of lysis and retain 0.5 ml of serum for use as a blank. For the measurement of lysis, deliver 0.3 ml volumes of the supernatants of the test and control series of cell–serum suspensions and of the blank serum and of the lysed cell suspension equivalent to 0% and 100% lysis, respectively, into 5 ml of 0.4 ml/l ammonia or Drabkin's reagent. Measure the lysis in a photoelectric colorimeter using a yellow–green (e.g. Ilford 625) filter or in a spectrometer at a wavelength of 540 nm.

If the test cells are from a patient with PNH, they will undergo definite, although incomplete, lysis in the acidified serum. Much less lysis or even no lysis at all, will be visible in the unacidified serum. No lysis will be brought about by the acidified inactivated serum. The normal control sample of cells should not undergo lysis in any of the three tubes.

In PNH, 10–50% lysis is usually obtained when lysis is measured as liberated haemoglobin. Exceptionally, there may be as much as 80% lysis or as little as 5%.

The red cells of a patient who has had a transfusion will undergo less lysis than they would have before the transfusion because the normal transfused cells do not have increased sensitivity to lysis. In PNH, it is characteristic that a young cell (reticulocyte-rich) population, such as the upper red cell layer obtained by centrifugation, undergoes more lysis than the red cells derived from mixed whole blood.

Acidified-Serum Test Lysis with Additional Magnesium (Modified Ham Test)

Principle

The sensitivity of the Ham test can be improved by the addition of magnesium to the test to enhance the activation of complement.

Method

The method is identical to that for the standard Ham test (see above) with the addition of 10 µl of 250 mmol magnesium chloride (final concentration = 4 mmol) to each tube prior to the incubation (Table 13.11).

Significance of the Acidified-Serum Lysis Test

A positive acidified-serum test, carried out with proper controls, denotes the PNH abnormality and PNH cannot be diagnosed unless the acidified-serum test is positive. The addition of magnesium chloride increases the sensitivity of the acidified-serum test.

When the acidified-serum test is positive, a direct antiglobulin test (see p. 500) should also be carried out. If this is positive, it could be the result of a lytic antibody that has given a false-positive acidified-serum test. This can be confirmed by appropriate serological studies. In such complex cases flow cytometry after reaction of the red cells with anti-CD59 is recommended because it is a more definitive test for PNH (see below).

The only disorder other than PNH that may appear to give a clear-cut positive test result is a rare congenital dyserythropoietic anaemia, congenital dyserythropoietic anaemia type II or HEMPAS.[95,96] In contrast to PNH, however, HEMPAS red cells undergo lysis in only a proportion (about 30%) of normal sera; moreover, they do not undergo lysis in the patient's own acidified serum and the sucrose lysis test is negative. In HEMPAS, the expression of glycosylphosphatidylinositol (GPI)-linked proteins, such as CD55 and CD59, is normal. Lysis in HEMPAS appears to be a result of the presence on the red cells of an unusual antigen, which reacts with a complement-fixing IgM antibody ('anti-HEMPAS') present in many, but not in all, normal sera.[96]

Heating at 56°C inactivates the lytic system and, if there is lysis in inactivated serum, the test cannot be considered positive. Markedly spherocytic red cells or effete normal red cells may lyse in acidified serum, probably owing to the lowered pH, and such cells may also lyse in acidified inactivated serum.

PNH red cells are not unduly sensitive to lysis by a lowered pH *per se*. The addition of the acid adjusts the pH of the serum–cell mixture to the optimum for the activity of the lytic system. As is shown in Figure 13.1, it is possible to construct pH–lysis curves, if different concentrations of acid are used. The optimum pH for lysis is between pH 6.5 and 7.0 (measurements made after the addition of the red cells to the serum).

Sucrose Lysis Test

An iso-osmotic solution of sucrose (92.4 g/l) is required.[97] This can be stored at 4°C for up to 3 weeks.

For the test, set up two tubes, one containing 0.05 ml of fresh normal group AB- or ABO-compatible serum diluted in 0.85 ml of sucrose solution and the other containing 0.05 ml of serum diluted in 0.85 ml of saline. Add to each tube 0.1 ml of a 50% suspension of washed red cells. After incubation at 37°C for 30 min, centrifuge the tubes and examine for lysis. If lysis is visible in the sucrose-containing tube, measure this in a photoelectric colorimeter or a spectrometer as described earlier, using the tube containing serum diluted in saline as a blank and a tube containing 0.1 ml of the red cells suspension in 0.9 ml of 0.4 ml/l ammonia in place of the sucrose–serum mixture as a standard for 100% lysis.

Interpretation

The sucrose lysis test is based on the fact that red cells absorb complement components from serum at low ionic concentrations.[94,98] PNH cells, because of their great sensitivity, undergo lysis but normal red cells do not. The red cells from some patients with leukaemia[72] or primary myelofibrosis may undergo a small amount of lysis, almost always <10%; in such cases, the acidified-serum test is usually negative and PNH should not be diagnosed. In PNH, lysis is usually between 10% and 80%, but exceptionally may be as little as 5%. Sucrose lysis and acidified-serum lysis of PNH red cells are fairly closely correlated. The sucrose lysis test is usually negative in HEMPAS.

Flow Cytometry Analysis of the GPI-Linked Proteins on Red Cells

Principle

The patient's red cells are stained with a fluorescein-labelled antibody that is specific for one of several GPI-linked proteins, for example CD55, CD58 (leucocyte function antigen-3) or CD59 ('protectin'), which are deficient in PNH red cells. The stained cells are then analysed with a flow cytometer. In some laboratories where facilities are available, flow cytometry has replaced the Ham test as the primary method for the diagnosis of PNH.

The patient's red cells can be obtained in any of the anticoagulants described for the Ham test. The cells, if taken into ACD, can be stored for 2–3 weeks prior to analysis. Fluorescein-conjugated anti-CD59 (MEM 43, Cymbus Bioscience Ltd, Southampton, UK) gives excellent results when used for red cell analysis. It is important to use the conjugated antibody because staining with unconjugated anti-CD59 followed by a fluorescein-conjugated second layer antibody may result in artefact, probably owing to red cell agglutination. There is no suitable anti-CD55 antibody commercially available at present. Anti-CD58 (BRIC5, Bioproducts Laboratories, UK, used at 20 µg/ml) gives reproducible results for red cell analysis, but the level of CD58 expression on PNH type-II cells is higher than that of many other GPI-linked proteins and thus studying CD58 expression is useful but not ideal.[99]

Method

Chill 1×10^6 cells in 50 µl of PBS on ice with 50 µl of monoclonal antibody for 30 min. Wash twice in PBS + azide (200 mg/l) and then chill with fluorescein-labelled goat antimouse antibody on ice in the dark for 30 min. Wash twice in PBS + azide and then fix with approximately 0.5 ml of 1% formaldehyde in Isoton II (Beckman Coulter). Analysis is performed using a flow cytometer. A negative control antibody should always be used to assess the fluorescence of cells lacking the antigen. The cells from a normal subject should be stained as an additional control to verify that negative cells in the test sample are true PNH cells and not artefactual.

Other Immunological Techniques

The GPI-linked proteins such as CD59 can also be studied by a modification of the gel technology used for blood grouping.

Flow Cytometry Analysis of the GPI-Anchor or GPI-Linked Proteins on Neutrophils

Principle

A proportion of the patient's neutrophils have been demonstrated to be part of the PNH clone in all patients with PNH. GPI-linked proteins that are suitable for analysis include CD16, CD24, CD55, CD59 and CD67.[100,101] There are available numerous fluorescein-conjugated antibodies to CD16 that are suitable for use in this analysis – for example, fluorescein-conjugated anti-Leu-11a (Beckman Coulter). Similarly, fluorescein-conjugated anti-CD59 (Cymbus Biosciences) and anti-CD55 are of value. FLAER (fluorescein-labelled pro-aerolysin) analysis can also be used, pro-aerolysin binding selectively and with high affinity to the GPI anchor.[102]

Method

The patient's neutrophils are obtained by collecting blood, anticoagulating with preservative-free heparin (10 μ/ml), and obtaining a buffy coat. The formation of a buffy coat can be accelerated by adding 1 ml of 6% hetastarch in 0.9% sodium chloride (Hespan, DuPont) to 10 ml of blood. Then $1–2 \times 10^6$ cells are analysed. It is important that all the subsequent staining and washing are performed at 4°C to minimize non-specific staining. Chill the cells in 50 μl of PBS on ice with 50 μl of mono-clonal antibody (MoAb) for 30 min. Wash twice in PBS + 0.1% BSA (PBS + BSA) and then chill with fluorescein-labelled goat antimouse antibody on ice in the dark for 30 min. Wash twice in PBS + BSA and then fix with approximately 0.5 ml of 1% formaldehyde in Isoton II (Beckman Coulter). For conjugated antibodies, a single incubation step only is required, followed by a wash and then fixing prior to analysis. Analysis is performed using a flow cytometer. Appropriate normal controls and negative controls should always be tested in parallel to the patient's samples.

A negative control antibody should always be used to assess the fluorescence of cells lacking the antigen. The cells from a normal subject should be stained as an additional control to verify that negative cells in the test sample are true PNH cells and not an artefact.

Significance of Flow Cytometric Analysis

The presence of a population of cells with a deficiency of more than one GPI-linked protein is diagnostic of PNH (Fig. 13.3). It is important to analyse more than one protein, because there are extremely rare cases in which an inherited deficiency of one protein has been described (i.e. the Inab phenotype,[103-105] a deficiency of CD55 owing to a defect of the structural gene encoding this protein, and inherited deficiency of CD59[106] due to a defect in the gene encoding CD59). Analysis of the expression of CD59 on erythrocytes allows the identification of PNH type II as well as PNH type III red cells. This is important because, although patients with only PNH type II red cells do not usually suffer from significant haemolysis, they may suffer some of the complications of PNH, such as thrombosis. The analysis of neutrophils for GPI-linked proteins is more difficult than red cell analysis. It is, however, probably more sensitive because the proportion of abnormal neutrophils is usually higher than the proportion of PNH red cells because of the reduced survival of PNH red cells compared to normal cells and because of the effect of transfusions. Thus, flow cytometry applied to neutrophils is a more sensitive method for the diagnosis of PNH than methods relying on the complement sensitivity of PNH red cells.

Figure 13.3 Expression of glycosylphosphatidylinositol (GPI)-linked proteins on the red cells in paroxysmal nocturnal haemoglobinuria (PNH). Flow cytometry of the erythrocytes from a normal control and three patients with PNH stained with a negative control antibody and antibodies to several GPI-linked proteins. M.B, two populations; normal and absent GPI-linked proteins. C.J, mainly reduced GPI-linked proteins, but there is also a very small normal component present. R.K, three populations; normal, reduced and absent GPI-linked proteins. Fl, fluorescence intensity.

PNH-Like Red Cells

By treating normal red cells with certain chemicals, it is possible to increase their complement sensitivity so that they take on many of the characteristics of PNH cells.[107] The chemicals include sulphydryl compounds such as L-cysteine, reduced glutathione, 2-aminoethyl-*iso*-thiouronium bromide (AET) and 2-mercaptobenzoic acid.[108] AET- and 2-mercaptobenzoic acid-treated cells can be used conveniently as a positive control for *in vitro* lysis tests for PNH.[109]

Preparation of AET Cells

Prepare an 8 g/l solution of AET and adjust its pH to 8.0 with 5 mol/l NaOH. Collect normal blood into ACD and wash it ×2 in 9 g/l NaCl. Add 1 volume of the packed cells to 4 volumes of the AET solution in a 75 × 12 mm tube, which is then stoppered. Mix the contents gently and place the tube at 37°C for 10–20 min; the optimal time of incubation varies between red cell samples. Then wash the cells repeatedly with large volumes of saline until the supernatant is colourless. The red cells are now ready to use.[110]

Summary of Testing for PNH

The Ham test is still an important diagnostic test in PNH. If carried out with additional magnesium chloride and performed with the necessary controls, it is more sensitive than the unmodified test and remains specific for the diagnosis of PNH. The inclusion of a further test, such as the sucrose lysis test, is optional. The use of flow cytometry permits a better estimate of the size of the PNH clone and identifies the type of red cell abnormality. However, more experience and expensive equipment are required to perform flow cytometry reliably than are necessary to perform a Ham test. Flow cytometry is a useful diagnostic test in certain circumstances, especially when the patient is heavily transfused and it becomes necessary to analyse neutrophils and when following a patient after bone marrow transplantation. Flow cytometry may also be useful in the follow-up of groups of patients with aplastic anaemia because clonal evolution into PNH may be detected at an earlier stage. For laboratories already using gel technology for blood grouping and antibody screening, this technique provides a simple method for screening red cells for deficiency of GPI-linked protein.

REFERENCES

1. Chen FE, Owen I, Savage D, et al. Late onset haemolysis and red cell autoimmunization after allogeneic bone marrow transplant. *Bone Marrow Transplant.* 1997;19: 491–495.

2. Sanz J, Arriaga F, Montesinos P, et al. Autoimmune hemolytic anemia following allogeneic hematopoietic stem cell transplantation in adult patients. *Bone Marrow Transplant.* 2007;39:555–561.

3. O'Brien TA, Eastlund T, Peters C, et al. Autoimmune haemolytic anaemia complicating haematopoietic cell transplantation in paediatric patients: high incidence and significant mortality in unrelated donor transplants for non-malignant diseases. *Br J Haematol.* 2004;127:67–75.

4. Arndt PA, Leger RM, Garratty G. Serology of antibodies to second and third generation cephalosporins associated with immune hemolytic anaemia and/or positive direct antiglobulin tests. *Transfusion.* 1999;39:1239–1246.

5. Dacie JV, Worlledge SM. Auto-immune hemolytic anaemias. *Prog Hematol.* 1969;6:82–120.

6. Sokol RJ, Hewitt S, Stamps BK. Autoimmune haemolysis: An 18-year study of 865 cases referred to a regional transfusion centre. *Br Med J.* 1981;282:2023–2027.

7. Sokol RJ, Hewitt S, Stamos BK. Autoimmune haemolysis: mixed warm and cold antibody type. *Acta Haematol.* 1983;69:266–274.

8. Dacie JV. Auto-immune hemolytic anemias. *Arch Intern Med.* 1975;135: 1293–1300.

9. Petz LD, Garratty G. *Acquired Immune Haemolytic Anaemias.* 2nd ed. New York: Churchill Livingstone; 2004.

10. Morselli M, Luppi M, Potenza L, et al. Mixed warm and cold autoimmune hemolytic anemia: Complete recovery after 2 courses of rituximab treatment. *Blood.* 2002;99: 3478–3479.

11. Shulman IA, Branch DR, Nelson JM, et al. Autoimmune hemolytic anemia with both cold and warm autoantibodies. *J Am Med Assoc.* 1985;253:1746–1748.

12. Win N, Tiwari D, Keevil VL, et al. Mixed-type autoimmune haemolytic anaemia: unusual cases and a case associated with splenic T cell angioimmuno-blastic A non-Hodgkins' lymphoma. *Hematology.* 2007;12:159–162.

13. Dacie J. *The Haemolytic Anaemias. Vol. 3. The Auto-Immune Haemolytic Anaemias.* 3rd ed. Edinburgh: Churchill Livingstone; 1992.

14. Pirofsky B. *Autoimmunization and the Autoimmune Hemolytic Anemias.* Baltimore: Williams & Wilkins; 1969.

15. Petz LD, Garratty G. *Acquired Immune Hemolytic Anemias.* New York: Churchill Livingstone; 1980.

16. Sokol RJ, Hewitt S. Autoimmune hemolysis: a critical review. *CRC Critical Reviews in Oncology/ Hematology.* 1985;4:125–154.

17. Sokol RJ, Hewitt S, Booker DJ, et al. Enzyme linked direct antiglobulin tests in patients with autoimmune haemolysis. *J Clin Pathol.* 1985;38: 912–914.

18. Issitt PD. Serological diagnosis and characterization of the causative autoantibodies. *Methods in Hematology.* 1985;12:1–45.

19. Engelfriet CP, von dem Borne AE, Beckers D, et al. Auto-immune haemolytic anaemia: serological and immunochemical characteristics of the auto-antibodies: mechanisms of cell destruction. *Ser Haematol.* 1974; VII:328–347.

20. Worlledge SM. The interpretation of a positive direct antiglobulin test. *Br J Haematol.* 1978;39:157–162.

21. Robertson VM, Dickson LG, Romond EH, et al. Positive antiglobulin tests due to intravenous immunoglobulin in patients who received bone marrow transplant. *Transfusion.* 1987;27:28–31.

22. Ramsey G. Red cell antibodies arising from solid organ transplants. *Transfusion.* 1991;31:76–86.

23. Petz LD. Immunohematologic problems associated with bone marrow transplantation. *Transfus Med Rev.* 1987;1:85–100.

24. Shulman JA, Petz LD. Red cell compatibility testing: clinical significance and laboratory methods. In: Petz LD, Swisher SN, Kleinman S, et al., eds. *Clinical Practice of Transfusion Medicine.* 3rd ed. New York: Churchill Livingstone; 1996:199–244.

25. Szymanski IO, Odgren PR, Fortier NL, et al. Red blood cell associated IgG in normal and pathologic states. *Blood*. 1980;55: 48–54.

26. Clark JA, Tranley PC, Wallas CH. Evaluation of patients with positive direct antiglobulin tests and non-reactive eluates discovered during pretransfusion testing. *Immunohaematol*. 1992;8:9–12.

27. Heddle NM, Kelton JG, Turchyn KL, et al. Hypergammaglobulinemia can be associated with a positive direct antiglobulin test, a nonreactive eluate and no evidence of hemolysis. *Transfusion*. 1988;28: 29–33.

28. Huh YO, Liu FJ, Rogge K, et al. Positive direct antiglobulin test and high serum immunoglobulin G levels. *Am J Clin Pathol*. 1988;90: 197–200.

29. Vianna JL, Khamashta MA, Ordi-Ros J, et al. Comparison of the primary and secondary antiphospholipid syndrome: A European Multicenter Study of 114 patients. *Am J Med*. 1994;96:3–9.

30. Win N, Islam SI, Peterkin MA, et al. Positive direct antiglobulin test due to antiphospholipid antibodies in normal healthy blood donors. *Vox Sang*. 1997;72:182–184.

31. Petz LD, Yam P, Wilkinson L, et al. Increased IgG molecules bound to the surface of red blood cells of patients with sickle cell anemia. *Blood*. 1984;64:301–304.

32. Toy PT, Chin CA, Reid ME, et al. Factors associated with positive direct antiglobulin tests in pretransfusion patients: a case control study. *Vox Sang*. 1985;49: 215–220.

33. Stratton F, Renton PH. Effect of crystalloid solutions prepared in glass bottles on human red cells. *Nature (London)*. 1955;175:727.

34. Gorst DW, Rawlinson VI, Merry AH, et al. Positive direct antiglobulin test in normal individuals. *Vox Sang*. 1980;38:99–105.

35. Bareford D, Longster G, Gilks L, et al. Follow-up of normal individuals with a positive antiglobulin test. *Scand J Haematol*. 1985;35:348–353.

36. Freedman J. False-positive antiglobulin tests in healthy subjects. *J Clin Pathol*. 1979;32: 1014–1018.

37. Lau P, Haesler WE, Wurzel HA. Positive direct antiglobulin reaction in a patient population. *Am J Clin Pathol*. 1976;65:368–375.

38. Sokol RJ, Booker DJ, Stamps R, et al. IgA red cell autoantibodies and auto-immune hemolysis. *Transfusion*. 1997;37:175–181.

39. Chaplin Jr H. Clinical usefulness of specific antiglobulin reagents in autoimmune hemolytic anemia. *Prog Hematol*. 1973;8:25–49.

40. Worlledge SM, Blajchman MA. The autoimmune haemolytic anaemias. *Br J Haematol*. 1972;23 (suppl):61–69.

41. Lai M, Rumi C, D'onofrio G, et al. Clinically significant auto-immune hemolytic anemia with a negative direct antiglobulin test by routine tube test and positive by column agglutination method. *Immunohematol*. 2002;18:112–116.

42. Sokol RJ, Hewitt S, Booker DJ, et al. Small quantities of erythrocyte bound immunoglobulins and auto-immune haemolysis. *J Clin Pathol*. 1987;40:254–257.

43. Garratty G, Arndt PA. Application of flow cytofluorometry to red blood cell immunology. *Cytometry*. 1999;38:259–267.

44. Sokol RJ, Booker DJ, Stamps R, et al. IgA red cell autoantibodies and autoimmune haemolysis. *Transfusion*. 1997;37:175–181.

45. Owen I, Hows J. Evaluation of the manual Polybrene technique in the investigation of autoimmune hemolytic anemia. *Transfusion*. 1990;30:814–818.

46. Lalezari P, Jiang AC. The manual Polybrene test: a simple and rapid procedure for detection of red cell antibodies. *Transfusion*. 1980;20: 206–211.

47. Branch DR, Petz LD. Detecting alloantibodies in patients with autoantibodies. *Transfusion*. 1999;39:6–10.

48. Landsteiner K, Miller Jr CP. Serological studies on the blood of primates. II. The blood groups in anthropoid apes. *J Exp Med*. 1925;42:853–862.

49. Eicher CA, Wallace ME, Frank S, et al. The Lui elution: a simple method of antibody elution. *Transfusion*. 1978;18:647–652.

50. Roelcke D. Cold agglutination. *Transfus Med Rev*. 1989;3:140–166.

51. Wiener AS, Unger LJ, Cohen L, et al. Type-specific cold auto-antibodies as a cause of acquired hemolytic anemia and hemolytic transfusion reactions: biologic test with bovine red cells. *Ann Intern Med*. 1956;44: 221–240.

52. Wolach B, Heddle N, Barr RD, et al. Transient Donath–Landsteiner haemolytic anaemia. *Br J Haematol*. 1981;48:425–434.

53. Worlledge SM, Rousso C. Studies on the serology of paroxysmal cold hemoglobinuria (PCH) with special reference to a relationship with the P blood group system. *Vox Sang*. 1965;10:293–298.

54. Freedman J, Masters CA, Newlands M, et al. Optimal conditions for the use of sulphydryl compounds in dissociating red cell antibodies. *Vox Sang*. 1976;30: 231–239.

55. Habibi B. Drug-induced immune haemolytic anaemias. *Baillières Clinical Immunology and Allergy*. 1987;1:343–356.

56. Petz LD, Branch DR. Drug-induced immune haemolytic anemias. *Methods in Haematology*. 1985;12: 47–94.

57. Habibi B. Drug induced red blood cell autoantibodies co-developed with drug specific antibodies causing haemolytic anaemias. *Br J Haematol*. 1985;61:139–143.

58. Salama A, Gottsche B, Mueller-Eckhardt C. Autoantibodies and drug- or metabolite-dependent antibodies in patients with diclofenac-induced immune haemolysis. *Br J Haematol*. 1991;77: 546–549.

59. Salama C, Mueller-Eckhardt C. Cianidanol and its metabolites bind tightly to red cells and are responsible for the production of auto- and/or drug-dependent antibodies against these cells. *Br J Haematol*. 1987;66:263–266.

60. Salama A, Mueller-Eckhardt C. Immune-mediated blood dyscrasias related to drugs. *Semin Hematol*. 1992;29:54–63.

61. Dacie JV, Lewis SM. Paroxysmal nocturnal haemoglobinuria: clinical

manifestations, haematology and nature of the disease. *Ser Haematol.* 1972;5:3–23.

62. Sirchia G, Lewis SM. Paroxysmal nocturnal haemoglobinuria. *Clin Haematol.* 1975;4:199–229.

63. Hansch GM, Schonermark S, Roeicke D. Paroxysmal nocturnal hemoglobinuria type III: lack of an erythrocyte membrane protein restricting the lysis by C5b–9. *J Clin Invest.* 1987;80:7–12.

64. Rosse WF, Dacie JV. Immune lysis of normal human and paroxysmal nocturnal hemoglobinuria (PNH) red blood cells. 1. The sensitivity of PNH red cells to lysis by complement and specific antibody. *J Clin Invest.* 1966;45:736–748.

65. Ham TH, Dingle JH. Studies on destruction of red blood cells. II. Chronic hemolytic anemia with paroxysmal nocturnal hemoglobinuria: certain immunological aspects of the hemolytic mechanism with special reference to serum complement. *J Clin Invest.* 1939;18:657–672.

66. Hartmann RC, Jenkins Jr DE, Arnold AB. Diagnostic specificity of sucrose hemolysis test for paroxysmal nocturnal hemoglobinuria. *Blood.* 1970;35: 462–475.

67. Crosby WH. Paroxysmal nocturnal hemoglobinuria. A specific test for the disease based on the ability of thrombin to activate the hemolytic factor. *Blood.* 1950;5:843–846.

68. Dacie JV, Lewis SM, Tills D. Comparative sensitivity of the erythrocytes in paroxysmal nocturnal haemoglobinuria to haemolysis by acidified normal serum and by a high-titre cold antibody. *Br J Haematol.* 1960;6: 362–371.

69. Brubaker LH, Schaberg DR, Jefferson DH, et al. A potential rapid screening test for paroxysmal nocturnal hemoglobinuria. *N Engl J Med.* 1973;288:1059–1060.

70. Kabakci T, Rosse WF, Logue GL. The lysis of paroxysmal nocturnal haemoglobinuria red cells by serum and cobra factor. *Br J Haematol.* 1972;23:693–705.

71. Logue GL, Rossi WF, Adams JP. Mechanisms of immune lysis of red blood cells in vitro. I. Paroxysmal nocturnal hemoglobinuria cells. *J Clin Invest.* 1973;52:1129–1137.

72. Catovsky D, Lewis SM, Sherman D. Erythrocyte sensitivity to in-vitro lysis in leukaemia. *Br J Haematol.* 1971;21:541–550.

73. Lewis SM, Dacie JV, Tills D. Comparison of the sensitivity to agglutination and haemolysis by a high-titre cold antibody of the erythrocytes of normal subjects and of patients with a variety of blood diseases including paroxysmal nocturnal haemoglobinuria. *Br J Haematol.* 1961;7:64–72.

74. Rosse WF. Variations in the red cells in paroxysmal nocturnal haemoglobinuria. *Br J Haematol.* 1973;24:327–342.

75. Rosse WF, Adams JP, Thorpe AM. The population of cells in paroxysmal nocturnal haemoglobinuria of intermediate sensitivity to complement lysis: significance and mechanism of increased immune lysis. *Br J Haematol.* 1974;28:281–290.

76. Oni SB, Osunkoya BO, Luzzatto L. Paroxysmal nocturnal hemoglobinuria: evidence for monoclonal origin of abnormal red cells. *Blood.* 1970;36:145–152.

77. Kinoshita T, Medof ME, Silber R, et al. Distribution of decay-accelerating factor in the peripheral blood of normal individuals and patients with paroxysmal nocturnal hemoglobinuria. *J Exp Med.* 1985;162:75–92.

78. Nicholson-Weller A, Spicier DB, Austen KF. Deficiency of the complement regulating protein 'decay accelerating factor' on membranes of granulocytes, monocytes and platelets in paroxysmal nocturnal hemoglobinuria. *N Engl J Med.* 1985;312:1091–1097.

79. Auditore JV, Hartmann RC. Paroxysmal nocturnal hemoglobinuria: II. Erythrocyte acetylcholinesterase defect. *Am J Med.* 1959;27:401–410.

80. Chow F-L, Telen MJ, Rosse WF. The acetylcholinesterase defect in paroxysmal nocturnal hemoglobinuria: evidence that the enzyme is absent from the cell membrane. *Blood.* 1985;66: 940–945.

81. De Sandre G, Ghiotto G. An enzymic disorder in the erythrocytes of paroxysmal nocturnal haemoglobinuria: a deficiency in acetylcholinesterase activity. *Br J Haematol.* 1960;6:39–42.

82. Beck WS, Valentine WN. Biochemical studies on leucocytes. II. Phosphatase activity in chronic lymphatic leucemia, acute leucemia and miscellaneous hematologic conditions. *J Lab Clin Med.* 1965;38: 245–253.

83. Hartmann RC, Auditore JV. Paroxysmal nocturnal hemoglobinuria I. Clinical studies. *Am J Med.* 1959;27:389–400.

84. Lewis SM, Dacie JV. Neutrophil (leucocyte) alkaline phosphatase in paroxysmal nocturnal haemoglobinuria. *Br J Haematol.* 1965;11:549–556.

85. Nicholson-Weller A, March JP, Rosenfield SI, et al. Affected erythrocytes of patients with paroxysmal nocturnal hemoglobinuria are deficient in the complement regulatory protein, decay accelerating factor. *Proc Natl Acad Sci U S A.* 1983;80:5066–5070.

86. Pangbum MK, Schreiber RD, Müller-Eberhard HF. Deficiency of an erythrocyte membrane protein with complement regulatory activity in paroxysmal nocturnal hemoglobinuria. *Proc Natl Acad Sci U S A.* 1983;80:5430–5434.

87. Zalman LS, Wood LM, Frank MM, et al. Deficiency of the homologous restriction factor in paroxysmal nocturnal hemoglobinuria. *J Exp Med.* 1987;165:572–577.

88. Davies A, Simmons DL, Hale G, et al. CD59 and LY-6-like protein expressed in human lymphoid cells, regulates the action of the complement membrane attack complex on homologous cells. *J Exp Med.* 1989;170:637–654.

89. Holguin MH, Wilcox LA, Bernshaw NJ, et al. Relationship between the membrane inhibitor of reactive lysis and the erythrocyte phenotypes of paroxysmal nocturnal hemoglobinuria. *J Clin Invest.* 1989;84:1387–1394.

90. Holguin MH, Fredrick NJ, Bernshaw LA, et al. Isolation and characterization of a membrane protein from normal human

erythrocytes that inhibits reactive lysis of the erythrocytes of paroxysmal nocturnal hemoglobinuria. *J Clin Invest.* 1989;84:7–17.

91. Rosse WF, Hoffman S, Campbell M, et al. The erythrocytes in paroxysmal nocturnal haemoglobinuria of intermediate sensitivity to complement lysis. *Br J Haematol.* 1991;79:99–107.

92. Shichishima T, Terasawa T, Hashimoto C, et al. Heterogenous expression of decay accelerating factor and CD59/membrane attack complex inhibition factor on paroxysmal nocturnal haemoglobinuria (PNH) erythrocytes. *Br J Haematol.* 1991;78:545–550.

93. May JE, Rosse WF, Frank MM. Paroxysmal nocturnal hemoglobinuria: alternative-complement-pathway-mediated lysis induced by magnesium. *N Engl J Med.* 1973;289:705–709.

94. Packman CH, Rosenfeld SI, Jenkins Jr DE, et al. Complement lysis of human erythrocytes. Differing susceptibility of two types of paroxysmal nocturnal hemoglobinuria cells to C5b-9. *J Clin Invest.* 1979;64:428–433.

95. Crookston JH, Crookston MC, Burnie KL, et al. Hereditary erythroblastic multinuclearity associated with a positive acidified-serum test: a type of congenital dyserythropoietic anaemia. *Br J Haematol.* 1969;17:11–26.

96. Verwilghen RL, Lewis SM, Dacie JV. HEMPAS: congenital dyserythropoietic anaemia (type II). *Q J Med.* 1973;42:257–278.

97. Hartmann RC, Jenkins Jr DE. The 'sugar water' test for paroxysmal nocturnal hemoglobinuria. *N Engl J Med.* 1966;275:155–157.

98. Mollison PL, Polley MJ. Uptake of γ-globulin and complement by red cells exposed to serum at low ionic strength. *Nature (London).* 1964;203:535.

99. Hillmen P, Hows JM, Luzzatto L. Two distinct patterns of glycosylphosphatidylinositol (GPI) linked protein deficiency in the red cells of patients with paroxysmal nocturnal haemoglobinuria. *Br J Haematol.* 1992;80:399–405.

100. Plesner T, Hansen NE, Carlsen K. Estimation of PI-bound proteins on blood cells from PNH patients by quantitative flow cytometry. *Br J Haematol.* 1990;75:585–590.

101. van der Schoot CE, Huizinga TW, van't Veer-Korthof ET, et al. Deficiency of glycosyl-phosphatidylinositol-linked membrane glycoproteins of leukocytes in paroxysmal nocturnal hemoglobinuria, description of a new diagnostic cytofluorometric assay. *Blood.* 1990;76:1853–1859.

102. Brodsky RA. Advances in the diagnosis and therapy of paroxysmal nocturnal hemoglobinuria. *Blood Rev.* 2008;22:65–74.

103. Merry AH, Rawlinson VI, Uchikawa M, et al. Studies on the sensitivity to complement-mediated lysis of erythrocytes (Inab phenotype) with a deficiency of DAF (decay accelerating factor). *Br J Haematol.* 1989;73:248–253.

104. Merry AH, Rawlinson VI, Uchikawa M, et al. Lack of abnormal sensitivity to complement-mediated lysis in erythrocytes deficient only in decay accelerating factor. *Biochem Soc Trans.* 1989;17:514.

105. Telen MJ, Green AM. The Inab phenotype: characterization of the membrane protein and complement regulatory defect. *Blood.* 1989;74:437–441.

106. Yamashina M, Ueda E, Kinoshita T, et al. Inherited complete deficiency of 20-kilodalton homologous restriction factor (CD59) as a cause of paroxysmal nocturnal hemoglobinuria. *N Engl J Med.* 1990;323:1184–1189.

107. Sirchia G, Ferrone S. The laboratory substitutes of the red cell of paroxysmal nocturnal haemoglobinuria (PNH): PNH-like red cells. *Ser Haematol.* 1972;5:137–175.

108. Francis DA. Production of PNH-like red cells using 2-mercaptobenzoic acid. *Med Lab Sci.* 1983;40:33–38.

109. Sirchia G, Marubini E, Mercuriali F, et al. Study of two in vitro diagnostic tests for paroxysmal nocturnal haemoglobinuria. *Br J Haematol.* 1973;24:751–759.

110. Sirchia G, Ferrone S, Mercuriali F. The action of two sulfhydryl compounds on normal human red cells. Relationship to red cells of paroxysmal nocturnal haemoglobinuria. *Blood.* 1965;25:502–510.

Chapter | 14 |

Investigation of abnormal haemoglobins and thalassaemia

Barbara J. Wild, Barbara J. Bain

THE HAEMOGLOBIN MOLECULE

Human haemoglobin is formed from two pairs of globin chains each with a haem group attached. Seven different globin chains are synthesized in normal subjects; four are transient embryonic haemoglobins referred to as Hb Gower 1, Hb Gower 2, Hb Portland 1 and Hb Portland 2. Hb F is the predominant haemoglobin of fetal life and comprises the major proportion of haemoglobin found at birth. Hb A is the major haemoglobin found in adults and children. Hb A_2 and Hb F are found in small quantities in adult life (approximately 2–3.3% and 0.2–1.0%, respectively). The adult proportions of Hbs A, A_2 and F are usually attained by 6–12 months of age.

The individual chains synthesized in postnatal life are designated α, β, γ and δ. Hb A has two α chains and two β chains ($\alpha_2\beta_2$); Hb F has two α chains and two γ chains ($\alpha_2\gamma_2$) and Hb A_2 has two α chains and two δ chains ($\alpha_2\delta_2$). The α chain is thus common to all three types of haemoglobin molecules.

α chain synthesis is directed by two α genes, $\alpha1$ and $\alpha2$, on chromosome 16 and β and δ chain synthesis by single β and δ genes on chromosome 11; γ chain synthesis is directed by two genes, $^G\gamma$ and $^A\gamma$, also on chromosome 11. The globin genes are shown diagrammatically in Figure 14.1.

The four chains are associated in the form of a tetramer: the $\alpha_1\beta_1$ (and equivalent $\alpha_2\beta_2$) contact is the strongest and involves many amino acids with many interlocking side chains; the $\alpha_1\beta_2$ (and equivalent $\alpha_2\beta_1$) contact is less extensive and the contacts between similar chains are relatively weak. The binding of a haem group into the haem pocket in each chain is vital for the oxygen-carrying capacity of the molecule and stabilizes the whole molecule. If the haem attachment is weakened, the globin chains dissociate into dimers and monomers.

There are many naturally occurring, genetically determined variants of human haemoglobin (>1000)[1] and although many are harmless, some have serious clinical effects. Collectively, the clinical syndromes resulting from disorders of haemoglobin synthesis are referred to as 'haemoglobinopathies'. They can be grouped into three main categories:

1. Those owing to structural variants of haemoglobin, such as Hb S.
2. Those owing to failure to synthesize one or more of the globin chains of haemoglobin at a normal rate, as in the thalassaemias.
3. Those owing to failure to complete the normal neonatal switch from fetal haemoglobin (Hb F) to adult haemoglobin (Hb A). The third category comprises a group of disorders referred to as hereditary persistence of fetal haemoglobin (HPFH).

An individual can also have a combination of two or more of these abnormalities.

STRUCTURAL VARIANTS OF HAEMOGLOBIN

Alterations in the structure of haemoglobin are usually brought about by point mutations affecting one or, in some cases, two or more bases, coding for amino acids of the globin chains. An example of such a point mutation is Hb S caused by the substitution of valine for glutamic acid in position 6 of the β-globin chain ($\beta6^{Glu \rightarrow Val}$). Less commonly, structural change is caused by shortening or lengthening of the globin chain. For example, five amino acids are deleted in the β chain of Hb Gun Hill, whereas in Hb Constant Spring 31 amino acids are added to the α chain. Mutations associated with a frame shift can also lead to synthesis of a structurally abnormal haemoglobin, which may be either shorter or longer than normal. There may also be combinations of segments of β and γ or δ chains resulting in hybrid haemoglobins; the β and δ combinations are known as the Lepore ($5'\delta3'\beta$) and anti-Lepore ($5'\beta3'\delta$) haemoglobins.

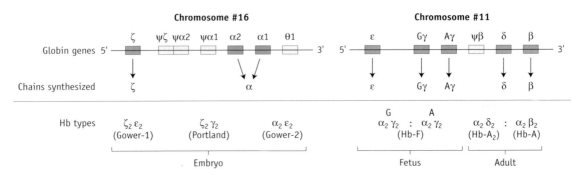

Figure 14.1 Location of the α-globin gene cluster on chromosome 16 and that of the β-globin gene cluster on chromosome 11. The black boxes represent functional genes. The α and γ globin genes are duplicated; the two α globin genes have the same product, whereas the products of the two γ globin genes are slightly different ($^G\gamma = \gamma$ 136Gly; $^A\gamma = \gamma$ 136Ala).

Many variant haemoglobins are haematologically and clinically silent because the underlying mutation causes no alteration in the function, solubility or stability of the haemoglobin molecule. Many of these variants are separated using electrophoresis or chromatography, but some are not and remain undetected. Some structural variants are associated with severe clinical phenotypes in the homozygous or even heterozygous state; these mutations affect the physical or chemical properties of the haemoglobin molecule, resulting in changes in haemoglobin solubility, stability or oxygen-binding properties. Some of these variants separate on electrophoresis or chromatography, whereas others do not. It is fortunate that the common haemoglobin variants that have clinical or genetic significance (e.g. Hbs S, C, D^{Punjab}, E and O^{Arab}) are readily detectable by electrophoretic and chromatographic techniques.

Haemoglobins with Reduced Solubility

Hb S

By far the most common haemoglobin variant in this group is sickle haemoglobin or Hb S. As a result of the replacement of glutamic acid by valine in position 6 of the β chain, Hb S has poor solubility in the deoxygenated state and can polymerize within the red cells. The red cell shows a characteristic shape change because of polymer formation and becomes distorted and rigid, the so-called sickle cell (see p. 90, Fig. 5.71). In addition, intracellular polymers lead to red cell membrane changes, generation of oxidant substances and abnormal adherence of red cells to vascular endothelium.

Clinical syndromes associated with common structural variants and those owing to their interaction with β thalassaemia are shown in Table 14.1.

Sickle Cell Disease

Sickle cell disease[2] (also called disorder) is a collective name for a group of conditions causing clinical symptoms that result from the formation of sickle red cells. It is common in people originating from Africa, but it is also found in considerable numbers of people of Indian, Arabic and Greek descent.

The homozygous state or sickle cell anaemia (β genotype SS) causes moderate anaemia resulting both from haemolysis and from the reduced oxygen affinity of haemoglobin S. The main clinical disability arises from repeated episodes of vascular occlusion by sickled red cells resulting in acute crises and eventually in end-organ damage. The clinical severity of sickle cell anaemia is extremely variable. This is partly due to the effects of inherited modifying factors, such as interaction with α thalassaemia or increased synthesis of Hb F and partly to socioeconomic conditions and other factors that influence general health.[2]

Sickle cell trait (β genotype AS), the heterozygous state, is very common, affecting millions of people worldwide. There are no associated haematological abnormalities. *In vivo* sickling occurs only at very high altitudes and at low oxygen pressures. Spontaneous haematuria, owing to sickling in the renal papillae, is found in about 1% of people with sickle cell trait.

Other Forms of Sickle Cell Disease

Sickle cell/Hb C disease is a compound heterozygous state for Hbs S and C. The abbreviation 'SC disease' is ambiguous and should be avoided; however, the term Hb SC disease is acceptable. This compound heterozygous state usually results in a milder form of sickle cell disease.

Sickle β/thalassaemia arises as a result of inheritance of one Hb S and one β thalassaemia gene. Africans and Afro-Caribbeans with this condition are often heterozygous for a mild β$^+$ thalassaemia allele resulting in the production of about 20% of Hb A. This gives rise to a mild sickling disorder. Inheritance of Hb S and β$^°$ thalassaemia trait is associated with severe sickle cell disease. Interaction of Hb S with haemoglobin D^{Punjab} (Hb D$^{Los\ Angeles}$) or with Hb O^{Arab} gives rise to severe sickle cell disease.[2]

Hb C

Hb C is the second most common structural haemoglobin variant in people of African descent. The substitution of glutamic acid in position 6 of the β chain by lysine results in a haemoglobin molecule with a highly positive charge, decreased solubility and a tendency to crystallize. However, Hb C does not give a positive sickle solubility test. Heterozygotes are asymptomatic, but target cells and irregularly contracted cells may be present in blood films. Homozygotes may have mild anaemia with numerous target cells and irregularly contracted cells (see Chapter 5, Fig. 5.32). Interaction with β$^°$ or β$^+$ thalassaemia trait results in mild or moderate haemolytic anaemia.

Other Sickling Haemoglobins

In addition to Hb S, there are at least nine haemoglobins (Hb S^{Antilles}, Hb C^{Ziquinchor}, Hb C^{Harlem}, Hb S^{Providence}, Hb S^{Oman}, Hb S^{Travis}, Hb S$^{South\ End}$, Hb S$^{Jamaica\ Plain}$, Hb S^{Cameroon}) that have both the β6 glutamic acid to valine mutation and an additional single point mutation in the β globin chain. These haemoglobins also have a positive solubility test because they have a reduced solubility but generally exhibit different electrophoretic and chromatographic properties from Hb S. They have clinical significance similar, but not necessarily identical, to Hb S: e.g. Hb S^{Antilles} is associated with an even greater propensity to sickling than Hb S.

Table 14.1 Clinical syndromes encountered with β^S and β^C variants

Hb	GENOTYPE	NAME	CLINICAL PROBLEMS
S	β^A/β^S	Sickle cell trait	None
	β^S/β^S	Sickle cell anaemia	Moderate haemolytic anaemia, vaso-occlusive episodes
C	β^A/β^C	C trait	None
	β^C/β^C	C disease	Occasional mild anaemia, increased incidence of gallstones
D^{Punjab}	β^A/β^D	D trait	None
	β^D/β^D	D disease	Occasional mild anaemia
O^{Arab}	$\beta^A/\beta^{o\ Arab}$	O trait	None
	$\beta^{o\ Arab}/\beta^{o\ Arab}$	O disease	Haemolytic anaemia
Interactions	β^S/β^C	Hb SC disease	Mild anaemia, vaso-occlusive problems
	$\beta^S/\beta^{D\ Punjab}$	SD disease	As for sickle cell anaemia
	$\beta^S/\beta^{o\ Arab}$	SO disease	As for sickle cell anaemia
	β^{othal}/β^S	Sickle-β^{othal}	As for sickle cell anaemia
	β^{+thal}/β^S	Sickle-β^{+thal}	Mild sickle cell disease
	β^{thal}/β^C	C/β thal	Mild haemolytic anaemia
	β^{thal}/β^D	D/β thal	Mild haemolytic anaemia
	$\beta^{thal}/\beta^{o\ Arab}$	O/β thal	Thalassaemia intermedia

Unstable Haemoglobins

Amino acid substitutions close to the haem group, or at the points of contact between globin chains, can affect protein stability and result in intracellular precipitation of globin chains. The precipitated globin chains attach to the red cell membrane giving rise to Heinz bodies, and the associated clinical syndromes were originally called the *congenital Heinz body haemolytic anaemias*. Changes in membrane properties may lead to haemolysis, often aggravated by oxidant drugs. There is considerable heterogeneity in the haematological and clinical effects of unstable haemoglobins. Many are almost silent and are detected only by specific tests, whereas others are severe, causing haemolytic anaemia in the heterozygous state. Hb Köln is the most common variant in this rare group of disorders.[3,4]

Haemoglobins with Altered Oxygen Affinity

Haemoglobin variants with altered oxygen affinity are a rare group of variants that result in increased or reduced oxygen affinity.[5] Mutations that increase oxygen affinity are generally associated with benign lifelong erythrocytosis. This may be confused with polycythaemia vera and may be inappropriately treated with cytotoxic drugs or ^{32}P.

Haemoglobin variants with decreased oxygen affinity are, with the exception of Hb S, even less common and are usually associated with mild anaemia and cyanosis.

However, owing to the reduced oxygen affinity, these patients are not functionally anaemic despite the reduced Hb. The low steady-state haemoglobin concentration in Hb S homozygotes is, at least in part, a result of its reduced oxygen affinity.

Measurement of oxygen dissociation is described on p. 269.

Hb M

The Hb M group is another rare group of variants.[6] Such haemoglobins have a propensity to form methaemoglobin, generated by the oxidation of ferrous iron in haem to ferric iron, which is incapable of binding oxygen. Despite marked cyanosis, there are few clinical problems. Most are associated with substitutions that disrupt the normal six-ligand state of haem iron.

Methaemoglobinaemia is also found in congenital NADH methaemoglobin reductase deficiency, as well as after exposure to oxidant drugs and chemicals (nitrates, nitrites, quinones, chlorates, phenacetin, dapsone and many others).

THALASSAEMIA SYNDROMES

The thalassaemia syndromes[7] are a heterogeneous group of inherited conditions characterized by defects in the synthesis of one or more of the globin chains that form the haemoglobin tetramer. The clinical syndromes associated with thalassaemia arise from the combined consequences of inadequate haemoglobin production and of unbalanced accumulation of one type of globin chain. The former causes anaemia with hypochromia and microcytosis; the latter leads to ineffective erythropoiesis and haemolysis. Clinical manifestations range from completely asymptomatic microcytosis to profound anaemia that is incompatible with life and can cause death *in utero* (Table 14.2). This clinical heterogeneity arises as a result of the variable severity of the primary genetic defect in haemoglobin synthesis and the coinheritance of modulating factors, such as the capacity to synthesize increased amounts of Hb F.

Thalassaemias are generally inherited as alleles of one or more of the globin genes located on either chromosome 11 (for β, γ and δ chains) or on chromosome 16 (for α chains). They are encountered in every population in the world but are most common in the Mediterranean littoral and near equatorial regions of Africa and Asia. Gene frequencies for the α and β thalassaemias on a global basis range from 1% to more than 80% in areas where malaria is endemic.[8]

Table 14.2 Clinical syndromes of thalassaemia

Clinically asymptomatic
  Silent carriers
    α⁺ thalassaemia heterozygotes (some cases)
    Rare forms of β thalassaemia trait
  Thalassaemia minor (low MCH and MCV, with or without mild anaemia)
    α⁺ thalassaemia heterozygotes (some cases)
    α° thalassaemia heterozygotes
    α⁺ thalassaemia homozygotes
    β° thalassaemia trait
    β⁺ thalassaemia trait
    Some cases of Hb E/β thalassaemia

Thalassaemia intermedia (transfusion independent)[a]
  Some β⁺/β⁺ thalassaemia homozygotes and compound heterozygotes
  Interaction of β°/β°, β°/β⁺ or β⁺/β⁺ with α thalassaemia
  Interaction of β°/β or β⁺/β with triple α
  Hb H disease
  α°/Hb Constant Spring thalassaemia
  β°/δβ or β⁺/δβ thalassaemia compound heterozygotes
  δβ/δβ thalassaemia
  Some cases of Hb E/β thalassaemia and Hb Lepore/β thalassaemia
  Rare cases of heterozygotes for β thalassaemia mutation, particularly involving exon 3 ('dominant β thalassaemia')

Thalassaemia major (transfusion dependent)
  β°/β° thalassaemia
  β⁺/β⁺ thalassaemia
  β°/β⁺ thalassaemia
  Some cases of β°/Hb Lepore and β⁺/Hb Lepore thalassaemia
  Some cases of β°/Hb E and β⁺/Hb E thalassaemia

MCH, mean cell haemoglobin; MCV, mean cell volume.
[a]β thalassaemia intermedia is defined as a symptomatic condition in which regular transfusion is not essential to maintain life; however some patients have a poor quality of life and may benefit from transfusion as their condition progresses.

β Thalassaemia Syndromes

Many different mutations cause β thalassaemia and related disorders.[9] These mutations can affect every step in the pathway of globin gene expression: transcription, processing of the messenger ribonucleic acid (mRNA) precursor, translation of mature mRNA and preservation of post-translational integrity of the β chain. More than 200 mutations have been described.[10] Most types of β thalassaemia are the result of point mutations affecting the globin gene, but some large deletions are also known. Certain mutations are particularly common in some communities. This helps to simplify prenatal diagnosis, which is carried out by detection or exclusion of a particular mutation in fetal DNA.

The effect of different mutations varies greatly. At one end of the spectrum are a group of rare mutations, mainly involving exon 3 of the β globin gene, which are so severe that they can produce the clinical syndrome of thalassaemia intermedia in the heterozygous state. At the other end are mild alleles that produce thalassaemia intermedia in the homozygous or compound heterozygous state and some that are so mild that they are completely haematologically silent, with normal mean cell volume (MCV) and Hb A_2 in the heterozygous state. In between are the great majority of β⁺ and β° alleles, which cause β thalassaemia major in the homozygous or compound heterozygous state and in the heterozygous state give rise to a mild anaemia (or Hb at the low end of the normal range), with microcytic, hypochromic indices and raised Hb A_2.[11]

β Thalassaemia major is a severe, transfusion-dependent, inherited anaemia. There is a profound defect of β chain production. Excess α chains accumulate and precipitate in the red cell precursors in the bone marrow resulting in ineffective erythropoiesis. The few cells that leave the marrow are laden with precipitated α chains and are rapidly removed by the reticuloendothelial system. The constant erythropoietic drive causes massive expansion of bone marrow and extramedullary erythropoiesis. If untreated, 80% of children with β thalassaemia die within the first 5 years of life.

Heterozygotes for β thalassaemia alleles usually have either a normal haemoglobin with microcytosis or a mild microcytic hypochromic anaemia; Hb A_2 is elevated and Hb F is sometimes also elevated. Laboratory features of various β thalassaemia syndromes are shown in Table 14.3.

α Thalassaemia Syndromes

There are four syndromes of α thalassaemia:[12] α^+ thalassaemia trait, where one of the two globin genes on a single chromosome fails to function; α° thalassaemia trait, where two genes on a single chromosome fail to function; Hb H disease, with three genes affected; and Hb Bart's hydrops fetalis, where all four are absent or defective. These syndromes are usually a result of deletions of one or more genes, although approximately 20% of the mutations described are non-deletional. α^+ thalassaemia is particularly common in Africa and α° thalassaemia is common in South-east Asia. The laboratory features are shown in Table 14.3.

Hb Bart's hydrops fetalis occurs mainly in people from South-east Asia but is also occasionally observed in people from Greece, Turkey and Cyprus. An affected fetus will be stillborn or will die shortly after birth. Severe anaemia and oedema are the hallmarks of this condition. Women carrying a hydropic fetus have a high incidence of complications of pregnancy. Prenatal diagnosis should be offered for women at risk of having a fetus with Hb Bart's hydrops fetalis.

Hb H disease gives rise to haemolytic anaemia; patients rarely require transfusion or splenectomy.

α° *thalassaemia trait* is characterized by microcytic, hypochromic indices. The haemoglobin level may be normal or slightly reduced. α^+ thalassaemia trait can be completely silent or there may be borderline microcytosis with a slightly reduced or normal mean cell haemoglobin concentration (MCHC). Haematologically, homozygosity for α^+ thalassaemia trait resembles heterozygosity for α° thalassaemia trait, but the genetic implications are very different. Both α^+ thalassaemia trait and α° thalassaemia trait are more difficult to diagnose than β thalassaemia trait because there is no characteristic elevation in Hb A_2, and Hb H bodies are frequently not demonstrated. Definitive diagnosis of the α thalassaemia trait is more reliably made with the use of DNA techniques or globin chain biosynthesis studies.

Thalassaemic Structural Variants

These are abnormal haemoglobins characterized by both a biosynthetic defect and an abnormal structure, such as the Lepore haemoglobins (Table 14.4).

Table 14.3 Laboratory findings in thalassaemia

PHENOTYPE	GENOTYPE	USUAL MCV	USUAL MCH	Hb A_2	Hb H INCLUSIONS
α Thalassaemia					
α thalassaemia trait	$-\alpha/\alpha\alpha$ (α^+/α)	N	N	N or ↓	−
α thalassaemia trait	$-\alpha/-\alpha$ or $-/\alpha\alpha$	N or ↓	N or ↓	N or ↓	+
Hb H disease					
Mild	$-/-\alpha$ (α°/α^+)	↓	↓	N or ↓	+++
Severe	$-/\alpha^T\alpha$ (α°/α^T)	↓	↓	N or ↓	+++
Hb Bart's hydrops fetalis (α thalassaemia major)	$-/-$ ($\alpha^\circ/\alpha^\circ$)	↓	↓	−	−
β Thalassaemia					
β thalassaemia trait	β°/β or β^+/β	↓	↓	↑	−
δβ thalassaemia trait	$\delta\beta^\circ/\beta$	↓	↓	N or ↓	−
β thalassaemia trait with normal Hb A_2	β^+/β	↓	↓	N	−
Hb Lepore trait	Hb Lepore/β	↓	↓	N or ↓	−
β thalassaemia intermedia	Heterogeneous	↓	↓	↑, N or ↓	−
β thalassaemia major	β°/β°, β°/β^+, β^+/β^+	↓	↓	↑, N or ↓	

MCV, mean cell volume; MCH, mean cell haemoglobin; N, normal.

Table 14.4 Thalassaemic structural variants[a]

HAEMOGLOBIN	STRUCTURE	WHEN HETEROZYGOUS	WHEN HOMOZYGOUS	IN COMBINATION WITH OTHER HAEMOGLOBINOPATHIES[17,18]
Lepore	Hybrid of part of δ and part of β chain owing to unequal crossover	Microcytosis, mild anaemia	Thalassaemia major or intermedia	With β thalassaemia gives thalassaemia major or intermedia
E[b]	$\beta^{26Glu \rightarrow Lys}$ resulting in abnormal messenger RNA and defective splicing	Microcytosis, mild anaemia	Microcytosis, mild anaemia	With β thalassaemia gives thalassaemia major or intermedia
Constant Spring or Paksé	Elongated α chain owing to incorporation of 31 extra amino acids	Microcytosis, mild anaemia	Microcytosis, mild anaemia	With α° thalassaemia gives Hb H disease

[a]Many other thalassaemic structural variants have been described but are much rarer than the three shown in this table.
[b]13–30% frequency in Cambodia, Thailand, Vietnam and some parts of China.

Increased Hb F in Adult Life

Haemoglobin production in man is characterized by two major switches in the haemoglobin composition of the red cells. During the first 3 months of gestation, human red cells contain embryonic haemoglobins (see p. 302), whereas during the last 6 months of gestation, red cells contain predominantly fetal haemoglobin. The major transition from fetal to adult haemoglobin synthesis occurs in the perinatal period and by the end of the first year of life red cells have a haemoglobin composition that usually remains constant throughout adult life. The major haemoglobin is then Hb A, but there are small amounts of Hb A_2 and Hb F. Only 0.2–1.0% of total haemoglobin in human red cells is Hb F and it is restricted to a few cells called 'F' cells. Both the number of F cells and the amount of Hb F per cell can be increased in various conditions, particularly if there is rapid bone marrow regeneration.[13]

The general organization of human globin gene clusters is shown in Figure 14.1. The products of two γ genes differ in only one amino acid: $^{G}\gamma$ has glycine in position 136, whereas $^{A}\gamma$ has alanine. In fetal red cells, the ratio of $^{G}\gamma$ to $^{A}\gamma$ is approximately 3:1; in adult red cells, it is approximately 2:3.

In recent years there has been much interest in the attempts to manipulate the fetal switch pharmacologically. If it was possible to reactivate Hb F synthesis reliably beyond the perinatal period, both β thalassaemia major and sickle cell disease would be ameliorated.

Inherited Abnormalities That Increase Hb F Concentration

More than 50 mutations that increase Hb F synthesis have been described.[13,14] They result in one of two phenotypes, HPFH or δβ thalassaemia; differentiation between these two types is not always simple but has clinical relevance. In general, HPFH has a higher percentage of Hb F and much more balanced chain synthesis. The most common, the African type of HPFH, is associated with a high concentration of Hb F (15–45%), pancellular distribution of Hb F on Kleihauer staining and normal red cell indices. Mutations causing increased synthesis of Hb F are mostly deletions, but some non-deletion mutations have also been described. In contrast, subjects with δβ thalassaemia have lower levels of Hb F accompanied by microcytic, hypochromic indices. The major clinical significance of these abnormalities is their interaction with β thalassaemia and Hb S. Compound heterozygotes for either of these conditions and HPFH have much milder clinical syndromes than the homozygotes for haemoglobin S or β thalassaemia. Compound heterozygotes for either of these conditions and δβ thalassaemia have a condition much closer in severity to the homozygous states.

Increased Hb F is also found in many other haematological conditions, including congenital red cell aplasia and congenital aplastic anaemia (Blackfan-Diamond and Fanconi anaemia, respectively), juvenile myelomonocytic leukaemia and some myelodysplastic syndromes. A small but significant increase in Hb F may occur in the presence of erythropoietic stress (haemolysis, bleeding, recovery from acute bone marrow failure) and in pregnancy.

INVESTIGATION OF PATIENTS WITH A SUSPECTED HAEMOGLOBINOPATHY

Investigation of a person at risk of a haemoglobinopathy encompasses the confirmation or exclusion of the presence of a structural variant, thalassaemia trait or both.

If a structural haemoglobin variant is present, it is necessary to ascertain the clinical significance of the particular variant so that the patient is appropriately managed. If it is confirmed that thalassaemia trait is present, it is not usually necessary to determine the precise mutation present because the clinical significance is usually negligible. The exception to this is an antenatal patient whose partner has also been found to have thalassaemia trait. If prenatal diagnosis is being considered, it may be necessary to undertake mutation analysis to predict fetal risk accurately and to facilitate prenatal diagnosis (see p. 146).

Because the inheritance of a haemoglobinopathy *per se* has genetic implications, it is important that genetic counselling is available for these patients.

In the majority of patients, the presence of a haemoglobinopathy can be diagnosed with sufficient accuracy for clinical purposes from knowledge of the patient's ethnic origin and clinical history (including family history) and the results of physical examination combined with relatively simple haematological tests. Initial investigations should include determination of haemoglobin concentration and red cell indices. A detailed examination of a well-stained blood film should be carried out. In some instances, a reticulocyte count and a search for red cell inclusions give valuable information. Assessment of iron status by estimation of serum iron and total iron binding capacity and/or serum ferritin is sometimes necessary to exclude iron deficiency. Other important basic tests are haemoglobin electrophoresis or high-performance liquid chromatography (HPLC), a sickle solubility test and measurement of Hb A_2 and Hb F percentage. In cases of common haemoglobin variants and classical β thalassaemia trait, accurate data from these tests will facilitate a reliable diagnosis without the need for more sophisticated investigations. However, definitive diagnosis of some thalassaemia syndromes can only be obtained using DNA technology (see p. 147 and p. 330). Similarly, in particular situations, haemoglobin variants will require unequivocal identification by the use of DNA technology or protein analysis by mass spectrometry.[15] Individuals or families who require such investigation must be carefully selected on the basis of family history and on the results of the basic investigations described later in this chapter. Large-scale screening programmes are increasingly being undertaken in some countries where individual case histories and the results of other laboratory tests are not usually available. The problems of such programmes are discussed on p. 318.

The majority of errors occurring in the detection and identification of a haemoglobinopathy are the result of either failure to obtain correct laboratory data or failure to interpret data correctly. In this chapter, a sequence of investigations is proposed based on procedures that should be available in the laboratory of any major hospital. Automated HPLC is increasingly replacing haemoglobin electrophoresis as the initial investigative procedure in laboratories analysing large numbers of samples. Isoelectric focusing (IEF) is, in general, used only to a limited extent, mainly for neonatal screening or in specialist laboratories and it is only briefly described here.

Laboratory investigation of a suspected haemoglobinopathy should follow a defined protocol, which should be devised to suit individual local requirements. The data obtained from the clinical findings, blood picture and electrophoresis or HPLC will usually indicate in which direction to proceed. The investigation for a structural variant is described in the first section and that for a suspected thalassaemia syndrome is described in the second section of this chapter. Screening tests for thalassemia trait and haemoglobin E trait that may be especially applicable in under-resourced areas are described in Chapter 26.

LABORATORY DETECTION OF HAEMOGLOBIN VARIANTS

A proposed scheme of investigation is shown in Figure 14.2 and a list of procedures follows:[15,16]

1. Blood count and film examination (see below)
2. Collection of blood and preparation of haemolysates (see p. 309)
3. Cellulose acetate electrophoresis, Tris buffer, pH 8.5 (see p. 310)
4. Citrate agar or acid agarose gel electrophoresis, pH 6.0 (see p. 312)
5. Automated HPLC (see pp. 314)
6. IEF (see p. 315)
7. Tests for Hb S (see p. 315)
8. Detection of unstable haemoglobins (see p. 318)
9. Detection of Hb Ms (see p. 319)
10. Detection of altered affinity haemoglobins (see p. 320)
11. Differentiation of common structural variants (see p. 320)
12. Neonatal screening (see p. 318)
13. Tests, such as zinc protoporphyrin estimation, to exclude iron deficiency as a cause of microcytosis (see Chapter 9)
14. Molecular techniques (see Chapter 8)
15. Procedures for use in under-resourced laboratories (see Chapter 26).

Globin chain electrophoresis, pH 8.0 and 6.3, is now rarely performed. Methods can be found in previous editions of this book.

Blood Count and Film

The blood count, including Hb and red cell indices, provides valuable information useful in the diagnosis of both α and β thalassaemia interactions with structural variants (see Chapter 3). A film examination may reveal characteristic

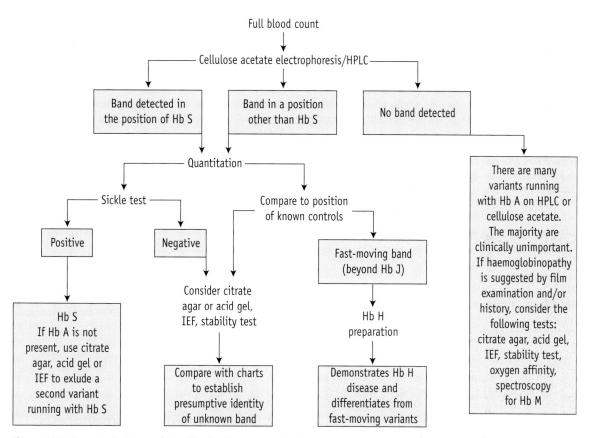

Figure 14.2 Suggested scheme of investigation for structural variants.

red cell changes such as target cells in Hb C trait, sickle cells in sickle cell disease and irregularly contracted cells in the presence of an unstable haemoglobin (see Chapter 5).

Discriminant functions using various formulae have been proposed as a basis for further testing for thalassaemia,[17,18] but we do not advise their use. Although such functions and formulae do indicate whether thalassaemia or iron deficiency is more likely, they may lead to individuals who have both iron deficiency *and* thalassaemia trait not being tested promptly. Generally this is not a problem and indeed it may be preferable to keep the patient under observation until iron deficiency has been treated and then to reassess the likelihood of thalassaemia trait. However, many of the patients who require testing for thalassaemia are women who are already pregnant. In such patients the likely delay in testing is unacceptable. Moreover, these formulae do not appear to have been validated for use during pregnancy. For these reasons, we advise that whenever genetic counselling might be required, testing for β thalassaemia trait should be carried out in all individuals with an MCH <27 pg and screening for α thalassaemia trait should be carried out in those individuals with an MCH <25 pg who belong to an ethnic group in which α° thalassaemia is prevalent.[11]

Collection of Blood and Preparation of Haemolysates

EDTA is the most convenient anticoagulant because it is used for the initial full blood count and film (see Chapter 1), although samples taken into any anticoagulant are satisfactory. Cells freed from clotted blood can also be used.

Preparation of Haemolysate for Qualitative Haemoglobin Electrophoresis

See individual methods.

Preparation of Haemolysate for the Quantification of Haemoglobins and Stability Tests

Preparation of haemolysate for the quantification of haemoglobins and stability tests can be used for qualitative electrophoresis and is necessary for quantitation of Hb A_2 and F or variant haemoglobins by elution. It is also essential for reliable stability tests.

Lyse 2 volumes of washed packed cells in 1 volume of distilled water and then add 1 volume of carbon tetrachloride (CCl_4). Alternatively, lyse by freezing and thawing, then add 2 volumes of CCl_4. Shake the tubes vigorously for approximately 1 min, then centrifuge at 1200 g (3000 rev/min) for 30 min at 4°C. Transfer the supernatant to a clean sample container and adjust the Hb to 100 ± 10 g/l with water. If an unstable Hb is suspected organic solvents should be avoided.

Note: Whole blood samples are best stored as washed, packed cells frozen as droplets in liquid nitrogen and subsequently stored at −20°C, −70°C or over liquid nitrogen. Alternatively, haemolysates may also be frozen at −20°C, −70°C or over liquid nitrogen.

Control Samples

Interpretation of migration patterns of test samples is undertaken by comparison to migration and separation of known abnormal haemoglobins used as control materials. Ideally, a mixture of Hbs A, F, S and C should be included on each electrophoretic separation. This material can be prepared as follows:

1. The control can be made from either the combination of a sickle cell trait sample (Hb A + Hb S) combined with a Hb C trait sample (Hb A + Hb C) and normal cord blood (Hb F + Hb A) or the combination of normal cord blood with a sample from a person with Hb SC disease (Hb S + Hb C).
2. Prepare lysates by the method given for a purified haemolysate.
3. Mix equal volumes of the lysates together and add a few drops of 0.3 mol/l KCN (20 g/l).
4. Analyse samples by electrophoresis to assess quality.
5. Aliquot and store frozen.

Note: Repeated freezing and thawing should be avoided.

Lyophilized controls are stable for considerably longer than liquid and can be purchased from commercial sources.

Quality Assurance

Because the haemoglobinopathies are inherited conditions, some of which carry considerable clinical and genetic implications, precise documentation and record-keeping are of paramount importance.[19] The use of cumulative records when reviewing a patient's data is very useful because it of itself constitutes an aspect of quality assurance. In some situations, repeat sampling, family studies or both may be required to elucidate the nature of the abnormality in an individual.

In-house standard operating procedures should be followed carefully, particularly in this field of haematology, where a small difference in technique can make a significant difference in the results obtained and can lead to misdiagnosis. Many of the techniques described have attention drawn to specific technical details that are important for ensuring valid results.[20]

It is necessary to use reference standards and control materials in each of the analyses undertaken and in some cases to use duplicate analysis to demonstrate precision. There are international standards for Hb F and Hb A_2 (see p. 591), whereas in some countries national reference preparations are also available from national standards institutions. These are extremely valuable because the target values have been established by collaborative studies. Control materials can be prepared in-house or obtained commercially. Samples stored as whole blood at 4°C can be used reliably for several weeks. All laboratories should confirm the normal range for their particular methods and the normal range obtained should not differ significantly from published data.

All laboratories undertaking haemoglobin analysis should participate in an appropriate proficiency testing programme (see p. 594). In the UK, the National External Quality Assessment Scheme (NEQAS) provides samples for sickle solubility tests; for detection and quantitation of variant haemoglobins; and for quantitation of Hbs A_2, F and S.

National and international guidelines have been published for all aspects of the investigations given here.[11,21–23,20,24,25]

Cellulose Acetate Electrophoresis at Alkaline pH

Haemoglobin electrophoresis at pH 8.4–8.6 using cellulose acetate membrane is simple, reliable and rapid. It is satisfactory for the detection of most common clinically important haemoglobin variants.[23–25]

Principle

At alkaline pH, haemoglobin is a negatively charged protein and when subjected to electrophoresis will migrate toward the anode (+). Structural variants that have a change in the charge on the surface of the molecule at alkaline pH will separate from Hb A. Haemoglobin variants that have an amino acid substitution that is internally sited may not separate and those that have an amino acid substitution that has no effect on overall charge will not separate by electrophoresis.

Equipment

Electrophoresis tank and power pack. Any horizontal electrophoresis tank that will allow a bridge gap of 7 cm. A direct current power supply capable of delivering 350 V at 50 mA is suitable for both cellulose acetate and citrate agar electrophoresis

Wicks of filter or chromatography paper

Blotting paper

Applicators. These are available from most manufacturers of electrophoresis equipment, but fine microcapillaries are also satisfactory

Cellulose acetate membranes. Plastic-backed membranes (7.6 × 6.0 cm) are recommended for ease of use and storage

Staining equipment.

Reagents

Electrophoresis buffer. Tris/EDTA/borate (TEB), pH 8.5. Tris-(hydroxymethyl)aminomethane (Tris), 10.2 g; EDTA (di-sodium salt), 0.6 g; boric acid, 3.2 g; water to 1 litre. The buffer should be stored at 4°C and can be used up to 10 times without deterioration

Wetting agent. For example, Zip-prep solution (Helena Laboratories): 1 drop of Zip-prep in 100 ml water

Fixative/stain solution. Ponceau S, 5 g; trichloroacetic acid, 7.5 g; water to 1 litre

Destaining solution. 3% (v/v) acetic acid, 30 ml; water to 1 litre

Haemolysing reagent. 0.5% (v/v) Triton X-100 in 100 mg/l potassium cyanide.

Method

1. Centrifuge samples at 1200 *g* for 5 min. Dilute 20 μl of the packed red cells with 150 μl of the haemolysing reagent. Mix gently and leave for at least 5 min. If purified haemolysates are used, dilute 40 μl of 10 g/dl haemolysate with 150 μl of lysing reagent.
2. *With the power supply disconnected,* prepare the electrophoresis tank by placing equal amounts of TEB buffer in each of the outer buffer compartments. Wet two chamber wicks in the buffer and place one along each divider/bridge support ensuring that they make good contact with the buffer.
3. Soak the cellulose acetate by lowering it slowly into a reservoir of buffer. Leave the cellulose acetate to soak for at least 5 min before use.
4. Fill the sample well plate with 5 μl of each diluted sample or control and cover with a 50 mm coverslip or a 'short' glass slide to prevent evaporation. Load a second sample well plate with Zip-prep solution.
5. Clean the applicator tips immediately prior to use by loading with Zip-prep solution and then applying them to a blotter.
6. Remove the cellulose acetate strip from the buffer and blot twice between two layers of clean blotting paper. Do not allow the cellulose acetate to dry.
7. Load the applicator by depressing the tips into the sample wells twice and apply this first loading onto

some clean blotting paper. Reload the applicator and apply the samples to the cellulose acetate.

8. Place the cellulose acetate plates across the bridges, with the plastic side uppermost. Place two glass slides across the strip to maintain good contact. Electrophorese at 350 V for 25 min.
9. After 25 min electrophoresis, immediately transfer the cellulose acetate to Ponceau S and fix and stain for 5 min.
10. Remove excess stain by washing for 5 min in the first acetic acid reservoir and for 10 min in each of the remaining two. Blot once, using clean blotting paper and leave to dry.
11. Label the membranes and store in a protective plastic envelope.

Interpretation and Comments

Figure 14.3 shows the relative electrophoretic mobilities of some common haemoglobin variants at pH 8.5 on cellulose acetate. Satisfactory separation of Hbs C, S, F, A and J is obtained (Fig. 14.4). In general, Hbs S, D and G migrate closely together, as do Hbs C, E and O^{Arab}. Differentiation between these haemoglobins can be obtained by using acid agarose gels, citrate agar electrophoresis, HPLC or IEF. However, there are slight differences in mobility

Cathode (−)

Origin --

------ Carbonic anhydrase

------ A$_2$'

C ------ A$_2$, E, C-Harlem, O-Arab

S ------ D, G, Q-India, Hasharon
------ Lepore

------ F

A ------

------ K-Woolwich

J ------

------ Bart's

N ------

------ I
------ H

Anode (+)

Figure 14.3 Schematic representation of relative mobilities of some abnormal haemoglobins. Cellulose acetate, pH 8.5.

AS

AD

AG

AC

AE

AJ

SS   (+F)

SC

+   **—**

Figure 14.4 Relative mobilities of some abnormal haemoglobins. Cellulose acetate, pH 8.5.

between Hbs S, Lepore and D^{Punjab} and also between Hbs C and E; optimization of the technique will facilitate detection of the difference. Generally, the Lepore Hbs and Hb D^{Punjab} migrate slightly anodal to Hb S (i.e. they are slightly faster than S); Hb C migrates slightly cathodal to Hb E (i.e. it is slightly slower than E).

All samples showing a single band in either the S or C position should be analysed further using acid agarose or citrate agar gel electrophoresis, HPLC or IEF to exclude the possibility of a compound heterozygote such as SD, SG, CE or CO^{Arab}.

The quality of separation resulting from this procedure is affected primarily by both the amount of haemoglobin

applied and the positioning of the origin. Also, delays between application of the sample and commencement of the electrophoresis, delay in staining after electrophoresis or inadequate blotting of the acetate prior to application will cause poor results. This technique is sensitive enough to separate Hb F from Hb A and to detect Hb A$_2$ variants.

If an abnormal haemoglobin is present, the detection of a Hb A$_2$ variant band in conjunction with the abnormal fraction is evidence that the variant is an α chain variant. Globin electrophoresis at both acid and alkaline pH is also useful in elucidating which globin chain is affected. However, with the more ready availability of HPLC, it is less often needed.

When an abnormal haemoglobin is found, it may be of diagnostic importance to measure the percentage of the variant; this can be done by the electrophoresis with elution procedure for Hb A$_2$ estimation given on p. 322. Quantitation of Hb S is often clinically useful, both in patients with sickle cell disease who are being treated by transfusion and for the diagnosis of conditions in which Hb S is coinherited with α and β thalassaemia, as outlined in Table 14.5. Quantitation of Hb S can be done with HPLC, electrophoresis with elution or by microcolumn chromatography.

Citrate Agar Electrophoresis at pH 6.0

Equipment[26,27]

Electrophoresis tank and power pack. Any horizontal electrophoresis tank that will allow a bridge gap of 7 cm. A direct current power supply capable of delivering 350 V at 50 mA is suitable for both cellulose acetate and citrate agar electrophoresis

Table 14.5 Results of laboratory investigations in interactions of Hb S and α or β thalassaemia in adults

	MCV	% S	% A	% A$_2$	% F
AS	N	35–38	62–65	<3.5	<1
SS	N	88–93	0	<3.5	5–10
S/β° thalassaemia	L	88–93	0	>3.5	5–10
S/β^+ thalassaemia	L	50–93	3–30	>3.5	1–10
S/HPFH	N	65–80	0	<3.5	20–35
AS/α^+ thalassaemia	N/L	28–35	62–70	<3.5	<1
AS/α° thalassaemia	L	20–30	68–78	<3.5	<1
SS/α thalassaemia	N/L	88–93	0	<3.5	1–10
MCV, mean cell volume; N, normal; L, low; HPFH, hereditary persistence of fetal haemoglobin.					

Cooling bars (*Helena Laboratories*)
Perspex trays, 80 × 100 × 2 mm
Wicks of sponge, filter paper or chromatography paper
Applicators. These are available from most manufacturers of electrophoresis equipment, but fine microcapillaries are also satisfactory.

Reagents

Difco Bacto-agar.
Lysing reagent. 0.5% (v/v) Triton X-100 in 100 mg/l potassium cyanide.

Buffer

Stock buffer. Trisodium citrate dihydrate, 73.5 g; 0.5 mol/l citric acid, 34.0 ml; water to 1 litre
Working buffer. Dilute stock buffer 1 in 5 with water. Prepare on day of use
5 g/dl potassium cyanide. Potassium cyanide, 0.5 g; distilled water to 100 ml
Dianisidine stain. 3% hydrogen peroxide (10 volumes), 1.0 ml; 1% sodium nitroprusside (nitroferricyanide), 1.0 ml; 3% acetic acid, 10.0 ml; 0.2% o-dianisidine in methanol, 5.0 ml. Prepare mixture just before use
Wetting agent. For example, Zip-prep solution (Helena Laboratories); 1 drop in 100 ml water.
3% Acetic acid. 120 ml glacial acetic acid made up to 4 litres with water
Gel-Bond or similar support.

Method

1. Centrifuge sample (1200 *g* for 5 min). Dilute 20 μl of packed red cells with 300 μl of haemolysing reagent. Mix gently and leave for at least 5 min. For cord blood samples, dilute 20 μl of packed red cells with 150 μl of the lysing reagent. For purified haemolysates, dilute 20 μl of 10 g/dl haemolysate with 150 μl of lysing reagent.
2. *With the power supply disconnected*, place equal volumes working buffer in each of the outer buffer compartments. Wet two sponge wicks in the buffer and place one in each compartment against the divider. Place two frozen cooling sticks in each central chamber. If cooling bars or ice packs are not available, run the electrophoresis at 4°C.
3. Add 0.5 g agar to 50 ml working buffer. Heat to approximately 95°C, stirring gently until the agar has dissolved. Allow to cool to 60°C; add 0.5 ml of 5 g/dl potassium cyanide. Pipette approximately 10 ml into each of four Perspex trays (80 × 100 × 2 mm) and allow to stand for about 15 min at room temperature until set. These gels may be kept for 1 week at 4°C in a sealed plastic bag. Allow gels to come to room temperature before use.

4. Fill the sample well plate with 5 μl of each sample and cover with a 6 cm coverslip or glass slide. Load a second sample well plate with Zip-prep solution. Clean the applicator tips by loading with Zip-prep solution and then applying them to blotting paper. Load the applicator and apply this first loading onto some clean blotting paper. Reload the applicator and apply the samples to the agar gel.
5. Place gel plate in an inverted position in the electrophoresis tank so that the gel is in contact with sponge wicks and run at a constant voltage of 50 V for 60 min.
6. After 60 min, disconnect from power supply, remove gel and apply the stain solution by layering onto the agar using a Pasteur pipette. Allow to stain for 10 min at room temperature.
7. Wash in three changes of 3% acetic acid, float gels onto the hydrophilic side of a piece of Gel Bond and leave to dry. These mounted gels may then be kept indefinitely.

Interpretation and Comments

Figure 14.5 shows the relative electrophoretic mobilities of some common haemoglobin variants at pH 6.0 on citrate agar.

Agarose Gel Electrophoresis

Agarose gels are commercially available as substitutes for both alkaline and acid separation systems. They are simple to use and particularly useful in laboratories that process small numbers of samples.

Reagents and Method

The manufacturer's method should be followed.

Anode (+)

C ------

S -----C-Harlem
-----Hasharon

Origin --------------O-Arab, Q-India --------------------------
A -----D, E, G, Lepore, H, I, N, J

F -----Bart's, K-Woolwich

Cathode (-)

Figure 14.5 Schematic representation of relative mobilities of some abnormal haemoglobins. Citrate agar pH 6.0.

Interpretation

With acid agarose systems, the principle of the test is the same as that of citrate agar electrophoresis at the same pH, but it should be noted that there are significant differences in mobility of some variant haemoglobins. With alkaline systems, in general the same separation patterns are obtained, but where individual application notes are available these should be used for reference. Because not all kits provide these, laboratories may need to build up their own data on known variants.

Automated High-Performance Liquid Chromatography

Automated cation-exchange HPLC[28] is being used increasingly as the initial diagnostic method in haemoglobinopathy laboratories with a high workload.[29] Both capital and consumable costs are higher than with haemoglobin electrophoresis, but labour costs are less; overall costs may be similar.[30] In comparison with haemoglobin electrophoresis, HPLC has four advantages:

1. The analysers are automated and thus utilize less staff time and permit processing of large batches.
2. Very small samples (5 μl) are sufficient for analysis; this is especially useful in paediatric work.
3. Quantification of normal and variant haemoglobins is available on every sample.
4. A provisional identification of a larger proportion of variant haemoglobins can be made.[31]

Principle

HPLC depends on the interchange of charged groups on the ion exchange material with charged groups on the haemoglobin molecule. A typical column packing is 5 μm spherical silica gel. The surface of the support is modified by carboxyl groups to have a weakly cationic charge, which allows the separation of haemoglobin molecules with different charges by ion exchange. When a haemolysate containing a mixture of haemoglobins is adsorbed onto the resin, the rate of elution of different haemoglobins is determined by the pH and ionic strength of any buffer applied to the column. With automated systems now in use, elution of the charged molecules is achieved by a continually changing salt gradient; fractions are detected as they pass through an ultraviolet/visible light detector and are recorded on an integrating computer system. Analysis of the area under these absorption peaks gives the percentage of the fraction detected. The time of elution (retention time) of any normal or variant haemoglobin present is compared with that of known haemoglobins, providing quantification of both normal haemoglobins (A, F and A₂) and many variants.

Figure 14.6 shows a schematic representation of an HPLC system and Figure 14.7 shows a chromatogram of

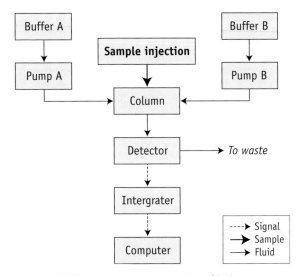

Figure 14.6 Diagrammatic representation of high-performance liquid chromatography (HPLC) showing the flow of sample and buffers.

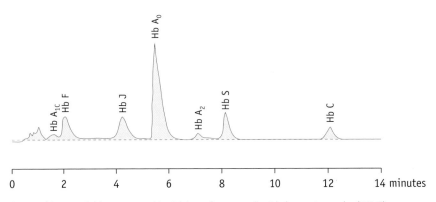

Figure 14.7 A mixture of haemoglobins separated by high-performance liquid chromatography (HPLC).

a mixture of different haemoglobins. Systems are available from various manufacturers.

Method

The manufacturer's procedure should be followed. To prolong the life of the column it is important to follow the manufacturer's instructions with regard to the concentration of haemoglobin in the sample to be injected.

Interpretation and Comments

Results are accurate and reproducible, but as with every method of haemoglobin analysis, controls should be run with every batch. If the system is being used for the detection of haemoglobin variants, elution times can be compared with those of known controls; actual times, however, are affected by the batch of buffer and column, the age of the column and the laboratory temperature. A better comparison may be obtained using the relative elution time, which is calculated by dividing the elution time of the variant with that of the main Hb A fraction. It should be noted that Hb A is separated into its component fractions of A_0 and A_1 and the A_1 fraction frequently subdivides into several peaks. Skill is required in interpretation of the results because various normal and abnormal haemoglobins may have the same retention time and a glycosylated variant haemoglobin will have a different retention time from the non-glycosylated form. HPLC usually separates Hbs A, A_2, F, S, C, D[Punjab] and G[Philadelphia] from each other.[29,32] However, both Hb E and Hb Lepore co-elute with haemoglobin A_2 (as other haemoglobins co-elute with A, S and F). The retention time of glycosylated and other derivatives of Hb S can be the same as those of Hb A_0 and A_2. For example, derivatives of haemoglobin S co-elute with haemoglobin A_2, so that percentages of A_2 by this method are inaccurate and therefore do not have the same significance as percentage of haemoglobin A_2 measured by alternative methods.[33] For these reasons, and because there are more than 1000 variants identified, HPLC can never definitively identify any haemoglobin. It is important to analyse variants found using second-line techniques, such as a sickle solubility test, alkaline and acid electrophoresis, or isoelectric focusing.

HPLC is also applicable for the quantification of Hb A_{1c} for the monitoring of diabetes mellitus; to make optimal use of staff and equipment, this procedure is sometimes carried out in haematology laboratories. In fact, an increased glycosylated fraction is not infrequently noted when HPLC is performed for investigation of a suspected haemoglobinopathy.[34] Unless the patient is already known to suffer from diabetes mellitus, this abnormality should be drawn to the attention of clinical staff.

Isoelectric Focusing

Principle

IEF utilizes a matrix containing carrier ampholytes of low molecular weight and varying isoelectric points (pIs). These molecules migrate to their respective pIs when a current is applied, resulting in a pH gradient being formed; for haemoglobin analysis, a pH gradient of 6–8 is usually used. Haemoglobin molecules migrate through the gel until they reach the point at which their individual pIs equal the corresponding pH on the gel. At this point, the charge on the haemoglobin is neutral and migration ceases. The pH gradient counteracts diffusion and the haemoglobin variant forms a discrete narrow band.[35,36]

Method

Pre-prepared plates of either polyacrylamide or agarose gel can be obtained from various manufacturers. For the exact method, the manufacturer's instructions should be followed.

Interpretation and Comments

IEF is satisfactory for analysis of haemolysates, whole blood samples or dried blood spots. The use of dried blood spots is suitable for samples that have to be transported long distances and where only a few drops of blood can be obtained. Whereas IEF has the advantage that it separates more variants than cellulose acetate, it also has the disadvantage that it separates haemoglobin into its post-translational derivatives. For instance, Hb F separates into F_1 (acetylated F) and F_{11}; Hb A can produce five bands – A_0, A_1, A(αmet), A(βmet) and A($\alpha\beta$met) – and similarly for other haemoglobins. This makes interpretation more difficult. Identification of variants is still only provisional using IEF, and second-line methods should be used for further analysis.

Figure 14.8 shows the relative isoelectric points of some common haemoglobin variants and Figure 14.9 shows the separation obtained.

TESTS FOR Hb S

Tests to detect the presence of Hb S depend on the decreased solubility of this haemoglobin at low oxygen tensions.

Sickling in Whole Blood

The sickling phenomenon may be demonstrated in a thin wet film of blood (sealed with a petroleum jelly/paraffin wax mixture or with nail varnish). If Hb S is present, the red cells lose their smooth, round shape and become

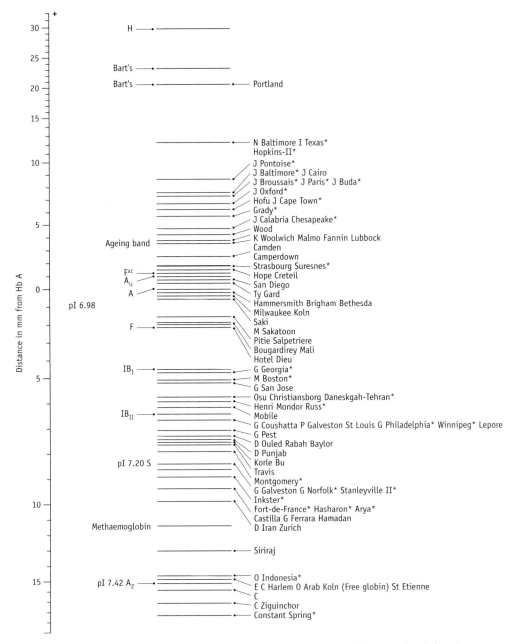

Figure 14.8 Schematic representation of relative mobilities of some abnormal haemoglobins. Isoelectric focusing. *Note* the presence of two bands for haemoglobin Bart's. The scale in mm is not linear. *Indicates α chain mutations. *(Reproduced with permission from Basset et al.[36])*

sickled. This process may take up to 12 h in Hb S trait, whereas changes are apparent in homozygotes and compound heterozygotes after 1 h at 37°C. These changes can be hastened by the addition of a reducing agent such as sodium dithionite as follows:

Reagents

Disodium hydrogen phosphate (Na_2HPO_4). 0.114 mol/l (16.2 g/l)
Sodium dithionite $(Na_2S_2O_4)$. 0.114 mol/l (19.85 g/l). Prepare freshly just before use

Figure 14.9 Relative mobilities of some abnormal haemoglobins. Isoelectric focusing. The controls are mixtures of various haemoglobins.

Figure 14.10 Photomicrograph of sickled red cells. Sickle cell anaemia. Sealed preparation of blood. Fully sickled filamentous forms predominate.

Working solution. Mix 3 volumes of Na_2HPO_4 with 2 volumes of $Na_2S_2O_4$ to obtain a pH of 6.8 in the resultant solution. Use immediately.

Method

Add 5 drops of the freshly prepared reagent to 1 drop of anticoagulated blood on a slide. Seal between slide and coverglass with a petroleum jelly/paraffin wax mixture or with nail varnish. Sickling takes place almost immediately in sickle cell anaemia and should be obvious in sickle cell trait within 1 h (Fig. 14.10). A test on a positive control of Hb A plus Hb S must be performed at the same time.

Hb S Solubility Test

Principle

Sickle cell haemoglobin is insoluble in the deoxygenated state in a high molarity phosphate buffer. The crystals that form refract light and cause the solution to be turbid.[37]

Reagents

Phosphate buffer. Anhydrous dipotassium hydrogen phosphate, 215 g; anhydrous potassium dihydrogen phosphate, 169 g; sodium dithionite, 5 g; saponin, 1 g; water to 1 litre.

Note: Dissolve the K_2HPO_4 in water before adding the KH_2PO_4, then add the dithionite and finally the saponin. This solution is stable for 7 days. Store refrigerated.

Method

1. Pipette 2 ml of reagent into three 12 × 75 mm test tubes.
2. Allow the reagent to warm to room temperature.
3. Add 10 μl of packed cells (from EDTA-anticoagulated blood) to one tube, 10 μl of packed cells from a known sickle cell trait subject as a positive control to the second tube and 10 μl packed cells from a normal subject as a negative control to the final tube.
4. Mix well and leave to stand for 5 min.
   Note: The blood reagent mixture should be light pink or red. A light orange colour indicates that the reagent has deteriorated.
5. Hold tube 2.5 cm in front of a white card with narrow black lines and read for turbidity, in comparison with the positive and negative control samples.

6. If the test appears to be positive, centrifuge at 1200 *g* for 5 min. A positive test will show a dark red band at the top, whereas the solution below will be pink or colourless.

Interpretation and Comments

A positive solubility or sickling test indicates the presence of Hb S and as such is useful in the differential diagnosis of Hbs D and G, which migrate with Hb S on cellulose acetate electrophoresis at alkaline pH. Positive results are also obtained on samples containing the rare haemoglobins that have both the Hb S mutation and an additional mutation in the β chain. A positive solubility test merely indicates the presence of a sickling haemoglobin and does not differentiate between homozygotes, compound heterozygotes and heterozygotes. In an emergency, it may be necessary to decide if an individual suffers from sickle cell disease before the haemoglobin electrophoresis results are available. In these circumstances, if the solubility test is positive, a provisional diagnosis of sickle cell trait can be made if the red cell morphology is normal on the blood film. If the blood film shows any sickle cells or numerous target cells, irrespective of the Hb, a provisional diagnosis of sickle cell disease should be made; many patients with sickle cell/Hb C compound heterozygosity will have a normal Hb. Remember that the sickle test is likely to be negative in infants with sickle cell disease.

False-positive results have been reported in severe leucocytosis; in hyperproteinaemia (such as multiple myeloma); and in the presence of an unstable haemoglobin, especially after splenectomy. The use of packed cells, as described in this method, minimizes the problem of false-positive results caused by hyperproteinaemia and hyperlipidaemia.

False-negative results can occur in patients with a low Hb and the use of packed cells will overcome this problem. False-negative results may also occur if old or outdated reagents are used and if the dithionite/buffer mixture is not freshly made. False-negative results are likely to be found in infants younger than age 6 months and in other situations (e.g. post-transfusion), in which the Hb S level is <20%.

All sickle tests, whether positive or negative, must be confirmed by electrophoresis or HPLC at the earliest opportunity.

NEONATAL (NEWBORN) SCREENING

Cord blood or a heel prick sample should be tested from all babies at risk of sickle cell disease or β thalassaemia major (i.e. where the mother has a gene for Hb S, C, D[Punjab], E, O[Arab], Lepore or β or δβ thalassaemia trait). If a cord-blood specimen is used, it is important that the sample is collected by venepuncture of the cleaned umbilical vein to avoid contamination with maternal blood because even small quantities of maternal blood can cause a case of sickle cell disease to be misdiagnosed as sickle cell trait.

In areas where the frequency of haemoglobinopathies is high, universal neonatal (newborn) screening should be undertaken where possible. Universal neonatal screening is now being carried out in England and will be gradually extended to the rest of the UK.[38] The screening programme is linked to the existing dried blood spot screening programme in place for phenylketonuria and congenital hypothyroidism. The same dried blood spot sample is tested for sickle cell disease. It must be emphasized that the main function of this screening is to detect sickle cell disease, although many cases of β thalassaemia major are also detected, dependent on the mutations present. Dried blood spot samples are tested using HPLC and IEF – HPLC is typically the first-line test and abnormalities are confirmed by IEF. Haemoglobin electrophoresis is not recommended for the analysis of dried blood spots. Analysis of cord blood samples is undertaken as a clinician-led request rather than for general screening. If umbilical cord blood samples are used, they can be examined by haemoglobin electrophoresis using cellulose acetate at alkaline pH or citrate agar at acid pH,[23] or by HPLC or IEF. If any abnormality is detected, a confirmatory technique should also be undertaken.

Babies provisionally diagnosed as having Hbs SS, SC, SD[Punjab], SO[Arab] or Sβ thalassaemia should be retested within 6–8 weeks of birth. After confirmation of the diagnosis, they should be followed in a paediatric clinic, immediately started on prophylactic penicillin to prevent pneumococcal infections, and appropriately managed in the long term.[3] β thalassaemia major is suspected when Hb A is either absent or greatly reduced at birth. Such babies are retested for confirmation. The diagnosis of β thalassaemia trait cannot be reliably made until 12 months of age unless DNA techniques are used (see p. 146).

DETECTION OF AN UNSTABLE HAEMOGLOBIN

Haemoglobin variants exhibit a wide range of instability but the clinically unstable haemoglobins can be detected by both the heat stability test and the isopropanol test.[39] However, minor degrees of instability that have little or no clinical significance may need other techniques. The unstable haemoglobins are frequently silent using electrophoretic or chromatographic techniques and tests for haemoglobin instability are essential in the detection or exclusion of an unstable haemoglobin.

Several methods are available for the demonstration of haemoglobin instability. Samples analysed should be as fresh as possible and certainly less than 1 week old. Controls should be of the same age as the test sample; a normal cord blood sample can be used as a positive control. The isopropanol test uses chemically prepared controls.

Heat Stability Test

Principle

When haemoglobin in solution is heated, the hydrophobic van der Waals bonds are weakened and the stability of the molecule is decreased.[40,41] Under controlled conditions, unstable haemoglobins precipitate, whereas stable haemoglobins remain in solution.

Reagent

Tris-HCl buffer, pH 7.4, 0.05 M. Tris, 6.05 g; water to 1 litre. Adjust the pH to 7.4 with concentrated HCl. (It is essential that Tris-sensitive electrodes are used.)

Method

1. Add 0.2 ml of lysate, freshly prepared by the purified haemolysate method (given on p. 309), to a tube containing 1.8 ml of buffer. The negative control is obtained from a fresh normal sample.
2. Place the tubes in a waterbath at 50°C. Examine the tubes at 60, 90 and 120 min for precipitation.

Interpretation and Comments

A major unstable haemoglobin will have undergone marked precipitation at 60 min and profuse flocculation at 120 min. The normal control may show some (fine) precipitation at 60 min, but this should be minimal.

Isopropanol Stability Test

Principle

When haemoglobin is dissolved in a solvent such as isopropanol, which is less polar than water, the hydrophobic van der Waals bonds are weakened and the stability of the molecule is decreased. Under controlled conditions, unstable haemoglobins precipitate, whereas stable haemoglobins remain in solution. This method has the advantage that it does not require a 37°C waterbath and positive controls can be made by modification of the reagent buffer.[42]

Reagents

Tris-HCl buffer, pH 7.4, 0.1 mol/l. Tris, 12.11 g; water to 1 litre. Adjust the pH to 7.4 with concentrated HCl. (It is essential that Tris-sensitive electrodes are used.)
Isopropanol buffer, 17%. Make 17 volumes of isopropanol up to 100 volumes with tris-HCl buffer. The 17% isopropanol buffer solution may be stored in a tightly stoppered glass bottle for 3 months at 4°C.
Positive controls. These are buffers produced by adding small amounts of zinc to the standard 17% isopropanol buffer. For the strongest positive control (5+), add

0.6 mmol/l zinc acetate and for the weaker positive control (1+), add 0.1 mmol/l zinc acetate to the buffer. Samples containing haemoglobin E or haemoglobin F can also be used as weak positive controls.

Method

1. Prepare oxyhaemoglobin haemolysates from test and normal control samples as given on p. 309.
2. Pipette 2.0 ml of the standard isopropanol buffer into two tubes, followed by 2.0 ml of the 1+ and 5+ control solutions, respectively, into two further tubes.
3. Add 0.2 ml of test sample to the first tube. Add 0.2 ml normal control sample into the three remaining tubes.
4. Place the tubes in a waterbath at 37°C for 30 min. Examine the tubes at 5, 20 and 30 min for turbidity and fine flocculation.

Interpretation and Comments

A normal sample will remain clear until 30 min, when a slight cloudiness may appear. Some unstable haemoglobins will show clearly observable precipitation even after 5 min incubation, whereas milder variants will not show precipitation until 20 min.

Positive results may be given by samples containing as little as 10% Hb F or by samples containing increased methaemoglobin as a result of prolonged storage. If the normal sample undergoes premature precipitation, check the temperature of the waterbath because it is likely to be higher than 37°C.

False-negative results should be avoided by continuing the incubation until the normal control undergoes precipitation.

DETECTION OF Hb Ms

Methaemoglobin (Hi) has iron present in the ferric form. Inherited variants of haemoglobin that undergo oxidation to methaemoglobin more readily than Hb A are referred to as Hb Ms. This is one of the causes of a very rare condition, congenital methaemoglobinaemia. The other cause of inherited methaemoglobinaemia is methaemoglobin reductase deficiency (see p. 240). Methaemoglobin levels vary, but may be as high as 40% of the total haemoglobin. Methaemoglobinaemia *per se* may also be caused by oxidant chemicals.

Methaemoglobin variants may be detected by haemoglobin electrophoresis at pH 7, but almost all can be distinguished from methaemoglobin A (Hi A) by their absorption spectra. Each methaemoglobin has its own distinct absorption spectrum. Hi A has two absorption peaks at 502 nm and 632 nm, whereas the peak absorbances for the variant Hb Ms are at different wavelengths (Fig. 14.11).

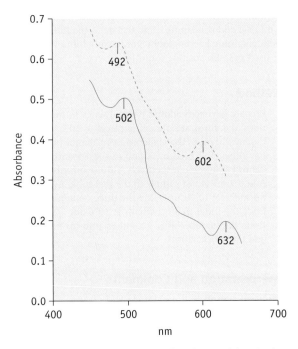

Figure 14.11 Absorption maxima of methaemoglobins in the range of 450–650 nm. Normal methaemoglobin is shown by a solid line; Hb M Saskatoon is shown by a dotted line.
(Reproduced with permission from Lehmann H, Huntsman KG 1974 Man's Haemoglobins, 2nd edition, p. 214. North-Holland, Amsterdam.)

Reagent

Potassium ferricyanide. 0.1 mol/l.

Method

1. Lyse washed red cells from a blood sample of known Hb A and of the test sample with water to give haemoglobin concentration of about 1 g/l.

2. Convert the haemoglobin to Hi by the addition of 5 μl of potassium ferricyanide solution to each ml of haemolysate.

3. Leave for 10 min at room temperature.

4. Record the spectrum of Hi A using an automatic scanning spectrometer.

5. Compare to the spectrum of Hi in the test sample.

DETECTION OF ALTERED AFFINITY HAEMOGLOBINS

Electrophoretic and chromatographic techniques are frequently unsuccessful in separating these abnormal haemoglobins and cannot be relied on for detection because the amino acid substitution often does not involve a change in charge.

The most informative investigation is the measurement of the oxygen dissociation curve (see p. 268). The most significant finding is a decreased Hill's constant ('n' value) because this can only come about by a change in the structure of the haemoglobin. The *p50* may be either increased (low-affinity haemoglobin) or decreased (high-affinity haemoglobin). High-affinity haemoglobins result in an increase in Hb level, whereas low-affinity haemoglobins result in a decrease in Hb level. The *p50* alone may be affected by other factors such as the high concentration of 2,3-DPG in pyruvate kinase deficiency. (Aspects of this are discussed in Chapter 11.)

DIFFERENTIAL DIAGNOSIS OF COMMON HAEMOGLOBIN VARIANTS

Suggested methods for differential diagnosis are given in Table 14.6 and Figure 14.12 gives a comparison of some common variants using different techniques.

Table 14.6 Methods helpful in the differential diagnosis of common structural variants

INITIAL FINDING ON CELLULOSE ACETATE ELECTROPHORESIS	MOST LIKELY VARIANT	DIFFERENTIATION
Band in position of Hb S	Hb S, D, G-Philadelphia, Lepore	Blood count, quantitation, solubility test, citrate agar/acid gel electrophoresis, IEF, HPLC
Band in position of Hb C	Hb C, E, O-Arab	Quantitation, citrate agar/acid gel electrophoresis, IEF, HPLC
Very fast band	Hb I, H	H bodies
IEF, isoelectric focusing; HPLC, high-performance liquid chromatography.		

Haemoglobin		Haemoglobins						Abnormal globin chains					
		Cellulose acetate pH 8.9			Agar gel pH 6.0			pH 8.0			pH 6.3		
		+A	S	C−	+C	S	A−	+β^A	β^S	α^A−	+β^A	β^S	α^A−
H	β_4	•											
I	$\alpha_2^I \beta_2$	•											
N	$\alpha_2 \beta_2^N$	•											
Bart's	γ_4	•											
J	$\alpha_2 \beta_2^J$	•											
K	$\alpha_2 \beta_2^K$	•											
F	$\alpha_2 \gamma_2$		•										
Lepore	$\alpha_2 \delta \beta_2$		•										
S	$\alpha_2 \beta_2^S$		•										
D	$\alpha_2 \beta_2^D$		•										
G	$\alpha_2^G \beta_2$		•										
G	$\alpha_2 \beta_2^G$		•										
E	$\alpha_2 \beta_2^E$			•									
O	$\alpha_2 \beta_2^O$			•									
C	$\alpha_2 \beta_2^C$			•									

Figure 14.12 Comparison of the relative mobilities of some abnormal haemoglobins by different methods. The position of Hbs A, S and C and their corresponding chains are indicated by the vertical lines. *(Adapted from ICSH.[23])*

INVESTIGATION OF SUSPECTED THALASSAEMIA

A suggested scheme of investigations is shown in Figure 14.13; the methods used are listed in the following.

1. Estimates of Hb A_2 between 3.3% and 3.8% need careful assessment and should be repeated.
2. Hb A_2 values in α thalassaemia trait are usually below 2.5%. Some types of β thalassaemia trait have normal Hb A_2 values.

Methods for Investigation of Thalassaemia

1. Full blood count with red cell indices and blood film and, in selected cases, reticulocyte count

2. Hb A_2 measurement by cellulose acetate electrophoresis with elution (see p. 322)
3. Hb A_2 measurement of microcolumn chromatography (see p. 323)
4. Automated HPLC (see p. 325)
5. Quantitation of Hb F (see p. 325 or HPLC)
6. Assessment of the distribution of Hb F (see p. 327)
7. Assessment of iron status (see p. 179)
8. Demonstration of red cell inclusion bodies (see p. 329)
9. DNA analysis (see p. 146).

Blood Count and Film

The blood count, including haemoglobin and red cell indices, provides valuable information useful in the diagnosis of both α and β thalassaemia. In classical cases, there will be an elevation in the red cell count, accompanied by a decrease in MCV and MCH. The MCHC and red cell distribution width (RDW) are often normal in thalassaemia trait,

(1) Values between 3.5% and 3.8% need careful assessment and should be repeated using a second method.
(2) A₂ values in α-thalassaemia are usually below 2.5%. some types of β-thalaessamia trait have normal Hb A₂ values

Figure 14.13 Suggested scheme of investigation for thalassaemia.

whereas in iron deficiency anaemia they are more likely to be abnormal. The blood film may show features such as target cells, basophilic stippling and microcytosis in the absence of hypochromia, which point to a diagnosis of thalassaemia trait. Anisochromasia, which is a feature of iron deficiency, is not usual in α and β thalassaemia trait, although it may be seen in haemoglobin H disease. Haemoglobin H disease is also characterized by marked poikilocytosis. The reticulocyte count is increased in haemoglobin H disease.

QUANTITATION OF Hb A₂

An increased Hb A₂ level is characteristic of heterozygous β thalassaemia and its accurate measurement is required for the diagnosis or exclusion of β thalassaemia trait. Estimations may be made by elution after cellulose acetate electrophoresis or by chromatography, either microcolumn or HPLC.

Measurement of Hb A₂ by Elution from Cellulose Acetate

Principle

Haemolysate is separated into its component fractions by alkaline electrophoresis on cellulose acetate membrane.

The relative proportions of the separated fractions are quantitated by spectrometry of the eluates of the separated fractions.[43,44]

Equipment

Electrophoresis tank and power pack. see p. 310
Wicks of double filter paper or chromatography paper
Cellulose acetate membranes (78 × 150 mm).

Reagent

TEB buffer, pH 8.5. Tris(hydroxymethyl) methylamine, 40.8 g; disodium EDTA, 2.4 g; orthoboric acid, 12.8 g; water to 4 litres.

Method

1. Prepare a purified haemolysate from washed red cells as described on p. 309. The haemolysate may be kept at 4°C for up to 1 week before analysis.
2. *With the power supply disconnected*, pour equal amounts of TEB buffer into both the anode and the cathode chambers. Cut lengths of filter or chromatography paper, soak them in the buffer chamber and place

them along the bridge supports as wicks. Set the bridge gap to 7 cm.

3. Soak the cellulose acetate by carefully floating the cellulose acetate sheet onto the surface of the buffer, making sure that no air bubbles are trapped underneath it. When the sheet has absorbed the buffer, submerge the sheet. Leave for at least 5 min, remove and blot carefully between two sheets of blotting paper.

4. Position the cellulose acetate across the bridge supports so that the long end of the sheet is on the anodal side. Using a ruler as a guideline, apply 30 μl of lysate to each sheet 1 cm from the cathode in a single line. Leave 1 cm margin at each end of the application line.

5. Run at a constant voltage of 250 V until separation is complete. This will take approximately 60 min and there should be at least a 1 cm gap between the A and A_2 bands at the end of the run. Check the separation at 40 min, ensuring that the Hb A (or variant such as Hb H, Hb J or Hb N) does not travel onto the wicks. Check again at 5–10 min thereafter. Samples with a variant band between the A and A_2 bands will take up to 30 min longer to obtain satisfactory separation.

6. Remove the sheet, holding it carefully at the anodal wick contact; do not place on a work surface. Cut off and discard the cellulose acetate that has been in contact with the cathodal wick. Cut a 'blank' strip of approximately 2 cm wide from the cathodal end of one sheet (do not use cellulose acetate that includes the application line). Cut out the Hb A_2 section, cutting the band into pieces approximately 1 cm square directly into a clean universal container. Cut out any variant band in the same way and finally cut out the Hb A band.

7. Add 4 ml of distilled water to both the blank and Hb A_2 containers and add 16 ml water to the Hb A container. Variant bands are usually eluted in 8 ml of water, although this may vary.

8. Mix the eluates for 20 min and mix again by inversion just before measuring the absorbance.

9. Read the absorbance of the blank against water at 415 nm. This reading should be <0.005. Read the absorbances of the haemoglobin solutions at 415 nm against the cellulose acetate blank.

Calculation

$$\%Hb\,A_2 = \frac{\text{Absorbance of Hb } A_2 \times 100}{\text{Absorbance of Hb } A_2 +}$$
$$(\text{Absorbance of Hb A} \times 4)$$

Interpretation and Comments

For interpretation of results and normal ranges, see p. 325. Duplicate values obtained should be within 0.2%. This

method is inaccurate in the presence of Hb C, Hb E and Hb O^{Arab} because they do not separate from Hb A_2.

The procedure is useful for the measurement of haemoglobin variants: in these cases, the volume of water used for elution should be adjusted to the apparent quantity of the variant as judged on electrophoresis. Particular care must be taken when cutting strips on which a variant of haemoglobin (e.g. Hb S) is present because the separation between Hb S and Hb A_2 is less certain.

To obtain accurate and precise results, use the same cuvette when reading the blank, Hb A_2 and Hb A absorbance of each sample. Read the blank, Hb A_2 and Hb A in that order to minimize the effects of carryover. Some types of cellulose acetate are unsuitable for elution; this can be detected by a very high blank reading. The haemoglobin concentration of the haemolysate is important: the absorbance reading of the haemoglobin A_2 must be at least 0.1 absorbance unit because low values will give inaccurately low Hb A_2 results.

Measurement of Hb A_2 by Microcolumn Chromatography

Principle

Microcolumn chromatography depends on the interchange of charged groups on the ion exchange cellulose with charged groups on the haemoglobin molecule. When a mixture of haemoglobins is adsorbed onto the cellulose, a particular haemoglobin component may be eluted from the column using a buffer (developer) with a specific pH and/or ionic strength, whereas other components (either a single haemoglobin or a mixture of haemoglobins) may be eluted by changing the pH or ionic strength of the developer. The separation of haemoglobin components depends on the pH and/or ionic strength of the developers used for the equilibration of the column and for the elution, the type of cellulose, the volume of the sample added, the size of the column, the gradient, flow rates and temperature. The following methods use the anion exchanger diethylaminoethyl (DEAE) cellulose (Whatman DE-52 microgranular pre-swollen), with Tris-HCl developers[45] or glycine-KCN developers.[46]

Measurement of Hb A_2 by Microcolumn Chromatography with Tris-HCl Buffers

Reagents

DE-52 ion exchange cellulose (*Whatman*)
Stock buffer 1.0 mol/l Tris. Tris, 121.1 g; water to 1 litre. It is essential that Tris-sensitive electrodes are used
Working buffer 1. KCN, 200 mg; stock buffer, 100 ml; water to 2 litres; adjust to pH 8.5 with concentrated HCl
Working buffer 2. KCN, 200 mg; stock buffer, 100 ml; water to 2 litres; adjust to pH 8.3 with concentrated HCl

Working buffer 3. KCN, 200 mg; stock buffer, 100 ml; water to 2 litres; adjust to pH 7.0 with concentrated HCl.
Important: If the buffers are stored at 4°C, they must be allowed to come to room temperature before use.[45]

Method

1. Prepare the slurry by adding 10 g of DE-52 to 200 ml of buffer 1. Mix gently and allow the cellulose to settle. Decant the supernatant and add a further 200 ml of buffer 1, mix gently for 10 min, then adjust the pH of the thoroughly suspended cellulose to 8.5 with concentrated HCl. Allow the cellulose to settle, remove the supernatant and resuspend in a further 200 ml of buffer 1. Mix gently for 10 min and ensure the pH is 8.5. Allow to settle and remove enough buffer so that the settled cellulose constitutes about half the total volume.
2. Secure short-form pipettes vertically in a support rack. Place either a 3 mm glass bead or a small piece of cotton wool in the tapered part of the pipette to act as a support for the slurry.
3. Fill the pipettes with thoroughly suspended cellulose slurry and allow the column to pack to a height of 5–6 cm.
4. Dilute 1 drop of haemolysate (100 g/l) with 5 drops of buffer 1.
5. When the excess buffer has drained from the column, gently apply the diluted lysate to the top of the column and allow it to be adsorbed onto the resin. Do not allow the surface of the column to dry out.
6. Apply 8 ml buffer 2 gently to the column with a 10–15 cm length of polythene tubing attached to the top of the pipette acting as a reservoir. Collect the eluate in a 10 ml flask and make the volume up to 10 ml with buffer 2.
7. Elute the remaining Hb A, using 10 ml of buffer 3; collect the eluate and make the volume up to 25 ml with the remaining buffer 3.
8. Read the absorbance of the eluted haemoglobins at 415 nm in a spectrometer, using water as a blank.

Calculate the Hb A_2 as follows:

$$\%\text{Hb A}_2 = \frac{A^{415}\text{Hb A}_2 \times 100}{A^{415}\text{Hb A}_2 + (2.5 \times A^{415}\text{Hb A})}$$

Interpretation and Comments

For interpretation and normal ranges, see p. 325. The technique is inappropriate in the presence of haemoglobin variants (see below). Factors affecting quality assurance include the concentration of haemoglobin applied to the column – excess haemoglobin will cause contamination of the Hb A_2 fraction with Hb A. An inadequate amount of haemoglobin will result in an eluate with an absorbance too low for accurate measurement.

The flow rate of the column may be adjusted by altering the height of the reservoir above the column. A flow rate of 10–20 ml/h is satisfactory. Raising the reservoir increases the flow rate but broadens the Hb A_2 band on the column, which will not affect quantitation providing there is adequate separation. To elute the Hb A_2 band, 8 ml of buffer 2 should be used; the greater part of that should elute between 4 and 6 ml.

Measurement of Hb A_2 by Microcolumn Chromatography with Glycine-Potassium Cyanide Developers

The method described as follows is suitable for samples containing variants such as Hb S. The elution of Hb A_2 is dependent on the pH of the ion exchanger and on the molarity of the developer.[46]

Reagents

Developer A. Glycine, 15.0 g; KCN, 0.1 g; water to 1 litre
Developer B. NaCl, 9.0 g; water to 1 litre
DE-52 ion exchange cellulose (Whatman).

Method

1. Prepare the slurry by adding 50 g of DE-52 to 250 ml of developer. Mix gently, then allow to settle and remove the supernatant. Repeat this process at least twice, then adjust the pH of the thoroughly suspended cellulose to 7.6 with 0.1 mol/l HCl. If the slurry is made too acidic, it should be discarded because any attempt to readjust it would increase the total ionic concentration and therefore alter the elution pattern. The slurry may be stored for up to 4 weeks, but the pH should be checked and, if necessary, readjusted before use.
2. Secure short-form pipettes vertically in a support rack. Place either a 3 mm glass bead or a small piece of cotton wool in the tapered part of the pipette to act as a support for the slurry.
3. Fill the pipette with thoroughly suspended DE-52 slurry and allow the column to pack under gravity to a height of about 6 cm.
4. Check each batch of columns with a Hb AS haemolysate. The Hb A_2 should elute in the first 3–4 ml and the Hb S should elute in the next 15–20 ml of the developer.
5. Dilute 1 drop of lysate (100 g/l) with 6 drops of water.
6. When all the excess buffer has drained from the column, gently apply the diluted lysate to the top of the column and allow it to be adsorbed onto the resin. Do not allow the surface of the column to dry out.
7. Apply developer A gently to the column with a piece of polythene tubing attached to the top of the pipette acting as a reservoir. About 3–4 ml of developer should be used to elute the Hb A_2 band. Collect the

eluate in a 5 ml flask and make the volume up to 5 ml with developer A.

8. Elute the remaining Hb A or Hb S + Hb A, using 15–20 ml of developer B; collect the eluate and make the volume up to 25 ml with developer B. If, at any stage, the flow through the column stops, it should be discarded.

9. Read the absorbance of the eluted haemoglobins at 415 nm in a spectrometer, using water as a blank.

Calculate the Hb A_2 as follows:

$$\%Hb\ A_2 = \frac{A^{415}Hb\ A_2 \times 100}{A^{415}Hb\ A_2 + (5 \times A^{415}Hb\ A)}$$

Modification for the Measurement of Hb S

To estimate the percentage of Hb S and the remaining haemoglobin as well as that of Hb A_2, Hb A_2 is eluted in the first 3–4 ml with developer A, Hb S is eluted in the next 15–20 ml of the same developer A, and the remaining haemoglobin is eluted with developer B. The eluate containing Hb A_2 is diluted to 5 ml and the eluates containing Hb S and the remaining haemoglobin are diluted to 25 ml. To ensure elution of all the Hb A_2 in the first 3–4 ml and all the Hb S in the next 15–20 ml, the pH of the ion exchanger may need adjustment following a test chromatogram.[46]

Interpretation and Comments

Hb A_2 percentages tend to be very slightly lower using the Tris buffer system, but with either procedure there should be a distinction between normal and classical β thalassaemia trait subjects.[45] An advantage of the glycine-KCN method is less sensitivity to minor changes in the pH of the developer; also it may be used for samples containing Hb S.

It should be noted that measurement of Hb A_2 in the presence of Hb S is not usually a very useful test. It is not necessary in order to distinguish sickle cell trait from sickle cell/β^+ thalassaemia and is not always reliable in distinguishing sickle cell anaemia from sickle cell/β° thalassaemia because there is often interaction with α thalassaemia trait. In these circumstances, family studies can be extremely helpful.

Measurement of Hb A_2 by High-Performance Liquid Chromatography

The principle of HPLC has been explained on p. 314. When this technology is used as the primary method for detecting variant haemoglobins, simultaneous quantitation of Hb A_2 and Hb F means that it can replace three separate traditional methods: haemoglobin electrophoresis, quantitation of Hb A_2 and quantification of Hb F. Each laboratory should establish its own reference range for the quantitation of Hb A_2 by this method, which should be similar to published ranges. Because the quantitation of Hb A_2 may be inaccurate in the presence of certain variant haemoglobins, such as Hb E, Hb Lepore and Hb S,[32] each chromatogram should always be inspected. Inspection will also permit identification of specimens with a split A_2 band as the result of heterozygosity for a δ chain variant. If the quantity of a haemoglobin with the retention time of Hb A_2 is higher than expected, an alternative technique should be applied to confirm its identity because a peak labelled as Hb A_2 can be Hb E or another haemoglobin that elutes with Hb A_2.

INTERPRETATION OF Hb A_2 VALUES

Hb A_2 values should be interpreted in relation to a reference range established in each individual laboratory using blood samples from the local population with a normal Hb and red cell indices.[11,47–50] The standard operating procedure for the relevant method should be strictly followed and 95% reference ranges should be determined. Ranges may differ slightly between methods and between laboratories. For example, in one of our laboratories the range determined for microcolumn chromatography was 2.2–3.3%, whereas in the other it was 2.3–3.5%. Technical variables affecting the range may include the use of packed cells rather than whole blood. Results obtained by HPLC analysis may be 0.1–0.2% higher than the results obtained by electrophoresis with elution. Once a reference range is determined, there is still a practical problem with borderline results, given that repeat estimates may vary by 0.1–0.2%. We recommend that Hb A_2 levels of 3.4–3.7% be regarded as borderline and that the assay should be repeated both on the same sample and on a fresh sample. There is also evidence that Hb A_2 is elevated in patients with HIV infection.[51,52]

When assays are being performed for genetic counselling, it can be useful to investigate the partner whenever borderline results are obtained.

The Hb A_2 percentage should be interpreted with knowledge of the Hb and red cell indices (Table 14.7).

QUANTITATION OF Hb F

Hb F may be estimated by several methods based on its resistance to denaturation at alkaline pH, by HPLC or by an immunological method.[53] Of the alkaline denaturation methods, that of Betke et al.[54] is reliable for small amounts (<10–15%) of Hb F, whereas for levels of more than 50% and in cord blood, the method of Jonxis and Visser[55] is preferable; however, this method is not reliable at levels of less than 10%.

Table 14.7 Interpretation of Hb A$_2$ values

Hb A$_2$ RANGE (%)	INTERPRETATION
>7.0	Hb A$_2$ values of >7.0% are extremely rare Exclude a structural variant Repeat Hb A$_2$ estimation Rare β thalassaemia mutations
3.8–7.0	β thalassaemia trait, unstable haemoglobin
3.4–3.7	Severe iron deficiency in β thalassaemia trait Additional δ chain variant with β thalassaemia trait (Total A$_2$ must be measured) Interaction of α and β thalassaemia Rare β thalassaemia mutations Presence of Hb S, making accurate measurement difficult Interaction of α thalassaemia and Hb S Analytical error, including carryover; repeat analysis
2.0–3.3	Normal δβ thalassaemia (if Hb F elevated) Rare cases of β thalassaemia trait, including coexisting β and δ thalassaemia and coexisting β and α thalassaemia α thalassaemia trait α or δ chain variant (total A$_2$ must be measured)
<2.0	δβ thalassaemia (if Hb F elevated) α thalassaemia trait Hb H disease Additional δ chain variant present (total Hb A$_2$ must be measured) δ thalassaemia Iron deficiency

Immunological methods have been devised to measure Hb F by immunodiffusion,[56] for which commercial kits are available (Helena Laboratories, Beaumont, Texas, USA) and by enzyme-linked immunoassay (ELISA).[57]

Modified Betke Method for the Estimation of Hb F

Principle

To measure the percentage of Hb F in a mixture of haemoglobins,[54] sodium hydroxide is added to a lysate and, after a set time, denaturation is stopped by adding saturated ammonium sulphate. The ammonium sulphate lowers the pH and precipitates the denatured haemoglobin. After filtration, the quantity of undenatured (unprecipitated) haemoglobin is measured. The proportion of alkali-resistant (fetal) haemoglobin is then calculated as a percentage of the total amount of haemoglobin present.

Equipment

Filter paper. Whatman No. 42
Vortex mixer
Glass tubes.

Reagents

Cyanide solution. Potassium cyanide, 25 mg; potassium ferricyanide, 100 mg. Dissolve in 500 ml distilled water. Store in a dark bottle
Saturated ammonium sulphate solution. Bring 1 litre of water to the boil and add ammonium sulphate until the solution is saturated. Cool and equilibrate at 20°C before use
Sodium hydroxide solution, 1.2 mol/l. Sodium hydroxide 4.8 g; distilled water to 100 ml. Prepare monthly. Equilibrate at 20°C before use.

Method

1. Prepare a lysate as described on p. 309. The lysate may be stored at 4°C for up to 1 week before use.
2. Add 0.25 ml lysate to 4.75 ml cyanide solution to make a solution of haemiglobincyanide (HiCN).
3. Transfer 2.8 ml of the haemiglobincyanide solution to a glass test tube and allow to equilibrate at 20°C.
4. Rapidly add 0.2 ml of 1.2 mol/l of NaOH and mix on a vortex mixer for 2–3 s.
5. After exactly 2 min, rapidly add 2 ml saturated ammonium sulphate solution and mix on a vortex mixer. Leave tubes to stand for 5–10 min at 20°C.
6. Filter twice through the same Whatman No. 42 filter paper, using a clean test tube to collect the filtrate each time. If the filtrate is not completely clear, filter again through the same paper. This filtrate contains the alkali-resistant haemoglobin.
7. To measure the total haemoglobin, transfer 0.4 ml of the haemiglobincyanide solution from step 2 into another tube and add 13.9 ml of water.
8. Read the absorbance of the alkali-resistant and total haemoglobin at 420 nm against a water blank.
9. Calculate the percentage alkali-resistant haemoglobin as follows:

$$\%\text{Alkali-resistant haemoglobin} = \frac{A^{420}\text{alkali-resistant Hb}}{A^{420}\text{total Hb} \times 20} \times 100$$

Interpretation and Comments

Elevation of Hb F has a variety of causes (see p. 307). In very exceptional situations, other abnormal haemoglobins will also exhibit resistance to alkali, giving high results. It is imperative that haemoglobin electrophoresis or HPLC is done on these samples tested for Hb F to exclude the possibility of an unusual variant being present.

A normal and a raised Hb F control should be tested with every batch of samples. The raised Hb F control should ideally contain between 5% and 15% Hb F and this can be prepared from a mixture of cord and adult blood. Each laboratory must verify its own normal range, which should not differ significantly from published values; for adults the range is 0.2–1.0%.

Zago et al.[58] reported variability in the capacity of different batches of filter paper to absorb haemoglobin from the filtrate, which caused low results. It is necessary to equilibrate the temperature of the reagents to 20°C and to control the reaction temperature to 20°C to obtain accurate and reproducible results.

Method of Jonxis and Visser

Principle

The increased resistance of Hb F to denaturation by alkali is detected by recording the change in absorption at 576 nm in each minute, caused by the addition of ammonium hydroxide.[55] At this wavelength, the absorption of oxyhaemoglobin differs from that of the alkali haemochromogen that is formed on denaturation.

When the logarithm of the percentage of haemoglobin remaining undenatured is plotted against time, a straight line is obtained. By extrapolation to time zero, the percentage of Hb F in the original sample can be calculated.

Reagents

Ammonium hydroxide solution. NH_4OH, 100 g; water to 1 litre
Sodium hydroxide solution, 0.06 mol/l. Sodium hydroxide, 2.4 g; water to 1 litre.

Method

1. All reagents should be allowed to reach room temperature before use. Add 0.1 ml of blood or lysate (100 g/l) to 10 ml of water and mix.
2. Add 2 drops of ammonium hydroxide solution and mix.
3. Measure the absorbance in a spectrophotometer at 576 nm (A_B).
4. Add 0.1 ml of the same blood or lysate to 10 ml of sodium hydroxide solution; then add 2 drops of ammonium hydroxide solution and mix thoroughly.
5. Measure the absorbance in a spectrometer at 576 nm at every minute for 15 min (A_T); then incubate the solution at 37°C for 15 min, cool to room temperature and measure the absorbance (A_E). The ratio $A_B:A_E$ should be constant.

6. Calculate the percentage of undenatured haemoglobin at each minute as follows:

$$\frac{A_T^{576} - A_E^{576}}{A_B^{576} - A_E^{576}}\,(\times 100)$$

Plot the percentage on the logarithmic scale of semilogarithmic paper against time. This should produce a straight line from which the original amount of Hb F at time zero can be found by extrapolation.

Interpretation and Comments

Comments regarding controls and normal ranges given for the Betke method are also applicable to this method. In addition, the Jonxis and Visser method requires an accurate spectrometer because the maximum absorption peak at 576 nm is very narrow and the difference in extinction between oxyhaemoglobin and alkali haemochromogen is relatively small. For interpretation of results, see p. 307.

Radial Immunodiffusion

The radial immunodiffusion procedure[56] can be used for the quantitation of Hb F. The principle is based on an antibody–antigen reaction; the anti-Hb F is incorporated into the gel support medium, resulting in the formation of a visible opaque precipitin ring.

The square of the diameter of this ring is directly proportional to the concentration of Hb F. A standard curve must be prepared from samples containing known levels of Hb F plotted against their haemoglobin concentrations. Helena Laboratories market a kit containing prepared plates, a microdispenser and a measuring device.

The method is simple, but the formation of the precipitin rings requires at least 18 h of incubation at room temperature. For this reason, rapid diagnostic work is not possible. Care must be taken with sample application because damage to the plate wells results in asymmetric precipitin rings and erroneous measurements.

ASSESSMENT OF THE INTRACELLULAR DISTRIBUTION OF Hb F

Differences in the intracellular distribution of Hb F are used to differentiate between heterozygotes for $\delta\beta$ thalassaemia and the classical African type of HPFH. In the former, it can be shown that not all red cells contain Hb F (heterocellular distribution), whereas in the latter every cell contains Hb F (pancellular distribution), although there is some variability in content from cell to cell. It has been suggested that a heterocellular distribution may be more apparent than real and merely reflects that high levels of Hb F tend to give a more pancellular distribution than lower levels. For this reason, results should be treated with caution and not used to make a diagnosis in isolation.

Two techniques have been widely used for demonstrating intracellular Hb F distribution. The most frequently used is the acid elution test of Kleihauer[59] that was originally developed for the detection of fetal red cells in the maternal circulation following transplacental haemorrhage. This method is described on p. 338. Less frequently used is the more sensitive immunofluorescent technique described in the following.

Immunofluorescent Method

Principle

Anti-Hb F antibody binds specifically and quantitatively to Hb F in fixed red cells. These cells can be identified after treatment with a second fluorescent-labelled antibody directed against the anti-Hb F.[14]

Equipment

Glass slides
Coplin jars
Microscope. Equipped with accessories for ultraviolet (UV) fluorescence
Moist chamber. Made from a Petri dish with moistened filter paper in the bottom.

Reagents

Phosphate buffered saline (PBS), pH 7.1. see p. 622
Rabbit antihuman Hb F serum. Dilute the antiserum 1 in 64 in PBS; store in small aliquots at $-20°C$. Stable for several months
Sheep (or goat) antirabbit immunoglobulin labelled with fluorescein isothiocyanate. Dilute 1 in 32 in PBS; store in small aliquots at $-20°C$. Stable for several months
Fixative. Acetone, 90 ml; methanol, 10 ml.

Method

1. Prepare thin blood films and allow to dry overnight.
2. Fix for 5 min at room temperature, shake off excess fixative and rinse immediately in PBS. If the films are too thick, they will peel off at this stage.
3. Rinse the slides in water and allow to dry.
4. Layer 5 μl of the anti-Hb F antisera onto the slide.
5. Incubate in the moist chamber at $37°C$ for 30 min or at room temperature for 60 min.
6. Rinse the slides thoroughly in PBS to remove any unbound antiserum.
7. Rinse the slides in water and allow to dry.
8. Layer 5 μl of the antirabbit antisera onto the slide.
9. Incubate in the moist chamber at $37°C$ for 30 min or at room temperature for 60 min.
10. Rinse the slides thoroughly in PBS to remove any unbound antiserum.
11. Rinse the slides in water and allow to dry.
12. Examine microscopically using a $×40$ objective and filters suitable for use with fluorescein isothiocyanate. To quantitate the number of Hb F-containing cells, count the total number of cells in a field under white light using an eyepiece grid, then the number of stained cells under the UV light. If the level of Hb F is less than 10%, at least 2000 cells should be counted.

Comments

In normal adults, from 0.1 to 7.0% of cells show detectable fluorescence. The proportion of positive cells correlates well with the percentage of Hb F as measured by alkali denaturation at levels between 0.5% and 5.0%. As little as 1 pg of Hb F per cell can be detected, giving much greater sensitivity than the acid elution method. This increased sensitivity, however, may make a heterocellular distribution appear pancellular if the proportion of Hb F is greater than 10%.[53]

Interpretation of Hb F values

See Table 14.8.[11,14]

ASSESSMENT OF IRON STATUS IN THALASSAEMIA

Concurrent iron deficiency makes the diagnosis of thalassaemia trait more difficult because it masks the typical blood picture and can reduce Hb A_2 synthesis.[47,48,50] In β thalassaemia trait, dependent on the severity of the anaemia, the Hb A_2 value may be reduced to borderline or even to normal levels (3.0–3.5%). However, in many patients with β thalassaemia trait and iron deficiency, the Hb A_2 will still be raised.

Whenever possible, individuals should not be investigated for the presence of thalassaemia trait if they are iron deficient. Iron stores are usually replete after 3–4 months of treatment with iron. However, if a pregnant woman is suspected of having a thalassaemia trait, it is not possible to wait for the correction of iron deficiency to establish the diagnosis. The woman and her partner should be tested without delay, with DNA analysis of globin genes being carried out if both are suspected of having thalassaemia trait (see Chapter 8, p. 146).

In addition to traditional methods for iron assessment, such as measurement of serum ferritin or serum iron plus total iron-binding capacity, estimation of zinc protoporphyrin (see pp. 192) is of potential value. This test can be carried out on an EDTA sample within a haematology

Table 14.8 Interpretation of Hb F values

Hb F RANGE (%)	INTERPRETATION
0.2–1.0	Normal results
1.0–5.0	In approximately 30% of β thalassaemia traits Some heterozygotes for a variant haemoglobin Some homozygotes for a variant haemoglobin Some compound heterozygotes for a variant haemoglobin and β thalassaemia Some individuals with haematological disorders (aplastic anaemia, myelodysplastic syndromes, juvenile myelomonocytic leukaemia) Some pregnant women (2nd trimester) Sporadically in the general population, particularly in Afro-Caribbeans (representing heterozygosity for non-deletional HPFH)
5.0–20.0	Occasional cases of β thalassaemia trait Some homozygotes for a variant haemoglobin including some sickle cell anaemia[a] Some compound heterozygotes for a variant haemoglobin and β thalassaemia Some types of heterozygous HPFH δβ thalassaemia
15.0–45.0	Heterozygous HPFH African type (usually >20%) Some cases of β thalassaemia intermedia
>45.0	β thalassaemia major Some cases of β thalassaemia intermedia Neonates
>95.0	Homozygous African-type (deletional) HPFH Some neonates (particularly if premature)

[a]Highest levels seen with Arab-Indian haplotype and in patients treated with hydroxycarbamide.

laboratory and is a measure of iron incorporation at the cellular level.

RED CELL INCLUSIONS

The most important red cell inclusions found in the haemoglobinopathies are Hb H inclusion bodies (precipitated β chain tetramers) found in α thalassaemia,[60] α chain inclusions found in β thalassaemia major[7,61] and Heinz bodies found in unstable haemoglobin diseases.[41,62]

Precipitated α chains are found in the cytoplasm of nucleated red cell precursors of patients with β thalassaemia major; they can be demonstrated by supravital staining of the bone marrow with methyl violet (as can Heinz bodies) and appear as irregularly shaped bodies close to the nucleus of normoblasts. After splenectomy they may also be found in the peripheral blood normoblasts and reticulocytes. Heinz bodies (insoluble denatured globin chains) form as a result of exposure to oxidant drugs or chemicals and develop spontaneously in glucose-6-phosphate dehydrogenase (G6PD) deficiency and in the unstable haemoglobin diseases. In unstable haemoglobin diseases, they are usually only seen in the peripheral blood after splenectomy but may be demonstrated in patients with an intact spleen if their blood is kept at 37°C for 24–48 h. The use of methyl violet and of brilliant cresyl blue in the demonstration of precipitated α chain and Heinz bodies is described on p. 336.

Demonstration of Hb H Inclusion Bodies

Reagent

Staining solution. 1.0% brilliant cresyl blue or New methylene blue. New batches of stain must be tested with a known positive control because the redox action of the dyes may vary from batch to batch.

Method

1. Mix 2 volumes of fresh blood (within 24 h of collection) with 1 volume of staining solution.
2. Incubate at 37°C for 2 h or at room temperature for 4 h.
3. Resuspend the cells and spread a thin blood film.
4. Examine the film as for a reticulocyte count. The inclusion bodies appear as multiple greenish-blue dots, like the pitted pattern on a golf ball (see p. 337). They can be readily distinguished from reticulocytes, which exhibit uneven reticular material or infrequent fine dots.

Interpretation and Comments

In α[+] thalassaemia trait, only a very occasional H body (1:1000 to 1:10 000) is usually seen; they are more numerous in α° thalassaemia, but the number of cells developing inclusions is not reliable in differentiating the various gene deletion patterns seen in α thalassaemia and the absence of demonstrable inclusions does not preclude a diagnosis of α thalassaemia trait. This test is most useful in Hb H disease, where inclusions are usually found in more than 30% of red cells.

FETAL DIAGNOSIS OF GLOBIN GENE DISORDERS

Prenatal diagnosis of globin gene disorders[21] is carried out if the fetus is at risk of thalassaemia major or a severe form of sickle cell disease such as sickle cell anaemia. Two approaches to fetal diagnosis are available: globin chain synthesis (used if the putative father is not available) and DNA analysis. DNA can be obtained from a chorionic villus sample or from amniotic fluid. Methods used for DNA analysis are described in Chapter 8.

When a potentially at-risk couple is detected, they will require counselling, and if a fetal diagnosis is requested, it is necessary to confirm the parental haemoglobin phenotype. The family or parental blood samples are sent to the diagnostic centre and the timing of fetal sampling is arranged.

Sample Requirements

Blood samples for globin chain synthesis have to be fresh (received within a few hours of collection) and transported at 4°C. Blood samples for DNA analysis can be sent by overnight delivery without refrigeration but must be processed, at the latest, within 3 days of collection. From each parent,

10 ml of blood in EDTA or heparin is required. If restriction fragment length polymorphism (RFLP) linkage analysis is required, the following additional samples are needed: blood from either a homozygous normal or affected child, or from a heterozygous child and one set of grandparents, or, if no child is available, blood from both sets of grandparents. The samples must be carefully and clearly labelled and the family tree must be drawn. Particulars of all haematological tests must be given.

Chorionic villus samples must be dissected free of any maternal tissue and sent by urgent overnight delivery in tissue culture medium or, preferably, in a special buffer obtainable from the DNA diagnostic laboratory. Amniotic fluid samples (15–20 ml are needed) and must be received within 24 h of collection. If a longer transit time is unavoidable, the amniocytes should be resuspended in tissue culture medium.

The laboratory performing DNA analysis for disorders of globin chain synthesis must be given accurate information on the precise ethnic origin of family members so that optimal use is made of the DNA available for diagnosis.

It is essential that follow-up data are obtained on all cases that have undergone fetal diagnosis. This should include tests on cord blood or heel prick sample at birth and a test at 6 months to confirm the carrier state. Whenever possible, DNA analysis of the child's globin genes should be carried out.

REFERENCES

1. Hardison R, Miller W. (Updated) *Globin gene server.* Available at:www.globin.cse.psu.edu.

2. Serjeant GR, Serjeant BE. *Sickle Cell Disease.* 3rd ed. Oxford: Oxford University Press; 2001.

3. Dacie JV. *The Haemolytic Anaemias, Vol. 2: The Hereditary Haemolytic Anaemias.* 3rd ed. Edinburgh: Churchill Livingstone; 1988: 322.

4. White JM. The unstable haemoglobin disorders. *Clin Haematol.* 1974;3:333–356.

5. Stephens AD. Annotation: Polycythaemia and high affinity haemoglobins. *Br J Haematol.* 1977;36:153–159.

6. Kiese M. *Methemoglobinemia: A Complete Treatise.* Cleveland, OH: CRC Press; 1974.

7. Weatherall DJ, Clegg JB. *The Thalassaemia Syndromes.* 4th ed. Oxford: Blackwell Science; 2001.

8. Flint J, Harding RM, Boyce AJ, et al. The population genetics of

haemoglobinopathies. *Baillières Clin Haematol.* 1998;11:1–51.

9. Thein SL. β-thalassaemia. *Baillières Clin Haematol.* 1998;11:91–126.

10. Thein SL. β thalassaemia. In: Green AR, ed. *Educational Book.* Birmingham: Fifth Congress of the European Haematology Association; 2000:132–137.

11. British Committee for Standards in Haematology. Guidelines for the investigation of the α and β thalassaemia traits. *J Clin Pathol.* 1994;47:289–295.

12. Higgs DR. β-Thalassaemia. *Baillières Clin Haematol.* 1993;6:117–150.

13. Wood WG. Increased HbF in adult life. *Baillières Clin Haematol.* 1993;6:177–213.

14. Wood WG, Stamatoyannopoulos G, Lim G, et al. F cells in the adult: normal values and levels in individuals with hereditary and acquired elevations of Hb F. *Blood.* 1975;46:671–682.

15. Wild BJ, Green BN, Cooper EK, et al. Rapid identification of hemoglobin

variants by electrospray ionization mass spectrometry. *Blood Cells Mol Dis.* 2001;27:691–704.

16. Wild BJ, Bain BJ. Detection and quantitation of normal haemoglobins: an analytical review. *Ann Clin Biochem.* 2004;41:1–15.

17. Lafferty JD, Crowther MA, Ali MA, et al. The evaluation of various mathematical RBC indices and their efficacy in discriminating between thalassemic and non-thalassemic microcytosis. *Am J Clin Pathol.* 1996;106:201–205.

18. Eldibany MM, Totonchi KF, Joseph NJ, et al. Usefulness of certain red blood cell indices in diagnosing and differentiating thalassemia trait from iron deficiency anemia. *Am J Clin Pathol.* 1999;111:676–682.

19. Stephens AD, Wild BJ. Quality control in haemoglobinopathy investigations. *Methods in Hematology.* 1990;22:72–85.

20. British Committee for Standards in Haematology Working Party of the

General Haematology Task Force. The laboratory diagnosis of haemoglobinopathies. *Br J Haematol.* 1998;101:783–792.

21. British Committee for Standards in Haematology. Guidelines for haemoglobinopathy screening. *Clin Lab Haematol.* 1988;10:87–94.

22. British Committee for Standards in Haematology. Guidelines for fetal diagnosis of globin gene disorders. *J Clin Pathol.* 1994;47:199–204.

23. International Committee for Standardization in Haematology. Recommendations for neonatal screening for haemoglobinopathies. *Clin Lab Haematol.* 1988;10:335–345.

24. International Committee for Standardization in Haematology. Simple electrophoretic system for presumptive identification of abnormal hemoglobins. *Blood.* 1978;52:1058–1064.

25. International Committee for Standardization in Haematology. Recommendations for a system for identifying abnormal hemoglobins. *Blood.* 1978;52:1065–1067.

26. Schneider RG. Identification of hemoglobin by electrophoresis. In: Schmidt RM, Huisman THJ, Lehmann H, eds. *The Detection of Hemoglobinopathies.* Cleveland, OH: CRC Press; 1974:11.

27. Marder VJ, Conley CL. Electrophoresis of hemoglobin on agar gel. Frequency of hemoglobin D in a Negro population. *Bulletin of the Johns Hopkins Hospital.* 1959;105:77–88.

28. Schroeder WA, Shelton JB, Shelton JR. Separation of hemoglobin peptides by high performance liquid chromatography (HPLC). *Hemoglobin.* 1980;4:551–559.

29. Wild BJ, Stephens AD. The use of automated HPLC to detect and quantitate haemoglobins. *Clin Lab Haematol.* 1997;19:171–176.

30. Phelan L, Bain BJ, Roper D, et al. An analysis of relative costs and potential benefits of different policies for antenatal screening for β thalassaemia trait and variant haemoglobins. *J Clin Pathol.* 1999;52:697–700.

31. Bain BJ, Wild BJ, Stephens AD, et al. *Variant Haemoglobins: a Guide to Identification.* Oxford: Blackwell Publishing; 2010.

32. Riou J, Godart CM, Hurtrel D, et al. Cation-exchange HPLC evaluated for presumptive identification of hemoglobin variants. *Clin Chem.* 1997;43:34–39.

33. Head CE, Conroy M, Jarvis M, et al. Some observations on the measurement of haemoglobin A_2 and S percentages by high performance liquid chromatography in the presence and absence of thalassaemia. *J Clin Pathol.* 2004;57:276–280.

34. Millar CM, Phelan L, Bain BJ. Diabetes mellitus diagnosed following request for haemoglobin electrophoresis. *Lancet.* 2002;117:778.

35. Righetti PG, Gianazza E, Bianchi-Bosisio A, et al. The hemoglobinopathies: conventional isoelectric focusing and immobilized pH gradients for hemoglobin separation and identification. *Methods in Hematology.* 1986;15:47–71.

36. Basset P, Beuzard Y, Garel MC, et al. Isoelectric focusing of human hemoglobins: its application to screening to characterization of 70 variants and to study of modified fractions of normal hemoglobins. *Blood.* 1978;51:971–982.

37. Evatt BL, Gibbs WN, Lewis SM, et al. *Fundamental Diagnostic Hematology: Anemia.* 2nd ed. Geneva: U.S. Department of Health and Human Services, Atlanta and World Health Organization; 1992.

38. *NHS Sickle cell and thalassaemia screening programme.* Available at: www.kcl-phs.org.uk/haemscreening.

39. Carrell RW. The hemoglobinopathies: methods of determining hemoglobin instability (unstable hemoglobins). *Methods in Haematology.* 1986;15:109–124.

40. Grimes AJ, Meisler A. Possible cause of Heinz bodies in congenital Heinz body anaemia. *Nature.* 1962;194:190–191.

41. Grimes AJ, Meisler A, Dacie JV. Congenital Heinz-body anaemia: further evidence on the cause of Heinz-body production in red cells. *Br J Haematol.* 1964;10:281–290.

42. Carrell RW, Kay R. A simple method for the detection of unstable haemoglobins. *Br J Haematol.* 1972;23:615–619.

43. Marengo-Rowe AJ. Rapid electrophoresis and quantitation of hemoglobins on cellulose acetate. *J Clin Pathol.* 1965;18:790–792.

44. International Committee for Standardization in Haematology. Recommendations for selected methods for quantitative estimation of Hb A2 and for Hb A2 reference preparation. *Br J Haematol.* 1978;38:573–578.

45. Efremov GD, Huisman THJ, Bowman K, et al. Microchromatography of hemoglobins: II A rapid method for the determination of Hb A2. *J Lab Clin Med.* 1974;83:657–664.

46. Huisman THJ, Schroeder WA, Brodie AR, et al. Microchromatography of hemoglobins III. A simplified procedure for the determination of hemoglobin A2. *J Lab Clin Med.* 1975;86:700–702.

47. Kattamis C, Lagos P, Metaxotou-Mavromati A, et al. Serum iron and unsaturated iron-binding capacity in the β-thalassaemia trait: their relation to the levels of haemoglobins A, A2 and F. *J Med Genet.* 1972;9:154–159.

48. Alperin JB, Dow PA, Peteway MB. Hemoglobin A2 levels in health and various hematological disorders. *Am J Clin Pathol.* 1977;67:219–226.

49. Efremov GD. The hemoglobinopathies: quantitation of hemoglobins by microchromatography. *Methods in Hematology.* 1986;15:72–90.

50. Wasi P, Na-Nakorn S, Pootrakul S, et al. Alpha- and beta-thalassemia in Thailand. *Ann N Y Acad Sci.* 1969;165:60–82.

51. Routy J, Monte M, Beaulieu R, et al. Increase of haemoglobin A2 in human immuno-deficiency virus-1-infected patients treated with zidovudine. *Am J Hematol.* 1993;43:86–90.

52. Howard J, Henthorn JS, Murphy S, et al. Implications of increased haemoglobin A2 values in HIV positive women in the antenatal

331

clinic. *J Clin Pathol*. 2005;58: 556–558.

53. Felice AE. The hemoglobinopathies: quantitation of fetal hemoglobin. *Methods in Hematology*. 1986;15: 91–108.

54. Betke K, Marti HR, Schlicht L. Estimation of small percentage of foetal haemoglobin. *Nature*. 1959;184:1877–1878.

55. Jonxis JHP, Visser HKA. Determination of low percentages of fetal hemoglobin in blood of normal children. *Am J Dis Child*. 1956;92: 588–591.

56. Chudwin DS, Rucknagel DL. Immunological quantification of hemoglobins F and A2. *Clin Chim Acta*. 1974;50:413–418.

57. Makler MT, Pesce AJ. ELISA assay for measurement of hemoglobin A and hemoglobin F. *Am J Clin Pathol*. 1980;74:673–676.

58. Zago MA, Wood WG, Clegg JB, et al. Genetic control of F-cells in human adults. *Blood*. 1979;53: 977–986.

59. Kleihauer E. Determination of fetal hemoglobin: elution technique. In: Schmidt RM, Huisman THJ, Lehmann H, eds. *The Detection of Hemoglobinopathies*. Cleveland, OH: CRC Press; 1974:20.

60. Weatherall DJ. The thalassemias: haematologic methods. *Methods in Haematology*. 1983;6:27–30.

61. Fessas P. Inclusions of hemoglobin in erythroblasts and erythrocytes of thalassemia. *Blood*. 1963;21: 21–32.

62. White JM, Dacie JV. The unstable hemoglobins – molecular and clinical features. *Prog Hematol*. 1971;7:69–102.

Chapter | **15** |

Erythrocyte and leucocyte cytochemistry

Barbara J. Bain, David Swirsky

ERYTHROCYTE CYTOCHEMISTRY

Siderocytes and Sideroblasts

Siderocytes are red cells containing granules of non-haem iron. They were originally described by Grüneberg[1] in small numbers in the blood of normal rat, mouse and human embryos and in large numbers in mice with a congenital anaemia. The granules are formed of a water-insoluble complex of ferric iron, lipid, protein and carbohydrate. This siderotic material (or haemosiderin) reacts with potassium ferrocyanide to form a blue compound, ferriferrocyanide; this reaction is the basis of a positive Prussian-blue (Perls') reaction. The material also stains with Romanowsky dyes and then appears as basophilic granules, which have been referred to as 'Pappenheimer bodies' (Fig. 15.1).[2] By contrast, ferritin, which is a water-soluble non-haem compound of iron with the protein apoferritin, is not detectable by Perls' reaction. Ferritin is normally present in all cells in the body, whereas, in health, haemosiderin is mainly found in macrophages in the bone marrow, liver (Kupffer cells) and spleen. When the body is overloaded with iron, as in haemochromatosis or transfusional haemosiderosis, excess iron is also found in other tissues.

Iron is transported in plasma attached to a β globulin, transferrin, and is taken up selectively by the bone marrow, where the iron–transferrin complex binds to transferrin receptors on the surface of the erythroblast; the iron is released from transferrin and enters the cell. Most of the iron is rapidly converted to haem, synthesis being partly in the cytosol and partly in the mitochondria. The non-haem residue is in the form of ferritin. Degradation of the ferritin turns some of it into haemosiderin, which can be visualized under the light microscope as golden-yellow refractile particles in phagocytic cells. When stained by Perls' reaction, haemosiderin is blue.

In health, siderotic granules can normally be seen, in preparations stained by Perls' reaction, in the cytoplasm of many of the erythroblasts of human bone marrow and in marrow reticulocytes.[3] However, they are not normally seen in human peripheral blood red cells. After splenectomy, siderocytes can always be found in the peripheral blood, often in large numbers. The reason for this is probably because reticulocytes, after delivery from the marrow, are normally sequestered for a time in the spleen and there they complete haem synthesis, utilizing, for this purpose, the iron stored in their cytoplasm within the siderotic granules. After splenectomy, this stage of reticulocyte maturation has to take place in the

Figure 15.1 Siderotic granules and Pappenheimer bodies. Photomicrographs of erythrocytes in a peripheral blood film from a splenectomized patient with a myelodysplastic syndrome (refractory anaemia with ring sideroblasts) showing Pappenheimer bodies: May–Grünwald–Giemsa (A); and siderotic granules: Perls' reaction (B).

bloodstream, with the result that, even in an otherwise healthy person, a small percentage of siderocytes can then be found in the peripheral blood. The spleen is also probably able to remove large siderotic granules – as may be found in disease – from red cells by a process of pitting,[4] and in its absence such granules persist in the red cells throughout their lifespan.

Method of Staining Siderotic Granules

Air dry films of peripheral blood or bone marrow and fix with methanol for 10–20 min. When they are dry, place the slides in a solution of 10 g/l potassium ferrocyanide in 0.1 mol/l HCl made by mixing equal volumes of 47 mmol/l (20 g/l) potassium ferrocyanide and 0.2 mol/l HCl immediately before use.

Leave the slides in the solution for about 10 min at about 20°C. Wash well in running tap water for 20 min, rinse thoroughly in distilled water and then counterstain with 1 g/l aqueous neutral red or eosin for 10–15 s. Care must be taken to avoid contamination by iron that may have been present on the slides or in staining dishes.

Prepare the glassware by soaking in 3 mol/l HCl before washing (see p. 623). For quality control, a positive bone marrow film should always be stained together with the test films.

Prussian-blue staining can be applied to films that have previously been stained by Romanowsky dyes, even after years of storage. It is advisable to let the films stand in methanol overnight to remove most of the Romanowsky stain. The film should be checked before carrying out Perls' reaction to ensure that there is no residual blue staining that could obscure Prussian-blue staining. Sundberg and Bromann described a technique whereby films were stained first by a Romanowsky dye (Wright's stain) and then overstained by the acid-ferrocyanide method.[5] This can give beautiful pictures, but the small blue-stained iron-containing granules tend to be masked in young erythroblasts by the general basophilia of the cell cytoplasm. Hayhoe and Quaglino described a method for combined periodic acid–Schiff (PAS) and iron staining.[6] This may be helpful in the investigation of abnormal erythropoiesis in which the erythroblasts give a positive PAS reaction (see p. 343). A rapid method has been described for demonstrating siderotic granules by staining with 1% bromochlorphenol blue for 1 min.[7] Iron-containing granules stain dark purple.

Significance of siderocytes

Siderocytes contain one or two (rarely many) small, unevenly distributed iron-containing granules that stain a Prussian-blue colour. There are normally a few very small scattered siderotic granules in about 40% of late erythroblasts.[3] They stain faintly and may be difficult to see by light microscopy. The percentage of erythroblasts recognizable as sideroblasts is increased in haemolytic anaemias and megaloblastic anaemias and in haemochromatosis and haemosiderosis, in proportion to the degree of saturation of transferrin (i.e. to the amount of iron available). A disproportionate increase in the percentage of erythroblasts that are sideroblasts occurs when the synthesis of haemoglobin is impaired, in which case the siderotic granules are both more numerous and larger than normal (Fig. 15.2). When there is a defect in haem synthesis, the granules are deposited in mitochondria and frequently appear to be arranged in a collar around the nucleus (Fig. 15.3) giving the 'ring sideroblasts' characteristic of sideroblastic anaemias. In contrast, the distribution of the granules within the cell tends to be mainly normal in conditions in which globin synthesis alone is affected (e.g. in thalassaemia) or when there is iron overload.

There are several types of sideroblastic anaemia. These include the congenital (hereditary) type, pyridoxine (vitamin B_6) deficiency (rarely), sideroblastic anaemia caused by B_6 antagonists (e.g. drugs used in antituberculosis therapy) and secondary sideroblastic anaemia in alcoholism and lead poisoning. The presence of ring sideroblasts is a defining feature of refractory anaemia with ring sideroblasts[8] and refractory cytopenia with multilineage dysplasia and ring sideroblasts, two of the World Health Organization (WHO) categories of myelodysplastic

Figure 15.3 Pathological sideroblasts. Sideroblastic anaemias. Accumulation of iron-containing granules in normoblasts, arranged characteristically around the nucleus. (A) Hereditary type; (B) myelodysplastic syndrome. Perls' reaction.

syndrome (MDS). They may also occur in other categories of MDS. Ring sideroblasts are not uncommon in other haematological neoplasms, including primary myelofibrosis and acute myeloid leukaemia (AML), particularly erythroleukaemia and the WHO categories of therapy-related AML and AML with multilineage myelodysplasia. Ring sideroblasts have been defined as erythroblasts with at least five siderotic granules surrounding at least one-third of the nucleus.[9,10]

In sideroblastic anaemia as a feature of a haematological neoplasm, erythroblasts at all stages of maturity may be loaded with siderotic granules, whereas in the secondary sideroblastic anaemias and in the hereditary types, the more mature cells seem most affected.

In addition to the siderotic granules within erythroblasts, haemosiderin can normally be seen in marrow films as accumulations of small granules, lying free or in macrophages in marrow fragments.[11] The amount of haemosiderin will be markedly increased in patients with increased iron stores, whereas haemosiderin is absent in iron deficiency anaemia (Fig. 15.4). In practice, staining to demonstrate iron stores in marrow fragments and siderotic granules in erythroblasts is a simple and valuable diagnostic procedure and should be applied as a routine to marrow films from the initial bone marrow aspirate of each patient.

Figure 15.2 Pathological sideroblasts. Thalassaemia. There is massive accumulation of iron-containing granules in normoblasts and phagocytic cells. Perls' reaction.

Figure 15.4 Prussian-blue staining (Perls' reaction) on aspirated bone marrow particles to demonstrate iron stores. (A) Normal, (B) absent, (C) increased and (D) grossly increased.

In chronic infections and in other examples of anaemia of chronic disease, the iron stores may be increased, with much siderotic material in macrophages but little or none visible in erythroblasts. Markedly excessive iron in macrophages is also a feature of thalassaemia intermedia and major and some dyserythropoietic anaemias. Conversely, absence of iron is diagnostic of iron deficiency or iron depletion (the latter term indicating the state in which storage iron is absent but anaemia is not yet evident). One study has shown that to establish the absence of stainable iron, at least seven particles must be examined, if necessary using more than one slide for this purpose.[12] There is no cytochemical method of demonstrating ferritin; methods of assay are described in Chapter 9.

Haemoglobin Derivatives

Heinz Bodies in Red Cells

Heinz, in 1890, was the first to describe in detail inclusions in red cells developing as the result of the action of acetyl-phenylhydrazine on the blood.[13] It is now known that Heinz bodies can be produced by the action on red cells of a wide range of aromatic nitro- and amino-compounds, as well as by inorganic oxidizing agents such as potassium

chlorate. They also occur when one or other of the globin chains of haemoglobin is unstable. In man, the finding of Heinz bodies is a sign of either chemical poisoning, drug toxicity, glucose-6-phosphate dehydrogenase (G6PD) deficiency or the presence of an unstable haemoglobin (e.g. Hb Köln). When of chemical or drug origin, Heinz bodies are likely to be visible in red cells only if the patient has been splenectomized previously or when large doses of the chemical or drug have been taken. When they are due to an unstable haemoglobin, they are rarely visible in freshly withdrawn red cells except after splenectomy. They may nevertheless develop *in vitro* in the blood of patients who have not been splenectomized if the specimen is incubated for 24–48 h.[14] Heinz bodies are a late sign of oxidative damage and represent an end-product of the degradation of haemoglobin. Reviews dealing with Heinz bodies include those by Jacob[15] and by White.[16]

Demonstration of Heinz Bodies

Unstained preparations

Heinz bodies may be seen as refractile objects in dry, unstained films, if the illumination is reduced by lowering the microscope condenser. They also can be seen by dark-ground illumination or phase-contrast microscopy. However, it is preferable to look for them in stained preparations (see below). In size they vary from 1 to 3 μm. One or more may be present in a single cell. They are usually close to the cell membrane and may cause a protrusion of the membrane; in wet preparations, they may move around within the cells in a slow Brownian movement.

The degradation product of an unstable haemoglobin (e.g. Hb Köln) exhibits green fluorescence when excited by blue light at 370 nm in a fluorescence microscope.[17]

Stained preparations

Dissolve approximately 0.5 g of methyl violet in 100 ml of 9 g/l NaCl and filter. Add 1 volume of blood (in any anticoagulant) to 4 volumes of the methyl violet solution and allow the suspension to stand for about 10 min at room temperature. Then prepare films and allow them to dry or view the suspension of cells between slide and coverglass. The Heinz bodies stain an intense purple (Fig. 15.5).

Heinz bodies also stain with other basic dyes. Brilliant green stains them well and none of the stain is taken up by the remainder of the red cell.[18] Rhodanile blue (5 g/l solution in 10 g/l NaCl) stains them rapidly[19] (i.e. within 2 min), at which time reticulocytes are only weakly stained. Compared with methyl violet, Heinz bodies stain less intensely with brilliant cresyl blue or New methylene blue. Nevertheless, they may be readily seen as pale blue bodies in a well-stained reticulocyte preparation, if the preparation is not counterstained.

If permanent preparations are required, fix the vitally stained films by exposure to formalin vapour for 5–10 min. Then counterstain the fixed films with 1 g/l eosin or neutral red, after thoroughly washing in water. If films are fixed in methanol, Heinz bodies are decolourized.

In β thalassaemia major, methyl violet staining of the bone marrow will demonstrate precipitated α chains. These appear as large irregular inclusions in late normoblasts, usually single and closely adhering to the nucleus. If such patients are splenectomized, inclusions are also found in reticulocytes and mature red blood cells, in the circulation as well as in the bone marrow.

Demonstration of Haemoglobin H Inclusions

Patients with α thalassaemia, who form haemoglobin H (β_4), have red cells in which multiple blue-green spherical inclusions develop on exposure to brilliant cresyl blue or New methylene blue as in reticulocyte preparations[20] (Fig. 15.6). This is mainly a feature of haemoglobin H disease, but small numbers of similar cells may be seen in α thalassaemia trait, particularly, but not only, in α° thalassaemia heterozygosity.

Method

Mix together in a small tube, as for staining reticulocytes (see p. 33), equal volumes of fresh blood or blood collected into ethylenediaminetetra-acetic acid (EDTA) and 10 g/l brilliant cresyl blue or 20 g/l New methylene blue in iso-osmotic phosphate buffer pH 7.4. Leave the preparation at 37°C for 3 h and make films at intervals during this time. Allow the films to dry and examine them without counter-staining. Haemoglobin H precipitates as multiple pale-staining greenish-blue, almost spherical, bodies

Figure 15.5 Glucose-6-phosphate dehydrogenase deficiency. Many of the cells contain large Heinz bodies. Stained supravitally by methyl violet.
(Courtesy of Mr David Roper.)

Figure 15.6 Denaturation of haemoglobin H by brilliant cresyl blue. The round bodies consist of precipitated Hb H.

Figure 15.7 Haemoglobin H disease. Almost every erythrocyte is affected.

Figure 15.8 Film of blood from patient with hereditary spherocytosis. There is an increased number of reticulocytes. Stained supravitally by brilliant cresyl blue.

of varying size (Fig. 15.7), which can be clearly differentiated from the darker-staining reticulofilamentous material of reticulocytes (Fig. 15.8).

The number of cells containing inclusions varies according to the type of α thalassaemia. In α° thalassaemia heterozygosity only 0.01–1.0% of the red cells contain inclusions, but this finding can provide a significant clue to diagnosis. In haemoglobin H disease (e.g. resulting from α° thalassaemia/α$^+$ thalassaemia compound heterozygosity, − −/−α), as a rule at least 10% of the cells develop inclusions and, in some cases, the percentage is considerably greater. Haemoglobin H inclusions are also detectable in patients with acquired haemoglobin H disease as a feature of a myelodysplastic syndrome.

It should be noted that a haemoglobin H preparation is not recommended when precise diagnosis of the type of α thalassaemia trait is required (e.g. in antenatal diagnosis). DNA analysis is then indicated (see p. 147).

Carboxyhaemoglobin and Methaemoglobin

Carboxyhaemoglobin- and methaemoglobin-containing cells can be demonstrated cytochemically. These methods are described by Kleihauer and Betke.[21] They have little practical value in modern practice.

Fetal Haemoglobin

An acid-elution cytochemical method that was introduced by Kleihauer et al.[22] is a sensitive procedure to identify individual cells containing haemoglobin F even when few are present. Their detection in the maternal circulation has provided valuable information on the pathogenesis of haemolytic disease of the newborn.

The identification of cells containing haemoglobin F depends on the fact that they resist acid elution to a greater extent than do normal cells; thus, in the technique described in the following, they appear as isolated, darkly stained cells among a background of palely staining ghost cells. The occasional cells that stain to an intermediate degree are less easy to evaluate; some may be reticulocytes because these also resist acid elution to some extent. The following method, in which elution is carried out at pH 1.5, is recommended.[23]

Reagents

Fixative. 80% ethanol
Elution solution. Solution A: 7.5 g/l haematoxylin in 90% ethanol. Solution B: $FeCl_3$, 24 g; 2.5 mol/l HCl, 20 ml; doubly distilled water to 1 litre.

For use, mix well 5 volumes of A and 1 volume of B. The pH is approximately 1.5. The solution can be used for about 4 weeks; if a precipitate forms, the solution should be filtered.

Counterstain. 1 g/l aqueous erythrosin or 2.5 g/l aqueous eosin.

Method

Prepare fresh air-dried films. Immediately after drying, fix the films for 5 min in 80% ethanol in a Coplin jar. Then rinse the slides rapidly in water and stand them vertically on blotting paper for about 10 min to dry. Next, place the slides for 20 s in a Coplin jar containing the elution solution. Then wash the slides thoroughly in water and finally place them in the counterstain for 2 min. Rinse in tap water and allow them to dry in the air. Fetal cells stain red and adult ghost cells stain pale pink (Fig. 15.9). Films prepared (a) from a mixture of cord blood and adult blood and (b) from normal adult blood should be stained

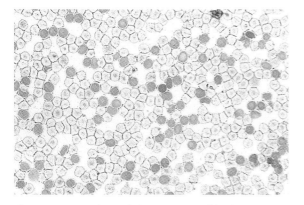

Figure 15.9 Cytochemical demonstration of fetal haemoglobin. Acid elution method. The preparation consists of a mixture of cord and normal adult blood. The darkly staining cells are fetal cells.

alongside the test films as positive and negative controls, respectively.

A number of modifications of the Kleihauer method have been proposed. In one, New methylene blue is incorporated in the buffer solution, the reaction time is prolonged and buffer is used for washing the films.[24] The advantage of this technique is that reticulocytes stain blue, whereas cells containing haemoglobin F stain pink.

An immunofluorescent staining method has been developed based on the use of a specific antibody against haemoglobin F, which does not react with haemoglobin A.[25] By using a double-labelling procedure with rhodamine-labelled antibody against γ globin and a fluorescein-labelled antibody against β globin, it is possible to detect the presence of haemoglobin F and haemoglobin A in the same cell.[26]

Haemoglobin S and Other Haemoglobin Variants

Immunodiffusion with specific antibodies has been used for the identification of haemoglobin S, haemoglobin A_2 and haemoglobin F in red cells.[27,28] An alternative method is by detection of cells after labelling the cells with fluorescein isothiocyanate (FITC).[27] By a double-labelling method similar to that described earlier, it is possible to identify haemoglobin S as well as another haemoglobin in individual cells.

LEUCOCYTE CYTOCHEMISTRY

Leucocyte cytochemistry encompasses the techniques used to identify diagnostically useful enzymes or other substances in the cytoplasm of haemopoietic cells. These techniques are particularly useful for the characterization

of immature cells in AML and the identification of maturation abnormalities in the myelodysplastic syndromes and myeloproliferative neoplasms. There are many variations in the staining techniques, as discussed in the recommendations of an Expert Panel of the International Committee (now Council) for Standardization in Haematology.[29,30] Detailed reference works discussing the theoretical and practical aspects of cytochemistry are available.[31] The use of cytochemistry to characterize lymphoproliferative disorders has been largely superseded by immunological techniques (see Chapter 16). The results of cytochemical tests should always be interpreted in relation to Romanowsky stains and immunological techniques. Control blood or marrow slides should always be stained in parallel to ensure the quality of the staining. The principal uses of cytochemistry are as follows:

1. To characterize the blast cells in acute leukaemia as myeloid (leading to a diagnosis of AML unless there is also evidence of lymphoid differentiation)
2. To demonstrate myeloperoxidase or non-specific esterase activity and thus contribute to a diagnosis of mixed-phenotype acute leukaemia, according to the criteria of the 2008 WHO Classification of Tumours of Haematopoietic and Lymphoid Tissues[32]
3. To identify granulocytic and monocytic components in AML
4. To identify unusual lineages occasionally involved in clonal myeloid disorders (e.g. basophils and mast cells)
5. To detect cytoplasmic abnormalities and enzyme deficiencies in myeloid disorders (e.g. myeloperoxidase-deficient neutrophils in myelodysplasia or acute leukaemia, neutrophil alkaline phosphatase-deficient neutrophils in chronic myelogenous leukaemia, CML)
6. To identify Auer rods in MDS (and thus classify a case as refractory anaemia with excess of blasts II in the WHO classification)
7. To confirm a diagnosis of hairy cell leukaemia.

It is particularly important that cytochemistry is not neglected in under-resourced countries when immunophenotyping is not readily available.

Myeloperoxidase

Myeloperoxidase (MPO) is located in the primary and secondary granules of neutrophils and their precursors, in eosinophil granules and in the azurophilic granules of monocytes. The MPO in eosinophil granules is cyanide resistant, whereas that in neutrophils and monocytes is cyanide sensitive. MPO splits H_2O_2 and in the presence of a chromogenic electron donor forms an insoluble reaction product. Various benzidine substitutes have been used, of which 3,3'-diaminobenzidine (DAB) is the preferred chromogen.[33,34] The reaction product is stable, insoluble and non-diffusible. Staining can be enhanced by immersing the slides in copper sulphate or nitrate, but this is generally not required in normal diagnostic practice. Alternative non-benzidine-based techniques use 4-chloro-1-naphthol (4CN)[35] or 3-amino-9-ethylcarbazole.[36] The former gives very crisp staining but is soluble in some mounting media and immersion oil; the latter shows some diffusibility and does not stain as strongly as DAB.

Method with 3,3′-Diaminobenzidine

Reagents

Fixative. Buffered formal acetone (BFA) (see p. 623)
Substrate. 3,3′-DAB (Sigma D-8001, Sigma-Aldrich, UK)
Buffer. Sorensen's phosphate buffer, pH 7.3 (see p. 622)
Hydrogen peroxide (H_2O_2, 30% w/v.)
Counterstain. Aqueous haematoxylin.

Method

1. Fix air-dried smears for 30 s in cold BFA.
2. Rinse thoroughly in gently running tap water and air dry.
3. Incubate for 10 min in working substrate solution. Thoroughly mix 30 mg DAB in 60 ml buffer, add 120 µl H_2O_2 and mix well.
4. Counterstain with haematoxylin for 1–5 min, rinse in running tap water and air dry.

Technical considerations

MPO is not inhibited by heparin, oxalate or EDTA anticoagulants. Films should be made within 12 h of blood collection. Staining is satisfactory on slides kept at room temperature for at least a week. The DAB should be stored frozen at −20°C in 1 ml aliquots of 30 mg in 1 ml of buffer. For optimum results, it is essential to dissolve the DAB thoroughly in the buffer and to ensure the reagents in the incubation mixture are well mixed. The stain is robust and not strictly pH dependent, with identical results being obtained when using buffers ranging in pH from 7.0 to 9.0. The counterstaining time should be adjusted to the minimum time to give clear nuclear detail. Methyl green is an alternative counterstain, giving excellent contrast with the DAB reaction product, but nuclear detail is more difficult to discern.

Results and interpretation

The reaction product is brown and granular (Fig. 15.10A). Red cells and erythroid precursors show diffuse brown cytoplasmic staining. The most primitive myeloblasts are negative, with granular positivity appearing progressively as they mature toward the promyelocyte stage. The positivity may be localized to the Golgi region.

Figure 15.10 (A) Myeloperoxidase (MPO) and (B) Sudan Black B (SBB). Bone marrow in acute myeloid leukaemia (French–American–British [FAB] M1). Myeloperoxidase staining shows Auer rods and cytoplasmic granular staining, whereas with SBB localized positive reaction in the blast cells is more definite and Auer rods are prominent.

Promyelocytes and myelocytes are the most strongly staining cells in the granulocyte series, with positive (primary) granules packing the cytoplasm. Metamyelocytes and neutrophils have progressively fewer positive (secondary) granules. Eosinophil granules stain strongly and the large specific eosinophil granules are easily distinguished from neutrophil granules. Eosinophil granule peroxidase is distinct biochemically and immunologically from neutrophil peroxidase. Monoblasts and monocytes may be negative or positive. When positive, the granules are smaller than in neutrophils and diffusely scattered throughout the cytoplasm. MPO activity is present in basophil granules but is not demonstrable in mature basophils by the DAB reaction described earlier.

Pathological variations

Some individuals have congenital deficiency of neutrophil MPO. All stages of the neutrophil lineage, from the myeloblast onward, are negative. In these individuals, the eosinophils stain normally. Other individuals have an MPO deficiency confined to eosinophils or monocytes. Dysplastic neutrophils may be MPO negative. Auer rods stain well with DAB and are seen more frequently on MPO staining than on Romanowsky-stained films.

Sudan Black B

Sudan Black B (SBB) is a lipophilic dye that binds irreversibly to an undefined granule component in granulocytes, eosinophils and some monocytes. It cannot be extracted from the stained granules by organic dye solvents and gives comparable information to that of MPO staining.[37] The currently used staining solution is essentially that described by Sheehan and Storey.[38]

Reagents

Fixative. Vapour from 40% formaldehyde solution
Stain. SBB (Sigma S-2380) 0.3 g in 100 ml absolute ethanol
Phenol buffer. Dissolve 16 g crystalline phenol in 30 ml absolute ethanol. Add to 100 ml distilled water in which 0.3 g $Na_2HPO_4.12H_2O$ has been dissolved
Working stain solution. Add 40 ml buffer to 60 ml SBB solution
Counterstain. May–Grünwald–Giemsa or Leishman stain (see p. 61).

Method

1. Fix air-dried smears in formalin vapour as follows. Place a small square of filter paper in the bottom of a Coplin jar. Add 2 drops of 40% formalin, put on the lid and leave for 15 min to allow vaporization. Place the slides in the Coplin jar and replace the lid. After 5–10 min, remove the slides and stand on end for 15 min to 'air wash'.
2. Immerse the slides in the working stain solution for 1 h in a Coplin jar with a lid on.
3. Transfer slides to a staining rack and immediately flood with 70% alcohol. After 30 s, tip the 70% alcohol off and flood again for 30 s. Repeat three times in total.
4. Rinse in gently running tap water and air dry.
5. Counterstain without further fixation with Leishman stain or May–Grünwald–Giemsa.

Technical Considerations

Buffered formal acetone fixation for 30 s is a satisfactory alternative to formalin vapour. The working stain solution should be replaced after 4 weeks. Bone marrow smears with fatty particles containing lipid-soluble SBB benefit from a 5-s swirl in xylene followed by rinsing in running tap water and air drying prior to counterstaining. The Romanowsky counterstain gives excellent cytological detail of all cells present.

Results and Interpretation

The reaction product is black and granular. The results are essentially similar to those seen with MPO staining, both in normal and leukaemic cells (Fig. 15.10B). MPO-negative neutrophils are also SBB negative. The only notable difference is in eosinophil granules, which have a clear core when stained with SBB. Rare cases (1–2%) of acute lymphoblastic leukaemia (ALL) show non-granular smudgy positivity not seen with MPO staining.[39] Basophils are generally not positive but may show bright red/purple metachromatic staining of the granules.

Neutrophil Alkaline Phosphatase

Alkaline phosphatase activity is found predominantly in mature neutrophils, with some activity in metamyelocytes. Although demonstrated as a granular reaction product in the cytoplasm, enzyme activity is associated with a poorly characterized intracytoplasmic membranous component distinct from primary or secondary granules.[40] Other leucocytes are generally negative, but rare cases of lymphoid malignancies show cytochemically demonstrable activity.[41] Bone marrow macrophages are positive. Early methods of demonstrating alkaline phosphatase relied on the use of glycerophosphate or other phosphomonoesters as the substrate at alkaline pH, with a final black reaction product of lead sulphide.[42] Azo-dye techniques are simpler, giving equally good results. These methods use substituted naphthols as the substrate and it is the liberated naphthol rather than phosphate that is used to combine with the azo-dye to give the final reaction product.[43–45]

Reagents

Fixative. 4% formalin methanol. Add 10 ml 40% formalin to 90 ml methanol. Keep at −20°C or in the freezer compartment of a refrigerator. Discard after 2 weeks
Substrate. Naphthol AS phosphate (Sigma N-5625). Store in freezer

Buffer. 0.2 mol/l Tris buffer, pH 9.0 (see p. 623)

Stock substrate solution. Dissolve 30 mg naphthol AS phosphate in 0.5 ml N,N-dimethylformamide (Sigma D-4551). Add 100 ml 0.2 mol/l Tris buffer, pH 9.1. Store in a refrigerator at 2–4°C. The solution is stable for several months

Coupling azo-dye. Fast Blue BB salt (Sigma F-0250). Store in freezer

Counterstain. Neutral red, 0.02% aqueous solution.

Method

1. Fix freshly made air-dried blood films for 30 s in cold 4% formalin methanol.
2. Rinse with tap water and air dry.
3. Prepare working substrate solution by allowing 40 ml of stock substrate solution to warm to room temperature. Add 24 mg of Fast Blue BB and mix thoroughly until dissolved. Incubate slides for 15 min.
4. Wash in tap water and air dry.
5. Counterstain for 3 min in 0.02% aqueous neutral red, rinse briefly and air dry.

Technical considerations

N,N-dimethylformamide may dissolve some types of plastic; therefore a glass tube should be used to dissolve the substrate. Blood films should be made soon after blood collection, preferably within 30 min because neutrophil alkaline phosphatase (NAP) activity decreases rapidly in EDTA-anticoagulated blood. Once spread, the blood film should be stained within 6 h. A control film with a predictably high score, e.g. from a patient with reactive neutrophilia or from a pregnant woman, should be processed together with the patient film. The technical aspects of blood film preparation and the effects of fixation on NAP activity are discussed by Kaplow.[46]

Results and Interpretation

The reaction product is blue and granular. The intensity of reaction product in neutrophils varies from negative to strongly positive, with coarse granules filling the cytoplasm and overlying the nucleus (Fig. 15.11). An overall score is obtained by assessing the stain intensity in 100 consecutive neutrophils, with each neutrophil scored on a scale of 1–4 as follows:

0 – Negative, no granules
1 – Occasional granules scattered in the cytoplasm
2 – Moderate numbers of granules
3 – Numerous granules
4 – Heavy positivity with numerous coarse granules crowding the cytoplasm, frequently overlying the nucleus.

The overall possible score will range between 0 and 400 (assessed on 100 neutrophils). Reported normal ranges show some variations, owing possibly in part to variations

Figure 15.11 Neutrophil alkaline phosphatase. A strongly positive (4+) and moderately positive (3+ and 2+) intensity of reaction are shown.

in scoring criteria and methodology: 13–160 (mean 61);[46] 14–100 (mean 46);[47] 37–98 (mean 68);[48] 11–134 (mean 48).[49] A normal range should therefore be established in each laboratory.

In normal individuals, it is rare to find any neutrophils with a score of 3 and a score of 4 should not be present. There is some physiological variation in NAP scores. Newborn babies, children and pregnant women have high scores and premenopausal women have, on average, scores one-third higher than those of men.[40] In pathological states, the most significant diagnostic use of the NAP score is in CML. In the chronic phase of the disease, the score is almost invariably low, usually zero. Transient increases may occur with inter-current infection. In myeloid blast transformation or accelerated phase, the score rises. Low scores are also commonly found in paroxysmal nocturnal haemoglobinuria (PNH) and the very rare condition of hereditary hypophosphatasia. There are many causes of a raised NAP score, notably in the neutrophilia of infection, polycythaemia vera, leukaemoid reactions and Hodgkin lymphoma. In aplastic anaemia, the NAP score is high, but it falls if PNH supervenes. With the greater use of cytogenetic and molecular genetic techniques to confirm the diagnosis of CML, the NAP score is rarely needed.

Acid Phosphatase Reaction, including Tartrate-Resistant Acid Phosphatase Reaction

Cytochemically demonstrable acid phosphatase is ubiquitous in haemopoietic cells. The staining intensity of different cell types is somewhat variable according to the method used. Its main diagnostic use is in the diagnosis of T-cell ALL and hairy cell leukaemia.[50,51] These diseases are more reliably diagnosed and characterized by immunophenotyping when this is available (see Chapter 16). The unmodified acid phosphatase stain is now largely redundant but the tartrate-resistant acid phosphatase stain is still useful for confirmation of the diagnosis of hairy cell leukaemia when immunophenotyping is not available. The pararosaniline method given in the following section, modified from Goldberg and Barka,[52] is recommended for demonstrating positivity in T lymphoid cells. Use of Fast Garnet GBC as coupler may be preferred for the demonstration of tartrate-resistant acid phosphatase activity.[29,51]

Reagents

Fixative. Methanol, 10 ml; acetone, 60 ml; water, 30 ml; and citric acid, 0.63 g. Adjust to pH 5.4 with 1 mol/l NaOH before use

Buffer pH 5.0. Sodium acetate trihydrate, 19.5 g; sodium barbiturate, 29.5 g; water to 1 litre (Michaeli's veronal acetate buffer)

Substrate solution. 25 mg naphthol AS-BI phosphate (Sigma N-2125) dissolved in 2.5 ml N,N-dimethylformamide

Sodium nitrite. 4% $NaNO_2$ aqueous solution

Coupling reagent

1. Stock pararosaniline. Dissolve 1 g pararosaniline (Sigma P-7632) in 25 ml warm 2 mol/l HCl. Filter when cool. Store at room temperature in the dark. Stable for 2 months
2. 4% sodium nitrite solution. Dissolve 200 mg sodium nitrite in 5 ml distilled water. Stable for 1 week at 4–10°C
3. Hexazotized pararosaniline. Mix equal volumes of pararosaniline and 4% sodium nitrite together 2 min before use.

Counterstain. 1% Aqueous methyl green or aqueous haematoxylin

Tartaric acid L(+) (Sigma T-1807)

Working solution A. Mix 92.5 ml of buffer with 2.5 ml of substrate solution. Add 32.5 ml of distilled water and then add 4 ml of hexazotized pararosaniline. Mix well and adjust pH to 5.0 using 1 mol/l NaOH

Working solution B. Add 375 mg of crystalline L(+)-tartaric acid to 50 ml of working solution A; the final concentration is then 50 mmol/l.

Method

1. Air dry films for several hours (24 h if possible).
2. Fix for 10 min in methanol/acetone/citric acid, rinse in tap water and air dry.
3. Incubate for 1 h at 37°C in working solutions A (acid phosphatase reaction) or incubate two films in working solutions A and B, respectively (tartrate-resistant acid phosphatase reaction).
4. Rinse in tap water and air dry.
5. Counterstain in 1% aqueous methyl green or aqueous haematoxylin for 5 min.
6. Rinse in tap water and mount wet in warmed glycerin jelly.

Results and Interpretation

The reaction product is red with a mixture of granular and diffuse positivity (Fig. 15.12). In T cells, acid phosphatase is an early differentiation feature. Almost all acute and chronic T-lineage leukaemias show strong activity. In T-lineage ALL, the activity is usually highly localized (polar). Granulocytes are strongly positive. Monocytes, eosinophils and platelets show variable positivity. In the bone marrow, macrophages, plasma cells and megakaryocytes are strongly positive.

In hairy cell leukaemia the majority of leukaemic cells react equally positively in the presence and absence of tartaric acid (Fig. 15.13).

When immunophenotyping is available, the unmodified acid phosphatase reaction is redundant. If a full range of appropriate monoclonal antibodies is available, the tartrate-resistant acid phosphatase reaction is also redundant.

Periodic Acid–Schiff Reaction

Periodic acid specifically oxidizes 1–2 glycol groups to produce stable dialdehydes. These dialdehydes give a red reaction product when exposed to Schiff's reagent (leucobasic fuchsin). Positive reactions occur with carbohydrates, principally glycogen, but also monosaccharides, polysaccharides, glycoproteins, mucoproteins, phosphorylated sugars, inositol derivatives and cerebrosides.[53] Glycogen can be distinguished from other positively reacting substances by its sensitivity to diastase digestion. In haemopoietic cells, the main source of positive reactions is glycogen.

Figure 15.12 Acid phosphatase. T-cell acute leukaemia with intense localized staining.

Figure 15.13 Acid phosphatase. Hairy cell leukaemia: acid phosphatase (A) and tartrate-resistant acid phosphatase (B).

Reagents

Fixative. Methanol

1% periodic acid. $HIO_4.2H_2O$, 10 g/l in distilled water

Schiff's reagent. Dissolve 5 g basic fuchsin in 500 ml of hot distilled water. Filter when cool. Saturate with SO_2 gas by bubbling for 1–12 h in a fume cupboard. Shake

vigorously with 2 g activated charcoal for 1 min in a conical flask in a fume cupboard and filter immediately through a large Whatman No. 1 filter into a dark bottle. The reagent is stable for 6 months at room temperature, stored in the dark

Counterstain. Aqueous haematoxylin.

Method

1. Fix films for 15 min in methanol.
2. Rinse in gently running tap water and air dry.
3. If required, expose fixed control films to digestion in diastase (100 mg in 100 ml of 0.9 g/l NaCl) for 20–60 min at room temperature.
4. Flood slides with 1% periodic acid for 10 min.
5. Rinse in running tap water for 10 min and air dry.
6. Immerse in Schiff's reagent for 30 min in a Coplin jar with a lid (the Schiff's reagent can be returned to the stock bottle after use).
7. Rinse in running tap water for 10 min and air dry.
8. Counterstain in aqueous haematoxylin for 5–10 min.

Technical Considerations

Formalin vapour (5 min), formalin/ethanol (10 ml 40% formalin/90 ml ethanol) (10 min) and buffered formal acetone (45 s) are satisfactory alternative fixatives. Previously fixed, iron-stained or Romanowsky-stained films can be overstained with the PAS reaction satisfactorily. Romanowsky-stained smears can be partly decolourized by soaking in methanol for 1 h prior to step 4. The intensity of the reaction product depends on the quality of the Schiff's reagent. Normal neutrophils should always stain intensely red and deterioration of the Schiff's reagent can be detected by examination of control normal films. Some methods recommend rinsing in a dilute sodium metabisulphite HCl solution ('SO_2 water') after step 6, but this is not necessary with good-quality Schiff's reagent.

Results and Interpretation

The reaction product is red, with intensity ranging from pink to bright red (Figs 15.14, 15.15). Cytoplasmic positivity may be diffuse or granular. Granulocyte precursors show diffuse weak positivity, with neutrophils showing intense confluent granular positivity. Eosinophil granules are negative, with diffuse cytoplasmic positivity. Basophils may be negative but often show large irregular blocks of positive material not related to the granules. Monocytes and their precursors show variable diffuse positivity with superimposed fine granules, often at the periphery of the cytoplasm. Normal erythroid precursors and red cells are negative. Megakaryocytes and platelets show variable, usually intense, diffuse positivity with superimposed fine granules, coarse granules and large blocks. Granular

Figure 15.14 Periodic acid–Schiff stain. (A) Dysplastic micromegakaryocytes with diffuse cytoplasmic staining and some coarse granules; (B) dyserythropoiesis with diffuse staining in a trinucleate normoblast and coarse granular and diffuse staining in a proerythroblast; and (C) acute lymphoblastic leukaemia with blasts showing block positivity.

positivity with negative background cytoplasm is found in 10–40% of peripheral lymphocytes, with no detectable differences between T and B cells.[54,55] Lymphoblasts show variable PAS-positive cytoplasmic granules or blocks on a clear background; it is block positivity on a clear background that is most characteristic of lymphoblasts rather than myeloblasts. When immunophenotyping is available, the PAS reaction is redundant for the diagnosis of ALL. It can still be useful in AML and MDS to identify abnormal erythroblasts and dysplastic megakaryocytes and to demonstrate the cytoplasmic blush that helps to confirm a diagnosis of acute promyelocytic leukaemia (Fig. 15.15).

Esterases

Leucocyte esterases are a group of enzymes that hydrolyse acyl or chloroacyl esters of α-naphthol or naphthol AS. Li et al.[56] identified nine esterase isoenzymes using polyacrylamide gel electrophoresis of leucocyte extracts from normal and pathological cells. The gels were stained in parallel with cell smears. The isoenzymes fell into two groups: bands 1, 2, 7, 8 and 9 corresponded to the 'specific' esterase of neutrophils, staining specifically with naphthol AS-D chloroacetate esterase (chloroacetate esterase, CAE), whereas bands 3, 4, 5 and 6 corresponded to 'non-specific' esterase (NSE), staining with α-naphthyl acetate esterase (ANAE) and α-naphthyl butyrate esterase (butyrate esterase, ANBE). Band 4 was best demonstrated by ANBE and band 5 by ANAE. The NSEs are inhibited by sodium fluoride (NaF). Naphthol AS acetate and naphthol AS-D acetate react with both specific and non-specific esterases, but only the reaction with the NSEs is inhibited by NaF. The methods using parallel slides with and without NaF are not generally used anymore because it is usually more informative to perform a combination of chloroacetate esterase and one of the 'non-specific' esterase stains on a single slide. The combined methods have the advantage of demonstrating pathological double staining of individual cells. All the esterase stains can be performed using a variety of coupling reagents, each of which gives a different coloured reaction product. The methods outlined as follows have been chosen for their simplicity and reliability.

Naphthol AS-D Chloroacetate Esterase

Reagents

Fixative. Buffered formal acetone (see p. 623)
Buffer. 66 mmol/l phosphate buffer, pH 7.4 (see p. 622)
Naphthol AS-D chloroacetate substrate solution.[29] Dissolve 0.1 g of naphthol AS-D chloroacetate (Sigma N-0758) in 40 ml N,N-dimethyl-formamide (Sigma D-4254). Keep refrigerated
Working substrate solution. Add 2 ml of naphthol AS-D chloroacetate stock solution to 38 ml of 66 mmol/l

Figure 15.15 Acute promyelocytic leukaemia. (A) May–Grünwald–Giemsa stain shows hypergranular promyelocytes with scattered Auer rods; (B) Sudan black B with strongly stained cytoplasm; (C) periodic acid–Schiff staining shows diffuse cytoplasmic blush; and (D) chloroacetate esterase gives strong cytoplasmic staining.

phosphate buffer, pH 7.4. Mix well. Add 0.4 ml of freshly prepared hexazotized New fuchsin. Mix well

Coupling reagent

1. Hexazotized New fuchsin. Dissolve 4 g of New fuchsin in 100 ml of 2N HCl.
2. Sodium nitrite solution 0.3 mol/l. Dissolve 2.1 g of sodium nitrite ($NaNO_2$) in 100 ml of water.
3. Immediately prior to using, add 0.2 ml of the hexazotized New fuchsin to 0.4 ml sodium nitrite, mix well and leave for 1 min before adding to substrate solution

Counterstain. Aqueous haematoxylin.

Method

1. Fix air-dried smears in cold buffered formal acetone for 30 s.
2. Rinse in gently running tap water and air dry.
3. Immerse the slides in the working substrate solution in a Coplin jar for 5–10 min.

4. Rinse in running tap water and air dry.
5. Counterstain in aqueous haematoxylin for 1 min.
6. 'Blue' in running tap water for 1 min and air dry.

Technical considerations

The CAE stain is robust and reliable. A satisfactory alternative to New fuchsin is 40 mg of Fast blue BB, but it requires thorough vigorous mixing with the substrate solution. The incubation time is important because most haemopoietic cells show some scattered granular staining if the incubation is prolonged. Hydrolysis of the substrate is rapid, with staining virtually complete within 3–5 min.

Results and interpretation

The reaction product is bright red (Fig. 15.15D). It is confined to cells of the neutrophil series and mast cells. Cytoplasmic CAE activity appears as myeloblasts mature to promyelocytes. Positivity in myeloblasts is rare, but promyelocytes and myelocytes stain strongly, with the reaction product filling the cytoplasm. More mature cells stain strongly but less intensely. It is therefore useful as a marker of cytoplasmic maturation in myeloid leukaemias. In acute promyelocytic leukaemia, the cells show heavy cytoplasmic staining. The characteristic multiple Auer rods stain positively, often with a hollow core. It is rare to see CAE-positive Auer rods in other forms of AML except in cases with the t(8;21) translocation.[57]

α-Naphthyl Butyrate Esterase

Reagents

Fixative. Buffered formal acetone
Buffer. 100 mmol/l phosphate buffer (Sorensen's), pH 8.0
Substrate stock solution. α-Naphthyl butyrate (Sigma N-8125) 100 µl in 5 ml acetone. The solution should be stored at −20°C and is stable for at least 2 months
Coupling reagent. Fast Garnet GBC (Sigma F-8761) 15 mg
Counterstain. Aqueous haematoxylin.

Method

1. Fix air-dried smears in buffered formal acetone for 30 s. Rinse in gently running tap water and air dry.
2. Add the Fast Garnet GBC to 50 ml buffer and mix well.
3. Add 0.5 ml of the α-naphthyl butyrate/acetone solution and mix well.
4. Pour the incubation medium into a Coplin jar containing the fixed slides and incubate for 20–40 min.
5. Rinse thoroughly by running tap water into the Coplin jar until clear.
6. Air dry and counterstain in aqueous haematoxylin for 1–5 min.

Technical considerations

The reaction product is soluble in immersion oil and synthetic mounting media. If slides are to be looked at repeatedly, they should be mounted in an aqueous mounting medium (e.g. Apathy's gum-arabic mountant or glycerin/gelatin). There may be batch-to-batch variation of the Fast Garnet GBC. Staining can be controlled by removing the control slide from the incubation medium after 20 min and examining it wet under a low-power (e.g. ×20) objective, returning it to the incubation medium while still wet. When the monocytes show as dark brown, staining is complete. Hexazotized pararosaniline is an alternative coupling reagent, which gives an insoluble brown reaction product and is suitable for mounting in synthetic mounting media.[56]

Results and interpretation

The reaction product is brown and granular (Fig. 15.16). The majority of monocytes (>80%) stain strongly, the remainder showing some weak staining. Negative monocytes are rare. Neutrophils, eosinophils, basophils and

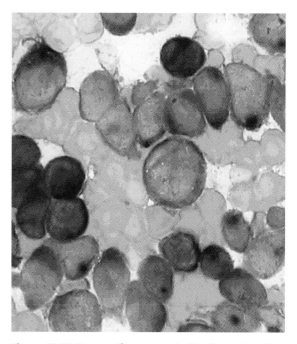

Figure 15.16 Non-specific esterase. Positive *(brown)* reaction in acute monocytic leukaemia (FAB M5).

platelets are negative. B lymphocytes are negative and T lymphocytes are more variably stained. In the bone marrow, monocytes, monocyte precursors and macrophages stain strongly. α-Naphthyl butyrate is more specific for identifying a monocytic component in AML than α-naphthyl acetate (see later).

α-Naphthyl Acetate Esterase

Reagents

Fixative. Buffered formal acetone
Buffer. 66 mmol/l phosphate buffer, pH 6.3
Substrate solution. Dissolve 100 mg α-naphthyl acetate (Sigma N-8505) in 5 ml ethylene monomethyl ether. Store at 4–10°C
Coupling reagent
1. Stock pararosaniline. Dissolve 1 g pararosaniline (Sigma P-7632) in 25 ml warm 2 mol/l HCl. Filter when cool. Store at room temperature in the dark. Stable for 2 months.
2. 4% sodium nitrite solution. Dissolve 200 mg sodium nitrite in 5 ml distilled water. This solution is stable for 1 week at 4–10°C.
3. Hexazotized pararosaniline. Mix equal volumes of pararosaniline and 4% sodium nitrite together 1 min before use.

Incubation medium. Add 2 ml of the α-naphthyl acetate solution to 38 ml of the 66 mmol/l phosphate buffer,

pH 6.3, and mix well. Add 0.4 ml of freshly prepared hexazotized pararosaniline and mix well
Counterstain. Aqueous haematoxylin.

Method

1. Fix air-dried smears in cold buffered formal acetone for 30 s.
2. Rinse in running tap water and air dry.
3. Immerse the slides for 30–60 min in the incubation medium in a Coplin jar.
4. Rinse in gently running tap water in the Coplin jar until clear and air dry.
5. Counterstain in aqueous haematoxylin for 2–5 min.

Technical considerations

Fast Blue BB 80 mg can be substituted as a coupling reagent. This gives a dark green/brown granular reaction product, which is soluble in mounting media and immersion oil. The haematoxylin staining time should be adjusted to give clear nuclear detail without overstaining to obscure nucleoli and chromatin texture.

Results and interpretation

The reaction product is diffuse red/brown in colour. Normal and leukaemic monocytes stain strongly. Normal granulocytes are negative, but in MDS or AML may give positive reactions of varying intensity. Megakaryocytes stain strongly and leukaemic megakaryoblasts may show focal or diffuse positivity. Most T lymphocytes and some T lymphoblasts show focal 'dot-like' positivity, but immunophenotyping has superseded cytochemistry for identifying and subcategorizing T cells. Leukaemic erythroblasts may show focal or diffuse positivity.

Sequential Combined Esterase Stain Using ANAE and CAE

Reagents

As earlier for ANAE and CAE stains.

Method

1. Follow the method and steps 1–4 listed earlier for α-naphthyl acetate esterase stain, rinse in tap water and air dry.
2. Without further fixation, prepare the naphthol AS-D chloroacetate incubation medium as explained previously, substituting 10 mg Fast Blue BB (Sigma F-0250) for hexazotized New fuchsin and incubate for 10 min.
3. Rinse in tap water and counterstain with aqueous haematoxylin for 1–3 min.

Technical considerations

Fast Blue BB is relatively insoluble and the chloroacetate incubation medium should be mixed vigorously before use.

Results and interpretation

The ANAE gives a brown reaction product and the CAE gives a granular bright blue product (Fig. 15.17). Staining patterns are identical to those seen with the two stains used separately. The double-staining technique avoids the need to compare results from separate slides and reveals aberrant staining patterns. In myelomonocytic leukaemias, cells staining with both esterases may be present. In MDS and AML with dysplastic granulocytes, double staining of individual cells may be present. This may be helpful when a diagnosis of MDS is not otherwise certain, but the same abnormal pattern may be seen in non-clonal dysplastic states such as megaloblastic anaemia.

Single Incubation Double Esterase (Naphthol AS-D Chloroacetate and α-Naphthyl Butyrate)[58]

Reagents

Fixative. Buffered formal acetone
Buffer. 100 mmol/l phosphate buffer, pH 8.0 (Sorensen's)
Substrates

1. 2.5 mg naphthol AS-D chloroacetate (Sigma N-0758) in 1 ml acetone
2. 4 mg α-naphthyl butyrate (Sigma N-8000) in 1 ml acetone

Coupling reagent. Fast Blue BB salt (Sigma F-0250)
Counterstain. Aqueous haematoxylin.

Method

1. Fix air-dried smears in buffered formal acetone for 30 s.
2. Rinse in tap water and air dry.

Figure 15.17 Combined esterase stain. Acute myelomonocytic leukaemia with almost equal numbers of chloroacetate esterase *(blue)* and non-specific esterase *(brown)* positive cells.

3. Dissolve 80 mg Fast Blue BB in 50 ml phosphate buffer by vigorous mixing.
4. Add naphthol AS-D chloroacetate and mix well.
5. Add α-naphthyl butyrate and mix well.
6. Incubate slides for 10–15 min in a Coplin jar in the dark.
7. Flush the Coplin jar with running tap water until clear.
8. Air dry the slides.
9. Counterstain in aqueous haematoxylin for 1 min, rinse and air dry.

Technical considerations

Steps 4 and 5 should be carried out rapidly. Staining can be extended to 30 min if necessary to ensure maximal ANBE staining, but at longer incubation times some non-specific granular CAE staining may occur.

Results and interpretation

The CAE reaction product is bright blue (granulocytes); the ANBE product is dark green/brown (monocytes). ANBE does not stain megakaryocytes or T cells as strongly as α-naphthyl acetate. Lam et al. suggest the use of hexazotized pararosaniline as coupling reagent in a single incubation combined esterase, which gives contrasting bright red and brown reaction products.[59]

In AML, the stain is useful for identifying monocytic and granulocytic components.

Toluidine Blue Stain

Toluidine blue staining is useful for the enumeration of basophils and mast cells. It binds strongly to the granules in these cells and is particularly useful in pathological states in which the cells may not be easily identifiable on Romanowsky stains. In AML and in CML and other myeloproliferative neoplasms, basophils may be dysplastic and poorly granular, as may the mast cells in systemic mastocytosis.

Reagents

Toluidine blue 1% w/v in methanol. Add 1 g of toluidine blue (BDH 34077) to 100 ml methanol and mix for 24 h on a roller or with a magnetic flea. The stain is stable indefinitely at room temperature. Keep tightly stoppered.

Method

1. Place air-dried smears on a staining rack and flood with the toluidine blue solution.
2. Incubate for 5–10 min.
3. Rinse briefly in gently running tap water until clear and air dry.

Results and Interpretation

The granules of basophils and mast cells stain a bright red/purple and are discrete and distinct (Fig. 15.18). Nuclei stain blue and cells with abundant RNA may show a blue tint to the cytoplasm. Although toluidine blue is said to be specific for these granules, with >10 min incubation, the primary granules of promyelocytes are stained red/purple. However, these are smaller and finer than the mast cell or basophil granules and easily distinguished.

Cytochemical Reactions and Leukaemia Classification

Myelodysplastic Syndromes and Acute Myeloid Leukaemia

MDS is an acquired clonal preleukaemic bone marrow disorder characterized largely by a cellular or hypercellular marrow, peripheral cytopenias and variable morphological abnormalities of the haemopoietic cells. The classification system proposed by the French-American-British (FAB) cooperative group in 1982[60] was widely used for many years but is now being superseded by the WHO classification (see Chapter 23). A Perls' reaction for haemosiderin is essential for the demonstration of ring sideroblasts. Other cytochemical evidence of dysplasia includes double staining of cells with chloroacetate and ANAE, the presence of SBB- or MPO-negative neutrophils and the presence of Auer rods (identified with SBB and MPO).

In AML, cytochemistry is helpful in defining monocytic cells (ANAE and ANBE), identifying Auer rods and demonstrating dysplasia (as mentioned earlier).

Figure 15.18 Toluidine blue. Chronic myelogenous leukaemia in accelerated phase. There are five strongly positive basophils.

Acute Lymphoblastic Leukaemia

The modern diagnosis and classification of ALL is by cytology, followed by immunophenotyping (see Chapter 16). If immunophenotyping is not available, cytochemistry remains important. It should be noted that, on Romanowsky staining, lymphoblasts may rarely contain fine azurophilic granules. However, Auer rods are never seen and MPO and CAE are negative, whether or not fine granules are present. Occasionally granules give a weak reaction with SBB. Although not lineage specific, the pattern of any PAS positivity may be helpful.[31] In ALL, 95% of cases show positive blocks or granules of bright red PAS-positive material. This may be present in very few blasts ($<$1%) or the majority. The critical difference from granular or block positivity in other leukaemic cells is the glass-clear background cytoplasm in lymphoblasts. Myeloblasts, monoblasts, leukaemic erythroblasts and megakaryoblasts all show some degree of diffuse cytoplasmic positivity and occasionally block positivity is seen. Acid phosphatase staining is more likely to give focal positivity in T-lineage than B-lineage acute leukaemias, but the difference is not clear enough to be of diagnostic certainty

and focal positivity is sometimes also seen in the erythroblasts of erythroleukaemia. Esterase staining is generally unhelpful; some T-cell cases show focal positivity with ANAE, but this is not specific.

Chronic Myeloproliferative Neoplasms

Although low NAP scores are typical in chronic phase CML and high scores are usually found in other myeloproliferative neoplasms, the finding of a high NAP score is too non-specific to be of diagnostic help.

Chronic Lymphoproliferative Disorders

Chronic lymphoproliferative disorders are now characterized by immunophenotyping (Chapter 16). The reactions for acid hydrolases (acid phosphatase, ANAE, β-glucuronidase and β-glucosaminidase) show focal positivity in most T-cell disorders but are negative in B-cell disorders. The tartrate-resistant acid phosphatase reaction for hairy cell leukaemia is the only cytochemical stain that is sufficiently specific to still be regarded as diagnostically useful (in the absence of immunophenotyping).

REFERENCES

1. Grüneberg H. Siderocytes: a new kind of erythrocyte. *Nature (London).* 1941;148:114–115.
2. Pappenheimer AM, Thompson KP, Parker DD, et al. Anaemia associated with unidentified erythrocytic inclusions after splenectomy. *Q J Med.* 1945;14:75–100.
3. Kaplan E, Zuelzer WW, Mouriquand C. Sideroblasts: a study of stainable nonhemoglobin iron in marrow normoblasts. *Blood.* 1954;9:203–213.
4. Crosby WH. Siderocytes and the spleen. *Blood.* 1957;12:165–170.
5. Sundberg RD, Bromann H. The application of the Prussian blue stain to previously stained films of blood and bone marrow. *Blood.* 1955;10:160–166.
6. Hayhoe FG, Quaglino D. Refractory sideroblastic anaemia and erythraemic myelosis: possible relationship and cytochemical observations. *Br J Haematol.* 1960;6:381–387.
7. Kass L, Eickholt MM. Rapid detection of ringed sideroblasts with bromchlorphenol blue. *Am J Clin Pathol.* 1978;70:738–740.

8. Bennett JM. Classification of the myelodysplastic syndromes. *Clin Haematol.* 1986;15:909–923.
9. Mufti GJ, Bennett JM, Goasgen J, et al. Diagnosis and classification of MDS: International Working Group on Morphology of MDS (IWGM-MDS) consensus proposals for the definition and enumeration of myeloblasts and ring sideroblasts. *Haematologica.* 2008;93:1712–1717.
10. Hasserjian RP, Gatterman N, Bennett JM, et al. Refractory anaemia with ring sideroblasts. In: Swerdlow SH, Campo E, Harris NL, et al., eds. *World Health Organization Classification of Tumours of Haematopoietic and Lymphoid Tissues.* Lyon: IARC Press; 2008:96–97.
11. Rath CE, Finch CA. Sternal marrow hemosiderin: a method for the determination of available iron stores in man. *J Lab Clin Med.* 1948;33:81–86.
12. Hughes DA, Stuart-Smith SE, Bain BJ. How should stainable iron in bone marrow films be assessed? *J Clin Pathol.* 2004;57:1038–1040.
13. Heinz R. Morphologische Veränderungen der rother

Blutkörperchen durche Gifte. *Virchows Archives.* 1890;122:112.
14. Dacie JV, Grimes AJ, Meisler A, et al. Hereditary Heinz-body anaemia: a report of studies on five patients with mild anaemia. *Br J Haematol.* 1964;10:388–402.
15. Jacob HS. Mechanisms of Heinz body formation and attachment to red cell membrane. *Semin Hematol.* 1970;7:341–354.
16. White JM. The unstable haemoglobins. *Br Med Bull.* 1976;32:219–222.
17. Eisinger J, Flores J, Tyson JA, et al. Fluorescent cytoplasm and Heinz bodies of hemoglobin Köln erythrocytes: evidence for intracellular heme catabolism. *Blood.* 1985;65:886–893.
18. Schwab ML, Lewis AE. An improved stain for Heinz bodies. *Am J Clin Pathol.* 1969;51:673.
19. Simpson CF, Carlisle JW, Mallard L. Rhodanile blue: a rapid and selective stain for Heinz bodies. *Stain Technol.* 1970;45:221–223.
20. Gouttas A, Fessas Ph, Tsevrenis H, et al. Description d'une nouvelle variété d'anémie hémolytique

congénitale. *Sang.* 1955;26: 911–919.

21. Kleihauer E, Betke K. Elution procedure for the demonstration of methaemoglobin in red cells of human blood smears. *Nature (London).* 1963;199:1196–1197.

22. Kleihauer E, Braun H, Betke K. Demonstration von fetalem Hämoglobin in den Erythrocyten eines Blutausstrichs. *Klin Wochenschr.* 1957;35:637–638.

23. Nierhaus K, Betke K. Eine vereinfachte Modifikation der säuren Elution für die cytologische Darstellung von fetalem Hämoglobin. *Klin Wochenschr.* 1968;46:47.

24. Clayton EM, Felhaus WD, Phythyon JM. The demonstration of fetal erythrocytes in the presence of adult red blood cells. *Am J Clin Pathol.* 1963;40:487–490.

25. Tomoda Y. Demonstration of foetal erythrocytes by immunofluorescent staining. *Nature (London).* 1964;202:910–911.

26. Thorpe SJ, Huehns EG. A new approach for the antenatal diagnosis of β-thalassaemia: a double labelling immunofluorescence microscopy technique. *Br J Haematol.* 1983;53:103–112.

27. Headings V, Bhattacharya S, Shukla S, et al. Identification of specific hemoglobins within individual erythrocytes. *Blood.* 1975;45:263–271.

28. Papayannopoulou Th, McGuire TC, Lim G, et al. Identification of haemoglobin S in red cells and normoblasts using fluorescent anti-Hb antibodies. *Br J Haematol.* 1976;34:25–31.

29. Shibata A, Bennett JM, Castoldi GL, et al. Recommended methods for cytological procedures in haematology. *Clin Lab Haematol.* 1985;7:55–74.

30. International Council for Standardization in Haematology. Procedures for the classification of acute leukaemias. *Leuk Lymphoma.* 1993;11:37–48.

31. Hayhoe FG, Quaglino D. *Haematological Cytochemistry.* 2nd ed. Edinburgh: Churchill Livingstone; 1988.

32. Borowitz MJ, Béné M-C, Harris NL, et al. Acute leukaemia of ambiguous lineage. In: Swerdlow SH, Campo E, Harris NL, et al., eds. *World Health Organization Classification of Tumours of Haematopoietic and Lymphoid Tissues.* Lyon: IARC Press; 2008:150–155.

33. Graham RC, Karnovsky MJ. The early stages of absorption of injected horseradish peroxidase in the proximal tubules of mouse kidney: ultrastructural cytochemistry by a new technique. *J Histochem Cytochem.* 1966;14:291–302.

34. Novikoff AB, Goldfischer S. Visualization of peroxisomes (microbodies and mitochondria with diaminobenzidine). *J Histochem Cytochem.* 1969;17: 675–680.

35. Elias JM. A rapid sensitive myeloperoxidase stain using 4-chloro-1-naphthol. *Am J Clin Pathol.* 1980;73:797–799.

36. Graham RC, Lundholm U, Karnovsky MJ. Cytochemical demonstration of peroxidase activity with 3-amino-9-ethylcarbazole. *J Histochem Cytochem.* 1965;13: 150–152.

37. Lillie RD, Burtner HJ. Stable sudanophilia of human neutrophil leucocytes in relation to peroxidase and oxidase. *J Histochem Cytochem.* 1953;1:8–26.

38. Sheehan HL, Storey GW. An improved method of staining leucocyte granules with Sudan Black B. *J Pathol Bacteriol.* 1974; 49:580.

39. Stass SA, Pui C-H, Melvin S, et al. Sudan black B positive acute lymphoblastic leukaemia. *Br J Haematol.* 1984;57:413–421.

40. Rosner F, Lee SL. Endocrine relationships of leukocyte alkaline phosphatase. *Blood.* 1965;5: 356–369.

41. Poppema S, Elema JD, Halie MR. Alkaline phosphatase positive lymphomas: a morphologic, immunologic and enzyme histochemical study. *Cancer.* 1981;47:1303–1312.

42. Gomori G. *Microscopic Histochemistry: Principles and Practice.* Chicago, IL: University of Chicago Press; 1952.

43. Kaplow LS. A histochemical procedure for localizing and evaluating leucocyte alkaline phosphatase activity in smears of blood and marrow. *Blood.* 1955;10:1023–1029.

44. Kaplow LS. Cytochemistry of leukocyte alkaline phosphatase: use of complex naphthol AS phosphates in azo-dye coupling technics. *Am J Clin Pathol.* 1963;39:439–449.

45. Rustin GJ, Wilson PD, Peters TJ. Studies on the subcellular localization of human neutrophil alkaline phosphatase. *J Cell Sci.* 1979;36:401–412.

46. Kaplow LS. Leukocyte alkaline phosphatase cytochemistry: applications and methods. *Ann N Y Acad Sci.* 1968;155:911.

47. Hayhoe FGJ, Quaglino D. Cytochemical demonstration and measurement of leucocyte alkaline phosphatase in normal and pathological states by modified azo-dye coupling technique. *Br J Haematol.* 1958;4:375–389.

48. Rutenberg AB, Rosales CL, Bennett JM. An important histochemical method for the demonstration of leukocyte alkaline phosphatase activity: clinical applications. *J Lab Clin Med.* 1965;65:698–705.

49. Bendix-Hansen K, Helleberg-Rasmussen I. I. Evaluation of neutrophil alkaline phosphatase: untreated myeloid leukaemia, lymphoid leukaemia and normal humans. *Scand J Haematol.* 1985;34:264–269.

50. Yam LT, Li CY, Lam KW. Tartrate-resistant acid phosphatase isoenzyme in the reticulum cells of leukemic reticuloendotheliosis. *N Engl J Med.* 1971;284:357.

51. Li CY, Yam LT, Lam KW. Acid phosphatase isoenzyme in human leucocytes in normal and pathologic conditions. *J Histochem Cytochem.* 1970;18:473–481.

52. Goldberg AF, Barka T. Acid phosphatase activity in human blood cells. *Nature.* 1962;195:297.

53. Hotchkiss RD. A microchemical reaction resulting in the staining of polysaccharide structures in fixed tissue preparations. *Arch Biochem.* 1948;16:131–141.

54. Higgy KE, Burns GF, Hayhoe FGJ. Discrimination of B, T and null lymphocytes by esterase cytochemistry. *Scand J Haematol.* 1977;18:437–438.

55. Quaglino D, Hayhoe FGJ. Observations on the periodic acid–Schiff reaction in lymphoproliferative diseases. *J Pathol Bacteriol.* 1959;78:521–532.

56. Li CY, Yam LT, Lam KW. Esterases in human leucocytes. *J Histochem Cytochem.* 1973;21:1.

57. Swirsky DM, Li YS, Matthews JG, et al. Translocation in acute granulocytic leukaemia: cytological, cytochemical and clinical features. *Br J Haematol.* 1983;56:199–213.

58. Swirsky DM. Single incubation double esterase cytochemical reaction using a single coupling reagent. *J Clin Pathol.* 1984;37:1187–1190.

59. Lam KW, Li CY, Yam LT. Simultaneous demonstration of non-specific esterase and chloro-acetate esterase in human blood cells. *Stain Technol.* 1985;60:169–172.

60. Bennett JM, Catovsky D, Daniel M-T, et al. Proposals for the classification of the myelodysplastic syndromes. *Br J Haematol.* 1982;51:189–199.

Chapter | **16** |

Immunophenotyping

Estella Matutes, Ricardo Morilla, Alison M. Morilla

INTRODUCTION

Since the development of the hybridoma technology in the 1970s, there have been major advances in the immunophenotypic characterization of haemopoietic malignancies and this, in turn, has resulted in a better understanding of normal haemopoietic differentiation. Prior to the availability of monoclonal antibodies (McAbs), it was possible to distinguish B and T lymphocytes from each other and both from early lymphoid precursor cells by the expression of surface or cytoplasmic (c) immunoglobulin in B lymphocytes; the ability to form rosettes with sheep erythrocytes (E-rosettes) in T lymphocytes; and the expression of the nuclear enzyme, terminal deoxynucleotidyl transferase (TdT), in lymphoid precursors. Over the last two decades, the application of new

technology has had a major impact on the diagnosis of acute and chronic leukaemias and has provided clues to the pathogenesis and prognosis of these disorders. Comparing patterns of expression between normal and neoplastic cells allows accurate detection of very small numbers of residual leukaemic cells. Beyond its diagnostic value, some chimeric McAbs, such as those recognizing the CD20, CD22, CD23, CD25, CD33 and CD52 antigens (CD = cluster of differentiation), are used *in vivo* as therapeutic agents; therefore, their estimation in the leukaemic cells has become an important clinical issue.

In addition to the increasing availability of a large number of McAbs that identify antigens in haemopoietic cells that are lineage-specific or restricted to particular levels of haemopoietic differentiation, a number of immunological techniques have been developed that allow the following:

1. Detection of both membrane and cytoplasmic or nuclear antigens by flow cytometry in previously fixed and stabilized cells
2. Simultaneous multicolour immunostaining with directly labelled McAb with different fluorochromes
3. Analysis of whole blood or bone marrow specimens without requiring the separation of mononuclear cells
4. Quantification of the number of molecules of an antigen at a single-cell level
5. Analysis or quantification of selected cell populations, such as the estimation of CD34-positive stem cells by the application of immunological gating strategies using CD45-labelled cells or gating on CD19-positive or CD3-positive cells for lymphoid disorders.

Although the diagnostic role of immunophenotyping is well-recognized, results should always be interpreted in the light of morphology and other relevant clinical and laboratory data.

This chapter includes descriptions of the following:

1. Techniques currently used for immunophenotyping
2. Panels of markers useful for the diagnosis of acute leukaemia, chronic lymphoproliferative disorders and plasma cell neoplasms and the rationale for their selection
3. Immunophenotypic profiles that characterize the different types of haematological neoplasms
4. New McAbs (e.g. against the tumour-suppressor gene product p53, CD38 and ZAP70), which are relevant for prognosis in lymphoid disorders
5. Multicolour immunophenotyping and gating strategies to detect minimal residual disease (MRD).

METHODS FOR THE STUDY OF IMMUNOLOGICAL MARKERS

There are several techniques for identifying antigens expressed by leucocytes:

1. Flow cytometry to test suspensions of viable cells or fixed cells
2. Immunocytochemistry to examine cells on cytospin-made slides or directly on blood or bone marrow films
3. Immunohistochemistry to study cells in frozen or paraffin-embedded sections from bone marrow biopsy specimens or other haemopoietic tissues.

The first two methods are used in haematology laboratories dealing with analysis of leukaemic samples, and the last is used, as a rule, in histopathology laboratories.

Preparation of the Specimens and Cell Separation

Nowadays, immunophenotyping is routinely performed on whole blood or bone marrow specimens incorporating a red cell lysis step, but isolated mononuclear cells can also be used.

The mononuclear cell fraction contains lymphocytes, monocytes and blasts and excludes neutrophils and erythrocytes. Methods for separating mononuclear cells include density gradient centrifugation with Ficoll-Triosil, Hypaque or Lymphoprep.

Ficoll-Gradient Method of Separation

Dilute 10 ml of anticoagulated (e.g. heparinized or ethylenediaminetetra-acetic acid, EDTA-anticoagulated) blood with an equal volume of phosphate buffered saline (PBS), pH 7.3 (see p. 622) or Hanks' solution. Add 10 ml of the diluted blood, drop by drop, to 7.5 ml of Lympho-prep (Nycomed) and then centrifuge for 30 min at

2000 rpm (approx. 500 g). This results in three visible layers: a top layer of plasma; an interphase layer of mononuclear cells; and a layer of red cells and neutrophils at the bottom. After removing the plasma, pipette the mononuclear cell layer into another tube and wash three times with Hanks' solution or tissue culture medium.

Red Blood Cell Lysing Methods

Blood and bone marrow samples are treated with a hypotonic erythrocyte lysing solution such as ammonium chloride-based (e.g. Easylyse Dako) or other commercially available solutions (e.g. FACS lysing solution, BD Biosciences). The red blood cells can be lysed either before or after incubation with the McAb (see below) without loss of fractions of mononuclear cells.

The time of incubation with the lysing reagent is important because prolonged exposure may alter the forward and side light scatter (FSC/SSC) patterns, whereas exposure that is too brief leaves red cells intact, resulting in excess debris and inaccurate results.

Prior to incubation with the lysing solution, the white cell count of the blood or bone marrow specimen should be estimated and, if necessary, the sample should be diluted to a maximum white cell concentration of $25–30 \times 10^9$ cells/l.

Multicolour Flow Cytometry Methods

There have been considerable improvements in flow cytometry instrumentation in recent years with the introduction of more lasers, more powerful computers and novel software for data acquisition and analysis

At the same time, the introduction of a large number of novel fluorochromes and the application of new McAbs has led to multiparametric immunophenotyping of cells, facilitating the accurate identification of normal and abnormal cell populations. Such advances have led to an increase in the complexity of data obtained and a subsequent increase in the comprehensiveness of the knowledge obtained by the flow cytometrist interpreting such data.[1]

Detection of membrane antigens

Multicolour flow cytometry:

1. Stain–Lyse–Wash (Fig. 16.1): Label tubes with the name of the patient, type of specimen, laboratory number and the combination of fluorochrome-conjugated McAb to be used including isotypic controls; isotypic controls are mouse immunoglobulin (Ig) of the same isotype as the McAbs but with no antigen specificity. Pipette 100 µl of the specimen (whole peripheral blood or bone marrow) into a tube.

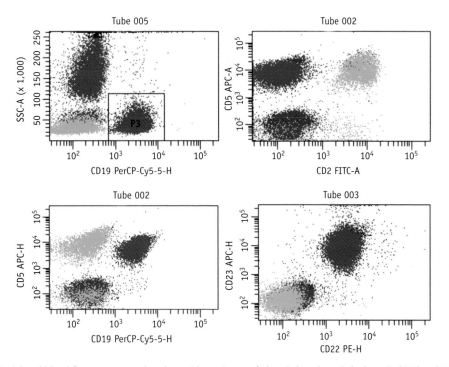

Figure 16.1 Peripheral blood flow cytometry dot plots with a mixture of chronic lymphocytic leukaemia (CLL) and T lymphocytes. P3 shows a gate on CD19-positive lymphocytes (blue). The CD19-positive lymphocytes also express CD5, CD22 and CD23. T lymphocytes (green) show positivity for CD2 and CD5. Red population correspond to granulocytes – they are negative for B and T markers.

Add the appropriate volume of McAb combination labelled with the specific fluorochrome conjugates stated in the laboratory protocol. There are more than a dozen fluorochrome conjugates that can be used for immunophenotyping and indeed some instruments and protocols can utilize up to 20–25 colours in the same tube. The limitations on which fluorochrome combination can be employed will depend on the number of lasers and detectors available in the instrument configuration. The volume of McAbs ranges from 5 to 20 μl, according to the manufacturer's instructions.

Incubate in the dark at room temperature for 15 min.

Add 1 ml of lysing solution (commercially available) and leave for 10 min in the dark at room temperature. Centrifuge for 5 min at 2000 rpm and discard the supernatant.

Add 2 ml of PBS (pH 7.3) containing 0.02% sodium azide, 0.02% bovine serum albumin (BSA) and 0.01% EDTA (PBS-azide-BSA). Centrifuge for 5 min at 2000 rpm and discard the supernatant. Repeat this step one more time.

Resuspend the cells in 0.2–0.5 ml of sheath fluid solution and acquire data on the flow cytometer.

2. Stain–Lyse–No Wash: This method utilizes the same procedure as the previous methodology but after incubation with the lysing solution, data from the sample are acquired on the flow cytometer. This method is ideal for samples with paucity of cells because it minimizes cell loss during the centrifugation of the washing step.

3. Lyse–Stain–Wash: Label tube with the patient's name, laboratory number and specimen. Add 5 to 10 ml of peripheral blood or bone marrow and add the same volume of ammonium chloride-based lysing solution; mix gently and incubate for 10 min at room temperature. After incubation, centrifuge the tube for 5 min at 300 g, discard supernatant after centrifugation and resuspend the cell pellet in 10 ml of PBS-azide-BSA. Repeat this washing procedure once more. If the cell pellet still contains red cells the lysing step can be repeated.

Finally, resuspend the cell pellet in 10 ml of PBS-azide-BSA and perform a white cell count. Aliquot a volume of cell suspension containing $1-2 \times 10^6$/tube. If the number of cells in the specimen is not enough for the ideal amount of cells per tube, aliquot the specimen equally between all the tubes. Add appropriate volume of McAb, incubate in the dark, repeat washing procedure and resuspend in 0.2–0.5 ml of sheath fluid. Acquire data on the flow cytometer.

Rationale for choosing antibody panels

There are different strategies for choosing which antibody panel to use, such as: (1) using a screening panel of McAbs followed by a more targeted panel according to the screening results; (2) choosing an acute leukaemia or a lymphoproliferative panel according to the suspected/referral diagnosis; (3) deciding on a specific panel of McAbs following morphological assessment of a film of the specimen after staining with May–Grünwald–Giemsa.

Detection of Surface Immunoglobulin

Lymphoproliferative disorders of mature B cells are distinguished from their normal counterparts by the identifications of two main types of phenotypic abnormalities: surface immunoglobulin light chain restriction and aberrant B-cell antigen expression (Fig. 16.2).

The method of detection of surface heavy and light chain immunoglobulins by flow cytometry differs from the one used to detect other surface antigens. This is because the interpretation of staining for kappa/lambda and heavy chains can be made more difficult by the presence of non-specific staining giving rise to either false positivity or negativity which can be misleading. This non-specific staining may be due to cytophilic antibodies binding to Fc receptors (monocytes and some lymphocytes) or to coating of antibodies to cell membranes of damaged or dying cells.

To overcome this problem, there are several options: the specimen can be washed with an isotonic solution prior to staining for the surface immunoglobulins. Non-specific staining can also be minimized by incubating the cells with serum prior to staining.

This phenomenon can be excluded by gating on B cells during data analysis, for instance assessing the surface immunoglobulins on a CD19+/CD45+ gate.

Finally, some B-cell lymphoproliferative disorders such as chronic lymphocytic leukaemia (CLL) may express surface immunoglobulin very weakly. It is preferable to use polyclonal antibodies to detect light chain restriction in these cases

There are two methods suitable for detecting surface Ig in blood and bone marrow cells, according to whether a PBS wash or a lysing procedure is used as the first step.

Method 1: Wash–Stain–Lyse–Wash

Label tubes with the name of the patient, type of specimen, laboratory number and the polyclonal or/and McAbs.

Pipette 100 µl of the specimen (blood or bone marrow) into a tube.

Add 2 ml of PBS-azide-BSA kept at 37°C and centrifuge for 5 min at 2000 rpm. Using a pipette, carefully remove and discard the supernatant. Repeat the procedure and resuspend the specimen in 50 µl of PBS-azide-BSA.

Add the appropriate McAb (or polyclonal antisera) combination, e.g. anti-kappa and anti-lambda, CD19,

Figure 16.2 Surface immunoglobulin light chain staining. (A) Dot plot showing strong expression of lambda light chain in a case of follicular lymphoma. (B) By contrast, weak/dim expression of lambda light chain in a case of CLL (mixture of CLL cells and T lymphocytes). Cells are negative with anti-kappa in both cases.

CD45; anti-kappa, CD19, CD45; anti-lambda, CD19, CD45; or (5-colour option) anti-kappa, anti-lambda CD19, CD5 and CD45. The volume of the McAb is usually between 5 and 20 µl, according to the manufacturer's instructions. Incubate in the dark at room temperature for 15 min. Add 1 ml of ammonium chloride-based lysing solution (commercially available) and incubate for 10 min at room temperature.

Add 1 ml of PBS-azide-BSA or Hanks' solution, centrifuge for 5 min at 2000 rpm and discard the supernatant. Repeat this step.

Resuspend cells in 0.2–0.5 ml of sheath fluid solution (e.g. Isoton).

Acquire data on a flow cytometer.

Method 2: Lyse–Stain–Wash

Label tubes with the name of the patient, type of specimen, laboratory number and the multicolour McAb combination as described above.

Pipette 100 μl of the specimen (whole blood or bone marrow).

Add 2 ml of ammonium chloride-based lysing solution, incubate for 10 min at room temperature and wash twice in PBS-azide-BSA as above.

Add the appropriate volume of McAb combination, according to the manufacturer's instructions.

Incubate in the dark for 15 min at room temperature. Add 2 ml of PBS-azide-BSA or Hanks' solution, centrifuge for 5 min at 2000 rpm and discard the supernatant. Repeat this step.

Resuspend cells in 0.2–0.5 ml of sheath fluid (e.g. Isoton) and acquire data on a flow cytometer.

Detection of Intracellular Antigens

This method is applied to the identification of antigens that are expressed within the cell, i.e. in the cytoplasm or nucleus. For example, intracellular immunoglobulins, MPO, lysozyme, CD3, CD79a, BCL2, TdT and Ki67 can all be detected by this method.

There are several commercially available kits containing solutions to fix and permeabilize cells to detect cytoplasmic or nuclear antigens. Overall, these reagents have little or no effect on the light scatter pattern, although their reliability and consistency for detecting particular nuclear and cytoplasmic antigens may vary.[2,3]

The kits contain two solutions: solution A is the fixing agent based on a paraformaldehyde solution and solution B is a lysing agent based on a combination of a lysing solution and a detergent.

The methods follow the manufacturer's kit instructions. Details that follow are for the method using Fix and Perm (Invitrogen).[4]

Method

Label tubes with the name of the patient, type of specimen, laboratory number and the McAb.

Pipette 100 μl of the specimen (whole blood or bone marrow) into a tube.

Add 100 μl of solution A (fixative) and incubate at room temperature for 15 min.

Wash twice in PBS-azide-BSA, centrifuging for 5 min at 2000 rpm.

Add 100 μl of solution B (lysing agent) and the appropriate amount of fluorochrome-conjugated McAb.

Incubate in the dark at room temperature for 15 min.

Wash twice in PBS-azide-BSA, centrifuging for 5 min at 2000 rpm.

Resuspend in 0.2–0.5 ml of sheath fluid solution (e.g. Isoton).

Acquire data on a flow cytometer.

Simultaneous Detection of Cytoplasmic/Nuclear and Membrane Antigens

Method

The first step in simultaneous detection of cytoplasmic/nuclear and membrane antigens (Fig. 16.3) involves immunostaining for membrane antigen detection, followed by cytoplasmic or nuclear antigen staining.

Label tubes with the name of the patient, type of specimen, laboratory number and the McAb.

Pipette 100 μl of specimen (whole blood or bone marrow) into a tube.

Add the appropriate fluorochrome-conjugated McAb, to detect the membrane antigen.

Incubate at room temperature for 15 min.

Without washing, add 100 μl of solution A (fixative) and incubate at room temperature for 15 min. Continue with the steps described earlier for cytoplasmic antigen detection.

Data Analysis Strategies with Multiparametric Flow Cytometry

Multiparametric data including staining with several fluorochromes and the scatter properties of cells is currently used to accurately identify different cell populations and distinct disease entities.

Flow cytometry immunophenotyping provides not only a screening for haemato-oncological disorders but also is an indispensable diagnostic tool. It can identify cells from different lineages, it can determine their stage of maturation, it can discriminate normal cells from abnormal by the assessment of antigen expression or the lack of it and it can quantify the tumour infiltration. It can estimate the presence of minimal residual disease by comparing patterns of expression with that seen in normal counterparts.

Traditionally flow cytometry data was analysed in bivariate plots of two- or three-colour analyses with the application of electronic gates based on the scatter characteristic of cells.

As computers became more powerful, other strategies have been developed employing 'immunological' and sequential gating associated with forward and side scatter properties. For instance, in cases of acute leukaemia the preferred routine practice is to gate blast populations based on the side scatter properties and CD45 expression rather than gating solely on forward and side scatter plots.

Similarly in cases of B-cell disorders, it is more informative to gate on CD19-positive cells and side scatter and for T-cell disorders to apply a gate on CD3-positive cells and side scatter. Multicolour flow cytometry gating of plasma cells is performed to differentiate between clonal and normal plasma cells by combining sequential gating on the CD45-negative/CD138-positive cells and then to look specifically at other antigen expression on these cells.

Figure 16.3 Flow cytometry dot plots showing CD45 gating and intracytoplasmic staining with the blast population (CD45 weak expression) highlighted in red and lymphocytes in green. TdT/CD19 plot showing simultaneous staining for membrane CD19 and intranuclear TdT. Cytoplasmic μ/CD22 plot showing simultaneous staining for intracytoplasmic markers; blasts are cμ-negative/cCD22-positive. Lysozyme/CD79a plot showing expression of CD79a in blasts.

Finally, a very important use of multicolour flow cytometry analysis strategies is in the detection of minimal residual disease of acute and chronic leukaemias. The sensitivity of these methods may be as good as 0.04% acquiring 50 000 events or 50 to 100 events of interest and increases as more events are acquired.

Until recently, advances made in computing capabilities, and the increased availability in fluorochrome conjugates, had not been matched by the developments in analysis software. However, new independent targeted analysis programmes to deal with these limitations have now been developed, which include novel tactics for the analysis of multiparametric flow cytometry data such as the software developed by the Euroflow consortium.[5]

Quantification of Antigens

Fluorescence quantification is defined as the measurement of the intensity of staining of cells by flow cytometry to provide an absolute value for the light intensity it measures.[6,7]

Quantification of fluorescence is performed by comparing cell fluorescence with an external standard by using different commercially available beads. The following areas will be covered in this section:

1. Staining of cells and beads
2. Acquisition of data
3. Quantification: calculation of the antigen binding capacity (ABC) or molecules of soluble fluorochrome (MESF) values.

Staining of cells and beads

There are three essential requirements for successful quantification: namely (a) the McAb has to be applied at saturating amounts both to the beads and to the cells in the specimen; (b) the same reagent from a specified company and at the same dilution should be used for the test and for any subsequent tests; and (c) the instrument fluorescence setting should be maintained unchanged once the beads have been run and analysis of the unknown sample should be carried out at the same settings.

The type of bead depends on the procedure used for the sample preparation. The beads are commercially available in kits, which usually comprise two tubes. One tube contains four types of beads with four different levels of fluorescence uptake: one very dim, one very bright and two intermediate; the other tube contains blank (non-fluorescent beads) (Fig. 16.4).

Acquisition of data

The first step involves acquisition of data relating to the beads on a flow cytometer. The data from a single tube

Marker	Left, Right	Events	% Gated	% Total	Peak	Peak Ch
All	1, 9910	1931	100.00	100.00	36	1
M1	2, 8	216	11.19	11.19	6	2
M2	25, 42	292	15.12	15.12	11	31
M3	71, 121	295	15.28	15.28	12	85
M4	262, 414	355	18.38	18.38	18	310
M5	730, 1114	340	17.61	17.61	19	842

Figure 16.4 Beads for antigen quantification. Upper: Gate used for the acquisition of the beads to eliminate doublets. Lower: Beads fluorescence intensity showing five peaks: blank (M1); dim (M2); bright (M5); and intermediate (M3 and M4).

with beads are sufficient for quantification with FCSC Quantum Cellular beads (Bangs Laboratories, IN, USA) and QIFIKIT beads (Dako, Glostrup, Denmark). With quantum simply cellular (QSC) beads (Bangs Laboratories, IN, USA), where a tube is run for each McAb, the tube with the beads for that particular McAb should be run first followed by all the relevant tubes with beads for each of the different McAbs.

To bring the beads into the FSC/SSC dot plot, the SSC voltage must be decreased more than that of the cells. There may be some doublets if the tube is not shaken vigorously and these are excluded by placing a tight gate around the beads and acquiring the data only for these gated beads.

The instrument should be set up so that the fluorescence signal of the tube with the blank (unlabelled) beads is located in the region between 0 and 10^1 and four other peaks of fluorescence are seen along the axis of the relevant fluorochrome. When the fluorescence voltage is established, these settings should be maintained throughout the rest of the analysis of the unknown samples. With QSC, the appropriate settings for each individual McAb must be used.

The data for the samples are then obtained. With the FCSC Quantum Cellular and QIFIKIT, only one set of beads is required because the same fluorescence standard curve can be used for the different McAbs to be quantified (e.g. CD5, CD19, CD4, CD8). With QSC, one set of fluorescence beads is stained for each McAb. The samples for a particular McAb should be run with the fluorescence settings obtained from beads stained with the corresponding McAb, so that one fluorescence standard curve should be obtained for each McAb. Thus, one curve is required with CD5-stained beads for all CD5-stained samples; one curve is required with CD19-stained beads for CD19-stained samples and so on.

Quantification: calculation of ABC or MESF values

Relevant software is provided with the quantification kits. These programs are user friendly and take into account the make of the instrument, the voltage used for the sample, the fluorochrome used and the source of the McAb. When the data obtained from the flow cytometer are entered, a standard curve is automatically produced. The standard calibration curve is produced when the values of the peak channels of the blank and the other four peaks obtained from the flow cytometer are entered into the program. The known number of molecules of fluorochrome obtained from the supplier of the beads is also entered into the program. The peak values for the unknown sample and one of the negative control samples are obtained by running them at the same fluorescence setting as the beads. When the peak value obtained with the sample is entered into the program, the ABC/MESF value of the unknown sample is calculated and the data are saved. For the final estimation of the ABC or MESF, the ABC or MESF value of the control tube is subtracted from the ABC or MESF value of the marker.

Immunocytochemistry

The most common immunocytochemical techniques are the immunoperoxidase (IP) and the alkaline phosphatase antialkaline phosphatase (APAAP) methods.[8,9] These detect both membrane and intracellular antigens prior to fixation of the preparation. The APAAP method is suitable for use on blood and bone marrow films and permits good preservation of cell morphology. IP is simpler than APAAP and is useful for the study of mature and immature lymphoid cells, but bone marrow samples containing myeloid cells with endogenous peroxidase may give a false-positive reaction unless steps are taken to inhibit the endogenous peroxidase activity. Unfortunately, these procedures may affect cell morphology and thus defeat one of the purposes of the test.

Immunoperoxidase

The IP method can be carried out with directly labelled antibodies (e.g. antihuman Ig conjugated with peroxidase) or by indirect methods using two or three layers. The first layer is a McAb (mouse Ig); the second layer is an antimouse Ig antibody conjugated with horseradish peroxidase; a third layer is a complex of peroxidase and antiperoxidase, which binds to the second layer and is used to reinforce the reaction. The reaction is completed by testing for peroxidase, using diaminobenzidine (DAB).

Method

Prepare cytocentrifuge slides and allow them to dry for at least 6–8 h at room temperature. If not used immediately, they should be wrapped in aluminium foil and stored at –20°C. Before testing, frozen material must be thawed at room temperature for 30 min. Make a ring around the chosen area using a diamond pencil.

Fix the slides in pure acetone for 10 min. If they have been kept at room temperature for more than 3 days, fix them for only 5 min.

Dry in air and then surround the marked area with a silicone ring (Dako pen, Dako Cytomation, or Sigmacote, Sigma-Aldrich).

Incubate for 30 min in a moist chamber with 30 µl of McAb diluted in PBS. The dilution of the McAb should be titrated in the individual laboratory for each batch of reagent, using known positive and negative controls.

Wash (flush) carefully with PBS (pH 7.3). Without allowing the slides to dry, add the second-layer antibody immediately after the second wash.

Incubate for 30 min with 30 µl of peroxidase-conjugated rabbit antimouse Ig antibody (Dako) diluted 1:20 in PBS (pH 7.3) containing 2% human AB serum.

Wash (flush) carefully with PBS (pH 7.3) twice as indicated earlier.

Incubate for 30 min in a moist chamber with 30 µl of peroxidase-labelled swine antirabbit antibody (Dako) diluted 1:20 in PBS (pH 7.3) containing 2% human AB serum.

Wash (flush) carefully with PBS (pH 7.3) twice as explained earlier.

Prepare an IP solution of 30 mg of DAB with 30% hydrogen peroxide in 50 ml of PBS; filter and pour into a coupling jar. Immerse the slides in this solution and incubate for 10 min at room temperature in the dark.

Note that the peroxidase substrate (DAB) is carcinogenic and must be handled with safety precautions, using a fume cupboard and gloves. As an alternative safer procedure, tablets of DAB, which are available commercially (Dako), can be dissolved in PBS.

Rinse in distilled water.
Counterstain with Harris haematoxylin for 10–20 s.
Wash in tap water for 2 min.
Wipe off excess water, let the slides dry in the air and mount with DPX (disterene resin dibutylphthalate in xylene).

For assessment of the reactivity with anti-TdT or other rabbit polyclonal antibodies, carry out an additional incubation for 30 min with a mouse anti-rabbit Ig antibody diluted 1:20 in PBS (pH 7.3) with 2% human AB serum prior to the incubation with the second layer of peroxidase-conjugated rabbit antimouse Ig antibody.

Interpretation

A positive reaction is identified by light microscopy as a dark brown deposit.

Immunoalkaline Phosphatase Antialkaline Phosphatase

The APAAP method involves several steps that can be applied to peripheral blood and bone marrow films. The stages include incubation with the McAb, incubation with a rabbit antimouse Ig antibody and incubation with immune complexes of APAAP. The second and third steps can be repeated to reinforce the reaction.

Method

Make films or cytocentrifuge slides and let them dry for at least 6–8 h. If not used immediately, wrap the slides in aluminium foil and store at −20°C. If frozen, thaw at room temperature for 30 min before carrying out the test. Make a ring around the chosen area using a diamond pencil. To test more than one McAb in the same slide, several rings can be marked.

Fix in pure cold acetone for 10 min. If the slides have been kept at room temperature for more than 72 h, fix them for only 5 min.

Allow to dry in the air.

When using peripheral blood or bone marrow films, wash around the encircled areas with a cotton stick wet with PBS to remove the adjacent red blood cells.

Surround the marked areas with a silicone ring (Dako pen or Sigmacote).

Incubate for 30 min with 30 µl of McAb diluted in Tris-buffered saline (TBS) 0.05 mol/l, pH 7.6. The appropriate dilution of the McAb must be determined by titrating each batch of reagent, using known positive and negative controls.

For all subsequent procedures, the slides must not be allowed to dry and incubation must be carried out in a moist chamber.

Wash (flush) carefully with TBS 0.05 mol/l and, immediately after the wash, add 20 µl of the second layer consisting of a rabbit antimouse Ig (Dako) diluted in TBS 0.05 mol/l with 2% human AB serum.

Incubate for 30 min at room temperature in a moist chamber. Wash (flush) again with TBS.

Incubate for 45 min with 100 µl of mouse APAAP complexes (Dako) diluted 1:60 in TBS 0.05 mol/l.

Wash (flush) again with TBS.

Cover the circles with the filtered APAAP developing solution for 15–20 min.

Rinse in distilled water.

Counterstain with Harris haematoxylin for 10–20 s.

Wash in tap water for 2 min.

Wipe off excess water and mount with Glycergel (Dako) or another water-soluble mounting medium.

Do not use DPX to cover preparations because the reaction will be faint or will become negative.

For estimation of the reactivity with anti-TdT or other polyclonal rabbit antibody, carry out a further incubation step with a mouse antirabbit Ig antibody diluted 1:20 in TBS prior to the incubation with the second layer.

Preparation of buffers and solutions

TBS 0.05 M, pH 7.6 (to wash and dilute McAb). Make a stock solution with 60.57 g of tris-hydroxymethyl-methylamine in 500 ml of distilled water. Adjust pH to 7.6 with 385 ml of 1 N HCl. Add distilled water to 1 litre and store at 4°C.

To prepare the working solution, dilute the stock solution 1:10 in 9 g/l NaCl.

TBS 0.1 M, pH 8.2 (to dilute the substrate). Make a stock solution with 1.21 g of Tris and 80 ml of water. Adjust pH to 8.2 with 4.8 ml of 1 N HCl. Add water to 100 ml (this solution can be stored for 1 month at 4°C).

Developing solution (substrate). Mix, in the following order, 20 mg of naphthol AS-MX phosphate (Sigma-Aldrich), 2 ml of N,N-dimethylformamide (Merck), 98 ml of Tris buffer 0.1 mol/l and 24 mg of levamisole (Sigma-Aldrich).

Store in glass flasks at −20°C in 5 ml aliquots.

Thaw immediately before use; add 5 mg of fast red TR salt (Sigma-Aldrich) per vial and filter.

The developing solution is also available commercially as a kit.

Immunological Markers in Acute Leukaemia

Panel of McAb Useful for Diagnosis and Classification

Although there are a large number of McAb-recognizing antigens of haemopoietic cells, for practical reasons a well-defined set of reagents needs to be selected for the study of cases of acute leukaemia. The set of markers described here have been largely selected in accordance with the recommendations of the European Group for the Immunological Classification of Leukaemias (EGIL), the British Committee for Standards in Haematology and the World Health Organization (WHO) classification.[10–12]

An initial McAb panel should help to distinguish acute myeloid leukaemia (AML) from acute lymphoblastic leukaemia (ALL) and further classify ALL into B- or T-cell lineage (Table 16.1). This panel is constituted as follows:

1. B-lymphoid markers: CD19, CD10, CD20 and cytoplasmic CD22 and CD79a
2. T-lymphoid markers: CD2, CD7 and cytoplasmic CD3
3. Myeloid markers: CD13, CD33, CD117 and cytoplasmic myeloperoxidase MPO
4. Non-lineage-specific markers, which are expressed in haemopoietic progenitor cells: CD34, HLA-Dr and TdT.

Table 16.1 Panel of monoclonal antibodies for the diagnosis of acute leukaemias

	ALL		AML
	B-lineage	**T-lineage**	
First-line	CD19, CD22, CD79a, CD10[a], CD20	CD7, CD2, cCD3	CD13, CD33, CD117, anti-MPO
		TdT, HLA-Dr, CD34	
Second-line	cμ,[a] SmIg	CD1a, CD5, CD4, CD8 anti-TCR	CD41, CD42, CD62p, anti-glycophorin A (CD235a)

[a]CD10 and cμ are not essential for a diagnosis of B-lineage ALL, but they can be useful in paediatric cases to identify common-ALL, pro-B-ALL and pre-B-ALL.

Optional markers: CD14, antilysozyme, CD36 and CD64 to identify a monocytic component in AML.

ALL, acute lymphoblastic leukaemia; AML, acute myeloid leukaemia; CD, cluster of differentiation; c, cytoplasmic; MPO, myeloperoxidase; TdT, terminal deoxynucleotidyl transferase; TCR, T-cell receptor.

Two aspects that need to be considered are the lineage specificity of the antigen and whether it is expressed in the membrane or the cytoplasm. Some markers are highly specific and sensitive for a particular lineage (e.g. CD3 for T cells and anti-MPO for myeloid cells), whereas others (e.g. CD10, CD13 and CD7) are less lineage specific. Nevertheless, the latter may support a lymphoid or myeloid commitment in cases that are negative with the most specific markers or when results are equivocal. The second aspect to take into account is that the most specific markers are either expressed earlier in the cytoplasm than in the membrane during cell differentiation (e.g. CD3),[13] or they are only detectable in the cytoplasm (e.g. MPO). Markers of haemopoietic precursors such as TdT or CD34, although not essential, are helpful when problems of differential diagnosis arise between acute leukaemias and lymphomas in leukaemia phase.

A second set of McAb is necessary to classify ALL further into the various subtypes and to identify rare cases of AML derived from cells committed to the megakaryocytic and erythroid lineages. This set comprises cμ staining in B-lineage ALL; CD1a, CD4, CD5, CD8 and anti-TCR in T-lineage ALL; and, in AML, antibodies that detect membrane glycoproteins present in platelets and megakaryocytes or glycophorin A expressed by erythroid precursors.

Identification of cell reactivity with other McAb may include CD14, antilysozyme, CD64 and CD36. Although CD14 and antilysozyme are not specific for acute monoblastic leukaemias, both are more frequently expressed during monocytic differentiation. CD36 is often expressed in poorly differentiated erythroid leukaemias. Although this marker is not specific for erythroid precursors, being expressed also in monoblasts and megakaryocytic cells, when considered together with reactivity with other McAb (e.g. negative for HLA-Dr, antiplatelet McAb and MPO), it is highly indicative of erythroid acute leukaemia.

McAbs against non-haemopoietic cells rarely need to be included when performing immunophenotyping for the diagnosis of acute leukaemias. However, rare cases of neuroblastoma or oat cell carcinoma can mimic acute leukaemia in the bone marrow and in such cases antineuroblastoma McAb and the pan-leucocyte marker CD45 may help in establishing the correct diagnosis.

Other markers that are useful for the characterization of acute leukaemias, although not routinely used, are the following:

1. A McAb that recognizes the altered distribution of promyelocytic protein (PML) in cases of acute promyelocytic leukaemia with t(15;17). Although PML is expressed in normal myeloid cells and in blasts from other subtypes of AML, the pattern of expression, e.g. multiparticulate or cytoplasmic in the cases with t(15;17), is different from that of normal myeloid cells or myeloblasts of other types of AML. The latter are either negative with anti-PML or have the protein expressed in larger nuclear bodies. The reactivity with anti-PML needs to be assessed under fluorescence microscopy or light microscopy with an immunocytochemical technique.[14]

2. The McAbs 7.1/NG2 and NG1 that are preferentially expressed in a subset of pro-B or early B-cell ALL with 11q23 rearrangement[15] and in a proportion of AML with features of monocytic differentiation (irrespective of the presence of 11q23 rearrangement).[16–18]

3. The McAb CD56, CD123 and CD94 to identify rare cases of blastic plasmacytoid dendritic cell neoplasm and natural killer (NK) cell leukaemia/lymphoma in cases without evidence of myeloid and lymphoid commitment with specific cell markers.[12]

Immunological Classification of Acute Leukaemias

There are two major differentiation lineages in the lymphoid system, B and T, and lymphoblastic leukaemias arise from B- or T-precursor cells. Table 16.2 illustrates that only a few McAbs react positively with the most immature lymphoblasts; with maturation, however, more McAbs become reactive. Thus, to demonstrate all cases of leukaemia of a particular lineage, it is always important to include in the battery of McAbs those that will detect the most immature cells. B-lineage ALL is defined by the expression of at least two B-cell antigens, CD79a, CD19, CD10 and/or CD22; T-lineage ALL is defined by the expression of nuclear TdT and CD3. CD7 is also consistently positive in T-ALL. However, the expression of CD7 does not by itself define T-ALL because this McAb is positive in about 20% of cases of AML.

B- and T-lineage ALL can be further subclassified on the basis of cell differentiation or maturation (Table 16.2). Although this subclassification is not essential for diagnosis, it can be useful because of the correlation between certain B-lineage subtypes and molecular cytogenetic and clinical features.

B-lineage ALL can be classified into three subtypes: pro-B-ALL (previously designated null-ALL), common-ALL and pre-B-ALL (Table 16.2). There is some correlation between these immunological subtypes and molecular genetics and prognosis. The majority of infant ALL with t(4;11)(q21;q23) and/or rearrangement of the MLL gene at 11q23 are pro-B-ALL and often express CD15, whereas the common-ALL phenotype is associated with hyperdiploidy or t(12;21) involving the ETV6 (TEL) gene, both associated with a good prognosis. The t(1;19)(q23;p13) is more common in the subset of pre-B-ALL. 'Mature B-ALL' (French-American-British, FAB, L3 ALL) is not classified as ALL in the WHO classification but is included in the group of high-grade, non-Hodgkin lymphomas

Table 16.2 Immunological classification of acute leukaemias[a]

Lymphoblastic leukaemia/lymphomas (ALL) (TdT+)

    B-cell precursor (CD19+ and/or CD79a+ and/or CD22+)

        pro-B-ALL (no expression of other B-cell markers)

        common-ALL (CD10+, cytoplasmic μ−)

        pre-B-ALL (cytoplasmic μ+)

    T-cell precursor (cytoplasmic CD3+, CD7+)[b]

        pro-T-ALL (no expression of other T-cell markers)

        pre-T-ALL (CD2+ and/or CD5+)

        cortical T-ALL (CD1a+)

        mature T-ALL (membrane CD3+)

Acute myeloid leukaemias (AML)

    AML (French-American-British [FAB] M0–M5) (anti-MPO+ and/or CD13+ and/or CD33+ and/or CD117+)

    Pure erythroid leukaemia (anti-glycophorin A+, anti-blood group antigen+, CD36+)

    Megakaryoblastic leukaemias (CD41+, CD42+, CD62P+).

    Blastic plasmacytoid dendritic cell neoplasm

Miscellaneous

    Mixed phenotype acute leukaemias (MPAL) (coexpression of myeloid and lymphoid markers)[c]

    Myeloid antigen positive ALL

    Lymphoid antigen positive AML

    Natural killer (NK) cell lymphoblastic leukaemia/lymphoma

    Acute undifferentiated leukaemia

[a]Adapted from the European Group for the Immunological Characterization of Leukemias (EGIL) classification.
[b]CD4 and CD8 are variably expressed.
[c]Definition of MPAL is described below.
TdT, terminal deoxynucleotidyl transferase; MPO, myeloperoxidase.

subclassified in two subgroups on the basis of the membrane expression of the T-cell receptor (TCR) complex molecules, αβ or γδ.

AML can be defined immunologically by the expression of two or more myeloid markers: CD13, CD33, CD117 and anti-MPO in the absence of lymphoid markers.[10] The most specific marker for the myeloid lineage is MPO followed by CD117; as a rule, both are negative in ALL.[19] There is no marker that allows the distinction between the various FAB subtypes of AML.[20] However, some McAb may be preferentially positive in certain AML subtypes such as CD14, CD64 and antilysozyme in cases with monocytic differentiation, absence of HLA-Dr and CD34 expression in M3 AML or expression of CD19 in M2 AML. Furthermore, immunological markers are essential for the diagnosis of poorly differentiated myeloid leukaemias or M0 AML in which blasts do not show myeloid features by morphology or cytochemistry.[21]

In poorly differentiated leukaemias in which the first panel of lymphoid and myeloid markers does not show positive results, McAb against platelet glycoproteins Ib, the complex IIb/IIIa and IIIa (e.g. CD41, CD42 and CD62P) should be tested to confirm or exclude the diagnosis of acute megakaryoblastic leukaemia,[10] and McAb to glycophorin A or to the red blood cell groups such as Gerbich should be used to confirm or exclude erythroid leukaemias. In addition, the WHO classification now considers a rare form designated blastic plasmacytoid dendritic neoplasm, previously included in the group of blastoid NK neoplasms, under the umbrella of AML. The neoplastic cells are CD4+, CD56+ and CD123+ and 50% of cases are CD68+. Rarely, they express T or myeloid associated markers.[12]

Immunophenotyping facilitates the diagnosis of an unusual form of acute leukaemia designated mixed phenotype acute leukaemia (MPAL). This leukaemia accounts for <5% of cases and is characterized by the coexpression of a constellation of myeloid and lymphoid antigens in the blast cells. The lack of agreement among various workers on the definition of MPAL has made it difficult to establish whether this constitutes a distinct clinicopathological entity. Until recently, the diagnosis of MPAL was based on a scoring system[22,23] proposed by the EGIL group,[10] which aimed to distinguish MPAL from cases of ALL or AML with aberrant expression of a marker from another lineage. In the 2008 WHO classification, the definition of this leukaemia was changed. The myeloid component is defined exclusively by positivity with anti-MPO or a positive cytochemical reaction for MPO and/or by clear evidence of a monocytic component by cytochemistry or immunophenotyping and the T-lymphoid component is defined by the expression of CD3 whether cytoplasmic or membrane. Since there is no marker specific for the B-lymphoid lineage, evidence of B-lymphoid differentiation should be based on the expression of CD19 plus another B-cell marker (CD10, CD22 or

(NHL) because it corresponds to the leukaemic manifestation of Burkitt lymphoma.[12]

T-lineage ALL can also be subdivided into several subgroups according to the stage of differentiation of the lymphoblasts. In the most immature form, or pro-T-ALL, blasts only express CD7 and cytoplasmic CD3; in pre-T-ALL, there is also expression of CD2 or CD5; cortical T-ALL is defined by the expression of CD1a; and in the rare mature T-ALL, blasts express membrane as well as cytoplasmic CD3 (Table 16.2). T-cell-associated antigens such as CD2, CD5, CD4, CD8 and TCR are expressed with variable frequency in the cortical and mature T-ALL; for instance, coexpression of CD4 and CD8, a phenotype characteristic of normal cortical thymocytes, is frequent in cortical T-ALL. In addition, mature T-ALL can be

CD79) or weak/negative CD19 and strong expression of two of the specified B-cell markers. The WHO does not distinguish cases with co-expression of lymphoid and myeloid antigens ('biphenotypic') from those with two separate populations ('bilineal'). Emphasis is made that some AML with recurrent chromosome abnormalities and those with a background of dysplasia should not be diagnosed as MPAL.[12]

In addition to MPAL, the WHO considers natural killer (NK) cell lymphoblastic leukaemia/lymphoma and acute undifferentiated leukaemia under the umbrella of acute leukaemias of ambiguous lineage.[12] NK cell lymphoblastic leukaemia/lymphoma is a provisional entity. The lack of specific NK markers has made establishing a diagnosis difficult in such cases. However, this diagnosis should be considered in cases that are CD56+, CD94+ and CD161+ that may express immature T-cell-associated antigens such as CD7 and even c CD3 epsilon chain but lack Ig and TCR gene rearrangement and provided blastic plasmacytoid dendritic cell neoplasm has been excluded.[12,24] The other rare subgroup is acute undifferentiated leukaemia in which the blasts lack T and myeloid specific markers, do not express B-lymphoid-associated markers and do not have features of other lineages (i.e. megakaryoblastic, erythroid or plasmacytoid dendritic cells). An extensive panel of McAb needs to be used for the diagnosis of this leukaemia. The blasts usually are HLA-Dr+, CD34+ and CD38+ and may be TdT+.

Immunological Markers in Chronic Lymphoproliferative Disorders

Immunophenotyping is essential for the diagnosis and characterization of the lymphoproliferative disorders. Immunological markers enable one to distinguish lymphoblastic leukaemias and lymphoblastic lymphomas, which are usually TdT-positive, from mature or chronic lymphoid neoplasms, which are consistently TdT-negative. Immunophenotyping also demonstrates whether the malignant cells are of B- or T-lymphoid nature and demonstrates clonality in the B-cell cases. Markers may also be useful to confirm or establish the diagnosis of certain entities that show distinct immunological profiles and others may provide prognostic information.

Panel of McAb for Diagnosis and Classification

The diagnosis of a B- or T-cell disorder requires a small but comprehensive battery of McAb. It is convenient to use a two-step procedure with an initial panel applicable to all cases and a second panel based on the results with the first panel and the tentative diagnosis by clinical features and/or cell morphology (Table 16.3).[11,25]

Table 16.3 Panel of monoclonal antibodies for the diagnosis of lymphoid disorders

	B CELL	T CELL
First-line	SmIg (kappa/lambda), CD19, CD23, FMC7, SmCD79b, SmCD22, CD5[a], CD20[b]	CD2, CD5[a]
Second-line	CD11c, CD25, CD103, CD123, CD38, CD138, cIg	CD3, CD4, CD7, CD8, CD57

[a]B-cell subset and T-cell marker.
Optional markers: CD79a and natural killer associated (e.g. CD16, CD56 and CD11b).
[b]Not in initial panel but added because of relevance to treatment.
c, cytoplasmic; Ig, immunoglobulin; Sm, surface membrane.

The first panel of markers is intended to distinguish B-cell from T-cell disorders, to demonstrate B-cell clonality, to confirm the diagnosis of CLL and to confirm or exclude a non-CLL B-cell neoplasm. It comprises immunostaining with anti-kappa and anti-lambda, CD2 or CD3 (T-cell marker), CD5 (a marker of T cells and a subset of B cells) and four McAbs that detect antigens in subsets of B cells: CD23, FMC7, CD79b against the β chain of the B-cell receptor and membrane CD22. With the two latter reagents, as well as surface Ig, assessment of the fluorescence intensity is important to distinguish between CLL and other B-cell disorders (Fig. 16.4). The results obtained with this set of McAbs can be combined into a scoring system (Table 16.4) to establish the diagnosis of CLL and to distinguish CLL cases with atypical morphology and CLL with increased numbers of prolymphocytes (CLL/PL) from other B-cell diseases such as B-cell prolymphocytic leukaemia (B-PLL) and B-cell lymphomas in

Table 16.4 Scoring system for the diagnosis of chronic lymphocytic leukaemia (CLL)[a]

MARKER	POINTS	
	1	0
CD5	Positive	Negative
CD23	Positive	Negative
FMC7	Negative	Positive
SmIg[b]	Weak	Moderate/strong
CD22/CD79b[b]	Weak/negative	Moderate/strong

[a]Scores for CLL range from 3 to 5, whereas in the other B-cell disorders they range from 0 to 2.
[b]Membrane expression.

leukaemic phase.[25–27] The characteristic profile of CLL is that of a clonal B-cell with weak surface immunoglobulin (SmIg) usually IgM+IgD±, CD5+, CD23+, FMC7− and weak or negative CD79b and CD22.[25–27] FMC7 has been shown to recognize an epitope of CD20 and it has been suggested that this marker could be replaced by CD20 in the diagnostic scoring system for CLL. However, data show that replacement of FMC7 by CD20 results in a decrease in sensitivity of the scoring because most cases of CLL express CD20 weakly.[28] Nevertheless, although CD20 is not particularly useful for diagnosis, it should be incorporated into the panel of markers for chronic lymphoid disorders because it is used increasingly as a therapeutic tool in these conditions. Other markers that may be used include CD200, which appears to be useful in the CD5+ B-cell disorders to distinguish cases of CLL (CD200+) from mantle-cell lymphomas (CD200-),[29] and Ki-67, which allows the estimation of the proliferative rate in cases of high-grade lymphoma.

When the marker profile using the first-line panel of McAb yields a B-cell phenotype not typical of CLL, a second panel of McAb can be used. This is selected in light of the review of the cell morphology, clinical information or other laboratory features. For example, estimation of the cell reactivity with four McAbs (CD11c, CD25, CD103 and CD123) is useful to distinguish hairy cell leukaemia (HCL) from other disorders with circulating villous cells that may be confused with HCL, such as splenic marginal zone lymphoma (SMZL) and the HCL variant. Cells from the majority of HCL cases coexpress three or four of the markers mentioned earlier, whereas SMZL and cells from HCL variant are positive with one or at most two of these markers.[30] Among the four HCL-associated markers, CD123, which recognizes the β chain of the interleukin 3 receptor is the most useful in distinguishing HCL from SMZL and the variant form of HCL. CD123 is consistently expressed in HCL cells, whereas it is negative in the other two conditions.[31]

When the first-line panel of markers suggests a T-cell phenotype (CD2+ or CD3+, CD5±), expression of other T-cell markers such as CD3 (if not already used), CD7, CD4, CD8 and CD57 may need to be investigated. CD25 may be used in cases of suspected adult T-cell leukaemia lymphoma but its expression is not pathognomonic of this disease as it may be positive in other mature T-cell neoplasms. When markers do not indicate either B lineage or T lineage, but cytology is consistent with a lymphoid lineage, testing for NK cell markers should be done.

Unusual situations may occur in the case of plasma cell leukaemia and myeloma, in which the cells are negative with all T-cell and the majority of B-cell markers including surface Ig expression; clonal plasma cells express Ig only in the cytoplasm (with light chain restriction) and are positive with two common antigens, i.e. CD38 bright and CD138 in conjunction with negativity for CD45.[32]

The best approach to differentiate normal from neoplastic plasma cells is a multicolour methodology using CD45 negativity versus CD138 strong positivity as gating strategy. Multicolour flow cytometry staining using CD45, CD38, CD138, CD19, CD56, CD20 and cytoplasmic Ig light chains provides the most sensitive and specific method to distinguish normal from clonal plasma cells. Normal plasma cells are characterized by the expression of CD45, CD19, CD38 and CD138 with polyclonal expression of light chains. Clonal plasma cells are characterized by the expression of CD38, CD138, CD56 and intracytoplasmic light chain restriction with no detection of surface light chains and lack of expression of CD45 and CD19 and often no expression of CD20.

Multiparametric flow cytometry generally recognizes fewer plasma cells than those found in the specimen films and trephine biopsy sections. This may be explained by patchy infiltration and by loss of plasma cells during sample processing for flow cytometry studies due to plasma cell clumping.

Other markers that have diagnostic and prognostic value in chronic lymphoid disorders are described below.

p53 protein

The p53 protein can be detected in cells by immunocytochemistry and flow cytometry with specific antibodies. There is a good correlation between p53 expression point mutation with or without deletion of TP53 genes. It therefore appears that there is no need for gene sequencing to be done on a routine basis because flow cytometry, fluorescence in situ hybridization (FISH) or both provide accurate information of the p53 status.[33] Although not essential for diagnosis, this test may be useful as a prognostic indicator because of its correlation with resistance to purine analogue therapy and disease progression in patients with B-cell disorders, particularly CLL.[33–35]

CD38 and ZAP70 expression

CD38 and ZAP70 are two markers shown to have a major prognostic impact in CLL. The expression of CD38 has emerged as a prognostic factor independent of the immunoglobulin heavy chain (IgHV) mutational status.[36,37] CD38 should be assessed by a triple colour flow cytometry method to ensure that the expression is evaluated in the leukaemic cells. Although the first reports used thresholds of 20–30% CD38+ cells to consider this marker as positive, it has become apparent that there is intra-clonal diversity and that a threshold of 7% is the most reliable and informative in terms of prognosis.[38,39] ZAP70 encodes a tyrosine kinase that is expressed in normal T cells, NK cells and a few B cells. Microarray studies in CLL have shown that the pattern of gene expression is very similar in cases with mutated or unmutated IgHV genes with only minor differences in a few genes. Among these, ZAP70 is preferentially expressed in the cases with unmutated IgHV; thus it was suggested that ZAP70 could be used as a surrogate marker for the IgHV mutational status. To this end, it is important to estimate its expression in purified B-CLL cells by RNA analysis or by a multicolour flow cytometric method that allows the simultaneous assessment of ZAP70 expression in T, NK and CLL cells (Fig. 16.5).[39,40] At present, it is uncertain which is the best threshold (10% or 20%) for ZAP70+ CLL cells to consider that this marker is positive. There is now evidence that ZAP70 is not a surrogate marker for the unmutated IgVH. Discrepant results are seen in up to 30% of cases and the combination of CD38, ZAP70 and IgVH mutations is needed to establish the prognosis of CLL more precisely.[39]

McAb against the Variable Regions of the β TCR and Killer Immunoglobulin Receptors

There is a set of McAb that identifies T lymphocytes that bear the various variable regions of the TCR β and hence might be useful to demonstrate clonality of the T-cell population, particularly in cases with large granular lymphocyte (LGL) lymphocytosis, when molecular studies (e.g. polymerase chain reaction, PCR) cannot easily be performed. There is also a potential role in identifying T-cell clones in patients with hypereosinophilia. A good correlation between flow cytometry and PCR has been demonstrated with flow cytometry able to predict clonality with a sensitivity of 93% and specificity of 80%.[41] McAb that recognize molecules belonging to the Ig superfamily, essentially the killer immunoglobulin receptors (KiRs) clustered under CD158a, CD158b, CD158c and CD158e, can also potentially recognize clonal LGL disorders and are particularly useful in those derived from NK cells in which clonality cannot be established by molecular tests.[42]

McAb Against CD20, CD52 and CD33

The expression of the CD20 and CD52 antibodies should be assessed in patients with lymphoid neoplasms and CD33 in AML in whom antibody therapy with rituximab, alemtuzumab or gemtuzumab ozogamicin, respectively, is contemplated.

Immunological Profiles of Chronic Lymphoproliferative Disorders

The most common immunophenotypes of the B- and T-cell disorders are shown in Tables 16.5 and 16.6. CLL has a phenotype that clearly distinguishes this disease from the other B-cell leukaemias. By contrast, there is overlap on the marker expression in the other B-cell malignancies; for this reason, in cases with a B-cell marker profile different from CLL, the immunophenotypic analysis needs to be interpreted in the light of morphology and other clinical and laboratory information such as histology or genetic analysis to establish the precise diagnosis.[27]

There is no specific immunological profile that distinguishes the various T-cell diseases (Table 16.6). However, expression of CD8 and CD57, with or without expression of NK-associated markers such as CD16 or CD56, is characteristic of T-cell LGL leukaemia, whereas such expression is rarely seen in other conditions.[42] By contrast, coexpression of CD4 and CD8 is almost exclusively seen in approximately 25% of T-cell prolymphocytic leukaemia (T-PLL) (Table 16.6).[43,44] Other markers may also be differentially expressed in various T-cell malignancies. Thus, for example, there is expression of CD25 in adult T-cell leukaemia lymphoma (ATLL); strong reactivity with CD7 in T-PLL;[43–45] expression of granzyme B, TIA-1 or perforins in T-cell or NK-cell LGL leukaemias and TCR γδ in hepatosplenic T-cell lymphoma.[42]

Immunological Markers for the Detection of Minimal Residual Disease

Immunophenotyping can be a useful tool to detect small numbers of residual leukaemic cells in peripheral blood or bone marrow specimens when such cells are not detected by standard morphology or histopathology. Detection of minimal residual disease (MRD) applies to both acute and chronic lymphoid leukaemias; it is likely to have prognostic significance in terms of probability of relapse and in some instances its detection directs further therapy.

This is carried out by multicolour immunofluorescent methods with a combination of McAbs aimed at identifying 'aberrant' phenotypes not present in normal haemopoietic cells and/or by considering the different density in normal and leukaemic cells.[46–48] For example, although normal bone marrows, particularly in infants or when regenerating after therapy, have a minor cell population with a B-cell precursor phenotype (e.g. TdT+, CD10+, CD19+), similar to that of ALL blasts, quantitative studies provide discrimination between the normal precursors (strong TdT and weak CD10 and CD19) and ALL blasts (weak TdT, strong CD10/CD19).[47,48] Similarly, there is a small B-cell population in normal blood and bone marrow that coexpresses CD5, a phenotype characteristic of CLL. However, by estimating the proportions of CD5+ cells within the whole B-cell population (CD19+), it is possible to demonstrate whether cells represent residual leukaemia or normal B-lymphocytes. More recently a standardized multiparameter flow cytometry method has been described for CLL minimal residual disease (MRD). This combines sequential gating, i.e. lymphocytes (G1), CD19+ lymphocytes (G2) and CD5+/CD19+ (G3), with a comparison of the pattern of expression of the following McAbs: CD79b, CD20, CD38, CD81 and CD43 between normal and CLL cells (Fig. 16.6); this has been shown to have a sensitivity of 0.01%.[49]

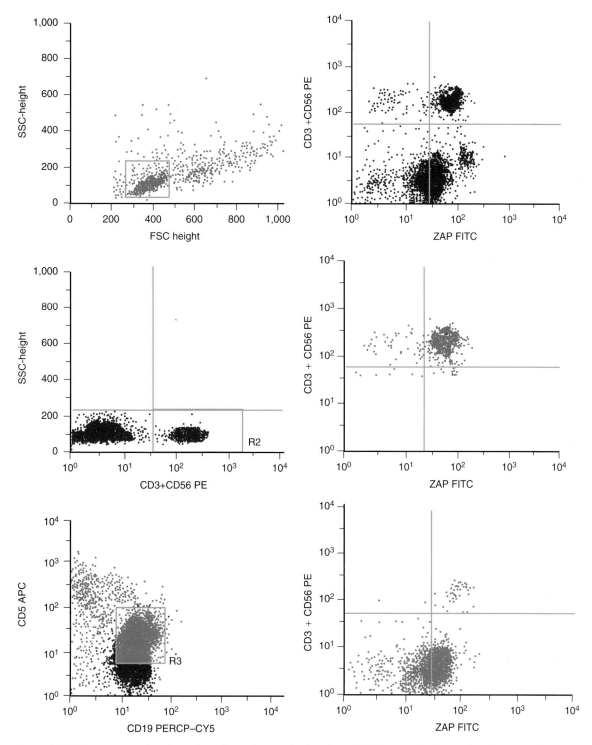

Figure 16.5 Flow cytometry dot plots using a four-colour method to detect ZAP70 expression in T/NK lymphocytes and CLL lymphocytes. Upper plots: Gate on the whole lymphocyte population (left) and the expression of ZAP70 (right). Middle plots: Gate on CD3/CD56-positive cells, which represent T and natural killer cells (left) and the expression of ZAP70 in this population (right). Lower plots: Gate on CD5/CD19 positive cells (CLL cells) (left) and the expression of ZAP70 in this subset (right).

Table 16.5 Membrane markers in mature B-cell disorders (CD2−)

DISEASE	SMlg	CD5	CD23	FMC7	CD22	CD79b
CLL	Weak	++	++	±	Weak/−	Weak/−
B-PLL	Strong	±	−	++	+	++
HCL	Strong	−	−	++	++	+
HCL-variant	Strong	−	−	++	++	+
SMZL	Strong	±	±	++	++	++
FL	Strong	±	±	++	++	++
Mantle cell	Strong	++	−	++	++	++
Large cell	Strong	±	±	++	++	++
MM/PCL[a]	Negative	−	−	−	−	−

[a]Express cytoplasmic immunoglobulin (light chain restricted), CD38, CD79a, CD138 and, with a variable frequency, other B-cell markers; CD19 and CD45 are negative. Scoring: (−), negative or positive in <10% of cases; (±), positive in 10–25% of cases; (+), positive in 25–75% of cases; and (++), positive in >75% of cases.
SmIg, surface immunoglobulin; CLL, chronic lymphocytic leukaemia; B-PLL; B-prolymphocytic leukaemia; HCL, hairy cell leukaemia; SMZL, splenic marginal zone lymphoma; FL, follicular lymphoma; MM/PCL, multiple myeloma/plasma cell leukaemia.

Table 16.6 Immunological markers in mature T-cell disorders (CD2+)

MARKER	T-PLL	LGL LEUKAEMIA[a]	ATLL	SS	PTCL-NOS
CD3	++	++	++	++	+
CD7	++	+	±	+	+
CD4+, CD8−	+	−	++	++	+
CD4+, CD8+	±	−	−	−	+
CD4−, CD8+	±	++	−	−	+
CD4−, CD8−	−	±	−	−	+

[a]A proportion of cases are CD3 negative and have a natural killer phenotype: CD56+, CD16+.
Scoring: (−), negative or positive in <10% of cases; (±), positive in 10–25% of cases; (+), positive in 25–75% of cases; and (++), positive in >75% of cases.
T-PLL, T-prolymphocytic leukaemia; LGL, large granular lymphocyte; ATLL, adult T-cell leukaemia lymphoma; SS, Sézary syndrome; PTCL-NOS, peripheral T-cell lymphoma, not otherwise specified.

Similar multicolour flow cytometry strategy is employed to detect MRD in HCL applying sequential gating making use of scatter properties and the co-expression of CD123 and CD103 to identify the hairy cells, followed by assessment of the expression of other HCL and B-cell markers such as CD11c, CD20, CD25 and light chains (identifying light chain restriction).

In bone marrow tissue sections, occasional residual abnormal leukaemic cells can be highlighted and easily recognized using immunohistochemistry with markers known to react with the leukaemic cells, e.g. CD72 (DBA44) in HCL.[50]

It is essential to identify any phenotypic aberrancy present at diagnosis in an individual patient in order to look for the same leukaemia-associated aberrancy during follow-up.

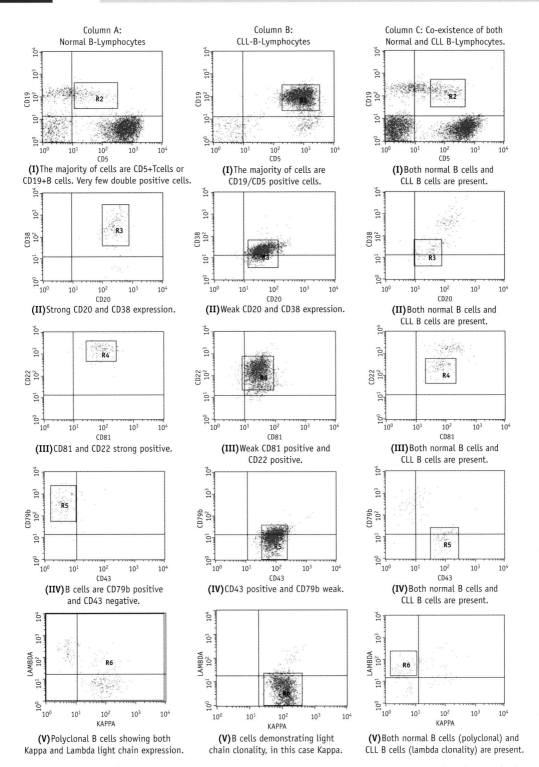

Figure 16.6 Flow cytometry dot plots showing pattern of expressions highlighted in boxes. Normal B lymphocytes (Column A), CLL lymphocytes (Column B) and a mixture of CLL MRD positivity (in the square regions) and normal B lymphocytes (Column C).

REFERENCES

1. Wood BL, Arroz M, Barnett D, et al. Bethesda International Consensus 2006 recommendations on the immunophenotypic analysis of hematolymphoid neoplasia by flow cytometry: optimal reagents and reporting for the flow cytometric diagnosis of hematopoietic neoplasia. *Cytometry B Clin Cytom.* 2007;72(suppl 1):S41–S42.

2. Groeneveld K, Temarvelde JG, van den Beemd MW, et al. Flow cytometry detection of intracellular antigens for immunophenotyping of normal and malignant leukocytes. BTS Technical Report. *Leukemia.* 1996;10:1383–1389.

3. Pizzolo G, Vincenzi C, Nadali G, et al. Detection of membrane and intracellular antigens by flow cytometry following ORTHO PermeaFix fixation. *Leukemia.* 1995;9:226–228.

4. da Costa ES, Peres RT, Almeida J, et al. Harmonization of light scatter and fluorescence flow cytometry profiles obtained after staining peripheral blood leucocytes for cell surface-only versus intracellular antigens with the Fix & Perm reagent. *Cytometry B Clin Cytom.* 2010;78:11–20.

5. Pedreira CE, Costa ES, Barrena S, et al. EuroFlow Consortium. Generation of flow cytometry data files with a potentially infinite number of dimensions. *Cytometry A.* 2008;73:834–846.

6. Bikoue A, George F, Poncelet LW, et al. Quantitative analysis of leukocyte membrane antigen expression: normal adult values. *Cytometry.* 1996;26:137–147.

7. Poncelet P, George F, Papa S, et al. Quantitation of haemopoietic cell antigens in flow cytometry. *Eur J Histochem.* 1996;40(suppl 1):15–32.

8. Erber WN, Mynheer LC, Mason DY. APAAP labelling of blood and bone-marrow samples for phenotyping leukaemia. *Lancet.* 1986;i:761–765.

9. Mason DY, Erber WN. Immunocytochemical labeling of leukemia samples with monoclonal antibodies by the APAAP procedure. In: Catovsky D, ed. *The Leukemic Cell.* Edinburgh: Churchill Livingstone; 1991:196.

10. Bene MC, Castoldi G, Knapp W, et al. Proposals for the immunological classification of acute leukemias. *Leukemia.* 1995;9:1783–1786.

11. Bain BJ, Barnett D, Linch D, et al. Revised guideline on immunophenotyping in acute leukaemias and chronic lymphoproliferative disorders. *Clin Lab Haematol.* 2002;24:1–13.

12. Swerdlow SH, Campo E, Harris NL, et al. *World Health Organization (WHO) Classification of Tumours of Haemopoietic and Lymphoid Tissues.* Lyon: IARC Press; 2008.

13. Janossy G, Coustan-Smith E, Campana D. The reliability of cytoplasmic CD3 and CD22 antigen expression in the immunodiagnosis of acute leukemia: a study of 500 cases. *Leukemia.* 1989;3:170–181.

14. O'Connor SJ, Forsyth PD, Dalal S, et al. The rapid diagnosis of acute promyelocytic leukaemia using PML (5E10) monoclonal antibody. *Br J Haematol.* 1997;99:597–604.

15. Behm FG, Smith FO, Raimondi SC, et al. Human homologue of the rat chondroitin sulfate proteoglycan, NG2, detected by monoclonal antibody 7.1 identifies childhood acute lymphoblastic leukemias with t(4;11)(q21;q23) or t(11;19)(q23;p13) and MLL rearrangements. *Blood.* 1996;87:1134–1139.

16. Wutchter C, Schnittger S, Schoch C, et al. Detection of acute leukemia cells with 11q23 rearrangements by flow cytometry: sensitivity and specificity of monoclonal antibody 7.1. *Blood.* 1998;92(suppl 1):228a.

17. Smith FO, Rauch C, Williams DE, et al. The human homologue of rat NG2, a chondroitin sulfate proteoglycan, is not expressed on the cell surface of normal hematopoietic cells but is expressed by acute myeloid leukemia blasts from poor-prognosis patients with abnormalities of chromosome band 11q23. *Blood.* 1996;87:1123–1133.

18. Mauvieux L, Delabesse E, Bourquelot P, et al. NG2 expression in MLL rearranged acute myeloid leukaemia is restricted to monoblastic cases. *Br J Haematol.* 1999;107:674–676.

19. Bene MC, Bernier M, Casasnovas RO, et al. The reliability and specificity of c-kit for the diagnosis of acute myeloid leukemias and undifferentiated leukemias. *Blood.* 1998;92:596–599.

20. Bennett JM, Catovsky D, Daniel MT, et al. Proposed revised criteria for the classification of acute myeloid leukemia. *Ann Intern Med.* 1985;103:620–625.

21. Bennett JM, Catovsky D, Daniel MT, et al. Proposals for the recognition of minimally differentiated acute myeloid leukaemia (AML-MO). *Br J Haematol.* 1991;78:325–329.

22. Buccheri V, Matutes E, Dyer MJS, et al. Lineage commitment in biphenotypic leukemia. *Leukemia.* 1993;7:919–927.

23. Matutes E, Morilla R, Farahat N, et al. Definition of acute biphenotypic leukemia. *Haematologica.* 1997;82:64–66.

24. Feulliard J, Jacob MC, Valensi F, et al. Clinical and biological features of CD4+ CD56+ malignancies. *Blood.* 2002;99:1556–1563.

25. Matutes E, Owusu-Ankomah K, Morilla R, et al. The immunological profile of B-cell disorders and proposal of a scoring system for the diagnosis of CLL. *Leukemia.* 1994;8:1640–1645.

26. Moureau EJ, Matutes E, A'Hern RP, et al. Improvement of the chronic lymphocytic leukemia scoring system with the monoclonal antibody SN8 (CD79b). *Am J Clin Pathol.* 1997;108:378–382.

27. Matutes E, Attygale A, Wotherspoon A, et al. Diagnostic issues in chronic lymphocytic leukaemia (CLL). *Best Pract Res Clin Haematol.* 2010;23:3–20.

28. Delgado J, Matutes E, Morilla A, et al. Diagnostic significance of CD20 and FMC7 expression in B cell disorders. *Am J Clin Pathol.* 2003;120:754–759.

29. Palumbo GA, Parrinello N, Fargione G, et al. CD200 expression may help in differential diagnosis between mantle-cell lymphoma and B-cell chronic lymphocytic leukaemia. *Leuk Res.* 2009;33: 1212–1216.

30. Matutes E, Morilla R, Owusu-Ankomah K, et al. The immunophenotype of hairy cell leukaemia (HCL): proposal for a scoring system to distinguish HCL from B-cell disorders with hairy or villous lymphocytes. *Leuk Lymphoma.* 1994;14(suppl 1):57–61.

31. del Giudice I, Matutes E, Morilla R, et al. The diagnostic value of CD123 in B-cell disorders with hairy or villous lymphocytes. *Haematologica.* 2004;89:303–308.

32. Craig FE, Foon KA. Flow cytometric immunophenotyping for hematologic neoplasms. *Blood.* 2008;111:3941–3967.

33. Thornton PD, Gruzka-Westwood AM, Hamoudi RA, et al. Characterization of TP53 abnormalities in chronic lymphocytic leukaemia. *Hematol J.* 2004;5:47–54.

34. Lens D, Dyer MJ, Garcia Marco JA, et al. p53 abnormalities in CLL are associated with excess of prolymphocytes and poor prognosis. *Br J Haematol.* 1997;99: 848–857.

35. Dohner H, Fischer K, Bentz M, et al. p53 gene deletion predicts for poor survival and non-response to therapy with purine analogs in chronic B-cell leukemias. *Blood.* 1995;85:1580–1589.

36. Damle RN, Walie T, Fais F, et al. Immunoglobulin V gene mutation status and CD38 expression as novel prognostic indicators in chronic lymphocytic leukemia. *Blood.* 1999;94:1840–1847.

37. Ibrahim S, Keating M, Do K-A, et al. CD38 expression as an important prognostic factor in B-cell chronic lymphocytic leukaemia. *Blood.* 2001;98:181–186.

38. Thornton PD, Fernandez C, Giustolisi G, et al. CD38 as a prognostic indicator in chronic lymphocytic leukaemia. *Hematol J.* 2004;5:145–151.

39. Morilla A, Gonzalez de Castro D, Del Giudice I, et al. Combinations of ZAP-70, CD38 and IGHV mutational status as predictors of time to first treatment in CLL. *Leuk Lymphoma.* 2008;49: 2108–2115.

40. Crespo M, Bosch F, Villamor N, et al. ZAP-70 expression as a surrogate for immunoglobulin-variable-gene region mutations in chronic lymphocytic leukemia. *N Engl J Med.* 2003;348: 1764–1775.

41. Lima M, Almeida J, Santos AH, et al. Immunophenotypic analysis of the TCR-Vbeta repertoire in 98 persistent expansions of CD3(+)/TCR-alphabeta(+) large granular lymphocytes: utility in assessing clonality and insights into the pathogenesis of the disease. *Am J Pathol.* 2001;159:1861–1868.

42. Matutes E. Immunological and clinical features of T-cell large granular lymphocyte leukaemia. The education programme for the annual congress of European Hematology Association. *Haematologica.* 2009;3:302–307.

43. Matutes E. Chronic T-cell lymphoproliferative disorders. *Rev Clin Exp Hematol.* 2003;6:401–420.

44. Matutes E, Brito-Babapulle V, Swansbury J, et al. Clinical and laboratory features of 78 cases of T-prolymphocytic leukemia. *Blood.* 1991;78:3269–3274.

45. Ginaldi L, Matutes E, Farahat N, et al. Differential expression of CD3 and CD7 in T-cell malignancies: a quantitative study by flow cytometry. *Br J Haematol.* 1996;93: 921–927.

46. Bene MC, Kaeda JS. How and why minimal residual disease studies are necessary in leukaemia: a review from WP10 and WP12 of the European Leukaemia Net. *Haematologica.* 2009;94:1135–1150.

47. Farahat N, Lens D, Zomas A, et al. Quantitative flow cytometry can distinguish between normal and B-cell precursors. *Br J Haematol.* 1995;91:640–646.

48. Campana D, Counstan-Smith E. Advances in the immunological monitoring of childhood acute lymphoblastic leukemia. *Best Pract Res Clin Haematol.* 2002;15: 1–19.

49. Rawston AC, Villarmor N, Ritgen M, et al. International standardized approach for flow cytometric residual disease monitoring in chronic lymphocytic leukaemia. *Leukemia.* 2007;21:956–964.

50. Matutes E, Meeus P, McLennan K, et al. The significance of minimal residual disease in hairy cell leukaemia treated with deoxycoformycin: a long-term follow-up study. *Br J Haematol.* 1997;98:375–383.

Chapter 17

Diagnostic radioisotopes in haematology

S. Mitchell Lewis, Peter Charles Cotton, Kuldip Nijran

CHAPTER CONTENTS

Radioactive isotopes must be distinguished from non-radioactive isotopes of the same chemical. The radioactive forms are usually referred to as *radionuclides* or *radioisotopes*. These terms are interchangeable and in this chapter, the latter term is used.

Methods using radioisotopes have an important place in haematological diagnosis. Tests that may be undertaken in haematology departments include total blood volume (TBV), red cell survival studies, vitamin B_{12} absorption (Schilling) tests (reagents not currently available) and, occasionally, ferrokinetic studies.

Other investigations that may have haematological interest are more likely to be referred to a department of medical physics or nuclear medicine. Even when the tests are not carried out directly in the haematology department, it is essential for the haematologist to understand their principles and limitations and to be able to interpret the results in clinical terms. Various textbooks[1,2] provide more complete accounts of the theory and practice of nuclear medicine techniques, as does a monograph on radioisotopes in haematology by Lewis and Bayly.[3]

The main properties of the radioisotopes useful in diagnostic haematology are shown in Table 17.1. The units used to express radioactivity and the effects of radiation on the body are given in the previous edition. Anyone handling radioisotopes must be aware of the potential radiation hazard. It is also important to be aware of the potential biohazard of handling blood products and administering them to patients (see Chapter 24).

Table 17.1 Radioisotopes used for diagnostic investigations in haematology

ELEMENT	HALF-LIFE ($T_{1/2}$)	ENERGIES (MeV)	PHARMACEUTICAL	APPLICATION	ACTIVITIES (MBq)	RADIATION DOSE (mSv)	CHEST X-RAY EQUIVALENCE[a]
^{57}Co	270 days	0.122 0.136	Vitamin B_{12}	Investigation of megaloblastic anaemias	0.02	0.05	3
^{58}Co	711.3 days	0.811 0.511			0.2	10	
^{51}Cr	27.8 days	0.320	Sodium chromate	Red cell volume	0.8	0.3	15
				Red cell lifespan	2	0.6	30
				Gastrointestinal bleeding	4	1	50
				Spleen scan	4	1	50
				Spleen pool	4	1	50
^{59}Fe	45 days	1.09	Ferric chloride or citrate	Oral iron absorption	0.4	4	200
		1.29		Ferrokinetic studies	0.4	4	200
^{125}I	60 days	0.035	Iodinated human serum albumin	Plasma volume	0.2	0.06[b]	3
^{111}In	2.81 days	0.247 0.173	Indium chloride → oxine/tropolone	Red cell volume	2	1	50
				Spleen scan	5	2	100
				Platelet lifespan	4	2	100
^{99m}Tc	6 h	0.141	Pertechnetate	Red cell volume	2	0.02	1
				Spleen scan	100	1	50
				Spleen pool	100	1	

MBq, megabecquerel; 1 MBq = 10^6 Bq = approximately 27 μCi; Sv, Sievert; 10^3 mSv = 1 Sv.
[a]The number of chest X-rays that would expose the subject to the same amount of radiation as the radioisotopes that are listed. A simple chest X-ray has a radiation dose of 0.02 mSv, but for some radiological investigations it is far greater. For example, for intravenous urography, computed tomography (CT) scan of the chest and a large bowel barium study the effective radiation doses are 4.0, 8.0 and 9.0 mSv, respectively.
[b]Provided that the thyroid is blocked and the label is excreted in the urine; if not blocked, about 20% will accumulate in the thyroid, resulting in a radiation dose of 1 mSv to the thyroid.

SOURCES OF RADIOISOTOPES

Radioisotopes that emit γ-rays are particularly useful because they have the advantage of emissions that penetrate tissues well, so they can be detected at the surface of the body when they have originated within organs. The radioisotope should have as short a half-life ($T_{1/2}$) as is compatible with the duration of the test. A radioisotope with a very short half-life can be administered in much higher amounts than those that are likely to remain active in the body for a considerably longer time.

The longer-lived radioisotopes that are used for haematological investigations are generally available from commercial suppliers. The usual way of obtaining certain short-lived radioisotopes is by means of a radioisotope generator, in which a moderately long-lived parent radioisotope decays to produce the required short-lived isotope. In this way ^{99m}Tc ($T_{1/2}$ = 6 h) can be derived from ^{99}Mo ($T_{1/2}$ = 66 h).

RADIATION PROTECTION

The quantity of radioactivity used in diagnostic work is usually small and good laboratory practice is all that is necessary for safe working. However, before using radioisotopes, workers should be familiar with the regulations concerning radiation protection for themselves, their fellow workers and patients.[4]

The effect of radiation on the body depends on the amount of energy deposited and is expressed in grays (Gy). The unit that describes the overall effect of radiation on the body, or the 'effective dose,' is measured in sieverts (Sv) or millisieverts (mSv). The annual whole-body dose limit for somebody working with radioisotopes is in the order of 20 mSv, whereas 1 mSv is the annual limit for the general public. To put this into perspective, 1 mSv is produced by normal background radiation in about 6 months and the radiation dose from a single chest X-ray is 0.02 mSv.[5] No statutory limit of total annual radiation dose has been set for patients, but it is an important requirement that radioisotopes should be handled only in approved laboratories under the direction of a trained person who holds a certificate from the appropriate authority specifying the radioisotopes that the individual is authorized to use and the dose limits that must not be exceeded. In the UK, this authority is the *Administration of Radioactive Substances Advisory Committee* (ARSAC).[5] Radioisotopes should not be given to pregnant women unless the investigation is considered imperative; if an investigation is necessary during lactation, breast-feeding should be discontinued until radioactivity is no longer detectable in the milk. When radioisotope investigations are necessary in children, the dose relative to that for an adult should be based on body weight (Table 17.2).

The laboratory (premises) using radioisotopes should be registered to store, handle and dispose of radioactive materials, and appropriate permits are obtained under the Environmental Permitting Regulations 2010.[5a]

In general, the radioactive waste from radioisotopes used in haematological diagnostic procedures may be poured down a single designated laboratory sink. It should be washed down with a large quantity of running water.

If the waste material exceeds the amount allowed for disposal in this way, it should be stored in a suitable place until its radioactivity has decayed sufficiently for it to be disposed of via the refuse system. All working and storage areas and disposal sinks should be clearly labelled with the internationally recognized trefoil symbol. Records should be kept of the amount of radioactive waste disposed down the drains and this should not exceed the permitted amount on the premises' registration.

Decontamination of working surfaces, walls and floors can usually be achieved by washing with a detergent such as Decon 90 (Decon Laboratories, Ltd). Glassware can be decontaminated by soaking in Decon 90 and plastic laboratory ware can be decontaminated by washing in dilute (e.g. 1%) nitric acid.

Protective gloves must always be worn when handling radioisotopes; any activity that does get on the hands can usually be removed by washing with soap and water or, if that fails, with a detergent solution. For each laboratory in which isotopes are used, a radiation protection supervisor (RPS) should be nominated to supervise protection procedures and to ensure that a careful record is kept of all administered radioisotopes. This RPS should work in association with the departmental safety officer (see p. 579) and must ensure that all personnel working with radioactive materials wear dosimetry badges (available from an approved dosimetry service provider, e.g. Landauer, Oxford; ISO Pharma, Norway), which must be checked at regular intervals.

APPARATUS FOR MEASURING RADIOACTIVITY *IN VITRO*

The radioisotopes used for most haematological tests are measured in a scintillation counter with thallium-activated sodium iodide crystals. These are available in various shapes and sizes. A 'well-type' crystal contains a cavity into which is inserted a small container or test tube holding up to 5 ml of fluid. Because the sample is almost surrounded by the crystal, counting is achieved with high efficiency. Because the geometric efficiency of a well-type counter depends on the position of the sample in relation to the crystal, it is important to use the same volume for each sample in a series. Another form of crystal detector is a solid circular cylinder, 2.5–10 cm in diameter. In this form, it is used for *in vivo* measurements and occasionally for the measurement of bulky samples (e.g. samples of faeces or 24-h urine specimens), thus avoiding the need to concentrate them to a smaller volume.

An alternative method for measuring bulky material is by using two opposed detectors in a single counting system. The sample is placed in a 450 ml waxed cardboard carton with a screw-top lid and is positioned between two counters placed above and below it with a plastic ring over the lower

Table 17.2 Radioisotope doses for children as a decimal fraction of the adult dose	
WEIGHT (kg)	**FRACTION OF ADULT DOSE**
10	0.3
15	0.4
20	0.5
30	0.6
40	0.75
50	0.9
60	0.95
70	1.0

counter to ensure that the specimen in the carton is approximately equidistant from both crystals. The counting system is surrounded by lead and the responses of both crystals are counted together. If a single detector system is used, it is essential to homogenize the samples.

APPARATUS FOR MEASURING RADIOACTIVITY *IN VIVO*

Surface Counting

Surface counting depends on shielding the crystals by means of a lead collimator to exclude as far as possible the radiation from outside a well-defined area of the body. It is thus possible to measure the radioactivity in individual organs such as the spleen and liver.

Imaging

The most widely used method for imaging is by the scintillation camera (gamma camera). It consists of a lead shielding, a large thin sodium iodide detector, an array of photomultiplier tubes, a collimator with multiple parallel holes and a system for pulse height analysis and for storage and display of the data. By scanning down the body, an image of the distribution of the label is built up and recorded. It can also be used to measure the quantity of the isotope in various organs. By rotating the scintillation camera around the body, single-photon emission computed tomography (SPECT) can be performed to produce sectional images. Positron emission tomography (PET) has augmented scintillation scanning and uses radioisotopes that are positron emitters.[6,7]

Measurement of Radioactivity with a Scintillation Counter

Standardization of Working Conditions

For each radioisotope, it is necessary to plot a spectrum of pulse height distribution and to identify a window corresponding to the energy at which the maximum number of pulses is emitted. Examples of spectra and selected settings are illustrated in Figure 17.1. The setting of the

Figure 17.1 Spectra of radioisotopes obtained on a scintillation spectrometer. (A) ^{51}Cr, (B) ^{99m}Tc, (C) ^{125}I and (D) ^{59}Fe. The radionuclides should be counted with the window set within the limits indicated by the vertical lines.

apparatus, once determined, should remain constant for many months.

Counting Technique

Measurement of radioactivity

Measurements are usually carried out for a fixed time period and the results are recorded as counts per second (cps) or counts per minute (cpm). Radioactivity is subject to random but statistically predictable variation similar to that in blood cell counts (see p. 612). The accuracy of the count depends on the total number of the counts recorded as the variance (σ) of a radioactive count $= \sqrt{}$ total count.

Thus, on a count of 100 the inherent error is 10%, whereas it is 1% on a count of 10 000. Any measured activity represents the difference between the sample count and the background count, in which the errors of both counts are cumulative. In practice, a net count of 2500 over background is adequate for the accuracy required for clinical studies.

Background counts should be measured alongside that of the radioactive material. If the count rate of the sample is not much above background, then the background should be counted for as long a time as the sample. If the sample-count rate is less than the background, accurate measurement requires extremely long counting times.

Correction for Physical Decay

Because physical decay is a continuous process that proceeds at an exponential rate, it is possible to correct mathematically for the loss of radioactivity and to convert any measurement back to the initial reference time. This is necessary when comparing successive observations made at different times after the administration of a radionuclide to a patient.[8]

Double Radioisotope Measurements

If more than one radionuclide is present in a sample, it is possible to measure the radioactivity of each radioisotope separately by one of the following techniques.

Differential decay

Differential decay is of value especially when one of the labels has a very short half-life (e.g. ^{99m}Tc, half-life 6 h). The method is to count the activity in the mixture twice – the second count when the short-lived label has effectively disappeared.

Physical separation

When the two radioisotopes produce γ rays of different energies, they can be identified by their characteristic features and separated using an energy analyser. Correction for any 'cross talk' is carried out by counting a standard of each radionuclide (A and B) at both channel settings.

The proportion of A (P_A) spilling over into channel B = channel B counts $\div$ channel A counts from the radionuclide A standard (both corrected for background) and the proportion of B (P_B) spilling over into channel A = channel A counts $\div$ channel B counts from the radionuclide B standard. The total counts obtained for labels A and B in their correct channels can then be corrected for the proportion of 'foreign' counts.

BLOOD VOLUME

The haemoglobin concentration (Hb), red cell count and packed cell volume or haematocrit (PCV/Hct) do not invariably reflect the total red cell volume (RCV). Whereas in most cases for practical purposes, there is adequate correlation between peripheral blood values and (total) RCV,[8] there will be a discrepancy if the plasma volume is reduced or increased disproportionately. Fluctuation in plasma volume may result in haemodilution, giving rise to pseudoanaemia, or conversely, haemoconcentration, giving rise to pseudopolycythaemia.

An increase in plasma volume occurs in pregnancy, returning to normal soon after delivery. Increased plasma volume may also be found in patients with cirrhosis, nephritis and congestive cardiac failure and when there is marked splenomegaly. Reduced plasma volume occurs with oedema, with dehydration, following the administration of diuretic drugs, in smokers and sometimes as a persistent unexplained phenomenon. It also occurs during prolonged bed rest.

In contrast to the fluctuations in plasma volume, RCV does not fluctuate to any extent if erythropoiesis is in a steady state.

Measurement of blood volume should thus be considered whenever the Hct is persistently higher than normal; demonstration of an absolute increase in RCV is necessary to diagnose polycythaemia and to assess its severity. However, it should be noted that the discovery of a recurring *JAK2* mutation (*JAK2* V617F) in the great majority of patients with polycythaemia vera means that blood volume studies are now rarely needed for the confirmation of this diagnosis. The component parts of the TBV (i.e. red cell and plasma volume) can also be measured separately in the elucidation of obscure anaemias when the possibility of an increase in plasma volume cannot be excluded.

Measurement of Blood Volume

Principle

The principle is that of dilution analysis. A small volume of a readily identifiable radioisotope is injected intravenously, either bound to the red cells or to a plasma component, and its dilution is measured after time has been allowed for the injected material to become thoroughly mixed in the circulation but before significant quantities have left the circulation or become unbound. The most practical method now available is to use a small volume of the patient's red cells labelled with radioactive chromium (^{51}Cr), technetium (pertechnetate) (^{99m}Tc) or indium (^{111}In). The labelled red cells are diluted in the whole blood of the patient and from their dilution the TBV can be calculated; the RCV, too, can be deduced from knowledge of the PCV. The plasma volume can be measured directly by injecting human albumin labelled with radioactive iodine (^{125}I) that is diluted in the plasma compartment.

In contrast to measurement of RCV, plasma volume measurements are only approximations because the labelled albumin undergoes continuous slow interchange between the plasma and extravascular fluids, even during the mixing period. For this reason, it is undesirable to attempt to calculate RCV from plasma volume on the basis of the observed PCV. However, because the RCV is generally more stable, calculation of TBV from RCV is usually more reliable, provided that the difference between whole-body and venous PCV is appreciated and allowed for (see p. 379). Measurement of red cell and plasma volumes separately by direct methods is to be preferred.

Red Cell Volume

Radioactive Chromium Method

For the radioactive chromium method,[9] add approximately 10 ml of blood to 1.5 ml of sterile National Institutes of Health (NIH)-A acid–citrate–dextrose (ACD) solution (see p. 619) in a sterile bottle with a screw cap. Centrifuge at 1200–1500 g for 5 min. Discard the supernatant plasma and buffy coat and slowly, with continuous mixing, add to the cells 8×10^3 Bq of Na$_2$^{51}CrO$_4$ per kg of body weight. The sodium chromate should be in a volume of at least 0.2 ml, being diluted in 9 g/l NaCl (saline). Allow the blood to stand for 15 min at 37°C for labelling to take place. Wash the red cells twice in 4–5 volumes of sterile saline: for all procedures requiring sterile saline, this should be 9 g/l (0.9%) sodium chloride BP (non-pyrogenic); 12 g/l NaCl should be used when red cell osmotic fragility is greatly increased (e.g. in cases of hereditary spherocytosis).

Finally, resuspend the cells in a volume of sterile saline sufficient for an injection of about 5 ml and the preparation of a standard. Take up the appropriate volume into a syringe that is weighed before and after the injection. The volume injected is calculated from the following formula:

$$\text{Volume injected (ml)} = \frac{\text{Weight of suspension injected (g)}}{\text{Density of suspension (g/ml)}}$$

The density of the suspension $= 1.0 + $ Hb of suspension (g/l) $\times 0.097/340$, assuming that packed red cells have

a mean cell haemoglobin concentration (MCHC) of 340 g/l and a density of 1.097.

Inject the suspension intravenously without delay and note the time; at 10, 20 and 30 min later, collect 5–10 ml of the patient's blood and add it to the appropriate amount of K$_2$ EDTA anticoagulant. This blood should preferably be drawn from a vein other than that used for the injection. However, it is often convenient to insert a self-retaining needle; in this case, care must be taken to ensure that the isotope is well-dispersed into the bloodstream when injected by flushing through with 10 ml of sterile saline. When the mixing time is likely to be prolonged, as in splenomegaly, cardiac failure or shock, another sample should be taken 60 min after the injection.

Measure the PCV of each sample. PCV should be obtained by microhaematocrit centrifugation for 5 min or for 10 min if the PCV is more than 0.50 and correcting for trapped plasma by deducting 2% from the measurement. A more accurate measurement of the PCV can be obtained by the International Council for Standardization in Haematology (ICSH) surrogate reference method (see p. 30).

Deliver 1 ml volumes into counting tubes and lyse with saponin; a convenient method is to add 2 drops of 2% saponin. Measure their radioactivity in a scintillation counter. Then dilute an aliquot of the original suspension that was not injected 1 in 500 in water (for use as a standard) and determine the radioactivity of a 1 ml volume. Then:

$$\text{Red cell volume (RCV) (ml)} = \frac{\begin{array}{l}\text{Radioactivity of standard (cpm/ml)} \\ \times \text{Dilution of standard} \times \text{Volume} \\ \text{injected (ml)}\end{array}}{\begin{array}{l}\text{Radioactivity of post-injection} \\ \text{sample (cpm/ml)}\end{array}} \times \begin{array}{l}\text{PCV (on} \\ \text{blood sample)}\end{array}$$

Technetium Method

^{99m}Tc is available as sodium pertechnetate. This passes freely through the red cell membrane and will become attached to the cells only if it is present in a reduced form as it enters the cells when it binds firmly to β chains of haemoglobin. For this to occur, the red cells must be treated with a stannous (tin) compound by the following *in vivo* procedure.

Dissolve a vial of Stannous Reagent (stannous fluoride and sodium medronate [Amerscan, Amersham International]) in 6 ml of sterile saline and inject intravenously 0.03 ml/kg body weight.

After 15 min, collect 5 ml of blood into a sterile container to which has been added 200 iu of liquid heparin. Add 2 MBq of freshly generated ^{99m}Tc in approximately 0.2 ml of saline or 100 MBq if measurement of splenic red cell pool and scanning are also required. Allow to stand at room temperature for 5 min. Centrifuge; wash twice in cold sterile saline and resuspend in a sufficient volume of cold sterile saline for an injection of 5–10 ml. Draw 5 ml into a syringe that is weighed before and after injection and carry out subsequent procedures as for the chromium method. Because of the short half-life of ^{99m}Tc, radioactivity must be measured on the day of the test. Because 5–10% of the radioactivity is eluted from the red cells within an hour, the method is less suitable than the chromium and indium methods when delayed mixing is suspected (e.g. in splenomegaly).

Indium is available as ^{111}In chloride. The labelling procedure is simpler than with ^{99m}Tc and, because there is less elution than with technetium during the first hour,[10] it is particularly suitable for delayed sampling. For labelling blood cells, the indium is complexed with oxine[11] or tropolone.[12]

Calculating Total Blood Volume

The TBV can be calculated by multiplying the value for RCV by 1/(whole-body PCV) (see below). Plasma volume can be calculated by subtracting RCV from TBV.

If a sample has been taken at 60 min in cases in which delayed mixing is suspected and there is a significant difference between the measurements at 10–30 min and 60 min, then the 60 min measurement should be used for calculating the RCV.

Plasma Volume

^{125}I-Human Serum Albumin Method

Human serum albumin (HSA) labelled with ^{125}I or ^{131}I is available commercially (from ISO Pharma, Norway; Mallinckrodt Medical (Nuclear Medicine Division), Northampton, UK). The albumin concentration should not be less than 20 g/l. The user must be reassured that only donors who are negative for human immunodeficiency virus (HIV) and hepatitis B and C have been used as the source of albumin. ^{125}I is readily distinguishable from ^{51}Cr, ^{99m}Tc and ^{111}In and this makes possible the simultaneous direct determination of RCV and plasma volume (see below). If further doses of the radioisotope are to be administered for repeat tests, it is advisable to block the thyroid by administering 30 mg of potassium iodide by mouth on the day before the test and daily for 2–3 weeks thereafter.

Withdraw approximately 20 ml of blood into a syringe containing a few drops of sterile heparin solution and transfer to a 30 ml sterile bottle with a screw cap. After centrifuging at 1200–1500 g for 5–10 min, transfer approximately 7 ml of plasma to a second sterile bottle and add 2.5 × 10^3 Bq of the radionuclide-labelled HSA per kg body weight (approx. 0.2 MBq in total). Inject a measured amount (e.g. 5 ml) and retain the residue for preparation of a standard.

After 10, 20 and 30 min, withdraw blood samples from a vein other than that used for the original injection

(or after flushing through with 10 ml of sterile 9 g/l NaCl [saline] if a butterfly needle has been used) and deliver into bottles containing EDTA or heparin.

Measure the PCV (see above), centrifuge the sample and separate the plasma. Prepare a standard by diluting part of the residue of the uninjected HSA 1 in 100 in saline.

Measure the radioactivity of the plasma samples in a scintillation counter and, by extrapolation on semilogarithmic graph paper, calculate the radioactivity of the plasma at zero time. If only a single sample is collected 10 min after the injection, the radioactivity at zero time may be approximated by multiplying by 1.015 to allow for early loss of the radioisotope from the circulation. Reliance on a single 10 min sample will lead to error if the mixing of the albumin in the plasma is delayed. After measuring the radioactivity of the standard, the plasma volume (ml) is calculated as follows:

$$\frac{\text{Radioactivity of standard (cpm/ml)} \times \text{Dilution of standard} \times \text{Volume injected (ml)}}{\text{Radioactivity of postinjection sample (cpm/ml, adjusted to zero time)}}$$

Calculating Total Blood Volume

As has already been indicated, the TBV is frequently calculated from the RCV and PCV. Before this can be done, however, the observed PCV has to be corrected for the difference between the whole-body and venous PCV.

Whole-body and venous packed cell volume ratio

PCV measured on venous blood is not identical to the average PCV of all the blood in the body. This is mainly because the red cell:plasma ratio is less in small blood vessels (capillaries, arterioles and venules) than in large vessels. The ratio between the whole-body PCV and venous blood PCV is normally about 0.9,[9] and it is thus necessary in the calculation of TBV from measurements of RCV to multiply the observed PCV by 0.9. Thus, TBV is given by the following:

$$\text{Red cell volume} \times \frac{1}{\text{PCV} \times 0.9}$$

However, the ratio varies in individuals, especially in splenomegaly and it is better to estimate RCV and plasma volume by separate measurements rather than to attempt to calculate one of these from an estimate of the other.

Simultaneous Measurement of Red Cell Volume and Plasma Volume

Collect blood and label the red cells by one of the methods described earlier. If ^{99m}Tc is used, it is necessary first to inject stannous reagent (see p. 378). Then add ^{125}I

HSA (see above) and mix it with the labelled red cell suspension. Inject an accurately measured amount and dilute the remainder 1 in 500 in water for use as a standard. Collect three blood samples at 10, 20 and 30 min, respectively, after the administration of the labelled blood and estimate the radioactivity of a measured volume of each sample and a similar volume of the standard.

When ^{99m}Tc has been used in combination with ^{125}I, count on the same day; then leave for 2 days to allow the ^{99m}Tc to decay and count again for ^{125}I activity. Because the radioactivity in the preparation from ^{125}I is much smaller than that from ^{99m}Tc, the count from the red cells is not likely to be significantly affected by interference from ^{125}I in the initial count. However, if necessary, a correction can be made by subtracting the ^{125}I counts on day 2 (corrected for decay) from the original counts to obtain a measurement of the counts owing only to the ^{99m}Tc.

When ^{51}Cr has been used in combination with ^{125}I and a multichannel counter is available, measure the radioactivity owing to the ^{51}Cr and ^{125}I at the appropriate settings for ^{51}Cr and ^{125}I.

Calculate the radioactivity owing to the red cell label in the blood from the mean of the 10-, 20- and 30-min samples and obtain that owing to ^{125}I from the value extrapolated to zero time. Calculate RCV as described on p. 378.

Plasma volume is calculated from the formula:

$$\frac{\text{Radioactivity of standard (cpm/ml)} \times}{\text{Dilution of standard} \times \text{Volume injected (ml)} \times (1 - PCV)} \frac{}{\text{Radioactivity of postinjection sample}} \\ \text{(cpm/ml, corrected to zero time)}$$

Total blood volume = RCV + plasma volume

Expression of Results of Blood Volume Estimations

RCV, plasma volume and TBV are usually expressed in ml/kg of body weight. Because fat is relatively avascular, low values are obtained in obese subjects and the relation between TBV and body weight varies according to body composition. Blood volume is more closely correlated with lean body mass (LBM).[13] Earlier methods for determination of LBM were not practical as a routine procedure and discounting excess fat by using an estimate of so-called 'ideal weight' is arbitrary and tends to overcorrect for the avascularity of fat. The International Council for Standardization in Haematology (ICSH) developed two formulae, based on body surface area, which provide normal reference values in men and women, respectively.[14] They are as follows.

Mean Normal Red Cell Mass (ml)

Men: $[1486 \times S] - 825$; ±25% includes 98% limits
Women: $[1.06 \times age\ (years)] + [822 \times S]$; ±25% includes 99% limits

Mean Normal Plasma Volume (ml)

Men: $1578 \times S$; ±25% includes 99% limits
Women: $1395 \times S$; ±25% includes 99% limits

$$S = [W^{0.425} \times H^{0.725} \times 0.007184]$$

where S = surface area (m²), W = weight (kg), H = height (cm).

However, the problem of establishing the LBM has been overcome to some extent because there are now instruments that are simple to use for estimating body composition by the different response of fat and other tissues to electrical impedance (body composition analyser, Holtain Ltd, Crosswell, Dyfed, Wales; body fat monitor, Tanita Corporation, IL, USA).[13,15]

Thus, RCV can now be obtained by a direct measurement that discounts the effect of fat. The graph in Figure 17.2 shows the normalization of the RCV in ml/kg LBM.[13] It is obtained as follows: on arithmetic graph paper with % fat on the horizontal (x) axis and RCV in ml/kg total body weight on the vertical (y) axis, plot the intercepts of the following:

Fat 20% with RCV 29 ml; Fat 50% with RCV 19 ml

Join these two points and extend the line to the right and left.

When the % fat is known in any individual (male or female), draw a line vertically from this reading on the x axis to the slope and where this line intersects the slope draw a horizontal line to the y axis. The reading of this line on the y axis is the normalized RCV for that individual. When the measured RCV is >120% of this figure, it is equivalent to 43 ml/kg LBM and a diagnosis of polycythaemia can be made with confidence in men or women.

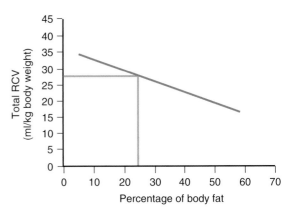

Figure 17.2 Normalization of red cell volume in ml/kg lean body mass. This example shows a patient with 25% body fat; from the slope of the graph the normalized red cell volume for that person should be 28 ml/kg body weight. A measurement of more than 120% of this value (i.e. 33.6 ml) would indicate polycythaemia.

Range in Health

The TBV is 250–350 ml at birth. After infancy, the volume increases gradually until adult life when the RCV in men is 30 ± 5 ml (2SD)/kg and in women it is 25 ± 5 ml (2SD)/kg. Plasma volume (for men and women) is 40–50 ml/kg; TBV is 60–80 ml/kg.

As a rule, the TBV remains remarkably constant in an individual and rapid adjustments take place within a few hours after blood transfusion or intravenous infusion. In pregnancy, both the plasma volume and TBV increase. The plasma volume increases especially in the 1st trimester and the total volume increases later; by full term the plasma volume will have increased by about 40% and TBV will have increased by 32% or even more. The blood volume returns to normal within a week postpartum.[16]

Bed rest causes a reduction in plasma volume and muscular exercise and changes in posture cause transient fluctuations. In practice, the patient should always be allowed to rest in a recumbent position for 15 min before measuring the blood volume.

Splenic Red Cell Volume

The red cell content of the normal spleen (the red cell 'pool') is <5% of the total RCV (i.e. <100–120 ml in an adult). In splenomegaly, the pool is increased (e.g. by perhaps as much as 5–10 times in myelofibrosis, polycythaemia vera and hairy cell leukaemia and other lymphoproliferative disorders).[17] An increase in the volume of the splenic red cell pool may itself be a cause of anaemia; measurement of the pool may be useful in investigating the anaemia in these conditions. It is also useful in determining the cause of erythrocytosis because the expanded pool in polycythaemia vera contrasts with that in secondary polycythaemia, which is normal.[18]

An approximate estimate of the splenic RCV can be obtained from the difference between the RCV calculated from the measurement of the blood sample that has been collected 2–3 min after the injection of labelled cells and that measured after mixing has been completed (i.e. after a delay of 20 min). The splenic RCV can be estimated more accurately by quantitative scanning, after injecting viable red cells labelled with ^{99m}Tc.[19] The blood volume is measured in the usual way using 100 MBq of ^{99m}Tc. The splenic area is scanned 20 min after the injection or after 60 min when there is splenomegaly. To delineate the spleen more precisely, it may be necessary to carry out a second scan after an injection of heat-damaged labelled red cells (see p. 388). From the radioactivity in the spleen, relative to that in a standard, and knowledge of the total RCV, the proportion of the total RCV contained in the spleen can be calculated. This technique has also been used for demonstrating localized accumulation of blood in haemangiomas in the liver,[20] telangiectasia and other vascular abnormalities.[21]

FERROKINETICS

Whereas much can be learned about the rate and efficiency of erythropoiesis from the red cell count and reticulocyte counts, studies of iron metabolism and measurement of red cell lifespan with radioactive isotopes may provide useful additional information.

Radioactive iron (^{59}Fe) has a moderately short half-life, 45 days, and labels haemoglobin after injection. It also labels the plasma iron pool and this allows the measurement of iron clearance and calculation of plasma iron turnover. Its subsequent appearance in haemoglobin permits the assessment of the rate of haemoglobin synthesis and the completeness of the utilization of iron. Because it is a γ-ray emitter, radioactivity can be measured *in vivo* and the sites of distribution of the administered iron and the probable sites of erythropoiesis can thus be determined. (^{59}Fe is not available at present from the former supplier, Amersham plc, but it may be available from POLATOM, www.polatom.pl.)

Iron Distribution

Principle

Iron is transported to the bone marrow bound to transferrin. The transferrin–iron complex binds to transferrin receptors of the erythroblast membrane and the complex enters the cell by endocytosis; iron is then released into the cytosol, with transferrin and its receptor being recycled to the cell surface where transferrin is released into the plasma. Iron not bound to transferrin finds its way to the liver and to other organs rather than to the bone marrow, whereas colloidal particles of iron are rapidly removed by phagocytic cells.

The ferrokinetic studies with ^{59}Fe that provide information on erythropoiesis include the rate of clearance of the radioiron from the plasma and iron incorporation into circulating red cells (iron utilization). These are relatively simple procedures but they do not take account of the recirculation of iron that returns to the plasma from tissues, nor of iron turnover resulting from dyserythropoiesis or haemolysis. To take account of these factors requires much more complex and time-consuming procedures with multiple sampling over an extended period,[22] but the simpler tests provide sufficiently reliable and useful measurements for clinical purposes.

In ferrokinetic studies, it is important to ensure that any iron administered is bound to transferrin. In most cases, plasma has an adequate amount of transferrin. However, the unsaturated iron-binding capacity (UIBC) or transferrin concentration of the patient's plasma should be measured before the test is carried out and, if the UIBC is <1 mg/l (20 µmol/l) or the transferrin concentration is <0.6 g/l, normal donor plasma (HIV and hepatitis B and C negative) should be used instead of that of the patient for the subsequent labelling procedure.

Method

Under sterile conditions, obtain 5–10 ml of plasma from freshly collected heparinized blood. Add 0.4 MBq of ^{59}Fe ferric citrate (specific activity >0.2 MBq/μg). Incubate at room temperature for 15 min. Fill a syringe with all but 1 ml of the mixture. Weigh the syringe to the nearest 10 mg. Inject its content intravenously into the patient, starting a stopwatch at the midpoint of the injection. Reweigh the empty syringe and calculate the volume injected:

$$\text{Volume of plasma (ml)} = \frac{\text{Weight of plasma (g)}}{1.015}$$

Dilute the residual portion of the dose (1 ml) 1 in 100 in water and use as a measure of the total amount of radioactivity and as a standard in subsequent measurements.

Plasma Iron Clearance

Take a sample at 3 min and four or five further samples over a period of 1–2 h, collecting them into heparin or EDTA. Retain a portion of one sample for measurement of plasma iron. Measure the radioactivity in unit volumes of plasma from the samples and plot the values obtained on log linear graph paper. A straight line will usually be obtained for the initial slope. The radioactivity at the moment of injection is inferred by extrapolation back to zero time and the time taken for the plasma radioactivity to decrease to half its initial value ($T_{1/2}$-plasma clearance) is read off the graph (Fig. 17.3).

Range of $T_{1/2}$-plasma clearance in health = 60–140 min.

The clearance rate is influenced by the intensity of erythropoiesis and also by the activity of the macrophages of the reticuloendothelial (RE) system, especially in the

Figure 17.3 Plasma iron clearance. ^{59}Fe activity in plasma at 10, 20, 30 and 60 min extrapolated to the vertical axis to obtain activity at zero time. The $T_{1/2}$ was 90 min.

liver, spleen and bone marrow, where the iron is retained as storage iron. Also, to a lesser extent, circulating reticulocytes may take up some of the iron. A rapid clearance indicates hyperactivity of one or more of these mechanisms, as for instance in iron deficiency anaemia, haemorrhagic anaemia, haemolytic anaemia and polycythaemia vera. The clearance rate is decreased in aplastic anaemia. In leukaemia and in myelofibrosis, the results are variable, depending on the amount of erythropoietic marrow and the extent of extramedullary erythropoiesis; in myelofibrosis, however, rapid clearance is by far the more common finding. In dyserythropoiesis, the clearance may be normal or accelerated.

Iron Utilization

Collect blood samples daily or at least on alternate days, for a period of about 2 weeks after the administration of the ^{59}Fe. Measure the radioactivity per ml of whole blood and calculate the percentage utilization on each day from the formula:

$$\frac{\text{cpm/ml daily whole blood sample} \times 100 \times f}{\text{cpm/ml whole blood sample at zero time}}$$

where f is a PCV/Hct correction factor

$$\text{i.e.,} \quad \frac{0.9\text{PCV}}{1 - 0.9\text{PCV}}$$

When there is reason to suspect that the body:venous PCV ratio is not 0.9, measure the RCV by a direct method (see p. 378). Note, however, that because calculation of plasma volume from extrapolation of the ^{59}Fe disappearance curve is often unreliable, it should not be used as the basis for calculation of RCV.

Calculate the percentage utilization on each day from the formula:

$$\text{Percentage utilization} = \frac{\text{Red cell volume (ml)} \times}{\text{cpm/ml red cells} \times 100}{\text{Total radioactivity injected (cpm)}}$$

Note: The radioactivity is adjusted for physical decay up to the day of measurement.

Plot the daily measured percentages against time on arithmetic graph paper. Record the maximum utilization (Fig. 17.4).

The calculation gives a measure of effective erythropoiesis. In normal subjects, red cell radioactivity increases steadily from 24 h and reaches a maximum of 70–80% utilization on the 10th to 14th day.

A rapid plasma clearance is usually associated with early and relatively complete utilization and the converse also applies. The results are inconsistent in megaloblastic anaemia and in haemoglobinopathies, in which there is ineffective erythropoiesis; they also are inconsistent in myelofibrosis, depending on the extent of extramedullary erythropoiesis and whether the red cell lifespan is reduced. If there is rapid haemolysis, the utilization curve

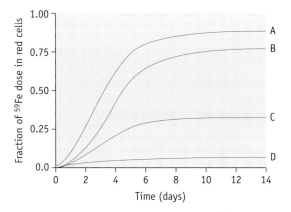

Figure 17.4 Iron utilization. Red-cell uptake of ^{59}Fe in (A) iron deficiency and polycythaemia, (B) a normal subject, (C) dyserythropoiesis and (D) severe aplastic anaemia.

will be distorted by destruction of some of the labelled red cells; this may be recognized if frequent (daily) samples are measured. In aplastic anaemia, the utilization is usually 10–15%; in ineffective erythropoiesis, it is as a rule 30–50%.

The ferrokinetic patterns in various diseases are shown in Table 17.3 and Figure 17.4.

Body Iron Distribution

An overall picture of ferrokinetics can be constructed from surface counting with a scintillation probe positioned over the liver, spleen, sacrum (for bone marrow) and heart (for blood pool) after an intravenous injection of ^{59}Fe. By counting over several days, it is possible to

Table 17.3 Ferrokinetic patterns in various diseases

	PLASMA CLEARANCE T$_{1/2}$	RED CELL UTILIZATION[a]
Normal	60–140 min	80%
Iron deficiency	Shortened	Increased (90%)
Aplastic anaemia	Prolonged	Decreased (10%)
Chronic infection	Slightly shortened	Normal
Dyserythropoiesis	Slightly shortened	Decreased (30%)
Myelofibrosis	Shortened	Decreased (50%)
Haemolytic anaemia	Shortened	Increased (85%)

[a]Average figures are shown, but there is a wide range, depending on the stage and severity of the disease.

identify sites of erythropoiesis from early counts and sites of red cell destruction from later counts. This test is rarely performed nowadays, although it has some clinical value for determining the extent of extramedullary erythropoiesis in the spleen before splenectomy.

Where there are facilities for using cyclotron-produced ^{52}Fe and positron emission tomography (PET), high-resolution images of the intramedullary and extramedullary distribution of erythropoietic tissue can be obtained. This is especially helpful in the myeloproliferative neoplasms for diagnosing transition of polycythaemia vera to myelofibrosis and for differentiating essential thrombocythaemia from reactive thrombocytosis.[23] It is also useful in identifying residual skeletal erythropoiesis in aplastic anaemia.

ESTIMATION OF THE LIFESPAN OF RED CELLS *IN VIVO*

There is extensive literature on the survival of red cells in haemolytic anaemias using radioisotope labelling of red cells (see review by Bentley and Miller[24]). Although now undertaken less frequently than in the past, measurement of red cell survival can still provide important data in cases of anaemia in which increased haemolysis is suspected but not clearly demonstrated by other tests. In the usual procedure, a population of circulating red cells of all ages is labelled ('random labelling'). By contrast, in 'cohort labelling' a radionuclide (e.g. ^{59}Fe) is incorporated into haemoglobin during its synthesis by erythroblasts and radioactivity is measured in red cells that appear in the circulation as a cohort of closely similar age. Red cell lifespan can be calculated from measurements of red cell iron turnover,[25] but the results have to be interpreted with caution because of the reutilization for haem synthesis of iron derived from red cells at the end of their lifespan. Random labelling is a much more practical method than cohort labelling.

Radioactive Chromium (^{51}Cr) Method

Radioactive chromium (^{51}Cr) is a γ-ray emitter with a half-life of 27.8 days. As a red cell label, it is used in the form of hexavalent sodium chromate. After passing through the surface membrane of the red cells, it is reduced to the trivalent form that binds to protein, preferentially to the β-globin chains of haemoglobin.[26] In this form, it is not reutilized or transferred to other cells in the circulation.

The main disadvantage of ^{51}Cr is that it gradually elutes from red cells as they circulate; there may be, too, an increased loss over the first 1–3 days and uncertainty as to how much has been lost makes it impossible to measure red cell lifespan accurately. Chromium, whether radioactive or non-radioactive, is toxic to red cells, probably by its oxidizing actions; it inhibits glycolysis in red cells when present at a concentration of 10 μg/ml or more[27] and blocks glutathione reductase activity at a concentration exceeding 5 μg/ml.[28] Blood should thus not be exposed to >2 μg of chromium per ml of packed red cells.

$Na_2{}^{51}CrO_4$ is available commercially at a specific activity of about 15–20 GBq/mg Cr. For administration, the stock solution usually must be dissolved in 9 g/l NaCl (saline) (see below). ACD must not be used as a diluent because this reduces the chromate to the cationic chromic form.

Care must be taken to avoid lysis when the red cells are washed; it may be necessary, especially if the blood contains spherocytes, to use a slightly hypertonic solution (e.g. 12 g/l NaCl). This should certainly be used if an osmotic fragility test has demonstrated lysis in 9 g/l NaCl. In patients whose plasma contains high-titre, high-thermal-amplitude cold agglutinins, the blood must be collected in a warmed syringe and delivered into ACD solution previously warmed to 37°C; the labelling and washing in saline should be carried out in a 'warm room' at 37°C.

Method

The technique of labelling red cells is the same as for TBV measurement (see p. 378).[29] To ensure as little damage to red cells as possible, with subsequent minimal early loss and later elution, it is important to maintain the blood at an optimal pH. This can be achieved by adding 10 volumes of blood to 1.5 volumes of NIH-A ACD solution (see p. 619).

For a red cell survival study, 0.02 MBq per kg body weight (an average total dose of c2 MBq) is recommended. If this is to be combined with a spleen scan or pool measurement, a higher dose (4 MBq) should be used, bearing in mind that <2 μg of chromium should be added per ml of packed red cells.

After injection, allow the labelled cells to circulate in the recipient for 10 min (or for 60 min in patients with cardiac failure or splenomegaly, in whom mixing may be delayed). Then collect a sample of blood from a vein other than that used for the injection (or after washing the needle through with saline if a butterfly needle is used) and mix with EDTA as anticoagulant. The radioactivity in this sample provides a baseline for subsequent observations. Retain part of the labelled cell suspension that was not injected into the patient to serve as a standard. This enables the blood volume to be calculated if required.

Take further 4–5 ml blood samples from the patient 24 h later (day 1) and subsequently at intervals, the frequency of the samples depending on the rate of red cell destruction: in general, three specimens between day 2 and day 7 and then two specimens per week for the

duration of the study. Measurements should be continued until at least half the radioactivity has disappeared from the circulation.

Measure the Hb or PCV in a part of each sample; then lyse the samples with saponin, mix well and deliver 1 ml into counting tubes, if possible in duplicate.

Measurement of Radioactivity

Estimate the percentage survival (of ^{51}Cr) on any day (t) by comparing the radioactivity of the sample taken on that day with that of the day 0 sample (i.e. the sample withdrawn 10 [or 60] min after the injection of the labelled cells). Thus, ^{51}Cr survival on day t (%) is given by the following:

$$\frac{cpm/ml \text{ of blood on day t}}{cpm/ml \text{ of blood on day 0}} \times 100$$

No adjustment is necessary for the physical decay of the isotope, provided that the standard is counted within a few minutes of the day t sample.

Carry out the measurements in any high-quality scintillation counter, at least 2500 counts being recorded to achieve a precision within ±2%.

Processing of Radioactivity Measurements

Before the data can be analysed and interpreted, factors, other than physical decay, that are involved in the disappearance of radioactivity from the circulation have to be considered. There are two processes: ^{51}Cr-labelled cells are lost from the circulation by lysis, phagocytosis or haemorrhage and, in addition, ^{51}Cr is eluted from intact red cells that still circulate.

Elution

The rate of elution differs to a small extent from one individual to another. It is thought to vary to a greater extent between different diseases, especially when the red cell lifespan is considerably reduced. However, in such cases, elution and variation in the rate of elution become unimportant. The rate of elution is also influenced by technique, especially by the anticoagulant solution into which the blood is collected prior to labelling. With the NIH-A ACD solution, the rate of elution is about 1% per day.[29]

Early Loss

Sometimes, in addition to the elution that occurs continuously and at a relatively low and constant rate, up to 10% of the ^{51}Cr may be lost within the first 24 h. The cause of this major early loss is obscure and several components may be involved. If this major loss does not continue beyond the first 2 days, it is often looked on as an artefact, in the sense that it does not denote an increased rate of lysis *in vivo*, and it can be, and typically is, ignored by replotting the figures as described on p. 387. This procedure is acceptable, at least for clinical studies, but it does not take into account the possibility that a small proportion of red cells are present that lyse rapidly. It is common practice to calculate the $T_{50}Cr$ (i.e. the time taken for the concentration of ^{51}Cr in the blood to fall to 50% of its initial value) after correcting the data for physical decay but not for elution. T_{50} is used rather than $T_{1/2}$ because the elimination of the label is not a constant exponential fraction of the original amount. The chief objection to the use of $T_{50}Cr$ is that it may be misleading without additional information on the pattern of the survival curve. Moreover, the mean red cell lifespan cannot be directly derived from it. With the technique described earlier, the mean value of T_{50} in normal subjects is 30 days, with a range of 25–33 days (Table 17.4).

Correction for Elution

When haemolysis is marked, elution is of minor importance and can be ignored. When haemolysis is not greatly increased, it is essential to correct for elution. This can be done by multiplying the measured survival by the factors given in Table 17.4.

Survival Curves

Normal red cell survival (corrected for elution) will be in the range shown in Figure 17.5. When survival is reduced, a survival curve should be drawn and from this the mean red cell lifespan can be derived.

Plot the % radioactivity figures or count rates per ml of whole blood (corrected for physical decay and for elution) on arithmetic and semilogarithmic graph paper and attempt to fit straight lines passing through the data points.

1. If a straight line can be fitted to the arithmetic plot, the mean red cell lifespan is given by the point in time at which the line or its extension cuts the abscissa (Fig. 17.6).
2. As a rule, however, a straight line is better fitted to the semilogarithmic plot; the mean red cell lifespan can be read as the exponential e^{-1} (that is, the time when 37% of the cells are still surviving [Fig. 17.7]) or calculated by multiplying the half-time of the fitted line by the reciprocal of the natural log of 2 (0.693) (i.e. multiplying by 1.44).

A computer programmed curve-fitting procedure is more precise but is not likely to improve overall accuracy of the results for clinical purposes.

Interpretation of Survival Curves

In the autoimmune haemolytic anaemias, the slope of elimination is usually markedly curvilinear when the data are plotted on arithmetic graph paper. Red cell

Table 17.4 Normal range for ^{51}Cr survival curves with correction for elution

DAY	% ^{51}Cr (CORRECTED FOR DECAY; NOT CORRECTED FOR ELUTION)	ELUTION CORRECTION FACTORS[a]
1	93–98	1.03
2	89–97	1.05
3	86–95	1.06
4	83–93	1.07
5	80–92	1.08
6	78–90	1.10
7	77–88	1.11
8	76–86	1.12
9	74–84	1.13
10	72–83	1.14
11	70–81	1.16
12	68–79	1.17
13	67–78	1.18
14	65–77	1.19
15	64–75	1.20
16	62–74	1.22
17	59–73	1.23
18	58–71	1.25
19	57–69	1.26
20	56–67	1.27
21	55–66	1.29
22	53–65	1.31
23	52–63	1.32
24	51–60	1.34
25	50–59	1.36
30	44–52	1.47
35	39–47	1.53
40	34–42	1.60

[a]To correct for elution, multiply the % ^{51}Cr by the elution factor for the particular day.

Figure 17.5 ^{51}Cr red cell survival. The hatched area shows the normal range.

Figure 17.6 ^{51}Cr red cell survival curve. Patient with hereditary spherocytosis. The results give a straight line when plotted on arithmetic graph paper. The mean cell lifespan is indicated by the point at which its extension cuts the abscissa (20 days).

Figure 17.7 ^{51}Cr red cell survival curve. Patient with autoimmune haemolytic anaemia. The results have been plotted on semilogarithmic graph paper and the mean cell lifespan was read as the time when 37% of the cells were still surviving (9–10 days). The T$_{50}$Cr was 6–7 days. MCL, mean cell lifespan.

destruction is typically random and the curve of elimination is thus exponential and the data give a straight line when plotted on semilogarithmic graph paper.

In some cases of haemolytic anaemia (possibly only when there are intracorpuscular defects), the survival curve appears to consist of two components, an initial steep slope followed by a much less steeply falling slope. This suggests the presence of cells of widely varying lifespan. This type of 'double population' curve is seen in paroxysmal nocturnal haemoglobinuria, in sickle cell anaemia, in some cases of hereditary enzyme-deficiency haemolytic anaemia and when the labelled cells consist of a mixture of transfused normal cells and short-lived patient's cells. The mean cell lifespan of the entire cell population can be deduced by plotting the points on semilogarithmic graph paper, as described earlier. The proportion of cells belonging to the longer-lived population can be estimated by plotting the data on arithmetic graph paper and extrapolating the less steep slope back to the ordinate; the lifespan of this population can be estimated by extending the same slope to the abscissa (Fig. 17.8). The lifespan of the short-lived cells can be deduced from the formula:

$$MCLs = \frac{\%S}{\dfrac{100}{MCL_T} - \dfrac{\%L}{MCL_L}}$$

where S = short-lived population, L = longer-lived population, T = entire cell population and MCL = mean cell lifespan.

Figure 17.8 ^{51}Cr red cell survival curve showing a 'double population'. By plotting the data on semilogarithmic graph paper as described in Figure 17.7, the mean cell lifespan (MCL) of the entire cell population was deduced as 5 days. When plotted on arithmetic graph paper, by extrapolation of the less steep slope to the ordinate it was deduced that approximately 30% of the red cells belonged to one population, and by extrapolation of the same slope to the abscissa the MCL of this population was deduced as 35 days. The lifespan of the remaining 70% of cells was calculated to be 3.6 days (see formula). The T$_{50}$Cr was 3–4 days.

Correction for Early Loss

The simplest method is to ignore the early loss by taking as 100% the radioactivity still present at the end of 24–48 h. Alternatively, the following method can be used; it has the advantage that the slope of the survival curve is not altered. Plot the data on arithmetic graph paper, extrapolate the line of the slope beyond the initial steep part back to the ordinate and take the point of intersection as 100%; then calibrate the ordinate scale accordingly.

Blood Volume Changes

There is no need to correct the measurements of radioactivity per ml of whole blood for alterations in PCV provided that the total blood volume remains constant throughout the study. However, if it is suspected that the TBV may be changing (e.g. in patients suffering from haemorrhage or being transfused), serial determinations of TBV should be carried out and the observed radioactivity should be multiplied by the observed TBV and divided by the initial TBV. In practice, if a patient receives a blood transfusion during a survival study, it can, as a general rule, be assumed that the TBV will have returned to its pretransfusion level within 24–48 h.

Correction of Survival Data for Blood Loss

When there is a relatively constant loss of blood during a red cell survival study, the true mean red cell lifespan can be obtained by the following equation:

$$\text{True MCL} = \frac{\text{Ta} \times \text{RCV}}{\text{RCV} - (\text{Ta} \times \text{L})}$$

where Ta = apparent time of MCL (days), RCV = red cell volume (ml) and L = mean rate of loss of red cells (ml/day).

Normal Red Cell Lifespan

The mean red cell lifespan in health is usually taken as 120 days.

Determination of Sites of Red Cell Destruction Using ^{51}Cr

Because ^{51}Cr is a γ-ray emitter, the sites of destruction of red cells, with special reference to the spleen and liver, can be determined by *in vivo* surface counting using a shielded scintillation counter placed, respectively, over the heart, spleen and liver. This procedure is laborious, but occasionally it may provide clinically useful information on the role of the spleen in various types of haemolytic anaemia, especially by predicting response to splenectomy.[30]

COMPATIBILITY TEST

The behaviour of labelled donor cells in a recipient will provide important information on the compatibility or otherwise of the donor blood:

1. When serological tests suggest that all normal donors are incompatible
2. When in the presence of an alloantibody no non-reacting donor can be found
3. When the recipient has had an unexplained haemolytic transfusion reaction.

Method

Remove 1–2 ml of blood from the tubing attached to donor bag using a sterile technique. Label 0.5 ml of the red cells with 0.8 MBq of ^{51}Cr, 2 MBq of ^{111}In or 2 MBq of ^{99m}Tc in the standard way (see p. 378) and administer to the recipient. Collect 5–10 ml of blood into EDTA or heparin at 3, 10 and 60 min after the injection from a vein other than that used for the injection. Prepare 1 ml samples in counting vials. Centrifuge the remainder of the specimens and pipette 1 ml of the plasma into counting vials. Measure the radioactivity in the usual way. Calculate the activity in the blood and plasma samples as a percentage of the 3 min blood sample.[29]

Interpretation

With compatible blood, the radioactivity in the 60 min sample is, on average, 99% of that of the 3 min sample, but it may vary between 94% and 104%. If the blood radioactivity at 60 min is not less than 70% and the plasma activity is not more than 3%, the donor cells may be transfused with minimal hazard.[29]

VISUALIZATION OF THE SPLEEN BY SCINTILLATION SCANNING

Anatomical features of organs, including the spleen, are usually studied in radiology or nuclear medicine departments by means of magnetic resonance imaging (MRI), computed tomography imaging (CT scans) or ultrasound imaging. Imaging of radioisotope-labelled red cells provides an alternative functional method. If red blood cells labelled with ^{99m}Tc are heat damaged, they will be selectively removed by the spleen. ^{99m}Tc-labelled colloid is also removed from the circulation by the spleen, but this is not as specific because it is also taken up by reticuloendothelial cells in the liver and elsewhere. The rate of uptake of the isotope by the spleen is a measure of its function (see below). Imaging by scintillation scanning is usually started about 1 h after the injection of the damaged cells, but it can be performed up to 3–4 h later. Accumulation of radioactivity within the spleen after administration of heat-damaged labelled cells thus provides a means of demonstrating its size and position, whether it is absent or has reduced function and the presence of splenunculi. Satisfactory scans can also be obtained with ^{51}Cr or ^{111}In.

Method

With ^{99m}Tc as the label, carry out pre-tinning *in vivo* by an injection of a stannous compound as described on p. 378. Then collect 5–10 ml of blood into a sterile bottle containing 100 iu of heparin. Wash twice in sterile 9 g/l NaCl (saline), centrifuging at 1200–1500 *g* for 5–10 min. Transfer 2 ml of the packed red cells to a 30 ml glass bottle with a screw cap; heat the bottle in a waterbath at a constant temperature of 49.5–50°C for exactly 20 min with occasional gentle mixing. Wash the cells in saline until the supernatant is free from haemoglobin and discard the final supernatant. Label with 40 MBq of ^{99m}Tc by the method described on p. 378. After it has stood for 5 min, wash twice in saline. Resuspend in about 10 ml of saline and inject as soon as possible. After about 1 h carry out a gamma camera scan.[31]

Spleen Function

Information on splenic activity may be obtained by measuring the rate of clearance of heat-damaged labelled red cells from the circulation. A blood sample is taken exactly 3 min after the midpoint of the injection and further samples are collected at 5-min intervals for 30 min, at 45 min and finally at 60 min. The radioactivity in each sample is measured and expressed as a percentage of the radioactivity in the 3-min sample. The results are plotted on semi-logarithmic graph paper, the 3-min sample being taken as 100% radioactivity. For consistent results, a carefully standardized technique is necessary to ensure that the red cells are damaged to the same extent.

The disappearance curve is, as a rule, exponential (Fig. 17.9). The initial slope reflects the splenic blood flow; the rate of blood flow is calculated as the reciprocal of the time taken for the radioactivity to fall to half the 3-min value (i.e. $\frac{0.693}{T_{1/2}}$),

where 0.693 is the natural log of 2.

When the spleen is functioning normally, the $T_{1/2}$ is 5–15 min and fractional splenic blood flow is 0.05–0.14 ml/min (i.e. 5–14% of the circulating blood per min). The clearance rate is considerably prolonged in some patients with thrombocythaemia and in other conditions associated with splenic atrophy such as sickle cell anaemia, coeliac disease and dermatitis herpetiformis.[17] It thus provides some indication of spleen function. However, the disappearance curve is a complex of at least two components. The first (mentioned earlier) reflects the splenic blood flow and the second component mainly measures cell trapping, the consequence of both transient

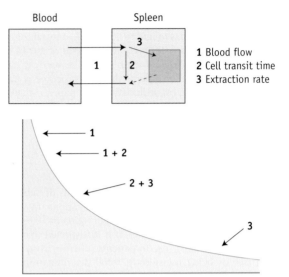

Figure 17.9 Curve of disappearance of heat-damaged red cells from the circulation. The curve shows the sequence of blood flow, transient pooling, sequestration and irreversible trapping of cells.

sequestration and phagocytosis with irreversible extraction of the cells from circulation.[32,33] Measurement of phagocytosis alone is obtained more reliably with immunoglobulin G (IgG) (anti-D)-coated red cells.[34]

LEUCOCYTE IMAGING

The main diagnostic value of ^{111}In-labelled granulocyte scintigraphy is to localize specific sites of infection and abscesses and, in investigation of patients with fever of unknown origin, to rule out an infectious cause for the fever.[35] For this it is necessary to prepare a granulocyte concentrate separated from other leucocytes (see p. 65). This is then labelled with ^{111}In in a procedure similar to that for labelling platelets (see p. 389)[36] and administered. The sites of granulocyte accumulation are shown by gamma camera scan.

MISCELLANEOUS IMAGING

In addition to the radioisotopes discussed earlier, there are other radioisotopes that can be used to provide information in haematological disorders. For example, ^{18}F-FDG (fluorine-18 fluorodeoxyglucose), a tracer of glucose metabolism, with position emission tomography (PET) can be useful in the assessment of tumour metabolism.[37,38] The information generated can assist in clinical staging of patients with malignancies, including lymphoma. Malignant tissue shows enhanced uptake of this tracer and this information can be used to monitor progress of patients receiving chemotherapy.

Similarly, other more mainstream radiological investigations can be useful in the management of haematological diseases. For example, MRI can assist in monitoring the progress of patients with lymphoma and myeloma. In the management of patients with iron overload, MRI scans (by specified imaging method T2) can provide important information on liver and cardiac iron that can be used to optimize iron chelation regimens.[39]

MEASUREMENT OF BLOOD LOSS FROM THE GASTROINTESTINAL TRACT

The ^{51}Cr method of red cell labelling can be used to quantitate blood lost into the gastrointestinal tract because ^{51}Cr is neither excreted nor more than minimally reabsorbed. Accordingly when the blood contains ^{51}Cr-labelled red cells, faecal radioactivity is at a very low level unless bleeding has taken place somewhere within the gastrointestinal tract. Measurement of the faecal radioactivity then gives a reliable indication of the extent of the blood loss.

Method

Label the patient's own blood with approximately 4 MBq of ^{51}Cr, as described on see p. 378. On each day of the test, collect the faeces in plastic or waxed cardboard cartons. Prepare a standard by adding a measured volume (3–5 ml) of the patient's blood, collected on each day, to approximately 100 ml of water in a similar carton. Compare the radioactivity of the faecal samples and the corresponding daily standard in a large-volume counting system (see p. 375). Then:

$$\text{Volume of blood in faeces (in ml)} = \frac{\text{cpm/24 hour faeces collection}}{\text{cpm/ml standard}}$$

Blood loss from any other source (e.g. surgical operation or menstruation) can be measured in a similar way by counting swabs, dressings and so on placed in a carton. It is not, however, possible to measure blood or haemoglobin loss in the urine (haematuria or haemoglobinuria) by this method because free ^{51}Cr is normally excreted in the urine.

An imaging procedure has also been described in which blood is labelled with ^{99m}Tc and a large-field scintillation scan is performed after 60–90 min and, if necessary, again at intervals for 24 h.[40]

MEASUREMENT OF PLATELET LIFESPAN

Principle

The procedure for measuring platelet lifespan is broadly similar to that for red cell survival (see p. 383). A method using ^{111}In-labelled platelets was recommended by ICSH.[41] A modification of this method especially for use with low platelet counts[42] is described in the following.

Method

Collect 51 ml of blood into 9 ml of NIH-A ACD (see p. 619); a proportionally lower amount is required if the platelet count is normal or high. Distribute the blood equally into three 30 ml polystyrene tubes, each containing 2 ml of 60 g/l hydroxyethyl starch (Hespan, Bristol Myers Squibb). Mix and immediately centrifuge at 150 g for 10 min. Transfer the supernatant platelet-rich plasma into clean centrifuge tubes and add ACD, 1 volume to 10 volumes of the platelet-rich plasma. If necessary, centrifuge again at 150 g for 5 min to remove residual red cells.[42]

Centrifuge the platelet-rich plasma at 640 g for 10 min to obtain platelet pellets. Carefully remove the supernatant plasma but do not discard. Add 1 ml of this platelet-poor plasma to the platelet pellets, gently tap the tubes to resuspend and pool the contents.

Prepare a solution of tropolone, 4.4 mmol/l (0.54 mg/ml) in HEPES-saline buffer, pH 7.6 (see p. 622). Mix 0.1 ml with 8 MBq (250 μCi) of ^{111}InCl in <50 μl of 40 mmol/l HCl. Add the platelet suspension with gentle mixing and leave at room temperature for 5 min. Then add 5 ml of platelet-poor plasma. Centrifuge at 640 g for 10 min. Remove the supernatant and resuspend the platelet pellet in 5 ml of platelet-poor plasma. Take up the platelet suspension into a 10 ml plastic syringe.

Add 0.5 ml of the platelet suspension to 100 ml of water in a volumetric flask as a standard. Weigh the syringe, inject the platelets into the patient through a butterfly needle and reweigh.

$$\text{Volume injected} = \text{Wt (g)} \times 1/1.015$$

where 1.015 is the specific gravity of plasma.

Collect 5 ml blood samples in EDTA at 45 min and at 2, 3 and 4 h after injection and then daily for up to 10 days.

Measure the PCV/Hct and centrifuge part of each sample at 1500 g for 10 min to obtain cell-free plasma.

Lyse part of the whole blood sample with 2% saponin and measure the radioactivity in 1 ml sample of whole blood, plasma and diluted standard.

From radioactivity in 1 ml of whole-blood sample subtract the radioactivity in 1 ml of plasma, corrected for the true volume of plasma in 1 ml of whole blood (i.e. 1 − PCV/Hct).

Calculation of Platelet Recovery at Each Sampling Time

$$\frac{\text{cpm/ml blood sample (corrected for plasma activity)} \times \text{Total BV (ml)}}{\text{cpm/ml standard} \times \text{dilution of standard} \times \text{volume injected}}$$

Note: If total blood volume is not measured, an approximate estimate can be obtained from the subject's height and weight.[43]

Analysis of Data

Plot the percentage survival against time on arithmetic graph paper and estimate the survival time as for red cell survival (see p. 385).

By this method, normal platelet lifespan is 8–10 days, but the validity of the analysis is based on the assumption that the blood volume is constant and the pattern of disappearance of platelets from the circulation remains constant during the course of the study.

Platelet Survival in Disease

In autoimmune (idiopathic) thrombocytopenia purpura, platelet lifespan is considerably reduced. It is also shortened in consumption coagulopathies and in thrombotic thrombocytopenic purpura. In thrombocytopenia, because of defective production of platelets, the lifespan should be normal, provided that platelets are not being lost by bleeding during the course of the study. In thrombocytopenia associated with splenomegaly, the recovery of injected labelled platelets is low, but their survival is usually almost normal. By quantitative scanning with ^{111}In, it is possible to measure the splenic platelet pool and to distinguish the relative importance of pooling and destruction of platelets in the spleen.[44–46] The splenic platelet pool is normally about 30% of the total platelet population and it is thought that each platelet spends one-third of its lifespan in the spleen. The size of the pool is increased in splenomegaly, resulting in thrombocytopenia but not necessarily in a reduced mean platelet lifespan.

REFERENCES

1. Wagner HN, Szabo Z, Buchanan JW. *Principles of Nuclear Medicine.* Philadelphia: Saunders; 1995.

2. Maisey MN, Britton KE, Collier BD. *Clinical Nuclear Medicine.* 3rd ed. London: Chapman and Hall; 1998.

3. Lewis SM, Bayly RJ, eds. *Methods in Hematology 14: Radionuclides in Haematology.* Edinburgh: Churchill Livingstone; 1986.

4. Allisy-Roberts P, ed. *Medical and Dental Guidance Notes. Good Practice Guide on All Aspects of Ionizing Radiation Protection in the Clinical Environment.* York, UK: Institute of Physics and Engineering in Medicine; 2002.

5. ARSAC. *Notes for guidance on the administration of radiopharmaceuticals and use of sealed radioactive sources.* Didcot Oxon: Health Protection Agency, Radiation Protection Division, Chilton; 2006. Available at: *www.arsac.org.uk.*

5a. *The Environmental Permitting (England and Wales) Regulations 2010 (SI 2010 No.675).* London: HMSO; 2010.

6. Alavi A, ed. Impact of FDG-PET imaging on the practice of medicine. *Semin Nucl Med.* 2002;32: 1–76.

7. Jamar F, Lonneux M. Positron emission tomography in haematology. In: Peters AM, ed. *Nuclear Medicine in Radiological Diagnosis.* London: Martin Dinitz; 2003:519–529.

8. Bentley SA, Lewis SM. The relationship between total red cell volume, plasma volume and venous haematocrit. *Br J Haematol.* 1976;33:301–307.

9. International Committee for Standardization in Haematology. Recommended methods for measurements of red-cell and plasma volume. *J Nucl Med.* 1980;21:793–800.

10. Ferrant A, Lewis SM, Szur L. The elution of ^{99m}Tc from red cells and its effect on red cell volume measurement. *J Clin Pathol.* 1974;27:983–985.

11. Goodwin DA. Cell labelling with oxine chelates of radioactive metal ions: techniques and clinical implications. *J Nucl Med.* 1978;19:557–559.

12. Osman S, Danpure HJ. A simple in vitro method of radiolabelling human erythrocytes in whole blood with ^{113m}In-tropolonate. *Eur J Haematol.* 1987;39:125–127.

13. Berlin NI, Lewis SM. Measurement of total red-cell volume relative to lean body mass for diagnosis of polycythaemia. *Am J Clin Pathol.* 2000;114:922–926.

14. International Council for Standardization in Haematology (Expert Panel on Radionuclides). Interpretation of measured red cell mass and plasma volume in adults. *Br J Haematol.* 1995;89:747–756.

15. Lukaski HC, Johnson PE, Bolunchuk WW, et al. Assessment of fat-free mass using bioelectrical impedance measurements of the human body. *Am J Clin Nutr.* 1985;41:810–817.

16. Lund CJ, Sisson TR. Blood volume and anemia of mother and baby. *Am J Obstet Gynecol.* 1958;76: 1013–1023.

17. Pettit JE. Spleen function. *Clin Haematol.* 1977;6:639–656.

18. Bateman S, Lewis SM, Nicholas A, et al. Splenic red cell pooling: a diagnostic feature in polycythaemia. *Br J Haematol.* 1978;40:389–396.

19. Hegde UM, Williams ED, Lewis SM, et al. Measurement of splenic red cell volume and visualization of the spleen with ^{99m}Tc. *J Nucl Med.* 1973;14:769–771.

20. Miller JH. Technetium-99m-labelled red blood cells in the evaluation of the liver in infants and children. *J Nucl Med.* 1987;28:1412–1418.

21. Front D, Israel O. Tc-99m-labelled red blood cells in the evaluation of vascular abnormalities. *J Nucl Med.* 1981;22:149–151.

22. Cavill I. Plasma clearance studies. *Methods in Hematology.* 1986;14: 214–244.

23. Peters AM, Swirsky DM. Blood disorders. In: Maisey MN, Britton KE, Collier BD, eds. *Clinical*

Nuclear Medicine. 3rd ed. London: Chapman and Hall; 1998.

24. Bentley SA, Miller DT. Radionuclide blood cell survival studies. *Methods in Hematology*. 1986;14:245–262.

25. Ricketts C, Cavill I, Napier JAF. The measurement of red cell lifespan using ^{59}Fe. *Br J Haematol*. 1977;37:403–408.

26. Pearson HA. The binding of ^{51}Cr to hemoglobin. I. In vitro studies. *Blood*. 1963;22:218–230.

27. Jandl JH, Greenberg MS, Yonemoto RH, et al. Clinical determination of the sites of red cell sequestration in hemolytic anemias. *J Clin Invest*. 1956; 35:842–867.

28. Koutras GA, Schneider AS, Hattori M, et al. Studies of chromated erythrocytes: mechanisms of chromate inhibition of glutathione reductase. *Br J Haematol*. 1965;11:360–369.

29. International Committee for Standardization in Haematology. Recommended methods for radioisotope red-cell survival studies. *Br J Haematol*. 1980;45:659–666.

30. International Committee for Standardization in Haematology. Recommended methods for surface counting to determine sites of red-cell destruction. *Br J Haematol*. 1975;30:249–254.

31. Royal HD, Brown ML, Drum DE, et al. Procedure guideline for hepatic and splenic imaging. *J Nucl Med*. 1998;39:1114–1116.

32. Peters AM, Ryan PF, Klonizakis I, et al. Analysis of heat-damaged erythrocyte clearance curves. *Br J Haematol*. 1981;49:581–586.

33. Peters AM, Ryan PFJ, Klonizakis I, et al. Kinetics of heat damaged autologous red blood cells. *Scand J Haematol*. 1982;28:5–14.

34. Peters AM, Walport MJ, Elkon KB, et al. The comparative blood clearance kinetics of modified radiolabelled erythrocytes. *Clin Sci*. 1984;66:55–62.

35. Kjaer A, Lebech A-M. Diagnostic value of ^{111}In-granulocyte scintigraphy in patients with fever of unknown origin. *J Nucl Med*. 2002; 43:140–144.

36. Buscombe J. Infection. In: Maisey MN, Britton KE, Collier BD, eds. *Clinical Nuclear Medicine*. 3rd ed. London: Chapman and Hall; 1998.

37. Weber WA, Schwaiger M, Avril N. Quantitative assessment of tumour metabolism using FDG-PET imaging. *Nucl Med Biol*. 2000;27:683–687.

38. Schöder H, Larson SM, Yeung HW. PET/CT in oncology: Integration into clinical management of lymphoma, melanoma and gastrointestinal malignancies. *J Nucl Med*. 2004;45:72S–81S.

39. Anderson LJ, Wonke B, Prescott E, et al. Comparison of effects of oral deferiprone and subcutaneous desferrioxamine on myocardial iron concentrations and ventricular function in beta-thalassaemia. *Lancet*. 2002;360:516–520.

40. Ford PV, Bartold SP, Fink-Bennett DM, et al. Procedure guideline for gastrointestinal bleeding and Meckel's diverticulum scintigraphy. *J Nucl Med*. 1999;40:1226–1232.

41. International Committee for Standardization in Haematology. Recommended methods for ^{111}In platelet survival studies. *J Nucl Med*. 1988;29:564–566.

42. Danpure HJ, Osman S, Peters AM. Labelling autologous platelets with ^{111}In tropolonate for platelet kinetic studies: limitations imposed by thrombocytopenia. *Eur J Haematol*. 1990;45:223–230.

43. Hurley PJ. Red cell and plasma volumes in normal adults. *J Nucl Med*. 1975;16:46–52.

44. Peters AM, Swirsky DM. Blood disorders. In: Maisey MN, Britton KE, Collier BD, eds. *Clinical Nuclear Medicine*. 3rd ed. London: Chapman and Hall; 1998:525–539.

45. Peters AM, Saverymuttu SH, Bell RN, et al. The kinetics of short-lived indium-111 radiolabelled platelets. *Scand J Haematol*. 1985; 34:137–145.

46. Peters AM, Saverymuttu SH, Wonke B, et al. The interpretation of platelet kinetic studies for the identification of site of abnormal platelet destruction. *Br J Haematol*. 1984;57:637–649.

Chapter | **18** |

Investigation of haemostasis

Michael A. Laffan, Richard Manning

COMPONENTS OF NORMAL HAEMOSTASIS

The haemostatic mechanisms have several important functions: (1) to maintain blood in a fluid state while it remains circulating within the vascular system; (2) to arrest bleeding at the site of injury or blood loss by formation of a haemostatic plug; (3) to limit this process to the vicinity of the damage; and (4) to ensure the eventual removal of the plug when healing is complete. Normal physiology thus constitutes a delicate balance between these conflicting tendencies and a deficiency or exaggeration of any one may lead to either thrombosis or haemorrhage. There are at least five different components involved: blood vessels, platelets, plasma coagulation factors and their inhibitors and the fibrinolytic system. In this chapter, a brief review of normal haemostasis is presented, followed by a discussion on the general principles of basic tests used to investigate haemostasis and bleeding disorders.

The Blood Vessel

General Structure of the Blood Vessel

The blood vessel wall has three layers: intima, media and adventitia. The intima consists of endothelium and subendothelial connective tissue and is separated from the media by the elastic lamina interna. Endothelial cells form a continuous monolayer lining all blood vessels. The structure and the function of the endothelial cells vary according to their location in the vascular tree, but in their resting state they all share three important characteristics: they are 'non-thrombogenic' (i.e. they promote maintenance of blood in its fluid state); they play an active role in supplying nutrients to the subendothelial structures; and they act as a barrier to cells, macromolecules and particulate matter circulating in the bloodstream. The permeability of the endothelium may vary under different conditions to allow various molecules and cells to pass.

Endothelial Cell Function

The luminal surface of the endothelial cell[1] is covered by the glycocalyx, a proteoglycan coat. It contains heparan sulphate and other glycosaminoglycans, which are capable of activating antithrombin, an important inhibitor of coagulation enzymes. Tissue factor pathway inhibitor (TFPI) is present on endothelial cell surfaces bound to these heparans but also tethered to a glycophosphoinositol (GPI) anchor. The relative importance of these two TFPI pools is not known. Endothelial cells express a number of coagulation active proteins that play an important regulatory role such as thrombomodulin and the endothelial protein C (PC) receptor. Thrombin generated at the site of injury is rapidly bound to a specific product of the endothelial cell, thrombomodulin. When bound to this protein, thrombin can activate PC (which degrades factors Va and VIIIa) and a carboxypeptidase which inhibits fibrinolysis (discussed later). Thrombin also stimulates the endothelial cell to produce tissue plasminogen activator (tPA). The endothelium can also synthesize protein S, the cofactor for PC. Finally, endothelium produces von Willebrand factor (VWF), which is essential for platelet adhesion to the subendothelium and stabilizes factor VIII within the circulation. VWF is both stored in specific granules called Weibel Palade bodies and secreted constitutively, partly into the circulation and partly toward the subendothelium where it binds directly to collagen and other matrix proteins. The expression of these and other important molecules such as adhesion molecules and their receptors are modulated by inflammatory cytokines. The lipid bilayer membrane also contains adenosine diphosphatase (ADPase), an enzyme that degrades adenosine diphosphate (ADP), which is a potent platelet agonist (see p. 434). Many of the surface proteins are found localized in the specialized lipid rafts and invaginations called 'caveolae', which may provide an important level of regulation.[2]

The endothelial cell participates in vasoregulation by producing and metabolizing numerous vasoactive substances. On the one hand, it metabolizes and inactivates vasoactive peptides such as bradykinin; on the other hand, it can also generate angiotensin II, a local vasoconstrictor, from circulating angiotensin I. Under appropriate stimulation the endothelial cell can produce vasodilators such as nitric oxide (NO) and prostacyclin or vasoconstrictors such as endothelin and thromboxane. These substances have their principal vasoregulatory effect via the smooth muscle but also have some effect on platelets.

The subendothelium consists of connective tissues composed of collagen (principally types I, III and VI), elastic tissues, proteoglycans and non-collagenous glycoproteins, including fibronectin and VWF. After vessel wall damage has occurred, these components are exposed and are then responsible for platelet adherence. This appears to be mediated by VWF binding to collagen. VWF then undergoes a conformational change and platelets are captured via their surface membrane glycoprotein Ib binding to VWF. Platelet activation follows and a conformational change in glycoprotein IIbIIIa allows further, more secure, binding to VWF via this receptor as well as to fibrinogen. At low shear rates ($<1000 \, s^{-1}$) platelet binding directly to collagen appears to dominate.[3]

Vasoconstriction

Vessels with muscular coats contract following injury, thus helping to arrest blood loss. Although not all coagulation reactions are enhanced by reduced flow, this probably assists in the formation of a stable fibrin plug by allowing activated factors to accumulate to critical concentrations. Vasoconstriction[1,4] also occurs in the microcirculation in vessels without smooth muscle cells. Endothelial cells themselves can produce vasoconstrictors such as angiotensin II. In addition, activated platelets produce thromboxane A_2 (TXA_2), which is a potent vasoconstrictor.

Platelets

Platelets[5,6] are small fragments of cytoplasm derived from megakaryocytes. On average, they are 1.5–3.5 μm in diameter but may be larger in some disease states. They do not contain a nucleus and are bounded by a typical lipid bilayer membrane. Beneath the outer membrane lies the marginal band of microtubules, which maintain the shape of the platelet and depolymerize when aggregation begins. The central cytoplasm is dominated by the three types of platelet granules: the δ granules, α granules and lysosomal granules. The contents of these various granules are detailed in Table 18.1. Finally there exist the dense tubular system and the canalicular membrane system; the latter communicates with the exterior. It is not clear how all these elements act together to perform such functions as contraction and secretion, which are characteristic of platelet activation.

Table 18.1 Some contents of platelet granules

DENSE (δ) GRANULES	α GRANULES	LYSOSOMAL VESICLES
ATP	PF4	Galactosidases
ADP	β-Thromboglobulin	Fucosidases
Calcium	Fibrinogen	Hexosaminidase
Serotonin	Factor V	Glucuronidase
Pyrophosphate	Thrombospondin	Cathepsin
P selectin (CD62P)	Fibronectin	Glycohydrolases
Transforming growth factor-beta (1)	PDGF	+ others
Catecholamines (epinephrine/ norepinephrine)	PAI-1	
GDP/GTP	Histidine-rich glycoprotein α_2 Macroglobulin Plasmin inhibitor P selectin (CD62)	

ADP, adenosine 5′-diphosphate; ATP, adenosine 5′-triphosphate; GDP, guanosine 5′-diphosphate; GTP, guanosine 5′-triphosphate; PAI-1, plasminogen activator inhibitor-1; PDGF, platelet-derived growth factor; PF4, platelet factor 4.

The platelet membrane is the site of interaction with the plasma environment and with the damaged vessel wall. It consists of phospholipids, cholesterol, glycolipids and at least nine glycoproteins, named GPI to GPIX. The membrane phospholipids are asymmetrically distributed, with sphingomyelin and phosphatidylcholine predominating in the outer leaflet and phosphatidyl-ethanolamine, -inositol and -serine in the inner leaflet. After platelet activation the membrane also expresses binding sites for several coagulation proteins, including factor XI and factor VIII.

The contractile system of the platelet consists of the dense microtubular system and the circumferential microfilaments, which maintain the disc shape. Actin is the main constituent of the contractile system, but myosin and a regulatory calcium-binding protein, calmodulin, are also present.

Platelet Function in the Haemostatic Process

The main steps in platelet function[7] are adhesion, activation with shape change and aggregation. When the vessel wall is damaged, the subendothelial structures, including basement membrane, collagen and microfibrils, are exposed. VWF binds to collagen and microfibrils and then captures platelets via initial binding to platelet GPIb, resulting in an initial monolayer of adhering platelets. Binding via GPIb initiates activation of the platelet via a G-protein mechanism. Once activated, platelets immediately change shape from a disc to a tiny sphere with numerous projecting pseudopods. After adhesion of a single layer of platelets to the exposed subendothelium, platelets stick to one another to form aggregates. Fibrinogen, fibronectin, further VWF released from platelets and the glycoprotein Ib-IX and IIbIIIa complexes are essential at this stage to increase the cell-to-cell contact and facilitate aggregation. Certain substances (agonists) react with specific platelet membrane receptors to promote platelet aggregation and further activation. The agonists include exposed collagen fibres, ADP, thrombin, adrenaline, (epinephrine) serotonin and certain arachidonic acid metabolites including TXA_2. In areas of non-linear blood flow, such as may occur at the site of an injury, locally damaged red cells release ADP, which further activates platelets.

Platelet Aggregation

Platelet aggregation may occur by at least two independent but closely linked pathways. The first pathway involves arachidonic acid metabolism. Activation of phospholipase enzymes (PLA_2) releases free arachidonic acid from membrane phospholipids (phosphatidyl choline). About 50% of free arachidonic acid is converted by a lipo-oxygenase enzyme to a series of products including leucotrienes, which are important chemoattractants of white cells. The remaining 50% of arachidonic acid is converted by the enzyme cyclooxygenase into labile cyclic endoperoxides, most of which are in turn converted by thromboxane synthetase into TXA_2. TXA_2 has profound biological effects, causing secondary platelet granule release and local vasoconstriction, as well as further local platelet aggregation via the second pathway below. It exerts these effects by raising intracellular cytoplasmic free calcium concentration and binding to specific granule receptors. TXA_2 is very labile with a half-life of <1 min before it is degraded into the inactive thromboxane B_2 (TXB_2) and malonyldialdehyde.

The second pathway of activation and aggregation can proceed completely independently from the first one: various platelet agonists, including thrombin, TXA_2 and collagen, bind to receptors and via a G-protein mechanism, activate phospholipase C. This generates diacylglycerol and inositol triphosphate, which in turn activate protein kinase C and elevate intracellular calcium, respectively. Calcium is released from the dense tubular system to form complexes with calmodulin; this complex and the free calcium act as coenzymes for the release reaction, for the activation of different regulatory proteins and of actin and myosin and the contractile system and also for the liberation of arachidonic acid from membrane phospholipids and the generation of TXA_2.

The aggregating platelets join together into loose reversible aggregates, but after the release reaction of the platelet granules, larger, firmer aggregates form. Changes in the platelet membrane configuration now occur; 'flip-flop' rearrangement of the surface brings the negatively charged phosphatidyl-serine and -inositol on to the outer leaflet, thus generating platelet factor 3 (procoagulant) activity. At the same time specific receptors for various coagulation factors are exposed on the platelet surface and help coordinate the assembly of the enzymatic complexes of the coagulation system. Local generation of thrombin will then further activate platelets.

Platelets are not activated if in contact with healthy endothelial cells. The 'non-thrombogenicity' of the endothelium is the result of a combination of control mechanisms exerted by the endothelial cell: synthesis of prostacyclin, capacity to bind thrombin and activate the PC system, ability to inactivate vasoactive substances and so on. Prostacyclin released locally binds to specific platelet membrane receptors and then activates the membrane-bound adenylate cyclase (producing cyclic adenosine monophosphate or cAMP). cAMP inhibits platelet aggregation by inhibiting arachidonic acid metabolism and the release of free cytoplasmic calcium ions.

Thus platelets have at least three roles in haemostasis:

1. Adhesion and aggregation forming the primary haemostatic plug
2. Release of platelet activating and procoagulant molecules
3. Provision of a procoagulant surface for the reactions of the coagulation system.

Blood Coagulation

The central event in the coagulation pathways[8] is the production of thrombin, which acts upon fibrinogen to produce fibrin and thus the fibrin clot. This clot is further strengthened by the crosslinking action of factor XIII, which itself is activated by thrombin. The two commonly used coagulation tests, the activated partial thromboplastin time (APTT) and the prothrombin time (PT), have been used historically to define two pathways of coagulation activation: the intrinsic and extrinsic paths, respectively. However, this bears only a limited relationship to the way coagulation is activated *in vivo*. For example, deficiencies of factor XII or of factor VIII both produce marked prolongation of the APTT, but only deficiency of the latter is associated with a haemorrhagic tendency. Moreover, there is considerable evidence that activation of factor IX (intrinsic pathway) by factor VIIa (extrinsic pathway) is crucial to establishing coagulation after an initial stimulus has been provided by factor VIIa-tissue factor (TF) activation of factor X (Fig. 18.1).[8]

Investigation of the coagulation system centres on the coagulation factors, but the activity of these proteins is also greatly dependent on specific surface receptors and

Intrinsic pathway

Extrinsic pathway

Figure 18.1 Schematic representation of the coagulation network. The major interactions are shown by the bold arrows. Inhibitory factors and clot limiting mechanisms are not shown. HMWK, high molecular weight kininogen; PL, phospholipid; TFPI, tissue factor pathway inhibitor.

phospholipids largely presented on the surface of platelets and also by activated endothelium. The necessity for calcium in many of these reactions is frequently used to control their activity *in vitro*. The various factors are described in the following sections, as far as possible in their functional groups; their properties are detailed in Table 18.2.

The Contact Activation System

The contact activation system[9] comprises factor XII (Hageman factor), high molecular weight kininogen (HMWK) (Fitzgerald factor) and prekallikrein/kallikrein (Fletcher factor). As mentioned earlier, these factors are not essential for haemostasis *in vivo*. Important activities are to activate the fibrinolytic system, to activate the complement system and to generate vasoactive peptides: in particular, bradykinin is released from HMWK by prekallikrein or FXIIa cleavage. Kallikrein and factor XIIa also function as chemoattractants for neutrophils. The contact activation system also has some inhibitory effect on thrombin activation of platelets and prevents cell binding to endothelium. Recent evidence implicates the contact system in thrombosis via activation by polyphosphate released from platelets.[10]

When bound to a negatively charged surface *in vitro*, factor XII and prekallikrein are able to reciprocally activate one another by limited proteolysis, but the initiating event is not clear. It may be that a conformational change in factor XII on binding results in limited autoactivation that triggers the process. HMWK acts as a (zinc-dependent) cofactor by facilitating the attachment of prekallikrein and factor XI, with which it circulates in a complex, to the negatively charged surface. It has been shown in *in vitro* studies that platelets or endothelial cells can provide the necessary negatively charged surface for this mechanism and also possess specific receptors for factor XI. The contact system can activate fibrinolysis by a number of mechanisms: plasminogen cleavage, urokinase plasminogen activator (uPA) activation and tissue plasminogen activator (tPA) release. Most importantly from the laboratory point of view, the contact activation system results in the generation of factor XIIa, which is able to activate factor XI, thus initiating the coagulation cascade of the intrinsic pathway.

Tissue Factor

TF is the cofactor for the extrinsic pathway and the physiological initiator of coagulation. It is a transmembrane protein and constitutively present in many tissues outside the vasculature and on the surface of stimulated inflammatory cells such as monocytes and, under some conditions, endothelial cells. Factor VIIa binds to TF in the presence of calcium ions and then becomes enzymatically active. Small amounts of factor VIIa are present in the circulation but have virtually no enzymic activity unless

Table 18.2 The coagulation factors

NO.	FACTOR	RMM (DALTONS)	HALF-LIFE	CONCENTRATION IN PLASMA	
				µg/ml	nmol/l
I	Fibrinogen	340 000	90 h	1.5–4 × 10	–
II	Prothrombin	70 000	60 h	100–150	1400
V	–	330 000	12–36 h	5–10	20
VII	–	48 000	6 h	0.5	10
VIII	–	200 000	12 h	0.2	0.7
VWF	–	800 000–140 000 000	10–24 h[a]	10	–
IX	–	57 000	24 h	4	90
X	–	58 000	40 h	10	170
XI	–	158 000	60 h	6	30
XII	–	80 000	48–52 h	30	375
Prekallikein	–	85 000	48 h	40	450
HMWK	–	120 000	6.5 days	80	700
XIII	–	32 000	3–5 days	30 (A+B)	900 (tetramer)

RMM, relative molecular mass (molecular weight); h, hours; HMWK, high molecular weight kininogen; VWF, von Willebrand factor.
[a]The half-life of VWF varies according the ABO blood group, being shortest in O, longest in AB and intermediate in A and B.

bound to TF. The factor VIIa–TF complex can activate both factor X and factor IX and therefore two routes to thrombin production are stimulated. Factor Xa subsequently binds to TFPI and then to factor VIIa to form an inactive quaternary (Xa–TF–VIIa–TFPI) complex. This mechanism therefore functions to shut off the extrinsic pathway after an initial stimulus to coagulation has been provided.

The Vitamin K-Dependent Factors

The vitamin K-dependent factors group includes coagulation factors II, VII, IX and X. However, it is important to remember that the anticoagulant proteins S, C and Z are also vitamin K-dependent. Each of these proteins contains a number of glutamic acid residues at its amino terminus that are γ-carboxylated by a vitamin K-dependent mechanism. This results in a novel amino acid, γ-carboxyglutamic acid, which by binding calcium is essential in promoting a conformational change in the protein and binding of the factor to negatively charged phospholipid. Because this binding is crucial for coordinating the interaction of the various factors, the proteins produced in the absence of vitamin K (PIVKAs) that are not γ-carboxylated are essentially functionless. The vitamin K-dependent factors are proenzymes or zymogens, which require cleavage, sometimes with release of a small peptide (activation peptide), to become functional. Measurement of these activation peptides has been used as a means of assessing coagulation activation.

Cofactors

Factors VIII and V are the two most labile of the coagulation factors and they are rapidly lost from stored blood or heated plasma. They share considerable structural homology and are cofactors for the serine proteases FIX and FX, respectively; they both require proteolytic activation by factor IIa or Xa to function. Factor VIII circulates in combination with VWF, which is present in the form of large multimers of a basic 200 kDa monomer. One function of VWF is to stabilize factor VIII and protect it from degradation. In the absence of VWF, the survival of factor VIII in the circulation is extremely short (i.e. <2 h instead of the normal 8–12 h). VWF may also serve to deliver factor VIII to platelets adherent to a site of vascular injury. Once factor VIII has been cleaved and activated by thrombin it no longer binds to VWF.

Fibrinogen

Fibrinogen[11] is a large dimeric protein, each half consisting of three polypeptides named Aα, Bβ and γ held together by 12 disulphide bonds. The two monomers are joined together by a further three disulphide bonds. A variant γ chain denoted γ' is produced by a variation in messenger RNA splicing. In the process a platelet binding site is lost and high-affinity binding sites for FXIII and thrombin are gained. The γ' variant constitutes approximately 10% of plasma fibrinogen. A less common (<2%) γ chain variant 'γE' is also produced by splice variation. Fibrinogen is also found in platelets, but the bulk of this is derived from glycoprotein IIbIIIa-mediated endocytosis of plasma fibrinogen, which is then stored in alpha granules, rather than synthesis by megakaryocytes. Fibrin is formed from fibrinogen by thrombin cleavage releasing the A and B peptides from fibrinogen. This results in fibrin monomers that then associate and precipitate forming a polymer that is the visible clot. The central E domain exposed by thrombin cleavage binds with a complementary region on the outer or D domain of another monomer. The monomers thus assemble into a staggered overlapping two-stranded fibril. More complex interactions subsequently lead to branched and thickened fibre formation, making a complex mesh that binds and stabilizes the primary platelet plug.

Factor XIII

The initial fibrin clot is held together by non-covalent interactions and can be deformed and resolubilized. Factor XIII, which is also activated by thrombin, is able to covalently crosslink these fibrin monomers. Factor XIII is a transglutaminase that joins a glutamine residue on one chain to a lysine on an adjacent chain. This loss of resolubility is the basis of the screening test for factor XIII deficiency.

Inhibitors of Coagulation

A number of mechanisms exist to ensure that the production of the fibrin clot is limited to the site of injury and is not allowed to propagate indefinitely.[12,13] First, there are a number of proteins that bind to and inactivate the enzymes of the coagulation cascade. Probably the first of these to become active is TFPI, which rapidly quenches the factor VIIa–TF complex that initiates coagulation. It does this by combining first with factor Xa, so that further propagation of coagulation is dependent on the small amount of thrombin that has been generated during initiation being sufficient to activate the intrinsic pathway.

The principal physiological inactivator of thrombin is antithrombin (AT, formerly ATIII), which belongs to the serpin group of proteins. This binds to factor IIa forming an inactive thrombin–antithrombin complex (TAT), which is subsequently cleared from the circulation by the liver. This process is greatly enhanced by the presence of heparin or vessel wall heparan. AT is responsible for approximately 60% of thrombin-inactivating capacity in the plasma; the remainder is provided by heparin cofactor II and less specific inhibitors such as α2 macroglobulin. AT is also capable of inactivating factors X, IX, XI and XII but to lesser degrees than thrombin.

As thrombin spreads away from the area of damage it is also bound by thrombomodulin on the surface of endothelial cells. In this way it is changed from a primarily procoagulant protein to an anticoagulant one. Although remaining available for binding to AT, thrombin bound to thrombomodulin no longer cleaves fibrinogen. It now has a greatly enhanced preference for PC as a substrate. PC is presented to the thrombin–thrombomodulin complex by the endothelial protein C receptor (EPCR) and when activated by thrombin cleavage acts to limit and arrest coagulation by inactivating factors Va and VIIIa. This action is further enhanced by its cofactor, protein S, which does not require prior activation. The role of EPCR is particularly important in larger vessels, where the effective concentration of thrombomodulin is low. PC is subsequently inactivated by its own specific inhibitor.

The Fibrinolytic System

The deposition of fibrin and its removal are regulated by the fibrinolytic system.[14] Although this is a complex multicomponent system with many activators and inhibitors, it centres around the fibrinogen- and fibrin-cleaving enzyme plasmin. Plasmin circulates in its inactive precursor form, plasminogen, which is activated by proteolytic cleavage. The principal plasminogen activator (PA) in humans is tissue plasminogen activator (tPA), which is another serine protease. tPA and plasminogen are both able to bind to fibrin via the amino acid lysine. Binding to fibrin brings tPA and plasminogen into close proximity so that the rate of plasminogen activation is markedly increased and thus plasmin is generated preferentially at its site of action and not free in plasma. The second important physiological PA in humans is called urokinase (uPA). This single chain molecule (scu-PA or pro-urokinase) is activated by plasmin or kallikrein to a two-chain derivative (tcu-PA), which is not fibrin-specific in its action. However, the extent to which this is important in vivo is not clear and the identification of cell surface receptors for uPA suggests that its primary role may be extravascular. The contact activation system also appears to generate some plasminogen activation via factor XIIa and bradykinin-stimulated release of tPA. The degradation products released by the action of plasmin on fibrin are of diagnostic use and are discussed later in this chapter. The activation of plasmin on fibrin is restricted by the action of a carboxypeptidase, which removes the amino terminal lysine residues to which plasminogen and tPA bind. This carboxypeptidase is activated by thrombomodulin-bound thrombin and is referred to as thrombin-activated fibrinolysis inhibitor (TAFI).

PAI-1 (plasminogen activator inhibitor-1) is a potent inhibitor of tPA, produced by endothelial cells, hepatocytes, platelets and placenta. Levels in plasma are highly variable. It is a member of the serpin family and is active against tPA and tcu-PA. A second inhibitor PAI-2 has also been identified, originally from human placenta, but its role and importance are not yet established.

The main physiological inhibitor of plasmin in plasma is plasmin inhibitor (α2-antiplasmin), which inhibits plasmin function by forming a 1:1 complex (plasmin–antiplasmin complex, PAP). This reaction in free solution is extremely rapid but depends on the availability of free lysine-binding sites on the plasmin. Thus, fibrin-bound plasmin in the clot is not accessible to the inhibitor. Deficiencies of the fibrinolytic system are rare but have sometimes been associated with a tendency to thrombosis or haemorrhage.

GENERAL APPROACH TO INVESTIGATION OF HAEMOSTASIS

This section begins with some general points regarding the clinical and laboratory approach to the investigation of haemostasis. Following this, the basic or first-line screening tests of haemostasis are described. These tests are generally used as the first step in investigation of an acutely bleeding patient, a person with a suspected bleeding tendency or as a precaution before an invasive procedure is carried out. They have the virtue that they are easily performed and the patterns of abnormalities obtained point clearly to the appropriate next set of investigations. It should be remembered, however, that these tests examine only a portion of the haemostatic mechanism and have limited sensitivity for the presence of significant bleeding diatheses such as von Willebrand disease (VWD) or disorders of platelets or vessels. Hence a normal 'clotting screen' should not be taken to mean that haemostasis is normal.[15]

Clinical Approach

The investigation of a suspected bleeding tendency may begin from three different points:

1. *Investigating a clinically suspected bleeding tendency.* The investigation properly begins with the bleeding history, which may suggest an acquired or congenital disorder of primary or secondary haemostasis. If the bleeding history or family history is significant, appropriate specific tests and assays should be performed, notwithstanding the results of screening tests such as the PT, APTT and so on. Considerable

effort has been put into defining those aspects of clinical history that predict a significant bleeding disorder and bleeding state questionnaires are now available.[16]

2. *Following up an abnormal first-line test.* The abnormalities already detected will determine the appropriate further investigations (discussed later).

3. *Investigation of acute haemostatic failure.* This is often required in the context of an acutely ill or postoperative patient. Investigations are therefore directed toward detecting disseminated intravascular coagulation (DIC) or a previously undetected coagulation defect (congenital or acquired). The availability of a normal premorbid coagulation screen and further questioning to determine a bleeding history can be extremely useful in this respect.

In all cases, comprehensive clinical evaluation, including the patient's history, the family history and the family tree, as well as the details of the site, frequency and the character of haemorrhagic manifestations (purpura, bruising, large haematomata, haemarthroses, etc.), are required to establish a definitive diagnosis. If considered in conjunction with laboratory results, they will help avoid misinterpretation. It is also desirable to undertake a series of screening tests before proceeding to more specific tests. The results of the screening investigations, taken in conjunction with clinical information, usually point to the appropriate additional procedure.

Principles of Laboratory Analysis

It is worth remembering that the tests of coagulation performed in the laboratory are attempts to mimic *in vitro* processes that normally occur *in vivo*. Not surprisingly, this may give rise to misleading results. One of the most striking is the gross prolongation of the APTT in complete factor XII deficiency in the absence of any bleeding tendency. Similarly, the amount of factor VII required to produce a normal PT is greatly in excess of the amount required for normal haemostasis. Conversely, normal screening tests do not necessarily imply that the patient has entirely normal haemostasis.

The more detailed investigations of coagulation proteins also require caution in their interpretation depending on the type of assay performed. These can be divided into three principal categories, as described in the following sections.

Immunological

Immunological tests include immuno-diffusion, immuno-electrophoresis, radioimmunometric assays, latex agglutination (immunoturbidimetric) tests and tests using enzyme-linked immunosorbent assays (ELISA). Fundamentally, all these tests rely on the recognition of the protein in question by polyclonal or monoclonal antibodies.

Polyclonal antibodies lack specificity but provide relatively high sensitivity, whereas monoclonal antibodies are highly specific but produce relatively low levels of antigen binding. Immunological assays are often easy to perform, particularly convenient for large batches and can be bought as kits with standardized controls. The obvious drawback of these assays is that they may tell you nothing about the functional capacity of the antigen detected. If possible they should always be carried out in parallel with a functional assay.

With advances in automation, latex agglutination kits are becoming more popular and replacing the more established ELISA assays. Latex microparticles are coated with antibodies specific for the antigen to be determined. When the latex suspension is mixed with plasma an antigen–antibody reaction takes place, leading to the agglutination of the latex microparticles. Agglutination leads to an increase in turbidity of the reaction medium and this increase in turbidity is measured photometrically as an increase in absorbance. Usually the wavelength used for latex assays is 405 nm, although for some assays a wavelength of 540 or 800 nm is used. Instrument-specific application sheets should be followed for each kit. This type of assay is referred to as immunoturbidimetric. Do not freeze latex particles because this will lead to irreversible clumping. An occasional problem with latex agglutination assays is interference from rheumatoid factor or other autoantibodies. These may cause agglutination and overestimation of the protein under assay. It is then preferable to resort to an ELISA assay.

Assays using chromogenic peptide substrates (amidolytic assays)

The serine proteases of the coagulation cascade have narrow substrate specificities.[17] It is possible to synthesize a short peptide specific for each enzyme that has a dye (p-nitroaniline, p-NA) attached to the terminal amino acid. When the synthetic peptide reacts with the specific enzyme, the dye is released and the rate of its release or the total amount released can be measured photometrically. This gives a measure of the enzyme activity present. Chromogenic substrate assays can be classified into direct and indirect assays. Direct assays can be further subclassified into primary assays, in which a substrate specific for the enzyme to be measured is used, and secondary assays, in which the enzyme or proenzyme measured is used to activate a second protease for which a specific substrate is available. Specific substrates are available for many coagulation enzymes. However, the substrate specificity is not absolute and most kits include inhibitors of other enzymes capable of cleaving the substrate to improve specificity. Indirect assays are used to measure naturally occurring inhibitors and some platelet factors.[15]

It should be remembered that the measurement of amidolytic activity is not the same as the measurement of

biological activity in a coagulation assay and in some cases may not accurately reflect this. This is particularly important when dealing with the molecular variants of various coagulation factors. The assays can be automated, carried out in a microtitre plate or in a tube when a spectrophotometer is used to measure the intensity of the colour development.

Coagulation assays

Coagulation assays are functional bioassays and rely on comparison with a control or standard preparation with a known level of activity. In the one-stage system optimal amounts of all the clotting factors are present except the one to be determined, which should be as near to nil as possible. The best one-stage system is provided by a substrate plasma obtained either from a patient with severe congenital deficiency or artificially depleted by immunoadsorption. The principles of bioassay, its standardization and its limitations are considered in detail on p. 417.

Coagulation techniques are also used in mixing tests to identify a missing factor in an emergency or to identify and estimate quantitatively an inhibitor or anticoagulant. The advantage of this type of assay is that it most closely approximates the activity *in vivo* of the factor in question. However, they can be technically more difficult to perform than the other types described earlier and their susceptibility to interference from other plasma components has a detrimental effect on their accuracy and precision.

Other Assays

Other assays include measurement of coagulation factors using snake venoms, assay of ristocetin cofactor and the clot solubility test for factor XIII. DNA analysis is becoming more useful and more prevalent in coagulation. However, this requires entirely different equipment and techniques (see Chapter 8).

NOTES ON EQUIPMENT

Waterbaths

A 37°C waterbath is required for manual coagulation tests, incubation steps and the rapid thawing of frozen specimens. Waterbaths set at 37°C should vary by no more than ± 0.5°C because slight variation in temperature will markedly affect the speed of clotting reactions. A waterbath with plastic or glass sides is preferable and some type of cross-illumination helps to determine the exact time of formation and appearance of the fibrin clot. Check that the temperature is 37°C before and during use. Distilled water should be used to fill the waterbath and maintain the water level.

Refrigerators and Freezers

Check that the temperature has not been out of the acceptable range of $4 \pm 2°C$ for refrigerators and $-20 \pm 2°C$ or $-80 \pm 2°C$ (as applicable) for freezers, rechecking during the day. Records must be kept.

Centrifuges

Check to ensure each machine is clean before and after use. Also do a visual inspection of rotors, buckets and liners for corrosion and cracks. Thorough maintenance records should be kept.

Reagents and Buffers

Attention must be paid to the age and condition of solutions. This is particularly important with the calcium chloride solution. Whenever a solution is prepared it should be correctly labelled and dated. Buffers should be inspected for bacterial growth before use: contamination with microorganisms can cause errors and assay failures as a result of the release of enzymes and other active biological substances into solution. Azide may be added as a preservative to some buffers but should not be used in reagents for platelet studies or ELISA substrates. Chromogenic substrates should be reconstituted with sterile distilled water; contamination with bacterial enzymes may cause para nitro-aniline (pNA) release and yellow discoloration of the reagent. Records of batch numbers and expiry dates should be kept.

Plastic and Glass Tubes

For clotting tests, $75 \times 10\,mm$ glass rimless test tubes should be used. Plastic tubes should be used for sample dilutions, storage and reagent preparation.

Pipettes

A range of graduated glass (certified Class A) and automatic pipettes must be obtained. The latter should be accurate and durable. Fluids should not be drawn into the pipette barrels and acids should not be pipetted with instruments containing metal piston assemblies, which may become pitted or corroded. Attention to technique is vital because contamination of reagents with used pipette tips may occur, there may be errors of volume as a result of fluid on the exterior of the pipette tip or the manner of addition of a reagent may alter the results obtained. The amount of fluid drawn into the tip should be inspected visually with each pipetting procedure. Records of pipette accuracy and precision should be kept.

Stopwatches and Stopclocks

Stopclocks are useful for timing incubation periods of several minutes or more, but stopwatches that may be held in the hand, and controlled rapidly, should be used for measuring clotting times and for short incubations. At least four stopwatches are needed unless an automated coagulometer is used.

Automated Coagulation Analysers

A wide variety of automated and semi-automated coagulation analysers are available. The choice of analyser depends on predicted workload, repertoire and cost implications. A thorough evaluation of the current range of analysers is recommended.

Modern analysers distributed in the European Economic Area must be CE marked, certifying that the product has met EU consumer safety, health or environmental requirements.

If coagulation analysers are used, it is important to ensure that their temperature control and the mechanism for detecting the endpoint are functioning properly. Although such instruments reduce observer error when a large number of samples are tested, it is important to apply stringent quality control at all times to ensure accuracy and precision.

Evaluating and choosing an automated analyser

The purchasing or leasing of new equipment is a complicated process and the most important factors to be considered will vary from one laboratory to another.

Specification standards may be classified into *Mandatory* and *Desirable*. An example classification is shown below:

Mandatory requirements

- Performance of clotting, chromogenic and immunological assays
- Reliable test results with acceptable levels of accuracy and precision
- Closed vial, cap piercing
- Positive barcode identification
- Effective flagging of abnormal results
- Storage of quality control data
- Reagents stable
- Sample throughput time appropriate for workload
- Rapid analysis of urgent samples
- Bidirectional interface
- Continual sample loading
- Conformity to national health and safety legislation.

Desirable additional requirements

- Good reputation of supplier and satisfaction of other users
- Acceptable level of service, telephone support and availability of engineer support
- Availability of independent evaluation report
- Satisfactory performance of analyser and reagent combinations in an external quality assessment scheme
- Satisfactory results of an on-site evaluation

- Ease of implementation in laboratory with minimal necessary changes to existing practice
- Ease of implementation of future requirements and increase in workload
- Guaranteed supply of reagents and consumables
- Post-sales support, training and education.

The final decision is usually made after competitive tenders are submitted to ensure fairness to all relevant commercial firms and after achieving the lowest appropriate cost. The selection process should take into account the following cost implications:

- Capital bid cost or leasing/rental cost
- Cost of reagents and consumables per year
- Cost of maintenance contracts per year
- Cost of computer interfacing.

The extent to which each analyser fulfils the *essential* and *desirable* attributes can be scored according to their relative importance. Thus, for example, the specification standard should be *weighted*, 10 for the most important, 1 for the least important criterion; compliance with the specification standard should be given a *mark*: 5 as the best and 1 as the worst score.

A total score is then calculated as Weighting × Mark and summed for each analyser.

Safety

Each laboratory should have its own safety recommendations and procedures to follow in case of accident or contamination (see Chapter 24).

PRE-ANALYTICAL VARIABLES INCLUDING SAMPLE COLLECTION

Many misleading results in blood coagulation arise not from errors in testing but from carelessness in the pre-analytical phase. Ideally, the results of blood tests should accurately reflect the values *in vivo*.

When blood is withdrawn from a vessel, changes begin to take place in the components of blood coagulation. Some occur almost immediately, such as platelet activation and the initiation of the clotting mechanism dependent on surface contact.

It is essential to take precautions at this early stage to prevent, or at least minimize, *in vitro* changes by conforming to recommended criteria during collection and storage. These criteria, as described below, have been established by the Clinical and Laboratory Standards Institute (CLSI).

Collection of Venous Blood

Venous blood samples should be obtained whenever possible, even from the neonate. Capillary blood tests require modification of techniques, experienced operators and

locally established normal ranges; they are not an easy alternative to tests on venous blood. All blood samples must be collected by personnel who are trained and experienced in the technique. Patients requiring venepuncture should be relaxed and in warm surroundings. Excessive stress and vigorous exercise cause changes in blood clotting and fibrinolysis. Stress and exercise will increase factor VIII, VWF and fibrinolysis.

Whenever possible, venous samples should be collected without a pressure cuff, allowing the blood to enter the syringe by continuous free flow or by the negative pressure from an evacuated tube (see p. 3). Venous occlusion causes haemoconcentration, increase of fibrinolytic activity, platelet release and activation of some clotting factors. In the majority of patients, however, light pressure using a tourniquet is required; this should be applied for the shortest possible time (e.g. <1 min). The venepuncture must be 'clean'; blood samples from an indwelling line or catheter should not be used for tests of haemostasis because they are prone to dilution and heparin contamination.

To minimize the effects of contact activation, good-quality plastic or polypropylene syringes should be used. If glass blood containers are used, they should be evenly and adequately coated with silicon.

The blood is thoroughly mixed with the anticoagulant by inverting the container several times. The samples should be brought to the laboratory as soon as possible. If urgent fibrinolysis tests are contemplated, the blood samples should be kept on crushed ice until delivered to the laboratory. Assays of tPA and of PA1-1 antigen are preferably performed on samples taken into trisodium citrate to prevent continued tPA–PA1-1 binding (see p. 621).

If an evacuated tube system is used for collecting samples for different tests, the coagulation sample should be the second or third tube obtained.

Patient identification is of utmost importance. Care must be taken in labelling the patient sample both at the bedside and within the laboratory.

Blood Sample Anticoagulation

The most commonly used anticoagulant for coagulation samples is trisodium citrate. A 32 g/1 (0.109 M) solution (see p. 621) is recommended. Other anticoagulants, including oxalate, heparin and ethylenediaminetetra-acetic acid (EDTA), are unacceptable. The labile factors (factors V and VIII) are unstable in oxalate, whereas heparin and EDTA directly inhibit the coagulation process and interfere with endpoint determinations. Additional benefits of trisodium citrate are that the calcium ion is neutralized more rapidly in citrate and APTT tests are more sensitive to the presence of heparin.

For routine blood coagulation testing, 9 volumes of blood are added to 1 volume of anticoagulant (i.e. 0.5 ml of anticoagulant for a 5 ml specimen). When the haematocrit is abnormal with either severe anaemia or polycythaemia, the blood:citrate ratio should be adjusted.[18] For a 5 ml specimen (total), the amount of citrate should be as follows:

HAEMATOCRIT	CITRATE (ml)
0.20	0.70
0.25	0.65
0.30	0.61
0.55	0.39
0.60	0.36
0.65	0.30
0.70	0.26

Time of Sample Collection

The time of day when the sample is collected can be an important factor in the interpretation of results. Fibrinolytic activity follows a definite circadian pattern with a trough at around 6 a.m.

The timing of the collection of the blood sample in relation to drug administration should also be taken into consideration (e.g. after subcutaneous heparin therapy).

The timing following administration of factor concentrate samples is very important. The following times are recommended:

Factor VIII: at 15 min
Factor IX: at 30 min
Desmopressin: at 30 min after intravenous infusion, 60 min after intranasal.

Transportation to the Laboratory

An efficient and regular collection service is necessary. It is important that samples are delivered as quickly as possible to prevent deterioration of the labile clotting factors such as factors V and VIII. Automated systems can facilitate rapid delivery, but should be avoided when platelet function tests are to be performed because the associated trauma may affect results. For certain investigations it is necessary for the samples to be placed on ice once taken and delivered immediately to the laboratory.

Centrifugation: Preparation of Platelet-Poor Plasma

Most routine coagulation investigations are performed on platelet-poor plasma (PPP), which is prepared by centrifugation at 2000 g for 15 min at 4°C (approx. 4000 rev/min

in a standard bench cooling centrifuge). The sample should be kept at room temperature if it is to be used for PT tests, lupus anticoagulant (LAC) or factor VII assays and it should be kept at 4°C for other assays; the testing should preferably be completed within 2 h of collection. Care must be taken not to disturb the buffy coat layer when removing the PPP.

Samples for platelet function testing, LAC and the activated PC resistance (APCR) test should not be centrifuged at 4°C. These samples should be prepared by centrifugation at room temperature to prevent activation of platelets and release of platelet contents such as phospholipid and factor V. For LAC testing and APCR it is very important that the number of platelets and the amount of platelet debris in the samples are minimized. The platelet count should be below 10×10^9/l. This is best achieved by double centrifugation or filtration of the plasma through a 0.2 μm filter.

Storage of Plasma and Sample Thawing

Some tests such as the PT and APTT are carried out on fresh samples. Certain coagulation assays, unless urgently required, can be performed in batches at a later date on deep frozen plasma. Storage of small aliquots of samples in liquid nitrogen (−196°C) is the optimum, although samples may be frozen at −40°C or −80°C for several weeks without significant loss of most haemostatic activities. Gentle but thorough mixing of samples is essential after thawing and before testing. Once thawed, the sample should never be refrozen.

Some Common 'Technical' Errors

A false abnormality of the clotting time may occur in the following situations:

1. Faulty collection of the sample, resulting in it undergoing partial clotting
2. Underfilling or overfilling of the bottle or high or low haematocrit (can cause the volume of citrate in relation to the plasma volume to be incorrect; see above)
3. An unsuitable anticoagulant, such as EDTA, used in collecting the sample
4. Collection of blood through a line that has at some stage been in contact with heparin
5. Contamination of the kaolin/platelet substitute reagent with a trace of thromboplastin
6. Undue delay in sample analysis
7. Use of inaccurate pipettes (documented proof of pipette calibration is essential)
8. Machine malfunction
9. Incorrect waterbath temperature
10. Calcium chloride at incorrect concentration or not freshly prepared.

CALIBRATION AND QUALITY CONTROL

Reference Standard (Calibrator)

International (WHO) and national standards are available for a number of coagulation factors (see p. 589). For diagnostic tests it is necessary to test a calibrated normal reference preparation alongside the patients' plasmas.

Because the concentration of some coagulation factors may vary as much as fourfold in different normal plasma samples, it is inadvisable to use plasma from any one person to represent 100% clotting activity. The larger the number of donors in the pool, the more likely the pool clotting activity will be 100% or 100 iu/dl. A suggested minimum for the normal pool is 20 donors. It is preferable to use a calibrated reference plasma for routine use with each assay. If this is not possible, then a locally prepared normal pool can be used provided it is itself calibrated against a reference preparation.

Calibration of Standard Pools and Suggested Calibration Procedure

Whenever possible, the normal pool should be calibrated as described in the following against a freeze-dried reference material already calibrated against the international standard. The reference material may be a national standard (e.g. National Institute for Biological Standards and Control) or a commercial standard. In the absence of reference materials the laboratory should obtain as large a normal pool as possible and assign it a value of 100 iu/dl.

The most important principle of calibration is repetition to minimize possible errors at each stage of calibration. It is necessary to carry out at least four independent assays and preferably six. An independent assay is an assay for which a new ampoule of standard is opened, or if a freeze-dried standard is not available, for which a new set of dilutions are prepared from frozen previous reference plasma. Each plasma must be tested in duplicate; two replicate assays should be carried out each day and the procedure should be repeated on at least 4 days (four independent assays). Whenever possible more than one operator should be involved.

Comparison should always be made with the previous normal pool. The potency of the new normal pool is calculated for each replicate assay on each day and an overall mean value is calculated. This calibration also enables an assessment of the precision of the method used.

Control Plasma

Controls are included alongside patient samples in a batch of tests. Inclusion of both normal and abnormal controls will enable detection of non-linearity in the standard curve. Whereas a reference standard (calibrator) is used for accuracy, controls are used for precision. Precision control, the recording of the day-to-day variation in control values, is an important procedure in laboratory coagulation. Participation in an external assessment scheme (see p. 594) is also important to ensure inter-laboratory harmonization. The use of lyophilized reference standard and control plasmas has become widespread, whereas locally calibrated standard pools are used especially in under-resourced countries. The results of participation in external qualitycontrol schemes require careful attention. The large number of different reagents, substrate plasmas, reference preparations and analysers available makes comparison of like with like difficult. Ideally all combinations should give similar results, but this is often not the case and the results should be used to carefully choose the combination used.

A control must be stable and homogeneous; the exact potency is not important, although the approximate value should be known to select a preparation at the upper or lower limit of the normal reference range.

Fresh control blood is required for procedures such as platelet aggregation and should be obtained from 'normal' healthy subjects. Fresh controls should be prepared in exactly the same way as the patient sample. Normal and abnormal controls are usually obtained from commercial companies.

Variability of Coagulation Assays

Within a laboratory, variability is most commonly the result of a dilution error, differences in the composition of reagents, failure to take the time-trend into account and differences in experience and technique between operators. A coefficient of variation of 15–20% is not uncommon for factor VIII assays but should be much lower for antigenic assays.

Variability between laboratories is much higher. Apart from the factors described for the within-laboratory variability, there is the major effect of differences in methods and in the composition of reagents. Comparability between laboratories improves if standardized reagents are used.

The unavoidable variability associated with coagulation assays makes the use of reliable reference materials imperative.

PERFORMANCE OF COAGULATION TESTS

Handling of Samples and Reagents

All plasma samples should be kept in plastic or siliconized glass tubes and placed on melting ice or at 4°C until used, except when cold activation of factor VII and platelets is to be avoided, in which case the plasma is kept at room temperature. All pipetting should be performed using disposable plastic pipettes or autodiluter pipette tips. The actual clotting tests are performed at 37°C in new round-bottom glass tubes of standard size (10 or 12 mm external diameter). Ideally, all glassware should be disposable. If the tubes have to be reused, scrupulous cleaning using chromic acid and a detergent such as 2% Decon 90 is essential.

Eliminating a Time Trend

The potential instability of biological reagents used in tests of haemostasis makes it desirable to arrange results so as to reduce time-related errors. Thus, if there is a significant length of time between the test with the patient's plasma and the test with the control sample, the difference may be the result of the deterioration of one or more of the reagents or of the plasma itself rather than a true defect or deficiency. In the simplest case, if there are two samples A and B, the readings should be carried out in the order A_1, B_1, B_2, A_2. Additional specimens are allowed for by inserting further letters into the design.

Assay Monitoring and Endpoint Detection

Manual Methods

Detecting clot formation as the endpoint depends to some extent on the rate of its formation: the shorter the clotting time the more opaque is the clot and the easier it is to detect. A slowly forming clot may appear as mere fibrin wisps, which are difficult to detect by eye or machine. In manual work, the observer must try to adopt a uniform convention in selecting the moment in clot formation that will be accepted as the endpoint. It is also important to ensure that the tube can be watched with its lower part under the water or while being quickly dipped in and out so as to avoid cooling and a slowing down of the clot formation. Bubbles also make the determination of the endpoint difficult.

Manual clotting techniques are still used in WHO calibration schemes and therefore should be viewed as an essential skill, despite the ever-increasing reliance on automation. It is worth remembering that not all results produced by an automated analyser are correct; dubious or inconsistent results should be checked manually.

In instrumental work the coagulometer must be shown to detect long clotting times reliably and reproducibly. The various coagulometers available have different means of detecting the endpoint, which may make comparison of results difficult. Some commonly used techniques are as follows.

Electromechanical

Impedance, steel ball

The sample cuvette rotates and a steel ball (e.g. Amelung KC4A) remains stationary in a magnetic field until the formation of fibrin strands around the ball produces

movement. This is detected by a change in the magnetic field and the coagulation time is recorded.

A steel ball (e.g. Axis-Shield Group; Thrombotrack) rotates under the influence of a magnet until the formation of fibrin strands around the ball stops it rotating. This is detected by a sensor and the coagulation time is recorded.

Photo-Optical Analysis

Scattered light detection for clotting assays (660 nm)

The turbidity during the formation of a fibrin clot is measured as an increase in scattered light intensity when exposed to light at a wavelength of 660 nm.

Transmitted light detection for chromogenic assays (405 nm, 575 nm, 800 nm)

Colour production leads to a change in light absorbance, which is detected as a change in transmitted light. Over time, the change in absorbance per minute is calculated ($\triangle OD/min$). Various wavelengths can be used such as 405 nm, 575 nm and 800 nm.

Transmitted light detection for immunoassays (405 nm, 575 nm, 800 nm)

The change in light absorbance caused by the antigen–antibody reaction is detected as the change in transmitted light. Over time, the change in absorbance per minute is calculated ($\triangle OD/min$). Some analysers detect light transmittance at multiple wavelengths between 395 and 710 nm.

Nephelometry

Nephelometry (IL ACL analysers) is the determination of the intensity of light scatter using a detector placed at right angles to the incident light path and detecting light of the same wavelength as the incident light. The procedure is particularly useful in measuring complexes of antigen and antibody produced by immunoprecipitation.

Photo-optical endpoint determination and analyses

A number of methods can be used to define the change in optical transmission that corresponds to the endpoint of the reaction.

Percentage Detection Method

After initiating the clotting reaction, the transmitted light is monitored and a baseline A/D value (bH) is determined for the reaction (bH = 0%) (Fig. 18.2). The reaction is then monitored until the clotting reaction is completed (dH = 100%). The time to an optionally set endpoint, usually 50%, is then determined. At this point the A/D value per unit time shows the greatest change and the fibrin monomer polymerization reaction rate is high.

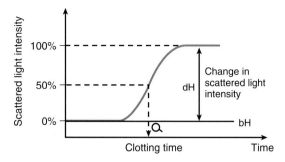

Figure 18.2 Endpoint determination: percentage detection method.
(Reproduced by permission of Sysmex UK Ltd.)

Detection based on this principle enables coagulation analysis to be more accurate at low fibrinogen concentrations in samples with low A/D values and those samples for which the initial amount of A/D value is higher than usual, such as lipaemic and haemolysed samples.

Rate Method

After the start of the reaction, the increase in absorbance per minute is monitored. At the predetermined end time, the final increase in absorbance per minute measurement is made. The rate of the absorbance increase per minute between these two time point measurements is calculated (Fig. 18.3). The calculated change in absorbance (dOD/min) is expressed as the raw data and used to construct a standard curve (i.e. there is no endpoint *per se*).

VLin Integral Method

The VLin integral method (Fig. 18.4) evaluates the absorbance per minute of an immunological reaction. This is monitored and mathematical analysis used to determine

Figure 18.4 Analysis of reaction: VLin integral method. This is used for immunological assays.
(Reproduced by permission of Sysmex UK Ltd.)

the peak rate of reaction (maximum velocity). Using this method allows for increase in analytical sensitivity, extended measuring range, reduced measurement time and improved antigen excess reliability when measuring an immunological reaction. The VLin integral evaluation method is used for immunological assays, including D-dimer and VWF antigen.

Analysis Time Over

The 'Analysis Time Over' check (Fig. 18.5) is used to detect whether the reaction endpoint is correct. If the sample reaction end angle is greater than the permitted angle at maximum detection time, the result will be flagged with an 'Analysis Time Over' error. The situation occurs when testing samples with prolonged clotting times and satisfactory endpoint has not been reached by the end of the time allotted for analysis. When this occurs the following checks should be performed:

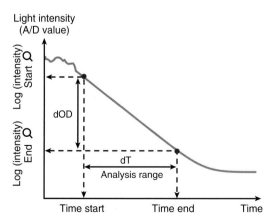

Figure 18.3 Analysis of reaction: rate method. This is used for chromogenic assays.
(Reproduced by permission of Sysmex UK Ltd.)

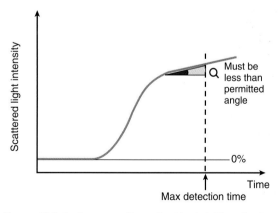

Figure 18.5 Analyser trace illustrating 'Analysis Time Over'. The reaction is incomplete at the end of the maximum allotted recording time.
(Reproduced by permission of Sysmex UK Ltd.)

1. Check the sample for possible anticoagulant contamination, haemolysis, lipaemia, hyperbilirubinaemia or turbidity.
2. Verify delivery of sample and reagent.
3. Set the 'Maximum Reading Time' to a longer time and reanalyse the sample.
4. If reanalysis of the sample results in a numeric value without an error flag, the result can be reported.
5. If reanalysis gives an 'Analysis Time Over' message again, the sample may not be capable of forming a firm clot. In these situations, the clotting time must be checked manually.

Turbidity Level Over

If the dH exceeds the detection capacity of the A/D converter, the result will not be reported and it may be suspected that sample plasma is turbid or lipaemic (Fig. 18.6). When this occurs, the following checks should be performed:

1. Check the sample for turbidity, lipaemia, haemolysis or hyperbilirubinaemia.
2. Verify delivery of sample and reagent.
3. For a fibrinogen assay, dilute the sample with Owren's veronal buffer and reanalyse.
4. If reanalysis of the sample results in a numeric value without an error flag, the result can be reported.
5. Clotting tests such as PT, APTT and thrombin time (TT) must be performed manually.

Clot Signatures: Normal and Abnormal APTT Clot Waveforms

Information on the dynamics of clot formation may also be extracted from the optical profiles generated when performing the PT or APTT tests. It has been demonstrated

Figure 18.6 The contributions of sample defects that may contribute to a 'Turbidity Level Over' error at different wavelengths.
(Reproduced by permission of Sysmex UK Ltd.)

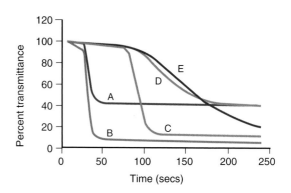

Figure 18.7 Clot signatures: normal and abnormal activated partial thromboplastin time (APTT) clot waveforms. (A) Normal specimen; APTT = 29 s, fibrinogen concentration = 2.89 g/l. (B) Biphasic response in a suspected disseminated intravascular coagulation (DIC) specimen with normal APTT (28.5 s) and elevated fibrinogen (6.74 g/l). (C) Patient treated with heparin (0.52 anti-Xa u/ml); prolonged APTT (81.2 s) and elevated fibrinogen concentration (5.54 g/l). (D) Factor VIII-deficient specimen (<1%), with prolonged APTT (84.1 s) and slightly reduced fibrinogen concentration (1.56 g/l). (E) Factor IX-deficient specimen (<1%) with prolonged APTT (83.4 s) and normal fibrinogen concentration (2.94 g/l).
(Reproduced by permission of Biomerieux.)

that such profiles (clot waveforms) show a different pattern in certain clinical conditions compared to normal (Fig. 18.7). Furthermore, the shape of this pattern is predictable for the particular abnormality and the term 'clot signature' has been used in this context.

The A2 Flag on the MDA system identifies the presence of a biphasic APTT waveform often seen in patients with DIC and a high sensitivity (98%), specificity (98%) and positive predictive value (74%) have been reported.[19]

It is important to note that the biphasic APTT waveform has also been observed in samples from patients not diagnosed as having DIC by standard criteria. In this respect, it may indicate an emerging or occult and potentially serious clinical condition associated with the activation of coagulation. Further clinical and laboratory investigation is then warranted.

Molecular Mechanism of the Biphasic Waveform: LC-CRP

The development of the biphasic waveform is a consequence of the formation of a divalent metal ion-dependent complex of C-reactive protein (CRP) and very low density lipoprotein (VLDL) and, to a lesser extent, intermediate density lipoprotein (IDL).

This lipoprotein-complexed CRP has been designated LC-CRP. In the APTT assay, when the citrated plasma is recalcified, the formation of this complex results in a reduction in light transmission, detected by the first slope of the biphasic waveform.

Commonly Used Reagents

Some reagents are common to the majority of first-line tests. They are described here, whereas the reagents specific for one particular test or assay only are described with the details of the relevant test.

CaCl₂

The working solution is best prepared from a commercial molar solution. Small volumes of 0.025 mol/l concentration should be prepared frequently and stored for short periods to avoid proliferation of microorganisms. Prewarmed $CaCl_2$ should always be discarded at the end of the working day.

Barbitone buffer

- 50 ml sodium diethyl barbiturate ($C_8H_{11}O_3N_2Na$) 0.2 M (41.2 g/l)
- Add 32.5 ml hydrochloric acid (HCl) 0.2 M
- Make up to 200 ml with water and correct pH to 7.4 with HCl

Barbitone buffered saline, pH 7.4

- NaCl: 5.67 g
- Barbitone buffer, pH 7.4, 1 litre
- Before use, dilute with an equal volume of 9 g/l NaCl.
- pH 7.3–7.4 is recommended for most clotting tests.

Glyoxaline buffer

Dissolve 2.72 g of glyoxaline (imidazole) and 4.68 g of NaCl in 650 ml of water. Add 148.8 ml of 0.1 mol/l HCl and adjust the pH to 7.4. Adjust the volume to 1 l with water.

Owren's veronal buffer

- Sodium acetate: 3.89 g
- Barbitone sodium: 5.89 g
- Sodium chloride: 6.8 g
- Dissolve the salts in 800 ml of water
- Add 21.5 ml of 1 mol/l HCl, then make up to 1 l with water, mix and check that the pH is 7.4.

Factor-Deficient Plasmas

Plasmas deficient in specific factors are required for many bioassays. They may be obtained from individuals with congenital deficiency of the factor, but frequently these patients will have been treated with plasma concentrates and there is a danger of infection. Many laboratories now use commercial plasmas rendered deficient in the factor by immunodepletion and then lyophilized. However, it is important to establish that these are completely deficient. Once reconstituted, lyophilized plasmas should be gently mixed and left to stand for 20 min before use.

If an automated coagulation analyser is used, the factor-deficient plasma should be placed in position 10 min prior to testing.

THE 'CLOTTING SCREEN'

Basic tests of coagulation are often performed with no specific diagnosis in mind and in the absence of any clinical indication of a haemostatic disorder. There may be numerous reasons for this and the tests performed may give clues to diagnosis or may detect an unsuspected hazard that increases the risk of postoperative bleeding. Equally, they may produce false-positive abnormalities that cause concern and confusion and delay procedures.[15] The choice and extent of tests performed in this screening process will vary between hospitals. Our current practice is to perform PT, APTT, TT and fibrinogen assay.

Prothrombin Time

Principle

The PT test measures the clotting time of recalcified plasma in the presence of an optimal concentration of tissue extract (thromboplastin) and indicates the overall efficiency of the extrinsic clotting system. Although originally thought to measure prothrombin, the test is now known to depend also on reactions with factors V, VII and X and on the fibrinogen concentration of the plasma.

Reagents

Patient and control plasma samples

Platelet-poor plasma (PPP) from the patient and control is obtained as described on p. 404. Note that plasma stored at 4°C may have a shortened PT as a result of factor VII activation in the cold.

Thromboplastin

Thromboplastins were originally tissue extracts obtained from different species and different organs containing tissue factor and phospholipid. Because of the potential hazard of viral and other infections from handling human brain, it should no longer be used as a source of thromboplastin. The majority of animal thromboplastins now in use are extracts of rabbit brain or lung. A laboratory method for a rabbit brain preparation, of use in under-resourced laboratories, is described on p. 613.

The introduction of recombinant thromboplastins has resulted in a move away from rabbit brain thromboplastin. They are manufactured using recombinant human tissue factor produced in *Escherichia coli* and synthetic phospholipids, which do not contain any other clotting factors such as prothrombin, factor VII and factor X. Therefore, they are highly sensitive to factor deficiencies and oral anticoagulant-treated patient plasma samples and have an International Sensitivity Index (ISI) close to 1.

Each preparation has a different sensitivity to clotting factor deficiencies and defects, in particular the defect induced by oral anticoagulants. For control of oral anticoagulation a preparation calibrated against the International Reference Thromboplastin should be used (see Chapter 20). It is important to remember that some thromboplastins are not sensitive to an isolated factor VII deficiency and that use of animal thromboplastin for analysis of human samples may produce abnormalities solely as a result of species differences.

$CaCl_2$

0.025 mol/l.

Method

Deliver 0.1 ml of plasma into a glass tube placed in a waterbath and add 0.1 ml of thromboplastin. Wait 1–3 min to allow the mixture to warm. Then add 0.1 ml of warmed $CaCl_2$ and start the stopwatch. Mix the contents of the tube and record the endpoint. Carry out the test in duplicate on the patient's plasma and the control plasma. When a number of samples are to be tested as a batch, the samples and controls must be suitably staggered to eliminate the time bias. Some thromboplastins contain calcium chloride, in which case 0.2 ml of thromboplastin is added to 0.1 ml plasma and timing is started immediately.

Expression of Results

The results are expressed as the mean of the duplicate readings in seconds or as the ratio of the mean patient's plasma time to the mean normal control plasma time. The control plasma is obtained from 20 normal men and women (not pregnant and not taking oral contraceptives) and the geometric mean normal PT (MNPT) is calculated. (For further details and a discussion of the importance of the PT in oral anticoagulant control, when results may be reported as an International Normalized Ratio [INR], see Chapter 20.)

Normal Values

Normal values depend on the thromboplastin used, the exact technique and whether visual or instrumental endpoint reading is used. With most rabbit thromboplastins the normal range of the PT is between 11 and 16 s; for recombinant human thromboplastin, it is somewhat shorter (10–12 s). Each laboratory should establish its own normal range.

Interpretation

The common causes of prolonged PTs are as follows:

1. Administration of oral anticoagulant drugs (vitamin K antagonists)
2. Liver disease, particularly obstructive jaundice
3. Vitamin K deficiency
4. Disseminated intravascular coagulation
5. Rarely, a previously undiagnosed factor VII, X, V or prothrombin deficiency or defect (see p. 418). *Note*: with prothrombin, factor X or factor V deficiency the APTT will also be prolonged.

Activated Partial Thromboplastin Time

Specific variations of the APTT test are known as the partial thromboplastin time with kaolin (PTTK) and the kaolin cephalin clotting time (KCCT), reflecting the methods used to perform the test.

Principle

The test measures the clotting time of plasma after the activation of contact factors and the addition of phospholipid and $CaCl_2'$, but without added tissue thromboplastin, and so indicates the overall efficiency of the intrinsic pathway. To standardize the activation of contact factors, the plasma is first preincubated for a set period with a contact activator such as kaolin, silica or ellagic acid. During this phase of the test, factor XIIa is produced, which cleaves factor XI to factor XIa, but coagulation does not proceed beyond this in the absence of calcium. After recalcification, factor XIa activates factor IX and coagulation follows. A standardized phospholipid is provided to allow the test to be performed on PPP. The test depends not only on the contact factors and on factors VIII and IX but also on the reactions with factors X, V, prothrombin and fibrinogen. It is also sensitive to the presence of circulating anticoagulants (inhibitors) and heparin.

Reagents

PPP. From the patient and a control, stored as described on p. 404

Kaolin. 5 g/l (laboratory grade) in barbitone buffered saline, pH 7.4 (see p. 621). Add a few glass beads to aid resuspension. The suspension is stable at room temperature. Other insoluble surface active substances such as silica, celite or ellagic acid can also be used.

Phospholipid. Many reagents are available; these contain different phospholipids. When choosing a reagent for the APTT, it is important to establish that the activator–phospholipid combination is sensitive to deficiencies of factors VIII, IX and XI at concentrations of 0.35–0.4 iu/ml. Reagents that fail to detect reductions of this degree are

too insensitive for routine use. The system should also be responsive to unfractionated heparin over the therapeutic range of approximately 0.3–0.7 iu/ml. In addition, some laboratories will wish the system to be sensitive to the presence of lupus-like anticoagulants.
$CaCl_2$. 0.025 mol/l.

Method

Mix equal volumes of the phospholipid reagent and the kaolin suspension and leave in a glass tube in the water-bath at 37°C. Place 0.1 ml of plasma into a second glass tube. Add 0.2 ml of the kaolin–phospholipid solution to the plasma, mix the contents and start the stopwatch simultaneously. Leave at 37°C for 10 min with occasional shaking. At exactly 10 min, add 0.1 ml of prewarmed $CaCl_2$ and start a second stopwatch. Record the time taken for the mixture to clot. Repeat the test at least once on both the patient's plasma and the control plasma. It is possible to do four tests at 2-min intervals if sufficient stopwatches are available.

Expression of Results

Express the results as the mean of the paired clotting times.

Normal Range

The normal range is typically 26–40 s. The actual times depend on the reagents used and the duration of the pre-incubation period, which varies in manufacturer's recom-mendations for different reagents. These variables also greatly alter the sensitivity of the test to minor or moder-ate deficiencies of the contact activation system. Labora-tories can choose appropriate conditions to achieve the sensitivity they require. Each laboratory should calculate its own normal range.

Interpretation

The common causes of a prolonged APTT are as follows:
1. Disseminated intravascular coagulation
2. Liver disease
3. Massive transfusion with plasma-depleted red blood cells
4. Administration of or contamination with heparin or other anticoagulants
5. A circulating anticoagulant (inhibitor)
6. Deficiency of a coagulation factor other than factor VII.

The APTT is also moderately prolonged in patients taking oral anticoagulant drugs and in the presence of vitamin K deficiency. Occasionally, a patient with previously undiag-nosed haemophilia or another congenital coagulation dis-order presents with an isolated prolonged APTT. If the patient's APTT is abnormally long, the equal mixture test must be set up (see below).

Deficiency or Circulating Anticoagulant?

In cases with a long APTT, a 50:50 mixture of normal and test plasma should be tested to distinguish between factor deficiency and the effect of an inhibitor (see p. 421).

Thrombin Time
Principle

Thrombin is added to plasma and the clotting time is measured. The TT is affected by the concentration and reaction of fibrinogen and by the presence of inhibitory substances, including fibrinogen/fibrin degradation pro-ducts (FDPs) and heparin. The clotting time and the appearance of the clot are equally informative.

Reagents

PPP. From the patient and a control
Thrombin solution. A commercial bovine thrombin is used. It is stored frozen as a 50 NIH unit solution and it is freshly diluted in barbitone buffered saline in a plastic tube so as to give a clotting time of normal plasma of 15 s (usually approx. 7–8 NIH thrombin units per ml). Shorter times with normal plasma may fail to detect mild abnormalities.

Method

Add 100 µl thrombin solution to 200 µl of control plasma in a glass tube at 37°C and start the stopwatch. Measure the clotting time and observe the nature of the clot (e.g. whether transparent or opaque, firm or wispy). Repeat the procedure with two tubes containing patient's plasma in duplicate and then with a second sample of control plasma.

Expression of Results

The results are expressed as the mean of the duplicate clot-ting times in seconds for the control and the test plasma.

Normal Range

A patient's TT should be within 2 s of the control (i.e. 15–19 s). Times of 20 s and longer are definitely abnormal.

Interpretation of Results

The common causes of prolonged TT are as follows:
1. Hypofibrinogenaemia as found in DIC and, more rarely, in a congenital defect or deficiency

2. Raised concentrations of FDP, as encountered in DIC or liver disease
3. Extreme prolongation of the TT is nearly always a result of the presence of unfractionated heparin. If the presence of heparin is suspected, a Reptilase time test can be carried out (see p. 417) or the test can be repeated after the addition of heparinase. Low molecular weight heparin (LMWH) produces only a slight prolongation at therapeutic levels
4. Dysfibrinogenaemia, either inherited or acquired, in liver disease or in neonates
5. Hypoalbuminaemia[20]
6. Paraproteinemia.

Shortening of the TT occurs in conditions of coagulation activation.

A transparent bulky clot is found if fibrin polymerization is abnormal, as is the case in liver disease and some congenital dysfibrinogenaemias.

A gross elevation of the plasma fibrinogen concentration may also prolong the TT. Correction can be obtained by diluting the patient's plasma with saline (see p. 417).

Measurement of Fibrinogen Concentration

Numerous methods of determining fibrinogen concentration have been devised, including clotting, immunological, physical and nephelometric techniques, and all tend to give slightly different results, presumably partly because of the heterogeneous nature of plasma fibrinogen.[21] Many automated analysers will now provide an estimate of fibrinogen concentration determined from the coagulation changes during the PT (PT-derived fibrinogen). This is simple, inexpensive and widely used. However, its use is not recommended because it is inaccurate (overestimates fibrinogen) in some disease states and in patients who are anticoagulated.[22,23] Guidelines on fibrinogen assays have been published and recommend the Clauss technique for routine laboratory use.[24]

Fibrinogen Assay (Clauss Technique)

Principle

Diluted plasma is clotted with a strong thrombin solution; the plasma must be diluted to give a low level of any inhibitors (e.g. FDPs and heparin). A strong thrombin solution must be used so that the clotting time over a wide range is independent of the thrombin concentration.[25]

Reagents

Calibration plasma. With a known level of fibrinogen calibrated against an International Reference Standard
PPP. From the patient and a control

Thrombin solution. Freshly reconstituted to 100 NIH u per ml in 9 g/l NaCl
Owren's veronal buffer. pH 7.4. see p. 398.

Method

A calibration curve is prepared each time the batch of thrombin reagent is changed or there is a drift in control results; this is used to calculate the results of unknown plasma samples.

Make dilutions of the calibration plasma in veronal buffer to give a range of fibrinogen concentrations (i.e. 1 in 5; 1 in 10; 1 in 20 and 1 in 40). Part (0.2 ml) of each dilution is warmed to 37°C, 0.1 ml of thrombin solution is added and the clotting time is measured. Each test should be performed in duplicate. Plot the clotting time in seconds against the fibrinogen concentration in g/l on log/log graph paper. The 1 in 10 concentration is considered to be 100% and there should be a straight-line connection between clotting times of 5 and 50 s. Make a 1 in 10 dilution of each patient's sample and clot 0.2 ml of the dilution with 0.1 ml of thrombin.

The fibrinogen level can be read directly off the graph if the clotting time is between 5 and 50 s. However, outside this time range, a different assay dilution and mathematical correction of the result will be required (i.e. if the fibrinogen level is low and a 1 in 5 dilution is required, divide answer by 2 and for a 1 in 20 dilution multiply answer by 2).

The clot formed in this method may be 'wispy' as a result of the plasma being diluted and endpoint detection may be easier with optical or mechanical automated equipment. These have been assessed with available substrates and give reasonably consistent results.[26] The high concentration of thrombin used raises the risk of carry over into subsequent tests.

Normal range

The normal range is approximately 1.8–3.6 g/l.

Interpretation

The Clauss fibrinogen assay is usually low in inherited dysfibrinogenaemia but is insensitive to heparin unless the level is very high (>0.8 u/ml). High levels of FDPs (>190 μg/ml) may also interfere with the assay.[27] Because the chronometric Clauss assay is a functional assay it will generally give a relevant indication of fibrinogen function in plasma. When an inherited disorder of fibrinogen is suspected, a physicochemical estimation should be obtained (e.g. clot weight estimate of fibrinogen or total clottable fibrinogen or an immunological measure; see p. 424). If a dysfibrinogenaemia is present, it will reveal a discrepancy between the (functional) Clauss assay and the physical amount of fibrinogen present.

Platelet Count

Before considering further investigation of a suspected bleeding disorder, always check the platelet count and the blood film (for size and staining characteristics of platelets).

Interpretation of First-Line Tests

The pattern of abnormalities obtained using the first-line tests described earlier often gives a reasonably clear indication of the underlying defect and determines the appropriate further tests required to define it. The patterns are outlined in Table 18.3. The further tests that include specific factor assays and tests for DIC are described in the following sections.

SECOND-LINE INVESTIGATIONS

Relevant second-line investigations are described with each of the patterns of abnormalities detected by the first-line tests.

1

PT	Normal
APTT	Normal
Thrombin time	Normal
Fibrinogen concentration	Normal
Platelet count	Normal

If all the first-line investigations are normal in a patient who continues to bleed from the site of an injury or after surgery (or has a history of such bleeding), there are several possible diagnoses:

1. A disorder of platelet function, either congenital or acquired
2. von Willebrand disease (VWD) in which the factor VIII is not sufficiently low to cause prolongation of the APTT. This is quite common in mild cases
3. A mild coagulation disorder that is below the sensitivity of the routine tests to detect or that has been masked by the administration of blood products or by high levels of other factors: for example, mild factor VIII deficiency of 30 iu/dl
4. Factor XIII deficiency
5. A vascular disorder of haemostasis
6. Bleeding from a severely damaged vessel or vessels with normal haemostasis
7. A disorder of fibrinolysis such as antiplasmin or PAI-1 deficiency
8. Administration of LMWH.

Second-line investigations required in this situation are specific factor assays for the suspected deficiencies or appropriate screening tests such as the PFA-100 system (see p. 425) or factor XIII assay. Note that some LMWH may be present at therapeutic levels without abnormality of the coagulation screening tests; an anti-Xa assay will reveal their presence.

2

PT	Long
APTT	Normal
Thrombin time	Normal
Fibrinogen concentration	Normal
Platelet count	Normal

This combination of results is found in the following:

1. Factor VII deficiency, congenital or secondary to liver disease or vitamin K deficiency
2. At the start of oral anticoagulant therapy
3. Some thromboplastins are sensitive to lupus-like anticoagulants and some APTT reagents are insensitive, giving rise to this pattern of results
4. Depending on reagents used, mild deficiencies of factor II, V or X may cause prolongation of the PT while the APTT remains in the normal range.

A mixing test should be performed. Factor VII assay is described later. It is usually, but not always, possible to establish from the history whether the patient has received oral anticoagulant drugs. Specific tests for lupus and specific factor assays should be performed, as indicated by the mixing test results. Biochemical measures of liver function should be obtained.

3

PT	Normal
APTT	Long
Thrombin time	Normal
Fibrinogen concentration	Normal
Platelet count	Normal

An isolated prolonged APTT is found in the following:

1. Congenital deficiencies or defects of the intrinsic pathway (i.e. factor VIII, factor IX, factor XI and factor XII deficiency), as well as in prekallikrein and HMWK deficiencies

Table 18.3 First-line tests used in investigating acute haemostatic failure

	TEST			FIBRINOGEN	PLATELET COUNT	CONDITION
	PT	APTT	TT			
1.	N	N	N	N	N	Normal haemostasis Disorder of platelet function Factor XIII deficiency Disorder of vascular haemostasis Mild/masked coagulation factor deficiency Mild von Willebrand disease Disorder of fibrinolysis
2.	Long	N	N	N	N	Factor VII deficiency Early oral anticoagulation Lupus anticoagulant (with some reagents) Mild factor II, V or X deficiency
3.	N	Long	N	N	N	Factor VIII, IX, XI, XII, prekallikrein or HMWK deficiency Circulating anticoagulant, e.g. lupus anticoagulant Mild factor II, V or X deficiency
4.	Long	Long	N	N	N	Vitamin K deficiency Oral anticoagulants Factor V, X or II deficiency Multiple factor deficiency, e.g. liver failure Combined factor V + VIII deficiency
5.	Long	Long	Long	N or Abnormal	N	Heparin (large amount) Liver disease Fibrinogen deficiency/disorder Inhibition of fibrin polymerization Hyperfibrinolysis
6.	N	N	N	N	Low	Thrombocytopenia
7.	Long	Long	N	N or Abnormal	Low	Massive transfusion Liver disease
8.	Long	Long	Long	Low	Low	Disseminated intravascular coagulation Acute liver disease

HMWK, high molecular weight kininogen; N, normal.

2. Depending on the reagents used, mild deficiencies of factors II, V or X may cause prolongation of APTT, whereas the PT remains in the normal range
3. VWD, owing to low levels of factor VIII
4. In the presence of circulating anticoagulants (inhibitors). These may be specific (e.g. anti-factor VIII) or non-specific, usually an antiphospholipid antibody
5. Heparin (a common cause), either because the patient is undergoing treatment or because of sample contamination. However, the TT is extremely sensitive to unfractionated heparin and will then also be prolonged. A Reptilase time will confirm this if necessary. Detecting LMWH may require an anti-Xa assay as noted earlier.

The next diagnostic step is to establish whether the patient has a deficiency or an inhibitor by performing the 50:50 mixture test described on p. 421. Mixing tests should be done immediately, followed by the specific assay or tests, as described later.

4

PT	Long
APTT	Long
Thrombin time	Normal
Fibrinogen concentration	Normal
Platelet count	Normal

The main causes of a prolonged PT and APTT are as follows:

1. Lack of vitamin K. In this case the PT is usually relatively more prolonged than is the APTT
2. The administration of oral anticoagulant drugs. The PT is usually relatively more prolonged than is the APTT
3. Liver disease giving rise to multiple factor deficiencies. (In some cases the fibrinogen is also abnormal.)
4. Rare congenital or acquired defects of factors V, X or prothrombin and combined factors V and VIII deficiency.

Mixing experiments using the PT may be useful if there is no history of anticoagulant therapy and no obvious reason for failure of vitamin K absorption (e.g. parenteral feeding, long-term antibiotic treatment). If correction is obtained, specific factor assays should be performed.

5

PT	Long
APTT	Long
Thrombin time	Long
Fibrinogen concentration	Normal/abnormal
Platelet count	Normal

Abnormalities in all three screening coagulation tests are found in the following:

1. In the presence of unfractionated heparin (TT usually disproportionately long)
2. In hypofibrinogenaemias, afibrinogenaemias and dysfibrinogenaemias
3. In some cases of liver disease
4. In systemic hyperfibrinolysis.

To distinguish between these conditions, perform a Reptilase or Ancrod time, measure the fibrinogen concentration and measure the level of FDPs or D-dimers in plasma. The pattern may also appear in incipient DIC, but usually the platelet count will also fall in this case.

6

PT	Normal
APTT	Normal
Thrombin time	Normal
Fibrinogen concentration	Normal
Platelet count	Low

If the only abnormality is a low platelet count, possible causes must be investigated. Premorbid counts and a clinical history should be sought to establish whether the thrombocytopenia is long-standing and possibly constitutional and a blood film should be examined. When it appears to be acquired, the usual approach is to perform a bone marrow aspirate to exclude marrow failure and establish whether megakaryocytes are present. If the number and morphology of megakaryocytes in the marrow is normal, further investigations are undertaken to establish the cause of the presumed peripheral destruction of platelets. Heparin and other drugs are common causes in hospital practice.

7

PT	Long
APTT	Long
Thrombin time	Normal
Fibrinogen concentration	Normal/abnormal
Platelet count	Low

This pattern of abnormalities of the screening tests is found:

1. After massive transfusion with stored/plasma reduced blood that is deficient in coagulation factors
2. In some cases of chronic liver disease, especially cirrhosis
3. In DIC. Although DIC will eventually result in depletion of fibrinogen, this is often a relatively late event.

Specific factor assays may be useful if the situation persists. Consider the possibility that the low platelet count has a separate aetiology and that the situation is in fact the same as in Section 4.

8

PT	Long
APTT	Long
Thrombin time	Long
Fibrinogen concentration	Low
Platelet count	Low

All the first-line tests are abnormal in the following:

1. Acute DIC
2. Some cases of acute liver necrosis with DIC.

It is only exceptionally necessary to confirm the diagnosis of DIC with additional tests (e.g. by estimating FDP or D-dimer concentration or by carrying out a screening test for the presence of fibrin monomers). Consider the possibility that more than one pathology is present.

Correction Tests Using the PT or APTT

Principle

Unexplained prolongation of the PT or APTT can be investigated with simple correction tests by mixing the patient's plasma with normal plasma. Correction indicates a possible factor deficiency, whereas failure to correct suggests the presence of an inhibitor, but interpretation should initially be cautious; see below.

Reagents

Plasmas for correction. Normal plasma contains all the coagulation factors; therefore mixing tests with normal plasma will identify the presence of an inhibitor or a factor deficiency. In previous editions the use of aged and adsorbed plasma is described, but these correction reagents may give misleading results if not used with great care. It is better to proceed directly to specific factor assays if appropriate factor-deficient plasmas are available.
PPP. From the patient and a control
Other reagents. As described on p. 409.

Method

Perform a PT and/or APTT on control, patient's and a 50:50 (0.05 ml of each) mixture of the control and patient plasma. Perform all the tests in duplicate using a balanced order to avoid time bias. Note that mixing experiments to detect factor VIII inhibitors may require incubation for 2 h (see p. 422).

Interpretation

If the prolongation is the result of a deficiency of a clotting factor, the PT or APTT of the mixture should return to within a few seconds of normal. It is then necessary to identify the specific factor(s) that are deficient.

If the APTT is prolonged and normal plasma fails to correct the APTT, an inhibitor should be suspected. An inhibitor screen and tests for an LAC should be performed.

However, mixing tests may be misleading in two particular circumstances:

1. Some inhibitors (usually anti-factor VIII antibodies) are time dependent in their action and testing immediately after mixing may show correction, whereas testing after 2 h of incubation reveals an inhibitory effect.
2. Some lupus-like anticoagulants are relatively weak and may only be apparent if 25:75 mixes of normal and test plasma are used. This makes confusion with factor deficiency possible. For details of testing for inhibitors, see p. 421.

Comment

Correction tests are sometimes not as clear-cut as the literature and theory would suggest. Incomplete correction can be difficult to interpret, especially if the initial prolongation is modest. If the correction tests fall into the 'grey' area, specific factor levels should be measured and tests for the presence of an LAC should be performed, checking for time-dependent effects and non-linearity.

Correction Tests Using the Thrombin Time

Principle

The tests use certain physicochemical properties of reagents to bind to inhibitors or abnormal molecules and normalize the prolonged TT. Protamine sulphate has a net electropositive charge and interacts with heparin, as well as binding to FDP, neutralizing the inhibitory effects of both. Toluidine blue is also a charged reagent that will neutralize heparin but has no effect on FDP. It is interesting that toluidine blue normalizes the TT in some dysfibrinogenaemias, probably by interacting with the excess of sialic acid attached to the fibrinogen molecules. Mixing with serum or albumin solution will correct the prolongation of the TT resulting from hypoalbuminaemia.

Reagents

Patient's and control plasma
Protamine sulphate. 1% and 10% in 9 g/l NaCl
Toluidine blue. 0.05 g in 100 ml of 9 g/l NaCl
Bovine thrombin. As described under thrombin time.

Method

Perform the test as described for TT, adding 0.1 ml of saline to the controls and replacing in the test with protamine sulphate or toluidine blue solution. Also perform a TT on a 50:50 mixture of control and test plasma.

Interpretation

See Table 18.4.

Comment

The endpoint may be difficult to see in samples with a low fibrinogen content in the presence of toluidine blue owing to the dark colour of the reagent. Grossly elevated fibrinogen concentrations or the presence of a paraprotein can cause a prolonged time not corrected by either protamine or toluidine blue. Diluting the test plasma in saline will shorten the TT.

Reptilase or Ancrod Time

Batroxobin (Reptilase), a purified enzyme from the snake *Bothrops atrox*, and ancrod (Viprinex), a similar enzyme from the snake *Agkistrodon rhodostoma*, may be used to replace thrombin in the TT test.[28]

The venoms are reconstituted as directed by the manufacturers and the test is performed exactly as described for the TT. The snake venoms are not inhibited by heparin and will give normal times for the clotting of normal plasma in the presence of heparin. The clotting times will, however, remain prolonged in the presence of raised FDP or abnormal or reduced fibrinogen or hypoalbuminaemia.

INVESTIGATION OF A BLEEDING DISORDER RESULTING FROM A COAGULATION FACTOR DEFICIENCY OR DEFECT

When the screening tests indicate that an individual has a coagulation defect, the plasma concentration of the coagulation factors should be assayed. Such assays establish the diagnosis of the deficiency or defect and they assess its severity; they also can be used to monitor replacement therapy and to detect the carrier state in families in which one or more members are affected by a congenital bleeding disorder.

An individual may have a congenital deficiency of a coagulation factor because of impaired synthesis or because a variant of the molecule that is deficient in clotting activity is synthesized. In both instances the results of assays based on coagulation tests will be subnormal, but when a variant molecule is being produced, the result of an immunological assay may be normal or near normal.

General Principles of Parallel Line Bioassays of Coagulation Factors

If two materials containing the same coagulation factor are assayed in a specific assay system in a range of dilutions and the clotting times are plotted against the plasma concentration on linear graph paper, curved dose–response lines are obtained. If the plot is redrawn on double-log paper, a sigmoid curve with a straight middle section is obtained (Fig. 18.8), although in some cases (e.g. factor VIII) semi-log paper is required. If the dilutions of the test and standard materials are chosen carefully, it should be possible to draw two straight parallel lines. The horizontal distance between the two lines represents the difference in potency ('strength' or concentration) of the factor assayed. If the test line is to the right of the standard, it contains less of the factor than the standard; if it is to the left, it contains more. The assay is based on the assumption that both test and control behave like simple dilutions of each other. This assumption has caused some problems when assaying samples containing factor VIII or IX concentrates (see below).

When setting up and performing a parallel line assay, a number of measures must be taken to ensure that the assay is valid and reliable.

1. *Dilution range.* This should be chosen so that the coagulation times lie on the linear portion of the sigmoid curve. For example, when assaying factor VIII by a one-stage assay, dilutions giving times between 60 and

Table 18.4 Interpretation of correction tests using the thrombin time (TT)

SALINE	TT OF TEST PLASMA CORRECTED WITH			INTERPRETATION
	Normal plasma	Protamine sulphate	Toluidine blue	
No	Yes	No	No	Deficiency
No	Var	No	Yes	Dysfibrinogenaemia of liver disease
No	Var	Yes	No	High concentration of FDPs

FDPs, fibrin degradation products; var, variable.
It is essential to exclude the possibility of heparin contamination.

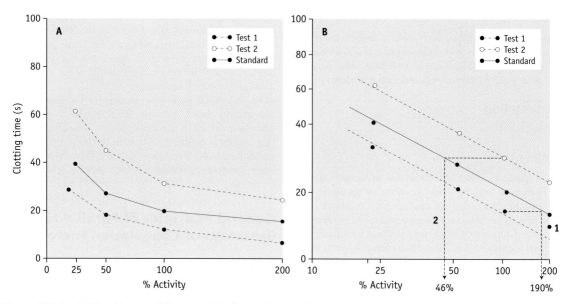

Figure 18.8 Parallel line bioassay of factor VII. (A) Clotting times with 1 in 5, 1 in 10, 1 in 20 and 1 in 40 dilutions of test and standard plasma plotted on linear graph paper. (B) The same data plotted on double-log paper. Three parallel straight lines are obtained. The horizontal shift of the test line represents the difference in potency. In this case, test 1 has a potency of 190 iu/dl and test 2 has a potency of 46 iu/dl. The 1 in 10 dilution of the standard plasma is assigned a potency of 100 iu/dl.

100 s are chosen if the blank clotting time is more than 120 s. (The blank consists of a mixture of buffer and substrate or deficient plasma, which provides all factors except the one to be measured.)

2. *Number of dilutions.* At least three dilutions of the standard and the test are assayed to give the best graphic or mathematical solution.
3. *Responses.* Dilutions of the test sample should be chosen so that the clotting times fall within the range obtained for the standard. If it transpires that the test result falls outside this range, the standard curve should not be extrapolated but the dilutions of the test and/or the standard must be adjusted.
4. *Duplicates and replicates.* Duplicates are obtained from the same dilution of the sample and sometimes by subsampling from the same incubation mixture. Replicates are true repeats involving a fresh dilution and fresh reagents. Normally, coagulation times are measured on duplicates. Replicates are sometimes used for particularly difficult assays.
5. *Temporal drift.* This has already been discussed. Duplicates in a coagulation assay should always be tested in a balanced order (e.g. ABCCBA).

Note on Single Point Factor Assays

Factor assay results are dependent on obtaining parallel lines for the test and reference plasmas. Many automated coagulation analysers will give an assay result obtained from a single dilution assuming that this condition is met. However, this is not always true and if an inhibitor is suspected, results from more than one dilution should be obtained for comparison and to determine parallelism. Similarly, if the result is above or below the linear part of the standard curve, further dilutions should be tested.

Assays Based on the Prothrombin Time

The investigation of an isolated prolonged PT (e.g. suspected factor VII deficiency or defect) in an individual with a lifelong history of bleeding includes a one-stage factor VII assay. If a reduced concentration of factor VII is found, further tests may include immunoassays of factor VII and, when possible, a family study.

One-Stage Assay of Factor VII
Principle

The assay of factor VII is based on the PT. The assay compares the ability of dilutions of the patient's plasma and of a standard plasma to correct the PT of a substrate plasma. It is easily adapted to assay of prothrombin, factor V or factor X.

Reagents

PPP from the patient
Standard/reference plasma. See p. 405

Factor VII-deficient plasma. Commercial or from a patient with known severe deficiency
Barbitone buffered saline. See p. 409
Thromboplastin. It is recommended that a recombinant human thromboplastin is used for the assay of human factor VII. Rabbit brain thromboplastin known to be sensitive to factor VII deficiency has been used, but there is a danger of the interspecies differences giving misleading results. The thromboplastin should be reconstituted according to the manufacturer's instructions and may have sufficient Ca for the assay. Warm sufficient thromboplastin for the assay to 37°C.
CaCl₂. 0.025 mol/l (if not present in the thromboplastin preparation).

Method

Prepare 1 in 5, 1 in 10; 1 in 20 and 1 in 40 dilutions of the standard and test plasma in buffered saline. Transfer 0.1 ml of each dilution to a glass tube and add to it 0.1 ml of deficient (substrate) plasma. Mix and allow to warm to 37°C. Add 0.1 ml of dilute thromboplastin and start the stopwatch. Record the clotting time. If the thromboplastin does not contain calcium, start the stopwatch after adding 0.1 ml of CaCl₂. A blank must be included with every assay and all tests must be carried out in duplicate and in balanced order.

Calculation of Results

Plot the clotting times of the test and standard against the concentration of factor VII on log-log graph paper. Read the concentration as shown in Figure 18.8.

Normal Range

The normal range is 50–150 iu/dl.

Interpretation

Patients with a congenital deficiency have factor VII levels of 30 iu/dl and less. The concentration measured may vary according to the thromboplastin used in the assay, so human thromboplastin is preferable. A small proportion of patients have normal factor VII antigen despite abnormal functional activity.

Assays Based on the Activated Partial Thromboplastin Time

An APTT-based assay (e.g. factor VIII) may be indicated after obtaining correction of a prolonged APTT by mixing with another plasma. An assay for factor VIII is described, but this is easily adapted to factor IX, factor XI or contact factor assays by substituting the relevant factor-deficient plasma.

One-Stage Assay of Factor VIII
Principle

The one-stage assay for factor VIII[29,30] is based on the APTT according to the bioassay principle described earlier.

Reagents

PPP. From the patient
Standard/reference plasma. See p. 405
Factor VIII-deficient plasma (substrate plasma). If using a commercial plasma, the reagent should be reconstituted according to the manufacturer's instructions. If a haemophiliac donor is used, his factor VIII concentration should be less than 1 iu/dl and his plasma should be free of inhibitors. The plasma should be stored in suitable volumes (e.g. 2 ml) at −20°C or lower until used. All samples obtained from patients must be considered potentially infective. Patient samples should be tested for antibodies to human immunodeficiency virus (HIV) and hepatitis C virus and for hepatitis B surface (HBs) antigen.
Barbitone buffered saline. See p. 409.
Reagents for APTT.
Plastic tubes. To avoid contact activation while preparing samples
Icebath.

Method

Place the APTT reagent and CaCl₂ at 37°C and the patient's, standard and substrate plasma in the icebath until used.

Make 1 in 10 dilutions of the test and standard plasma in buffered saline in plastic tubes in the icebath. Using 0.2 ml volumes, make doubling dilutions in buffered saline to obtain 1 in 20 and 1 in 40 dilutions. Place 0.1 ml of the three dilutions (1 in 10, 1 in 20 and 1 in 40) in glass tubes. If the test plasma is suspected of having a very low factor VIII content, make 1 in 5, 10 and 20 dilutions of the test instead.

Add to each dilution 0.1 ml of freshly reconstituted or thawed substrate plasma and warm up at 37°C. Perform APTTs according to the laboratory protocol following a balanced order of duplicates.

The dilutions should be tested at 2-min intervals on the master watch. The assay must end with a blank consisting of 0.1 ml of buffered saline and 0.1 ml of substrate plasma.

Calculation of Results

Plot the clotting times of the test and standard against the concentration of factor VIII on semi-log paper. Read the concentration as shown in Figure 18.8. It is important to obtain straight and parallel lines if the result is to be

419

accurate. The reasons for non-parallelism and curvature are as follows:

1. Technical error. Repeat the assay with fresh dilutions.
2. Activation of the plasma by poor collection. A new sample should be collected.
3. A low concentration of factor VIII in the test plasma giving rise to non-parallel lines. Stronger concentration of plasma should be prepared and tested.
4. The presence of an inhibitor. The tests described on p. 421 should be carried out.

Some automated coagulometers produce computed values using mathematical formulae. If the standard plasma is calibrated in terms of international units, the result can be expressed in iu. For example, if the standard plasma has a factor VIII concentration of 65 iu/dl and the test is shown to have 20 iu/dl of the activity of the standard, the test plasma will have a factor VIII concentration of 13 iu/dl (20% of 65 iu/dl).

Normal Range

The normal range is 45–158 iu/dl. Each laboratory should determine its own normal range.

Interpretation

Some clinically normal people have factor VIII concentrations of 35–50 iu/dl. Values below 30 iu/dl are unequivocally abnormal; values below 50 iu/dl are significant in carriers of haemophilia (heterozygotes).

A reduced factor VIII concentration is found in the following:

1. Haemophilia A
2. Some carriers of haemophilia A (heterozygotes)
3. VWD, types I and III and some cases of type II
4. Congenital combined deficiency of factors VIII and V (rare)
5. Disseminated intravascular coagulation
6. Acquired haemophilia (anti-factor VIII antibodies).

Further Tests in Haemophilia A

Reduction in factor VIII secondary to VWD should be excluded. VWF:Ag and VWF:RCo (described later) should be measured and the patient's family history should be investigated. A low factor VIII with normal VWF:Ag and VWF:RCo may also result from the Normandy type VWD (Type 2N), which should be suspected when there is not a clear sex-linked family history and which can be confirmed by a VWD–factor VIII binding assay.[31]

Two-Stage and Chromogenic Assays for Factor VIII

The one-stage factor VIII assay is sensitive to preactivation of coagulation factors in the patient sample. The two-stage and chromogenic assays circumvent this problem by preactivating all the available factor VIII and then assaying this in a separate system by its ability to generate Xa. In the chromogenic assay this is measured using a chromogenic Xa substrate; in the two-stage assay it is measured by a clotting endpoint. In general these have proved too cumbersome or expensive for widespread use and preactivation is rarely a significant problem. However, a clinically significant discrepancy between the two types of assay has been reported in some cases of mild haemophilia. In these cases mutations destabilizing the interaction between the A_1 and A_2 domains result in a one-stage assay result that is higher than that obtained by two stage. Most significantly, the patient's clinical problem is more in keeping with the two-stage assay result.[32,33] The reverse phenomenon (two-stage higher than one stage) can also occur but is not associated with bleeding.[34] The chromogenic assay has also found utility in avoiding some of the problems encountered assaying factor VIII concentrates.

Monitoring Replacement Therapy in Coagulation Factor Defects and Deficiencies

Estimations of factor VIII levels in patients with haemophilia treated with factor VIII concentrates often yield discrepant results. This is primarily because the factor VIII concentrate (diluted in haemophilic plasma) is compared with a plasma standard. In general, two-stage or chromogenic assays reveal greater potency than one-stage assays in this situation. This has been particularly noted in patients who have been treated with B domainless factor VIII (Refacto, Wyeth). In this case a product-specific reference preparation is available from the company. It is recommended that this is used in conjunction with a chromogenic assay, but this may not be necessary.[35-37] In most other cases the clinical experience of using results from one-stage assays remains valid.

Assays of factor VIII concentrates are fraught with difficulty and a detailed discussion is beyond the scope of this chapter.[35,38] The difficulties arise from several problems. First, the concentrate potency may be assigned using either a one-stage assay (as in the USA) or the chromogenic assay (as in Europe). Second, many concentrates, even when diluted in haemophilic plasma, behave differently in one-stage and chromogenic assays. As a result, there are separate WHO standards for factor VIII measurement: a plasma for measurement of factor VIII in plasma samples and a concentrate for measurement of factor VIII in concentrates. This is based on the principle of assaying like against like, although there are so many different concentrates with different characteristics that this is difficult to truly achieve and all must eventually be calibrated against a single plasma pool.[37]

Investigation of a Patient Whose APTT and PT are Prolonged

A prolonged APTT and PT but a normal TT in a patient with a bleeding disorder may be the result of a defect or deficiency of one of the factors of the common pathway: factor X, factor V or prothrombin. In addition, the patient could be suffering from the much rarer combined deficiency of factors V and VIII. Liver disease and vitamin K deficiency should always be excluded, even in the presence of a family history of bleeding. Mixing tests illustrated on p. 422 may help to pinpoint the defect; the missing factor or factors should be estimated quantitatively. Factor X, factor V and prothrombin can all be assayed satisfactorily using a prothrombin-based assay as described for factor VII. The Taipan venom assay for prothrombin and the Russell's viper venom assay for factor X are described in the 8th edition of this book.

INVESTIGATION OF A PATIENT WITH A CIRCULATING ANTICOAGULANT (INHIBITOR)

Circulating anticoagulants or acquired inhibitors of coagulation factors are immunoglobulins arising either in congenitally deficient individuals as a result of the administration of the missing factor or in previously haemostatically normal subjects as a part of an autoimmune process. Usually, an inhibitor is suspected when a prolonged clotting test does not correct after mixing 50:50 with normal plasma or if an apparent factor deficiency does not fit with a patient's clinical history.

The most common anticoagulant in haemostatically normal people is the LAC, but despite the prolongation of clotting tests *in vitro*, this anticoagulant predisposes to thrombosis and its diagnosis and investigation therefore are considered on p. 448. Of the anticoagulants that cause a bleeding tendency, antibodies to factor VIII are most common, either in haemophiliacs or as autoantibodies in previously normal individuals. Patients with haemophilia usually develop antibodies with simple kinetics; this inhibitor reacts with factor VIII in a linear fashion and the antigen–antibody complex has no factor VIII activity. Antibodies in non-haemophilic individuals or patients with mild/moderate haemophilia usually develop antibodies with complex kinetics: inactivation of factor VIII is at first rapid, but it then slows as the antigen–antibody complex either dissociates or displays some residual factor VIII activity. Addition of further factor VIII results to the same residual (equilibrium) factor VIII activity.

Inhibitors directed against other coagulation factors are very rare, but an acquired form of VWD may arise in this way, usually from a paraprotein. Hypoprothrombinaemia owing to autoantibodies is a rare complication of systemic lupus erythematosus.[39] Only the factor VIII inhibitor assays are described in detail in this section.

Confusion may arise in the presence of an inhibitor if different clotting factors are assayed. For instance, if a patient's plasma contains an inhibitor directed against factor VIII and the factor IX level in that plasma is assayed using factor IX-deficient plasma, the clotting times in the factor IX assay may be prolonged. This may lead to the mistaken conclusion that the patient has factor IX deficiency, particularly if a single dilution of test plasma is used. Clotting factors should always be assayed at multiple dilutions. If the inhibitor is specifically directed against one clotting factor, that factor will appear to be equally deficient at all dilutions of the patient's plasma. The assayed level of other clotting factors will increase with increasing dilution as the inhibitor is diluted out.

Circulating Inhibitor (Anticoagulant) Screen Based on the APTT

Principle

Circulating anticoagulants or inhibitors affecting the APTT may act immediately or be time dependent. Normal plasma mixed with a plasma containing an immediately acting inhibitor will have little or no effect on the prolonged clotting time. In contrast, if normal plasma is added to a plasma containing a time-dependent inhibitor, the clotting time of the latter will be substantially shortened. However, after 1–2 h, correction will be abolished and the clotting time will become long again. To detect both types of inhibition, normal plasma and test plasma samples are tested immediately after mixing and also after incubation together at 37°C for 120 min.

Reagents

Normal plasma. Commercial lyophilized normal plasma or a plasma pool from 20 donors as described on p. 405
PPP. From the patient
Reagents for the APTT. See p. 410.

Method

Prepare three plastic tubes as follows: place 0.5 ml of normal plasma in one tube, 0.5 ml of the patient's plasma in a second tube and a mixture of 0.25 ml of normal and 0.25 ml of patient's plasma in a third tube. Incubate the tubes for 120 min at 37°C and then place all three tubes in an icebath or on crushed ice. Next, make a 50:50 mixture of the contents of tubes 1 and 2 into a fourth tube, which serves to check for the presence of an immediate inhibitor. Perform APTTs in duplicate on all four tubes.

Results and Interpretation

See Table 18.5. Note that the incubation period results in a prolongation of the normal plasma APTT.

Method for Detecting Inhibitors in Patients with Haemophilia

A simple inhibitor screen has been reported to be more sensitive than a Bethesda assay in monitoring for the development of inhibitors in haemophilia A and B. Add 0.4 ml patient plasma (or factor-deficient control plasma) to 0.1 ml of 5 iu/ml factor VIII or IX concentrate, giving a final concentration of 1 iu/ml. Mix gently and incubate at 37°C for 60 min for haemophilia A patients and 10 min for haemophilia B patients. Perform appropriate factor assay for the patient and control sample; if the factor level in the patient sample is less than 90% of the control sample the inhibitor screen is positive.[40]

Quantitative Measurement of Factor VIII and Other Inhibitors

Principle

Factor VIII inhibitors[41] are usually time dependent.[38] Thus if factor VIII is added to plasma containing an inhibitor and the mixture is incubated, factor VIII will be progressively neutralized. If the amount of factor VIII added and the duration of incubation are standardized, the strength of the inhibitor may be measured in units according to how much of the added factor VIII is destroyed.

In the Bethesda method, the unit is defined as the amount of inhibitor that will neutralize 50% of 1 unit of factor VIII in normal plasma after 2 h of incubation at 37°C.

Dilutions of test plasma are incubated with an equal volume of the normal plasma pool at 37°C. The normal plasma pool is taken to represent 1 unit of factor VIII. Dilutions of a control normal plasma containing no inhibitor are treated in the same way. An equal volume of normal plasma mixed with buffer is taken to represent the 100% value.

At the end of the incubation period, the residual factor VIII is assayed and the inhibitor strength is calculated from a standard graph of residual factor VIII activity versus inhibitor units.

Inhibitor Assay Modifications

The Bethesda assay and Nijmegen modification give similar results at high levels of factor VIII inhibition. Reports have shown that shifts in pH and protein concentrations will lead to changes in factor VIII stability and inactivation. Factor VIII inactivation increases with pH and reduced protein concentration leads to further inactivation of factor VIII activity. This can result in false-positive results using the unmodified Bethesda method. The Nijmegen modification prevents these discrepancies by buffering normal plasma with 0.1 M imidazole buffer at pH 7.4 and using immunodepleted factor VIII-deficient plasma in the control mixture.[42] The assay can also be modified to use factor VIII concentrate (Oxford method) or by increasing the incubation time to 4 h (New Oxford method).

Reagents

Glyoxaline buffer. See p. 409
Kaolin. 5 mg/ml and platelet substitute. Phospholipid or preferred APTT reagent
Factor VIII-deficient plasma
Standard plasma. Normal plasma pool.

Method

Pipette into each of a series of plastic tubes 0.2 ml of normal pool plasma. Add 0.2 ml of glyoxaline buffer to the first tube (this tube serves as the 100% value); add 0.2 ml of test plasma dilutions in glyoxaline buffer to each

TUBE	CONTENT	CLOTTING TIME		
1	Normal plasma	Normal	Normal	Normal
2	Patient's plasma	Long	Long	Long
3	50:50 mixture, patient: normal; incubated 2 h	Normal	Long	Long
4	50:50 mixture, patient: normal; no incubation	Normal	Long	Normal
Interpretation		Deficiency	Immediately acting inhibitor	Time-dependent inhibitor

Table 18.5 Interpretation of the inhibitor screen based on the activated partial thromboplastin time

of the other tubes. If the patient's inhibitor has been assayed previously, this can be used as a guide to the dilutions that should be used. If the patient has not been tested before, a range of dilutions should be set up ranging from undiluted plasma to a 1 in 50 dilution.

Cap, mix and incubate all the tubes for 2 h at 37°C. Then immerse all the tubes in an icebath. Perform factor VIII assays on all the incubation mixtures.

Calculation of Results

Record the residual factor VIII percentage for each mixture assuming the assay value of the control to be 100%. The dilution of test plasma that gives the residual factor VIII percentage nearest to 50% (between 30% and 60%) is chosen for calculating the strength of inhibitor. Results are calculated as shown in Figure 18.9 and in Table 18.6 for three different patients with a mild inhibitor only detected in undiluted plasma, a stronger inhibitor with simple kinetics and an inhibitor with complex kinetics, respectively.

Interpretation

If the residual factor VIII activity is between 80% and 100%, the plasma sample does not contain an inhibitor. If the residual activity is less than 60%, the plasma unequivocally contains an inhibitor. Values between 60% and 80% are borderline and repeated testing on additional samples is needed before the diagnosis can be established.

Tests for Other Inhibitors

Factor IX inhibitors can be measured in a system identical to that described earlier. Because factor IX inhibitors act immediately, there is no need for prolonged incubation; the mixtures can be assayed after 5 min at 37°C. The activity of the inhibitor against porcine factor VIII can be measured by substituting porcine factor VIII concentrate, appropriately diluted in factor VIII-deficient plasma, for normal plasma.

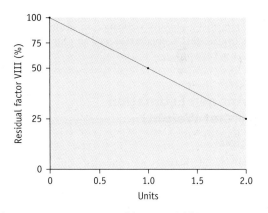

Figure 18.9 Measurement of factor VIII inhibitors. Relationship between the residual factor VIII activity in normal plasma and the inhibitor activity of the test plasma can be read off this plot. At 50% inhibition the test plasma contains, by definition, 1 Bethesda inhibitor unit per ml. Note that the y-axis is a logarithmic scale.

Table 18.6 Example of the calculation of Bethesda units (u) in three plasma samples

PATIENT	PLASMA DILUTION	% RESIDUAL VIII	CALCULATION u × DILUTION	INHIBITOR IN BETHESDA u
A	Undiluted	61	0.70 × 1	= 0.07
B	1 in 5	33	1.60 × 5	= 8.0
	1 in 10	55	0.85 × 10	= 8.5
	1 in 15	68	0.55 × 15	= 8.3
C	1 in 5	40	1.30 × 5	= 6.5
	1 in 10	55	0.85 × 10	= 8.5
	1 in 15	61	0.70 × 15	= 10.5
	1 in 20	65	0.60 × 20	= 12

Patient A has a mild inhibitor, patient B an inhibitor with simple kinetics and patient C an inhibitor with complex kinetics. All values are chosen for the percent residual factor VIII activity close to 50%. The units for the calculation are read from Figure 18.9 using the % residual VIII. (Modified from Kasper CK, Ewing NP 1982 The haemophilias: measurement of inhibitor to factor VIII C (and IX C). *Methods in Haematology* 5:39).

Note. In patients B and C the results should be reported as 8.5 Bethesda units (u); in C, the calculated level of inhibitor may continue to rise with increasing dilution.

INVESTIGATION OF A PATIENT SUSPECTED OF AFIBRINOGENAEMIA, HYPOFIBRINOGENAEMIA OR DYSFIBRINOGENAEMIA

A patient suspected of afibrinogenaemia, hypofibrinogenaemia or dysfibrinogenaemia[43] usually has a prolonged APTT, PT and TT. The prolongation of the PT is usually less marked than that of the APTT and TT. There may be either a history of bleeding or of recurrent thrombotic events but many patients (c50%) are asymptomatic. It is important that a physical estimation of fibrinogen (such as the clot weight) is obtained as well as a function-based assay (e.g. Clauss).

Fibrinogen Estimation (Dry Clot Weight)

Principle

Fibrinogen in plasma is converted into fibrin by clotting with thrombin and calcium. The resulting clot is weighed and may include other proteins such as some FDPs. It is, however, simpler than the total clottable protein method used for the international standard[44] and provides a useful comparison for the Clauss.

Reagents

Platelet-poor plasma (PPP)
$CaCl_2$. 0.025 mol/l
Bovine thrombin. 50 NIH u/ml.

Method

Pipette 1 ml of plasma into a 12×75 mm glass tube and warm to 37°C. Place a wooden applicator or swab stick in the tube, add 0.1 ml of $CaCl_2$ and 0.9 ml of thrombin and mix. Incubate for 15 min at 37°C.

Gently wind the fibrin clot onto the stick, squeezing out the serum. Wash the clot in a tube containing at first 9 g/l NaCl, then water. Blot the clot carefully with filter paper, remove the fibrin from the stick and put into acetone for 5–10 min. Dry the clot in a hot air oven or over a hot lamp for 30 min. Allow it to cool and then weigh it.

Results

The fibrinogen level is expressed as g/l (i.e. the weight of fibrin obtained from 1 ml of plasma ×1000).

Normal Range

Normal range is 1.8–3.6 g/l.

Further Investigations

Whenever a congenital fibrinogen abnormality is suspected, DIC and hyperfibrinolysis must be excluded; FDP should not be in excess and there should be no evidence of the consumption of other coagulation factors and platelets (see p. 440). Immunological or chemical determination of fibrinogen concentration is the next step in investigation. In dysfibrinogenaemias there is often a normal or even raised plasma fibrinogen concentration using these methods, although the functional assays indicate a deficiency. Other tests that may be helpful are the Reptilase time, fibrinopeptide release, factor XIII cross-linking, tests of polymerization, binding to thrombin and lysis by plasmin. DNA analysis to detect the mutation responsible may be useful to allow comparison with other reported phenotypes. Testing the parents or other family members is sometimes a useful means for establishing whether a hereditary fibrinogen abnormality is present.

DEFECTS OF PRIMARY HAEMOSTASIS

Investigation of the Vascular Disorders of Haemostasis

Vascular disorders of haemostasis are those that arise as a result of a defect or deficiency of the vessel wall. This may result from one of the inherited disorders of collagen or from an acquired disorder such as amyloid or scurvy.

In general, the tests of coagulation available in the laboratory will be of little help in elucidating such defects. The only test of possible use is the bleeding time. Tests of capillary resistance are of little value. A careful clinical history and physical examination are most likely to provide the basis for diagnosis. Particular attention should be paid to previous scars, associated signs of the inherited syndromes and evidence of systemic disease. In some cases a tissue biopsy may be useful, but confirmation of the diagnosis requires analysis of collagen from cultured fibroblasts or DNA analysis of the relevant candidate genes.[45]

Bleeding Time

A standard incision is made on the volar surface of the forearm and the time the incision bleeds is measured. Cessation of bleeding is dependent on an adequate number of platelets, the ability of the platelets to adhere to the subendothelium directly and via adhesion molecules such as VWF and fibrinogen. However the test has poor sensitivity for disorders such as VWD, is a poor predictor of bleeding risk and is poorly reproducible. Consequently, it is now rarely performed and readers are referred to previous editions for details.

Laboratory Tests of Platelet–von Willebrand Factor Function

The PFA-100 System

The *in vitro* system for measuring platelet–VWF function, PFA-100 (Dade Behring), was introduced as a substitute for the bleeding time. The instrument aspirates a citrated whole-blood sample under constant vacuum from the sample reservoir through a capillary and a microscopic aperture cut into a membrane. The membrane is coated with collagen and either epinephrine or adenosine 5′-diphosphate (ADP). It therefore attempts to reproduce under high shear rates VWF binding, platelet attachment, activation and aggregation, which slowly build a stable platelet plug at the aperture. The time required to obtain full occlusion of the aperture is reported as the 'closure time'. Collagen/epinephrine is the primary screening cartridge and the collagen/ADP is used to identify possible aspirin use.

Studies have shown this system to be sensitive to platelet adherence and aggregation abnormalities and to be dependent on normal VWF, glycoprotein Ib and glycoprotein IIbIIIa levels but not on plasma fibrinogen or fibrin generation.[46]

The PFA-100 system may reflect VWF function better than the bleeding time, but it is not sensitive to vascular-collagen disorders.[47,48] Studies have shown that many patients with minor platelet disorders such as secretion defects are not detected by the PFA-100.[49]

INVESTIGATION OF SUSPECTED VON WILLEBRAND DISEASE

A diagnosis of VWD[50,51] should be considered in individuals with a relevant history or family history of bleeding, particularly of the mucosal type. Although a prolonged bleeding time and APTT in screening tests is suggestive, these are normal in many patients with VWD and specific assays must be performed. Preliminary screening with a test such as the PFA-100 may be useful in excluding borderline cases. All relevant activities (i.e. factor VIII concentration; VWF:Ag concentration; collagen binding activity, VWF:CB; and ristocetin cofactor activity, VWF:RiCoF) should be measured. When interpreting the results, the very wide range of VWF levels in the normal population and the effect of ABO blood group should be borne in mind. It is apparent that many individuals with levels down to 30% of normal do not have any significant

bleeding tendency and caution should be exercised in diagnosing VWD on the basis of moderately low VWF levels alone.[50–53]

Thus, if an abnormality is detected it should be considered in relation to the clinical history. When a discrepancy between antigen and function is found (i.e. function is <70% of the antigen) multimer analysis of the plasma should be performed. In normal plasma, each multimer of VWF (a large molecule consisting of 2 to >20 subunits of VWF) is seen to be composed of a 'triplet,' a dark central band sandwiched between two lighter bands; high molecular weight multimers predominate. In VWD, the multimer analysis may be superficially normal, there may be no VWF:Ag detectable, the high molecular weight forms necessary for normal platelet adhesion may be lacking or the triplet pattern may be abnormal. On the basis of these results VWD can be classified as shown in Table 18.7.[50,51]

Enzyme-Linked Immunosorbent Assay for Von Willebrand Factor Antigen

Principle

ELISA involves coating a special microtitre plate with a primary antibody to von Willebrand factor antigen (VWF:Ag).[52] A suitable dilution of the test plasma is added to the wells, allowing the VWF:Ag to bind to the primary antibody. After removal of excess antigen by washing the plate, a second antibody, conjugated to an enzyme, usually peroxidase and called the 'tag' antibody, is added and this binds to the VWF:Ag already bound to the plate. On addition of a specific substrate, a colour change occurs. After the reaction has been stopped with acid, the optical density (OD) of each well can be measured using an electronic plate reader; the OD is directly proportional to the amount of VWF:Ag present in the test plasma.

Reagents

0.05 M Carbonate buffer. 1.59 g Na_2CO_3, 2.93 g $NaHCO_3$, 0.2 g NaN_3 in 1 litre of distilled water (pH 9.6)
0.01 M Phosphate buffered saline. 0.39 g $NaH_2PO_4.2H_2O$, 2.68 g $Na_2HPO_4.12H_2O$, 8.47 g NaCl in 1 litre distilled water (pH 7.2)
0.1 M Citrate phosphate buffer. 8.8 g citric acid, 24.0 g $Na_2HPO_4.12H_2O$ in 1 litre distilled water (pH 5.0)
Anti VWF:Ag antiserum
Anti VWF:Ag conjugated with peroxidase
Platelet-poor (100%) calibration plasma
PPP (tests and control)
1,2-o-Phenylenediamine dihydrochloride (orthophenylenediamine, OPD)
1 M Sulphuric acid
Hydrogen peroxide 20 vol
Tween 20.

Table 18.7 Classification of von Willebrand disease

TYPE	INHERITANCE	VIII	VWF:Ag	RiCoF	MULTIMER ANALYSIS	COMMENTS
1	Autos. dominant	L/N	L	L	Normal pattern	–
2A	Autos. dominant	L/N	L/N	L	Absent large and intermediate-size multimers; some forms have abnormal triplets	–
2B	Autos. dominant	L/N	L	L/N	Large multimers absent; normal triplets	Aggregation with low-dose ristocetin in platelet-rich plasma, thrombocytopenia
2M	Autos. dominant	N	N	L*	Normal pattern; some forms have ultra-large multimers	–
2N	Autos. recessive	L	N	N	Normal pattern	Abnormal factor VIII binding
3	Autos. recessive	L	L	L	Virtually absent	–

Autos., autosomal; L, low; N, normal; RiCoF, ristocetin cofactor; VWF, von Willebrand factor.
Note. Following reports of VWD in which the only abnormality is a defect in collagen binding, it has been suggested that the 2M category be extended to include these patients.[51] VWD is extremely varied and recessive forms of Type 1 and Type 2 are occasionally encountered.

Method

Dilute the antihuman-VWF:Ag 1:500 in 0.05 M carbonate buffer (i.e. 40 μl antibody in 20 ml buffer) and add 100 μl to each well of the microtitre plate. Incubate for 1 h at room temperature in a moist chamber. Discard antibody and wash three times by immersion in a trough of phosphate buffered saline (PBS) with 0.5 ml/l Tween for 2 min, followed by inversion onto absorbent paper.

Prepare dilutions of the 100% standard 1:10, 1:20, 1:40 and 1:60 in PBS with 1 ml/l Tween. Dilute patient's and control plasmas 1:10, 1:20 and 1:40 in the same way and add 100 μl of each dilution in duplicate to the wells of the microtitre plate. Incubate for 1 h as before and repeat washing.

Dilute the antihuman-VWF:Ag-peroxidase conjugate 1:500 in 1 ml/l PBS-Tween (i.e. 40 μl antibody in 20 ml buffer) and add 100 μl to each well. Incubate for 1 h. Wash twice in 0.5 ml/l PBS Tween and once in 0.1 M citrate phosphate buffer.

Dissolve 40 mg of substrate (OPD) in 15 ml citrate phosphate buffer. Add 10 μl of 20 volume hydrogen peroxide to the substrate solution immediately before use and then add 100 μl to each well.

When the yellow colour has reached an intensity at which a mid-yellow ring is clearly visible in the bottom of the wells, stop the reaction by the addition of 150 μl of 1 M sulphuric acid. Read the optical density across the plate at 492 nm using a microtitre plate reader. Plot the standard curve on log-linear graph paper. VWF:Ag levels are obtained by reading from the reference curve.

Normal Range

The normal range is approximately 50–200 iu/dl.

Interpretation

The results must be interpreted in conjunction with the results of factor VIII assay and the ristocetin cofactor assay (Table 18.7). VWF:Ag can also be measured by an immunoelectrophoretic assay. (The Laurell rocket method for this is described in the 7th edition of this book.)

von Willebrand Factor Antigen Immunoturbidimetric Assay

Latex microparticles, coated with antibodies specific for VWF, are incubated with plasma; an antigen–antibody reaction occurs, resulting in agglutination of the latex microparticles. Agglutination of the microparticles leads to an increase in turbidity and hence absorbance, which is measured photometrically. Using a standard curve, the VWF concentration can be calculated (Instrumentation Laboratories, Stago; Siemens, Dade). Falsely elevated results may be obtained in the presence of rheumatoid factor or in acquired von Willebrand syndrome.

Ristocetin Cofactor Assay

Principle

Washed platelets do not 'agglutinate' in the presence of ristocetin unless normal plasma is added as a source of VWF. 'Agglutination' follows a dose–response curve dependent on the amount of plasma/VWF added. Freshly washed platelets or formalin-fixed platelets can be used in the assay. Fixed platelets take longer to prepare but are not susceptible to aggregation (as distinct from 'agglutination') with ristocetin and they can be stored so that they are available for emergency use. Freshly washed platelets are quicker to prepare and retain a functional platelet membrane, but they cannot be retained for later use. Commercial lyophilized, fixed, washed platelet preparations are available. Once reconstituted these preparations are stable for several weeks and should enhance assay standardization.[54]

Assay Using Fresh Platelets

Reagents

K_2EDTA. 0.134 mol/l
Citrate–saline. One volume of 31.1 g/l trisodium citrate + 9 volumes of 9 g/l NaCl
EDTA–citrate–saline. One volume of 0.134 mol/l K_2EDTA + 9 volumes of citrate–saline.

Method

Collect 40–60 ml of normal blood into a one-tenth volume of EDTA–saline in flat-bottom plastic universal containers. Do not use conical bottom containers. Centrifuge at 150–200 g at room temperature (about 20°C) for 15 min.

Pipette, using a plastic pipette, the platelet-rich plasma (PRP) into a plastic container. Mark the level of plasma on the tube. Centrifuge at 1500–2000 g to obtain a platelet button.

Discard the PPP. Resuspend the platelet button in a 2 ml volume of EDTA–citrate–saline by gently squeezing the liquid up and down a pipette until a smooth suspension is formed. Add EDTA–citrate–saline to the 20 ml mark.

Centrifuge at 1500–2000 g for 15 min. Discard the supernatant. Resuspend in EDTA–citrate–saline and leave at room temperature for 20 min to elute the ristocetin cofactor off the platelets.

Centrifuge again, discard the supernatant and resuspend in EDTA–citrate–saline two more times to a total of four washes.

Centrifuge at 1500–2000 g for 15 min. Discard the supernatant and resuspend in citrate–saline using a volume slightly under the original plasma volume (marked on the container). Centrifuge at 800 g for 5 min to remove platelet clumps, white cells and red cells.

Remove the platelet-rich supernatant carefully. Perform a platelet count and dilute the platelet-rich suspension with citrate–saline until the platelet count is about 200×10^9/l.

Leave the platelets at room temperature for 30–45 min to allow the platelets to recover from the trauma of washing and centrifugation.

Reagents for Assay

Citrate–saline

Ristocetin. 100 mg/ml. Stored frozen in 1 ml volumes.

Plasma standard

PPP. From the patient(s).

Assay method

Confirm that the washed platelets do not 'agglutinate' with ristocetin in the absence of added plasma. Deliver 0.5 ml of citrate–saline into an aggregometer cuvette and 0.4 ml of the platelet suspension + 0.1 ml of citrate–saline into another cuvette. Place in the warming block and leave it there for 3 min to warm. Add 5 µl of ristocetin and record at 1 cm/min for 2 min. The absorbance resulting from citrate–saline alone is taken to represent 100% agglutination and that resulting from platelets alone represents zero (%) agglutination (blank). The absorbance resulting from the platelet suspension must not exceed five divisions on the chart paper. If it is greater, the platelets must be washed again and the procedure must be repeated. The reading of this blank must be repeated every hour.

All plasma samples and ristocetin should be kept in an icebath.

Standard Curve

A standard curve is obtained by making doubling dilutions, 1 in 2 to 1 in 32 in citrate–saline, of the standard plasma (donor pool, commercial reference plasma or other reference materials). Frozen plasma standards may be preferred because lyophilization can result in pH changes which affect lyophilized platelets. The absorbance resulting from a mixture of 0.4 ml of citrate–saline and 0.1 ml of plasma dilution is taken to represent 100% agglutination and that resulting from the mixture of 0.4 ml of platelet suspension and 0.1 ml of plasma dilution represents zero (0%) agglutination.

Add 5 µl of ristocetin to the cuvette containing the mixture giving zero agglutination and record the agglutination for 2 min. Test each dilution of the standard plasma in a similar way.

The patient's plasma is tested at two dilutions, depending on the expected concentration of VWF in the plasma. Both dilutions should give agglutination within the range of that of the standard curve.

Reset 100% and zero aggregation for each patient.

A reading of the platelet blank should be repeated at hourly intervals. If the reading differs from the original, the difference must be subtracted from the results of subsequent tests.

Results

Measure 'agglutination' at 1 or 2 min depending on the strength of agglutination. All responses must be compared on the same time scale and not read at maximum agglutination.

Plot the standard curve on semi-log paper with agglutination on the linear scale and the concentration of VWF in iu/dl on the log scale (Fig. 18.10). For assay purposes, assign the 1 in 2 dilution of standard plasma a value of 0.50 iu/ml. (Each batch of standard is precalibrated and may not necessarily be 1.0 iu/ml.)

Read the patient's VWF concentration directly off the standard curve, correct for the dilution factor and average the two results from the different dilutions.

Figure 18.10 Ristocetin cofactor assay. The standard curve is plotted on semi-log paper. Each test plasma is assayed in two dilutions. Plasma 1 (+) produced the following readings: 1 in 4 dilution: 16 divisions of the chart paper = 7 iu (four times [dilution factor] = 28 iu/dl); 1 in 2 dilutions: 22 divisions = (13 iu/dl [twice dilution factor] = 26 iu/dl). The mean of the two readings is 27 iu/dl. Plasma 2 (*) gave the following results: 1 in 2 dilution: 7 divisions = (2.5 iu [twice dilution factor] = 5 iu/dl). 1 in 4 dilution: 5 divisions (not shown). This result was similar to the blank and the plasma was next tested undiluted, giving a reading of 10 divisions = 4 iu/dl. The mean is 4.5 iu/dl (very low).

Normal Range

The normal range is approximately 50–200 iu/dl.

Interpretation

The VWF concentration measured by ristocetin cofactor assay should be interpreted in conjunction with other factor VIII and VWF:Ag assays, as shown in Table 18.7.

Assay Using Formalin-Fixed Platelets
Reagents

Sodium citrate solution. 32 g/l trisodium sodium citrate ($Na_3C_6H_5O_7.2H_2O$)
K_2EDTA. 0.134 mol/l
2% formalin (40% formaldehyde). In 9 g/l NaCl
0.05% sodium azide. In 9 g/l NaCl.

Method

Suitable preparations can be obtained from citrated blood in a blood donation bag, from a normal individual or from a therapeutic venesection carried out on a patient with a normal platelet count. Acid–citrate–dextrose or citrate–phosphate–dextrose solution from the donor bag is ejected through the taking needle and replaced by the equivalent volume of sodium citrate. Collect *c* 500 ml of blood.

Centrifuge the blood at 300 *g* for 15 min at room temperature. Separate the PRP and add 9 volumes of PRP to 1 volume of EDTA solution. Incubate for 1 h at 37°C to reverse the effect of ADP released during the preparation. Add an equal volume of 2% formalin and leave at 4°C for 1 h. Centrifuge at 200 *g* for 10 min at 4°C. Decant the supernatant and recentrifuge it at 250 *g* for 20 min at 4°C. Discard the supernatant and resuspend the platelet sediment in chilled (4°C) 9 g/l NaCl. Wash the platelets twice more. After the final wash, resuspend the platelets in the sodium azide solution. Adjust the platelet count to $300–500 \times 10^9/l$. The suspension is stable for 1 month at 4°C.

Fixed platelets are also available commercially.

Reagents for Assay

Buffer for plasma dilutions. Barbitone buffer, pH 7.4, containing 40 mg/ml of bovine serum albumin (see p. 409)
Ristocetin, plasma standard and patient's PPP. As described in the previous assay.

Assay Method

Follow the method described for washed fresh platelets. Prepare all plasma dilutions in the albumin containing buffer.

Results, interpretation and normal range are as described for the washed platelet assay.

Collagen Binding Assay (ELISA)

The ELISA-based VWF collagen binding assay (VWF:CB) was developed as an alternative to VWF:RiCoF as a measure of VWF functional activity. It has the advantage over VWF:RiCoF of using an ELISA-based system, giving greater precision. Clearly, because it measures a different ligand binding property of ristocetin, it should be seen as a complementary rather than alternative assay of VWF function. Indeed, some cases of VWD have reduced VWF:RiCoF but normal VWF:CB and vice versa. The assay conditions have been adjusted to make the result sensitive to the presence of high molecular weight multimers of VWF and thus to its functional activity *in vivo*.

The collagen binding assay ELISA method is based on the ability of VWF to bind collagen. The source of collagen is an important variable and wells of the ELISA test strips are coated with human collagen type III although type I and type I/III mixtures have also been used.[55] After incubation with the test plasma, the amount of VWF bound is detected using an anti-VWF peroxidase-conjugated antibody. Antibody-peroxidase binding is quantified in the usual way and the intensity of the colour generated is directly proportional to the VWF:CB concentration. Using a reference curve, the VWF:CB is quantified.

Collagen binding assay kits can be obtained through companies such as Technoclone UK Ltd and Gradipore. Assay details can be found in the manufacturer's instructions. They may vary with manufacturer and even from batch to batch of the same kit. Particular attention should be paid to the shelf life of the kits. Each laboratory should establish its own normal range.

Multimeric Analysis of von Willebrand Factor Antigen in Plasma Samples

Non-Radioactive Multimer Method

Multimeric analysis of von Willebrand factor antigen is important in the diagnosis and treatment of VWD.[56] The gold standard method is the autoradiographic method described by Enayat and Hill.[56] This method uses radioactive iodine (I^{125}) and is performed in only a few specialized centres.

The non-radioactive method described here uses a peroxidase-conjugated antibody to VWF:Ag to replace the radioactive antibody described in previous editions.

Plasma samples are diluted in a buffer containing 8 M urea and sodium dodecyl sulphate (SDS) and are heated to ensure mobility of protein is related to size and not molecular charge. Samples are electrophoresed through an agarose stacking gel at pH 6.8 and then through a running gel of higher agarose concentration at pH 8.8. After running overnight on a cooling plate, the protein is fixed in the gel, washed and incubated with a peroxidase-conjugated antibody to VWF:Ag followed by extensive washing. The VWF:Ag multimers are revealed by adding a colour substrate reagent and scanning the gel. The scanned image is modified using photographic editing software (e.g. Microsoft Picture It or Corel Draw Graphics Suite) to produce a black-and-white image suitable for presentation.

The technique described here uses an agarose gel in a discontinuous buffer system. The method appears less prone to technical problems than an acrylamide/agarose system and yet can distinguish clearly the known patterns of VWD subtypes.

Reagents

Horseradish peroxidase-conjugated rabbit antihuman-VWF:Ag. DAKO Laboratories
Agarose, ultra-pure DNA grade. Seakem, code No. LE 49052-5
SDS. BDH
Glycine. BDH
Sodium EDTA. BDH
Hydrochloric acid. BDH
Propan-2-ol. BDH
Acetic acid. BDH
Tris base (T1503). BDH
Bromophenol blue. Sigma
Marvel or Baby Milk. Mothercare
Deionized water.

Preparation of Stock Solutions

2 M Tris. 242.2 g per litre water (121.1 g/500 ml deionized water)
3 M HCl. 26.2 ml (1 N HCl, SG 1.18)/100 ml deionized water
0.01 M Na_2EDTA. 3.3624 g/l or 0.336 g/100 ml deionized water.

These three reagents may be stored at 4°C for up to 3 months.

Preparation of Buffers

Stacking buffer

25.0 ml 2 M Tris
15.8 ml 3 M HCl
Make up to 100 ml with deionized water
Check pH is 6.8
May be stored at 4°C for up to 2 weeks.

Running buffer

75.0 ml 2 M Tris
8.9 ml 3 M HCl
Make up to 100 ml with deionized water
Check pH is 8.8
May be stored at 4°C for up to 2 weeks.

Sample buffer

500 µl 2 M Tris
10 ml stock EDTA
Make up to 100 ml with deionized water
May be stored at 4°C for up to 4 weeks.

For use:

9.61 g urea
0.4 g SDS
Dissolve in sample buffer and make up to 20 ml
May need to warm to dissolve
Carefully adjust the pH to 8.0 with 1 M HCl
Use within 1 day of preparation.

10% SDS

1 g SDS dissolved in deionized water to a final volume of 10.0 ml. Store at 4°C to prevent bacterial growth; warm to room temperature just before use. Discard after 4 weeks of storage.

Electrophoresis buffer

57.6 g glycine
12.0 g Tris base
2.0 g SDS

Dissolve and make up to 2 litres with deionized water. Make up fresh on day of use. Cool to 4°C prior to electrophoresis.

Acid/alcohol fixative

100 ml propan-2-ol
40 ml acetic acid
Make up to 400 ml with deionized water
Washing solutions (0.5 ml/l Tween 20 PBS).

0.01 M phosphate buffered saline, pH 7.2

0.39 g $NaH_2PO_4.2H_2O$
2.68 g $Na_2HPO_4.12H_2O$
8.474 g NaCl
Make up to 1 litre with deionized water
The washing solution is prepared by adding 0.5 ml/l Tween 20.

Colour Buffer (0.1 M Citrate Phosphate Buffer, pH 5.0)

8.8 g Citric acid
24.0 g $Na_2HPO_4.12H_2O$
Make up to 1 litre with deionized water.

Colour reagent

60 mg ortho-phenylenediamine (OPD)
120 ml 0.1 M citrate phosphate buffer
40 µl hydrogen peroxide (20 vol). Add just before use.

Preparation of Gels

Running gel (1.6% agarose, 0.1% SDS)

1.6 g agarose
25.0 ml running buffer
74.0 ml deionized water
1.0 ml 10% SDS (add last to prevent frothing).

Dissolve the agarose by boiling in a conical flask using a microwave oven. Place a thick glass slide over the top of the conical flask to keep the loss of water to a minimum, thus maintaining the correct agarose concentration. Ensure that the agarose has fully dissolved. Add the SDS to the molten agarose last to prevent excessive frothing. Keep at 60°C in a waterbath.

Stick the hydrophilic side of standard gel bond (Pharmacia LKB) to a clean glass slide (10 × 205 mm) using a few drops of water. Cast the gel between the hydrophobic side and a clean glass plate separated by a 1 mm spacer, using Bulldog clips to clamp the mould together. Warm the mould prior to addition of molten agarose by standing it in a 37°C oven. Allow the resultant gel (183 × 100 mm) to set at 4°C in a refrigerator.

Stacking gel (0.8% agarose, 0.1% SDS)

0.32 g agarose
10.0 ml stacking buffer four times
29.6 ml deionized water
0.4 ml 10% SDS
Dissolve by boiling as explained earlier.

Addition of the stacking gel to the running gel

Carefully disassemble the running gel mould and remove the top 1.5 cm of gel using a clean scalpel blade. After reassembly, pour the stacking gel to fill the mould. Allow gel to set at 4°C in a fridge for several hours.

Preparation of samples

Dilute plasma samples in sample buffer as follows:
250 µl sample
700 µl sample buffer
15 µl 1% bromophenol blue dye
Place diluted samples at 60°C for exactly 30 min, then keep them at 4°C for not more than 30 min prior to electrophoresis.

Electrophoresis (Day 1 Evening)

Set the cooling system used at 8°C to achieve a gel temperature of 13°C. Prepare wicks from J-cloths (Johnson and Johnson) and Whatman No.1 24 cm filter papers. Fold a filter paper in half and mark the folded edge 27 mm from each end. From these marks draw lines at right angles and join the points where they cut the arc. Cut out the rectangle thus drawn and it will act as part of one wick. Also cut two double-thickness J-cloth rectangles 183 × 120 mm. Place

500 ml of cold electrophoresis buffer in each reservoir of the electrophoresis tank.

Once again, carefully disassemble the mould; remove the gel bond, leaving the gel on the glass plate. Using a template, cut 10 wells 10 × 2 mm in the stacking gel 8 mm from the interface of running and stacking gels. Place the gel on the cooling platen. Soak two filter paper wicks in electrophoresis buffer and position over the gel by 5 mm at either end. Soak two J-cloth wicks in electrophoresis buffer, placing one completely over the paper wick at the running gel end and the other over the paper wick at the stacking gel end, leaving a small portion of the paper wick visible.

Pipette 35–40 μl of diluted sample into each well, taking care not to touch the wick. Electrophorese the gel at a constant current of 5 mA per gel (approximately 65 V). Stop the electrophoresis when the blue dye has migrated 1 cm from each well. Carefully remove residual liquid from each well and refill each well with molten stacking gel. Start electrophoresis at the same current. After a total of 18–20 h, the dye will have run off the gel into the wick and electrophoresis is complete.

Gel Fixation (Day 2 Morning)

Remove the gel gently from the glass plate and fix for 1 h using the acid/alcohol fixative solution in a suitable container.

Gel Washing (Day 2)

Once fixed, wash the gel in three changes of distilled water for a total of 3 h. Transfer the gel to a small plastic tray and wash with 1% milk powder for 20 min followed by 10% milk powder for 20 min. Wash the gel extensively in 0.5 ml/l Tween 20 PBS for the remainder of the day.

Addition of the Peroxidase-Conjugated Rabbit Antihuman-VWF:Ag (Day 2 Evening)

Dilute 400 μl of the peroxidase-conjugated rabbit antihuman-VWF in 400 ml of 0.5 ml/l Tween 20 PBS. Then add this to the gel in the tray and mix gently overnight. Place a plastic sheet over the plastic tray to prevent evaporation.

Extensive Washing (Two Days and Nights)

Pour the peroxidase-conjugated rabbit antihuman-VWF mixture to waste. Remove the gel from the plastic tray and place into another flat-bottomed tray. Then wash the gel extensively with frequent changes of 0.5 ml/l Tween 20 PBS for the next 2 days and 2 nights.

Addition of the Colour Substrate (Day 5)

Prepare the colour reagent by adding 6 × 10 mg OPD tablets to 120 ml 0.1 M citrate phosphate buffer. Add 40 μl of hydrogen peroxide just before use. Place the gel into a plastic tray, pour the colour reagent over the gel and mix gently. Ensure the colour reagent gets underneath the gel. When the colour begins to develop, remove the gel from the plastic tray and place between two sheets of gel bond, draining off any excess substrate reagent.

Scanning the Developing Gel

When the multimer patterns become visible, the gel is ready to scan. The gel will continue to develop colour for several minutes and eventually the background gel will become too dark to see the multimer patterns clearly. Scan the gel several times as the colour develops to get the best image of the multimer patterns.

The scanned gel will appear as shown as in Figure 18.11A. The top section is the stacking gel where the samples were added prior to electrophoresis; the main body of the gel is the running gel showing the multimer patterns. The scan is manipulated using photographic editing software (see Fig. 18.11C,D) and the final result shown in Figure 18.11E.

Interpretation

See Figure 18.12.[57]

INVESTIGATION OF A SUSPECTED DISORDER OF PLATELET FUNCTION, INHERITED OR ACQUIRED

(For investigation assays of VWD, see p. 425; for diagnosis of thrombocytopenia, see p. 610.)

Abnormalities of platelet function all lead to signs and symptoms characteristic of defects of primary haemostasis: bleeding into the mucous membranes, epistaxes, menorrhagia and skin ecchymoses. The patient may also suffer from abnormal intraoperative or postoperative bleeding and oozing from small cuts or wounds.

Laboratory Investigation of Platelets and Platelet Function

The peripheral blood platelet count and, for some laboratories, PFA-100 are first-line tests of platelet function.[58,59] However, some disorders of platelet function are not detected by these tests. Additional information may be obtained by inspecting a fresh blood film, which may show abnormalities of platelet size or morphology that may be of diagnostic importance.

If the screening procedures or clinical history suggest a disorder of primary haemostasis and VWF function is normal, further tests should be organized. Drugs and certain foods (Table 18.8) may affect platelet function tests and the patient must be asked to refrain from taking such substances for at least 7 days before the test.

Figure 18.11 von Willebrand factor multimer gel. See text for preparation. (A) Scan of the original stained gel. (B) Adjustment of image tint. (C) Conversion to monochrome image. (D) Adjustment of brightness and contrast. (E) Final gel image.

The usual sequence of investigation is shown in Figure 18.13. Platelet function tests can be divided into six main groups (Table 18.9): adhesion tests, aggregation tests, assessment of the granular content, assessment of the release reaction, investigation of the prostaglandin pathways and tests of platelet coagulant activity. Expression of platelet glycoproteins can be assessed by flow cytometry, although this does not necessarily correlate with functional activity.

The *granular content* of the platelets can be assessed by electron microscopy or by measuring the substances released. Adenine nucleotide and serotonin release from the dense granules are best measured by a specialist laboratory. The release of β-thromboglobulin and platelet factor 4 can be measured using commercial radioimmunoassay kits, but there are problems with reproducibility and interpretation of the results. The release from the α granules is mostly investigated as a marker of *in vivo* platelet activation and thrombotic tendency. Platelet VWF is measured to diagnose some variants of VWD.

If the initial aggregation studies suggest a defect in the prostaglandin pathways, TXB_2 can be estimated quantitatively by radioimmune assay. Highly specific assays of various steps in arachidonic acid metabolism are also available but are outside the scope of a routine laboratory.

Platelet coagulant activity – the completion of the membrane 'flip-flop' – can be indirectly measured using the prothrombin consumption index. This test is rarely performed now but is abnormal in Scott syndrome, a rare bleeding disorder; it was described in the 7th edition of this book. Alternatively, phosphatidyl serine exposure can be directly assessed by flow cytometry (see later).

Platelet Aggregation

Principle

The light absorbance of PRP decreases as platelets aggregate. The amount and the rate of fall are dependent on platelet reactivity to the added agonist provided that other

1 2 3 4 5 6 7

Figure 18.12 Autoradiograph of the electrophoretic analysis of von Willebrand factor (VWD) multimer patterns. The largest multimer appear at the top of the gel. The normal pattern with numerous large multimers and a triplet pattern visible in the smaller multimers are shown in lane 7. Lanes 1 and 6 are compatible with type 1 VWD in which there is a generalized decrease in multimer numbers but the normal triplet pattern is retained. In lane 2 there is virtually no VWF detected, indicating type 3 VWD. Lanes 3 and 5 show both abnormality of VWF amount and multimer pattern, indicating type 2A. In lane 4 there is a selective loss of the large multimers typical of type 2B VWD.

variables, such as temperature, platelet count and mixing speed, are controlled. The absorbance changes are monitored on a chart recorder.

Reagents

Test and control platelet-rich plasma

The patient and control subject should not have ingested any drugs, beverages or foods that may affect aggregation for at least 10 days (Table 18.8) and preferably should have fasted overnight because the presence of chylomicra may also disturb the aggregation patterns. Collect 20 ml of venous blood with minimal venous occlusion and add to a one-tenth volume of trisodium citrate (see p. 621) contained in a plastic or siliconized container. The blood should not be chilled because cold activates the platelets. PRP is obtained by centrifuging at room temperature (c 20°C) for 10–15 min at 150–200 g. Carefully remove the PRP, avoiding contamination with red cells or buffy coat, and place in a stoppered plastic tube. Store at room temperature until tested. This is stable for about 3 h. It is important to test all samples after a similar interval of time (say 1 h) and to store them at the same temperature to minimize variation.

Table 18.8 Substances that commonly affect platelet function

Agents that affect prostanoid synthesis
    Aspirin
    Non-steroidal anti-inflammatory drugs
    Corticosteroids

Agents that bind to platelet receptors and membranes
    α-antagonists
    β-blockers
    Antihistamines
    Tricyclic antidepressants
    Local anaesthetics
    Ticlopidine
    Clopidogrel
    IIbIIIa blocking agents
    Selective serotonin reuptake inhibitors (SSRIs)

Antibiotics
    Penicillin
    Cephalosporins

Agents that increase cyclic adenosine monophosphate levels
    Dipyridamole
    Aminophylline
    Prostanoids

Others
    Heparin
    Chondroitin sulphate and glucosamine
    Dextran
    Ethanol
    Clofibrate
    Phenothiazine
    Garlic

Test and control platelet-poor plasma

Centrifuge the remaining blood at 2000 g for 20 min to obtain PPP.

Use of platelet-rich plasma

A platelet count is performed on the PRP. Adjustment of the platelet count in the PRP is not recommended because this inhibits platelet activation.[60] PRP should always be stored in tightly stoppered tubes that are filled nearly to the top to avoid changes in pH, which also affect platelet aggregation and tests of nucleotide release.

Aggregating agents

The five aggregating agents listed in the following should be sufficient for the diagnosis of most functional disorders. A recent study recommended a minimal screening panel of

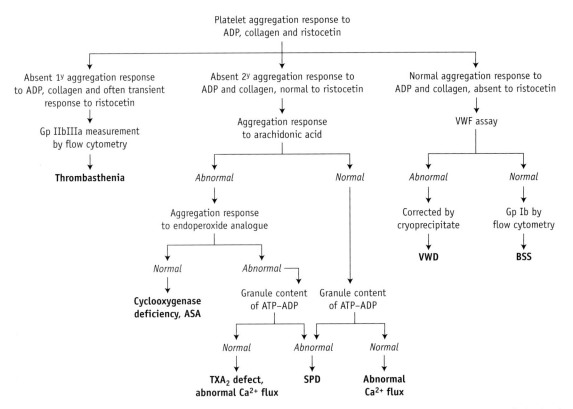

Figure 18.13 Flowchart for investigation of suspected platelet dysfunction. SPD, storage pool defect; ITP, coating of platelets by autoantibodies in idiopathic thrombocytopenic purpura; VWD, von Willebrand disease; BSS, Bernard–Soulier syndrome; ASA, effect of aspirin ingestion.

1.25 µg/ml collagen, 6 µM epinephrine, 1.6 mM arachidonic acid and 1.0 µM U44619 (endoperoxide analogue).[61] This combination had high specificity but relatively poor sensitivity and was frequently coupled with additional tests such as nucleotide release. For research purposes and when investigating unusual kindreds, other agonists listed in Table 18.9 may also be used.

Adenosine 5′-diphosphate

The anhydrous sodium salt of ADP is used. Prepare a stock solution by dissolving 4.93 mg of the trisodium salt or 4.71 mg of the disodium salt in 10 ml of 9 g/l NaCl, pH 6.8. This makes a 1 mmol/l solution. Store in 0.5 ml volumes at –40°C until use; they remain stable for up to 3 months at this temperature. Once thawed, the solution must be used within 3 h and then discarded. For aggregation testing, prepare 100, 50, 25, 10 and 5 µmol/l solutions.

Collagen 1 mg/ml (Mascia Brunelli, Sigma, Helena)

This collagen is a 1 mg/ml stock solution. For use, dilute in the buffer supplied with the collagen or in 5% dextrose to obtain concentrations of 10 and 40 µg/l. When diluted 1:10 in PRP (see below), the final concentrations will be 1 and 4 µg/ml.

Ristocetin sulphate (American Biochemical & Pharmaceutical Corporation, Marlton, NJ, USA)

Each vial of ristocetin sulphate contains 100 mg of ristocetin and should be stored at 4°C until dissolved; 8 ml of 9 g/l NaCl are added to each vial so as to obtain a 12.5 mg/ml solution. Store at –40°C in 0.5 ml volumes until used. Ristocetin may be refrozen after use. It should never be used in concentrations of greater than 1.4 mg/ml because protein precipitation may occur in plasma and give rise to false results.

Arachidonic acid

Arachidonic acid is Na-salt, 99% pure. Dissolve the contents of a 10 mg vial in 1.5 ml of sterile water by gentle mixing to give a 20 mmol/l stock solution. This may be frozen in 0.5 ml volumes at –20°C for later use. Prepare a working solution by making doubling dilutions of the stock in saline to give 5 and 10 mmol/l solutions.

Table 18.9 Platelet function tests

Adhesion tests
    Retention in a glass-bead column
    Baumgartner's technique
    PFA-100

Aggregation tests
    Turbidometric technique using
    ADP
    Collagen
    Ristocetin
    Adrenaline (epinephrine)
    Thrombin
    Arachidonic acid
    Endoperoxide analogues
    Calcium ionophore

Investigation of granule content and release
    Dense bodies
    Electron microscopy
    ADP and ATP content (bioluminescence)
    Serotonin release
Granules
    β-thromboglobulin
    Platelet factor 4
    VWF
    Fluorescence by flow cytometry

Prostaglandin pathways
    TXB_2 radioimmunoassay

Platelet coagulant activity
    Prothrombin consumption index

Flow cytometry
    Glycoprotein surface expression
    Activation
    P selectin (CD62) surface expression
    Fibrinogen binding
    Annexin binding (to phosphatidyl serine)
    Conformational changes in Gp IIbIIIa
    Platelet granule fluorescence

ADP, adenosine 5'-diphosphate; ATP, adenosine 5'-triphosphate; VWF, von Willebrand factor. Gp, glycoprotein.

Adrenaline (epinephrine)

Dissolve 1-epinephrine bitartrate, 3.33 mg, in 10 ml of water to prepare a 1 mmol/l stock solution. Store in 0.5 ml volumes at −40°C. Solutions of 20 and 200 μmol/l are prepared for use in barbitone buffered saline, pH 7.4.

Note

All aggregation reagents should be kept on ice until used.

Method

Centrifugation may cause cellular release of ADP and platelet refractoriness to aggregation and the actual aggregation test should not be started within 30 min of preparing the PRP. However, the tests should be completed within 3 h and whenever possible within 2 h of preparing the PRP. Platelets left standing at room temperature (*c* 20°C) become increasingly reactive to adrenaline and in some cases to collagen; the rate of change increases after 3 h.

Switch the aggregometer on 30 min before the tests are to be performed to allow the heating block to warm up to 37°C. Set the stirring speed to 900 rpm. Pipette the appropriate volume of PRP (this varies depending on the make of the aggregometer used) into a plastic tube or cuvette. Place the tube in the heating block. After 1 min insert the stirrer into the plasma. Set the transmission to 0 on the chart recorder. Replace with a cuvette containing PPP and set the transmission to 100%. Repeat this procedure until no further adjustments are needed and the pen traverses most of the width of the chart paper in response to the difference in absorbance between the PRP and PPP.

Allow the PRP to warm up to 37°C for 2 min and then add 1:10 volume of the agonist. Record the change in transmission until the response reaches a plateau or for 3 min (whichever is sooner). Repeat this procedure for each agonist. The starting amount for each agonist is the lowest concentration prepared as described earlier. If no release is obtained, increase the concentration until a satisfactory response is obtained.

Interpretation

Normal and abnormal platelet aggregation curves are shown in Figures 18.14 and 18.15.

Adenosine 5'-diphosphate

Low concentrations of ADP (<0.5 to 2.5 μmol/l) cause primary or reversible aggregation. First, ADP binds to a membrane receptor and releases Ca^{2+} ions. A reversible complex with extracellular fibrinogen forms and the platelets undergo a shape change reflected by a slight increase in absorbance. After this, the bound fibrinogen adds to the cell-to-cell contact and reversible aggregation occurs. At very low concentrations of ADP, platelets may disaggregate after the first phase. In the presence of higher concentrations of ADP an irreversible secondary wave aggregation is associated with the release of dense and α-granules as a result of activation of the arachidonic acid pathway. If only high doses of ADP are used, defects in the primary wave (measuring the second pathway as described on p. 396) will be missed.

Figure 18.14 Traces obtained during the aggregation of platelet-rich plasma. a, Shape change; b, primary wave aggregation; c, secondary wave aggregation; x, angle of the initial aggregation slope; y, height of the aggregation trace; d, lag phase.
(Redrawn from Yardumian DA, Mackie IJ, Machin SJ 1986 Laboratory investigation of platelet function: a review of methodology. Journal of Clinical Pathology 39:701–712.)

Collagen

The aggregation response to collagen is preceded by a short 'lag' phase lasting between 10 and 60 s. The duration of the lag phase is inversely proportional to the concentration of collagen used and to the responsiveness of the platelets tested. This phase is succeeded by a single wave of aggregation resulting from the activation of the arachidonic acid pathway and the release of the granules. Higher doses of collagen (>2 µg/ml) cause a sudden increase in intraplatelet calcium concentration and this may bring about the release reaction without activating the prostaglandin pathway. Collagen responses should therefore always be measured using 1 and 4 µg/ml concentrations.

Ristocetin

Ristocetin reacts with VWF and the membrane receptor to induce platelets to clump together ('agglutination'). It does not activate any of the three aggregation pathways and does not initially cause granule release. The response is assessed on the basis of the angle of the initial slope. The platelet response to 1.2 mg/ml is initially studied. Concentrations above 1.4 mg/ml may cause non-specific platelet 'agglutination' as a result of an interaction between ristocetin and fibrinogen and protein precipitation.

Arachidonic acid

Arachidonic acid induces TXA_2 generation and granule release even if there is a defect of agonist binding to the surface membrane or of the phospholipase-induced release of endogenous arachidonate. If steps further along the pathway are impaired, such as absence or inhibition of cyclooxygenase (e.g. aspirin effect), arachidonic acid will not produce normal aggregation.

Adrenaline (epinephrine)

No shape change precedes aggregation, but the response thereafter resembles the ADP response. Such a response is usually obtained with concentrations of 2–10 µmol/ml. Some clinically normal people have severely reduced responses to epinephrine.

Calculation of Results

Results can be expressed in one of three ways:[59,60]

1. As a percentage decrease in absorbance measured at 3 min after the addition of an agonist (Fig. 18.14) or the percentage of maximum aggregation. This does not provide any information on the shape of the curve.
2. By the initial slope of the aggregation tracing (Fig. 18.14). This indicates the rate of aggregation but does not show whether secondary aggregation has occurred.
3. By the minimum amount of agonist required to induce a secondary response.

Normal Range

The platelets of normal subjects usually produce a single reversible primary wave with 1 µmol/l ADP or less, biphasic aggregation with ADP at 2.5 µmol/l and a single irreversible wave at 5 or 10 µmol/l. A single-phase response is observed after a lag phase lasting not more than 1 min with 1 and 4 µg/ml of collagen. A single-phase or biphasic response is seen with 1.2 mg/ml of ristocetin and after 50 and 100 µmol/l of arachidonic acid. Normal ranges have been compiled for the common agonists.[62] Interpretation can be difficult but reduced maximal

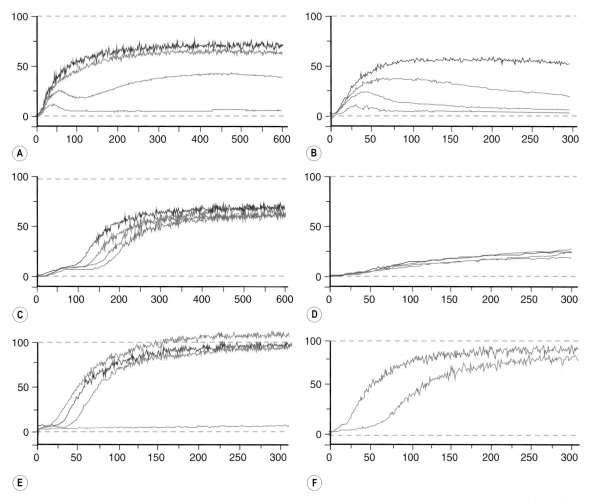

Figure 18.15 (A–F) Some examples of platelet aggregation analyses.
(A) Normal and (B) abnormal, responses to adenosine diphosphate.

Blue	0.5 μmol/l
Yellow	1.0 μmol/l
Green	2.0 μmol/l
Black	5.0 μmol/l

(C) Normal and (D) abnormal, responses to epinephrine.

Blue	0.5 μmol/l
Yellow	1.0 μmol/l
Green	2.0 μmol/l
Black	5.0 μmol/l

(E) Responses to collagen and ristocetin.

Blue	Low-dose ristocetin	0.75 mg/ml
Yellow	High-dose ristocetin	1.5 mg/ml
Green	Low-dose collagen	5 μg/ml
Black	High-dose collagen	10 μg/ml

(F) Responses to arachidonic acid.

Blue	High-dose arachidonic acid	0.5 mg/ml
Yellow	Low-dose arachidonic acid	0.25 mg/ml

aggregation with two or more agonists is highly indicative of a bleeding disorder.[61] Biphasic aggregation is observed with 2–10 μmol/l of adrenaline. A response to a low concentration of ristocetin (0.5 mg/ml) is abnormal and is a feature of type 2B VWD (see below).

Interpretation and Technical Artefacts

The volumes of PRP used will depend on the aggregometer and cuvette used. The smaller the cuvette, the more responses can be tested with a given volume of PRP, but the poorer the optical quality (because of a shorter lightpath) and the more likely the influence of factors such as debris or air bubbles.

Care should be taken to exclude red cells and granulocytes from PRP because these will interfere with the light transmittance and cause reduced response heights, which can be mistaken for abnormal aggregation. In diseases such as thalassaemia, where there may be red cell fragments and membranes, these may be removed by further centrifugation of PRP at $150\,g$ for 2 min or after settling has occurred.

If cryoglobulins are present, they may cause changes in transmittance which resemble the appearance of spontaneous aggregation. Warming the PRP to 37°C for 5 min allows aggregation to be tested in the normal way.

Lipaemic plasma may cause problems in adjusting the aggregometer and the responses may be compressed owing to the small difference in transmitted light between PRP and PPP. Care should be taken in the interpretation of results from such samples.

The pattern of responses in various disorders of platelet function is shown in Table 18.10. For a discussion of hyperaggregability, see p. 461.

Some common technical problems associated with platelet aggregation are described in Table 18.11.

Further Investigation of Platelet Function

If an abnormal aggregation pattern is observed, it is advisable to check the assessment on at least one further occasion. If the aggregation tests are persistently abnormal and the patient is not taking any drugs or substances known to interfere with platelet function, the following tests should be done (Fig. 18.13 and Table 18.10):

1. If thrombasthenia or the Bernard–Soulier syndrome is suspected, an analysis of membrane glycoproteins is necessary; most conveniently by flow cytometry.

2. If a release abnormality is suspected, additional agonists including synthetic endoperoxide analogues and calcium ionophores should be used in testing for aggregation. Release products can be measured directly or concurrently with aggregation in a lumiaggregometer. In addition, the total adenine nucleotide content of the platelets or the amount released after maximal stimulation should be

Table 18.10 Differential diagnosis of disorders of platelet function

CONDITION	PLATELET		AGGREGATION WITH					COMMENT/FURTHER TESTS
	Count	Size	ADP	Col	Ri	AA	A23187	
Thrombasthenia	N	N	0	0	1	0	0	IIbIIIa expression
Bernard–Soulier syndrome	Low	Large	N	N	0	N	N	Gp Ib expression
Storage pool defect (δ)	N	N	1	R	1	N	R	ATP:ADP pools
Cyclooxygenase deficiency	N	N	1/N	R	N	R	R	Responds to endoperoxide
Thromboxane synthetase deficiency	N	N	1/N	R	N	R/0	N	
Aspirin ingestion	N	N	1	R	N	R/0	N/R	Stop aspirin/NSAID and retest
Ehlers–Danlos syndrome	N	N	N	N	N	N	N	
von Willebrand disease	N	N	N	N	0/R	N	N	Assay VWF:Ag and RiCoF

N, normal; 0, absent; 1, primary wave only; R, reduced; Col, collagen; Ri, ristocetin; AA, arachidonic acid; A23187, calcium ionophore; ATP, adenosine 5′-triphosphate; ADP, adenosine 5′-diphosphate; NSAID, non-steroidal anti-inflammatory drug; RiCoF, ristocetin cofactor; VWF, von Willebrand factor.
Note that many other defects, such as found in oculocutaneous albinism, Chédiak–Higashi syndrome and grey platelet syndrome, have also been described.

Table 18.11 Technical factors that may influence platelet aggregation tests

Centrifugation	At room temperature, *not* at 4°C. Should be sufficient to remove red cells and white cells but not the largest platelets. Residual red cells in the PRP may cause apparently incomplete aggregation.
Time	For 30 min after the preparation of the PRP, platelets are refractory to the effect of agonists. Progressive increase in reactiveness occurs thereafter; more marked from 2 h onward.
Platelet count	Slow and weak aggregation observed with platelet counts below 150 or over 400×10^9/l.
pH	<7.7 inhibits aggregation; pH >8.0 enhances aggregation.
Mixing speed	<800 rpm or >1200 rpm slows aggregation.
Haematocrit	>0.55 is associated with less aggregation, especially in the secondary phase owing to the increased concentration of citrate in PRP. Use a lower citrate:blood ratio. It may also be difficult to obtain enough PPP. Centrifuging twice may help.
Temperature	<35°C causes decreased aggregation except to low-dose ADP, which may be enhanced.
Dirty cuvette	May cause spontaneous platelet aggregation or interfere with the optics of the system.
Air bubbles in the cuvette	Cause large, irregular oscillations, even before the addition of agonists.
No stir bar	No response to any agonist obtained.

PPP, platelet-poor plasma; PRP, platelet-rich plasma.

measured using a firefly bioluminescence technique; see lumiaggregometry below.[63]

3. When possible, electron microscopic studies of platelet ultrastructure should be carried out.
4. Factor VIII, VWF:Ag and ristocetin cofactor assay should be carried out on all patients investigated for an abnormality of platelet function who show abnormal ristocetin 'agglutination' or in whom all platelet function tests are normal.

Platelet Lumiaggregometry

The Chrono-log aggregometers (Chrono-log Corporation) measure platelet function using electrical impedance in whole blood or optical density in platelet-rich plasma; with simultaneous measurement of ATP release by luminescence.

Whole-blood aggregation measures platelet function in anticoagulated blood without the need to isolate them from other blood components. Without the necessity for centrifugation, the entire platelet population is tested and labile factors in the blood (e.g. prostacyclin and thromboxane A_2) that may influence platelet function are preserved.

Results of impedance aggregation tests are quantified by:

Ohms of aggregation at a given time in the test
Slope or rate of the reaction, in ohms change per min
Maximum extent of aggregation, in ohms.

The increase in impedance is directly proportional to the mass of the platelet aggregate. Impedance aggregation in blood is not dependent on optical characteristics of the sample, so tests can be performed on lipaemic and thrombocytopenic samples. The method is also useful in situations where sample volume is critical.

ATP secreted by dense granules is measured by a visible light range luminescence technique in either PRP or whole blood. The Lumi-aggregometer measures secretion by a sensitive luminescent (firefly luciferin-luciferase) assay for extracellular ATP in combination with the simultaneous measurement of aggregation. Luminescence measurement of ATP secretion provides unequivocal evidence of normal or impaired dense granule release (as in secretion defects and storage pool deficiency).

CLOT SOLUBILITY TEST FOR FACTOR XIII

Principle

Fibrin clots formed in the presence of factor XIII and thrombin are stable (as a result of crosslinking) for at least 1 h in 5 mol/l urea, whereas clots formed in the absence of factor XIII dissolve rapidly. Quality assurance surveys in the UK have shown that the solubility test for XIII is more sensitive when the sample is clotted with thrombin rather than calcium. Thrombin preparations containing calcium should not be used. The use of 5 M urea as described here will detect factor XIII deficiency of up to 5 iu/dl. One study suggested that deficiency of up to 10% could be detected by using 2% acetic acid as the lysing solution.[64]

Reagents

PPP. From the patient and a control subject
Thrombin. 10 NIH unit solution
Urea. 5 mol/l in 9 g/l NaCl.

Method

In duplicate, 0.2 ml patient plasma is mixed with 0.2 ml 10 NIH unit thrombin solution in a glass test tube and incubated at 37°C for 20 min. Set up a normal plasma control in the same way; EDTA-plasma can be included as a negative control. Each tube is filled with approximately 3 ml of urea solution, carefully dislodging the clot, and is left undisturbed at 37°C for 24 h. Inspect each tube for the presence of a clot at regular intervals.

Interpretation

The control clot, if normal, shows no sign of dissolving after 24 h. However, in the absence of factor XIII, the clot will have dissolved. The test is reported as normal if the clot is present and abnormal if the clot is absent. The clot solubility test has poor sensitivity and may only detect levels below approximately 5 iu/dl. The relationship between factor XIII level and adequate haemostasis is uncertain, but there is some evidence that levels of 5–40 iu/dl may also be associated with bleeding. In suspected cases photometric and ELISA assays of factor XIII are available for quantitative measurements.[65] The introduction of these assays into routine practice may clarify the significance of intermediate levels of factor XIII activity.

DISSEMINATED INTRAVASCULAR COAGULATION

The term DIC encompasses a wide range of clinical phenomena of varying degrees of severity. It is also sometimes referred to as consumptive coagulopathy because its characteristic feature is excessive and widespread activation of the coagulation mechanism with consequent consumption of clotting factors and inhibitors with loss of the normal regulatory mechanisms. In acutely ill patients this usually results in defibrination and a haemorrhagic diathesis. In some situations, however, the activation may be less marked and partially compensated, resulting in a tendency to thrombosis. This latter phenomenon is typical of the coagulation activation seen in association with malignancy and may be associated with slightly shortened clotting times.

The diagnosis of acute DIC can generally be made from abnormalities of the basic first-line screening tests described earlier occurring in an appropriate clinical context. Characteristically, the PT, APTT and TT are all prolonged and the fibrinogen level is markedly reduced. In association with the consumption of clotting factors responsible for these abnormalities there is also a fall in platelet count also resulting from consumption. As DIC develops, a decrease in platelet count is an early sign and hypofibrinogenaemia may be relatively late. This distinguishes it from dilutional coagulopathy in which the reverse is usually the case. Concomitantly there is activation of the fibrinolytic system and an increase in circulating fibrin(ogen) degradation products. These abnormalities form the basis for the diagnosis of DIC. Diagnostic guidelines are available but are most useful in clinical trials rather than routine practice.[66] More elaborate tests are not usually performed but can demonstrate reductions in individual clotting factors, antithrombin and antiplasmin and increased levels of thrombin–antithrombin and plasmin–antiplasmin complexes and of activation peptides such as prothrombin F1+2. Some analysers provide a waveform analysis that can detect early stages of DIC.[67]

Detection of Fibrinogen/Fibrin Degradation Products Using a Latex Agglutination Method

Principle

A suspension of latex particles is sensitized with specific antibodies to the purified FDP fragments D and E. The suspension is mixed on a glass slide with a dilution of the serum to be tested. Agglutination indicates the presence of FDP in the sample. By testing different dilutions of the unknown sample, a semiquantitative assay can be performed.[68]

Reagents

Venous blood. Collected into a special tube (provided with the kit) containing the antifibrinolytic agent and thrombin
Test kit. Oxoid Ltd, Basingstoke, Hampshire, UK.
Positive and negative controls. Provided by the manufacturer
Glycine buffer. Part of the kit.

Method

Allow the tube with blood to stand at 37°C until clot retraction commences. Then centrifuge the tube and withdraw the serum for testing. It is important that the fibrinogen in the sample is completely clotted or this will be detected by the test. This may be a problem in the presence of heparin or a dysfibrinogenaemia or high levels of FDPs. Addition of a few drops of 100 u (NIH)/ml thrombin will enhance clotting in these cases.

Make 1 in 5 and 1 in 20 dilutions of serum in glycine buffer. Mix 1 drop of each serum dilution with 1 drop of latex suspension on a glass slide. Rock the slide gently for 2 min while looking for macroscopic agglutination. If a positive reaction is observed in the higher dilution, make doubling dilutions from the 1 in 20 dilution until macroscopic agglutination can no longer be seen.

Interpretation

Agglutination with a 1 in 5 dilution of serum indicates a concentration of FDP in excess of 10 μg/ml; agglutination in a 1 in 20 dilution indicates FDP in excess of 40 μg/ml.

Normal Range

Healthy subjects have an FDP concentration of less than 10 μg/ml. Concentrations between 10 and 40 μg/ml are found in a variety of conditions, including acute venous thromboembolism, acute myocardial infarction and severe pneumonia, and after major surgery. High levels are seen in systemic fibrinolysis associated with DIC and thrombolytic therapy with streptokinase.

Screening Tests for Fibrin Monomers

Principle

When thrombin acts on fibrinogen, some of the monomers do not polymerize but give rise to soluble complexes with plasma fibrinogen and FDP. These complexes can be associated *in vitro* by ethanol or protamine sulphate. Now rarely used: see previous editions for method.

Detection of Crosslinked Fibrin D-Dimers Using a Latex Agglutination Method

Principle

The latex agglutination method used to detect crosslinked fibrin D-dimers is identical to the test previously described for FDP, but in this case the latex beads are coated with a monoclonal antibody directed specifically against fibrin D-dimer in human plasma or serum. Because there is no reaction with fibrinogen, the need for serum is eliminated and measurements can be performed on plasma samples.

Reagents

Several manufacturers market kits for the measurement of D-dimers. These usually contain the latex suspension, dilution buffer and positive and negative controls.

Method

The manufacturer's protocol should be followed. Undiluted plasma is mixed with one drop of latex suspension on a glass slide and the slide is gently rocked for the length of time recommended in the kit. If macroscopic agglutination is observed, dilutions of the plasma are made until agglutination can no longer be seen.

Interpretation

Agglutination with the undiluted plasma indicates a concentration of D-dimers in excess of 200 mg/l. The D-dimer level can be quantified by multiplying the reciprocal of the highest dilution showing a positive result by 200 to give a value in mg/l.

Normal Range

Plasma levels in normal subjects are <200 mg/l. There has been much study of D-dimer assays as a useful way of excluding thrombosis, but there is naturally a compromise between sensitivity and specificity, especially when a rapid turnaround time is required. The lack of an international standard and the poor correlation between kits mean that the use of kits for this purpose should be validated individually. A number of kits using ELISA methods for the detection of D-dimers are now available that have greater sensitivity but are more cumbersome to perform. Latex tests using automated analysers may provide an acceptable compromise.[69] These tests have now been incorporated into clinical guidelines according to their sensitivity.[70]

INVESTIGATION OF CARRIERS OF A CONGENITAL COAGULATION DEFICIENCY OR DEFECT

Carrier detection is important in genetic counselling and antenatal diagnosis may enable heterozygotes to consider termination of pregnancy with a severely affected fetus and may optimize management of the pregnancy and delivery. The information of value in carrier detection is derived from family studies, phenotype investigations and determination of genotype.

Family Studies

Haemophilia A and B (factor VIII and factor IX deficiency) are inherited by X-linked genes. This means that all the sons of a person with haemophilia will be normal and all of his daughters will be carriers. The children of a carrier have a 0.5 chance of being affected if they are sons and a 0.5 chance of being carriers if they are daughters. The other coagulation factor defects are inherited as autosomal traits. Heterozygotes possess approximately half the normal concentration of the coagulation factor and are generally not affected clinically; only homozygotes have a significant bleeding tendency. Factor XI is an exception to this where heterozygotes sometimes bleed excessively after trauma or surgery. The most common form of VWD (type 1) is inherited as an autosomal dominant trait.

A detailed family study is important in all coagulation factor defects to establish the true nature of the defect and its severity. Patients often describe any familial bleeding tendency as haemophilia and it is therefore essential to prove the exact defect in every new patient and family. In inbred kindreds, the likelihood of homozygotes emerging is increased.

PHENOTYPE INVESTIGATION

Theoretically, one might expect the concentration of the affected coagulation factor in the heterozygote or carrier to be roughly half that of normal. However, in the case of factor VIII and factor IX, this is complicated by the phenomenon of X chromosome inactivation. Women possess two X chromosomes, but in each cell only one of these two is used and the other is largely inactivated. In each cell the choice of which X is active is essentially random and varies over a normal distribution. Thus, in carriers of haemophilia A or B, the level of factor VIII or IX also varies over roughly a normal distribution depending on the proportions of the normal and haemophiliac containing Xs that are used. As a result, some carriers may have an entirely normal level of factor VIII or factor IX and others may be significantly deficient. This chromosome inactivation is sometimes referred to as Iyonization after Mary Lyon, by whom it was first described.

In the case of factor VIII, the level of VWF has sometimes been found to be useful. The ratio of VIII to VWF: Ag is reduced in most carriers and can be used in conjunction with the family history to determine a probability that the subject is a carrier. These estimations are further complicated by the fact that factor VIII behaves as an acute-phase reactant and may be elevated by a number of intercurrent factors including pregnancy, stress and exercise.

When a detailed family study has been carried out it may be possible to establish the statistical chance of inheriting a coagulation defect. (For a review, see Graham et al.[71])

GENOTYPE ASSIGNMENT

The advent of molecular biology and the cloning of many of the genes for coagulation factors, especially factor VIII and factor IX, have revolutionized the approach to carrier determination. The discovery of genetic polymorphisms, some of which are multi-allelic, within the coagulation factor genes, has meant that in most families the affected gene can be tracked and the carrier state can be determined with a high degree of probability. Increasingly, the genetic defect itself can be identified, resulting in unequivocal genotypic assignment in every member of a family. This must now be regarded as the standard of care, removing the ambiguity and uncertainty of preceding methods.

The techniques required for these analyses are described in Chapter 21. The problem of carrier determination and antenatal diagnosis has been dealt with in a comprehensive World Health Organization/World Federation of Hemophilia review.[72] Although the options for affected families increase,[73,74] approximately one-third of cases arise with no preceding family history.

REFERENCES

1. Cines DB, Pollak ES, Buck CA, et al. Endothelial cells in physiology and in the pathophysiology of vascular disorders. Blood. 1998;91(10): 3527–3561.

2. Frank PG, Woodman SE, Park DS, et al. Caveolin, caveolae and endothelial cell function. Arterioscler Thromb Vasc Biol. 2003;23(7): 1161–1168.

3. Ruggeri ZM. Von Willebrand factor, platelets and endothelial cell interactions. J Thromb Haemost. 2003;1(7):1335–1342.

4. May AE, Neumann FJ, Preissner KT. The relevance of blood cell-vessel wall adhesive interactions for vascular thrombotic disease. Thromb Haemost. 1999;82(2): 962–970.

5. Nurden AT. Inherited abnormalities of platelets. Thromb Haemost. 1999;82(2):468–480.

6. Ruggeri ZM. Mechanisms initiating platelet thrombus formation. [published erratum appears in Thromb Haemost. 1997;78(4):1304] [see comments]. Thromb Haemost 1997;78(1):611–616.

7. Wei AH, Schoenwaelder SM, Andrews RK, et al. New insights into the haemostatic function of platelets. Br J Haematol. 2009;147(4):415–430.

8. Mann KG. Biochemistry and physiology of blood coagulation. Thromb Haemost. 1999;82(2): 165–174.

9. Colman R, Schmaier A. Contact system: a vascular biology modulator with anticoagulant, profibrinolytic, antiadhesive and proinflammatory attributes. Blood. 1997;90 (10):3819–3843.

10. Muller F, Mutch NJ, Schenk WA, et al. Platelet polyphosphates are proinflammatory and procoagulant

mediators in vivo. *Cell*. 2009;139(6): 1143–1156.

11. Lord ST. Fibrinogen and fibrin: scaffold proteins in hemostasis. *Curr Opin Hematol*. 2007;14(3):236–241.

12. van Boven HH, Lane DA. Antithrombin and its inherited deficiency states. *Semin Hematol*. 1997;34(3):188–204.

13. Rezende SM, Simmonds RE, Lane DA. Coagulation, inflammation and apoptosis: different roles for protein S and the protein S-C4b binding protein complex. *Blood*. 2004;103(4): 1192–1201.

14. Rijken DC, Lijnen HR. New insights into the molecular mechanisms of the fibrinolytic system. *J Thromb Haemost*. 2009;7(1):4–13.

15. Chee YL, Crawford JC, Watson HG, et al. Guidelines on the assessment of bleeding risk prior to surgery or invasive procedures. British Committee for Standards in Haematology. *Br J Haematol*. 2008;140(5):496–504.

16. Bowman M, Mundell G, Grabell J, et al. Generation and validation of the Condensed MCMDM-1VWD Bleeding Questionnaire for von Willebrand disease. *J Thromb Haemost*. 2008;6(12):2062–2066.

17. Witt I. Test systems with synthetic peptide substrates in haemostaseology. *Eur J Clin Chem Clin Biochem*. 1991;29 (6):355–374.

18. Ingram GI, Hills M. The prothrombin time test: effect of varying citrate concentration. *Thromb Haemost*. 1976;36(1): 230–236.

19. Toh CH. Transmittance waveform of routine coagulation tests is a sensitive and specific method for diagnosing non-overt disseminated intravascular coagulation. *Blood Rev*. 2002;16(suppl 1):S11–S14.

20. Mumford AD, O'Donnell J, Gillmore JD, et al. Bleeding symptoms and coagulation abnormalities in 337 patients with AL-amyloidosis. *Br J Haematol*. 2000;110(2):454–460.

21. Palareti G, Maccaferri M, Manotti C, et al. Fibrinogen assays: a collaborative study of six different methods. C.I.S.M.E.L. Comitato Italiano per la Standardizzazione dei Metodi in Ematologia e Laboratorio. *Clin Chem*. 1991;37(5):714–719.

22. De Cristofaro R, Landolfi R. Measurement of plasma fibrinogen concentration by the prothrombin-time-derived method: applicability and limitations. *Blood Coagul Fibrinolysis*. 1998;9(3):251–259.

23. Lawrie AS, McDonald SJ, Purdy G, et al. Prothrombin time derived fibrinogen determination on Sysmex CA-6000. *J Clin Pathol*. 1998;51(6): 462–466.

24. Mackie IJ, Kitchen S, Machin SJ, Lowe GD. Haemostasis and Thrombosis Task Force of the British Committee for Standards in Haematology. Guidelines on fibrinogen assays. *Br J Haematol*. 2003;121(3):396–404.

25. Clauss A. Rapid physiological coagulation method in determination of fibrinogen. *Acta Haematologica (Basel)*. 1957;17:237.

26. Mackie J, Lawrie AS, Kitchen S, et al. A performance evaluation of commercial fibrinogen reference preparations and assays for Clauss and PT-derived fibrinogen. *Thromb Haemost*. 2002;87(6):997–1005.

27. Jespersen J, Sidelmann J. A study of the conditions and accuracy of the thrombin time assay of plasma fibrinogen. *Acta Haematologica*. 1982;67(1):2–7.

28. Funk C, Gmur J, Herold R, et al. Reptilase-R, a new reagent in blood coagulation. *Br J Haematol*. 1971;21(1):43–52.

29. Kirkwood TB, Snape TJ. Biometric principles in clotting and clot lysis assays. *Clin Lab Haematol*. 1980;2(3):155–167.

30. Williams KN, Davidson JM, Ingram GI. A computer program for the analysis of parallel-line bioassays of clotting factors. *Br J Haematol*. 1975;31(1):13–23.

31. Zhukov O, Popov J, Ramos R, et al. Measurement of von Willebrand factor-FVIII binding activity in patients with suspected von Willebrand disease type 2N: application of an ELISA-based assay in a reference laboratory. *Haemophilia*. 2009;15(3):788–796.

32. Keeling DM, Sukhu K, Kemball-Cook G, et al. Diagnostic importance of the two-stage factor VIII:C assay demonstrated by a case of mild haemophilia associated with His1954–>Leu substitution in the factor VIII A3 domain. *Br J Haematol*. 1999;105(4):1123–1126.

33. Pipe SW, Eickhorst AN, McKinley SH, et al. Mild hemophilia A caused by increased rate of factor VIII A2 subunit dissociation: evidence for nonproteolytic inactivation of factor VIIIa in vivo. *Blood*. 1999;93(1):176–183.

34. Mumford AD, Laffan M, O'Donnell J, et al. A Tyr346–>Cys substitution in the interdomain acidic region a1 of factor VIII in an individual with factor VIII:C assay discrepancy. *Br J Haematol*. 2002;118(2):589–594.

35. Prowse CV. In vivo recovery of factor VIII following transfusion: a survey of recent data and publications to assess the influence of standards used for potency assignment. On behalf of the Subcommittee on Factor VIII and IX of the Scientific and Standardization Committee of the ISTH. *Thromb Haemost*. 1995;74(4):1191–1196.

36. Sukhu K, Harrison P, Keeling D. Factor VIII assays in haemophilia a patients treated with ReFacto. *Br J Haematol*. 2003;121(2):379–380.

37. Ingerslev J, Jankowski MA, Weston SB, et al. Collaborative field study on the utility of a BDD factor VIII concentrate standard in the estimation of BDDr Factor VIII:C activity in hemophilic plasma using one-stage clotting assays. *J Thromb Haemost*. 2004;2(4):623–628.

38. Barrowcliffe TW, Raut S, Hubbard AR. Discrepancies in potency assessment of recombinant FVIII concentrates. *Haemophilia*. 1998;4(4):634–640.

39. Galli M, Barbui T. Antiprothrombin antibodies: detection and clinical significance in the antiphospholipid syndrome. *Blood*. 1999;93(7):2149–2157.

40. Keeling D, Beavis J, Sukhu K. A simple inhibitor screen is more sensitive than a Bethesda assay in monitoring for the development of inhibitors in haemophilia A and B. *Br J Haematol*. 2005;128(6):885.

41. Verbruggen B, van Heerde WL, Laros-van Gorkom BAP. Improvements in factor VIII

inhibitor detection: From Bethesda to Nijmegen. *Semin Thromb Hemost.* 2009;35(8):752–759.

42. Verbruggen B, Novakova I, Wessels H, et al. The Nijmegen modification of the Bethesda assay for factor VIII:C inhibitors: improved specificity and reliability. *Thromb Haemost.* 1995; 73(2):247–251.

43. Hill M, Dolan G. Diagnosis, clinical features and molecular assessment of the dysfibrinogenaemias. *Haemophilia.* 2008;14(5):889–897.

44. Gaffney PJ, Wong MY. Collaborative study of a proposed international standard for plasma fibrinogen measurement. *Thromb Haemost.* 1992;68(4):428–432.

45. Callewaert B, Malfait F, Loeys B, et al. Ehlers-Danlos syndromes and Marfan syndrome. *Baillières Best Pract Res Clin Rheumatol.* 2008; 22(1):165–189.

46. Favaloro EJ. Clinical utility of the PFA-100. *Semin Thromb Hemost.* 2008;34(8):709–733.

47. Cattaneo M, Federici AB, Lecchi A, et al. Evaluation of the PFA-100 system in the diagnosis and therapeutic monitoring of patients with von Willebrand disease. *Thromb Haemost.* 1999;82(1):35–39.

48. Fressinaud E, Veyradier A, Truchaud F, et al. Screening for von Willebrand disease with a new analyzer using high shear stress: a study of 60 cases. *Blood.* 1998; 91(4):1325–1331.

49. Quiroga T, Goycoolea M, Munoz B, et al. Template bleeding time and PFA-100 have low sensitivity to screen patients with hereditary mucocutaneous hemorrhages: comparative study in 148 patients. *J Thromb Haemost.* 2004; 2(6):892–898.

50. Laffan M, Brown SA, Collins PW, et al. The diagnosis of von Willebrand disease: a guideline from the UK Haemophilia Centre Doctors' Organization. *Haemophilia.* 2004;199–217.

51. Nichols WL, Hultin MB, James AH, et al. von Willebrand disease (VWD): evidence-based diagnosis and management guidelines, the National Heart, Lung and Blood Institute (NHLBI) Expert Panel report (USA). *Haemophilia.* 2008;14 (2):171–232.

52. Bartlett A, Dormandy KM, Hawkey CM, et al. Factor-VIII-related antigen: measurement by enzyme immunoassay. *Br Med J.* 1976;1(6016):994–996.

53. Riddell AF, Gomez K, Millar CM, et al. Characterization of W1745C and S1783A: 2 novel mutations causing defective collagen binding in the A3 domain of von Willebrand factor. *Blood.* 2009; 114(16):3489–3496.

54. Macfarlane DE, Stibbe J, Kirby EP, et al. Letter: A method for assaying von Willebrand factor (ristocetin cofactor). *Thromb Diath Haemorrh.* 1975;34(1):306–308.

55. Favaloro EJ. Collagen binding assay for von Willebrand factor (VWF: CBA): detection of von Willebrands Disease (VWD) and discrimination of VWD subtypes, depends on collagen source. *Thromb Haemost.* 2000;83(1):127–135.

56. Enayat MS, Hill FG. Analysis of the complexity of the multimeric structure of factor VIII related antigen/von Willebrand protein using a modified electrophoretic technique. *J Clin Pathol.* 1983; 36(8):915–919.

57. Sadler JE, Budde U, Eikenboom JCJ, et al. Update on the pathophysiology and classification of von Willebrand disease: a report of the Subcommittee on von Willebrand Factor. *J Thromb Haemost.* 2006;4(10):2103–2114.

58. Bolton-Maggs PH, Chalmers EA, Collins PW, et al. A review of inherited platelet disorders with guidelines for their management on behalf of the UKHCDO. *Br J Haematol.* 2006;135(5):603–633.

59. BCSH. Guidelines on platelet function testing. The British Society for Haematology BCSH Haemostasis and Thrombosis Task Force. *J Clin Pathol.* 1988;41(12):1322–1330.

60. Cattaneo M, Lecchi A, Zighetti ML, et al. Platelet aggregation studies: autologous platelet-poor plasma inhibits platelet aggregation when added to platelet-rich plasma to normalize platelet count. *Haematologica.* 2007;92(5):694–697.

61. Hayward CP, Pai M, Liu Y, et al. Diagnostic utility of light transmission platelet aggregometry: results from a prospective study of individuals referred for bleeding disorder assessments. *J Thromb Haemost.* 2009;7(4):676–684.

62. Dawood BB, Wilde J, Watson SP. Reference curves for aggregation and ATP secretion to aid diagnose of platelet-based bleeding disorders: effect of inhibition of ADP and thromboxane A(2) pathways. *Platelets.* 2007;18(5):329–345.

63. David JL, Herion F. Assay of platelet ATP and ADP by the luciferase method: some theoretical and practical aspects. *Adv Exp Med Biol.* 1972;34:341–354.

64. Jennings I, Kitchen S, Woods TA, et al. Problems relating to the laboratory diagnosis of factor XIII deficiency: a UK NEQAS study. *J Thromb Haemost.* 2003; 1(12):2603–2608.

65. Oertel K, Hunfeld A, Specker E, et al. A highly sensitive fluorometric assay for determination of human coagulation factor XIII in plasma. *Anal Biochem.* 2007;367(2): 152–158.

66. Levi M, Toh CH, Thachil J, et al. Guidelines for the diagnosis and management of disseminated intravascular coagulation. British Committee for Standards in Haematology. *Br J Haematol.* 2009;145(1):24–33.

67. Toh CH, Samis J, Downey C, et al. Biphasic transmittance waveform in the APTT coagulation assay is due to the formation of a Ca(++)-dependent complex of C-reactive protein with very-low-density lipoprotein and is a novel marker of impending disseminated intravascular coagulation. *Blood.* 2002;100(7):2522–2529.

68. Garvey MB, Black JM. The detection of fibrinogen-fibrin degradation products by means of a new antibody-coated latex particle. *J Clin Pathol.* 1972;25(8):680–682.

69. Keeling DM, Wright M, Baker P, et al. D-dimer for the exclusion of venous thromboembolism: comparison of a new automated latex particle immunoassay (MDA D-dimer) with an established enzyme-linked fluorescent assay (VIDAS D-dimer). *Clin Lab Haematol.* 1999;21(5):359–362.

70. Keeling DM, Mackie IJ, Moody A, Watson HG. Haemostasis, Thrombosis Task Force of the British Committee for Standards in Haematology. The diagnosis of deep vein thrombosis in symptomatic outpatients and the potential for clinical assessment and D-dimer assays to reduce the need for diagnostic imaging. *Br J Haematol*. 2004;124(1):15–25.

71. Graham J, Elston R, Barrrow E, et al. The hemophilias: statistical methods for carrier detection in hemophilias. *Methods in Hematology*. 1982;5:156.

72. Peake IR, Lillicrap DP, Boulyjenkov V, et al. Report of a joint WHO/WFH meeting on the control of haemophilia: carrier detection and prenatal diagnosis. *Blood Coagul Fibrinolysis*. 1993; 4(2):313–344. [Erratum in: *Blood Coagul Fibrinolysis*. 1994;5(1):148] .

73. Oyesiku JO, Turner CF. Reproductive choices for couples with haemophilia. *Haemophilia*. 2002;8(3):348–352.

74. Pruthi RK. Hemophilia: a practical approach to genetic testing. *Mayo Clin Proc*. 2005;80(11):1485–1499.

Chapter | 19 |

Investigation of a thrombotic tendency

Michael A. Laffan, Richard Manning

INTRODUCTION TO THROMBOPHILIA

Investigations to identify an acquired or inherited increase in thrombotic tendency are frequently carried out in patients who develop venous or arterial thrombosis at a young age, in those who have a strong family history of such events or have thrombosis at an unusual site and in individuals of all ages with recurrent episodes of thromboembolism. In recent years, the utility of these tests, as judged by their ability to alter management, has come under scrutiny. In most cases the results of individual assays have a limited effect on decisions made on the basis of clinical history alone. This is partly because they are initiated in patients who have already had a thrombosis and have thus demonstrated their thrombotic tendency. Nonetheless, there is still a need to identify those individuals whose risk of further thrombosis is sufficiently high to warrant long-term anticoagulation and attention has turned to global tests of thrombotic potential and combinations of single traits as well as details of the clinical history. It should be remembered that many thromboses are almost entirely the result of circumstantial factors; these include trauma, fractures, operations and an acute-phase inflammatory response. Further investigation of coagulation is often unnecessary in these circumstances. The investigations described here are most commonly instituted in venous thrombosis, but some unexplained arterial events, especially in young people or when paradoxical embolism is suspected, are also studied. In general, the contribution of the inherited plasma coagulation factors is less evident for arterial than venous thrombosis because their effect is then often obscured by atherosclerosis.

In this chapter, the investigations to detect an acquired thrombotic tendency are presented first, followed by a simplified battery of tests needed to establish the diagnosis of the more important inherited 'thrombophilias'. Although the number of coagulation factors known to contribute to a thrombotic tendency has increased greatly in the last few years, it remains clear that not all factors have been identified. Hence, the failure to detect one of the traits described does not imply that the individual's risk of thrombosis is normal. An acquired thrombotic tendency is common and occurs in many conditions but is usually complex, multifactorial and not easily identifiable by a single laboratory test. The large number of traits identified, often with a small associated relative risk, makes their individual utility equally small. Until the interactions of these numerous factors are more completely understood, the clinical history remains a dominant factor in clinical management. The British Committee for Standards in Haematology has published guidelines on the investigation of inherited thrombophilia.[1]

TESTS FOR THE PRESENCE OF A LUPUS ANTICOAGULANT

The lupus anticoagulant (LAC) is an acquired autoantibody found in various autoimmune disorders and sometimes in otherwise healthy individuals.[2] LACs are immunoglobulins that bind to certain proteins when bound to phospholipid. The effective sequestration of phospholipid can then cause prolongation of phospholipid-dependent coagulation tests such as the prothrombin time (PT) or activated partial thromboplastin time (APTT). The name 'anticoagulant' is misleading because, despite the *in vitro* effects, patients do not have a bleeding tendency. Instead, there is a clear association with recurrent venous thromboembolism, cerebrovascular accidents and other arterial events and, in women, with recurrent abortions, fetal loss and other complications of pregnancy.[3] Therefore, tests for the presence of the LAC should be carried out in all young individuals with unexplained venous or arterial thrombosis and also in women with recurrent-early or late pregnancy loss.[4] Antibodies of this class are members of a larger group called antiphospholipid or anticardiolipin antibodies. (Although not precisely the same these terms

are used interchangeably.) Tests for lupus anticoagulant are usually performed in parallel with tests for the presence of antiphospholipid antibodies, usually by ELISA. In general these tests are not performed by haematology laboratories and are therefore not described here. Serological tests for antiphospholipid antibodies are not standardized and agreement between laboratories is poor. A large number of target proteins have been described but the most important, and the only one for which there is evidence of a pathogenic effect, is β_2-glycoprotein 1.[5] Increasingly, tests specifically for anti-β_2-glycoprotein 1 antibodies are performed and possible mechanisms for their prothrombotic activity are being elucidated.[6]

The presence of a LAC may be detected by the clotting screen and, depending on the reagents and methods used as well as on the potency and avidity of the antibody, either the PT or APTT may be prolonged. However, the sensitivity of both APTT and PT to LAC varies considerably, so that these tests may well be normal and, if clinically suspected, specific tests should always be performed.[4] The unmodified test for activated protein C (APC) resistance (see p. 456) is also sensitive to the presence of a LAC.

Patients with a LAC may show other abnormalities, including thrombocytopenia, a positive direct antiglobulin test and a positive antinuclear antibody test. Another frequent target for antiphospholipid antibodies is prothrombin but only rarely are these antibodies sufficient to inhibit or deplete prothrombin activity. Such patients may have a bleeding tendency. A recent international guideline on detection of lupus anticoagulants has been published[4] and recommended the following tests:

1. Dilute Russell's viper venom time (DRVVT) in conjunction with the platelet neutralization test.
2. An APTT test that has a low concentration of phospholipid and uses silica as an activator, thus making it sensitive to the presence of LAC.

There are a large number of additional tests which have in the past been successfully used for the detection of LAC, several of which are no longer recommended due to poor reproducibility, technical problems and lack of standardization.[4] The kaolin clotting time (KCT) and the dilute thromboplastin inhibition test are retained here because they are still widely used and thought to have some advantages by some authors. Although no single test is sufficiently sensitive to detect all LAC, readers are counselled against performing an excessive (more than two) number of tests because a large number of false positives will be generated. The most recent guidelines for the optimal performance of testing for LAC have been well laid out and are summarized in Box 19.1.[4]

Sample Preparation

It is essential that all the samples of plasma tested for an LAC should be as free of platelets as possible. This is achieved by further centrifugation of plasma at 2500 *g* for 10 min. A platelet count of $<10 \times 10^9/l$ should be achieved. The plasma is centrifuged at room temperature to avoid platelet activation because platelet microvesicles may also invalidate the test. After separation, the plasma should be frozen at $-70°C$ as soon as possible to prevent deterioration. Prior to testing, the frozen sample should be rapidly warmed to 37°C in a water bath.

Dilute Russell's Viper Venom Time

Principle

Russell's viper venom (RVV) activates factor X, leading to a fibrin clot in the presence of factor V, prothrombin, phospholipid and calcium ions. A LAC prolongs the clotting time by binding to the phospholipid and preventing the action of RVV. As the following test describes, dilution of the venom and phospholipid makes it particularly sensitive for detecting a LAC.[7] Because RVV activates factor X directly, defects of the contact system and factor VIII, IX and XI deficiencies do not influence the test. The DRVVT should be combined with a platelet/phospholipid neutralization procedure to add specificity and this is incorporated into several commercial kits.

Reagents

Platelet-poor plasma. From the patient and a control (depleted of platelets by second centrifugation or microfiltration) (see p. 404)
Glyoxaline buffer. 0.05 mol/l, pH 7.4 (see p. 409)
RVV (American Diagnostica Inc). Stock solution: 1 mg/ml in saline. For working solution, dilute approximately 1 in 200 in buffer. The working solution is stable at 4°C for several hours
Phospholipid. Platelet substitute; also available commercially
CaCl2. 0.025 mol/l (see p. 409).

Reagent Preparation

The RVV concentration is adjusted to give a clotting time of 30–35 s when 0.1 ml of RVV is added to the mixture of 0.1 ml of normal plasma and 0.1 ml of undiluted phospholipid. The test is then repeated using doubling dilutions of phospholipid reagent. The last dilution of phospholipid before the clotting time is prolonged by 2 s or more is selected for the test (thus giving a clotting time of 35–37 s).

Method

Place 0.1 ml of pooled normal plasma and 0.1 ml of dilute phospholipid reagent in a glass tube at 37°C. Add 0.1 ml of dilute RVV and, after warming for 30 s, add 0.1 ml of CaCl2. Record the clotting time. Repeat the sequence using the test plasma. Calculate the ratio of the clotting times of the test and control (normal pool) plasma.

Interpretation

The normal range for the ratio should be determined in each laboratory; it is usually between 0.9 and 1.05. Ratios >1.05 suggest the presence of a LAC but could also arise from an abnormality of factors II, V or X, fibrinogen; or some other inhibitor. The presence of an inhibitor can be confirmed by testing a mixture of equal volumes of patient's and control plasma, whereas phospholipid dependence can be confirmed by using the platelet neutralization test described next. Mixing with normal plasma corrects an abnormal dilute RVV test result as a result of factor deficiency or defect, but it does not do so in the presence of the LAC. The platelet or phospholipid neutralization procedure shortens the clotting time in the dilute RVV test when this is prolonged due to a LAC (see below).

Platelet Neutralization Test

Principle

When an excess of phospholipid, originally in the form of lysed platelets, is added to clotting tests, the tests become insensitive to the presence of a LAC. This appears to be a result of the ability of the platelets/phospholipid to adsorb the LAC. Platelet neutralization reagents are available commercially and are usually provided in DRVVT kits. Commercial reagents are preferred for consistency but a method for preparation is provided below. To utilize this property of platelets, they must be washed to remove contaminating plasma proteins and activated or 'fractured' to expose their coagulation factor binding sites.

Reagents for preparation of platelet neutralization reagent

Commercial platelet extract reagent or washed normal platelets
Acid–citrate–dextrose (ACD) anticoagulant solution (see p. 619), pH 5.4, is required for washed platelets. For use, 6 parts of blood is added to 1 part of this anticoagulant
Na₂EDTA. 0.1 mol/l in saline
Calcium-free Tyrode's buffer. Dissolve 8 g NaCl, 0.2 g KCl, 0.625 g Na₂HPO₄, 0.415 g MgCl₂ and 1.0 g NaHCO₂ in 1 litre of water. Adjust pH if necessary to 6.5 with 1 mol/l HCl.

Method

Collect normal blood into ACD and centrifuge at 270 *g* for 10 min. Pipette the supernatant platelet-rich plasma (PRP) into a plastic container and centrifuge again to obtain more PRP, which is added to the first lot. Dilute the PRP with an equal volume of the calcium-free buffer and add one-tenth volume of EDTA to give a final concentration of 0.01 mol/l. Centrifuge the mixture in a conical or round-bottom tube at 2000 *g* for 10 min and discard the supernatant. Gently resuspend the platelet pellet in buffer and 0.01 mol/l EDTA. Centrifuge again, discard the supernatant and resuspend the pellet in buffer alone. Then centrifuge the platelets a third time and resuspend the pellet in buffer without EDTA to give a platelet count of at least 400×10^9/l. The washed platelets may be stored below

$-20°C$ in volumes of 1–2 ml. Before use, they must be activated by thawing and refreezing 3–4 times.

Use the washed platelets or the commercial reagent in the dilute RVV test or in the APTT in place of the usual phospholipid reagent. First, determine a suitable dilution by testing a range of doubling dilutions in the test system with control plasma. A suitable dilution gives a similar clotting time to that obtained using control plasma and the phospholipid reagent.

Interpretation

The addition of platelets or a commercial 'confirm' phospholipid reagent to the DRVVT system corrects the clotting time when a LAC is present. It does not correct the time when the prolongation is due to a factor deficiency or an inhibitor directed against a specific coagulation factor. However, the ability of different batches of platelets to perform this correction is variable and may vary further with storage. Accordingly, each time the test is performed a plasma sample known to contain a LAC should be tested in parallel to establish the efficacy of the platelets.

Many commercial kits are now available for performing the tests described above. As with all such tests, there is an inevitable trade-off between sensitivity and specificity. This varies with different techniques, kits and coagulometer. One survey of reagents found that the best discriminator of positivity was by using a normalized correction ratio (CR) of DRVVT clotting times as follows:

$$CR = \frac{\left(\frac{P_D}{N_D}\right) - \left(\frac{P_C}{N_C}\right)}{\frac{P_D}{N_D}} \times 100\%$$

where P is patient's clotting time and N is the clotting time of normal plasma and D represents the detection procedure and C represents the confirmation (platelet/phospholipid neutralization) procedure.[7] A correction of >10% is regarded as positive, but care should be taken to establish a local normal range. Other calculations may also be used such as a simple ratio of P_D/P_C or percentage correction: $[(P_D - P_C)/P_D] \times 100\%$.[4]

False-positive results may be obtained in patients receiving intravenous heparin although some reagents contain neutralizing agents. Interpretation may be difficult in patients receiving oral anticoagulants; this can sometimes be overcome by performing the test on a 50:50 mix with normal plasma.

Interpretation of Tests for Lupus Anticoagulant

Detailed instructions for the interpretation of LAC testing have been published.[4] No single test detects all lupus-like anticoagulants and, if suspected clinically, then two specific tests should be performed before concluding that a LAC is not present.[4,8] Conversely, a single positive test should be repeated 12 weeks later because a transient positive may arise as the result of intercurrent illness or medication. It is crucial to distinguish LAC from specific anti-factor VIII antibodies, which are more typically time dependent but may have some immediate effect as well. Specific factor assays can be useful in discrimination but note that a LAC may result in non-parallelism and spuriously low results in these assays. Similarly, some weak LAC are neutralized by 50:50 mixing with normal plasma and sometimes exhibit a time-dependent effect. Some transient non-specific coagulation inhibitors are not detected by tests for LAC. Tests may be falsely negative while taking warfarin.

Kaolin Clotting Time

Principle

When the APTT is performed in the absence of platelet substitute reagent, it is particularly sensitive to a LAC. If the test is performed on a range of mixtures of normal and patient's plasma, different patterns of response are obtained, indicating the presence of a LAC, deficiency of one or more of the coagulation factors or the 'lupus cofactor' effect.[9]

There are commercially available kits based on the KCT, such as Kaoclot (Life Therapeutics USA). This method uses a low-turbidity colloidal kaolin solution, making this reagent slow to settle and therefore suitable for use on automated coagulation analysers. Kaoclot shows high sensitivity to LACs but is not suitable for testing patients undergoing heparin therapy

Reagents

Kaolin. 20 mg/ml in Tris buffer, pH 7.4. This may need to be reduced to 5 mg/ml in some automated analysers (see p. 410)
Normal platelet-poor plasma. Depleted of platelets by second centrifugation
Patient's plasma. Also platelet depleted
CaCl$_2$. 0.025 mol/l.

Method

Mix normal and patient plasma in plastic tubes in the following ratios of normal to patient's plasma: 10:0, 9:1, 8:2, 5:5, 2:8, 1:9 and 0:10. Pipette 0.2 ml of each mixture into a glass tube at 37°C. Add 0.1 ml of kaolin and incubate for 3 min, then add 0.2 ml of CaCl$_2$ and record the clotting time.

Results

Plot the clotting times against the proportion of normal to patient's plasma on linear graph paper as shown in Figure 19.1.

Interpretation

The pattern obtained for each patient must be critically assessed. A convex pattern (Pattern 1) indicates a positive result, whereas a concave pattern (Pattern 4) indicates a negative result. Pattern 2 indicates a coagulation factor deficiency and a LAC. Pattern 3 is found in plasma that contains a LAC but is also deficient in a cofactor necessary for the full inhibitory effect. The initial rate of slope is important because a steep slope indicates a positive result. This allows the test to be simplified so that only the tests of 100% normal and of 80% normal/20% test plasmas need be performed. The slope can be calculated using the ratio of KCT at 20% test plasma and KCT at 100% normal control plasma (N). For a positive result the ratio at this point should be ≥1.2.

Thus,

$$\frac{KCT\ (80\%N:20\%Test)}{KCT\ (100\%N)} \geq 1.2$$

A control KCT of <60 s may indicate contamination of the control plasma with phospholipid.

Dilute Thromboplastin Inhibition Test

Principle

When the thromboplastin used for the PT is diluted, the PT becomes prolonged. At a certain point (usually 1:50–1:500 dilution) the concentration of phospholipid is low enough for the test to become sensitive to phospholipid binding antibodies and when a LAC is present the ratio of the test plasma to normal plasma clotting time increases. This test is now considered more useful because some thromboplastin reagents (e.g. Innovin) are more sensitive to LACs. However, it should be noted that diluting thromboplastin makes the system sensitive to low levels of factor VIII as are encountered in mild haemophilia, acquired haemophilia and low levels of factor V or factor VII. Care should be taken that these disorders are not confused. In one study, the test was determined to be positive when the dilute PT ratio (test/mean normal) using Innovin at 1:200 dilution was >1.15.[10]

OTHER ACQUIRED THROMBOPHILIC STATES

There are numerous other disorders that are associated with an increased risk of thrombosis but are not usually diagnosed using coagulation-based tests. Appropriate tests for some of these such as myeloproliferative neoplasms and

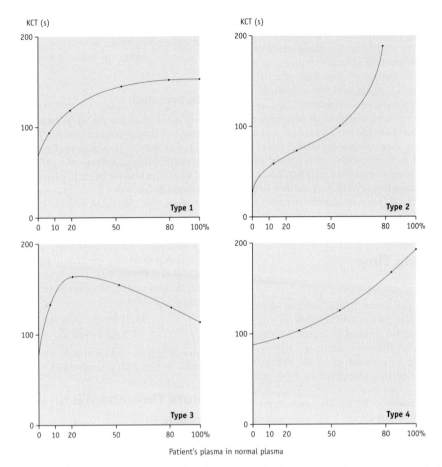

Figure 19.1 Curves obtained using the kaolin clotting time (KCT) to test for the presence of a lupus anticoagulant (see text).

paroxysmal nocturnal haemoglobinuria are found elsewhere in this book. One of the most important factors precipitating thrombosis is malignancy. However, the value of extensive testing for possible malignancy in patients with thrombosis remains contentious; some studies have shown that a history and examination combined with a few simple tests detect the large majority of malignancy and other systemic disorders. Other studies suggest that more intensive screening including abdominal and pelvic scans are required to achieve this. Large numbers of 'tumour marker' analyses result in numerous false positives. Even when tests have been effective in detecting occult malignancy it is not clear there is any improvement in outcome.[11,12]

INVESTIGATION OF INHERITED THROMBOTIC STATES

Testing for thrombotic syndromes remains frequent, despite doubts about its clinical utility.[1] Patients with disorders of pregnancy and those with thrombotic disorders

are often referred for investigation. Prior to testing for thrombophilia consideration should be given to the likely benefits including alteration in management that can be achieved. This requires a carefully taken history, noting in particular the circumstances of any previous thrombotic event, a family history of thrombosis and identification of any coexisting disorders. The relevant tests are described below.

Antithrombin (AT)

AT[13] (previously known as antithrombin III) is the major physiological inhibitor of thrombin and factors IXa, Xa and XIa. AT deficiency is found in approximately 2% of cases of thrombosis and may be acquired or congenital. Various methods are available for measuring either functional activity or antigenic quantity of AT. The functional methods are based on the reaction with thrombin or factor Xa and can be coagulation based or chromogenic assays. A chromogenic assay is described below.

Antithrombin (AT) Measurement Using a Chromogenic Assay

Principle

In the presence of heparin, AT reacts rapidly to inactivate thrombin by forming a 1:1 complex. The chromogenic AT assay is a two-step procedure. In the first step, the plasma sample is incubated with a fixed quantity of thrombin and heparin. In the second step the residual thrombin is measured spectrometrically by its action on a synthetic chromogenic substrate, which results in the release of p-nitro-aniline (pNA) dye. The use of bovine thrombin avoids interference in the assay by heparin cofactor II; this can also be achieved by measuring the Xa-neutralizing capacity of the AT and an appropriate chromogenic substrate. The assay thus measures heparin cofactor activity rather than progressive AT activity and may therefore also detect AT variants with altered heparin binding.

Method

Carry out the procedure on dilutions of a standard plasma to construct a standard graph. Then test dilutions of the test plasma in an identical manner and read the results directly from the standard graph.

The reagents provided and details of the method vary among manufacturers and should be closely followed. There may also be variation between different batches of the same reagent.

Normal range

The normal range is generally between 0.75 and 1.25 iu/ml. Some manufacturers suggest a slightly narrower range (i.e. 0.8–1.20 iu/ml), but it is preferable for each laboratory to establish its own normal range. Repeated freezing and thawing of samples, as well as storage at or above $-20°C$, results in a reduction in AT concentration.

Interpretation

In an inherited deficiency, the AT concentration is usually <0.7 iu/ml. Most cases are heterozygotes for null mutations (type I deficiency) and have levels of approximately 50% of normal. Be aware that numerous type 2 variants have been described affecting the reactive site, the heparin binding site or having pleiotropic effects, sometimes resulting in assay results that are close to normal. The clinical significance of heterozygous heparin-binding site mutations is probably low. Further tests such as AT antigen, crossed immunoelectrophoresis or mutation analysis may be required to identify variant molecules.[14,15] A low level of AT may be acquired as a result of active thrombosis, liver disease, heparin therapy, nephrotic syndrome or asparaginase therapy; very low values are sometimes encountered in fulminant disseminated intravascular coagulation (DIC) or liver failure. Normal newborns have a lower AT concentration (0.60–0.80 iu/ml) than adults.

In neonates who are congenitally deficient, very low values (0.30 iu/ml and lower) may be found. It is also important to remember that oral anticoagulant therapy may increase the AT concentration by approximately 0.1 iu/ml in cases of congenital deficiency.

Antithrombin Antigen Determination

AT antigen can be assessed using various methods such as enzyme-linked immunosorbent assay (ELISA), immuno-electrophoresis assays and latex agglutination (nephelometry).

Principle

Latex agglutination assays are based on the agglutination of a suspension of antibody-coated, micro-latex particles in the presence of plasma containing AT antigen (the antibody is attached by covalent bonding). The wavelength is such that light can pass through the latex suspension unabsorbed. However, in the presence of AT antigen, the antibody-coated latex particles agglutinate to form aggregates of diameter greater than the wavelength of the light; the latter is then absorbed. There is a direct relationship between the observed absorbance value and the concentration of the antigen being measured. The convenience of this form of test is that it can be performed on automated analysers.

Protein C (PC)

PC[16,17] is a vitamin K-dependent protein. After activation by thrombin, which is accelerated in the presence of thrombomodulin on the vascular endothelium, PC complexes with phospholipids and protein S (PS) to degrade factors Va and VIIIa. Inherited heterozygous PC deficiency is found in 2–4% of first-episode thromboses and 5–7% of all recurrent thromboembolic episodes in young adults.[18–20] The importance of the PC–PS system is evidenced by the catastrophic syndrome of purpura fulminans in neonates with homozygous PC or PS deficiency.[21] Acquired PC deficiency is found in all conditions associated with vitamin K deficiency or defect, including oral anticoagulant therapy. A low plasma concentration is also found in DIC, sepsis (especially meningococcal septicaemia), in liver disease, sickle cell disease and in the early postoperative period.

PC can be measured using a chromogenic assay, a coagulation assay or an antigenic method.[22]

Measurement of Functional Protein C by the Protac Method

Principle

In the presence of a specific snake venom activator, PC is converted into its active form. This allows the activation to be carried out in whole plasma without separation of

PC. Activated PC is measured by its action on one of the specific synthetic substrates (e.g. S-2366, CBS 65.25). The reaction is stopped by the addition of 50% acetic acid and the *p*-nitro-alanine produced is measured in a spectrometer at 405 nm.

Reagents

Platelet-poor plasma. Standard and test samples are centrifuged at 1500–2000 *g* for 15 min. After centrifugation, plasma can be stored indefinitely at −40°C or below

Protac. This is an activator derived from the venom of *Agkistrodon contortrix contortrix* (Southern copperhead snake). It is obtained commercially; each vial contains lyophilized powder, which is reconstituted and stored according to the manufacturer's instructions

Specific chromogenic substrate. Reconstituted and stored according to the manufacturer's instructions

Barbitone buffered saline. See p. 409

Acetic acid. 50%.

Method

Construct the standard curve according to the instructions using a calibrated reference plasma.

The assay is carried out by a two-step method. In the first step, plasma and activator are incubated for an exact period of time. In the second step, the specific chromogenic substrate is added and the reaction is stopped with acetic acid, again at a precise point in time. Read the amount of the dye produced at 405 nm against a blank obtained as follows: acetic acid, activator and chromogenic substrate are first mixed, then activated standard or patient's plasma is added to the mixture and the absorbance is measured at 405 nm. The manufacturer's instructions must be closely followed. Plot the PC activity against the corresponding absorbance reading on linear graph paper.

Normal range

The normal range is 0.70–1.40 iu/ml. Preferably, each laboratory should establish its own normal range.

Further Investigation for Protein C Deficiency

If inherited PC deficiency is suspected, an immunological assay may also be carried out with an ELISA-based kit, which will distinguish a type 1 or type 2 deficiency. The amidolytic assay described here does not detect the rare type 2 PC deficiency due to mutations in the Gla domain, although they can be detected by a coagulation-based assay.[22] The specificity of the chromogenic substrate is limited and is augmented by the inclusion of substances that inhibit other enzymes capable of cleaving the substrate. In some circumstances, this can fail and spuriously high PC activities can be obtained, which may obscure PC deficiency.[23] PC activity and antigen are reduced in patients taking oral vitamin K antagonists, although it is sometimes possible to make a provisional diagnosis of PC deficiency by using a PC:VIIc ratio.[24] It is also important to exclude vitamin K deficiency and/or liver disease by assaying other vitamin K-dependent factors. Family studies should be carried out whenever possible.

Clotting-Based Protein C Assay

Principle

PC clotting assays use an APTT reagent incorporating a PC activator derived from the Southern copperhead snake venom (*Agkistrodon contortrix contortrix*), PC-deficient plasma and calcium chloride. The APTT reagent activates both PC and the factors of the intrinsic pathway. The clotting time of normal plasma is long (>100 s), whereas that of PC-deficient plasma is normal (30 s). The degree of prolongation of the clotting time when patient plasma is mixed with PC-deficient plasma is proportional to the concentration of PC in the patient plasma.

Unlike chromogenic PC assays, PC clotting assays are sensitive to functional PC defects such as phospholipid binding (mutations in the Gla domain) and calcium binding. However, they are also sensitive to anticoagulants, Factor V Leiden, LACs and raised factor VIII levels. A functional protein C activity assay can also be performed using the DRVVT which may be less sensitive to these effects.[25]

Protein C Antigen

PC antigen can be measured using a conventional ELISA. Commercial kits are available.

Protein S (PS)

PS is also a vitamin K-dependent protein that acts as a cofactor for activated PC. It is similar to the serine proteases of the coagulation system in having a Gla domain and four EGF domains; however, instead of a protease domain it has a large terminal domain closely homologous to sex hormone-binding globulin (SHBG). In plasma, 60% of PS is bound to C4b-binding protein (C4bBP) via the SHBG[26] and does not possess any APC cofactor activity; the remaining 40% is free and available to interact with APC. Functional assays of PS are based on the capacity of PS to augment the prolongation of a clotting test time by APC. However, PS has some APC-independent anticoagulant activity that can also be measured in coagulation assays and it can also act as a cofactor for TFPI.[27,28] Measurement of the total and free PS antigen is possible using enzyme-linked immunoassays. All three measurements are considered together here but usually measurement of free PS is adequate.

Enzyme-Linked Immunosorbent Assay of Free and Total Protein S

Principle

The total PS in plasma is detected by a standard ELISA using polyclonal antibodies.[29] The analysis is then repeated using plasma in which C4bBP-bound PS has been removed by polyethylene glycol (PEG) precipitation. This gives a measure of free PS.

Reagents

Polytheneglycol (PEG) precipitation solution. Dissolve 100 g of PEG 8000 in 200 ml of sterile water. Prepare approximately 50 ml of working PEG by diluting the stock solution to exactly 18.75% with sterile water. Store in 2-ml aliquots at $-20°C$.

Coating buffer (phosphate buffered saline, pH 7.2). 0.39 g $Na_2HPO_4.2H_2O$, 2.68 g $Na_2HPO_4.12H_2O$, 8.474 g NaCl. Make up to 1 litre and adjust to pH 7.2; store at $4°C$.

Wash buffer. This is the same as the coating buffer, but it contains 0.5 M NaCl and 0.2% v/v Tween 20. Add 10.37 g of NaCl to 1 litre of coating buffer and 0.2% Tween 20. (Mix well.) Store at $4°C$.

Dilution buffer. This is the washing buffer with 30 g/1 PEG 8000. Store at $4°C$.

Substrate buffer Na_2HPO_4 (citrate phosphate buffer, pH 5.0). 7.3 g citric acid, 23.87 g. $Na_2HPO_4.12H_2O$. Make up to 1 litre with water. Adjust pH to 5.0.

o-phenylenediamine

Anti-PS and anti-PS peroxidase conjugated. (Dako Ltd)

Sulphuric acid, 1 M

Microtitre plates. (Greiner Labortechnick Ltd)

Standards and controls

Hydrogen peroxide. 30% w/v.

Methods

Dilute the antihuman PS immunoglobulin 1:1000 in coating buffer (i.e. 20 μl in 20 ml of buffer). Add 0.1 ml to each well of a microtitre plate, cover with Parafilm and leave overnight in a moist chamber at $4°C$. On the day the assay is to be performed, warm an aliquot of working PEG solution to $30°C$. Accurately pipette 200 μl of standard, patient's and control plasma samples into conical Eppendorf tubes; warm for 5 min at $37°C$. Add exactly 50 μl of warmed PEG, immediately cap and vortex mix twice for exactly 5 s each time. Place in a water/crushed ice mixture. In turn, treat all the samples identically. Leave for 30 min on the melted ice. Centrifuge for 30 s in the Eppendorf centrifuge. Then return to ice and remove 100 μl into a labelled tube (taking care not to remove any precipitate).

Prepare dilutions of control and patient's samples in PEG dilution buffer as follows. For total PS, dilute 0.05 ml of reference plasma in 8 ml of diluent. Use the

PEG precipitated reference plasma for measuring free PS; add 0.1 ml to 4 ml of dilution buffer.

Prepare a range of standards from these stock solutions using the same dilution schedule for free and total PS.

A. Stock solution = 1.25 iu/ml.
B. 0.8 ml stock + 0.2 ml buffer = 1.0 iu/ml.
C. 0.6 ml stock + 0.4 ml buffer = 0.75 iu/ml.
D. 0.4 ml stock + 0.6 ml buffer = 0.5 iu/ml.
E. 0.2 ml stock + 0.8 ml buffer = 0.25 iu/ml.
F. 0.1 ml stock + 0.9 ml buffer = 0.125 iu/ml.
G. 0.05 ml stock + 0.95 ml buffer = 0.0625 iu/ml.

Control and patient's samples are tested at two dilutions – total PS plasma: 1:200 and 1:400 and free PS PEG supernatants: 1:50 and 1:100. Shake out the contents of the previously prepared plate and blot on tissue. Wash the plate three times in wash buffer by filling all the wells, leaving for 2 min, shaking out the contents, blotting and repeating. Add 100 μl of each dilution of standard, control or patient's plasma in duplicate across the plate. Cover and incubate for 3 h in a wet box at room temperature. Wash the plate as described earlier. Dilute 2 μl of peroxidase-labelled antibody in 24 ml of dilution buffer. Add 100 μl of diluted tag (peroxidase-conjugated) antibody to each well and leave in a wet box for 2–3 h at room temperature. Wash the plate as described earlier. Make up the substrate solution by adding 8 mg of o-phenylenediamine to 12 ml of citrate phosphate buffer. Immediately before use add 10 μl of hydrogen peroxide. Add 100 μl of substrate solution to each well. When the weakest standard has a visible yellow colour, add 150 μl of 1 M sulphuric acid to each well. Read the optical densities on a plate reader at 492 nm. Plot the optical densities against plasma dilutions on double-log graph paper and read the patient's values from the corresponding calibration curve (i.e. total against total and free against free).

The polyclonal antibody should have similar affinities for free and bound PS; high plasma dilutions and long incubation times help to avoid differential affinity leading to error. Alternatively, two monoclonal antibodies (capture and tag) with the same affinity for free and bound PS can be used (Asserachrom).

Automated assays using antibodies to distinguish free and total PS are now available.[30–32]

Protein S Functional Assay

Principle

Functional PS can be assessed using coagulation-based assays activated by different means. In one commercial assay (American Diagnostica Inc) dilutions of normal and test plasmas are mixed with PS-deficient plasma. Activation of these mixtures is achieved by a reagent containing factor Xa, activated PC and phospholipid. After a 5 min activation time, clot formation is initiated by the addition of calcium chloride. Under these conditions, the prolongation of the clotting time is directly proportional to the concentration of PS in the patient plasma. The use of factor Xa as the activator minimizes the potential interference by high levels of factor VIII.

A PS function assay may also be based on the PT, in which case the effect of factor VIII is again bypassed. The PT-based PS assay uses PS-depleted plasma activated by Protac, thus providing activated PC. The PT is increased by the APC–PS-mediated destruction of factor Va, which occurs in the presence of PS from the test and control plasmas. The PT is measured using bovine thromboplastin and prolongation is proportional to PS activity.

These tests are performed according to the manufacturer's instructions and many tests can be automated.

Because the assays are subject to interference by other plasma factors, it is recommended that the test plasma is assayed at two different dilutions to ensure parallelism with the standard curve.

PS functional assays are designed to measure the PC cofactor activity of PS, but as discussed earlier, this is not its only anticoagulant activity. PS that is bound to C4bBP, is inadequately γ-carboxylated or has been cleaved by thrombin does not have PC cofactor activity but its effect on the assays is unknown.

Interpretation of Protein S Functional and Antigenic Assays

PS deficiency has been classified into three subtypes according to the pattern of results obtained in functional and antigenic assays (Table 19.1).

Studies have suggested that the type I and type III patterns are both the result of the same genetic defect and that the difference may be the result of an age-related increase in C4bBP.[33,34]

Although an estimate of PS functional activity would be ideal for diagnosing PS deficiency, the functional PS assays available are problematic. Like other functional assays they are prone to external influences: factor V Leiden (FVL), LAC and levels of other coagulation factors. Fortunately type II PS defects appear to be extremely rare; many previously diagnosed cases proved to be due to FVL. Thus

measurement of free PS is the preferred method for detecting PS deficiency.[35,36] Low levels of PS may be an acquired phenomenon during pregnancy and with oral anticoagulation, nephrotic syndrome, use of oral contraceptives, systemic lupus erythematosus, HIV infection and liver disease. Catastrophically low levels have been reported in children after varicella infection owing to autoantibody production.[37] It is important to note that the normal range for premenopausal women is significantly lower than in other groups and local normal ranges should be determined to avoid misinterpretation, paying attention to the additional effects of hormonal therapy and artefactual reduction in PS as described earlier.[38,39] Although C4bBP is elevated during an acute-phase reaction, the PS-binding β chain does not increase and as a result free PS does not decrease.[40]

Activated Protein C Resistance

In 1993, Dahlback et al.[41] described an inherited tendency to thrombosis characterized by a defective plasma response to activated PC. This became known as activated PC resistance (APCR) and was subsequently shown in >90% of cases to result from a polymorphism encoding the amino acid change Arg506Glu subsequently named factor V Leiden.[42] This mutation destroys a cleavage site for APC, which greatly slows APC inactivation of factor Va. It also blocks the conversion by APC of factor V into factor Vi, which acts as a cofactor for APC degradation of factor VIIIa. APCR is found in approximately 20% of patients with a first episode of venous thrombosis.

Principle[43]

When activated PC (APC) is added to plasma and an APTT is performed, there is normally a prolongation of the clotting time as a result of factor V and factor VIII degradation. The original detection of this phenomenon was by means of a modified APTT, but it can also be detected using modifications of the PT, DRVVT and factor Xa clotting time. These tests all vary somewhat in their sensitivity and specificity for the FVL mutation, which is generally improved by mixing the test plasma with factor V-deficient plasma. This reduces the effect of other factors such as factor VIII and prothrombin, which can alter estimation of APCR[44] and restores the sensitivity of the test in patients who are taking oral anticoagulants. However, the test remains sensitive to interference by LACs. Numerous commercial kits are available for these tests.

Expression of Results

APCR was originally reported as a simple ratio of clotting times with and without APC. The result can be normalized by expressing this as a ratio of the same result obtained with normal plasma, i.e.

Table 19.1 Classification of protein S deficiency			
CATEGORY	TOTAL PS	FREE PS	FUNCTIONAL PS
Type I	Low	Low	Low
Type II	Normal	Normal	Low
Type III	Normal	Low	Low

$$\text{Normalized APCR} = \frac{T + APC}{T - APC} \div \frac{N + APC}{N - APC}$$

when T = test and N = normal.

The use of a normalized ratio improves day-to-day precision and may also improve accuracy. However, it is extremely important that the pooled normal plasma does not contain FVL because very small amounts (2.5%) markedly affect the response to APC. A normal range should be established locally and its relationship to the presence of FVL should be determined.

Interpretation

The Leiden thrombophilia survey estimated the relative risk of thrombosis for APCR to be approximately 7.[45] Studies using DNA analysis alone have generally found slightly lower relative risks.[46] Most testing strategies have been directed toward producing tests that have a high sensitivity and specificity for FVL to avoid the need for DNA analysis. It seems that 'acquired APCR' or APCR resulting from other causes represents a prothrombotic state even in the absence of FVL,[47] as does the presence of acquired APCR in prothrombotic states such as pregnancy. These are not (except LACs) detected after mixing with factor V-deficient plasma. Some laboratories use a combination of plasma and DNA testing to assess patients' status but increasingly DNA analysis alone is performed and this can be combined with analysis of the prothrombin gene (below).

Increased Prothrombin, Factor VIII and Other Factors

A later finding from the Leiden thrombophilia survey was that elevated levels of prothrombin were significantly associated with thrombosis.[48] Most elevated levels were associated with a mutation in the 3' untranslated region of the gene (G20210A). The mutation is detected by a simple polymerase chain reaction-based test (see p. 148). Subsequently, other factors, including factor VIII, factor IX and factor XI, have been shown to have an association with thrombosis when elevated.[49–51]

Heparin Cofactor II

There is no clear evidence that heparin cofactor II (HCII) deficiency is more prevalent in patients with thrombosis than in the normal population; consequently, testing is not recommended as part of thrombophilia investigation.[52] (A method for measuring HCII is described in previous editions of this book.)

FIBRINOLYTIC SYSTEM

Investigation of Suspected Dysfibrinogenaemia

Congenital dysfibrinogenaemia, which may be associated with thrombosis, should be suspected in individuals with a prolonged thrombin time and a slightly or moderately reduced fibrinogen concentration in plasma. The presence of a dysfibrinogen is proved when a significant (usually two-fold) discrepancy is found between the Clauss and clot weight assays. (For details of investigation see p. 412.)

Investigation of the Fibrinolytic System: General Considerations

The investigation of fibrinolysis has an uncertain place in haemostasis. It seems well-established that uncontrolled fibrinolytic capacity as a result of plasmin inhibitor or plasminogen activator inhibitor (PAI-1) deficiency can lead to a haemorrhagic tendency, although these are rare.[53,54] Conversely it has been difficult to demonstrate that an impaired fibrinolytic capacity results in a tendency to venous thrombosis. This may be attributed in part to the poor reproducibility of the global tests such as euglobulin clot lysis or fibrin plate lysis but it has not been resolved by use of either specific assays or genetic polymorphic markers.[55] More recently a plasma clot lysis time has been developed which has been shown to detect a reduced fibrinolytic potential associated with an increased risk of first and recurrent thrombosis.[56,57] Moreover, this defect was associated with levels of thrombin-activatable fibrinolysis inhibitor (TAFI), PAI-1, plasminogen and tissue plasminogen activator (tPA), although for the latter two the association was lost after adjusting for other variables. This test is not yet in routine clinical use. High levels of tPA were shown to be predictive of myocardial infarction in the ECAT (European Concerted Action on Thrombosis and Disabilities) study, but it is possible that this unexpected association can be interpreted as demonstrating an abnormality of endothelial function rather than a problem with fibrinolysis *per se*.[58–61]

Fibrinolysis shows considerable diurnal variation as well as interference from plasma lipids and stress. It is therefore generally recommended that these tests be performed in the morning after an overnight fast, after a period of no smoking and after the subject has lain resting for ≥15 min (the plasma half-life of tPA is approximately 5 min). Great care is required in obtaining and handling samples for the assays described later.[62] Tests for fibrin and fibrinogen degradation products are described in Chapter 18.

Investigation of 'Fibrinolytic Potential'

The 'fibrinolytic potential' is measured as the combined effect of plasminogen activators and inhibitors. The concentration of activators may be increased by venous occlusion or by the administration of desmopressin (1-deamino-8-D-arginine vasopressin). The global tests, euglobulin lysis time and fibrin plate lysis are described first followed by assays for specific components of the fibrinolytic system.

Euglobulin Clot Lysis Time

Principle

When plasma is diluted and acidified, the precipitate (euglobulin) that forms contains plasminogen activator (mostly tPA), plasminogen and fibrinogen. Most of the plasmin inhibitors are left in the solution. The precipitate is redissolved, the fibrinogen is clotted with thrombin and the time for clot lysis is measured.

Reagents

Acetic acid. 0.01%
Bovine thrombin. 10 NIH u/ml
Fresh platelet-poor plasma from the patient and control. Because tPA is very labile, blood must be collected into cooled sample tubes, placed on ice and processed immediately
Glyoxaline buffer. pH 7.4. See p. 409.

Method

Place venous blood in a plastic tube containing citrate; after mixing, keep the tube in an icebath. Centrifuge the sample as soon as possible (never later than 30 min after collection) at 4°C at 1200–1500 g. Pipette 1.0 ml of plasma into 9 ml of acetic acid. Mix well and keep on ice for 15 min. Centrifuge at 4°C for 15 min, at 1500 g, to deposit the white euglobulin precipitate. Discard the supernatant, invert the tubes, then wipe the walls with cotton wool on an applicator stick until completely dry inside. Add 0.5 ml of glyoxaline buffer and dissolve the precipitate. Place duplicate 0.3 ml volumes of the dissolved euglobulin fractions from the patient and control in glass tubes and obtain clotting by adding 0.1 ml of thrombin. Leave undisturbed at 37°C and inspect for clot lysis at 15 min intervals.

Normal range

The normal range is 90–240 min.

Interpretation

A technical problem leading to an artefactually long lysis time is the failure to maintain a low temperature throughout all the stages of the test. Furthermore, the fact that a variable amount of PAI-1 precipitates in the euglobulin fraction makes it essential to analyse a normal control on each occasion the test is performed. Exercise and prolonged venous stasis shorten the lysis times. There is also a significant diurnal variation; lysis time is longer in the morning than at noon or in the afternoon. Prolonged fibrinolysis (as found during fibrinolytic therapy) may result in plasminogen depletion and give rise to a falsely long lysis time. In DIC, a low fibrinogen concentration in the patient's plasma gives a wispy clot, which dissolves rapidly and results in a falsely short lysis time. Conversely, high levels of fibrinogen result in a prolonged lysis time.

Long lysis times are found in the last trimester of pregnancy, in the postoperative period, after myocardial infarction, in individuals who are obese and in many cases of recurrent venous thrombosis. Very short lysis times are seen in some haematological or disseminated malignancies and in cirrhosis. A short lysis time is also seen in factor XIII deficiency.

Lysis of Fibrin Plates

Principle

Most commercially available fibrinogen preparations are contaminated with plasminogen. If a standard fibrinogen solution is poured into a Petri dish and clotted with $CaCl_2$ and thrombin, a solid fibrin plate is obtained. If the euglobulin fraction under test is placed on the plate, the plasminogen in the plate is converted into plasmin and a zone of lysis appears around the sample. The area of lysis is proportionate to the concentration of plasminogen activator in the euglobulin fraction.[63]

Reagents

Bovine fibrinogen
Bovine thrombin. 50 NIH u/ml
Calcium chloride. 0.025 mol/l
Barbitone buffered saline. (see p. 409)
Platelet-poor plasma. From the patient and a control; collected as described for euglobulin lysis time.

Equipment

Equipment includes plastic Petri dishes.

Method

To prepare the fibrin plate, dilute the fibrinogen in buffered saline to obtain a final concentration of 1.5 g/l. Pipette 10 ml of diluted fibrinogen into a Petri dish. Place it on a level tray. Add 0.5 ml of $CaCl_2$ and 0.2 ml of thrombin solution. Mix the contents by swirling quickly. The plate clots within 10 to 20 s; it must clot evenly to be suitable for the test. Leave the plate undisturbed for 20 min. The prepared plates can then be kept for 3–4 days at 4°C.

Carefully apply 30 µl of the euglobulin fraction, prepared as described in the previous test, to the surface of the plate. There is no need to cut a well. Place in an incubator at 37°C for 24 h. This preparation time can be shortened by the addition of exogenous plasminogen.[63]

Perform all tests (patient and control) in duplicate.

Results

Calculate the zone of lysis by measuring two diameters in mm at right angles to each other. Multiply the two values to obtain the approximate area of lysis in mm^2.

Normal range

The normal range is variable but is usually between 40 and 60 mm^2.

Interpretation

The area of lysis may be difficult to define because of incomplete lysis. Only areas of complete, clear lysis should be measured. In other respects the interpretation is as for the euglobulin clot lysis time except that the levels of plasminogen and fibrinogen in the test plasma do not affect the result. The same problems in preparing the euglobulin fraction apply as does the necessity for a normal control.

Venous Occlusion Test

Principle

Localized venous occlusion[64] of an arm for a standardized period is used as a stimulus for release of tPA from the vessel wall. The original intention was that this would be a better measure of functional defects in fibrinolysis than a resting sample. Preocclusion and postocclusion lysis times, using the previously described euglobulin lysis or the fibrin plate lysis tests, are measured. In normal subjects fibrinolysis is greatly enhanced by occlusion. However, given the problems associated with global assays of fibrinolysis, it seems preferable to perform specific measurements of tPA before and after occlusion.

Method

Withdraw blood from the arm to be tested without stasis, place it in a citrate-containing tube and keep in an icebath. Inflate the sphygmomanometer cuff to a pressure midway between the systolic and diastolic pressure. Leave the inflated cuff on for 10 min. Take a sample of venous blood from below the cuff immediately before deflation and place on ice. Measure the lysis in both samples, as described previously. This test is uncomfortable and some patients may not be able to tolerate as much as 10 min of occlusion. Petechiae are commonly seen after the test is completed.

Results

The postocclusion lysis times should be shorter than the preocclusion times. Shortening by at least 30 min is found in most normal subjects.

Interpretation

Failure to enhance lysis is found in some cases of recurrent venous thrombosis, in people who are obese, after surgery, trauma or severe illness and in Behçet's syndrome. It may also result from a failure to release the activator because insufficient pressure was applied or the occlusion time was too short. Normal people vary in the degree of response: 'good' responders increase the concentration of tPA by three-fold to four-fold, whereas 'poor' responders may consistently show only a very slight enhancement of fibrinolysis even with longer occlusion times. When comparing plasma levels of proteins preocclusion and postocclusion, an adjustment for changes in haematocrit may be required.[65] The effect of the venous occlusion test and the levels of tPA are very variable over time.[66,67]

Investigation of Suspected Plasminogen Defect or Deficiency

Inherited plasminogen deficiency or defect may be found in 2–3% of unexplained thromboses in young people.[68,69] However, there is no good evidence that deficiency is associated with an increase risk of thrombosis. The only consistent clinical finding appears to be ligneous conjunctivitis.[70] The laboratory screening should be carried out using a functional assay based on full transformation of plasminogen into plasmin by activators. Such assays can be caseinolytic, fibrin substrate or chromogenic.

Chromogenic Assay for Plasminogen

Principle

In this two-step amidolytic assay, plasminogen is first complexed with excess streptokinase. In the second step, the plasmin-like activity of the streptokinase–plasminogen complex is measured by its effect on a plasmin-specific peptide (e.g. S-2251). The amount of the dye released is proportional to the amount of plasminogen available in the sample for complexing with streptokinase. The streptokinase–plasminogen complex is not significantly inhibited by the plasma plasmin inhibitors. An excess of plasminogen-free fibrinogen can be added to maximize the activity and avoid confounding by the presence of fibrin degradation products (FDPs).

Reagents and method

Details can be found in the manufacturer's instructions.

Normal range

The normal range is usually approximately 0.75–1.60 iu/ml.

Interpretation

Plasminogen concentration is reduced in the newborn, in patients with cirrhosis, in DIC and during and after thrombolytic therapy, but the assay is less reliable in these circumstances when fibrinogen/fibrin degradation products may augment plasmin activity. A high concentration of fibrinogen can also augment plasmin activity and make the assay less reliable. Plasminogen is an acute-phase reactant and an increased concentration is found in infection, trauma, myocardial infarction and malignant disease. Hereditary plasminogen deficiency is most commonly due to a type I deficiency and so an antigenic test is usually sufficient. If suspicion remains high then a functional assay will be required.

Tissue Plasminogen Activator Amidolytic Assay

Principle

Different amidolytic assays for tPA have been described.[71,72] One relies on the activation of purified plasminogen to plasmin in the presence of fibrinogen fragments, which stimulate the tPA activity in the test plasma. The plasmin is measured using a specific chromogenic substrate. In the second method, tPA is captured on specific antibodies bound to a solid-phase matrix such as a microtitre plate; the various plasma inhibitors of tPA and plasmin are washed away, plasminogen is added together with a stimulator of tPA activity and the plasmin produced is measured with chromogenic substrates. Alternatively, chromogenic substrates specific for tPA may be used, but there are specificity problems, especially in the plasma assays.

Interpretation

tPA is secreted into plasma in its active form but rapidly complexes with its principal inhibitor PAI-1. The amount of active tPA in the plasma is a result of this equilibrium and represents only a small fraction of the total (antigenic) tPA. This process continues after blood sampling unless blood is taken into an appropriate acidic anticoagulant (see above).

tPA can also be measured by ELISA using monoclonal antibodies on microtitre plates, although concentration closely parallels the PAI-1 concentration and says little about the proportion of free, active tPA.

Plasminogen Activator Inhibitor Activity Assay

Principle

Plasma anti-plasminogen activator activity is almost entirely due to PAI-1. A fixed amount of tPA is added in excess to undiluted plasma and part of it rapidly complexes with PAI-1. Plasminogen in plasma is then activated into plasmin by the residual, uncomplexed tPA. The amount of plasmin formed is directly proportional to the residual tPA activity and inversely proportional to the PAI activity of the sample. The amount of plasmin generated is measured using a plasmin-specific substrate.

Reagents are available in kit form and the manufacturer's instructions must be closely followed. The normal range, in particular the lower limit, is not clearly defined and many normal subjects have levels below the assay's lower limit of detection.[73,74] Each laboratory should establish its own range until reliable normal values become available.

The time of sampling must be standardized. Early morning (7 a.m.) samples have much greater levels of activity than those done later in the day. Rapid sample processing is extremely important because PAI leaks from platelets in sampled blood and PAI-1 in plasma rapidly converts to a latent (inactive) form. An ELISA assay is also available to measure the total PAI-1 present.

Plasminogen Activator Inhibitor Antigen Assay

Principle

Microplate wells coated with an anti-PAI-1 monoclonal antibody are incubated with samples and standards. PAI-1 present in the samples and standards is bound to the solid phase during this incubation. Unbound substances are then removed by washing. An enzyme-labelled anti-PAI-1 monoclonal antibody (conjugate) is added. The conjugate binds to the antibody–antigen complexes formed in the previous incubation. Unbound conjugate is then removed by washing. Finally, enzyme substrate is added. The action of the bound enzyme on the substrate produces a blue colour, which turns yellow after stopping the reaction with acid. The absorbances are read in a microplate reader at 450 nm. The amount of colour is proportional to the concentration of PAI-1. The assay is specific for total PAI-1, including both free and complexed forms.

Specimen Collection

Blood should be collected into CTAD tubes or Diatube H (Stago) and immediately cooled on ice; CTAD is a buffered tri-sodium citrate solution with theophylline, adenosine and dipyridamole. Vacutainer coagulation tubes with

CTAD (Becton-Dickinson) samples can be stored on ice for up to 7 h in the collection tubes. If the sample is not tested immediately, it should be separated and frozen as soon as possible.

Reagents and Method

This is available in a kit based on an ELISA (Chromogenix).

Normal Range

The normal range is usually 11–69 ng/ml. However, each laboratory should establish its own normal range.

Plasmin Inhibitor (α_2 Antiplasmin) Amidolytic Assay

Principle

Plasma dilutions are incubated with excess plasmin, a proportion of which are inhibited by antiplasmins. The residual, uninhibited plasmin is measured using a specific chromogenic substrate. Plasmin inhibitor is the major circulating inhibitor of plasmin and forms complexes much faster than other inhibitors; if the reaction times are short, the assay effectively measures plasmin inhibitor only.

Different commercial kits are available containing all the necessary reagents. The manufacturer's instructions should be carefully followed. Care is required when aliquoting the plasmin solution, which has a high viscosity because of its glycerol content. Note that plasmin bound to α_2 macroglobulin may escape inhibition, thus underestimating inhibitor activity.

The usual normal range is between 0.80 and 1.20 iu/ml. Congenital plasmin inhibitor deficiency is associated with a severe bleeding tendency. A reduced concentration is also found in liver disease, in DIC and during thrombolytic therapy. Plasmin inhibitor increases with age and is higher in Caucasians than in Africans.

PLATELET 'HYPERREACTIVITY' AND ACTIVATION

Platelets may be more reactive than normal as a consequence of *in vivo* activation by thrombin or non-endothelial surfaces, such as prosthetic valves or Dacron grafts. This can sometimes be detected by a lowered threshold (increased sensitivity) for aggregating agents. Because there is considerable variation in response to aggregating agents in normal people, the attempts to show platelet hyperaggregability are rarely successful and the results are frequently inconsistent. Spontaneous aggregation of platelets in the blood can also be demonstrated.[75]

Platelets that have formed a part of a platelet thrombus and have been released into the circulation may show a measurable decrease in their ability to aggregate because of a loss of some granular content. The released contents can be measured in plasma; the α-granule proteins, β-thromboglobulin and platelet factor 4 are the constituents most commonly measured. Overall the problems with these tests make them of doubtful utility;[59] they are described in previous editions of this book.

Several genetic polymorphisms have been reported to affect the reactivity of platelet glycoproteins and P selectin. Although they may be important in population studies, their clinical significance for individual patients remains unclear.[76,77]

Platelet Activation: Flow Cytometry

The problems associated with previous tests of platelet activation have been circumvented to some extent by the application of flow cytometric analysis of platelets in whole-blood samples.

Principle

The activation of platelets is associated with the appearance of new antigenic determinants on the platelet surface. Some of these are molecules present in platelet granules brought to the surface during degranulation (e.g. CD62P, CD63, LAMP-1 and CD40L) and others are new conformations of existing molecules (e.g. the ligand-induced binding site on GpIIbIIIa). These can be detected using fluorescein-conjugated antibodies and the degree of expression can be quantified by flow cytometry. This gives a measure of platelet activation with a much greater degree of sensitivity than platelet factor 4 or β-thromboglobulin estimation and may still be successful in the presence of thrombocytopenia. Samples may need to be collected into inhibitors of platelet activation such as PGE_1. Numerous alternative surface molecules are available (Table 19.2). These tests have not yet entered routine laboratory practice but are proving increasingly useful in research.[78] An alternative approach is offered by the PFA-100 (see p. 425) in which short closure times may be indicative of platelet hyperreactivity and/or hyperreactive von Willebrand factor species.

HOMOCYSTEINE

Following the observation that patients with homocystinuria have venous and arterial thromboses with accelerated vascular damage, there has been considerable interest in patients with less marked elevation of plasma homocysteine (hyperhomocysteinaemia). This has been

Table 19.2 Indicators of platelet activation detectable by flow cytometry

NAME	CD DESIGNATION	COMMENT
Gplb, IX, V	CD42	Decreases
GpIIbIIIa	CD41	Increases
Phosphatidyl serine	–	Increases Detected by Annexin V binding
Lysosomal Integral membrane protein (gp53, granulophysin)	CD63	Indicates lysosomal degranulation
P selectin	CD62P	Indicates α granule release, subsequently cleaved and measurable in plasma
Fibrinogen	–	Surface-bound fibrinogen increases
IIbIIIa activation	–	Conformation change in IIbIIIa produced by activation, detected by PAC-1 antibody

shown to have an association with arterial and venous thrombosis but the assay has little clinical utility and dietary interventions have been ineffective.[79,80] Until recently, homocysteine has been measured by high-performance liquid chromatography or mass spectroscopy, but an ELISA-based assay is now available that allows it to fit more easily into coagulation laboratory practice. To standardize study results, homocysteine is measured either while fasting or after a methionine load. Rapid processing of samples is required because homocysteine quickly leaches out of red blood cells.

MARKERS OF COAGULATION ACTIVATION

Numerous commercial kits are available for measuring molecules produced by coagulation activation.

Principle

The activation of many proteins active in coagulation is mediated by proteolytic cleavage with the release of small peptides: activation peptides. The most frequently measured of these is prothrombin fragment 1 + 2, which is released when prothrombin is converted to thrombin. It has an appreciable half-life of approximately 45 min, which allows a measurable concentration to accumulate in plasma and provides an indication of the rate at which thrombin is being generated.

An alternative is to measure the concentration of thrombin–antithrombin complexes (TAT), which provides similar information. Plasmin–antiplasmin complexes provide corresponding information about fibrinolysis. These can all be measured using commercially available ELISA kits but are not used routinely and are not required for normal diagnostic work.[81] Other tests such as fibrinopeptide A require exceptional care and the use of special anticoagulants to prevent *in vitro* activation of the sample.

A plasmin cleavage product of crosslinked fibrin, D-dimer (see p. 441) is another measure of activity in the coagulation system. Several studies have shown that elevated levels of D-dimer are an indicator of future risk of thrombosis. It is not yet certain whether they have on their own, or in conjunction with other factors, sufficient predictive value to alter management but they are currently being incorporated into management protocols. The test is usually performed after oral anticoagulants have been discontinued.

GLOBAL ASSAYS OF COAGULATION

As a response to the failure of reductive approaches to identify assays that reliably predict thrombosis or thrombotic risk, some workers have moved in the opposite direction and devised global assays that assess the overall coagulation potential of a blood or plasma sample. These tests include the endogenous thrombin potential (ETP) and the thromboelastograph. While use of thromboelastography has increased in the management of haemorrhage, their ability to assess thrombotic risk is less well described. There is some evidence that increased ETP can predict patients at increased risk of first or recurrent thrombosis.[82] However, neither of these techniques is in routine diagnostic use. Some manufacturers have developed kits for global assessment of the PC–PS pathway.

REFERENCES

1. Baglin T, Gray E, Greaves M, et al. Clinical guidelines for testing for heritable thrombophilia. *Br J Haematol.* 2010;149(2):209–220.

2. Devreese K, Hoylaerts MF. Laboratory diagnosis of the antiphospholipid syndrome: a plethora of obstacles to overcome. *Eur J Haematol.* 2009;83(1):1–16.

3. Palomo I, Segovia F, Ortega C, et al. Antiphospholipid syndrome: a comprehensive review of a complex and multisystemic disease. *Clin Exp Rheumatol.* 2009;27(4):668–677.

4. Pengo V, Tripodi A, Reber G, et al. Update of the guidelines for lupus anticoagulant detection. Subcommittee on Lupus Anticoagulant/Antiphospholipid Antibody of the Scientific and Standardization Committee of the International Society on Thrombosis and Haemostasis. *J Thromb Haemost.* 2009;7(10):1737–1740.

5. de Laat B, Pengo V, Pabinger I, et al. The association between circulating antibodies against domain I of beta2-glycoprotein I and thrombosis: an international multicenter study. *J Thromb Haemost.* 2009;7(11):1767–1773.

6. Agar C, van Os GMA, Morgelin M, et al. β2-Glycoprotein I can exist in 2 conformations: implications for our understanding of the antiphospholipid syndrome. *Blood.* 2010;116(8):1336–1343.

7. Thiagarajan P, Pengo V, Shapiro SS. The use of the dilute Russell viper venom time for the diagnosis of lupus anticoagulants. *Blood.* 1986;68(4):869–874.

8. Brandt JT, Barna LK, Triplett DA. Laboratory identification of lupus anticoagulants: results of the Second International Workshop for Identification of Lupus Anticoagulants. On behalf of the Subcommittee on Lupus Anticoagulants/Antiphospholipid Antibodies of the ISTH. *Thromb Haemost.* 1995;74(6):1597–1603.

9. Exner T, Rickard KA, Kronenberg H. A sensitive test demonstrating lupus anticoagulant and its behavioural patterns. *Br J Haematol.* 1978;40(1):143–151.

10. Arnout J, Vanrusselt M, Huybrechts E, et al. Optimization of the dilute prothrombin time for the detection of the lupus anticoagulant by use of a recombinant tissue thromboplastin. *Br J Haematol.* 1994;87(1):94–99.

11. Monreal M, Lensing AW, Prins MH, et al. Screening for occult cancer in patients with acute deep vein thrombosis or pulmonary embolism. *J Thromb Haemost.* 2004;2(6):876–881.

12. Piccioli A, Lensing AW, Prins MH, et al. Extensive screening for occult malignant disease in idiopathic venous thromboembolism: a prospective randomized clinical trial. *J Thromb Haemost.* 2004;2(6):884–889.

13. van Boven HH, Lane DA. Antithrombin and its inherited deficiency states. *Semin Hematol.* 1997;34(3):188–204.

14. Lane DA, Olds RJ, Conard J, et al. Pleiotropic effects of antithrombin strand 1C substitution mutations. *J Clin Invest.* 1992;90(6):2422–2433.

15. Kottke-Marchant K, Duncan A. Antithrombin deficiency: issues in laboratory diagnosis. *Arch Pathol Lab Med.* 2002;126(11):1326–1336.

16. Castellino FJ, Ploplis VA. The protein C pathway and pathologic processes. *J Thromb Haemost.* 2009;7(suppl 1):140–145.

17. Bertina RM. Specificity of protein C and protein S assays. *La Ricerca in Clinica e in Laboratorio Journal.* 1990;20(2):127–138.

18. Lane DA, Mannucci P, Bauer K, et al. Inherited thrombophilia: part 1. *Thromb Haemost.* 1996;76(5):651–662.

19. Lane DA, Mannucci P, Bauer K, et al. Inherited thrombophilia: part 2. *Thromb Haemost.* 1996;76(6):824–834.

20. Rosendaal FR, Reitsma PH. Genetics of venous thrombosis. *J Thromb Haemost.* 2009;7(suppl 1):301–304.

21. Marlar RA, Neumann A. Neonatal purpura fulminans due to homozygous protein C or protein S deficiencies. *Semin Thromb Hemost.* 1990;16(4):299–309.

22. Khor B, Van Cott EM. Laboratory tests for protein C deficiency. *Am J Hematol.* 2010;85(6):440–442.

23. Mackie IJ, Gallimore M, Machin SJ. Contact factor proteases and the complexes formed with alpha 2-macroglobulin can interfere in protein C assays by cleaving amidolytic substrates. *Blood Coagul Fibrinolysis.* 1992;3(5):589–595.

24. Jones DW, Mackie IJ, Winter M, et al. Detection of protein C deficiency during oral anticoagulant therapy – use of the protein C:factor VII ratio. *Blood Coagul Fibrinolysis.* 1991;2(3):407–411.

25. Cooper PC, Cooper SM, Goodfellow KJ, et al. Evaluation of a new venom-based clotting assay of protein C. *International Journal of Laboratory Hematology.* 2008;30(5):437–443.

26. Rezende SM, Simmonds RE, Lane DA. Coagulation, inflammation and apoptosis: different roles for protein S and the protein S-C4b binding protein complex. *Blood.* 2004;103(4):1192–1201.

27. Hackeng TM, Rosing J. Protein S as cofactor for TFPI. *Arterioscler Thromb Vasc Biol.* 2009;29(12):2015–2020.

28. Castoldi E, Hackeng TM. Regulation of coagulation by protein S. *Curr Opin Hematol.* 2008;15(5):529–536.

29. Comp PC, Doray D, Patton D, et al. An abnormal plasma distribution of protein S occurs in functional protein S deficiency. *Blood.* 1986;67(2):504–508.

30. Deffert C, Esteve F, Grimaux M, et al. A direct, automated, immuno-turbidimetric assay of free protein S antigen in plasma. *Blood Coagul Fibrinolysis*. 2001;12(2):137–141.

31. Serra J, Sales M, Chitolie A, et al. Multicentre evaluation of IL Test Free PS: a fully automated assay to quantify free protein S. *Thromb Haemost*. 2002;88(6):975–983.

32. Aillaud MF, Pouymayou K, Brunet D, et al. New direct assay of free protein S antigen applied to diagnosis of protein S deficiency. *Thromb Haemost*. 1996;75 (2):283–285.

33. Simmonds RE, Zoller B, Ireland H, et al. Genetic and phenotypic analysis of a large (122-member) protein S-deficient kindred provides an explanation for the familial coexistence of type I and type III plasma phenotypes. *Blood*. 1997;89 (12):4364–4370.

34. Zoller B, Garcia dFP, Dahlback B. Evaluation of the relationship between protein S and C4b-binding protein isoforms in hereditary protein S deficiency demonstrating type I and type III deficiencies to be phenotypic variants of the same genetic disease. *Blood*. 1995;85 (12):3524–3531.

35. Lawrie AS, Lloyd ME, Mohamed F, et al. Assay of protein S in systemic lupus erythematosus. *Blood Coagul Fibrinolysis*. 1995;6(4):322–324.

36. Persson KE, Dahlback B, Hillarp A. Diagnosing protein S deficiency: analytical considerations. *Clin Lab*. 2003;49(3–4):103–110.

37. Levin M, Eley BS, Louis J, et al. Postinfectious purpura fulminans caused by an autoantibody directed against protein S. *J Pediatr*. 1995;127 (3):355–363.

38. Faioni EM, Valsecchi C, Palla A, et al. Free protein S deficiency is a risk factor for venous thrombosis. *Thromb Haemost*. 1997;78 (5):1343–1346.

39. Gari M, Falkon L, Urrutia T, et al. The influence of low protein S plasma levels in young women, on the definition of normal range. *Thromb Res*. 1994;73(2): 149–152.

40. Garcia de Frutos P, Alim RI, Hardig Y, et al. Differential regulation of alpha and beta chains of C4b-binding protein during acute-phase response resulting in stable plasma levels of free anticoagulant protein S. *Blood*. 1994;84(3):815–822.

41. Dahlback B, Carlsson M, Svensson PJ. Familial thrombophilia due to a previously unrecognized mechanism characterized by poor anticoagulant response to activated protein C: prediction of a cofactor to activated protein C [see comments]. *Proc Natl Acad Sci U S A*. 1993;90 (3):1004–1008.

42. Bertina RM, Koeleman BP, Koster T, et al. Mutation in blood coagulation factor V associated with resistance to activated protein C [see comments]. *Nature*. 1994;369(6475):64–67.

43. Bertina RM. Laboratory diagnosis of resistance to activated protein C (APC-resistance). *Thromb Haemost*. 1997;78(1):478–482.

44. Laffan MA, Manning R. The influence of factor VIII on measurement of activated protein C resistance. *Blood Coagul Fibrinolysis*. 1996;7(8):761–765.

45. Koster T, Rosendaal FR, de RH, et al. Venous thrombosis due to poor anticoagulant response to activated protein C: Leiden Thrombophilia Study [see comments]. *Lancet*. 1993;342(8886–8887): 1503–1506.

46. Ridker PM, Glynn RJ, Miletich JP, et al. Age-specific incidence rates of venous thromboembolism among heterozygous carriers of factor V Leiden mutation. *Ann Intern Med*. 1997;126(7):528–531.

47. de Visser MC, Rosendaal FR, Bertina RM. A reduced sensitivity for activated protein C in the absence of factor V Leiden increases the risk of venous thrombosis. *Blood*. 1999;93 (4):1271–1276.

48. Poort SR, Rosendaal FR, Reitsma PH, et al. A common genetic variation in the 3'-untranslated region of the prothrombin gene is associated with elevated plasma prothrombin levels and an increase in venous thrombosis. *Blood*. 1996;88 (10):3698–3703.

49. Koster T, Blann A, Briet E, et al. Role of clotting factor VIII in effect of von Willebrand factor on occurrence of deep vein thrombosis. *Lancet*. 1995;345:152–155.

50. Meijers JC, Tekelenburg WL, Bouma BN, et al. High levels of coagulation factor XI as a risk factor for venous thrombosis. *N Engl J Med*. 2000;342 (10):696–701.

51. O'Donnell J, Tuddenham EG, Manning R, et al. High prevalence of elevated factor VIIIc levels in patients referred for thrombophilia screening: role of increased synthesis and relationship to the acute phase reaction. *Thromb Haemost*. 1997;77: 825–828.

52. Tollefsen DM, van Boven HH, Lane DA. Laboratory diagnosis of antithrombin and heparin cofactor II deficiency. Antithrombin and its inherited deficiency states. *Semin Thromb Hemost*. 1990;16 (2):162–168.

53. Fay WP, Parker AC, Condrey LR, Shapiro AD. Human plasminogen activator inhibitor-1 (PAI-1) deficiency: characterization of a large kindred with a null mutation in the PAI-1 gene. *Blood*. 1997;90 (1):204–208.

54. Lind B, Thorsen S. A novel missense mutation in the human plasmin inhibitor (alpha2-antiplasmin) gene associated with a bleeding tendency. *Br J Haematol*. 1999;107 (2):317–322.

55. Lane D, Grant P. Role of hemostatic gene polymorphisms in venous and arterial thrombotic disease. *Blood*. 2000;95(5):1517–1532.

56. Lisman T, de Groot PG, Meijers JC, et al. Reduced plasma fibrinolytic potential is a risk factor for venous thrombosis. *Blood*. 2005;105 (3):1102–1105.

57. Meltzer ME, Bol L, Rosendaal FR, et al. Hypofibrinolysis as a risk factor for recurrent venous thrombosis; results of the LETS follow-up study. *J Thromb Haemost*. 2010;8 (3):605–607.

58. Juhan VI, Pyke SD, Alessi MC, et al. Fibrinolytic factors and the risk of myocardial infarction or sudden death in patients with angina pectoris. ECAT Study Group. European Concerted Action on Thrombosis and Disabilities. *Circulation*. 1996;94(9):2057–2063.

59. Pyke SD, Thompson SG, Buchwalsky R, et al. Variability over time of haemostatic and other

cardiovascular risk factors in patients suffering from angina pectoris. ECAT Angina Pectoris Study Group. *Thromb Haemost.* 1993;70(5):743–746.

60. Ridker PM, Vaughan DE, Stampfer MJ, et al. Endogenous tissue-type plasminogen activator and risk of myocardial infarction [see comments]. *Lancet.* 1993;341 (8854):1165–1168.

61. Thompson SG, Kienast J, Pyke SD, et al. Hemostatic factors and the risk of myocardial infarction or sudden death in patients with angina pectoris. European Concerted Action on Thrombosis and Disabilities Angina Pectoris Study Group [see comments]. *N Engl J Med.* 1995;332(10):635–641.

62. Kluft C, Meijer P. Update 1996: Blood collection and handling procedures for assessment of plasminogen activators and inhibitors (Leiden fibrinolysis workshop). *Fibrinolysis.* 1996;10 (suppl 2):171–179.

63. Marsh NA, Gaffney PJ. The rapid fibrin plate – a method for plasminogen activator assay. *Thromb Haemost.* 1977;38(2):545–551.

64. Juhan VI, Valadier J, Alessi MC, et al. Deficient t-PA release and elevated PA inhibitor levels in patients with spontaneous or recurrent deep venous thrombosis. *Thromb Haemost.* 1987;57(1):67–72.

65. Wieczorek I, Ludlam CA, MacGregor I. Venous occlusion does not release von Willebrand factor, factor VIII or PAI-1 from endothelial cells – the importance of consensus on the use of correction factors for haemoconcentration [letter] [see comments]. *Thromb Haemost.* 1993;69(1):91–93.

66. Marckmann P, Sandstrom B, Jespersen J. The variability of and

associations between measures of blood coagulation, fibrinolysis and blood lipids. *Atherosclerosis.* 1992;96 (2–3):235–244.

67. Stegnar M, Mavri A. Reproducibility of fibrinolytic response to venous occlusion in healthy subjects. *Thromb Haemost.* 1995;73(3): 453–457.

68. Dolan G, Greaves M, Cooper P, et al. Thrombovascular disease and familial plasminogen deficiency: a report of three kindreds. *Br J Haematol.* 1988;70(4):417–421.

69. Heijboer H, Brandjes DP, Buller HR, et al. Deficiencies of coagulation-inhibiting and fibrinolytic proteins in outpatients with deep-vein thrombosis [see comments]. *N Engl J Med.* 1990;323(22): 1512–1516.

70. Mehta R, Shapiro AD. Plasminogen deficiency. *Haemophilia.* 2008;14(6): 1261–1268.

71. Holvoet P, Cleemput H, Collen D. Assay of human tissue-type plasminogen activator (t-PA) with an enzyme-linked immunosorbent assay (ELISA) based on three murine monoclonal antibodies to t-PA. *Thromb Haemost.* 1985;54(3): 684–687.

72. Mahmoud M, Gaffney PJ. Bioimmunoassay (BIA) of tissue plasminogen activator (t-PA) and its specific inhibitor (t-PA/INH). *Thromb Haemost.* 1985;53(3): 356–359.

73. Agren A, Wiman B, Stiller V, et al. Evaluation of low PAI-1 activity as a risk factor for hemorrhagic diathesis. *J Thromb Haemost.* 2006;4(1): 201–208.

74. Santamaria A, Borrell M, Mateo J, et al. What is the clinical impact of low plasminogen activator inhibitor-1 (PAI-1) activity? A case

report and study of the incidence of low PAI-1 antigen in a healthy population. *J Thromb Haemost.* 2007;5(7):1565–1566.

75. Wu KK, Hoak JC. Spontaneous platelet aggregation in arterial insufficiency: mechanisms and implications. *Thromb Haemost.* 1976;35(3):702–711.

76. Afshar-Kharghan V, Li CQ, Khoshnevis-Asl M, Lopez JA. Kozak sequence polymorphism of the glycoprotein (GP) Ibalpha gene is a major determinant of the plasma membrane levels of the platelet GP Ib-IX-V complex.[see comment]. *Blood.* 1999;94(1): 186–191.

77. Bennett JS, Catella-Lawson F, Rut AR, et al. Effect of the Pl(A2) alloantigen on the function of beta(3)-integrins in platelets. *Blood.* 2001;97(10):3093–3099.

78. Harrison P. Progress in the assessment of platelet function. *Br J Haematol.* 2000;111 (3):733–744.

79. Gatt A, Makris M. Hyperhomocysteinemia and venous thrombosis. *Semin Hematol.* 2007;44(2):70–76.

80. Undas A, Brozek J, Szczeklik A. Homocysteine and thrombosis: from basic science to clinical evidence. *Thromb Haemost.* 2005;94(5): 907–915.

81. Bauer KA, Rosenberg RD. Activation markers of coagulation. *Baillières Clin Haematol.* 1994;7(3):523–540.

82. Besser M, Baglin C, Luddington R, et al. High rate of unprovoked recurrent venous thrombosis is associated with high thrombin-generating potential in a prospective cohort study. *J Thromb Haemost.* 2008;6(10):1720–1725.

Chapter | **20** |

Laboratory control of anticoagulant, thrombolytic and antiplatelet therapy

Michael A. Laffan, Richard Manning

Anticoagulant and antithrombotic therapy is given in various doses to prevent formation or propagation of thrombus. Anticoagulant drugs, unlike fibrinolytic agents, have little if any effect on an already-formed thrombus. There are five main classes of drugs that require consideration:

1. Coumarins and indanediones, which are orally active and act by interfering with the γ-carboxylation step in the synthesis of the vitamin K-dependent factors (see p. 398).
2. Heparin, heparinoids (low molecular weight and synthetic compounds) and the heparin pentasaccharide (fondaparinux), which have a complex action on haemostasis; the main effect being the potentiation and acceleration of the effect of antithrombin.
3. Defibrinating agents such as ancrod (Viprinex) and batroxobin (Reptilase) which induce hypocoagulability by the removal of fibrinogen from the blood.
4. Direct thrombin and Xa inhibitors. These include hirudin and its derivatives (natural or recombinant) and a number of orally active synthetic compounds which are now entering clinical use.
5. Antiplatelet drugs such as aspirin, non-steroidal anti-inflammatory drugs, dipyridamole, inhibitors of the P2Y12 ADP receptor and inhibitors of IIb IIIa function, some of which are antibodies.

ORAL ANTICOAGULANT TREATMENT USING VITAMIN K ANTAGONISTS

It has not yet proved possible to produce a therapeutic reduction in thrombotic tendency without increasing the risk of haemorrhage. The purpose of laboratory control is to maintain a level of hypocoagulability that effectively minimizes the combined risks of haemorrhage and thrombosis: the therapeutic range. Individual responses to oral anticoagulant treatment with vitamin K antagonists[1] are extremely variable and so must be regularly and frequently controlled by laboratory tests to ensure that the anticoagulant effect remains within the therapeutic range.

Selection of Patients

Before starting oral anticoagulant treatment it is advisable to perform the first-line coagulation screen – a prothrombin time (PT), an activated partial thromboplastin time (APTT), a thrombin time (TT) and a platelet count. Any abnormality of these tests must be investigated because a contraindication to the use of oral anticoagulants may be revealed and an abnormality will confound their use for controlling anticoagulant effect. History and clinical examination should be assessed to ensure that no local or general haemorrhagic diathesis exists.

Methods Used for the Laboratory Control of Oral Anticoagulant Treatment

The one-stage PT of Quick is the most commonly used test. Originally, lack of standardization of the thromboplastin preparations and methods of expressing the PT results led to great discrepancies in the reported results and hence also in anticoagulant dosage. The use of the International Sensitivity Index (ISI), to assess the sensitivity of any given thromboplastin and the International Normalized Ratio (INR), to report the results, has minimized these difficulties and greatly improved uniformity of anticoagulation throughout the world.

Chromogenic substrate assays of factors X, VII or II have been used for the control of anticoagulant treatment and might be necessary when baseline tests are abnormal. Although it is possible to use such a single factor measurement, it must be remembered that the PT measures the effect of three vitamin K-dependent factors (factors VII, X and II) and is also affected by the presence of PIVKAs (proteins induced by vitamin K absence or antagonism), which are the acarboxy forms of vitamin K-dependent factors. It thus gives a better assessment of the situation *in vivo*: in addition, data on the appropriate individual factor levels corresponding to a given INR are limited.[2,3]

The Thrombotest of Owren and the prothrombin and proconvertin (P&P) method of Owren and Aas were used in the past, but they are no longer recommended for oral anticoagulant control.

Standardization of Oral Anticoagulant Treatment

Standardization of oral anticoagulant therapy comprises the following steps:

1. A thromboplastin is chosen and its ISI is determined by comparison with a reference thromboplastin.

2. The geometric mean normal PT is determined for that thromboplastin.

3. PTs are performed on patient samples and the results are converted to an INR.

Reference thromboplastins (rabbit and bovine) are available as World Health Organization (WHO) Reference Preparations via the National Institute for Biological Standards and Control (NIBSC) (www.nibsc.ac.uk), the Institute for Reference Materials and Measurements (IRMM) (Irc-irmm-rm-sales@ec.europa.eu) or certified reference materials from commercial suppliers (see p. 588). All the reference preparations have been calibrated, now sometimes indirectly, against a primary WHO reference of human brain thromboplastin, which was established in 1967.[4,5]

The following terms are used in the calibration procedure described below:

International Sensitivity Index (ISI).[4,6] This is the slope of the calibration line obtained when the PTs obtained with the reference preparation are plotted on the vertical axis of log-log paper and the PTs obtained by the test thromboplastin are plotted on the horizontal axis. The same normal and anticoagulated patients' plasma samples are used for both sets of results.

International Normalized Ratio (INR). This is the PT ratio for a sample, which, by calculation, would have been obtained had the original primary, human reference thromboplastin been used to perform the PT. Its calculation is shown below.

Calibration of Thromboplastins

Principle

The test thromboplastin should be calibrated against a reference thromboplastin of the same species (rabbit versus rabbit, bovine versus bovine) although reference plasmas from different species must at some stage be compared with each other.[3] All reference preparations are calibrated in terms of the primary material of human origin and have an ISI, which is assigned after a collaborative trial involving many laboratories from different countries.

Reagents

Normal citrated plasma. From 20 healthy donors
Anticoagulated plasma. From 60 patients stabilized on oral anticoagulant treatment for at least 6 weeks. The tests need not all be done at the same time but may be carried out on freshly collected samples on successive days
Reference and test thromboplastins
$CaCl_2$. 0.025 mol/l.

Method

Carry out PT tests as described on p. 409. Allow the plasma and thromboplastin to warm up to 37°C for at least 2 min before mixing or adding $CaCl_2$. Test each plasma in duplicate with each of the two thromboplastins in the following order with minimum delay between tests.

	REFERENCE THROMBOPLASTIN	TEST THROMBOPLASTIN
Plasma 1	Test 1	Test 2
	Test 4	Test 3
Plasma 2	Test 5	Test 6
	Test 8	Test 7, etc.

Record the mean time for each plasma. If there is a discrepancy of more than 10% in the clotting times between duplicates, repeat the test on that plasma.

Calibration

Plot the PTs on log-log graph paper, with results using the reference preparation (y) on the vertical axis and results with the test thromboplastin (x) on the horizontal axis (Fig. 20.1). On arithmetic paper, it is necessary to plot

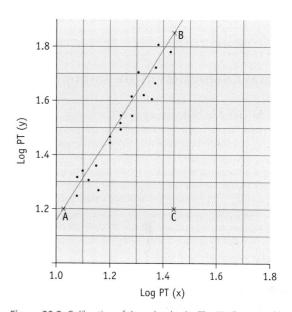

Figure 20.2 Calibration of thromboplastin. The PTs (in seconds) are converted to their logarithms, which are plotted on arithmetic graph paper. The slope is calculated as in Figure 20.1. In this example, A to C = 42 mm, B to C = 65 mm, $b = 65/42 = 1.54$. Therefore, ISI $= 1.11 \times 1.54 = 1.71$.

the logarithms of the PTs (Fig. 20.2). The relationship between the two thromboplastins is determined by the slope of the line (b).

An estimate of the slope can be obtained as shown in Figures 20.1 and 20.2; this can then be used to obtain an approximation of the ISI of the test thromboplastin.

Whenever possible, however, to obtain a reliable measurement, the following more complicated calculation should be used instead.

Calculation of International Sensitivity Index

The natural logarithms of the PTs obtained using the reference thromboplastin and the test thromboplastin are called y_i and x_i, respectively, where $i = 1,2,3\ldots$ N for N pairs of results.

The following designations are then made:

x_0 and y_0 are the arithmetic means of the N values of x_i and y_i, respectively;

Q_1 and Q_2 are the sums of the squares of (x_i-x_0) and (y_i-y_0), respectively;

P is the sum of their products $\Sigma(x_i-x_0)(y_i-y_0)$

$E = (Q_2-Q_1)^2 + 4P^2$

$$\text{And } b = \frac{Q_2 - Q_1 + E^{1/2}}{2P}$$

where b is the slope of the graph. The ISI of the preparation under test (ISI_t) is then given by the following:

Figure 20.1 Calibration of thromboplastin. The PTs (in seconds) with the test thromboplastin are plotted on the horizontal axis (x) and with the reference thromboplastin on the vertical axis (y) on double-log graph paper. The best-fit line is drawn by eye and the slope is obtained as follows: Points (A) and (B) are marked on the line just below the lowest recorded PT and just above the longest recorded PT, respectively, (C) and a vertical through (B) meet. The distance between (B) and (C) is measured accurately in mm. The slope $b = $ (B to C)/(A to C). In this example B to C = 55 mm, A to C = 35 mm, $b = 55/35 = 1.57$. The ISI of the reference thromboplastin was 1.11. Therefore, the ISI of the test thromboplastin $= 1.11 \times 1.57 = 1.74$.

$$ISI_t = ISI_{IRP} \times b$$

where IRP stands for International Reference Preparation.

Local Calibration of Thromboplastins

Although the ISI system has been very effective in standardizing anticoagulant control and improving agreement between laboratories, it is not perfect. One reason is that the ISI of a thromboplastin may vary according to the technique or coagulometer used and even with different models of the same instrument. To circumvent this, a system of local calibration has been suggested. In this system, a set of plasmas with an assigned INR are tested with the local thromboplastin–machine combination. These results are plotted on log-log paper against the assigned INR. The INR for subsequent patient samples can then be read off the graph using the locally measured PT.[3,4] Thus, the PT is converted directly into an INR without the need for measurement of the ISI.

Geometric Mean Normal Prothrombin Time

The geometric mean normal PT (GMNPT) for each batch of thromboplastin should be determined by testing 20 normal samples or blood donors. An equal number of males and females should be tested.

Calibration Audits

External quality-assurance surveys (e.g. UKNEQAS, see p. 594) will reflect differences regarding thromboplastin–machine combinations but not differences in blood sampling techniques (i.e. capillary and venous blood sampling). This can be a problem when capillary blood sampling is used in an outpatient setting, whereas venous samples are taken for inpatient anticoagulant monitoring. Regular audits comparing results from a range of patients whose blood has been sampled by both capillary and venous techniques will provide information not provided by NEQAS surveys.[4,5]

Determination of the International Normalized Ratio

If a local calibration scheme is not used, then it is essential to use a thromboplastin whose ISI has been determined either by the commercial supplier or (preferably) according to a local, regional or national procedure. The PT result can then be expressed as an INR. Using the INR/ISI system, the patient's INR should be the same in any laboratory in the world. To ensure safety and uniformity of anticoagulation, the results should be reported as an INR, either alone or in parallel with the locally accepted method of reporting.

INR = prothrombin time ratio obtained using the test thromboplastin to the power of the ISI of the test reagent.

The PT ratio is calculated using the patient's test result and the geometric mean normal prothrombin time (GMNPT) from 20 normal donors: INR = (PT patient/GMNPT)^{ISI}.

For example, a ratio of 2.5 using a thromboplastin with ISI of 1.4 can be calculated from the formula to be $2.5^{1.4} = 3.61$, which is either read from a logarithmic table or calculated on an electronic calculator.

The GMNPT is the logarithmic mean normal PT (i.e. $e^{(\Sigma lnPT)/N}$). In this way, the level of anticoagulation in all plasma samples can be compared and a meaningful therapeutic range can be established regardless of the thromboplastin used.

Capillary Reagent

Reagents are commercially available for monitoring the INR using samples of capillary blood. These are usually a mixture of thromboplastin, calcium and adsorbed plasma so that when whole blood is added the reagent measures the overall clotting activity; it is sensitive to deficiency of factors II, VII and X. The reagents have an ISI assigned to them in the same way as individual thromboplastins and the INR is calculated from the PT ratio. These reagents are frequently used in anticoagulant clinics, when a large number of INRs need to be performed rapidly, and in point-of-care testing (see p. 471).

Therapeutic Range and Choice of Thromboplastin

Several authorities have now published recommended therapeutic ranges denoting the appropriate degree of anticoagulation in different clinical circumstances.[7,8] These are largely based on controlled clinical trials but to some extent also represent a consensus on practice that has emerged over many years.

The choice of thromboplastin largely determines the accuracy with which anticoagulant control can be maintained. If the ISI of the thromboplastin is high, then a small change in PT represents a large change in the degree of anticoagulation. This affects the precision of the analysis and the coefficient of variation for the test increases with the ISI. Moreover, the target prothrombin ratio range becomes very small for any given range of INR. This is illustrated in Figure 20.3 and Table 20.1. For these reasons, it is strongly recommended that a thromboplastin with a low ISI (i.e. close to 1) is used.

Management of Overanticoagulation

The approach to management of a patient whose INR exceeds the therapeutic range with or without bleeding is shown in Table 20.2.[7]

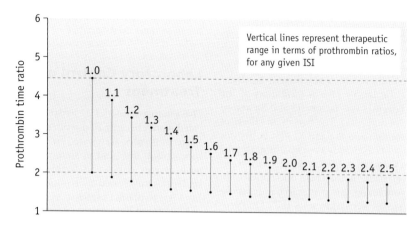

Figure 20.3 The ratios obtained with thromboplastins with given ISI values equivalent to INR therapeutic range of 2.0–4.5. *(Slightly modified, from Poller L 1987 Oral anticoagulant therapy. In: Bloom AL, Thomas DP (eds) Haemostasis and Thrombosis, 2nd edition. Churchill Livingstone, Edinburgh, with permission.)*

Table 20.1 Therapeutic ranges equivalent to an INR of 2.0–4.0 using different commercial thromboplastins

THROMBOPLASTIN	ISI	RATIOS EQUIVALENT TO INR 2.0–4.0
Thrombotest	1.03	2.0–3.8
Thromborel	1.23	1.7–3.1
Dade FS	1.35	1.65–2.8
Simplastin	2.0	1.3–2.0
Boehringer	2.1	1.35–1.9
Ortho	2.3	1.3–1.8

ISI, International Sensitivity Index; INR, International Normalized Ratio. (Modified from Poller L 1987 Oral anticoagulant therapy. In: Bloom AL, Thomas DP (eds) *Haemostasis and Thrombosis*, p. 870, 2nd edition. Churchill Livingstone, Edinburgh.)

Table 20.2 Recommendations for management of bleeding and excessive anticoagulation[7]

3.0<INR<6.0 (target INR 2.5)	1. Reduce warfarin dose or stop
4.0<INR<6.0 (target INR 3.5)	2. Restart warfarin when INR <5.0
6.0<INR<8.0 No bleeding or minor bleeding	1. Stop warfarin 2. Restart when INR <5.0
INR >8.0 No bleeding or minor bleeding	1. Stop warfarin 2. Restart warfarin when INR <5.0 3. If other risk factors for bleeding give 0.5–2.5 mg of vitamin K (oral or i.v.)
Major bleeding	1. Stop warfarin 2. Give PCC 30–50 u/kg or FFP 15 ml/kg if PCC not available 3. Give 5 mg of vitamin K (i.v.)

FFP, fresh-frozen plasma; INR, International Normalized Ratio; PCC, prothrombin complex concentrate.

Point-of-Care Testing

There are now schemes for monitoring INR at point of care outside the hospital clinic. These require selection and standardization of appropriate analysers and a quality-control programme that includes participation in an external quality assessment scheme. It is essential to have liaison with the local laboratory for training of staff and supervision of the quality-control programme. There should be an established procedure for checking any problems of instrument performance and for referring to the specialist centre patients who are difficult to control.[9,10]

Self-management of warfarin treatment akin to home glucose monitoring may also be an effective point-of-care procedure for selected patients. They should first attend two or more training sessions on the use and quality control of the appropriate analyser, interpretation of INR, adjustment of warfarin dosage and guidance on when it is necessary to be seen at the specialist clinic.[10]

HEPARIN TREATMENT

The anticoagulant action of heparin is primarily a result of its ability to bind to antithrombin (AT), thereby accelerating and enhancing the latter's rate of inhibition of the major coagulation enzymes (i.e. factors IIa and Xa and to lesser extents IXa, XIa and XIIa). The two main effects of heparin, the antithrombin and the anti-Xa effects, are differentially dependent on the size of the heparin molecule. The basic minimum sequence needed to promote anticoagulant activity has been identified as a pentasaccharide unit. Of the molecules containing this pentasaccharide, those comprising fewer than 18 saccharide units and of molecular weight <5000 Da can only augment the inhibitory activity of AT against Xa. In contrast, longer chains can augment anti-IIa activity as well by formation of a tertiary complex bridging both AT and thrombin molecules.

Hence, low molecular weight heparins (LMWHs), which have an average molecular mass of 5000 Da, have a ratio of anti-Xa to antithrombin effect of 2–5 compared with that of unfractionated heparin (UFH), which is defined as having a ratio of 1. However, all heparin preparations are heterogeneous mixtures of molecules with different molecular weight and many do not contain the crucial pentasaccharide sequence. Heparin also produces some anticoagulant effect by promoting the release of tissue factor pathway inhibitor (TFPI) from the endothelium (see p. 399).

Selection of Patients

It is advisable to perform the first-line tests of haemostasis (as described in Chapter 18) before starting treatment. In the presence of a reduced platelet count or deranged coagulation, heparin may be contraindicated or, if used, the dose must be reduced.

Laboratory Control of Heparin Treatment

The pharmacokinetics of heparins are extremely complicated, partly because of the variation in molecule size.[11,12] Large molecules are cleared by a rapid saturable cellular mechanism and bind to numerous acute-phase proteins such as von Willebrand factor and fibronectin. Smaller molecules are cleared by a non-saturable renal route and bind less to plasma proteins. As a result, therapeutic doses of UFH result in a variable degree of anticoagulation and require close monitoring (Table 20.3). The dose–response relationship is much more predictable for the LMWHs and most trials have not monitored therapy with these agents, which are simply given on a 'units per kg' dosing regimen. Thus the approach to monitoring heparin therapy varies according to the type of heparin used and the clinical circumstance.

Prophylactic therapy with either UFH or LMWH is given by subcutaneous injection and is usually not monitored. However, LMWHs may be monitored in some circumstances when it is expected that pharmacokinetics may be altered, such as during pregnancy and in renal failure. A blood sample is taken 4 h after subcutaneous injection to detect the peak heparin level. Some authors have also measured trough levels prior to injection.

Therapeutic treatment with UFH is given by continuous intravenous infusion and is usually monitored using the APTT, which is repeated 6 h after every dose change. Rarely, therapeutic UFH is given twice daily by subcutaneous injection, in which case samples for testing should be taken at

Table 20.3 Tests used in the laboratory control of heparin treatment

TEST	ADVANTAGES	DISADVANTAGES
Whole-blood clotting time	Simple, inexpensive, no equipment needed	Time consuming, can only be carried out at the bedside, one at a time, insensitive to <0.4 iu/ml anti-Xa and to LMW heparins
APTT	Simple, many tests can be carried out in parallel	Not all reagents sensitive to heparin, insensitive to <0.2 iu/ml anti-Xa and to LMW heparins, affected by variables other than heparin
TT	Simple, many tests can be carried out in parallel	Insensitive to <0.2 iu/ml and to LMW heparins. Steep dose–response
Protamine neutralization	Sensitive to all concentrations	Time consuming and insensitive to LMW heparins
Anti-Xa assays	Sensitive to all concentrations and to LMW heparins	Expensive if commercial kits used; time consuming if home-made reagents used. Not clear that anti-Xa is the clinically relevant measure

APTT, activated partial thromboplastin time; LMW, low molecular weight; TT, thrombin time.

the midpoint between injections. If heparin resistance is suspected, then an anti-Xa assay must be performed.

LMWHs have relatively little effect on the APTT and if monitoring is required, a specific heparin assay must be used. The result will then be reported as heparin activity in u/ml. In general, unless stated otherwise, this is measured as anti-Xa activity. International standards for UFH[13] and for LMWH are now available and the assay results reported in iu/ml.[14]

It is important to note that therapeutic levels of LMWH may be present without producing prolongation of PT, APTT or TT. The dose–response curve of the TT is too steep to make it useful for monitoring heparin therapy. However, it is very sensitive to the presence of UFH and is a useful laboratory indicator of its presence.

Activated Partial Thromboplastin Time for Heparin Monitoring

Principle

The APTT is the most widely used test for monitoring unfractionated heparin therapy. It is very sensitive to heparin but has a number of shortcomings that must be kept in mind. First, different APTT reagents have different sensitivities to heparin. It is important to establish that the reagent in use has a linear relationship between clotting times and heparin concentration in the therapeutic range (0.35–0.7 anti-Xa iu/ml). An example of different responses is shown in Figure 20.4. The result is expressed as a ratio of the time obtained with that for the normal pool containing no heparin (often called 'the heparin ratio').

The second shortcoming of the APTT in the control of heparin treatment is that the APTT is affected by a number of variables not related to heparin. The most important of these are fibrinogen and factor VIII concentration and the presence of fibrinogen/fibrin degradation products (FDPs). When these factors are abnormal, there may be dissociation of the APTT and heparin level causing 'apparent heparin resistance'. In these circumstances a heparin assay must be performed. Last, the use of the APTT may be rendered invalid by the presence of inhibitors, factor deficiency (including liver disease) or other coagulation-active drugs. In severely ill patients a significant prolongation of the APTT may arise from disseminated intravascular coagulation (DIC) or haemodilution, giving a misleading impression of heparin effect. It has not proved possible to develop for APTT reagents a calibration system equivalent to the ISI employed for thromboplastins in the PT.

Reagents and Method

The reagents and method are described on p. 410.

Figure 20.4 APTT response to heparin added to plasma *in vitro*. APTT response expressed as ratio (APTT of heparinized plasma/APTT of plasma without heparin). Three different reagents and methods are shown.
(Slightly modified from Thomson JM (ed) 1985 Blood Coagulation and Haemostasis. A Practical Guide, p. 370. Churchill Livingstone, Edinburgh, with permission.)

Therapeutic Range

The therapeutic range for heparin is 0.35–0.7 iu/ml by anti-Xa assay and 0.2–0.4 iu/ml by protamine titration. The prolongation of the APTT achieved with these concentrations varies between reagents according to the reagents and coagulometer used. The results may be expressed as clotting time in seconds or as a ratio. For the majority of sensitive reagents, ratios of 1.5–3.0 cover the therapeutic range, but this must be determined for each reagent and, ideally, each batch of reagent. It is important that samples from patients treated with heparin are used for calibration because these give significantly different results from those obtained when normal plasma is 'spiked' with heparin. Regression analysis is used to determine the normal range and a better fit may be obtained using logarithmically transformed APTT values. Plasma from samples for heparin monitoring should be separated within 2 hours because heparin activity is lost with time.

Near-Patient Heparin Monitoring

The whole-blood activated clotting time (ACT) is routinely used to assess heparin effects during cardiac surgery. However, the ACT is not a specific assay for heparin and may be influenced by several other factors such as hypothermia, haemodilution and platelet dysfunction. For these reasons the ACT may be misleading with regard to the proper administration of heparin and protamine.[15]

Principle

The ACT is determined by using one of several different clotting cascade activators, such as kaolin or celite (diatomaceous earth activator) to which a sample of whole blood is added and a method of endpoint detection such as optical or electromagnetic. No additional phospholipid is added. A number of commercial devices are available suitable for use in operating theatres. The ACT is thus primarily a system with little laboratory involvement.

Anti-Xa Assay for Heparin

Principle

Plasma anti-Xa activity as a result of antithrombin is enhanced by the addition of heparin and either a coagulation or amidolytic (chromogenic) assay of anti-Xa activity can be adapted to measure this effect. A standard curve is constructed by adding varying amounts of heparin to a normal plasma pool, which provides the source of the antithrombin. A known amount of Xa is added and, after incubation, the amount of Xa remaining is assayed by chromogenic or coagulation-based assay. A number of commercial kits based on clotting or chromogenic substrate methods are in use but although they give linear and reproducible responses, studies have shown considerable variation between kits.[16] A standard curve should be constructed that is appropriate for the level of heparin expected. Some but not all assays add an exogenous source of antithrombin to the test sample, but it is not clear how important this is in patients with low antithrombin levels.

Chromogenic Method

The assay is performed as instructed with the kit. The concentration of heparin is read off a standard curve constructed according to the manufacturer's instructions.

Clotting Method

Principle

The anti-Xa activity of antithrombin is enhanced by the addition of heparin. The inhibition of factor Xa induced by heparin is measured in a modified factor-X assay.

Reagents

Pooled normal plasma. From 20 normal donors

Patient's plasma. Citrated platelet-poor plasma (PPP) should be collected 4 h after subcutaneous injection of LMWH, 6 h after subcutaneous injection of UFH and 6 h after a dose change of UFH infusion; it should be tested as soon as possible after the collection and kept at 4°C or on crushed ice until tested

Buffer. Trisodium citrate 30 volumes, glyoxaline buffer (see p. 409) 150 volumes and 20% bovine albumin 1 volume

Commercially prepared artificial factor X-deficient plasma. Reconstitute according to instructions

Platelet substitute. Mix equal volumes of factor X-deficient plasma and platelet substitute. This is the working reagent and is kept at 37°C

Factor Xa. Reconstitute as instructed by the manufacturer. Dilute further in the buffer to give a 1 in 100 dilution. Keep on crushed ice until used

Heparin. 1000 iu/ml or as supplied by the manufacturer. Dilute in 9 g/l NaCl to 10 iu/ml. Ideally, the same batch of heparin as the patient is receiving should be used

$CaCl_2$. 0.025 mol/l.

Method

A standard curve is constructed as shown in Table 20.4. Add 0.05 ml of each dilution to 0.45 ml of the normal plasma pool. This will give final concentrations of heparin from 0.05 to 0.30 iu/ml in 0.05 iu steps.

Pipette 0.3 ml of diluted factor Xa into a large glass tube at 37°C.

Add 0.1 ml of the first standard dilution. Start the stopwatch. At 1 min and 30 s exactly transfer duplicate 0.1 ml volumes of the mixture into two tubes each containing 0.1 ml of prewarmed $CaCl_2$.

Table 20.4 Preparation of a standard curve for an anti-Xa assay

REAGENT	TUBE					
	1	2	3	4	5	6
Heparin (10 iu/ml) (ml)	0.05	0.10	0.15	0.20	0.25	0.30
Saline (ml)	0.95	0.90	0.85	0.80	0.75	0.70
Concentration of heparin (iu/ml)	0.5	1.0	1.5	2.0	2.5	3.0
Final conc. of heparin after addition to normal plasma pool	0.05	0.10	0.15	0.20	0.25	0.30

At 2 min after subsampling add 0.2 ml of the mixture of factor X-deficient plasma and platelet substitute, start the stopwatch, mix and record the clotting time.

Repeat for each dilution of standard. The patient's sample is tested undiluted in pooled normal plasma if the clotting time is longer than the times used to construct the standard curve.

Calculation

Plot the clotting times against the heparin concentration on log-linear graph paper, with the clotting times on the linear axis. The concentration of heparin in the patient's sample can be read directly from the standard curve. It is multiplied by the dilution factor if necessary.

Protamine Neutralization Test

Principle

This test is an extension of the TT, varying amounts of protamine sulphate being added to the plasma before the addition of thrombin. When all the heparin present in plasma has been neutralized, the clotting time should become normal. The concentration of heparin in the plasma can be calculated from the amount of protamine sulphate required to produce this effect. The protamine neutralization test is used mainly to calculate the dose of protamine sulphate needed to neutralize circulating heparin after cardiopulmonary surgery or haemodialysis, but it can also be used to control treatment or to calculate the dose of protamine to be administered if the patient needs rapid reversal of heparinization.

Reagents

Protamine sulphate. Dilute protamine in barbitone buffer, pH 7.4. Dilute 5 ml of protamine sulphate (10 mg/ml) 1 in 20 with buffer to give 1 dl of a stock solution containing 500 μg/ml. Then make working solutions to cover the range of 0–500 μg/ml in 50 μg steps from the stock solution by dilution with buffer. The solutions keep indefinitely at 4°C

Thrombin. Dilute thrombin in barbitone buffer to a concentration of about 20 National Institutes of Health (NIH) u/ml. Adjust the concentration so that 0.1 ml of thrombin solution clots 0.2 ml of normal plasma at 37°C in 10 ± 1 s. Keep the thrombin in a plastic tube in melting ice during the assay

Plasma. Citrated PPP from the patient.

Method

Place 0.2 ml of test plasma and 20 μl of barbitone buffer in a glass tube kept in a waterbath at 37°C. Allow the mixture to warm and then add 0.1 ml of thrombin. Record the clotting time. If this is *c* 10 s, there is no demonstrable heparin in the plasma. If the TT is prolonged, repeat the test using 20 μl of the 500 μg/ml protamine solution instead of buffer. Repeat the test if necessary, until a concentration of protamine is found that gives a clotting time of *c* 10 s.

Calculation

If 20 μl of 150 μg/ml protamine sulphate produce a normal TT (whereas the clotting time is prolonged with 100 μg/ml protamine), then the concentration of 15 μg of protamine is sufficient to neutralize the heparin in 1 ml of plasma. Assuming weight-for-weight neutralization, the patient's plasma contains 15 μg of heparin per ml or 1.5 iu, assuming that 1 mg of heparin is equivalent to 100 iu. This figure can be further converted to concentration of heparin per ml of whole blood by multiplying by 1 − haematocrit (Hct).

In the previous example, for *in vivo* neutralization of heparin by protamine sulphate, assuming a total blood volume of 75 ml per kg body weight, the required dose of protamine (in mg) would be as follows:

$$\frac{15 \times 75 \times \text{bodyweight} \times (1 - \text{Hct})}{1000}$$

Heparin-Induced Thrombocytopenia

Most patients receiving unfractionated heparin experience a small and immediate drop in their platelet count. In the past this has been referred to as type 1 heparin-induced thrombocytopenia (HIT) and is completely harmless. It is thought to arise as a result of heparin binding to platelets. The term HIT is now used more generally to describe a second more serious thrombocytopenia (type II HIT) seen in approximately 5% of patients receiving UFH and which is a result of development of antibodies against heparin-platelet factor 4 (PF4) complexes. The antigen–antibody complexes bind to and activate platelets via the FCRγII, resulting in accelerated clearance. Type II HIT develops 5–12 days after starting heparin therapy and causes a profound decrease in platelets to <50% of preheparin value and usually $<50 \times 10^9$/l. The process of activation sometimes results in arterial, or more frequently venous, platelet thrombus formation particularly in patients who are ill or septic and skin necrosis has also been reported. This syndrome of heparin-induced thrombocytopenia and thrombosis (HITT) has a high mortality. Heparin must be stopped immediately and alternative immediate-acting anticoagulation must be instituted.[17]

The diagnosis of HIT is primarily clinical and there is no test that can be performed with sufficient speed, sensitivity and specificity to positively guide the primary decision to stop heparin. The decision to perform laboratory tests and the interpretation of the results should always be performed after consideration of the clinical likelihood or pre-test probability.[18] A simple scoring scheme (the 4 Ts system) has been devised and tested for this purpose (Table 20.5).[19]

However, antibody tests do have sufficient sensitivity to reliably exclude the diagnosis while lacking the specificity to positively identify it. Thus confirmatory information is useful and a number of tests can be performed to substantiate the diagnosis.[20,21] These may be either *functional* tests in which platelet activation is detected or *immunological* tests in which the presence of PF4–heparin-dependent antibodies are detected. Examples of the former include what is regarded as the 'gold standard' test, the serotonin release assay,[22] but this is too cumbersome and inconvenient for routine use. Alternatives are heparin-induced platelet aggregation and flow cytometry-based tests.[23] The simplest for routine use is a modified platelet aggregation test as described in the following section.[24] Although the immunological tests appear to have greater sensitivity and are more easily reproducible, they do not demonstrate the functional significance of the antibodies.

Heparin-Induced Thrombocytopenia: Detection by Platelet Aggregation

Addition of heparin to the patient's PPP results in heparin–PF4 complexes that are bound by the pathological antibody. The antibody-heparin–PF4 complexes then bind to and activate the platelets. Platelet activation is detected as aggregation.

Principle

Blood is centrifuged gently to obtain platelet-rich plasma (PRP), which is stirred in a cuvette at 37°C, between a light source and a photocell.

Reagents

Normal control platelet-rich plasma (PRP). Preferably blood group O or the same group as the patient should be used. (For method see p. 433.) A platelet count is performed on the PRP. The number of platelets will influence aggregation response if the count falls outside a range of 200–400 × 10^9/l. If necessary the PRP is adjusted to give a platelet count of 300 × 10^9/l by diluting with control platelet-poor plasma (PPP).

Patient and normal control PPP. Are obtained by centrifuging at 2000 *g* for 20 min. Check that the platelet count is zero.

Heparin. A sample of the type (batch identical) of heparin previously given to the patient is required. The heparin is diluted to give working concentrations of 10 and 20 iu/ml (final concentration of 1.0 and 2.0 iu/ml).

Method

Following the scheme shown in Table 20.6, four aggregation cuvettes are set up. Add 300 µl of normal PRP to each cuvette. Then add 200 µl of the appropriate patient or control PPP, along with a magnetic stir bar. Set the 100% baselines with the normal control PPP and the 0% baselines with PRP and PPP. Set the stir rate at 1200 rpm. Observe the baselines for 1 min. Initiate aggregation by the addition of 50 µl of either heparin or saline. Observe aggregation for a minimum of 15 min (Fig. 20.5).

1. If aggregation (>20%) is observed in cuvette 4 with a final heparin concentration of 1.0 and 2.0 iu/ml, the test is repeated using normal platelets, patient plasma and a final heparin concentration of 0.2 iu/ml.

2. Aggregation observed in cuvette 4 only, with subsequent demonstration of heparin-induced

---

Table 20.5 Pre-test clinical scoring system to assess the likelihood of HIT

SCORE	2	1	0
Thrombocytopenia	>50% Platelet count fall to nadir >20 × 10^9/l	30–50% Platelet count fall or nadir 10–19 × 10^9/l	<30% Platelet count fall or nadir <10 × 10^9/l
Time of platelet fall (or other sequelae)[a]	Days 5–10 or day 1 with recent prior heparin (previous 30 days)	Day 10 or later or timing unclear; or day 1 with less recent heparin (previous 31–100 days)	Day 4 or earlier (but no recent prior heparin)
Thrombosis	Proven new thrombosis, skin necrosis or acute systemic reaction after intravenous UFH bolus	Progressive or recurrent thrombosis; erythematous skin lesions; suspected thrombosis (not proven)	None
Other explanation equally plausible	None evident	Possible	Definite

UFH, unfractionated heparin. Pre-test probability score: 6–8 indicates high; 4–5, intermediate; and 0–3, low.
[a]First day of heparin exposure is counted as day 0. Sequelae such as thrombosis or skin necrosis.

Table 20.6 The combinations of platelets, plasma and heparin required to test for heparin-induced thrombocytopenia

	CUVETTE 1	CUVETTE 2	CUVETTE 3	CUVETTE 4
Normal control PRP	300 µl	300 µl	300 µl	300 µl
Patient PPP	None	200 µl	None	200 µl
Normal control PPP	200 µl	None	200 µl	None
Heparin (10 or 20 iu/ml)	None	None	50 µl	50 µl
Saline (0.85%)	50 µl	50 µl	None	None

PRP, platelet-rich plasma; PPP, platelet-poor plasma.

	Black	Green	Red	Purple
Normal control PRP	300 µl	300 µl	300 µl	300 µl
Patient PPP	None	200 µl	None	200 µl
Normal control PPP	200 µl	None	200 µl	None
Heparin (10 or 20 iu/ml)	None	None	50 µl	50 µl
Saline (0.85%)	50 µl	50 µl	None	None

Figure 20.5 The combinations of platelets, plasma and heparin required to test for heparin-induced thrombocytopenia shown in Table 20.6. The aggregation traces show that platelet aggregation occurs only when the patient plasma is exposed to heparin (purple trace).

aggregation at a final concentration of 0.2 iu/ml, is considered positive for heparin-induced platelet aggregation.

3. A confirmatory step can be performed by repeating the test using a much higher final concentration of heparin (10–100 iu/ml). Inhibition of aggregation is suggestive of heparin-induced platelet aggregation.

4. Aggregation observed in cuvettes 1, 2 or 3 indicates that the reaction may be a result of something other than heparin-induced platelet aggregation and the test is repeated using different normal donor platelets and control PPP.

With experience, subjective assessment of aggregation responses is usually sufficient for clinical interpretation. A positive test result is shown in Figure 20.5. The total amount of aggregation seen may be reported.

Interpretation

See platelet aggregation (see p. 432).

Reported studies using platelet aggregation tests indicate they have a high specificity for HIT that is >90%. However, the sensitivity of the test is more variable and, although >80% on some occasions,[24] it is frequently much nearer 50–60% and therefore cannot reliably exclude HIT. The literature suggests that test sensitivity can be improved by the use of the patient's own platelets, platelets from selected donors known to be reactive in the assay or washed platelets.[25] The reactivity of the donor platelets can be established by using a known positive serum. Test specificity is enhanced by including neutralization of the reaction by a high dose of heparin but this is not always observed.

Immunological Tests for Heparin–PF4 Antibodies

Several commercial kits are available for detection of antibodies directed against the heparin–platelet factor 4 complex. These include enzyme immunoassays; 'PF4 enhanced' (GTI Diagnostics, Waukesha, WI, USA) and 'Zymutest HIA IgG' (Hyphen BioMed, Neuville-Sur-Oise, France), an immunofiltration kit (Akers Biosciences, Inc, Thorofare, NJ, USA) and a particle gel immunoassay which is described below. The first two of these have reported high sensitivity (>90%) for the presence of antibodies and although they lack specificity, have reasonable utility. The test performance can be improved by using the optical density (OD) to assign a probability of a true positive result.[26] The immunofiltration assay did not perform so well in one study[27] but subsequent reports were more encouraging.[28] These tests are performed according to the manufacturers' instructions.

Diamed Heparin–PF4 Antibody Test

The Diamed Heparin–PF4 antibody test[28] is a particle gel immunoassay consisting of red-coloured polymer particles coated with heparin–PF4 complex. When the patient's serum is mixed with the polymer particles, specific antibodies react with the heparin–PF4 complex on the particle surface, resulting in particle agglutination. The particles are centrifuged through a gel filtration matrix, agglutinated particles are trapped on top of the gel or within the gel and non-agglutinated particles form a button at the bottom of the tube. The result can be read visually.

HIRUDIN

Recombinant manufactured hirudin is now available and licensed for both prophylactic and therapeutic use in some indications. It is a direct thrombin inhibitor and is given intravenously or subcutaneously. It is most easily monitored using the APTT with the same target range as for heparin. The TT may be prolonged but the Reptilase time will be normal. An alternative measure is the ecarin clotting time (ECT). This is thought to be more accurate at high doses of hirudin but may give falsely high results when the amount of prothrombin in the sample is reduced below 50%. It is also useful when other factors such as antiphospholipid antibodies are causing prolongation of the APTT.

After 5 days therapy, 45% of patients will develop anti-hirudin antibodies, which may enhance or reduce the therapeutic effect. Hirudin is excreted via the kidneys and close monitoring is necessary, with dose reduction if renal impairment is present.

Ecarin Clotting Time

Ecarin[29] is a snake venom (*Echis carinatus*) that directly activates prothrombin to meizothrombin. This action is not dependent on phospholipid membranes and so is not impaired by the presence of lupus anticoagulant or by inadequate prothrombin carboxylation due to warfarin therapy. The activity of meizothrombin is not inhibited by heparin-antithrombin and can be detected by a clotting or chromogenic assay.

Reagents

Ecarin solution. Reconstituted according to manufacturer's instructions and diluted to 4 u/ml with buffer
Buffer. HEPES buffered saline (0.2 M) containing 0.025 M calcium chloride
Patient PPP.

Warm the reagents to 37°C.

Add 50 μl of ecarin reagent to 100 μl of PPP and record clotting time.

The clotting time for normal plasma is approximately 50 s. A standard curve can be created using appropriate dilutions of the thrombin inhibitor in question added to normal plasma. Commercial ecarin activity tests using chromogenic substrates for meizothrombin are also available.

ORAL ANTI-IIA AND ANTI-XA AGENTS

A number of orally active direct inhibitors of IIa and Xa are entering clinical use. The implications for laboratory practice are unclear because clinical trials have been carried out without monitoring of anticoagulant effect. However, it is likely that some measurement, or at least detection, of their effect will be required in some circumstances such as bleeding or renal failure. Anti-Xa activity can be measured as described for heparin but anti-IIa activity appears to be best measured using the ecarin clotting time (ECT). This test has previously been employed to measure high levels of hirudin because the ECT has a linear relationship with hirudin concentration over a greater range than the APTT.[30]

THROMBOLYTIC THERAPY

The thrombolytic agents currently in use are principally streptokinase and recombinant tissue-type plasminogen activator (rtPA). Tenecteplase and reteplase are genetically modified forms of tPA.

Streptokinase

Streptokinase is a purified fraction of the filtrate from cultures of *Streptokinase haemolyticus*. Streptokinase interacts with plasminogen or plasmin to form a plasminogen activator in plasma. The activator complex in turn cleaves a bond in the plasminogen molecule to give rise to free plasmin. Streptokinase therefore results in systemic fibrinogenolysis as well as lysis of fibrin clot. Streptokinase is a foreign protein and induces antibody production in humans, limiting a course of treatment to 3–5 days. It is recommended that 2 years should elapse before repeated administrations of streptokinase. It also cross-reacts with antistreptococcal antibodies, which may cause resistance to therapy, although this is usually overcome with large doses.

Tissue-Type Plasminogen Activator

The tissue-type plasminogen activator is a single- or double-chain polypeptide obtained by recombinant techniques or from tissue cultures. Plasminogen and tPA both have a high affinity for fibrin which acts a cofactor bringing the two molecules together and greatly accelerating plasmin formation. tPA thus causes less systemic fibrinogenolysis than any of the previously mentioned agents, although some decrease in circulating fibrinogen does occur, particularly with prolonged administration. It induces a thrombolytic state of longer duration than either streptokinase or urokinase infusion.

Selection of Patients

Thrombolytic treatment carries a serious risk of bleeding and thrombolytic agents should not be given to individuals after surgery or trauma or who are at a high risk of bleeding. In addition, each patient should have haemostatic function and platelet count measured before treatment is started.

Laboratory Control of Thrombolytic Therapy

Many laboratory tests are abnormal during thrombolytic therapy,[31] but a perfect and specific procedure for monitoring is not available. In practice, thrombolytic therapy is given rapidly according to protocol, with no time or need for adjustment of dosage. During thrombolytic therapy all screening tests of coagulation are prolonged, reflecting the hyperplasminaemic state with the reduction in the fibrinogen concentration and the presence of FDP. The prolongation is most marked with streptokinase and streptokinase–plasminogen complex; it is less marked with urokinase and least with tPA. The fibrinogen concentration commonly decreases to below 0.05 g/l and the FDP concentration may increase to more than 1000 ng/l.

Monitoring of therapy is only recommended for treatment lasting longer than 24 h. If possible, a sample should be obtained prior to treatment. Samples taken after fibrinolysis has begun should be taken into citrate plus an inhibitor of fibrinolysis such as aprotinin (250 u/ml) or ε-aminocaproic acid (EACA: 0.07 mol/l). The fibrinolytic state will affect several tests.

Activated Partial Thromboplastin Time

With effective fibrinolysis the APTT is likely to be prolonged >1.5 times control. This is a result of fibrinogen, factor V and factor VIII depletion and interference from FDPs. There are, however, no data to correlate APTT with therapeutic effect.

Thrombin Time

The TT can be used to monitor therapy. A few hours after the start of the infusion, the TT is prolonged to 40 s or more (control 15 ± 1 s); it then settles to approximately 20–30 s. Very long TTs carry a high risk of bleeding and are indicative of severe hyperplasminaemia.

Plasma Fibrinogen

Depending on duration of therapy and the specific plasminogen activator used, there is a variable decrease in fibrinogen. The fibrinogen should be measured by a method dependent on clottable fibrinogen (e.g. Clauss technique, see p. 412). The PT-derived fibrinogen is likely to be unreliable. Fibrin(ogen) degradation products will be elevated, but this is unlikely to be helpful.

Investigation of a Patient Who Bleeds While Taking Thrombolytic Agents or Immediately Afterwards

Haemorrhage is an inevitable risk associated with fibrinolytic therapy and may occur despite normal coagulation tests. When severe, bleeding will necessitate cessation of fibrinolysis and administration of tranexamic acid to inhibit its activity. Coagulation tests may guide replacement therapy with plasma or cryoprecipitate.

ANTIPLATELET THERAPY

Many drugs inhibit platelet function *in vitro*, but only a few have antiplatelet activity in acceptable doses. Each category of drugs has a different pharmacological action and requires different methods to demonstrate its effect on platelets. Antiplatelet agents are used in primary and secondary prevention of coronary heart disease, in unstable angina, in certain forms of cerebrovascular disease, to prevent thromboembolism associated with valvular disease and prosthetic heart valves and to prevent thrombosis in arteriovenous shunts. Haematology laboratories are only rarely asked to monitor these aspects of antiplatelet therapy. Indeed, it is said that the advantage of these agents is that monitoring is unnecessary.

Interest has been revived in the observation that some patients do not respond to aspirin. 'Aspirin resistance' is poorly defined and sometimes apparent resistance may be merely the result of a failure to take the medication. Otherwise this term may refer either to a failure to inhibit platelet function or a failure to suppress thromboxane A_2 production. The first may be detected by platelet function analysers such as the PFA-100 (see p. 425) or by platelet aggregation responses; the second may be detected by serum thromboxane B_2 levels or the metabolite 11-dehydro TXB_2 in the urine. A similar 'resistance' has been identified in patients taking clopidogrel, which blocks the platelet P2Y12 receptor. The effect of clopidogrel can be detected by demonstrating a reduced response to ADP in a modification of the standard platelet light transmission aggregometry (see p. 432). In addition a number of commercial assays are available to monitor antiplatelet therapy or to detect resistance. The PFA-100 is sensitive to aspirin but not clopidogrel effect. Monitoring antiplatelet therapy has not reached routine hospital practice: first, because the clinical utility of these assessments and the appropriate responses are not established;[32,33] and second, because a series of new antiplatelet agents with more reliable dose–response characteristics have been introduced.

REFERENCES

1. Ansell J, Hirsh J, Hylek E, et al. Pharmacology and management of the vitamin K antagonists: American College of Chest Physicians Evidence-based Clinical Practice Guidelines, 8th edition. *Chest*. 2008;133(supp 6):160S–198S.

2. Costa IM, Serralheiro AI, Rodrigues M, et al. Usefulness of factor II and factor X as therapeutic markers in patients under chronic warfarin therapy. *Biomed Pharmacother*. 2010;64(2):130–132.

3. Lind SE, Callas PW, Golden EA, et al. Plasma levels of factors II, VII and X and their relationship to the international normalized ratio during chronic warfarin therapy. *Blood Coagul Fibrinolysis*. 1997;8(1):48–53.

4. World Health Organization. Guidelines for thromboplastins and plasma used to control oral anticoagulant therapy. *World Health Organ Tech Rep Ser*. 1999;889:64–93.

5. Chantarangkul V, van den Besselaar AM, Witteveen E, et al. International collaborative study for the calibration of a proposed international standard for thromboplastin, rabbit, plain. *J Thromb Haemost*. 2006;4(6):1339–1345.

6. WHO. Guidelines for thromboplastins and plasma used to control oral anticoagulant therapy. *World Health Organ Tech Rep Ser*. 1999;889: Annex 3.

7. Baglin TP, Keeling DM, Watson HG. British Committee for Standards in Haematoogy. Guidelines on oral anticoagulation (warfarin), 3rd edition – 2005 update. *Br J Haematol*. 2006;132(3):277–285.

8. Hirsh J, Guyatt G, Albers GW, et al. Executive summary: American College of Chest Physicians Evidence-based Clinical Practice Guidelines, 8th edition. *Chest*. 2008;133(supp 6):71S–109S. [Erratum in *Chest* 2008; 134(4):892].

9. ISO. Clinical laboratory testing and in vitro medical devices – requirements for in vitro monitoring systems for self testing of oral anticoagulant therapy. *BS ISO*. 2007;17953.

10. Briggs C, Guthrie D, Hyde K, et al. Guidelines for point-of-care testing: haematology. *Br J Haematol*. 2008;142(6):904–915.

11. Hirsh J, Bauer KA, Donati MB, et al. Parenteral anticoagulants: American College of Chest Physicians Evidence-Based Clinical Practice Guidelines, 8th edition. *Chest*. 2008;133(supp 6):141S–159S. [Erratum in *Chest* 2008; 134(2):473].

12. Baglin T, Barrowcliffe TW, Cohen A, et al. Guidelines on the use and monitoring of heparin. *Br J Haematol*. 2006;133(1):19–34.

13. Gray E, Walker AD, Mulloy B, et al. A collaborative study to establish the 5th International Standard for Unfractionated Heparin. *Thromb Haemost*. 2000;84(6):1017–1022.

14. Gray E, Heath AB, Mulloy B, et al. A collaborative study of proposed European Pharmacopoeia reference preparations of low molecular mass heparin. *Thromb Haemost*. 1995;74(3):893–899.

15. Popma JJ, Prpic R, Lansky AJ, et al. Heparin dosing in patients undergoing coronary intervention. *Am J Cardiol*. 1998;82(8b):19–24.

16. Kitchen S, Iampietro R, Woolley AM, et al. Anti Xa monitoring during treatment with low molecular weight heparin or danaparoid: inter-assay variability. *Thromb Haemost*. 1999;82(4):1289–1293.

17. Keeling D, Davidson S, Watson H, et al. The management of heparin-induced thrombocytopenia. *Br J Haematol*. 2006;133(3):259–269. [Erratum in *Br J Haematol* 2006; 134(3):351].

18. Warkentin TE. New approaches to the diagnosis of heparin-induced thrombocytopenia. *Chest*. 2005;127(supp 2):35S–45S.

19. Warkentin TE, Heddle NM. Laboratory diagnosis of immune heparin-induced thrombocytopenia. *Curr Hematol Rep*. 2003;2(2):148–157.

20. Greinacher A, Warkentin TE. Recognition, treatment and prevention of heparin-induced thrombocytopenia: review and update. *Thromb Res*. 2006;118(2):165–176.

21. Warkentin TE, Greinacher A, Koster A, et al. Treatment and prevention of heparin-induced thrombocytopenia: American College of Chest Physicians Evidence-based Clinical Practice Guidelines, 8th edition. *Chest*. 2008;133(supp 6):340S–380S.

22. Sheridan D, Carter C, Kelton JG. A diagnostic test for heparin-induced thrombocytopenia. *Blood*. 1986;67(1):27–30.

23. Amiral J, Meyer D. Heparin-induced thrombocytopenia: diagnostic tests and biological mechanisms. *Bailliéres Clin Haematol*. 1998;11(2):447–460.

24. Chong BH, Burgess J, Ismail F. The clinical usefulness of the platelet aggregation test for the diagnosis of heparin-induced thrombocytopenia. *Thromb Haemost*. 1993;69(4):344–350.

25. Griffiths E, Dzik WH. Assays for heparin-induced thrombocytopenia. *Transfus Med*. 1997;7(1):1–11.

26. Warkentin TE, Sheppard JI, Moore JC, et al. Quantitative interpretation of optical density measurements using PF4-dependent enzyme-immunoassays. *J Thromb Haemost*. 2008;6(8):1304–1312.

27. Warkentin TE, Sheppard JI, Raschke R. Performance characteristics of a rapid assay for anti-PF4/heparin antibodies: the particle immunofiltration assay. *J Thromb Haemost*. 2007;5(11):2308–2310.

28. Bryant A, Low J, Austin S, et al. Timely diagnosis and management of heparin-induced thrombocytopenia in a frequent request, low incidence single centre using clinical 4T's score and particle gel immunoassay. *Br J Haematol*. 2008;143(5):721–726.

29. Potzsch B, Hund S, Madlener K, et al. Monitoring of recombinant hirudin: assessment of a plasma-based ecarin clotting time assay. *Thromb Res*. 1997;86(5):373–383.

30. Nowak G. The ecarin clotting time, a universal method to quantify direct thrombin inhibitors. *Pathophysiol Haemost Thromb.* 2003;33(4): 173–183.

31. Ludlam CA, Bennett B, Fox KA, et al. Guidelines for the use of thrombolytic therapy. Haemostasis and Thrombosis Task Force of the British Committee for Standards in Haematology. *Blood Coagul Fibrinolysis.* 1995;6(3):273–285.

32. Patrono C. Aspirin resistance: definition, mechanisms and clinical read-outs [see Comment]. *J Thromb Haemost.* 2003;1(8):1710–1713.

33. Harrison P, Frelinger 3rd AL, Furman MI, et al. Measuring antiplatelet drug effects in the laboratory. *Thromb Res.* 2007;120(3): 323–336.

Chapter | **21** |

Blood cell antigens and antibodies: erythrocytes, platelets and granulocytes

Fiona Regan

CHAPTER CONTENTS

ERYTHROCYTES

Red Cell Antigens

Since Landsteiner's discovery in 1901, that human blood groups existed, a vast body of serological, genetic and biochemical data on red cell (blood group) antigens has been accumulated. More recently, the biological functions of some of these antigens have been appreciated.

A total of 30 blood group systems have been described (Table 21.1). Each system is a series of red cell antigens, determined either by a single genetic locus or very closely linked loci. In addition to the blood group systems, there are six 'collections' of antigens (e.g. Cost), which bring together other genetically, biochemically or serologically related sets of antigens and a separate series of low-frequency (e.g. Rd) and high-frequency (e.g. Vel) antigens, which do not fit into any system or collection. A numeric catalogue of red cell antigens is being maintained by an International Society of Blood Transfusion (ISBT) Working Party.[1]

Apart from those of the ABO system, most of these antigens were detected by antibodies stimulated by transfusion or pregnancy.

Alternative forms of a gene coding for red cell antigens at a particular locus are called alleles and individuals may inherit identical or non-identical alleles. Most blood group genes have been assigned to specific chromosomes (e.g. ABO system on chromosome 9, Rh system on chromosome 1). The term genotype is used for the sum of the inherited alleles of a particular gene (e.g. AA, AO) and most red cell genes are expressed as codominant antigens (i.e. both genes are expressed in the heterozygote). The phenotype refers to the recognizable product of the alleles and there are many racial differences in the frequencies of red cell phenotypes, as shown in Table 21.2.

Red cell antigens are determined either by carbohydrate structures or protein structures. Carbohydrate-defined antigens are indirect gene products (e.g. ABO, Lewis, P). The genes code for an intermediate product, usually an enzyme that creates the antigenic specificity by transferring sugar molecules onto the protein or lipid. Protein-defined antigens are direct gene products and the specificity is determined by the inherited amino acid sequence and/or the

Table 21.1 Blood group systems recognized by the ISBT Working Party

ISBT NO.	SYSTEM NAME	SYSTEM SYMBOL	EPITOPE	CHROMOSOME
001	ABO	ABO	Carbohydrate (*N*-acetyl-D-galactosamine, galactose). A, B and H antigens mainly elicit IgM antibody reactions, although anti-H is very rare, see the Hh antigen system (Bombay phenotype, ISBT 018)	9
002	MNS	MNS	GPA/GPB (glycophorins A and B). Main antigens M, N, S, s	4
003	P	P_I	Glycolipid. Antigen P1	22
004	Rh	RH	Protein. C, c, D, E, e antigens (there is no 'd' antigen; lowercase 'd' indicates the absence of D)	1
005	Lutheran	LU	Protein (member of the immunoglobulin superfamily). Set of 21 antigens	19
006	Kell	KEL	Antibodies to glycoprotein. K_1 can cause haemolytic disease of the newborn (anti-Kell), which can be severe	7
007	Lewis	LE	Carbohydrate (fucose residue). Main antigens Le^a and Le^b – associated with tissue ABH antigen secretion	19
008	Duffy	FY	Protein (chemokine receptor). Main antigens Fy^a and Fy^b. Individuals lacking Duffy antigens altogether are immune to malaria caused by *Plasmodium vivax* and *Plasmodium knowlesi*	1
009	Kidd	JK	Protein (urea transporter). Main antigens Jk^a and Jk^b	18
010	Diego	DI	Glycoprotein (band 3, AE1 or anion exchange). Positive blood is found only among North-Central and East Asians and Native Americans	17
011	Yt or Cartwright	YT	Protein (AChE, acetylcholinesterase)	7
012	XG	XG	Glycoprotein	X
013	Scianna	SC	Glycoprotein	1
014	Dombrock	DO	Glycoprotein (fixed to cell membrane by GPI or glycosyl-phosphotidylinositol)	12
015	Colton	CO	Aquaporin 1. Main antigens Co(a) and Co(b)	7
016	Landsteiner-Wiener	LW	Protein (member of the immunoglobulin superfamily)	19
017	Chido/Rogers	CH/RG	C4A C4B (complement fractions)	6
018	Hh/Bombay	H	Carbohydrate (fucose residue)	19
019	Kx	XK	Glycoprotein	X
020	Gerbich	GE	GPC/GPD (glycophorins C and D)	2
021	Cromer	CROM	Glycoprotein (DAF or CD55, regulates complement fractions C3 and C5, attached to the membrane by GPI)	1
022	Knops	KN	Glycoprotein (CR1 or CD35, immune complex receptor)	1
023	Indian	IN	Glycoprotein (CD44 adhesion function?)	11

Table 21.1 Blood group systems recognized by the ISBT Working Party – cont'd

ISBT NO.	SYSTEM NAME	SYSTEM SYMBOL	EPITOPE	CHROMOSOME
024	Ok	OK	Glycoprotein (CD147)	19
025	Raph	MER2	Transmembrane glycoprotein	11
026	JMH	JMH	Protein (fixed to cell membrane by GPI)	6
027	li	I	Branched (I)/unbranched (i) polysaccharide	6
028	Globoside	GLOB	Glycolipid. Antigen P	3
029	GIL	GIL	Aquaporin 3	9
030	Rh-associated glycoprotein	RHAG	Rh-associated glycoprotein	6

IgM, immunoglobulin M; ISBT, International Society of Blood Transfusion.

Table 21.2 Frequencies of red cell phenotypes in US Black and White populations

SYSTEM	PHENOTYPE	US BLACK POPULATION (%)	US WHITE POPULATION (%)
ABO	O	49	43.7
	A	26	41.7
	B	20.5	10.6
	AB	4.5	4
Lewis	Le (a−b−)	28.5	6
Rh	Dce	47.8	2.1
	DCcEe	4.2	13.4
	dce	5.6	14.6
	DCe	2.6	18.9
MNSs	S−s+	68.1	45
	S+s+	24.5	44
	S+s−	5.9	11
	S−s−	1.5	Rare
Duffy	Fy (a−b−)	63.7	Rare
	Fy (a−b+)	18.8	34
	Fy (a+b+)	2	44
	Fy (a+b−)	15.5	17
Kidd	Jk (a+b−)	50	27.5
	Jk (a+b+)	41.4	49.4
	Jk (a−b+)	8.6	23.1

conformation of the protein. Proteins carrying red cell antigens are inserted into the membrane in one of three ways: single pass, multipass or linked to phosphatidylinositol (GPI-linked). Only a few red cell antigens are erythroid-specific (Rh, LW, Kell and MNSs), the remainder being expressed in many other tissues. The structure and functions of the membrane proteins and glycoproteins carrying blood group antigens have been reviewed by Daniels.[2] An illustration of the putative functions of molecules containing blood group antigens is provided in Table 21.3.

However, the main clinical importance of a blood group system depends on the capacity of alloantibodies (directed against the antigens not possessed by the individual) to cause destruction of transfused red cells or to cross the placenta and give rise to haemolytic disease in the fetus or newborn. This in turn depends on the frequency of the antigens and the alloantibodies and the characteristics of the latter: thermal range, immunoglobulin class and ability to fix complement. On these criteria, the ABO and Rh systems are of major clinical importance. Anti-A and anti-B are naturally occurring and are capable of causing severe intravascular haemolysis after an incompatible transfusion. The RhD antigen is the most immunogenic red cell antigen after A and B, being capable of stimulating anti-D production after transfusion or pregnancy in the majority of RhD-negative individuals.

ABO System

Discovery of the ABO system by Landsteiner marked the beginning of safe blood transfusion. The ABO antigens, although most important in relation to transfusion, are

Table 21.3 Putative functions of molecules containing blood group antigens

CLASS	BLOOD GROUP SYSTEM	STRUCTURE	FUNCTION
Transporter/channel	Kidd	Multipass GP	Urea transporter
	Colton	Aquaporin 1 Multipass CP	Water channel
	Diego	Band 3, multipass GP	Anion exchanger
Receptors	Duffy	DARC, multipass GP	Chemokine (*Plasmodium vivax* receptor)
	Indian	Single-pass GP	Hyaluronate receptor
Complement pathway	Chido/Rogers	Complement absorbed onto red cells	Complement component
	Cromer	DAF	Complement regulator
	Knops	Complement receptor 1	Complement regulator
Adhesion	LW	IgSF	Binds CD11/CD18 Integrins
Molecule	Lutheran	IgSF	? Laminin receptor
Enzyme	Yt	GPI-linked GP Acetylcholinesterase	Unknown on red cells
	Kell	Single-pass GP	? Endopeptidase
Structural protein	Gerbich	Glycophorins C and D Single-pass GP	Attachment to membrane skeleton

also expressed on most endothelial and epithelial membranes and are important histocompatibility antigens.[3] Transplantation of ABO-incompatible solid organs increases the potential for hyperacute graft rejection, although ABO-incompatible renal transplantation can be successfully carried out with plasmapheresis in addition to immunosuppression of the recipient.[4] Major ABO-incompatible stem cell transplants (e.g. group A stem cells into a group O recipient) will provoke haemolysis, unless the donation is depleted of red cells.

ABO Antigens and Encoding Genes

There are four main blood groups: A, B, AB and O (Table 21.4). In the British Caucasian population, the frequency of group A is 42%, B 9%, AB 3% and O 46%, but there is racial variation in these frequencies.[5] The epitopes of ABO antigens are determined by carbohydrates (sugars), which are linked either to polypeptides (forming glycoproteins) or to lipids (glycolipids).

The expression of ABO antigens is controlled by three separate genetic loci: *ABO* located on chromosome 9 and *FUT1* (*H*) and *FUT2* (*Se*), both of which are located on chromosome 19. The genes from each locus are inherited in pairs as Mendelian dominants. Each gene codes

Table 21.4 ABO blood group system

BLOOD GROUP	SUBGROUP	ANTIGENS ON RED CELLS	ANTIBODIES IN PLASMA
A	A_1	$A + A_1$	Anti-B
	A_2	A	(Anti-A_1)*
B	–	B	Anti-A, Anti-A_1
AB	A_1B	$A + A_1 + B$	None
	A_2B	$A + B$	(Anti-A_1)*
O	–	(H)†	Anti-A
			Anti-A_1
			Anti-B
			Anti-A,B‡

*Anti-A_1 found in 1–2% of A_2 subjects and 25–30% of A_2B subjects.
†The amount of H antigen is influenced by the ABO group; O cells contain most H and A_1B cells least. Anti-H may be found in occasional A_1 and A,B subject (see text).
‡Crossreactivity with both A and B cells.

Table 21.5 Glycosyltransferases produced by genes encoding antigens within the ABO, H and Lewis blood group systems

GENE	ALLELE	TRANSFERASE
FUT1	H	α-2-L-fucosyltransferase
	h	None
A	A	α-3-N-acetyl-D-galactosaminyltransferase
B	B	α-3-D-galactosyltransferase
O	O	None
FUT2	Se	α-2-L-fucosyltransferase
	se	None
FUT3	Le	α-3/4-L-fucosyltransferase
	le	None

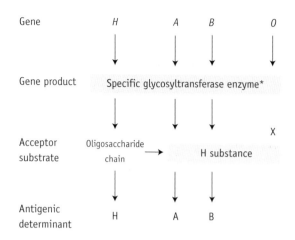

Figure 21.1 Pathways from HAB blood group genes to antigens. *Glycosyltransferase H transfers L-fucose; A transfers N-acetyl-D-galactosamine; B transfers D-galactose; O is inactive.

for a different enzyme (glycosyltransferase), which attaches specific monosaccharides onto precursor disaccharide chains (Table 21.5). There are four types of disaccharide chains known to occur on red cells, on other tissues and in secretions. The Type 1 disaccharide chain is found in plasma and secretions and is the substrate for the FUT2 (Se) gene, whereas Types 2, 3 and 4 chains are only found on red cells and are the substrate for the FUT1 (H) gene. It is likely that the O and B genes arose by mutation of the A gene. The O gene does not encode for the production of a functional enzyme; group O individuals commonly have a deletion at nucleotide 261 (the O1 allele), which results in a frame-shift and premature termination of the translated polypeptide and the production of an enzyme with no catalytic activity. The B gene differs from A by consistent nucleotide substitutions.[6] The expression of A and B antigens is dependent on the H and Se genes, which both give rise to glycosyltransferases that add L-fucose, producing the H antigen. The presence of an A or B gene (or both) results in the production of further glycosyltransferases, which convert H substance into A and B antigens by the terminal addition of N-acetyl-D-galactosamine and D-galactose, respectively (Fig. 21.1). Because the O gene produces an inactive transferase, H substance persists unchanged as group O. In the extremely rare Oh Bombay phenotype, the individual is homozygous for the h allele of FUT1 and hence cannot form the H precursor of the A and B antigen. Their red cells type as group O, but their plasma contains anti-H, in addition to anti-A, anti-B and anti-A,B, which are all active at 37°C. As a consequence, individuals with an Oh Bombay phenotype can only be safely transfused with other Oh red cells.

Serologists have defined two common subgroups of the A antigen. Approximately 20% of group A and group AB individuals belong to group A_2 and group A_2B, respectively, the remainder belonging to group A_1 and group A_1B. These subgroups arise as a result of inheritance of either the A^1 or A^2 alleles. The A_2 transferase is less efficient in transferring N-acetyl-D-galactosamine to available H antigen sites and cannot utilize Types 3 and 4 disaccharide chains. As a consequence, A_2 red cells have fewer A antigen sites than A_1 cells and the plasma of group A_2 and group A_2B individuals may also contain anti-A_1. The distinction between these subgroups can be made using the lectin *Dolichos biflorus*, which only reacts with A_1 cells. The H antigen content of red cells depends on the ABO group and, when assessed by agglutination reactions with anti-H, the strength of reaction tends to be graded $O > A_2 > A_2B > B > A_1 > A_1B$. Other subgroups of A are occasionally found (e.g. A_3, A_x) that result from mutant forms of the glycosyltransferases produced by the A gene and are less efficient at transferring N-acetyl-D-galactosamine onto H substance.[6]

The A, B and H antigens are detectable early in fetal life but are not fully developed on the red cells at birth. The number of antigen sites reaches 'adult' level at around 1 year of age and remains constant until old age, when a slight reduction may occur.

Secretors and Non-Secretors

The ability to secrete A, B and H substances in water-soluble form is controlled by FUT2 (dominant allele Se). In a Caucasian population, about 80% are secretors (genotype SeSe or Sese) and 20% are non-secretors (genotype sese) (Table 21.6). Secretors have H substance in the saliva and other body fluids together with A substances, B substances or both, depending on their blood group. Only traces of these

Table 21.6 Secretor status in the Caucasian population			
GENES	BLOOD GROUP OF RED CELLS	ABH SUBSTANCE PRESENT IN SALIVA	INCIDENCE (%)
Secretor *SeSe or Sese*	A	A + H	80
	B	B + H	
	AB	A + B + H	
	O	H	
Non-secretors *sese*	A, B, AB or O	None	20

substances are present in the secretions of non-secretors, although the antigens are expressed normally on their red cells and other tissues.

An individual's secretor status can be determined by testing for ABH substance in saliva (see p. 504).

ABO Antigens and Disease

Group A individuals rarely may acquire a B antigen from a bacterial infection that results in the release of a deacetylase enzyme. This converts N-acetyl-D-galactosamine into α-galactosamine, which is similar to galactose, the immunodominant sugar of group B, thereby sometimes causing the red cells to appear to be group AB. In the original reported cases, five out of seven of the patients had carcinoma of the gastrointestinal tract. Case reports attest to the danger of individuals with an acquired B antigen being transfused with AB red cells, resulting in a fatal haemolytic transfusion reaction following the production of hyperimmune anti-B.[7]

The inheritance of ABH antigens is also known to be weakly associated with predisposition to certain diseases. Group A individuals have 1.2 times the risk of developing carcinoma of the stomach than group O or B; group O individuals have 1.4 times more risk of developing peptic ulcer than non-group O individuals; and non-secretors of ABH have 1.5 times the risk of developing peptic ulcer than secretors.[8] The ABO group also affects plasma von Willebrand factor (VWF) and factor VIII levels; group O healthy individuals have levels around 25% lower than those of other ABO groups.[9] ABO blood group appears to mediate its effect by accelerating clearance of VWF but the mechanism is not yet clear[10] ABH antigens are also frequently more weakly expressed on the red cells of persons with leukaemia.

ABO Antibodies

Anti-A and anti-B

ABO antibodies, in the absence of the corresponding antigens, appear during the first few months after birth, probably as a result of exposure to ABH antigen-like substances in the diet or the environment (i.e. they are 'naturally occurring') (Table 21.4). This allows for reverse (serum/plasma) grouping as a means of confirming the red cell phenotype. The antibodies are a potential cause of dangerous haemolytic transfusion reactions if transfusions are given without regard to ABO compatibility. Anti-A and anti-B are always, to some extent, immunoglobulin M (IgM). Although they react best at low temperatures, they are nevertheless potentially lytic at 37°C. Hyperimmune anti-A and anti-B occur less frequently, usually in response to transfusion or pregnancy, but they may also be formed following the injection of some toxoids and vaccines. They are predominantly of IgG class and are usually produced by group O and sometimes by group A_2 individuals. Hyperimmune IgG anti-A and/or anti-B from group O or group A_2 mothers may cross the placenta and cause haemolytic disease of the newborn (HDN). These antibodies react over a wide thermal range and are more effective haemolysins than the naturally occurring antibodies. Group O donors should always be screened for high-titre anti-A and anti-B antibodies, which may cause haemolysis when group O platelets or plasma are transfused to recipients with A and B phenotypes.

Plasma-containing blood components from such high-titre universal donors should be reserved for group O recipients.

Anti-A₁ and anti-H

Anti-A_1 reacts only with A_1 and A_1B cells and is occasionally found in the serum of group A_2 individuals (1–8%) and not uncommonly in the serum of group A_2B subjects (25–50%). However, anti-A_1 normally acts as a cold agglutinin and is very rarely reactive at 37°C, when it is only capable of limited red cell destruction. There have been a few reports of red cell haemolysis ascribed to anti-A_1, which some authors have questioned because, although the antibodies reacted only with A_1 red cells, no attempts were made to absorb them with A_2 cells, which would have revealed their anti-A specificity.

Anti-H reacts most strongly with group O and A_2 red cells and also normally acts as a cold agglutinin. A notable, but rare, exception is the anti-H that occurs in the Oh Bombay phenotype, which is an IgM antibody and causes lysis at 37°C (Table 21.4) so that Oh Bombay phenotype blood would be required for transfusion.

Lewis System

Lewis Antigens and Encoding Genes

The Lewis antigens (Le^a and Le^b) are located on soluble glycosphingolipids found in saliva and plasma and are secondarily absorbed into the red cell membranes from the plasma.

The Le gene at the *FUT3* (*LE*) locus is located on chromosome 19 and codes for a fucosyltransferase, which acts on an adjacent sugar molecule to that acted on by the *Se* gene. Where *Se* and *Le* are present, the Le^b antigen is produced; where *Le* but not *Se* is present, Le^a is produced; and where *Le* is not present, neither Le^a nor Le^b is produced. After transfusion of red cells, donor red cells convert to the Lewis type of the recipient owing to the continuous exchange of glycosphingolipids between the plasma and red cell membrane.

Neonates have the phenotype Le(a−b−) because low levels of the fucosyltransferase are produced in the first 2 months of life.

Lewis Antibodies

Lewis antibodies are naturally occurring and are usually IgM and complement binding. *In vitro*, their reactivity is enhanced with the use of enzyme-treated red cells, when lysis may occur. However, only rare examples of anti-Le^a that are strictly reactive at 37°C have given rise to haemolytic transfusion reactions and there is no good evidence that anti-Le^b has ever caused a haemolytic episode. Explanations for the relative lack of clinical significance include their thermal range, neutralization by Lewis antigens in the plasma of transfused blood and the gradual elution of Lewis antigens from the donor red cells. Consequently, it is acceptable to provide red cells for transfusion that have not been typed as negative for the relevant Lewis antigen but are compatible with the recipient plasma when the compatibility test is performed strictly at 37°C.

Lewis antibodies have not been implicated in haemolytic disease of the fetus or newborn. The role of Lewis in influencing the outcome of renal transplants is unclear.

The P System and Globoside Collection

Antigens

The P$_1$ antigen of the P system and the P and P^k antigens of the globoside collection are related. Little is known of the genes involved or their products, but all are derived from the precursor, lactosyl ceramide dihexoside. Carbohydrate products related to the P system are widely distributed in nature.

Expression of P$_1$ varies considerably between individuals. One in 100 000 individuals is p (negative for P) and is resistant to parvovirus B19 infection.

Antibodies

Anti-P$_1$ is a common naturally occurring antibody of no clinical significance and red cells for transfusion can be provided that are crossmatch compatible at 37°C. Alloanti-P is also a naturally occurring antibody found in individuals with the rare P^k phenotype. Auto-anti-P is the specificity attributed to the Donath–Landsteiner antibody; it is a potent biphasic haemolysin, responsible for paroxysmal cold haemoglobinuria.

Anti-PP$_1$P^k is a naturally occurring high-titre IgM or IgG antibody and it is found only in individuals with the rare p phenotype. It is reactive at 37°C and is capable of causing intravascular haemolysis and HDN. It is also associated with spontaneous miscarriage in early pregnancy.

Rh System

The Rh system, formerly known as the Rhesus system, was so named because the original antibody that was raised by injecting red cells of rhesus monkeys into rabbits and guinea pigs reacted with most human red cells. Although the original antibody (now called anti-LW) was subsequently shown to be different from anti-D, the Rh terminology has been retained for the human blood group system. The clinical importance of this system is that individuals who are D negative are often stimulated to make anti-D if transfused with D-positive blood or, in the case of pregnant women, if exposed to D-positive fetal red cells that have crossed the placenta.

Rh Antigens and Encoding Genes

This is a very complex system. At its simplest, it is convenient to classify individuals as D positive or D negative, depending on the presence of the D antigen. This is largely a preventive measure, to avoid transfusing a D-negative recipient with the cells expressing the D antigen, which is the most immunogenic red cell antigen after A and B. At a more comprehensive level, it is convenient to consider the Rh system as a gene complex that gives rise to various combinations of three alternative antigens – C or c, D or d and E or e – as originally suggested by Fisher. The *d* gene was thought to be amorphic without any corresponding antigen on the red cell. Subsequently it was confirmed that the *RH* locus is on chromosome 1 and comprises two highly homologous, very closely linked genes, *RHD* and *RHCE*, each with 10 exons. Each gene codes for a separate transmembrane protein with 417 residues and 12 putative transmembrane domains. The D and CE proteins differ at 35 residues. The *RHCE* gene has four main alleles; *CE*, *Ce*, *ce* and *cE*. Positions 103 and 226 on the CE polypeptide, situated in the external loops, determine the C/c (serine/proline) and E/e (proline/alanine) polymorphisms, respectively. This concept of D and CcEe genes linked closely and transmitted together is consistent with the Fisher nomenclature.

In Caucasian, D-negative individuals, the *RHD* gene is deleted, whereas in Black races and other populations, single-point mutations, partial deletions or recombinations have been described. In individuals with a weak D antigen (D^u), there is a quantitative reduction in D antigen sites, believed to arise from an uncharacterized transcriptional defect. These individuals do not make anti-D antibodies following a D antigen challenge. Partial D individuals lack one or more epitopes of the D antigen, defined using panels of monoclonal reagents. D^{VI} is perhaps the most important partial D phenotype because such individuals not infrequently make anti-D. Partial D phenotypes arise from DNA exchanges between *RHD* and *RHCE* genes and from other rearrangements. Comprehensive reviews of this system have been provided by Avent and Reid[11] and Daniels et al.[12]

The Rh haplotypes are named either by the component antigens (e.g. CDe, cde) or by a single shorthand symbol (e.g. R^1 = CDe, r = cde). Thus, a person may inherit *CDe* (R^1) from one parent and *cde* (*r*) from the other and have the genotype *CDe/cde* (R^1r). The haplotypes in order of frequency and the corresponding shorthand notation are given in Table 21.7. Although two other nomenclatures are also used to describe the Rh system, namely, Wiener's Rh-Hr terminology and Rosenfield's numeric notation, the CDE nomenclature, derived from Fisher's original theory, is recommended by a World Health Organization Expert Committee[13] in the interest of simplicity and uniformity. The Rh antigens are defined by corresponding antisera, with the exception of 'anti-d', which does not exist. Consequently, the distinction between homozygous *DD* and the heterozygous *Dd* cannot be made by direct serological testing but may be resolved by informative family studies. It is still routine practice to predict the genotype from the phenotype on the basis of probability tables for the various Rh genotypes in the population (Table 21.7). However, in women with immune anti-D and a history of an infant affected by HDN, *RH* DNA typing is used in prenatal testing for the fetal D status to decide on the clinical management of the pregnancy, e.g. the need for monitoring for fetal anaemia using middle cerebral artery Doppler ultrasound. Suitable sources include amniotic fluid (amniocytes) and trophoblastic cells (chorionic villi) or after 15 weeks' gestation, maternal blood can be used because it contains fetal DNA.[14,15] In practice, multiplex polymerase chain reaction (PCR) is used, with more than two primer sets, to detect the different molecular bases for D-negative phenotypes in non-Caucasians. *RH* DNA typing also has applications in paternity testing and forensic medicine. There are racial differences in the distribution of Rh antigens, e.g. D negativity is more common in Caucasians (approximately 15%), whereas R^o (*cDe*) is found in approximately 48% of Black Americans but is uncommon (approximately 2%) in Caucasians. The Rh antigens are present only on red cells and are a structural part of the cell membrane. Complete absence of Rh antigens (Rh-null phenotype) may be associated with a congenital haemolytic anaemia with spherocytes and stomatocytes in the blood film, increased osmotic fragility and increased cation transport. This phenotype arises either as a result of homozygosity for silent alleles at the *RH* locus (the amorph type) or more commonly by homozygosity for an autosomal suppressor gene (X), genetically independent of the *RH* locus (the regulator type). Rh antigens are well-developed before birth and can be demonstrated on the red cells of very early fetuses.

Antibodies

Fisher's nomenclature is convenient when applied to Rh antibodies, and antibodies directed against all Rh antigens, except d, have been described: anti-D, anti-C, anti-c, anti-E and anti-e. Rh antigens are restricted to red cells and Rh antibodies result from previous alloimmunization by previous pregnancy or transfusion, except for some naturally occurring forms of anti-E and anti-C^W. Immune Rh antibodies are predominantly IgG (IgG1 and/or IgG3), but may have an IgM component. They react optimally at 37°C, they do not bind complement and their detection is often enhanced by the use of enzyme-treated red cells. Haemolysis, when it occurs, is therefore extravascular and predominantly in the spleen.

Anti-D is clinically the most important antibody; it may cause haemolytic transfusion reactions and was a common cause of fetal death resulting from haemolytic disease of the newborn before the introduction of anti-D prophylaxis. Anti-D is accompanied by anti-C in 30% of cases and anti-E in 2% cases. Primary immunization following a transfusion of D-positive cells becomes apparent within 2–5 months, but it may not be detectable following exposure to a small dose of D-positive cells in pregnancy. However, a second exposure to D-positive cells in a subsequent pregnancy will provoke a prompt anamnestic or secondary immune response.

Of the non-D Rh antibodies, anti-c is most commonly found and can also give rise to severe haemolytic disease of the fetus and newborn. Anti-E is less common, whereas anti-C is rare in the absence of anti-D.

Table 21.7 The Rh haplotypes in order of frequency (Fisher nomenclature) in Caucasians and the corresponding short notations

FISHER	SHORT NOTATIONS	APPROXIMATE FREQUENCY (%)
CDe	R^1	41
cde	r	39
cDE	R^2	14
cDe	R^0	3
C^WDe	R^{1w}	1
cdE	r''	1
Cde	r'	1
CDE	R^Z	Rare
CdE	r^y	Rare

Kell and Kx Systems

Antigens and Encoding Genes

A total of 34 antigens have been identified (K1–K34), but three very closely linked sets of alleles are clinically important: *K* (KEL1) and *k* (KEL2); *Kp^a* (KEL3), *Kp^b* (KEL4) and *Kp^c* (KEL21); and *Js^a* (KEL6) and *Js^b* (KEL7). These antigens are encoded by alleles at the *KEL* locus on chromosome 7, but their production also depends on genes at the *KX* locus on the X chromosome. The K antigen is present in 9% of the English population. The Kp^b antigen has a high frequency in Caucasians; the Js^b antigen is universal in Caucasians and almost universal in black races.

The Kell protein is a single-pass glycoprotein and is believed to be complexed by a disulphide bridge to the Kx protein, which is multipass with 10 putative transmembrane domains. It has considerable sequence homology to other neutral endopeptidases.

In the McLeod phenotype, red cells lack Kx and there is a marked decrease in all Kell antigens, an acanthocytic morphology and compensated haemolysis. The McLeod syndrome is X-linked with slow progression to cardiomyopathy, skeletal muscle wasting and neurological defects.

Kell Antibodies

Immune anti-K is the most common antibody found outside the ABO and Rh systems. It is commonly IgG1 and occasionally complement binding. Other immune antibodies directed against Kell antigens are less common. The presence of some of these antibodies, such as anti-k, anti-Kp^b and anti-Js^b, may cause extensive difficulties in the selection of antigen-negative units for transfusion.

Duffy System

Duffy antigens and encoding genes

The Duffy (Fy) locus is on chromosome 1 and encodes a multipass protein with seven or nine putative transmembrane domains.

The locus has the following alleles: *Fy^a*, *Fy^b*, which code for the co-dominant Fy^a and Fy^b antigens, respectively; *Fy^x*, which is responsible for a weak Fy^b antigen; and *Fy*, which is responsible when homozygous for the Fy(a−b−) phenotype in black races. This *Fy* gene is identical to the *Fy^b* gene in its structural region but has a mutation in the promoter region, resulting in the lack of production of red cell Duffy glycoprotein.

The Fy glycoprotein (also known as Duffy antigen receptor for chemokines, DARC) is a receptor for the CC and CXC classes of proinflammatory chemokines and is expressed on vascular endothelial cells and Purkinje cells in the cerebellum, but its precise role as a potential scavenger of excess chemokines is unknown. The Fy glycoprotein is also a receptor for *Plasmodium vivax*.

Duffy antibodies

Anti-Fy^a is much more common than anti-Fy^b and all other Duffy antibodies are rare apart from anti-Fy^3 (to both Fy^a and Fy^b), which occurs in some African/Afro-Caribbean patients, in whom Fy(a−b−) antigen status is common. They are predominantly IgG1 and are sometimes complement binding.

Kidd (JK) System

Kidd antigens and encoding genes

Genes at the *HUT 11(JK)* locus on chromosome 18 encode for a multipass protein, which carries both the Kidd antigens and the human erythroid urea transporter. The codominant alleles, *Jk^a* and *Jk^b*, represent a polymorphism on *HUT 11*, which differs by a single amino acid substitution at position 280 (Asp/Asn).

The Jk(a−b−) phenotype is very rare and is caused by homozygous inheritance of the silent allele, *Jk*, at the *JK* locus or by inheritance of the dominant inhibitor gene *In* (*Jk*) unlinked to the *JK* locus. These Jk(a−b−) cells are resistant to lysis by solutions of urea and have a selective defect in urea transport.

Kidd antibodies

Anti-Jk^a is more common than anti-Jk^b; both are usually IgG. Kidd antibodies are usually complement binding, which is thought to be because most of them contain an IgG3 fraction. Anti-Jk3 is produced by individuals of the rare Jk(a−b−) phenotype.

Kidd antibodies can be difficult to detect because they often show dosage (may only react with cells showing homozygous expressions of *Jk^a* or *Jk^b*), they fall to undetectable levels in plasma and they are often present in mixtures of alloantibodies. A previous history of antibodies is therefore important, to avoid a post-transfusion haemolytic reaction, due to an anamnestic response by an antibody that was below the level of detection before transfusion.

MNSs System

MNSs antigens and encoding genes

GYPA and *GYPB* are closely linked genes on chromosome 4 and encode glycophorin A (GPA) and glycophorin B (GPB), respectively. Both GPA and GPB are single-pass membrane sialoglycoproteins. *M* and *N* are alleles of *GYPA* (encoding the M and N antigens on GPA) and *S* and *s* are alleles of *GPYB* (encoding the S and s antigens on GPB). Many rare variants have been described owing to gene deletions, mutations and segmental exchanges.

The U antigen is found on the red cells of Caucasians and 99% of black races. U-negative individuals are, with rare exceptions, S−s− and lack GPB or have an altered form of GPB.

MNSs antibodies

Anti-M is a relatively common antibody that may be IgM or IgG. Rare examples are reactive at 37°C when they can give rise to haemolytic transfusion reactions. Anti-M very rarely gives rise to HDN.

Anti-N is uncommon and of no clinical significance.

Anti-S and anti-s are usually IgG; both rarely have been implicated in haemolytic transfusion reactions and HDN.

Anti-U is a rare immune antibody, usually containing an IgG1 component. It has been known to cause fatal haemolytic transfusion reactions and occasional severe HDN.

Other Blood Group Systems

Lutheran system

The antigens in the Lutheran system are not well-developed at birth and as a consequence there are no documented cases of clinically significant haemolytic disease owing to Lutheran antibodies.

Anti-Lu^a is uncommon and rarely of clinical significance. Anti-Lu^b has caused extravascular haemolysis.

Yt (Cartwright) system

The antigens Yt^a and Yt^b are found on GPI-linked acetylcholinesterase. Some examples of anti-Yt^a have caused accelerated red cell destruction.

Colton system

The antigens in the Colton system, Co^a and Co^b, are carried on the water-transport protein, channel-forming integral protein (CHIP-1). Anti-Co^a and the rarer anti-Co^b are both sometimes clinically significant.

Dombrock system

The antigens in the Dombrock system include Do^a and Do^b and also include the high-incidence antigens Gy^a, Hy and Jo^a. Antibodies of this system are usually weak, but all should be considered as potentially significant.

Clinical Significance of Red Cell Alloantibodies

The significance of the alloantibodies described, with respect to the nature of the haemolytic transfusion reaction they produce, is provided in Table 21.8. The majority of haemolytic transfusion reactions, however, are the result of ABO incompatibility.[16]

Mollison et al.[17] analysed the significance of blood group antigens other than those of the ABO system and D by looking at the prevalence of transfusion-induced red cell alloantibodies, excluding anti-D, -CD and -DE (Table 21.9). Rh antibodies, mainly anti-c or anti-E, accounted for 53% of the total and anti-K and anti-Fy^a accounted for a further 38%, leaving only about 9% for all other specificities.

Table 21.8 Antibody specificities related to the mechanism of immune haemolytic destruction

BLOOD GROUP SYSTEM	INTRAVASCULAR HAEMOLYSIS	EXTRAVASCULAR HAEMOLYSIS
ABO,H	A, B, H	
Rh		All
Kell	K	K, k, Kp^a, Kp^b, Js^a, Js^b
Kidd	Jk^a	Jk^a, Jk^b, Jk^3
Duffy		Fy^a, Fy^b
MNS		M, S, s, U
Lutheran		Lu^b
Lewis	Le^a	
Cartwright		Yt^a
Colton		Co^a, Co^b
Dombrock		Do^a, Do^b

A similar distribution of the different red cell antibodies was found in a smaller group of patients who experienced immediate haemolytic transfusion reactions (HTR). However, the figures for delayed HTR showed a striking increase in the relative frequency of Jk antibodies, which reflects the outlined characteristics of Jk antibodies.

Haemolytic disease of the fetus and newborn has not been associated with antibodies directed against Lewis antigens and only very mild disease is produced by anti-Lu^a and anti-Lu^b. With these exceptions, all other IgG antibodies directed against antigens in the systems mentioned should be considered capable of causing haemolysis in this setting.

The significance of the many other blood group antigens not referred to in the text is summarized in Table 21.10. However, it should be noted that the antibodies listed are usually wholly or predominantly IgG and would be detectable in routine pretransfusion testing using the indirect anti-globulin test (IAT).

It is difficult to find suitable blood for transfusion to a patient whose plasma contains an antibody, such as anti-Vel, which has a specificity for a high-frequency antigen and which can cause severe haemolytic transfusion reactions. In addition to using blood from a frozen blood bank and calling up rare phenotype donors, autologous blood could be considered for planned elective procedures and if necessary, the compatibility of red cells from close relatives (particularly siblings) can be investigated. Antibodies such as anti-Kn^a are commonly found and not clinically important, but their presence may cause delay in the provision of blood until their specificity has been determined.

Table 21.9 Relative frequency of immune red cell alloantibodies*

PATIENT GROUP	NO. STUDIED	BLOOD GROUP ALLOANTIBODIES (% OF TOTAL)				
		Rh[†]	K	Fy	Jk	Other
Transfused (some pregnant)	5228	53.1	28.1	10.2	4.0	4.7
Immediate HTR[‡]	142	42.2	30.3	18.3	8.5	0.7
Delayed HTR[‡]	82	34.2	14.6	15.9	32.9	2.4

*Excluding antibodies of ABO, Lewis, P systems and anti-M and anti-N.
[†]Excluding anti-D (or -CD or -DE); almost all were anti-c or anti-E.
[‡]Haemolytic transfusion reaction.
Adapted from Mollison PL, Engelfriet CP, Contreras M 1997 Blood transfusion in clinical medicine, 9th ed. Blackwell Scientific, Oxford, p. 112, based on published data from several sources.

Table 21.10 'Minor' blood group antigens

ANTIGEN	ANTIGEN FREQUENCY, (%) CAUCASIANS	ASSOCIATED HTR	ASSOCIATED HDN	COMMENTS
Di[a]	0	Yes	Yes	Part of DI system. Di[a]
Di[b]	100	Yes	Yes	More common in American Indians and North-Central and East Asians
Wr[a]	<0.1	Yes	Yes	
Xg[a]	65 (males); 88 (females)	Rarely	Rarely	Xg[a] only antigen in system
Sc1	>99.9	No	No	3 antigens in SC system
Sc2	<0.1	No	Mild	
Ge2	100	Some	No	7 antigens in GE system
Ge3	>99.9	Some	No	
Cr[a]	100	Some	No	10 antigens in CR system
Ch1	96	No	No	9 antigens in CH/RG systems, reside on chromosome 4
Rg1	98	No	No	reside on C4
Kn[a]	98	No	No	Belong to KN system of 5 antigens
McC[a]	98	No	No	
Yk[a]	92	No	No	
In[a]	0.1	Yes	No	In[a] has incidence of 4% in Asian Indians
In[b]	99	Yes	No	Asian Indians
LW[a]	100	Some	Mild	–
JMH	>99.9	No	No	One of 901 series* of high-incidence antigens
Vel	>99.9	Yes	No	One of 901 series;* complement binding
Bg[a]	approx. 15	No	No	Corresponds to HLA-B7, detectable on red cells

HTR, haemolytic transfusion reactions; HDN, haemolytic disease of the newborn.
*901 series refers to 11 red cell antigens with a frequency of >99%, based on ISBT terminology.[1]

Mechanisms of Immune Destruction of Red Cells

Immune-mediated haemolysis of red cells depends on the following:[18]

1. The immunoglobulin class of the antibody (for all practical purposes, antibodies directed against red cell antigens are either IgM or IgG or both)
2. The ability of the antibody to bind complement.
3. Interaction with the reticuloendothelial system (mononuclear phagocytic system). The most important phagocyte participating in immune haemolysis is the macrophage, predominantly in the spleen.

The mechanism of immune haemolysis also determines the site of haemolysis:

a. *Intravascular haemolysis* owing to sequential binding of complement components (C1 to C9) cascade and the formation of the membrane attack complex (MAC; $C5b678(9)_n$). This is characteristic of IgM antibodies, but some IgG antibodies can also act as haemolysins. Red cells are usually destroyed by intravascular complement lysis in ABO incompatible transfusion reactions (see p. 543). Most other alloimmune red cell destruction is extravascular and mediated by the mononuclear-phagocytic system.

Red cell autoantibodies may also cause intravascular lysis, especially the IgG autoantibody of PCH (see p. 277) and some autoantibodies of the cold haemagglutinin disease (CHAD) (see p. 277). Complement-mediated intravascular lysis may also occur in drug-induced immune haemolysis (see p. 289).

b. *Extravascular haemolysis* by the mononuclear phagocytic system is characteristic of IgG antibodies and occurs predominantly in the spleen. This is caused by non-complement-binding IgG antibodies or those that bind sublytic amounts of complement. Macrophages have Fcγ receptors for cell-bound IgG and sensitized red cells may be wholly phagocytosed or lose part of the membrane and return to the circulation as microspherocytes Spherocytes are less deformable and more readily trapped in the spleen than normal red cells; this shortens their lifespan. In addition to Fc receptor-mediated phagocytosis, antibody-dependent cell-mediated cytotoxicity (ADCC) may also contribute to cell damage during the close contact with splenic macrophages. Red cells are destroyed external to the monocyte membrane by lysosomal enzymes secreted by the monocyte.[19]

Complement components may enhance red cell destruction. Complement activation by some IgM and most IgG antibodies is not always complete and the red cell escapes intravascular lysis. The activation of complement stops at the C3 stage and, in these circumstances, complement can be detected on the red cell by the antiglobulin test using appropriate anticomplement reagents. The first activation product of C3 is membrane-bound C3b, which is constantly being broken down to C3bi. Red cells with these components on their surface adhere to phagocytes (monocytes, macrophages and neutrophils), which have complement receptors, CR1 (CD35) and CR3 (CD 11b/CD 18). These sensitized cells are rapidly sequestered in the liver because of its bulk of phagocytic cells (Küpffer cells) and large blood flow, but no engulfment occurs. When C3bi is cleaved, leaving only C3dg on the cell surface, the cells tagged with 'inactive' C3dg return to the circulation, as in chronic cold haemagglutinin disease. However, when IgG is also present on the cell surface, C3b enhances phagocytosis and under these circumstances both liver and spleen are important sites of extravascular haemolysis. Hence, C3b and C3bi augment macrophage-mediated clearance of IgG-coated cells and antibodies binding sublytic amounts of complement (e.g. Duffy and Kidd antibodies) often cause more rapid destruction and more marked symptoms than non-complement binding antibodies (e.g. Rh antibodies).

Macrophage activity is an important component of cell destruction and further study of cellular interactions at this stage of immune haemolysis may provide an explanation for the differing severity of haemolysis in patients with apparently similar antibodies. *In vitro* macrophage (monocyte) assays have been used sometimes to supplement conventional serological techniques to assess this aspect of immune haemolysis.[20]

Factors that may affect the interaction between sensitized cells and macrophages include the following:

1. *IgG subclass.* IgG1 and IgG3 antibodies have a higher binding affinity to mononuclear Fcγ receptors than IgG2 and IgG4 antibodies.
2. *Antigen density.* This affects the number of antibody molecules bound to the cell surface.
3. *Fluid-phase IgG.* Serum IgG concentration is a determinant of Fc-dependent mononuclear-phagocytic function. Normal levels of IgG block the adherence of sensitized red cells to monocyte Fc receptors (particularly FcγR1) *in vitro*. Haemoconcentration within the splenic sinusoids is probably a major factor in minimizing this effect *in vivo*, which may explain why the spleen is about 100 times more efficient at removing IgG-sensitized cells than the liver despite the greater macrophage mass and higher blood flow of the latter organ.

The initial effect of high-dose intravenous IgG is to cause blockade of macrophage FcγR. This reduces the immune clearance of antibody-coated cells and has particular application in the management of autoimmune thrombocytopenia and post-transfusion purpura.

4. *Regulation of macrophage activity.* Cytokines are known to be important in the upregulation of macrophage receptors. Interferon gamma enhances macrophage phagocytic activity by increasing the expression of FcγRI *in vitro* and *in vivo* and also activates FcγII without increasing the number of these receptors.[21]

Interleukin-6 also enhances FcγRII activation and increased activity of the CR1 receptor occurs through the action of T-cell cytokines and through chemotactic agents released in the inflammatory response.[22] The increased levels of proinflammatory cytokines and other biological mediators and their effects on the activity of the monocyte phagocytic system have been monitored in patients with systemic inflammatory response syndrome.[23] It is therefore possible that release of cytokines during viral and bacterial infections could, at least in part, trigger some episodes of autoimmune cell destruction.

The rate of immune destruction is therefore determined by antigen and antibody characteristics and the level of activation of the monocyte phagocytic system.

Antigen–Antibody Reactions

The red cell is a convenient marker for serological reactions. Agglutination or lysis (owing to complement action) is a visible indication (endpoint) of an antigen–antibody reaction. The reaction occurs in two stages: in the first stage the antibody binds to the red cell antigen (sensitization) and the second stage involves agglutination (or lysis) of the sensitized cells.

The *first stage* (i.e. association of antibody with antigen – sensitization) is reversible and the strength of binding (equilibrium constant) depends on the 'exactness of fit' between antigen and antibody. This is influenced by the following:

1. *Temperature.* Cold antibodies (usually IgM) generally bind best to the red cell at a low temperature (e.g. 4°C), whereas warm antibodies (usually IgG) bind most efficiently at body temperature (i.e. 37°C).
2. *pH.* There is relatively little change in antibody binding over the pH range 5.5–8.5, but to ensure comparable results, it is preferable to buffer the saline in which serum or cells are diluted to a fixed pH, usually 7.0. Some antibody elution techniques depend on altering the pH to <4 or >10.
3. *Ionic strength of the medium.* Low ionic strength increases the rate of antibody binding. This is the basis of antibody detection tests using low ionic strength saline (LISS).

The *second stage* depends on various laboratory manipulations to promote agglutination or lysis of sensitized cells. The cell surface is negatively charged (mainly owing to sialic acid residues), which keeps individual cells apart; the minimum distance between red cells suspended in saline is about 18 nm. Agglutination is brought about by antibody crosslinking between cells. The span between antigen-binding sites on IgM molecules (30 nm) is sufficient to allow IgM antibodies to bridge between saline-suspended red cells (after settling) and so cause agglutination. IgG molecules have a shorter span (15 nm) and are usually unable to agglutinate sensitized red cells suspended in saline; notwithstanding this, heavy IgG sensitization owing to high-antigen density lowers intercellular repulsive forces and is able to promote agglutination in saline (e.g. IgG anti-A, anti-B). The agglutination of red cells coated by either IgM or IgG antibodies is enhanced by centrifugation. However, it is standard procedure to promote agglutination of IgG-sensitized red cells by the following:

1. Reducing intercellular distance by pretreatment of red cells with protease enzymes (e.g. papain or bromelin), which reduce the surface charge of red cells (see p. 498)
2. Adding polymers (e.g. albumin), although the mechanism by which albumin or other water-soluble polymers enhance agglutination is uncertain
3. Bridging between sensitized cells with an anti-globulin reagent in the antiglobulin test (see p. 500).

Some complement-binding antibodies (especially IgM) may cause lysis *in vitro* (without noticeable agglutination), which can be enhanced by the addition of fresh serum as a source of complement. However, complement activation may only proceed to the C3 stage; in these circumstances cell-bound C3 can be detected by the antiglobulin test using an appropriate anticomplement reagent (see p. 500).

Quality Assurance within the Laboratory

It has long been appreciated that the test systems used for routine pre-transfusion testing are of the utmost importance because errors can and do lead to patient morbidity and mortality. It is therefore of little surprise that within the European Union all reagents, calibrators and control materials for red cell typing and for determining the presence of 'irregular anti-erythrocytic antibodies' have been included under the In-vitro Diagnostics (IVD) Medical Devices Directive[24] (see p. 588). This means that all reagents sold within the European Union must display the CE mark to show that they conform to the agreed Common Technical Specifications (CTS). In each European country, a Competent Authority will be able to withdraw or suspend certification of any reagent, depending on the information received from its Notified Body, which will perform batch release approval and monitor the performance of the manufacturer and the product.

The arrival of this Directive further reinforces the potential liabilities of an individual laboratory, which takes on the product liability of a manufacturer if reagents are made 'in-house' or if the manufacturer's recommended method is not strictly adhered to.

The majority of the following points are taken from the British Committee for Standards in Haematology (BCSH) guidelines[25] for pre-transfusion compatibility testing:

1. General aspects
   a. The laboratory should document its Quality System, appropriate to its requirements.
   b. Attention should be given to the sensible inclusion of internal controls in all the tests undertaken.
   c. The laboratory should participate in External Quality Assessment exercises.
   d. The laboratory should only make use of systems that have been validated against its documented requirements.
   e. The laboratory should ensure that they have procedures to cover the failure of automated equipment and computer(s). The laboratory should develop procedures to build in checks for all critical points in transfusion testing (e.g. preserving the identity of patient samples, transcribing results).

2. Reagents
   a. The head of the laboratory should refer to available specifications for reagents given by, for example, the International Society of Blood Transfusion (ISBT), the American Association of Blood Banks (AABB) or the Guidelines for the Blood Transfusion Services.[26,27]
   b. All reagents or systems should be used in accordance with the manufacturer's instructions. Where this is not possible, the procedure should be validated in accordance with the BCSH Guidelines on evaluation, validation and implementation of new techniques for blood grouping, antibody screening and crossmatching.[28]
   c. There should be a record of all batch numbers and expiry dates of all reagents used in the laboratory.

3. Techniques
   a. All procedures used should be in accordance with recommended practice as outlined here.
   b. It is essential that the antiglobulin technique chosen has been validated against the documented requirements of the laboratory and has been subjected to a thorough field trial before being introduced into the laboratory.[29]

   c. All changes in techniques must be thoroughly validated in accordance with the BCSH Guidelines on evaluation, validation and implementation of new techniques before being introduced into routine use.
   d. Written authorized standard operating procedures (SOPs) which cover all aspects of the laboratory work must be available and reviewed regularly.
   e. The regular checking and maintenance of all laboratory equipment must be documented. In particular, there should be a documented quality-assurance procedure for cell washers (e.g. using the National Institute of Biological Standards and Control, NIBSC anti-D standard).[30]

4. Staff training and proficiency
   a. There should be a documented programme for training laboratory staff, which covers all SOPs in use and which fulfils the documented requirements of the laboratory.
   b. Laboratory tasks should only be undertaken by appropriately trained staff.
   c. There must be a documented programme for assessing staff proficiency (e.g. replicate testing for the IAT), which should include details of the action limits for retraining.[31]

5. Auditing and reviewing practice
   a. There should be a system in place for documenting and reviewing all incidents of non-compliance with procedures.
   b. The systems should enable a full audit trail of laboratory steps, including the original results, interpretations, authorizations and all staff responsible for conducting each step.
   c. A programme of independent audits should be conducted to assess compliance with documented 'in-house' procedures.

6. Health and safety
   When appropriate, reagents should have been screened for human immunodeficiency virus and hepatitis B and C virus. All high-risk samples must be handled in accordance with the laboratory safety code (see Chapter 25).

General Points of Serological Technique

Serum versus Plasma

Serum is preferred to plasma for the detection of red cell alloantibodies. Nevertheless, plasma is being used increasingly for convenience in microplate technology and in automated systems.

When plasma is used, complement is inactivated by the ethylenediaminetetra-acetic acid (EDTA) anticoagulant.

This is relevant for the detection of some complement-binding antibodies (e.g. of Kidd specificity) that may be missed or give only weak reactions with anti-IgG in the routine antiglobulin test but can be readily detected by anti-complement (see p. 500). It is therefore essential, before using plasma, to optimize the sensitivity of techniques for detecting weak IgG antibodies and to validate the procedure (see p. 500). For example, in antibody screening, increased sensitivity can be achieved by using panel cells with homozygous expression of selected antigens (see p. 528).

Collection and Storage of Blood Samples

Positive identification of the patient and careful labelling of blood samples are essential to avoid misidentification errors. Venous blood is desirable for blood-grouping purposes and 5–10 ml of blood should be taken and either allowed to clot at room temperature or anticoagulated with EDTA in a sterile plastic tube. This will provide serum or plasma and red cells. If serum is required urgently, the specimen may be placed in a 37°C waterbath and centrifuged as soon as the clot can be seen to have started to retract.

Storage of Sera or Plasma

Great care must be taken to identify and label correctly any serum or plasma separated from the patient's original sample.

Whole blood samples will deteriorate over time. Problems associated with storage include red cell lysis; loss of complement in the serum; decrease in potency of red cell antibodies, particularly IgM antibodies; and bacterial contamination. However, in the absence of evidence, it has been suggested that whole blood can be stored at room temperature for up to 48 h and up to 7 days at 4°C. It has also been recommended that laboratories evaluate the stability of weak antibodies before making local decisions for storage conditions. Patient's serum or plasma is best stored frozen at −20°C or below in 1–2 ml volumes in plastic vials. Repeated thawing of a sample is harmful. If the sera are stored at −20°C or below, no precautions are necessary with respect to sterility. Complement deteriorates rapidly on storage, but sera separated from blood as quickly as possible and stored at −20°C retain most of their complement activity for 1–2 weeks. For compatibility tests, samples of serum should be separated from the red cells as soon as possible and stored at −20°C until used because the content of complement may be important for the detection of some antibodies.

Red Cell Suspensions

Normal ionic strength saline

A 2–3% suspension of washed red cells in phosphate buffered saline (PBS), pH 7.0, is generally recommended. Cells suspended in normal ionic strength saline (NISS) are routinely used for antibody titrations, but their use in routine pretransfusion testing has declined over the last decade as observations from external quality assessment exercises have demonstrated that laboratories using NISS have a significantly lower detection rate of antibodies than those using other technologies.[32]

Low ionic strength saline

It is known that the rate of association of antibodies with red cell antigens is enhanced by lowering the ionic strength of the medium in which the reactions take place. Hence, a major advantage of low ionic strength saline (LISS) is that the incubation period in the IAT (see p. 529) can be shortened while maintaining or increasing sensitivity to the majority of red cell antibodies. The LISS solution can be made up in the laboratory (see p. 620) or purchased commercially.

There was historical reluctance to use low ionic strength media in routine laboratory work for two reasons: first, nonspecific agglutination may occur when NaCl concentrations <2 g/l (0.03 mol/l) are used and second, complement components are bound to the red cells at low ionic strengths.

To avoid false-positive results, the following rules should be followed:

a. Red cells resuspended in LISS and serum or plasma should be incubated together in equal volumes: 2 volumes of cells to 2 volumes of serum are recommended to ensure the optimal molarity in the test of the order of 0.09 mol. Doubling the serum to cell ratio (by halving the cell concentration from 3% to 1.5%) will enhance the detection of some antibodies (e.g. anti-K) that might otherwise be missed.[33]

b. The red cells should be washed in saline twice and then once in LISS before suspending in LISS at 1.5–2% cell suspension.

c. The working solution of LISS should be freshly made and kept at room temperature.

d. Centrifugation force and time should be optimal to give maximum sensitivity with freedom from false-positive or false-negative reactions (see p. 501).

False-positive reactions may still infrequently occur with some sera/plasma. If plasma is used, subsequent serological work may be performed using NISS; if serum is used, anti-IgG should replace the polyspecific antiglobulin reagent.

Reagent Red Cells

Red cells of selected phenotypes are required for ABO and RhD grouping, Rh phenotyping and antibody screening and identification (see Chapter 20). Such cells are available commercially or from blood transfusion centres.

Use of Enzyme-Treated Cells

Enzyme-treated red cells are useful reagents in the detection and investigation of autoantibodies and alloantibodies. Papain and bromelin are currently used for this purpose. Enzyme treatment is known to increase the avidity of both IgM and IgG antibodies. The receptors of some red cell antigens, however, may be inactivated by enzyme treatment (e.g. M, N, S, Fy^b).

The most sensitive techniques are those using washed enzyme-pretreated red cells (two-stage), which should match the performance of the spin-tube LISS antiglobulin test (see p. 501) One-stage mixtures and papain inhibitor techniques are relatively insensitive and are not recommended. An ISBT/International Council for Standardization in Haematology (ICSH) protease enzyme standard and an agreed method for its use are available.

Methods for the preparation of papain solution (Low's method and the two-stage method) and for preparation of bromelin solution have been described.[34–36]

Agglutination of Red Cells by Antibody: A Basic Method

Agglutination tests are usually carried out in tubes, microtitre plates or column agglutination (gel) technology, using centrifugation or sedimentation. Slide tests are rarely used for emergency ABO and D grouping (see p. 524). For microplate tests, see p. 525.

Tube Tests

Add 1 volume of a 2% red cell suspension to 2–3 volumes of plasma in a disposable plastic tube. Mix well and leave undisturbed for the appropriate time (see later).

Tubes

For agglutination tests, use medium-sized (75×10 or 12 mm) disposable plastic tubes. Similar tubes should be used for lysis tests when it is essential to have a relatively deep layer of serum to look through, if small amounts of lysis are to be detected. The level of the fluid must rise much higher than the concave bottom of the tubes.

Glass tubes should always be used if the contents are to be heated to 50°C or higher or if organic solvents are being used. Glass tubes, however, are difficult to clean satisfactorily, particularly small-bore tubes and cleaning methods such as those given on p. 623 should be followed carefully.

Temperature and Time of Exposure of Red Cells to Antibody

In blood group serology, tube tests are generally done at 37°C, room temperature or both. There is some advantage in using a 20°C waterbath rather than relying on 'room temperature', which in different countries and seasons may vary from 15°C (or less) to 30°C (or more).

Sedimentation tube tests are usually read after 1–2 h have elapsed. Strong agglutination will, however, be obvious much sooner than this. In spin-tube tests, agglutination can be read after only 5–10 min incubation if the cell–plasma mixture is centrifuged.

Slide Tests

These are used rarely in a few parts of the world. Because of evaporation, slide tests must be read within about 5 min. Reagents that produce strong agglutination within 1–2 min are normally used for rapid ABO and RhD grouping. Because the results are read macroscopically, strong cell suspensions should be used (35–45% cells in their own serum or plasma)

Reading Results of Tube Tests

Only the strongest complete (C) grade of agglutination seems to be able to withstand a shake procedure without some degree of disruption, which may downgrade the strength of reaction. The BCSH Blood Transfusion Task Force has therefore recommended the following reading procedure.[37]

Microscopic reading

It is essential that a careful and standardized technique be followed. Lift the tube carefully from its rack without disturbing the button of sedimented cells. Holding the tube vertically, introduce a straight-tipped Pasteur pipette. Carefully draw up a column of supernatant about 1 cm in length and then, without introducing an air bubble, draw up a 1–2 mm column of red cells by placing the tip of the pipette in the button of red cells. Gently expel the supernatant and cells onto a slide over an area of about 2×1 cm. It is important not to overload the suspension with cells and the method described earlier achieves this.

A scheme of scoring the results is given in Table 21.11.

Macroscopic reading

A gentle agitation tip-and-roll 'macroscopic' method is recommended. It is possible to read agglutination tests macroscopically with the aid of a hand reading glass or concave mirror, but it is then difficult to distinguish reactions weaker than + (microscopic reading) from the normal slight granular appearance of unagglutinated red cells in suspension. Macroscopic reading thus gives lower titration values than does microscopic reading, but the former is recommended. Follow the system of scoring in Table 21.11.

A good idea of the presence or absence of agglutination can often be obtained by inspection of the deposit of sedimented cells: a perfectly smooth round button suggests no agglutination, whereas agglutination is shown by varying

Table 21.11 Scoring of results in red cell agglutination tests

SYMBOL	AGGLUTINATION SCORE*	DESCRIPTION
4+ or C (complete)	12	Cell button remains in one clump, macroscopically visible
3+	10	Cell button dislodges into several large clumps, macroscopically visible
2+	8	Cell button dislodges into many small clumps, macroscopically visible
1+	5	Cell button dislodges into finely granular clumps, macroscopically just visible
(+) or w (weak)	3	Cell button dislodges into fine granules, only visible microscopically[†]
−	0	Negative result – all cells free and evenly distributed

*Titration scores are the summation of the agglutination scores at each dilution.
[†]May be further classified depending on the number of cells in the clumps (e.g. clumps of 12–20 cells [score 3]; 8–10 cells [score 2]; 4–6 cells [score 1]. This is the minimum agglutination that should be considered positive.

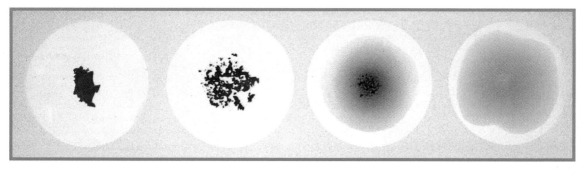

Figure 21.2 Macroscopic appearances of agglutination in round-bottom tubes or hollow tiles. Agglutination is shown by various degrees of 'graininess'; in the absence of agglutination, the sedimented cells appear as a smooth round button, as on the extreme right.

degrees of irregularity, 'graininess', or dispersion of the deposit (Fig. 21.2).

Demonstration of Lysis

Many blood-group antibodies lyse red cells under suitable conditions in the presence of complement. This is particularly true of anti-A and anti-B, anti-P, anti-Le^a and Le^b, anti-PP$_1$P^k (anti-Tj^a) and certain autoantibodies (see p. 284). If it is necessary to add fresh complement, this should be mixed with the serum being tested before the addition of red cells. Otherwise, agglutination occurs and could block complement access. Lysis should be looked for at the end of the incubation period before the tubes are centrifuged, if the cells have sedimented sufficiently; lysis may be scored semiquantitatively after centrifuging the suspensions and comparing the colour of the supernatant with that of the control.

If the occurrence of lysis is of interest, then the final volume of the cell–serum suspension has to be greater than is required for the reading of agglutination. Tubes (75 × 10 or 12 mm) should be used and the level of the cell–serum suspension must rise much higher than the concave bottom of the tubes.

In testing for lytic activity, a high concentration of complement may be required. Therefore, in contrast to tests for agglutination, it is advantageous to use a stronger red cell suspension (c5%).

Lysis tests are usually carried out at 37°C, but with cold antibodies a lower temperature (e.g. 20°C or 30°C) would be appropriate, depending on the upper thermal range of activity of the antibody or, in the case of the Donath–Landsteiner antibody, 0°C followed by 37°C (see p. 277).

With certain antibodies the pH of the cell–serum suspension affects the occurrence of lysis. In these, optimal pH is 6.5–6.8.

Controls

It is necessary to be sure that any lysis observed is not arte-factual (i.e. that lysis is brought about by the serum under test and not by the serum added as complement) and that the added complement is potent. A complement control (no test serum) is thus necessary, as is a control using a serum known to contain a lytic antibody.

In lysis tests, great care should be taken to deliver the cell suspension directly into the serum. If the cell suspension comes into contact with the side of the tube and starts to dry, this in itself will lead to lysis.

Antiglobulin Test

The antiglobulin test (Coombs test) was introduced by Coombs and colleagues in 1945[38] as a method for detect-ing 'incomplete' Rh antibodies (i.e. IgG antibodies capable of sensitizing red cells but incapable of causing agglutina-tion of the same cells suspended in saline), as opposed to 'complete' IgM antibodies, which do agglutinate saline-suspended red cells.

Direct and indirect antiglobulin tests can be carried out. In the *direct* antiglobulin test (DAT), the patient's cells, after careful washing, are tested for sensitization that has occurred *in vivo*; in the *indirect* antiglobulin test (IAT), nor-mal red cells are incubated with a serum suspected of con-taining an antibody and subsequently tested, after washing, for *in vitro*-bound antibody.

The antiglobulin test is probably the most important test in the serologist's repertoire. The DAT is used to demonstrate *in vivo* attachment of antibodies to red cells, as in autoim-mune haemolytic anaemia (see p. 275), alloimmune HDN (see p. 535) and alloimmune haemolysis following an incompatible transfusion (see p. 542). The IAT has wide application in blood transfusion serology, including anti-body screening and identification and crossmatching.

Antiglobulin Reagents

Polyspecific (broad-spectrum) reagents

The majority of red cell antibodies are non-complement-binding IgG; anti-IgG is therefore an essential component of any polyspecific reagent. Anti-IgA is not required because IgG antibodies of the same specificity almost always occur in the presence of IgA antibodies. Anti-IgM is also not required because clinically significant IgM alloantibodies that do not cause agglutination in saline are much more easily detected by the complement they bind.

Anticomplement has also traditionally been considered essential – namely, anti-C3c and anti-C3d. However, if plasma is used, only anti-IgG is necessary because EDTA prevents complement activation. In addition, it seems that most, if not all, antibodies detected by the C3-anti-C3 reac-tion in normal ionic strength tests can be detected with anti-IgG in polybrene, polyethylene glycol (PEG) and LISS.

Laboratories using techniques other than NISS have adopted the use of anti-IgG alone, supported by changes to guidelines from the AABB in 1990 and from the BCSH in 1996. Nevertheless, the BCSH guidelines stress the importance of having screening cells with homozygous expression of Jk[a] before deciding to use anti-IgG rather than a polyspecific antiglobulin reagent. Anti-C3 will certainly be required for DATs for the diagnosis of autoimmune haemolytic anaemia.

Monospecific reagents

Monospecific reagents can be prepared against the heavy chains of IgG, IgM and IgA and are referred to as anti-γ, anti-μ and anti-α; antibodies against IgG subclasses are also available. Specific antibodies against the complement com-ponents C4 and C3 and C3 breakdown products can be prepared as mentioned earlier.

The main clinical application of these monospecific reagents is to define the immunochemical characteristics of antibodies. This is relevant to the mechanisms of *in vivo* cell destruction and, in the case of IgG, the subclasses have different biological properties (see p. 494).

Quality Control of Antiglobulin Reagents

This is not commonly done in UK hospital laboratories, as they use commercial antiglobulin reagents. The quality control of antiglobulin reagents must always be carried out by the exact technique by which they are to be used. All reagents should be used according to the manufacturer's instructions, unless appropriately standardized for other methods.

An ISBT/ICSH freeze-dried reference reagent is available for evaluating either polyspecific antihuman globulin reagents or those containing their separate monospecific components.[26] The validation of a new antiglobulin reagent should assess the following qualities of the reagent:

1. *Specificity.* The reagent should only agglutinate red cells sensitized with antibodies and/or coated with significant levels of complement components
2. *Potency of anti-IgG by serological titration*
3. *Specificity and potency of anticomplement antibodies.* A polyspecific reagent should contain anti-C3c and anti-C3d at controlled levels to avoid false-positive reactions or a suitable potent monoclonal anti-C3d (e.g. BRIC-8). It should contain little or no anti-C4. The assessment of these qualities requires red cells specifically coated with C3b, Cb3i, C3d and C4. Details of the procedures recommended for the preparation of such cells have been published by an ISBT/ICSH Working Party.[39]

It is appreciated that some hospital blood banks worldwide will be unable to evaluate an antiglobulin reagent as com-prehensively as outlined earlier. They should, however, carry out the following minimal assessment of all new antiglobulin reagents:

1. Test the antiglobulin reagent for freedom from false-positive results by simulated crossmatch tests:

   a. Test for excess anti-C3d by incubating fresh serum at 37°C by NISS or LISS tests with 6 ABO-compatible cells from CPD-A1 donor unit segments (10–30 days old). This is a critical test for false-positive results owing to C3d uptake by stored blood, which is further augmented by incubation with fresh serum

   b. Tests for contaminating red cell antibodies (against washed A_1, B and O cells) must be negative.

Only proceed further if the antiglobulin reagent passes the previously listed tests.

2. Compare the antiglobulin reagent with the current reagent using a selection of weak antibodies. These antibodies may be selected from those encountered in routine work or can be obtained from a transfusion centre or reference laboratory. Store such antibodies in small volumes at 4°C for repeated tests.

3. Dilute a weak IgG anti-D (0.8 iu/ml), as used for routine antiglobulin test controls, from undiluted (neat) to 1 in 16 and sensitize R_1r red cells with each dilution of anti-D. These sensitized cells (washed four times) should then be tested with neat to 1 in 8 dilutions of the antiglobulin reagents. The antiglobulin reagent should not show prozones by immediate spin tests using 2 volumes of antiglobulin per test. The potency of the test antiglobulin should at least match the current antiglobulin reagent.

The ISBT/ICSH antiglobulin reference reagent can be used to calibrate an 'in-house' antiglobulin reagent for use as a routine standard.

The quality control of Ig class and subclass specific antiglobulin reagents, although following the previously listed general principles, is more complex. Details of the appropriate techniques are beyond the scope of this chapter; the reader should consult the review by Engelfriet et al.[40]

Recommended Antiglobulin Test Procedure

A spin-tube technique is recommended for the routine antiglobulin test; the procedure described here is based on BCSH *Guidelines for Compatibility Testing in Hospital Blood Banks*.[27,37] Reliable performance depends on the correct procedure at each stage of the test and appropriate quality-control measures.

The test is preferably carried out in glass tubes (75 × 10 or 12 mm), as plastic tubes may adsorb IgG, which could neutralize anti-IgG of the antiglobulin reagent.

1. *Sensitize red cells* (not relevant to the direct test) by using the following serum:cell ratios:

   a. For NISS, use at least 2 volumes of serum (preferably 4) and 1 volume of a 3% suspension of red cells washed (3 times) and suspended in PBS or 0.15 mol/l NaCl (see p. 621).

   b. For LISS, use 2 volumes of serum and 2 volumes of a 1.5% suspension of red cells washed twice in PBS or 0.15 mol/l NaCl and washed once in LISS and then suspended in LISS (see p. 621).

   c. For commercial low ionic strength additive solutions, the manufacturer's instructions must be followed.

   Because the volume of 'a drop' varies according to the type of pipette or dropper bottle, a measured or known drop volume should be used to ensure that appropriate serum:cell ratios are maintained. Mix the reactants by shaking, then incubate at 37°C, preferably in a waterbath, for a minimum period of 15 min for LISS tests and 45 min for NISS tests.

2. *Wash the test cells* four times with a minimum of 3 ml of saline per wash. Vigorous injection of saline is necessary to resuspend the cells and achieve adequate mixing. As much of the supernatant as possible should be removed after each wash to achieve maximum dilution of residual serum.

3. *Add 2 volumes of a suitable antiglobulin reagent* to each test tube and centrifuge without delay after thorough mixing. The combinations of centrifugal force (RCF) and time for spin-tube tests are as follows:

RCF (g)	100	200–220	500	1000
Time (s)	60	25–30	15	8–10

4. *Read agglutination* as previously described (see p. 498).

5. *Quality control of the test* should be monitored by the following:

   a. An IgG anti-D diluted to give 1+ or 2+ reactions with RhD-positive (R_1r) cells as a *positive control*.

   b. An inert group AB serum with the same RhD-positive cells as a *negative control*; this is not essential because most tests are negative.

   c. The addition of sensitized cells to all negative tests. This is widely used to detect neutralization of the antiglobulin reagent owing to incomplete removal of serum by the wash step. The value of this test as a control depends on the strength of reaction of the sensitized cells. Appropriate control cells sensitized with IgG anti-D should give a 3+ reaction when tested directly with the antiglobulin reagent and should still be positive (if the reagent is potent) when added to negative tests but downgraded (1+ or 2+) owing to the 'pooled-cell' effect of the non-sensitized cells. The reaction will, of course, be negative if the antiglobulin has been neutralized by residual serum.

The production of satisfactory antiglobulin control cells can be achieved by limiting the level of anti-D sensitization to that which gives a negative test in the presence of 1 in 1000 parts serum in saline.[37]

The suitability of the antiglobulin control cells can be checked as follows:

i. Prepare two tubes (10 × 75 mm) with 1 volume of 3% unsensitized cells; wash four times.

ii. Add 2 volumes of antiglobulin to each of the tubes, mix well, spin and read the tubes to confirm the tests are negative.

iii. Add 1 volume of 1 in 1000 serum in saline to one tube and 1 volume of saline as a control to the other tube. Mix and incubate for 1 min at room temperature.

iv. Add 1 volume of control cells to each tube, mix, spin and read the tests.

The test containing 1 in 1000 serum in saline should be negative and the control tube should give at least 2+ reaction. A negative reaction with the control tube suggests a washing deficiency and demands corrective action. If an automated cell-washing centrifuge is used, the washing efficiency should be checked.[30,37]

Alternative Technology for Antibody Detection by the Antiglobulin Test

Alternative techniques, now commonly in use, have a simpler reading phase than the manually read spin-tube IAT. These are of two main types: solid-phase red cell adherence methods[41] and column agglutination techniques. A well-performed spin-tube IAT, as described earlier, is the standard against which any new system should be compared.

Solid-phase red cell adherence methods involve systems in which known red cells, which may also be sensitized, are immobilized on a solid matrix. In the method referenced, ABO and D typing plates are prepared by immobilizing A_1-, B- and D-positive red cells to chemically modified U-bottom strips. The cells are then exposed to the appropriate antibody and the sensitized red cell monolayers are then dried. The unknown test cells are added and the plates are centrifuged after incubation. In a positive reaction, the cells spread over the surface of the well because they have adhered to the bound antibody. In a negative reaction, there is no adherence and the cells form a small button in the centre of the well when the plates are centrifuged.

For reverse typing and antibody screening, A_1, B and O screening cell monolayers are prepared and dried. The test serum is added and, if antibodies to any of the immobilized antigens are present, they attach to the monolayer. The tests are read by the addition of A_1B cells that are coated with anti-IgG.

Solid-phase methods are highly suited for automated reading by passing a light beam through the well at a point at which it will not be interrupted by the button of cells in a negative test but will be dispersed by the layer of red cells spread across the well in a positive test.

With *column agglutination techniques* very small volumes of serum and cells are mixed in a reservoir at the top of a narrow column that contains either a Dextran gel (DiaMed, AG, Switzerland) or glass beads (Bio Vue, Ortho-Clinical Diagnosis, NJ).[42] The columns with the integral reservoirs are supplied in card or cassette form, respectively. After a suitable incubation period, the cards/cassettes containing the tests are spun in a centrifuge in which the axis of the column is strictly in line with the centrifugal force. The red cells, but not the medium in which they are suspended, enter the column. Agglutinated red cells are trapped at the top of the column and unagglutinated red cells form a pellet at the bottom of the column (see Fig. 22.6, see p. 526).

The columns can also contain an antiglobulin reagent for performing DATs or IATs. Because, during centrifugation, the red cells but not the suspending fluid pass through the gel, the red cells do not have to be washed before coming into contact with the antiglobulin reagent. The columns can also include an antibody (e.g. anti-D) for cell typing. Antigen positive cells are agglutinated and trapped in the upper portion of the column.

The advantages of column agglutination technology are as follows:

1. Ease of use and reading and can theoretically be performed by relatively unskilled staff.
2. There is less chance of aerosol contamination from infected samples because of no cell washing before IATs.
3. The cards can be kept for up to 24 h, enabling the results to be reviewed by experienced staff.
4. Ease of automation and positive sample identification.

However, the technology is relatively expensive and its performance does not always compare favourably with the standard LISS-IAT in experienced hands.

Assessment of Individual Worker Performance

It is recommended that all staff (including 'on-call' staff who do not routinely work in the blood bank) should be assessed at regular intervals. A procedure based on 'blind' replicate antiglobulin tests may be used for this purpose.[31,37]

The procedure is as follows:

1. A low-titre (8–16) IgG anti-D, as used for the control of the antiglobulin test, should be titrated against OR_1r or pooled O RhD-positive cells to find the dilution of anti-D that gives 1+ or 2+ sensitized cells (most workers use around 0.3 iu/ml). A standard BCSH-NIBSC anti-D

reference reagent[43] is available for this purpose (available from NIBSC).

2. A batch of sensitized cells is prepared (e.g. by incubating 16 ml of the selected anti-D dilution with 8 ml of 3% washed OR_1 red cells at 37°C for 45 min).

3. Twelve tubes are labelled for blind tests by another person. One volume of 3% 1+ or 2+ sensitized cells and 2 volumes of group AB inert serum (to simulate the volumes of serum used in routine tests) are placed in 9 random tubes and then 1 volume of unsensitized cells + 2 volumes of group-AB inert serum are placed in the remaining tubes. The position of the various tests is recorded.

4. The cells are washed thoroughly four times, anti-globulin is added and the tubes are spun and read.

5. The number of false-negative (and false-positive) results are recorded for each worker and analysed in relation to reading and/or washing technique. It is advisable to give immediate tuition to any workers with washing or reading test faults, followed by further blind replicate trials to demonstrate improvement in procedure and to restore confidence.

Titration of Antibodies

A method for preparing primary dilutions of serum and subsequent antibody titration is illustrated in Figure 21.3.

External quality assessment exercises have demonstrated the wide range of titres reported for a single sample, reflecting the differing sensitivities of technologies in use and have also highlighted the lack of reproducibility.[44] The following points are taken from an addendum to the BCSH guidelines.[45]

Preparation of serial dilutions of patient's or other sera

1. All dilutions and titrations should be made using calibrated pipettes and a separate tip for each step.

2. The diluent should be buffered saline, pH 7.0, for agglutination tests; for lysis tests undiluted ABO-compatible fresh normal human serum should be acidified so that the pH of the cell–serum mixture is c 6.8. The normal serum serves as a source of complement.

3. Tube sizes and assay volumes should be chosen to permit thorough mixing of the dilutions.

4. When assaying high-titre samples, an initial dilution should be made to reduce the number of doubling serial transfers to less than 10. A sufficient range of dilutions should be chosen to ensure that two negative results can be observed.

5. The endpoint should be macroscopic and well-defined. The use of visual comparator aids should be considered where possible.

6. Wherever possible, each sample should be tested in parallel with the previous sample.

7. Titrations should be repeated if there is more than a one-tube difference in the titres obtained from sequential samples.

Addition of red cell suspensions to dilutions of serum

It is conventional to add 1 volume of red cell suspension to 1 volume of serum or serum dilution. This means that each antibody dilution, and hence the 'final' titre, will be twice

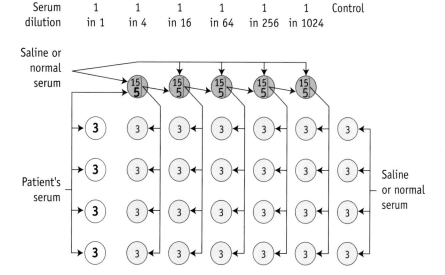

Figure 21.3 Diagram illustrating method of preparing four sets of four-fold dilutions of a serum. The large circles at the top represent the large tubes in which the primary dilutions are made; the smaller circles represent the tubes in which the titrations are carried out. The figures represent drops or volumes. The patient's neat serum is indicated by the bold type.

that of the original serum dilution. Because red cell antigen expression varies with the source and age of the sample, wherever possible, the same cell sample should be used.

Test for ABH Substance Secretion

In the majority of the population, substances with the appropriate A, B and H antigenic activity are distributed widely in saliva and all body fluids, controlled by a regulator secretor gene (*Se*), which is inherited independently of *ABH* genes. Only about 20% of people are non-secretors. Although rarely used, an individual's secretor status can be determined by testing saliva.

Method

Dilute an anti-A or anti-B serum so that it gives good visible agglutination with A_2 or B cells at the end of 1 h at room temperature (e.g. if the titre of the serum is 128, use it at a dilution of 1 in 16).

Collect several millilitres of saliva in a centrifuge tube. Place the tube in boiling water for 10 min and then centrifuge. Serially dilute the clear supernatant in saline so as to give dilutions ranging from 1 in 2 to 1 in 32. Use a tube containing saliva alone as a control. Add an equal volume of the diluted anti-A (or anti-B) serum to each tube and, after shaking the rack of tubes, allow them to stand at room temperature for 10–15 min. Then add an equal volume of a 2% suspension of A_2 (or B) red cells in saline to each tube. Mix the contents and allow to stand at room temperature for 1–2 h; then inspect for agglutination. If the saliva contains A or B substances, agglutination is usually inhibited in all the tubes except the saline control tube.

H substance can be demonstrated in a similar way using an extract of Ulex, eel serum or the naturally occurring 'incomplete' cold antibody as the source of anti-H.

Red Cell Genotyping

Red cell genotyping is not currently in widespread use, but is emerging as a potential alternative to serological provision of compatible blood for patients in future and is currently used occasionally in situations when serological techniques prove difficult, e.g. phenotyping of a recently transfused patient or in a patient with autoimmune haemolytic anaemia.[46]

PLATELET AND NEUTROPHILS

Platelet and Neutrophil Alloantigen Systems

Platelet and neutrophil alloantigens may be exclusive to each cell type (cell-specific) or shared with other cells. The currently recognized human platelet antigens (HPA) and human neutrophil antigens (HNA) are shown in Tables 21.12–21.14.[47–49] The historical nomenclature for granulocyte antigens used the letter N to indicate neutrophil specificity and this has been retained, although it is recognized that many studies used granulocytes rather than pure neutrophils and many 'neutrophil-specific' antibodies can also target granulocyte precursors. In the HPA nomenclature, HPA-1, -2, -3, -4 and -5 were designated as separate diallelic alloantigen systems. The high-frequency allele of a system was designated with the letter 'a' and the low-frequency allele was designated with the letter 'b'. However, this system is difficult to reconcile with recent molecular genetic knowledge, which suggests that each new base exchange does not constitute a new diallelic alloantigen system but rather defines a single allele that expresses a single new epitope. Currently, nine different GpIIIa alleles have been found in the human gene pool,[50] four allelic variants have been described for GpIa and GpIIb and two allelic variants have been found for the GpIbα and GpIbβ subunits[50] (a database of human platelet antigens is available at: www.ebi.ac.uk/ipd/hpa).[51] Of the shared antigens, the HLA system is the most important clinically; only class 1 antigens (HLA-A, -B and to a lesser extent -C) are expressed on platelets and granulocytes. ABH antigens are also expressed on platelets (in part absorbed from the plasma) but cannot be demonstrated on granulocytes.

Clinical Significance of Platelet and Neutrophil Antibodies

Platelet and neutrophil antibodies may be classified on the basis of the antigenic stimulus (e.g. allo-, iso-, auto- and drug-induced antibodies).

Alloantibodies

Alloimmunization to platelet and neutrophil antigens is most commonly a result of transfusion or pregnancy. The associated clinical problems depend on the specificity of the antibody, which determines the target cell involved. Cell-specific alloantibodies are associated with well-defined clinical conditions, which are summarized in Tables 21.15 and 21.16.

Alloimmune fetal and neonatal thrombocytopenia are commonly caused by anti-HPA-1a and less frequently by anti-HPA-5b. The chance of HPA-1a alloimmunization is strongly associated with maternal HLA class-II DRB3*0101 (DR52a) type.[56] Partners should be offered HPA genotyping and, if heterozygous, with a severely affected previous child, fetal HPA grouping should be considered in the first trimester of the next pregnancy using amniocyte DNA. Potential strategies for routine antenatal screening and the acceptability and cost-effectiveness of such a programme are discussed in several publications.[57,58]

Post-transfusion purpura is most commonly caused by anti-HPA-1a but can be associated with HPA antibodies with

Table 21.12 Molecular genetics of human platelet antigens (HPA)

SYSTEM	ANTIGEN	ORIGINAL NAMES	GLYCOPROTEIN	CD
HPA-1	HPA-1a	Zw^a, Pl^{A1}	Gpllla	CD61
	HPA-1b	Zw^b, Pl^{A2}		
HPA-2	HPA-2a	Ko^b	Gplbα	CD42b
	HPA-2b	Ko^a, Sib^a		
HPA-3	HPA-3a	Bak^a, Lek^a	Gpllb	CD41
	HPA-3b	Bak^b		
HPA-4	HPA-4a	Yuk^b, Pen^a	Gpllla	CD61
	HPA-4b	Yuk^a, Pen^b		
HPA-5	HPA-5a	Br^b, Zav^b	Gpla	CD49b
	HPA-5b	Br^a, Zav^a, Hc^a		
	HPA-6bw	Ca^a, Tu^a	Gpllla	CD61
	HPA-7bw	Mo^a	Gpllla	CD61
	HPA-8bw	Sr^a	Gpllla	CD61
	HPA-9bw	Max^a	Gpllb	CD41
	HPA-10bw	La^a	Gpllla	CD61
	HPA-11bw	Gro^a	Gpllla	CD61
	HPA-12bw	ly^a	Gplbβ	CD42c
	HPA-13bw	Sit^a	Gpla	CD49b
	HPA-14bw	Oe^a	Gpllla	CD61
HPA-15	HPA-15a	Gov^b	CD109	CD109
	HPA-15b	Gov^a		
	HPA-16bw	Duv^a	Gpllla	CD61

HPA, human platelet antigens; GP, glycoprotein location of epitopes.

Table 21.13 Human platelet antigen frequencies (%) in different populations

ANTIGEN	DUTCH	FINNS	AMERICAN CAUCASIAN	JAPANESE	KOREAN
HPA-1a	97.9	99.0	98.0	100.0	99.5
HPA-1b	28.8	26.5	20.0	0.3	2.0
HPA-2a	100.0	99.0	97.0	99.2	99.0
HPA-2b	13.5	16.5	15.0	19.7	14.0
HPA-3a	81.0	83.5	88.0	85.1	82.5
HPA-3b	69.8	66.5	54.0	66.2	71.5
HPA-4a	100.0		100.0	100.0	100.0
HPA-4b	0.0		0.0	2.0	2.0
HPA-5a	100.0	99.5	98.0	99.0	100.0
HPA-5b	19.7	10.0	21.0	7.0	4.5
HPA-6a		100.0		99.7	100.0
HPA-6b		2.4		4.8	4.0

Table 21.14 The human neutrophil antigen systems

ANTIGEN SYSTEM	ANTIGEN PHENOTYPE	LOCATION	ACRONYM	CAUCASIAN FREQUENCY (%)
HNA-1	HNA-1a	FcγRIIIb	NA1	58
	HNA-1b	FcγRIIIb	NA2	88
	HNA-1c	FcγRIIIb	SH	5
HNA-2	HNA-2a	gp50-64	NB1	97
HNA-3	HNA-3a	gp70-95	5b	97
HNA-4	HNA-4a	CD11b	MART	99
HNA-5	HNA-5a	CD11a	OND	96
HNA, human neutrophil antigen.				

Table 21.15 Clinical significance of platelet-specific alloantibodies[52]

1. Neonatal alloimmune thrombocytopenia

2. Post-transfusion purpura

3. Refractoriness to platelet transfusion
   Usually as a result of human leucocyte antigen antibodies.

Table 21.16 Clinical significance of neutrophil-specific alloantibodies[53–55]

1. Neonatal alloimmune neutropenia

2. Febrile reactions following transfusion (HLA antibodies also involved)

3. Transfusion-related acute lung injury (TRALI) (transfusion of high-titre antibody)

4. Poor survival and function of transfused neutrophils (HLA antibodies also involved)

5. Autoimmune neutropenia – some autoantibodies have allospecificity for HNA system antigens.

HLA, human leucocyte antigen; HNA, human neutrophil antigen.

other specificities against HPA-1b, HPA-2b, HPA-3a, HPA-3b, HPA-4a and HPA-5b.[59]

Immunological refractoriness to platelet transfusions is usually the result of anti-HLA antibodies. However, in multitransfused patients with HLA immunization, up to 25% may also have anti-HPA antibodies.[60,61]

Isoantibodies

Rarely, after blood transfusion or pregnancy, patients with type I Glanzmann's disease make antibodies that react with platelet glycoprotein (Gp) IIb/IIIa not present on their own platelets but present on normal platelets (i.e. isotypic determinants).[62–65] Similarly, patients with Bernard–Soulier syndrome may make antibodies against isotypic determinants on GpIbVIX not present on their own platelets.[66] This may present a serious clinical problem because no functional compatible donor platelets can be found to treat severe bleeding episodes.

Autoantibodies

Autoimmune thrombocytopenia may be idiopathic or secondary in association with other conditions. Demonstration of a platelet autoantibody is not required; even with the most suitable techniques now available, platelet autoantibodies remain elusive in a variable proportion (10–20%) of patients. The autoreactive antibodies target epitopes on certain glycoproteins. In 30–40% of patients these are directed against epitopes on the αIIbβ3 integrin heterodimer, platelet glycoprotein GpIIbIIIa (CD41) and in 30–40% against the von Willebrand receptor or complex GpIbα/GPIbβ/IX (CD42).[67–70]

In the diagnosis of autoimmune thrombocytopenia it is important to consider and exclude three other immunological conditions:

1. *Post-transfusion purpura (PTP).* A blood transfusion within 2 weeks will suggest this possibility, although it is very rare in the UK since leucodepletion of blood components.[59,16]

2. *Drug-induced immune thrombocytopenia.* A drug history is essential. Heparin-induced thrombocytopenia (HIT) is the most frequent drug-induced thrombocytopenia and can be confirmed by the demonstration of antibodies

to the heparin/platelet factor 4 (PF4) complex by ELISA (enzyme-linked immunosorbent assay).[71]

3. *Pseudothrombocytopenia.* The patient has an EDTA-dependent platelet antibody that is active only *in vitro*. The antibody (IgG and/or IgM) reacts with hidden (cryptic) antigens on platelet GpIIbIIIa, which are exposed owing to confirmational changes in the complex caused by the removal of Ca^{2+} by EDTA.[72] The antibody causes platelet agglutination in the EDTA blood sample associated with large platelet clumps on the blood film or platelet satellitism around neutrophils, both of which lead to a falsely low platelet count. To overcome this, blood should be taken into a tube containing citrate instead.

Autoimmune neutropenia may be idiopathic or secondary. Idiopathic autoimmune neutropenia is more common in infants than in adults, in whom it is usually associated with other disorders that have in common a postulated imbalance of the immune system.[73] However, it is the least well-studied of the autoimmune cytopenias because it is rare and performing granulocyte assays is difficult, lengthy, labour-intensive and expensive.

Neutrophil autoantibodies (which are usually IgG) are unusual in that they often have well-defined specificity for alloantigens, especially NA1 or NA2.[74] These autoantibodies may suppress granulocyte precursors in the bone marrow and cause more severe neutropenia. The investigation of suspected autoimmune neutropenia should, when possible, include granulocyte immunology and studies of colony growth (e.g. CFU-GM) to identify any suppression of bone marrow precursors, as a result of interaction with autoantibodies.

Drug-Induced Antibodies

Drug-induced antibodies may cause selective haemolytic anaemia (see p. 289), thrombocytopenia or neutropenia or various combinations of these in the same patient.[75,76]

A drug may cause an immune cytopenia by stimulating production of either an *autoantibody* (which reacts directly with the target cell independently of the drug itself) or a *drug-dependent antibody* (which destroys the target cell by reacting with a drug–membrane complex on the target cell).[77] Laboratory tests may demonstrate both types of antibody in some patients.[78]

Demonstration of Platelet and Neutrophil Antibodies

No single method will detect all types of platelet and neutrophil antibodies equally well. In practice, it is useful to have a basic screening method that will detect most commonly occurring antibodies, both cell-bound (direct test) and in serum (indirect test), and to supplement this with other selected methods for demonstrating particular properties of an antibody and for measuring the amount of cell-bound antibody.

Alloantibodies

Reports of national and international workshops make it possible to formulate guidelines for *platelet immunological tests*. The basic procedure for demonstrating platelet alloantibodies should include the following:

1. *A platelet test for platelet-reactive antibodies.* The ISBT/ICSH Working Party on Platelet Serology[79] recommended the platelet suspension immunofluorescence test[80] as the standard for assessment of other platelet antibody techniques.

   It is important to combine a sensitive binding assay, such as the platelet immunofluorescence test (PIFT), with an antigen-capture method, such as the monoclonal antibody immobilization of platelet antigens (MAIPA),[81] to increase the chance of detecting weak antibodies or those that react with relatively few antigen sites.

2. *A lymphocyte test for detecting HLA antibodies.* Because HLA antibodies also react with platelets, a lymphocyte cytotoxicity and/or ELISA assay should be included in the basic antibody screening procedure.

3. *Tests to differentiate platelet-specific from HLA antibodies.* The MAIPA technique using appropriate monoclonal antibodies is particularly useful for resolving mixtures of platelet-reactive antibodies (see p. 512). The chloroquine-'stripping' technique to inactivate HLA Class I molecules on platelets[52] is also helpful in this respect (see p. 511). Conventional serological techniques (e.g. differential reactions with a panel of normal lymphocytes and platelets; differential absorption of HLA antibodies) can also be used to differentiate cell-specific and HLA antibodies, but these are less suitable for rapid screening than the chloroquine-'stripping' technique.

Further characterization of platelet-specific antibodies will require referral to a reference laboratory. Identification of allospecificity should be carried out as for red cell antibodies by reaction with a selected genotyped panel of group O platelets, preferably with reference to the patient's platelet genotype.

An important consideration in platelet serology is the occasional occurrence of antibodies against hidden (cryptic) antigens of the GpIIbIIIa complex, which are exposed by EDTA and paraformaldehyde (PFA) fixation.[82] These antibodies, which are only active *in vitro*, are unpredictable but when suspected can be avoided by using unfixed test platelets from citrated blood.

The detection and identification of granulocyte alloantibodies should be left to experienced reference laboratories, but should follow a similar schedule with the use of monoclonal antibody immobilization of granulocyte antigens (MAIGA)[83,84] or adsorption of the sera with pooled platelets to differentiate between granulocyte-specific and HLA antibodies.

Autoantibodies

The detection of autoantibodies and drug-induced antibodies requires special consideration.

It can be misleading, when looking for platelet (or granulocyte) autoantibodies, only to test the patient's serum against normal platelets (granulocytes) because positive reactions may result from the presence of alloantibodies (e.g. HLA or cell-specific) induced by previous transfusion or pregnancy. It is important to show that an autoantibody in the patient's serum reacts with the patient's own cells. Ideally a DAT (e.g. PIFT) should be performed, before treatment is given, to detect antibody bound *in vivo*. Where a severe cytopenia exists, it may not be possible to harvest enough cells for the test; nevertheless, serum samples should be stored at −20°C and tested retrospectively against the patient's cells when the peripheral platelet (or neutrophil) count has increased in response to treatment.

A major interest in platelet autoimmunity has been the quantitative measurement of platelet-associated immunoglobulins as an indication of *in vivo* sensitization. A criticism of these quantitative methods is that they detect not only platelet autoantibody but also Ig nonspecifically trapped or bound to platelets and platelet fragments,[85] and are therefore generally nonspecific in the diagnosis of autoimmune thrombocytopenia.[86] It is now customary to use the direct PIFT,[87,88] using flow cytometry. The patient's platelets are incubated with isotype-specific fluorescein-isothiocyanate (FITC)-labelled conjugates (anti-IgG, anti-IgM and anti-IgA) and the test is reported as positive when the fluorescence intensity is >mean + 2SD when compared with the results obtained with pooled (10 or more) normal donor platelet suspensions. In a study of 75 patients with idiopathic thrombocytopenic purpura, using microscopy rather than flow cytometry, von dem Borne and colleagues[89] found a weak positive (± to +) direct PIFT in 60% of patients and strong reactions (++ to ++++) in only 26% of patients. In the same study, the indirect PIFT was positive with the patient's serum in 66% of cases who had a positive direct PIFT and it was positive with an ether eluate of the patient's platelets in 94% of the same cases. Although these results may be a reflection of the relative insensitivity of the method, they may result from a low-affinity antibody that is easily eluted during the assay procedure[85] or indicate an alternative immune mechanism for thrombocytopenia in some cases.

The Ig class of platelet autoantibodies is similar in idiopathic and secondary autoimmune thrombocytopenia; mostly it is IgG (92%), but often (also) it is IgM (42%) and sometimes (also) IgA (9%).[89] All IgG subclasses occur, but IgG1 and/or IgG3 are the most frequent.

A combination of the granulocyte immunofluorescence test (GIFT)[90] and the granulocyte agglutination test (GAT)[91] provides the most effective means of granulocyte antibody detection. However, immune complexes and aggregates in a patient's serum can still cause false-positive results. This can cause a problem for sera from adult patients with secondary autoimmune neutropenia, which should also be investigated for immune complexes (e.g. Clq-enzyme-linked immunosorbent assay). The granulocyte chemiluminescence test (GCLT)[92] is relatively insensitive to the presence of immune complexes when inactivated serum is used, but it is unable to detect antibodies of the IgM. Several reviews provide an appraisal of the techniques available for detecting granulocyte-specific antibodies and antigens,[93,94] including a recent review of investigations for transfusion-related acute lung injury (TRALI).[95]

Drug-Induced Antibodies

The serological investigation of drug-induced immune thrombocytopenia (neutropenia) follows the same pattern as for haemolytic anaemia (see p. 289), with the exception that it is not always possible to collect enough cells to test at the nadir of thrombocytopenia or neutropenia. The following blood samples are therefore necessary:

1. *Acute-phase blood sample when the cell count is at the nadir.* If there are too few cells to test for cell-bound antibody and complement at this time, it is necessary to test the acute-phase serum against the patient's cells during remission. These tests will demonstrate the immune basis of the cytopenia.

   If the patient's acute-phase serum is tested against *normal* donor cells, it is essential to take account of positive reactions owing to HLA or cell-specific alloantibody in the patient's serum. Furthermore, negative results with normal donor cells may be the result of absence of the antigen for the particular drug-dependent antibody (e.g. owing to genetic restriction of the antigen concerned).[96]

2. *Subsequent samples after stopping the drug.* Ideally, sampling should be done when the drug has been eliminated and the antibody is still detectable. Tests using this sample with and without the drug in the assay system are necessary to demonstrate the part played by the drug in causing the immune cytopenia. The drug may be added directly to the assay system (and included in the wash solution) or the cells may be pretreated with the drug. For some drugs, a metabolite and not the native drug is the appropriate antigen for testing; in these cases an 'ex vivo' drug antigen from urine or plasma may be used.[97]

Methods of Demonstrating Antibodies

The basic immunofluorescent antiglobulin method and the MAIPA assay will be described in detail. Only brief mention will be made of other methods.

The Immunofluorescent Antiglobulin Methods

The immunofluorescent antiglobulin methods are based on the conventional antiglobulin technique (see p. 500) and are suitable for platelet,[80] granulocyte[90] and lymphocyte[98] serology. The PIFT and GIFT (Fison Ltd, Loughborough, UK) are described in detail in this chapter.

These tests can either be read by direct examination of a cell suspension using fluorescence microscopy or by flow cytometry. These tests can detect allo-, auto- and drug-induced antibodies and, by using appropriate monospecific antiglobulin reagents, can determine the Ig class and subclass of the antibody and cell-bound complement components. Both tests can be used with chloroquine-treated cells to differentiate cell-specific from HLA antibodies.[99]

Patient's and Screening Panel Cells

Platelets and granulocytes are prepared from venous blood taken into 5% (w/v) Na_2EDTA in water (9 volumes blood:1 volume anticoagulant).

Screening panel cells should be obtained from group O donors for platelet serology to avoid positive reactions owing to anti-A and anti-B, but this is not necessary for granulocyte serology because A and B antigens cannot be demonstrated on granulocytes. If a patient's serum must be tested with ABO-incompatible platelets, anti-A and/or anti-B can be absorbed with corresponding red cells or A or B substance.

The best results are obtained with the freshest cell preparations, but some delay is tolerable (see later). Neutrophils are more susceptible to storage damage than platelets; cells should be fixed (see later) on the day of collection, but serology may be delayed to the following day. Platelets are more resilient and an anticoagulated blood sample may be satisfactory for testing for up to 2 days at ambient temperature ($c20°C$). Once fixed, platelets may be kept for 3–4 days at 4°C before serological testing. For longer storage, platelet-rich plasma may be kept at −40°C for at least 2 months; however, there is some membrane damage after recovery of frozen platelets, which causes increased background fluorescence that may limit the sensitivity of the test.[100,101] For longer-term storage a cryoprotectant (e.g. DMSO) may be used.[101]

Patient's Serum

Serum from clotted venous blood should be heated at 56°C for 30 min to inactivate complement and stored in 1–2 ml volumes at −40°C (to avoid repeated thawing of a stock).

Control Sera

Negative control serum is prepared from a pool of 10 sera from normal group AB male donors who have never been transfused. *Positive control* sera containing platelet-specific antibodies (e.g. anti-HPA-1a), granulocyte-specific antibodies or multispecific HLA antibodies should be obtained from reference centres.

Eluate from Patient's Sensitized Cells

Elution is important to confirm the antibody nature of cell-bound immunoglobulin and to determine the specificity of antibodies. This applies especially when no antibody is demonstrable in the patient's serum, which often occurs in patients with autoimmune thrombocytopenia and neutropenia.

Elution by lowering the pH of the medium, by ether (or DMSO) and by heating to 56°C, has been used.[102] For routine platelet serology, ether elution for platelet autoantibodies or heating to 56°C for platelet-specific alloantibodies could be used.

Heat Eluate

Incubate platelets or granulocytes suspended in 0.5 ml of 0.2% bovine serum albumin (BSA) in PBS for 60 min at 56°C. Centrifuge and remove the supernatant that contains the eluted antibody.

Platelet Preparation

1. Prepare platelet-rich plasma (PRP) by centrifugation of anticoagulated blood (200 g, 10 min).
2. Wash the platelets three times (2500 g, 5 min) in PBS/EDTA buffer (8.37 g of Na_2 EDTA dissolved in 2.5 1 of PBS, pH 7.2); resuspend the platelets thoroughly each time.
3. Fix the platelets in 3 ml of 1% paraformaldehyde solution for 5 min at room temperature. A stock solution of PFA is prepared by dissolving 4 g of PFA (BDH) in 100 ml of PBS by heating to 70°C with occasional mixing. Add 1 mol/l NaOH dropwise with continuous mixing until the solution clears. This 4% stock solution may be stored at 4°C protected from light for several months. Prepare a 1% PFA working solution by adding 1 volume of the 4% PFA stock solution to 3 volumes of PBS and by correcting the pH if necessary to 7.2–7.4 with 1 mol/l HCI.
   Wash the platelets twice as before and resuspend in PBS/EDTA buffer at a concentration of 250–500 × 10^9/ l for use in the PIFT.

Granulocyte Preparation

1. Mix anticoagulated blood or blood retained from platelet preparation after removal of PRP (and made up to its original volume with PBS) with 2 ml of Dextran solution per 10 ml of blood (Dextran 150 injection BP in 5% dextrose). Incubate this mixture at 37°C for

30 min at an angle of about 45° to accelerate red cell sedimentation and then remove the leucocyte-rich supernatant (LRS).

2. Granulocytes can be separated by double-density sedimentation (Fig. 21.4). The LRS is underlayered with 2 ml of lymphocyte separating medium (LSM) (LSM = Ficoll-Hypaque sp gr 1.077), which is then underlayered with 2 ml of mono-poly resolving medium (MPRM) (MPRM = Ficoll-Hypaque sp gr 1.114) (LSM and MPRM supplied by Flow Labs Ltd). The density gradient tube is then centrifuged at 2500 g for 5 min. Granulocytes form an opaque layer at the LSM/MPRM interface from which they are harvested by careful pipetting (microscopic examination shows that the cells from this layer are predominantly neutrophil polymorphs). Lymphocytes can similarly be harvested from the plasma/lSM interface (e.g. for use in the lymphocyte immunofluorescence test or LIFT).[98]

Leucocyte-rich
supernatant

Layer 1
Mononuclear cells
± platelets

Solution I
Ficoll–Hypaque
(sp gr 1.077)

Layer 2
Granulocytes

Solution II
Ficoll–Hypaque
(sp gr 1.114)

Layer 3
Red cells

Figure 21.4 Double-density separation of lymphocytes and granulocytes. A leucocyte-rich supernatant is underlayered with Ficoll–Hypaque with a specific gravity of 1.077 (Solution I) and 1.114 (Solution II) and then centrifuged at 2500 g for 5 min. Lymphocytes concentrate in layer 1; granulocytes concentrate in layer 2.

3. Wash the granulocytes three times at 400 g for 5 min) in PBS/BSA buffer (PBS pH 7.2 with 0.2% BSA).
4. Fix the granulocytes in 3 ml of 1% PFA for 5 min at room temperature.
5. Wash the granulocytes twice as before and resuspend in PBS/BSA buffer at a concentration of about 10×10^9/l for use in the GIFT.

Platelet and Granulocyte Immunofluorescence Tests

The serological methods for testing platelets and granulocytes in the suspension immunofluorescence test are similar, except that platelets are washed throughout in PBS/EDTA buffer and granulocytes are washed in PBS/BSA buffer. A flow diagram of the PIFT is shown in Figure 21.5.

FITC-labelled antiglobulin reagents are used as follows: anti-Ig (polyspecific), anti-IgG, anti-IgM and anti-C3. $F(ab)_2$ fragments of these reagents should be used to minimize nonspecific membrane fluorescence owing to Fc receptor binding, which is a particular problem with granulocytes. The optimal dilution for each reagent should be determined by chequer-board titration. Centrifuge the FITC conjugates at 2500 g for 10 min before use to remove fluorescent debris and reduce background fluorescence.

Positive and negative controls (as described earlier) should be included with each batch of tests.

Indirect Test

1. In plastic precipitin tubes (50 × 7 mm), mix 0.1 ml of serum and 0.1 ml of the appropriate cell suspension, as prepared earlier. (The method can also be adapted for use with microtitre plates, which has the advantage of using smaller volumes.)
2. Incubate for 30 min at 37°C (for IgG and C3 tests) and at room temperature (for IgM tests). For C3 tests *only*, sediment cells (1000 g, 5 min), remove the supernatant and resuspend the cell button in 0.1 ml of freshly thawed human serum as a source of complement. Incubate for 30 min at 37°C.
3. Wash the cells three times at 1000 g, for 5 min with appropriate buffer – PBS/EDTA for platelets, PBS/BSA for granulocytes; decant the final supernatant. This and subsequent steps are common for both the *indirect* test (i.e. patient's serum with donor cells) and the *direct* test (i.e. patient's own cells to detect *in vivo* sensitization).
4. Add the fluorescent antiglobulin reagent (0.1 ml of the appropriate dilution determined by chequer-board titration), mix with the cell button and leave at room temperature for 30 min in the dark.
5. Wash twice as before and remove the supernatant.
6. Mix 0.5 ml of glycerol – PBS (3 volumes glycerol:1 volume PBS) with the cell button and mount on a glass slide under a coverslip.

Figure 21.5 Platelet immunofluorescence test. PRP, platelet-rich plasma; PBS, phosphate buffered saline; PFA, paraformaldehyde; RBC, red blood cells.

7. Examine microscopically using ×40 objective and epifluorescent ultraviolet illumination.

Scoring Results

Reactions in the PIFT and GIFT may be scored on a scale from negative (−) through graded positives + to + + + +. Although subjective, this method of scoring in experienced hands can produce semiquantitative results in the PIFT.[103]

In general, normal platelets and granulocytes incubated with AB serum do not fluoresce after incubation with an appropriately diluted FITC antiglobulin reagent. Sometimes the negative control may show weak fluorescence (up to two fluorescing points on some cells); in these cases, the test result is classified as positive only if it is clearly stronger than the negative control (AB serum). Stronger fluorescence in the negative control should raise doubts about the performance of the test.

Use of Flow Cytometry

With simplification of flow cytometers and improved software, more platelet reference laboratories are using them for primary analysis in PIFT because sensitivity is improved. Nevertheless, platelets are more difficult to work with flow cytometrically than other cells and particular attention has to be paid to prevent aggregation and to ensure single cell suspensions. Presence of platelet particles and debris may also cause confusion. The technical considerations of applying flow cytometry to platelet work are the subject of several reviews.[87,88]

Chloroquine Treatment of Platelets and Granulocytes

Platelets for chloroquine treatment should be prepared from fresh blood or blood stored overnight at 4°C; granulocytes are suitable only if freshly prepared.[52,104] An important consideration is the extent of chloroquine-induced cell membrane damage, which is minimal with fresh cells.

1. Cells are prepared as already described. Two-thirds of the cells are treated with chloroquine; the remaining one-third are not treated. After washing and before PFA fixation, the cell button is incubated with 4–5 ml of chloroquine diphosphate in PBS (200 mg/ml, pH adjusted to 5.0 with 1 mol/l NaOH) for 2 h at room temperature with occasional mixing or overnight at 4°C without mixing, if this is more convenient for the laboratory routine.
2. Wash three times in the appropriate buffer and fix in 1% PFA as previously described. Cell clumping during washing may be a problem after chloroquine treatment, especially with granulocytes; cell clumps should be dispersed by repeated gentle aspiration with a Pasteur pipette. The final cell suspension for serological testing should be prepared as previously described.

When reading the test by fluorescence microscopy, it is important to recognize and allow for any fluorescence owing to chloroquine-induced cell damage, which is more likely to occur with granulocytes than platelets. Damaged cells are easily recognized by bright homogeneous fluorescence. Such cells should be excluded from assessment; only cells showing obvious punctuate fluorescence should be considered positive.

Chloroquine-treated cells were tested initially in the fluorescent antiglobulin method, but they may also be used in enzyme and radionuclide-labelled antigen methods.

Interpretation of Results with Chloroquine-Treated Cells

Typical results with HLA- and cell-specific antibodies are shown in Table 21.17. If a serum that has been shown to contain HLA antibodies by LCT and/or LIFT gives equal or stronger reactions with chloroquine-treated cells than with untreated cells, then a cell-specific antibody is also present. The Second Canadian Workshop on Platelet

Serology[100] concluded that a weaker reaction with chloroquine-treated platelets should be interpreted with caution; this could indicate residual HLA reactivity, especially in the presence of high-titre multispecific HLA antibodies. If a platelet-specific antibody is nevertheless still suspected, other methods should be used to confirm this (e.g. MAIPA using appropriate monoclonal antibodies for capture; see later).

Similar caution should be observed in interpreting the GIFT results with chloroquine-treated cells.

MAIPA Assay

The principle of the MAIPA assay is shown in Figure 21.6. The test is based on the use of monoclonal antibodies, such as anti-IIbIIIa, anti-IbIX, anti-IaIIa and anti-HLA class I, to 'capture' specific platelet membrane glycoproteins. The availability of appropriate monoclonal antibodies has led to the wider clinical application of this method.[81] The same principle can be used with granulocytes, depending on the availability of appropriate monoclonal antibodies.[81,105]

The following assay protocol was developed from the original method described by Kiefel.[81,106]

1. Prepare platelets as for the PIFT (see p. 510), except that paraformaldehyde fixation is omitted.
2. Resuspend a pellet of $50–100 \times 10^6$ platelets in 30 μl of human serum or plasma to be tested and incubate at 37°C for 30 min in a U-well microplate.
3. Wash platelets twice in PBS/EDTA buffer (8.37 g of Na_2EDTA in 2.5 l of phosphate buffered saline, see p. 622). Resuspend the platelets in 30 μl of mouse monoclonal antibody (anti-GpIIbIIIa, IaIIa, IbIX or HLA at 20 μg/ml) and incubate at 37°C for 30 min.
4. Wash platelets twice in PBS/EDTA buffer, lyse by the addition of 100 μl of Tris buffered saline (TBS) containing 0.5% Nonidet P-40 and leave at 4°C for 30 min.
5. Transfer the platelet lysate to a 2 ml conical tube and centrifuge at 11 600 g for 30 min at 4°C to remove particulate matter.

Table 21.17 Platelet and granulocyte antibody reactions using cells prepared with and without treatment with chloroquine

SERA	UNTREATED CELLS		CHLOROQUINE-TREATED CELLS	
	Platelets	Granulocytes	Platelets	Granulocytes
Negative	−	−	−	−
Multispecific HLA antibodies	+++	++	−	−
Granulocyte-specific antibody	−	++	−	+++
Platelet-specific antibody	+++	−	+++	−
HLA, human leucocyte antigen.				

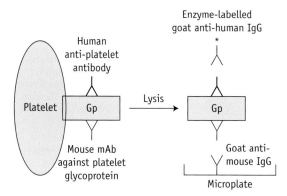

Figure 21.6 Monoclonal antibody immobilization of platelet antigens (MAIPA): principle of the method. gp, platelet membrane glycoprotein; mAb, monoclonal antibody.

6. Dilute 60 μl of the resulting supernatant with 180 μl of TBS wash buffer (0.5% Nonidet P-40, 0.05% Tween 20 and 0.5 mmol $CaCl_2$). Transfer 100 μl of diluted platelet lysate, in duplicate, to a flat-well microplate previously coated with goat antimouse IgG.* Leave at 4°C for 90 min.
7. Wash the microplate well four times with 200 μl of TBS wash buffer and then add 100 μl of alkaline phosphatase-labelled antihuman IgG (Jackson, code 109-055-008) diluted 1:4000 in TBS wash buffer. Leave at 4°C for a further 90 min, then wash the wells four times with TBS wash buffer and add 100 μl of substrate solution (1 mg/ml *p*-nitrophenyl phosphate in diethanolamine buffer, pH 9.8) to each well.
8. Measure the resulting colour change at 30 min using a dual-wavelength spectrometer (e.g. Bio-Rad model 450).

Express results as the mean absorbance at 405 nm of duplicate tests minus the mean of eight blanks containing TBS wash buffer instead of platelet lysate.

Use pooled AB serum as a negative control.

Other Methods

Several other methods have been developed for the detection of platelet antibodies.

Solid-phase red cell adherence (SPRCA) techniques (some commercially available) evolved as alternatives to the microscopic reading initially required for the PIFT. These assays combine traditional red cell serology technology with platelet serology. Platelets are captured on microtitre wells; test antibodies are applied; and, after washing and addition of antihuman globulin, platelet or HLA alloantibody binding is detected using tanned sheep red cells[107] or anti-D sensitized RhD-positive red cells.[108] SPRCA are robust, sensitive tests that lend themselves to automation and the chloroquine treatment of platelets can be used effectively to screen out HLA antibodies.

GTI PakPlus is a platelet antibody kit based on an ELISA principle (Quest Biomedical, Solihull, UK). Microwells coated with platelet glycoproteins or HLA class I antigens are incubated with test serum. After incubation, followed by washing to remove unbound proteins, any antibody bound to the microwell is detected using an alkaline-phosphatase-conjugated antihuman globulin reagent (anti-immunoglobulin or anti-IgG) and the appropriate substrate. Results are considered positive when the ratio of the mean absorbance of the test sample to that of the normal control sera is ≥ 2.0.[109]

With respect to testing for granulocyte antibodies when working with the GIFT or GAT, elucidation of the alloantibody requires panels of typed granulocytes, which cannot be preserved for more than a few hours. A technique has been reported that uses extracted granulocyte antigens coated onto U-well Terasaki plates and a micromixed passive haemagglutination test. Patient's serum and appropriate controls (sera known to contain granulocyte-specific antibodies, monoclonal antibodies, such as anti-CD16 and anti-NA1 and sera from normal donors) are added to the wells and, following incubation and washing, indicator blood cells are added (sheep red blood cells coated with antihuman IgG and antimouse IgG).[110]

Molecular Genotyping of Platelet Alloantigens

The application of DNA technology for platelet genotyping is based on the knowledge that the platelet antigen systems are the result of single DNA base changes, which lead to single amino acid substitutions in the platelet membrane glycoproteins (Table 21.13).

Molecular genotyping involves amplification of the relevant segments of genomic DNA from any nucleated cell by the PCR in combination with sequence-specific primers[111] or by allele-specific restriction enzyme analysis[112] or allele-specific oligonucleotide dot blot hybridization.[113]

Of the variety of PCR-based techniques available, the PCR with sequence-specific primers (PCR-SSP) is still the most widely used in the UK for the determination of HPA 1 to 5. Molecular genotyping has now been accepted to be an essential part of confirming the specificity assigned to platelet alloantibodies, as well as allowing the investigation of patients with severe thrombocytopenia and making possible the determination of the fetal platelet genotype in early pregnancy to assess the risk of alloimmune thrombocytopenia.

---

*The microplate is prepared by adding to each well 100 μl of goat antimouse IgG (Sera-Lab, code SBA 1030–01) at 3 μg/ml in carbonate coating buffer, pH 9.6. Leave the plate to stand overnight at 4°C. Next morning, wash the plate four times with TBS wash buffer. Leave the last wash supernatant for 30 min to 'block' nonspecific protein adsorption to the plastic and then decant.

REFERENCES

1. International Society of Blood Transfusion (ISBT) Working Party. Available at: http://ibgrl.blood.co.uk; Accessed 01.06.10.

2. Daniels G. Functions of red cell surface proteins. *Vox Sang.* 2007;93 (4):331–340.

3. Eastlund T. The histo-blood group ABO system and tissue transplantation. *Transfusion.* 1998;38:975–988.

4. Galliford J, Charif R, Chan KK, et al. ABO incompatible renal transplantation in a steroid sparing protocol. *Transplantation.* 2008;86(7):901–906.

5. Mourant AE, Kopec AC, Domaniewska-Sobczak K. *The Distribution of the Human Blood Groups and Other Biochemical Polymorphisms.* 2nd ed. Oxford: Oxford University Press; 1976.

6. Yainamoto F. Molecular genetics of the ABO histo-blood group system. *Vox Sang.* 1995;69:1–7.

7. Garratty G, Arndt P, Co S. Fatal ABO haemolytic transfusion reaction resulting from acquired B antigen only detectable by some monoclonal grouping reagents. *Transfusion.* 1993;33(suppl):47S.

8. Garratty G. Association of blood groups and disease: do blood group antigens and antibodies have a biological role? *Hist Philos Life Sci.* 1996;18:321–344.

9. O'Donnell J, Laffan M. The relationship between ABO histo-blood group, factor VIII and von Willebrand factor. *Transfus Med.* 2001;11:343–351.

10. Jenkins PV, O'Donnell JS. ABO blood group determines plasma von Willebrand factor levels: a biologic function after all? *Transfusion.* 46 (10):1836–1844..

11. Avent ND, Reid ME. The Rh blood group system: a review. *Blood.* 2000;95:375–387.

12. Daniels G, Poole G, Poole J. Partial D and weak D: can they be distinguished? *Transfus Med.* 2007;17(2):145–146.

13. World Health Organization (WHO). *Twenty-eighth Report of WHO Expert Committee on Biological Standardization.* Technical Report Series 610. Geneva: WHO; 1977.

14. Lo YM, Bowell PJ, Selinger M, et al. Prenatal determination of fetal rhesus D status by DNA amplification of peripheral blood of rhesus-negative mothers. *Ann N Y Acad Sci.* 1994;731:229–236.

15. Lo YM, Tein MS, Lau TK, et al. Quantitative analysis of fetal DNA in maternal plasma and serum: implications for noninvasive prenatal diagnosis. *Am J Hum Genet.* 1998;62:768–775.

16. Serious Hazards of Transfusion Annual Report . Available at: www. shotuk.org; 2008: ▨▨▨▨▨▨▨

17. Mollison PL. ▨▨▨▨ Contreras M. ▨▨ *Clinical Medicine.* ▨▨▨▨ Blackwell Scientific; 1997.▨▨.

18. Engelfriet CP. The immune destruction of red cells. *Transfus Med.* 1992;2:1–6.

19. Horsewood P, Kelton JG. Macrophage-mediated cell destruction. In: Garratty G, ed. *Immunobiology of Transfusion Medicine.* New York: Marcel Dekker; 1994:434–464.

20. Zupanska BA. Cellular bioassays and their use in predicting the clinical significance of antibodies. In: Garratty G, ed. *Immunobiology of Transfusion Medicine.* New York: Marcel Dekker; 1994:465–492.

21. Guyre PM, Miller R. Recombinant immune interferon increases immunoglobulin G Fc receptors on cultured human mononuclear phagocytes. *J Clin Invest.* 1983;72: 393–397.

22. Griffin JA, Griffin FM. Augmentation of macrophage complement receptor function in vitro. *J Exp Med.* 1979;150:653–675.

23. Volk HD, Reinke P, Krausch D. Monocyte deactivation-rationale for a new therapeutic strategy in sepsis. *Intensive Care Med.* 1996;22: S474–S481.

24. EU . In-vitro diagnostics IVD Medical Devices Directive 1998. *Official Journal of the European Communities.* 1998;1331. (7.12.98).

25. British Committee for Standards in Haematology. Guidelines for compatibility procedures in blood transfusion laboratories. *Transfus Med.* 2004;14:59–73.

26. Case J, Ford DS, Chung A. International reference reagents: antihuman globulin. *Vox Sang.* 1999;77:121–127.

27. Department of Health. *Guidelines for the blood transfusion services in the United Kingdom.* 4th ed. London: HMSO; 1998.

28. British Committee for Standards in Haematology . Recommendations for the evaluation, validation and implementation of new techniques for blood grouping antibody ▨▨▨▨ and crossmatching. ▨▨▨ *Med.* 1995;5:145–150.

▨▨. ▨▨▨ Validation of new ▨▨▨▨ gy for antibody detection by antiglobulin tests. *Transfus Med.* 1992;2:177–179.

30. Phillips PK, Voak D, Whitton CM, et al. BCSH-NIBSC anti-D reference reagent for antiglobulin tests: the in-house assessment of red cell washing centrifuges and of operator variability in the detection of weak macroscopic agglutination. *Transfus Med.* 1993;3:143–148.

31. Voak D, Downie DM, Moore BP. Replicate tests for the detection and correction of errors in anti-human globulin AHG tests: optimum conditions and quality control. *Haematologia (Budap).* 1988;2:3–16.

32. Knowles SM, Milkins CE, Chapman JF, et al. The United Kingdom National External Quality Assessment Scheme (Blood Transfusion Laboratory practice): trends in proficiency and practice between 1985 and 2000. *Transfus Med.* 2002;12:11–23.

33. Voak D, Downie DM, Haigh T, et al. Improved antiglobulin tests to detect difficult antibodies: detection of anti-Kell by LISS. *Med Lab Sci.* 1982;39: 363–370.

34. Scott ML, Voak D, Downie DM. Optimum enzyme activity in blood grouping and a new technique for antibody detection: an explanation for the poor performance of the

one-stage mix technique. *Med Lab Sci.* 1988;45:7–18.

35. Scott ML, Phillips PK. A sensitive two-stage papain technique without cell washing. *Vox Sang.* 1987;52:67–70.

36. Pirofsky B. The use of bromelin in establishing a standard cross-match. *Am J Clin Pathol.* 1959;32:350–356.

37. British Committee for Standards in Haematology. In Roberts B, ed. *Standard Haematology Practice.* Oxford: Blackwell Scientific; 1991:150–163.

38. Coombs RR, Mourant AE, Race RR. A new test of the detection of weak and 'incomplete' Rh agglutinins. *Br J Exp Pathol.* 1945;26:255–266.

39. Voak D, Downie DM, Moore PB, et al. Antihuman globulin reagent specification: the European and ISBT/ICSH view. *Biotest Bulletin.* 1986;1:7.

40. Engelfriet CP, Overbeeke MA, Voak D. The antiglobulin test, Coombs test and the red cell. In: Cash JD, ed. *Progress in Transfusion Medicine.* Vol. 2. Edinburgh: Churchill Livingstone; 1987:74–98.

41. Sinor LT. Advances in solid-phase red cell adherence methods and transfusion serology. *Transfus Med Rev.* 1992;6:26–31.

42. Lapierre Y, Rigel D, Adams J, et al. The gel test: a new way to detect red cell antigen–antibody reactions. *Transfusion.* 1990;30:109–113.

43. Phillips P, Voak D, Downie M. New reference reagent for the quality assurance of anti-D antibody detection. *Transfus Med.* 1998;8:225–230.

44. O'Hagan J, Milkins CE, Chapman JF, et al. Antibody titres – results of a UK NEQAS BGS exercise and accompanying questionnaire. *Transfus Med.* 1997;7(suppl 1).

45. British Committee for Standards in Haematology. Addendum for guidelines for blood grouping and red cell antibody testing during pregnancy. *Transfus Med.* 1999;9:99.

46. Van der Schoot CE, de Haas M, Engelfriet CP, et al. Genotyping for red cell polymorphisms. *Vox Sang.* 2009;96(2):167–179.

47. Santoso S. Human platelet-specific alloantigens: update. *Vox Sang.* 1998;74(suppl 2):249–253.

48. Bux J, von dem Borne AEG, de Haas L. ISBT Working Party on Platelet and Granulocyte Serology, Granulocyte Antigen Working Party: Nomenclature of granulocyte alloantigens. *Vox Sang.* 1999;77:251.

49. Lucas GF, Metcalfe P. Platelet and granulocyte polymorphisms. *Transfus Med.* 2000;10:157–174.

50. Metcalfe P, Watkins NA, Ouwehand WH, et al. Nomenclature of human platelet antigens (HPA). *Vox Sang.* 2003;85:240–245.

51. IPD–HPA Database. Available at: www.ebi.ac.uk/ipd/hpa; Accessed 30.07.10.

52. Nordhagen R, Flaathen ST. Chloroquine removal of HLA antigens from platelets for the platelet immunofluorescence test. *Vox Sang.* 1985;48:156–159.

53. Engelfriet CP, Tetteroo PA, van der Veen JP, et al. Granulocyte-specific antigens and methods for their detection. In: McCullough J, Sandler SG, Sweeney GE, eds. *Advances in Immunobiology: Blood Cell Antigens and Bone Marrow Transplantation.* New York: Liss; 1984:121.

54. McCullough J. The clinical significance of granulocyte antibodies and in vivo studies of the fate of granulocytes. In: Garraty G, ed. *Current Concepts in Transfusion Therapy.* Arlington, VA, USA: American Association of Blood Banks; 1985:125.

55. Minchinton RM, Waters AH. The occurrence and significance of neutrophil antibodies. *Br J Haematol.* 1984;56:521–528.

56. Decary F, L'Abbe D, Tremblay L, et al. The immune response to the HPA-1a antigen: association with HLA-DRw52a. *Transfus Med.* 1991;1:55–62.

57. Williamson LW, Hackett G, Rennie J, et al. The natural history of fetomaternal alloimmunization to the platelet-specific antigen HPA-1a PI^{A1} Zw^a as determined by antenatal screening. *Blood.* 1998;92:2280–2287.

58. Flug F, Karpatkin M, Karpatkin S. Should all pregnant women be tested for their platelet PLA Zw HPA-1 phenotype? *Br J Haematol.* 1994;86:1–5.

59. Mueller-Eckhardt C, Kroll H, Kiefel V, et al. European PTP Study Group: post-transfusion purpura. In: Kaplan-Gouet C, Schlegel N, Salmon C, et al. *Platelet Immunology: Fundamental and Clinical Aspects.* INSERM/John Libbey, Eurotext; 1991.

60. Schnaidt M, Northoff H, Wernet D. Frequency and specificity of platelet-specific allo-antibodies in HLA-immunised haematologic-oncologic patients. *Transfus Med.* 1996;6:111–114.

61. Kurz M, Hildegard G, Hocker P, et al. Specificities of anti-platelet antibodies in multitransfused patients with haemato-oncological disorders. *Br J Haematol.* 1996;95:564–569.

62. Bierling P, Fromont P, Elbez A, et al. Early immunization against platelet glycoprotein IIIa in a new born Glanzmann type I patient. *Vox Sang.* 1988;55:109–113.

63. Brown 3rd CH, Weisberg RJ, Natelson EA, et al. Glanzmann's thrombasthenia: assessment of the response to platelet transfusion. *Transfusion.* 1975;15:124–131.

64. Ribera A, Martin-Vega C, Pico M, et al. *Sensitization against platelet antigens in Glanzmann disease.* Manchester: Congress of the International Society of Blood Transfusion in Association with British Blood Transfusion Society (BBTS); 1988: Abstract XX, 240.

65. Van Leeuwen EF, von dem Borne AE, von Riesz LE, et al. Absence of platelet specific alloantigens in Glanzmann's thrombasthenia. *Blood.* 1981;57:49–54.

66. Degos L, Tobelem G, Lethielliux P, et al. A molecular defect in platelets of patients with Bernard-Soulier syndrome. *Blood.* 1977;50:899–903.

67. Van Leeuwen EF, Helmerhorst FM, Engelfriet CP, et al. Specificity of auto-antibodies in autoimmune thrombocytopenia. *Blood.* 1982;59:23–26.

68. Fujisawa K, Tani P, O'Toole TE, et al. Different specificities of platelet-associated and plasma auto-antibodies to platelet GPIIb-IIIa in patients with chronic immune thrombocytopenic purpura. *Blood.* 1992;79:1441–1446.

69. Fujisawa K, Tani P, McMillan R. Platelet-associated antibody to glycoprotein IIb/IIIa from chronic immune thrombocytopenic purpura patients often binds to divalent cation-dependent antigens. *Blood*. 1993;81:1284–1289.

70. Hou M, Stockelberg D, Kutti J, et al. Glycoprotein IIb/IIIa autoantigenic repertoire in chronic idiopathic thrombocytopenic purpura. *Br J Haematol*. 1995;91:971–975.

71. Kelton JG, Sheridan DP, Santos AV, et al. Heparin-induced thrombocytopenia: laboratory studies. *Blood*. 1988;72:925–930.

72. Pegels JG, Bruynes EC, Engelfriet CP, et al. Pseudothrombocytopenia: an immunologic study on platelet antibodies dependent on ethylene diamine tetra-acetate. *Blood*. 1982;59:157–161.

73. Shastri KA, Logue GL. Autoimmune neutropenia. *Blood*. 1993;81:1984–1995.

74. McCullough J, Clay ME, Thompson HW. Autoimmune granulocytopenia. *Baillière's Clinical Immunology and Allergy*. 1987;1:303.

75. Bux J, Mueller-Eckhardt C. Autoimmune neutropenia. *Semin Hematol*. 1992;29:45–53.

76. Mueller-Eckhardt C. Drug-induced immune thrombocytopenia. *Baillière's Clinical Immunology and Allergy*. 1987;1:369.

77. Mueller-Eckhardt C, Salama A. Drug-induced immune cytopenias: a unifying pathogenetic concept with special emphasis on the role of drug metabolites. *Transfus Med Rev*. 1990;4:69–77.

78. Salama A, Schutz B, Kiefel V, et al. Immune-mediated agranulocytosis related to drugs and their metabolites: mode of sensitization and heterogeneity of antibodies. *Br J Haematol*. 1989;72:127–132.

79. Metcalfe P, Waters AH. Report on the fourth ISBT/ICSH platelet serology workshop. *Vox Sang*. 1990;58:170–175.

80. Von dem Borne AE, Verheught FW, Oosterhof F, et al. A simple immunofluorescence test for the detection of platelet antibodies. *Br J Haematol*. 1978;39:195–207.

81. Kiefel V. The MAIPA assay and its applications in immunohaematology. *Transfus Med*. 1992;2:181–188.

82. von dem Borne AE, van der Lelie J, Vos JJ, et al. Antibodies against crypt antigens of platelets. Characterization and significance for the serologist. *Curr Stud Hematol Blood Transfus*. 1986;52:33.

83. Bux J, Kober B, Kiefel V, et al. Analysis of granulocyte-reactive antibodies using an immunoassay based upon monoclonal-antibody-specific immobilization of granulocyte antigens. *Transfus Med*. 1993;3:157–162.

84. Minchinton RM, Noonan K, Johnson TJ. Examining technical aspects of the monoclonal antibody immobilization of granulocyte antigen assay. *Vox Sang*. 1997;73:87–92.

85. Shulman NR, Leissinger CA, Hotchkiss AJ, et al. The non-specific nature of platelet associated IgG. *Trans Assoc Am Physicians*. 1982;95:213–220.

86. Von dem Borne AE. Autoimmune thrombocytopenia. *Baillière's Clinical Immunology and Allergy*. 1987;1:269.

87. Goodall AH, Macey MG. Platelet-associated molecules and immunoglobulins. In: Macey MR, ed. *Flow Cytometry – Clinical Applications*. London: Blackwell Scientific; 1994:148–191.

88. Ault KA. Flow cytometric measurement of platelet-associated immunoglobulin. *Pathol Immunopathol Res*. 1988;7:395–408.

89. Von dem Borne AE, Vos JJ, van der Lelie J, et al. Clinical significance of positive platelet immunofluorescence test in thrombocytopenia. *Br J Haematol*. 1986;64:767–776.

90. Verheugt FW, von dem Borne AE, Decary F, et al. The detection of granulocyte allo-antibodies with an indirect immunofluorescence test. *Br J Haematol*. 1977;36:533–544.

91. McCullough J, Clay ME, Press C, et al. *Granulocyte serology. A clinical and laboratory guide*. Chicago: ACSP; 1988.

92. Lucas GF. Prospective evaluation of the chemiluminescence test for the detection of granulocyte antibodies: comparison with the immunofluorescence test. *Vox Sang*. 1994;66:141–147.

93. Bux J. Challenges in the determination of clinically significant granulocyte antibodies and antigens. *Transfus Med Rev*. 1996;10:222–232.

94. Stroncek DF. Granulocyte immunology: is there a need to know? *Transfusion*. 1997;37:886–888.

95. ISBT Working Party . Recommendations of the ISBT Working Party on granulocyte immunobiology for leukocyte antibody screening in the investigation and prevention of antibody mediated transfusion related acute lung injury. *Vox Sang*. 2009;96:266–269.

96. Claas FH, Langerak J, de Beer LL, et al. Drug-induced antibodies: interaction of the drug with a polymorphic platelet antigen. *Tissue Antigens*. 1981;17:64–66.

97. Salama A, Mueller-Eckhardt C, Kissel K, et al. Ex vivo antigen preparation for the serological detection of drug-dependent antibodies in immune haemolytic anaemias. *Br J Haematol*. 1984;58:525–531.

98. Decary F, Vermeulen A, Engelfriet CP. *A look at HLA antisera in the indirect immunofluorescence technique LIFT. Histocompatibility testing*. Copenhagen: Munksgaard; 1975:380.

99. Metcalfe P, Minchinton RM, Murphy MF, et al. Use of chloroquine-treated granulocytes and platelets in the diagnosis of immune cytopenias. *Vox Sang*. 1985;49:340–345.

100. Decary F. Report on the second Canadian workshop on platelet serology. *Curr Stud Hematol Blood Transfus*. 1988;54:1.

101. Helmerhorst FM, Ten Boerge ML, van der Plas-van Dalen C, et al. Platelet freezing for serological purposes with and without a cryopreservative. *Vox Sang*. 1984;46:318–322.

102. Helmerhorst FM, van Oss CJ, Bruynes ECE, et al. Elution of granulocyte and platelet antibodies. *Vox Sang*. 1982;43:196–204.

103. Vos JJ, Huisman JG, Winkel IN, et al. Quantification of platelet-bound allo-antibodies by radioimmunoassay: a study on some variables. *Vox Sang*. 1987;53:108–116.

104. Minchinton RM, Waters AH. Chloroquine stripping of HLA antigens from neutrophils without removal of neutrophil specific antigens. *Br J Haematol.* 1984;57: 703–706.

105. Metcalfe P, Waters AH. Location of the granulocyte-specific antigen LAN on the Fc-receptor III. *Transfus Med.* 1992;2:283–287.

106. Kiefel V, Santoso S, Weisheit M, et al. Monoclonal antibody specific immobilization of platelet antigens MAIPA: a new tool for the identification of platelet-reactive antibodies. *Blood.* 1987;70: 1722–1726.

107. Shibata Y, Juji T, Nishizawa Y, et al. Detection of platelet antibodies by a newly developed mixed agglutination with platelets. *Vox Sang.* 1981;41:25–31.

108. Lown JA, Ivey JG. Evaluation of solid phase red cell adherence technique for platelet antibody screening. *Transfus Med.* 1991;1: 163–167.

109. Lucas GF, Rogers SE. Evaluation of an enzyme-linked immunosorbent assay kit GTI PakPlus® for the detection of antibodies against human platelet antigens. *Transfus Med.* 1999;9:63–67.

110. Araki N, Nose Y, Kohsaki M, et al. Antigranulocyte antibody screening with extracted granulocyte antigens by a micro-mixed passive haemagglutination method. *Vox Sang.* 1999;77:44–51.

111. Metcalfe P, Waters AH. HPA-1 typing by PCR amplification with sequence-specific primers PCR-SSP: a rapid and simple technique. *Br J Haematol.* 1993;85: 227–229.

112. Simsek S, Faber NM, Bleeker PM, et al. Determination of human platelet antigen frequencies in the Dutch population by immunophenotyping and DNA allele-specific restriction enzyme analysis. *Blood.* 1993;81: 835–840.

113. McFarland JG, Aster RH, Bussel JB, et al. Prenatal diagnosis of neonatal alloimmune thrombocytopenia using allele-specific oligonucleotide probes. *Blood.* 1991;78: 2276–2282.

Chapter | 22 |

Laboratory aspects of blood transfusion

Megan Rowley, Carol Cantwell, Clare Milkins

Safe and effective blood transfusion requires the combined efforts of blood transfusion services, biomedical scientists and clinicians to ensure the highest standards are applied to all the systems in a complex process from 'vein to vein'. This chapter provides a description of the laboratory framework required to provide the right blood components to the right patients at the right time. The increased awareness of what can go wrong with blood transfusion comes from a number of sources including the Serious Hazards of Transfusion UK haemovigilance scheme, which was started in 1996.[1,2] This confidential reporting scheme, using detailed root cause analysis of errors, has provided data that have

Figure 22.1 Cumulative data from SHOT (Serious Hazards of Transfusion) 1996–2009[2] showing distribution of errors, according to the main reporting categories, a total of 6653 completed case reports. IBCT, incorrect blood component transfused; I and U inappropriate and unnecessary; HSE, handling and storage errors; Anti-D, anti-D administration errors; ATR, acute transfusion reaction; HTR, haemolytic transfusion reaction; TRALI, transfusion-associated acute lung injury; TACO, transfusion-associated circulatory overload; PTP, post-transfusion purpura; TTI, transfusion transmitted infection; Autologous, autologous transfusion.

informed both national bodies and local transfusion services of measures to introduce in order to reduce risk (Fig. 22.1). It is clear that multiple errors can contribute to a single adverse event and that many of these are outside the control of the transfusion laboratory.

Within the laboratory setting, the application of strict protocols for sample labelling and testing, robust laboratory procedures, reliable documentation, frequent staff training and competency assessment should be used. Recently, the UK Transfusion Collaborative, comprising representatives of the professional bodies involved in UK transfusion practice, has produced some recommendations to reduce laboratory errors in transfusion. These address issues such training, competency, staffing levels and automated systems.[3]

This chapter is concerned with the testing of patient samples prior to the provision of appropriate compatible blood components including identification of red cell antibodies. It also covers compatibility testing and investigation of transfusion reactions and the testing required in other special situations including the antenatal and postnatal settings. National professional bodies such as the British Committee for Standards in Haematology (BCSH)[4] and the AABB[5] issue guidance to transfusion laboratories and this has been referenced where appropriate.

There is a new regulatory framework governing hospital transfusion laboratory practice which was implemented after the publication of two European Union Directives: 2002/98/EC and 2004/33/EC.[6] In the UK these are the Blood Safety and Quality Regulations 2005 (Statutory Instruments 2005/50, 2005/1098 and 2006/2013) and they set standards for quality and safety of human blood and blood components in hospital 'blood banks' as well as 'blood establishments' (the UK Blood Services).[7] 'Blood

banks' are regulated in their roles of storing, distributing and performing compatibility tests, on blood and blood components for use in hospitals. The implications for hospital transfusion practice are the requirement for 'vein to vein' traceability of blood components, the importance of maintaining the 'cold chain' for all therapeutic blood components, the need to store transfusion records for 30 years and the requirement for a quality management system.[6,7] UK laboratories have to assess themselves and submit an annual compliance report to the competent authority, which is the Medicines and Healthcare Products Regulatory Agency (MHRA).[8] The MHRA carries out laboratory inspections to assess compliance with these regulations.

The UK government, through the National Blood Transfusion Committee, continues to promote the safe and effective transfusion of blood components and has published three Health Service Circulars.[9] These documents aim to ensure that a team approach to blood transfusion safety is taken via the local clinical governance arrangements and to promote good transfusion practice via Hospital Transfusion Committees and Hospital Transfusion Teams supported by Regional Transfusion Committees.

TECHNOLOGY AND AUTOMATION IN BLOOD TRANSFUSION LABORATORIES

Important changes have taken place in the blood transfusion laboratory in the last 10–15 years, as outlined in the previous edition of this book. As a result transfusion laboratory practice is safer, largely as a result of the implementation of new technologies for testing, automated systems to replace manual systems and the widespread use of information technology (IT) systems to support transfusion laboratory practice.

Barcoded labels on blood components, reagents, patient samples and equipment are now commonplace and these result in safer transfer of information, free from the transcription errors associated with manual methods.

Column agglutination (CAT) and solid-phase technology can both be used on automated machines and CAT can also be used by manual techniques. In UK hospital transfusion laboratories these technologies have replaced tube techniques and liquid-phase microplates for antibody screening and crossmatching (Figs 22.2, 22.3).[10]

The currently available CAT systems include Ortho BioVue, which comprises a six-well cassette containing a glass microbead matrix, ID DiaMed cards utilizing Sephadex gel matrix, also with six wells, and an eight-well Sephadex gel matrix card from Grifols. Each offers a wide range of profiles and reagent systems.

The currently available solid-phase systems are Immucor Capture-R and Bio-Rad Solidscreen II. The Immucor system utilizes a range of red cell antigens adhered to the surface of a U-shaped microplate well. Sensitized red cells are then used as a marker. The Bio-Rad Solidscreen II is a solid-phase method for antibody screening and identification. The wells of the microplates are coated with protein A to allow the reaction to bind to the plate forming a solid-phase cell layer.

Individual laboratories need to make careful and informed decisions when selecting reagents for pre-transfusion testing. It is vital that any abbreviated testing in an automated or semiautomated system is carefully evaluated for the risks that could ensue if important controls were omitted when using this technology for blood grouping.[11]

Laboratory information management systems (LIMS) store patient details and results of laboratory tests, allowing timely and accurate access to important information. In the transfusion department, IT systems have a much broader use and the updated BCSH guidelines for the specification and use of Information Technology (IT) systems in blood transfusion practice (2006) reflect this.[12] Where possible, using bidirectional or unidirectional interfaces to automated blood grouping analysers, IT systems are used to eliminate errors that can arise when a manual step is employed, including interpretation of test results.

Computer algorithms support the 'electronic issue' of blood to patients with a negative antibody screen without the need to perform an antiglobulin crossmatch and, in the UK in 2009, 46% of laboratories were using this system for some or all of their patients (Fig. 22.4). The use of automation for all aspects of compatibility testing is now

Figure 22.2 Change in indirect antiglobulin test (IAT) technology for antibody screening. Data from UK NEQAS surveys 1998–2009.[10] These surveys of UK practice show that technology used for antibody screening and serological crossmatching is now predominantly column agglutination (CAT) with very few laboratories using tube techniques. LPM, liquid-phase microplate.

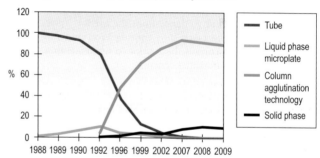

Change in IAT technology for antibody screening 1988–2009

- Tube
- Liquid phase microplate
- Column agglutination technology
- Solid phase

Figure 22.3 Change in technology for serological compatibility testing. Data from UK NEQAS surveys 1998–2009.[10] These surveys of UK practice show that technology used for antibody screening and serological crossmatching is now predominantly column agglutination with very few laboratories using tube techniques.

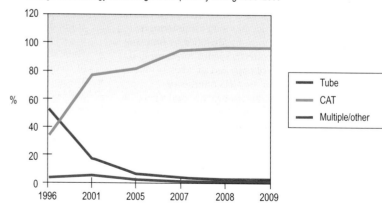

Change in technology for serological compatibility testing 1996–2009

- Tube
- CAT
- Multiple/other

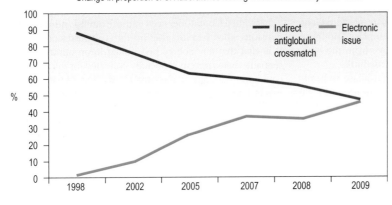

Change in proportion of UK laboratories issuing blood electronically 1998–2009

Figure 22.4 Change in proportion of UK laboratories issuing blood electronically 1998–2009. Data from UK NEQAS surveys indicating the increased use of electronic issue for compatibility testing in UK transfusion laboratories.

recommended practice as it is recognized that it is safer.[3] Automation brings several or all of the discrete activities of compatibility testing into a single platform process. It provides various levels of increased security over manual testing and may provide justification for abbreviated pre-transfusion testing (e.g. abandoning duplicate D, previously termed 'RhD', typing or reverse ABO grouping in the presence of a valid historical group). A risk assessment must be made and documented prior to any abbreviation of an established procedure, with consideration being given to the presence or absence of key functions in the automated equipment. The BCSH guidelines for compatibility procedures[12] and guidance from the MHRA[13] give a list of factors to be taken into consideration and the reader is advised to consult these prior to implementing automated or semiautomated systems.

PRE-TRANSFUSION COMPATIBILITY SYSTEMS

The process of providing blood for transfusion involves many steps, all of which have to be reliably completed. These include the following:

- Blood samples have to be taken from the correct patient and labelled at the bedside in a single uninterrupted procedure. The sample must be identified by four core patient identifiers: the correctly spelled forename and surname, the exact date of birth and an accurate unique patient number (such as the NHS number or equivalent). The sample should be dated and signed by the person taking the sample.[14] Some guidelines recommend that addressograph labels should not be accepted on blood samples for compatibility testing because it increases the risk of 'wrong blood in tube'(WBIT).[15] In an international study from the BEST collaborative, it was estimated that miscollected samples demonstrating WBIT occurred at a median rate of 0.5 per 1000, although there was great variation worldwide in the reported frequency of mislabelled samples, probably resulting from variation in policies for sample acceptance.[16] Labels printed at the bedside using barcoded patient wristband and hand-held scanners are acceptable.[14] The laboratory should have a policy for rejecting badly labelled samples, although in 2004 a survey of hospitals in England and North Wales showed considerable variation in the content and application of these policies.[17]

- A request for services should include the previously outlined four core patient identifiers as well as clear information about the source of the request and the location of the patient and clinical details including a detailed justification for the request. Previous transfusion history and any special considerations for the selection of blood (e.g. antigen negative if the patient has a clinically significant antibody, cytomegalovirus [CMV] tested or irradiated for certain groups of immunosuppressed patients) are also needed.

- An ABO and D group of the patient sample must be accurately performed.

- An antibody screen of the patient's plasma (or mother's plasma in the case of a neonate) should be able to detect any clinically significant red cell antibodies. In the event of a positive red cell antibody screen, antibody identification should be undertaken to assist the selection of compatible blood.

- There should be a check of existing transfusion records to compare current and historical results.

- The appropriate blood component should be selected and issued to a named patient using a serological crossmatch or electronic issue.

- Traceable documentation should exist to ensure that the results of laboratory compatibility procedures are available at the patient's bedside to allow a check before transfusing the blood component. This should include a blood bag compatibility label (Fig. 22.5) and may include a compatibility form. The patient must be

Figure 22.5 A unit of red cells showing the compatibility label.

identified with a wristband and the blood component should be prescribed on a drug or fluid administration chart.[14] In some countries, an additional bedside check of the patient's blood group is undertaken prior to commencing the transfusion.

Documentation of the Transfusion Process

All stages of the transfusion process must be clearly documented and these records must be kept. In addition to guidance from the UK Royal College of Pathologists on the retention of documents,[18] the BSQR 2005 regulations stipulate that the records must be accessible for 30 years.[7] This allows any blood component to be traced from the donor to the recipient should information come to light about any potential infective risks to the recipient.

Computer records are easier to search than paper records, but laboratory information systems are likely to become obsolete and be replaced several times within this mandatory 30-year period, so provision must be made to store historical data in an accessible format when procuring a replacement computer system.[12] Patient-held records are useful for patients who are treated in more than one institution, particularly if they have red cell antibodies and require phenotyped blood or if they have special requirements because of their underlying disease or its treatment. Credit card-sized records with corresponding patient information leaflets are issued by some transfusion centres to patients with red cell antibodies and similar cards exist for patients who require irradiated cellular blood components.[19]

Identification and Storage of Blood Samples

Depending on laboratory practice, blood transfusion tests use a clotted (serum) sample or EDTA-anticoagulated blood (plasma). Most laboratories using automated systems will use a plasma sample.

The reason for automated systems requiring plasma is because incompletely clotted blood samples may contain small fibrin clots that trap red cells into aggregates that could resemble agglutinates which could be falsely interpreted as a positive reaction. Clotted samples should be taken into a plain tube but not a tube with a separating gel.

The presence of complement in serum can cause lysis. If laboratory staff are used to recognizing agglutination as an indicator of a positive reaction they may fail to interpret the lysed red cells as an equally valid positive reaction. Therefore, when using serum for blood grouping and compatibility testing, any red cells in the test system should be washed and resuspended in saline which contains ethylenediamine tetra-acetic acid (EDTA) (see later). In addition, false-negative reactions may occur in immediate spin crossmatching with potent ABO antibodies, where rapid complement fixation causes a prozone effect (bound C1 inhibits agglutination). EDTA saline is not necessary when using plasma.

> Throughout this chapter, for the sake of brevity, 'plasma' is used as the majority of UK laboratories are automated and therefore anticoagulated (plasma) samples are required. If serum samples are specifically required, this will be indicated in the text.

On being received in the laboratory, the details on the request form must be checked against the blood sample. Each blood sample must be labelled with a unique sample number. Barcode labels offer the advantage of positive sample identification and reduce the number of transcription errors. Samples inadequately or inaccurately labelled should NOT be used for pre-transfusion testing.[11]

Great care must be taken to select and identify the sample prior to any testing. Transposition of samples in the laboratory can lead to an incorrect blood group being assigned to a patient, with serious consequences, including ABO incompatible transfusions. Where possible, the primary sample should be used for testing. If samples are separated, the plasma must be clearly and accurately identified and special precautions must be taken. If repeated testing on this sample is anticipated, storing separate small aliquots reduces the risk of sample deterioration, which occurs with repeated thawing/freezing of larger samples.

Whole blood samples should be tested as soon as possible because they will deteriorate over time. Problems associated with storage include lysis of the red cells, loss of complement in the serum and decrease in potency of antibodies. The BCSH guidelines[11] indicate working limits as outlined in Table 22.1. If separated plasma or serum samples are stored for later serological crossmatch, care must be taken to ensure that the patient has not been transfused in

Table 22.1 Recommended limits for storage of samples used for compatibility testing[11]

SAMPLE	18–25°C	4°C	−30°C
EDTA-anticoagulated whole blood	Up to 48 h	Up to 7 days	Not applicable
Separated plasma	Not applicable	Up to 7 days	Up to 6 months

the interim. It has been recommended that samples should be kept for a minimum of 7 days from group and screen, stored at 4°C. Samples should be retained post-transfusion for investigation of acute transfusion reactions and preferably stored for 7 days post-transfusion to enable investigation of delayed transfusion reaction.[18]

ABO AND D GROUPING

ABO and D grouping must be performed by a validated technique with appropriate controls. Before use, all new batches of grouping reagents should be checked for reliability by the techniques used in the laboratory. Grouping reagents should be stored according to manufacturer's instructions.

ABO Grouping

ABO grouping is the single most important serological test performed in compatibility testing; consequently, it is imperative that the sensitivity and security of the test system are not compromised. The fact that anti-A and anti-B are naturally occurring antibodies allow the patient's plasma to be tested against known A and B cells in a 'reverse' group.

This is an excellent built-in check for the 'forward' or cell group and has always been considered to be an integral part of ABO grouping, allowing the reading and recording of test results to be split into two discrete tasks. However, with secure, fully automated systems, linked to secure laboratory information management systems that, in combination, have the ability to prevent procedural ABO grouping errors, some laboratories now omit the reverse group when testing samples for which a historical group is available.[11] This should only be considered following a careful risk assessment and taking into account that the first sample taken may have been from the wrong patient. This may be in the order of 1:2000 samples.[16] Any discrepancy between the forward and reverse groups should be investigated further and any repeat tests should be undertaken using cells taken from the original sample rather than from a prepared cell suspension.

Reagents for ABO Grouping

Monoclonal anti-A and anti-B reagents have replaced polyclonal reagents in routine grouping tests. A_1 and B cells are used for reverse grouping; group O cells or an auto control may be included to ensure that reactions with A and B cells are not a result of the presence of cold autoantibodies. A diluent control should be included where recommended by the manufacturer.

D Grouping

D grouping is usually undertaken at the same time as ABO grouping for convenience and to minimize clerical errors that may arise through repeated handling of patients' samples. In the absence of secure automation, testing should be undertaken in duplicate because there is no counterpart of the 'reverse' grouping of ABO testing.

Reagents for D Grouping

Monoclonal reagents do not have the problem of possible contamination with antibodies of unwanted specificities, as was the case with polyclonal reagents. Therefore, the duplicate testing may be undertaken using the same anti-D reagent, although this should be dispensed as though it were two separate reagents.

DVI is the partial D with the fewest epitopes; therefore of all the D variants, DVI individuals are those most likely to form anti-D and a case of severe haemolytic disease of the fetus and newborn (HDFN) has been described.[20] For this reason, anti-D monoclonal reagents that do not detect DVI should be selected for testing patients' samples.[21,22] The use of anti-CDE reagents has led to the misinterpretation of r′ and r″ cells in UK National External Quality Assessment Scheme (NEQAS) exercises and, because they are of no value in routine patient typing, their use is not recommended.[10,11] Selection of high-avidity monoclonal anti-D reagents will allow detection of all but the weakest examples of weak D, negating the need to use more sensitive techniques to check the D status of apparent D negatives.

Some anti-D reagents have high levels of potentiator (e.g. polyethylene glycol) and should be used with caution; a diluent control is essential to demonstrate that the diluent does not promote agglutination of the test red cells as may happen if the patient's cells are coated *in vivo* with immunoglobulin G (IgG); any positive reaction seen with the control, however weak, invalidates the test result. Anti-D reagents are provided in many different kits and those responsible for selection and purchase should make themselves aware of the content, specificity and potentiation of the chosen reagent.

Methods

There are several techniques available for routine ABO and D grouping including tube test, slide test, liquid-phase and solid-phase microplates and columns. Other techniques for blood grouping have been described but they are not in routine use. For example, molecular ABO typing is reserved for investigating anomalous ABO groups, in organ transplantation where red cells from the donor are not available, forensic practice and paternity testing.[23] Care should be taken to use the appropriate reagent because not all reagents have been validated by the manufacturer for all techniques.

Tube and slide tests

Spin-tube tests may be used for urgent testing, where small numbers of tests are performed at once. Slide or tile techniques are widely used in under-resourced countries for ABO and D grouping. Spin-tube tests should be performed in 75×10 or 75×12 mm plastic tubes. Immediate spin tests may be used in an emergency, whereas routine tests are usually left for 15 min at room temperature (about 20°C) before centrifugation for 1 min at 150 g. Equal volumes (1 or 2 drops from either a commercial reagent dropper or a Pasteur pipette) of liquid reagents or plasma and 2% cell suspensions are used. The patient's red cells (diluted in phosphate buffered saline, PBS) should be tested against monoclonal anti-A and anti-B grouping reagents. The patient's plasma should be tested against A_1 and B reagent red cells (reverse grouping). In addition, the plasma should be tested against either the patient's own cells or group O cells (i.e. a negative control) to exclude reactions with A and B cells as a result of cold agglutinins other than anti-A or anti-B in the patient's sample. Mix the suspensions by tapping the tubes and leave them undisturbed for 15 min. Agglutination should be read as described on p. 498. Any discrepancy between the results of the red cell grouping and the reverse grouping should be investigated further and any repeat tests should involve cells taken from the original sample rather than the prepared suspension. Reverse grouping is not carried out for infants younger than 4 months of age because the corresponding antibodies are normally absent or maternal in origin.

EDTA for diluents

Stock solution. Prepare a 0.1 mol/l solution of EDTA (dipotassium salt) in distilled water. Adjust the pH to 7.0 using 5 mol/l NaOH.
Working solution. Mix 1 volume of stock solution with 9 volumes of saline or low ionic strength saline solution (LISS). Check the pH and adjust to 7.0 if necessary.

Slide method

In an emergency, rapid ABO grouping may be carried out on slides or tiles. The method is satisfactory if potent grouping reagents are used (p. 498). An immediate spin-tube test is preferable.

Liquid-phase microplate methods

Liquid-phase microplate technology provides a cheap and secure method for batch testing when semiautomation is utilized for dispensing and reading but it is no longer

the grouping technique of choice in the UK (see Fig. 22.2). In 2009, a UK NEQAS survey showed that only 13% of responding laboratories were using microplates for grouping, down from 41% in a similar survey in 2002.[10]

ABO and D grouping may be performed in a single microplate if monoclonal reagents are used. A resuspension technique using untreated U-well rigid polystyrene microplates is recommended for grouping. If microplates are to be reused they should be cleaned in mild detergent, rinsed thoroughly in distilled water and left to dry face down; alternatively, an ultrasonic bath may be used. Scored or otherwise damaged plates should be discarded.

The plate is usually laid out as 12×8 (12 tests and 8 reagents) but may be used in the opposite orientation (8×12), depending on the number of reagents and controls required. Particularly if performing this technique manually, the anti-D reagents should be kept away from the anti-A and anti-B reagents because splashing between wells can occur when dispensing reagents and handling the plates during testing if insufficient care is taken. The following method is recommended:[24]

1. Add 1 drop of reagent and diluent control (if required) to each appropriate well.
2. Add 1 or 2 drops of test plasma to the appropriate wells for reverse grouping and auto controls (if required).
3. Make a visual check to ensure that there are no empty wells.
4. Add 1 drop of a 3% cell suspension of test cells to the appropriate wells containing reagent, diluent control and auto control.
5. Add 1 drop of 3% reagent red cells to the appropriate wells containing test plasma.
6. Agitate carefully to mix, preferably using a microplate shaker.
7. Leave the plate to incubate at ambient temperature for 15 min and then centrifuge at 100 g for 40 s.
8. Resuspend the red cells using a microplate shaker. Excessive agitation will reduce the strength of agglutination. It should be remembered that agglutinates formed by some weaker examples of weak D may be disrupted and interpreted as D negative in microplate methods.
9. Results may be read visually or using an automated plate reader.

Column agglutination techniques

CAT techniques (see Chapter 21, p. 502) are now the commonest method for grouping in the UK (80% of laboratories who responded to a UK NEQAS survey in 2009, see Fig. 22.2), especially where automated systems are in place; these should always be performed in accordance with the manufacturer's instructions. There are several different profiles to choose from and some cards/cassettes include monoclonal antibodies to other blood group antigens (e.g. K) in

Figure 22.6 Column agglutination technology: blood group O D positive. First box, α. Second box, β. Third box, D. Fourth box, Control. Fifth box, A₁. Sixth box, B.

addition (see Chapter 21, p. 502 and Fig. 22.6). Forward and reverse grouping may be undertaken in separate cards/cassettes.

Solid-phase techniques

ABO/D grouping using solid-phase techniques would usually be part of a fully automated system and testing should be accordance with the manufacturer's instructions. Bio-Rad Erytype employs a standard agglutination technique for blood grouping performed in a microtitre plate. The reagents for the forward group are dried onto the wells. Uncoated empty wells are used with standard liquid red cells for a reverse group.

Controls

Positive and negative controls should be included with every test or batch of manual tests. In fully automated systems, the controls should be set up at least twice in a 24-h period. The timings should coincide with machine startup and changing of reagents, taking account of the length of time that reagents have been kept at room temperature on the machine. The control samples should be loaded in the same way as the test samples. The required controls are shown in Table 22.2. Where controls do not give the expected reactions, investigations should be undertaken to determine the validity of all tests undertaken subsequent to the most recent valid control results.

Table 22.2 Control cells for blood grouping

REAGENT	POSITIVE CONTROL	NEGATIVE CONTROL
Anti-A	A cells	B cells
Anti-B	B cells	A cells
Anti-D	D positive cells	D negative cells
A₁ cells	Anti-A	Anti-B
B cells	Anti-B	Anti-A

Causes of Discrepancies in ABO/D Grouping
False-Positive Reactions
Rouleaux

Rouleaux may occur in various clinical conditions, where the ratio of normal albumin to globulin is altered in plasma (e.g. multiple myeloma) and in the presence of plasma substitutes such as dextrans. The stacking of red cells on top of one another in columns may be misinterpreted as weak agglutination by inexperienced workers. Rouleaux will usually disperse on a slide if a drop of saline is added; alternatively, the reverse grouping can be repeated using plasma diluted 1 in 2 or 1 in 4 with saline.

Cold autoagglutination and cold reacting alloantibodies

Cold autoantibodies (usually anti-I) that are reactive at room temperature may lead to autoagglutination in the cell group (ABO and D) and panagglutination in the reverse group, causing a grouping anomaly (p. 277). The tests should be repeated using cells washed in warm saline and plasma pre-warmed to 37°C. An auto control should be included.

Cold reacting alloantibodies (e.g. anti-P₁) may cause agglutination of reverse grouping cells and, if this is suspected, reverse grouping should be repeated using pre-warmed plasma or grouping cells that lack the implicated antigen.

T-activation/polyagglutination

Polyagglutination[25] describes agglutination of red cells by all or most normal adult sera but not by the patient's own serum. This is as the result of IgM antibodies reacting with an antigen on the red cells which is usually hidden but can be exposed by enzyme activity. The most common form is T-activation, which occurs when the bacterial enzyme neuraminidase cleaves *N*-acetyl neuraminic acid from the red cell membrane, exposing the T antigen.

This used to be a problem when grouping with polyclonal reagents, which contain anti-T, but tests using monoclonal reagents are not affected by this phenomenon.

Acquired B

This arises in group A_1 patients where the expected reaction with anti-A is noted but an *additional* weak reaction with anti-B occurs. The blood group appears to be 'AB' but with anti-B in the reverse group. This discrepancy between the forward and reverse grouping may be overlooked if the patient's own anti-B is weak or if the reverse group is omitted.

The acquired B antigen is usually caused by a bacterial deacetylase enzyme acting on A_1 red cells and producing a B-like substance. Some anti-B reagents react strongly with the acquired B antigen (e.g. those derived from the ES4 clone).[26] Such anti-B reagents are rare but should be avoided in routine blood grouping.

Potentiators

Red cells may be coated with IgG as a result of *in vivo* sensitization. The use of potentiated techniques, such as the antiglobulin test for D typing, or of potentiated reagents for ABO or D typing, may result in a false-positive reaction; the latter would also result in a positive reaction with the diluent control, but UK NEQAS data have shown that some laboratories fail to include an appropriate control or fail to understand the significance of a positive control.[27] For this reason, use of potentiated techniques or reagents for blood grouping is not advised.

In vitro *bacterial contamination*

In vitro bacterial contamination of reagents, patients' red cells or reverse grouping cells may cause false-positive agglutination.

False-Negative Reactions

Failure to add reagents

The most likely cause of a false-negative grouping result is failure to add the reagent or test plasma. For this reason, in liquid-phase tube and plate tests, the serum or plasma should always be added first to the reaction chamber and a visual check should be made before red cells are added. The use of colour-coded reagents for ABO grouping is helpful in this respect. Automated systems have liquid level sensors resulting in an alert of the failure to add a reagent or test plasma.

Loss of potency

Inappropriate storage or freezing and thawing may cause a loss of potency of blood grouping reagents. The use of regular controls will alert the user to this problem.

Failure to identify lysis

In the presence of complement, anti-A and anti-B may cause *in vitro* lysis of reagent red cells. If lysis is not recognized as a positive reaction, falsely negative results may be recorded in reverse grouping tests. To avoid this, reverse grouping cells should be resuspended in EDTA saline, where serum rather than plasma is used.

Mixed-field appearance

This describes a dual population of agglutinated and non-agglutinated red cells which may be observed in both ABO and D grouping. It is important to recognize this as a mixed-field picture and not to confuse it with weak agglutination. The most likely cause of a mixed-field picture is the transfusion (either deliberate or accidental) of non-identical ABO or D red cells. Investigation will be required to determine the actual blood group of the patient, who may have been transfused in an emergency, at a different establishment or may have received an intrauterine transfusion. A mixed-field ABO group may be the first indication of a previous ABO-incompatible transfusion.

An ABO or D incompatible haemopoietic progenitor cell transplant will result in a mixed-field picture until total engraftment has occurred; the mixed-field picture may subsequently reappear when a graft is failing. Rarely, a dual population of cells is permanent and results from a weak subgroup of A (A_3) or a blood group chimerism.

Interpretation of a dual population of red cells will depend on the technique used. In a tube, microscopic reading will reveal strong agglutinates in a background sea of free cells. In column agglutination techniques there will be a line of agglutinated cells at the top of the column, with the non-agglutinated cells travelling through to the bottom of the column. In liquid-phase techniques if the reaction grade is not a strong positive or an obvious negative then the reactions requires further investigation, which may include microscopic examination. In a solid-phase technique a mixed field is seen as a dual population of cells, with the agglutination being surrounded by free cells. Automated systems should be set up to detect mixed-field pictures and this should be used in conjunction with local policies.

D variant phenotypes

Weak D phenotypes are where the entire D antigen is present but there are fewer D antigen sites per cell and most weak D types group as D positive with the currently available high-avidity commercial monoclonal anti-D reagents. Where differing reactions are obtained with two reagents, the patient may be a partial D (i.e. one or more of the epitopes of the D antigen is missing). It was generally thought that patients who are weak D are unable to make anti-D and may be treated as D positive whereas some patients with partial D may be capable of making immune anti-D following sensitization with the missing epitope. This concept has been challenged by reports of weak D patients with anti-D.[28]

Detailed genotypic analysis combined with structural modelling of the D antigen in D variants have demonstrated change in the amino acid sequence in the extracellular domain in partial D, whereas weak D is associated with mutations resulting in change to the amino acid sequence in the intracellular or membrane-spanning domain.

A weak reaction with a single anti-D reagent should be investigated with a second anti-D reagent before assigning a result of D positive. It is essential to be able to distinguish between a weak reaction and a mixed-field reaction because the latter may be the result of a patient who is being transfused with blood of a different D type.

If in doubt, it is safer to call the patient D negative, at least until investigations have been undertaken by a reference centre. This will be of no clinical consequence because it is safe to transfuse D negative blood to a patient who is D positive, and a pregnant woman who is D positive and her unborn child would be unlikely to be harmed by the injection of prophylactic anti-D immunoglobulin.

Current advice about choice of D-typing reagents is that because DVI lacks the most epitopes, such individuals are likely to make anti-D when challenged by transfusion or pregnancy. For this reason, anti-D reagents for routine grouping of patients' samples should not detect DVI.[11] There is little evidence to suggest that a DVI donor would elicit an immune response in a recipient who is D negative; however, weak D positive and partial D donors, including DVI donors, should be classified as D positive.[29] There are some important ethnic differences in the frequency of different Rh haplotypes, as shown in Table 22.3. Resolution of anomalous D grouping where a partial D is suspected now includes both serological testing and genotypic studies.[30]

ANTIBODY SCREENING

Antibody screening is usually undertaken at the same time as blood grouping and in advance of selecting blood for transfusion. Antibody screening may be more reliable and sensitive than crossmatching against donor cells because some antibodies react more strongly with red cells with homozygous expression (double dose) of the relevant

Table 22.3 Approximate frequencies of common haplotypes in selected populations[30]

HAPLOTYPE	APPROXIMATE FREQUENCIES		
	English	Nigerian	Chinese
DCe R^1	0.421	0.060	0.730
dce r	0.389	0.203	0.023
DcE R^2	0.141	0.115	0.187
Dce R^0	0.026	0.591	0.033
dcE r''	0.012	0	0
dCe r'	0.010	0.031	0.019

antigen than with those with heterozygous expression (single dose) – most notably anti-Jk^a/Jk^b but also anti-Fy^a, -Fy^b, -S and -s. Screening cells can be selected to reflect this, whereas donor cells are usually of unknown zygosity. In addition, reagent red cells are easier to standardize than donor cells and there is potentially less opportunity for procedural error, particularly in automated systems.

Clinically significant antibodies are those that are capable of causing patient morbidity as a result of accelerated destruction of a significant proportion of transfused red cells. With few exceptions, clinically significant antibodies are those that are reactive in the indirect antiglobulin test at 37°C; however, it is not possible to predict serologically which of these antibodies will definitely be of clinical significance, so the term 'of potential clinical significance' is often used.

Red Cell Reagents

The patient's plasma should be tested against at least two individual screening cells, used individually, not pooled. The screening cells should be group O and encompass the common antigens of the indigenous population.

In the UK, the following antigens should be expressed as a minimum: C, c, D, E, e, K, k, Fy^a, Fy^b, Jk^a, Jk^b, S, s, M, N and Le^a; one cell should be R_2R_2 and another R_1R_1 or $R_1^wR_1$. The following phenotypes should also be represented in the screening set: Jk(a+b−), Jk(a−b+), S+s−, S−s+, Fy (a+b−) and Fy(a−b+) (Table 22.4). These recommendations for homozygosity are based on UK data regarding the incidence of delayed haemolytic transfusion reactions, the need for high sensitivity in the detection of Kidd antibodies and the poorer performance of column agglutination techniques in the detection of some examples of Kidd antibodies using heterozygous cells.[11,29] The requirement for the expression of C^w and Kp^a antigens on screening cells has been the cause of much debate but in the UK and the USA detection of anti-C^w or anti-Kp^a is not a requirement even in the absence of an antiglobulin crossmatch.[11,29] This is because these are low-frequency antigens and the antibodies rarely cause delayed haemolytic transfusion reactions or severe haemolytic disease of the newborn.

Methods

Antibody screening should always be carried out by an indirect antiglobulin test as the primary method. Additional methods (e.g. two-stage enzyme or Polybrene) may also be used but are inferior for the detection of some clinically significant antibodies and should not be used alone. A large retrospective study showed that the vast majority of antibodies reactive only by enzyme technique are of no clinical significance.[31] In Issitt's study of 10 000 recently transfused patients, only one anti-c, initially unreactive by indirect antiglobulin test, caused a delayed haemolytic transfusion reaction.[32] There has been one SHOT report (1998–1999) of an enzyme-only anti-E that became detectable by indirect

Table 22.4 Expression of red cell antigens on screening cells[11]

BLOOD GROUP SYSTEM	ANTIGEN	HOMOZYGOUS CELLS RECOMMENDED
Rh	C	Yes (R_1R_1 or $R_1{}^wR_1$)
	c	Yes (R_2R_2)
	D	Yes (R_1R_1 and R_2R_2)
	E	Yes (R_2R_2)
	e	Yes (R_1R_1 or $R_1{}^wR_1$)
Kell	K	No[a]
	k	No
Duffy	Fy[a]	Yes
	Fy[b]	Yes
Kidd	Jk[a]	Yes
	Jk[b]	Yes
MNSs	M	No
	N	No
	S	Yes
	s	Yes
Lewis	Le[a]	No

[a]Although desirable, KK cells are unlikely to be available.

antiglobulin test 7 days following the transfusion, causing a delayed haemolytic transfusion reaction and subsequent death of the patient due to renal failure.[1]

For liquid-phase techniques, BCSH guidelines[11] recommend the use of red cells suspended in LISS, rather than in standard normal ionic strength saline (NISS), because LISS increases the speed and sensitivity of detection of many potentially clinically significant antibodies. There are conflicting reports about whether sensitivity can also be improved by adding polyethylene glycol.[33]

Indirect Antiglobulin Techniques

Column Agglutination

In many countries, including the UK, column agglutination is now more commonly used than traditional tube or liquid-phase microplate techniques (see Figs 22.2 and 22.3) because it has been shown to be at least as sensitive as a standard LISS spin-tube technique,[33,34] it is simpler to perform because it requires no washing phase, it uses small volumes of plasma and reagents, it has a more objective reading phase and it is easy to automate. The antihuman globulin (AHG) incorporated in the matrix is available as either a polyspecific or anti-IgG reagent. Red cell concentrations and volumes can be critical and it is important to follow manufacturers' instructions at all times.

Column agglutination crossmatching tests have been shown to be less sensitive than standard tube techniques in detection of weak ABO antibodies such as anti-A with A_2B cells and Kidd antibodies with heterozygous red cells.[27,35–37] It has been suggested that these failures may be the result of shear forces occurring during centrifugation, which cause weak agglutinates to be disrupted, especially when the antigen site density is low.[38]

Solid-Phase Systems

Solid-phase techniques (e.g. Immucor Capture-R and Bio-Rad Solidscreen II) are also becoming more popular because they have been shown to have a high level of sensitivity and they also lend themselves to full automation. In 2009 10% of UK laboratories were routinely using solid phase for antibody screening (see Fig. 22.3).

Liquid-Phase Techniques – Tubes and Microplates

Tube techniques are still used for antibody screening in some parts of the world. With LISS-suspension techniques it is important to keep a high serum:cell ratio, without affecting the ionic strength. Equal volumes of serum and 1.5–2% cells suspended in LISS will result in a serum:cell ratio of >60:1, ensuring optimal sensitivity. Reagents should be incubated for 15–20 min at 37°C and the cells then should be washed in PBS. After adding AHG, the red cells should be examined using a careful 'tip and roll' procedure to prevent disruption of weak agglutinates. Reading aids such a light box or concave mirror may also be used with this technique.

Liquid-phase microplate technology has never achieved a huge popularity for antibody screening because it is relatively difficult to introduce and standardize and it cannot be automated. Because it is becoming increasingly difficult to obtain AHG reagents standardized for use in microplates, no method is detailed here. However, further information is available in the BCSH guidelines, including a recommended method for screening in V-well plates, using a streaming technique.[11,24]

Controls

A weak anti-D should be used on a regular basis to ensure the efficacy of the whole procedure, although the exact frequency will depend on work patterns as described in the blood grouping section. Additional weak controls are also recommended to confirm the sensitivity of the procedure and the integrity of the red cell antigens throughout their shelf life; anti-Fy^a and/or anti-S are good examples because Fy^a and S antigens are protease labile and may deteriorate more quickly on reagent cells than the D antigen and their use will also ensure that enzyme-treated cells have not been used by mistake. Consideration should also be given to selecting controls which demonstrate that the correct screening cell has been added to the batch of tests. Anti-S can be used as a control following the use of bleach to clean automated blood grouping analysers to check no cleaning fluid remains; the S antigen is very sensitive to Clorox.

The use of red cells weakly sensitized with anti-D is essential to control the washing phase of every negative liquid-phase test because inadequate washing may result in complete or partial neutralization of AHG by unbound globulin. Any test that does not give a positive reaction at the expected strength, following addition of these cells (and subsequent centrifugation), indicates insufficient free anti-IgG and should be repeated. The washing phase of solid-phase systems is difficult to control and it may be necessary to add a weak control to every column to ensure that every probe has dispensed wash solution during each wash cycle.

ANTIBODY IDENTIFICATION

When an antibody is detected in the antibody screen, its specificity should be determined and its likely clinical significance should be assessed before blood is selected for transfusion or relevant advice is given during pregnancy. It is essential to use a systematic approach to antibody identification to ensure that all specificities of potential clinical significance are identified. It may be tempting to match a reaction pattern immediately and look no further, but this is likely to result in additional specificities being missed.

Principles

As a starting point, the test plasma should be tested against an identification panel of reagent red cells by the technique with which it was detected in the screen. The next section on reagents outlines the minimum requirements for the panel. Inclusion of an autoantibody test is helpful in distinguishing between an autoantibody, an antibody directed against a high-frequency antigen and a complex mixture of alloantibodies. The positive and negative reactions should be compared with the panel profile in conjunction with the screening results.

Each antibody specificity should be taken in turn and its presence should be systematically excluded, by identifying antigen-positive cells that have given negative reactions. Wherever possible a negative reaction should be obtained with a red cell with homozygous expression of the relevant antigen. For example, if a negative reaction has been recorded against a Jk(a+b−) cell, then the presence of anti-Jk^a can be excluded, but if the only negative reactions are against Jk(a+b+) cells, then anti-Jk^a cannot immediately be safely excluded. This will leave a list of potential specificities, which should be considered by matching the positive reactions to the antigen-positive cells to determine if any are definitely present. Once this process is complete with the initial screen and identification panel, further cells and techniques may need to be used to complete the exclusion process. For example, where anti-S has been identified as being present, an enzyme-treated panel may be required to exclude the presence of anti-E, where all of the E-positive cells were also S positive or a K+S− cell may need to be selected to exclude the presence of anti-K.[39] The more specificities present, the more complicated the process, and where resources are limited, samples may need to be sent to a reference centre to elucidate all specificities. If the reagents are available, phenotyping the patient's red cells early on in the process will allow exclusion of specificities for which the patient is antigen positive.

The specificity of an antibody should only be assigned when it is reactive with at least two examples of reagent red cells carrying the antigen and non-reactive with at least two examples of reagent red cells lacking the antigen. This is because a single positive reaction could occur if the panel cell unexpectedly expressed a low-frequency antigen and a single negative reaction could occur if the panel cell lacked a high-frequency antigen.

Phenotyping

When an antibody has been identified, the patient's own red cells should be phenotyped for the relevant antigen. If the patient's red cells are negative for the antigen, this confirms that the patient is capable of making an antibody of that particular specificity. If the patient's red cells are positive for the antigen this suggests one of the following:

1. The antibody is an autoantibody, in which case the direct antiglobulin test should be positive.
2. The patient has been transfused recently and the reagent is detecting transfused cells rather than the patient's own cells. Care should be taken to look for a mixed-field reaction. Evidence of a delayed transfusion reaction should be sought.
3. The initial antibody identification result is incorrect.
4. The patient's red cells are immunoglobulin-coated (positive DAT). Care should be taken, particularly when using reagents potentiated with PEG, to recognize this to prevent reporting a false-positive result.

Extended phenotyping can be helpful where a mixture of antibodies is present because it allows the exclusion of antibodies specific for antigens for which the patient is positive, reducing the number of additional reagent cells required.

Additional Panels/Techniques

The chances of identifying antibodies, where two specificities are present, are significantly improved by using a two-stage enzyme technique, where at least one of the relevant antigens is affected by enzymes.[27] For example, Rh antibodies are enhanced by proteolytic enzymes in routine use, whereas M, N, S, Fy^a and Fy^b antigens are destroyed. Similarly, two different panels of reagent cells provide an increased chance of excluding further specificities where a mixture of two antibodies has been identified.

Direct agglutination at room temperature or $4°C$ may be helpful to distinguish between an antibody of potential clinical significance and a cold reacting antibody; again this is particularly useful where a mixture of antibodies is present. Weak examples of Kidd antibodies are often enhanced by the use of an indirect antiglobulin test using enzyme-treated cells and this can be particularly helpful where the antibody is only reacting against homozygous cells by indirect antiglobulin test.

Reagents

An identification panel should consist of red cells from at least eight group O donors, although 10 is more common in commercial panels and allows easier elucidation of antibody mixtures. To be functional, the panel must permit confident identification of the most commonly encountered, clinically significant antibodies. The UK guidelines[11] can be summarized as follows:

1. For each of the commonly encountered clinically significant red cells antibodies, there should be at least two examples of phenotypes lacking, and at least two examples of phenotypes carrying, the corresponding antigen.
2. There should be at least one example of each of the phenotypes R_1R_1 and $R_1^wR_1$. Between them, these two samples should express the antigens K, k, Fy^a, Fy^b, Jk^a, Jk^b, M, N, S and s.
3. There should be at least one example of each of the phenotypes R_2R_2, r'r and r''r and at least two examples of the phenotype rr.
4. The following phenotypes should be expressed in those samples lacking both D and C antigens: K+, K−, Jk(a+b−), Jk(a−b+), S+s−, S−s+, Fy(a+b−) and Fy(a−b+). The panel should be able to resolve as many likely antibody mixtures as possible.

Antibody Cards

Delayed haemolytic transfusion reactions can occur when antibodies have not been detected in the current antibody screen or have been *incorrectly* identified, maybe by a different establishment.[1,2] It has been suggested that antibody cards, produced either by the hospital or the reference centre, could be carried by the patient for presentation on admission to hospital. To be effective, such cards have to be accompanied by patient information leaflets, explaining the significance of the antibodies and preferably handed personally to the patient by someone with a clear understanding of blood transfusion practice. There are potential pitfalls with this suggestion, not least that the level of proficiency in identifying antibodies and appreciating clinical significance varies between establishments. A better long-term approach may be to have a national database of patients who have been identified to have clinically significant antibodies.

SELECTION AND TRANSFUSION OF RED CELLS

Once the blood group of a patient has been established and any antibodies have been identified, a set of procedures is required to select units of red cells that are appropriate for transfusion. These include selecting ABO/D compatible units, which will also need to be negative for antigens to which the recipient has clinically significant red cell alloantibodies (Table 22.5); It is also important that consideration is given to certain clinical criteria dictating special requirements (e.g. the requirement for CMV-negative, irradiated or washed red cells). Selection according to these criteria depends on good clinical information, accurate ABO and D typing and a sensitive antibody screen.

Some patients are identified as definitely needing transfusion of blood, but others may be undergoing surgery where blood is crossmatched to 'stand by'. Audits have shown that blood is often crossmatched but not transfused. The transfusion ratio, or crossmatch index, can be used to assess how well blood stocks are managed. One option is to perform a blood group and antibody screen on a patient and then save the sample, only crossmatching blood if certain pre-agreed transfusion triggers are met. Local policy should define a maximum surgical blood ordering schedule, indicating which surgical procedures can be 'group and screen/group and save' and how many units of blood need to be crossmatched for procedures with a high likelihood of intraoperative transfusion.[41] The decision as to whether blood is crossmatched in advance may relate to local factors including the proximity of the blood transfusion laboratory to the operating theatre (or other location where blood is to be transfused) and the time it takes to provide compatible blood following a request.

Once the appropriate red cells have been selected, compatibility needs to be ensured. This is usually referred to as crossmatching, which may include an indirect antiglobulin test to check for incompatibility as a result of IgG antibodies and ABO antibodies or an immediate spin test to check for ABO incompatibility only. Instead of a

Table 22.5 Recommendations for the selection of blood for a patient with red cell antibodies

SYSTEM	ANTIBODY	RECOMMENDATION
ABO	Anti-A$_1$	IAT crossmatch compatible at 37°C
Rh	Anti-D, -C, -c, -E, -e	Antigen negative*
Rh	Anti-C^w	IAT crossmatch compatible[†]
Kell	Anti-K, -k	Antigen negative*
Kell	Anti-Kp^a	IAT crossmatch compatible[†]
Kidd	Anti-Jk^a, -Jk^b	Antigen negative*
MNS	Anti-M (active at 37°C)	Antigen negative*
MNS	Anti-M (not active at 37°C)	IAT crossmatch compatible at 37°C
MNS	Anti-N	IAT crossmatch compatible at 37°C
MNS	Anti-S, -s, -U	Antigen negative*
Duffy	Anti-Fy^a, -Fy^b	Antigen negative*
P	Anti-P$_1$	IAT crossmatch compatible at 37°
Lewis	Anti-Le^a, -Le^b, Le^{a+b}	IAT crossmatch compatible at 37°C
Lutheran	Anti-Lu^a	IAT crossmatch compatible at 37°C
Diego	Anti-Wr^a (anti-Di3)	IAT crossmatch compatible[†]
H	Anti-HI (in A$_1$ and A$_1$B patients)	IAT crossmatch compatible at 37°C
All	Other active by IAT at 37°C	Seek advice from blood centre

IAT, indirect antiglobulin test.
*Antigen negative and crossmatch compatible.
[†]These recommendations apply when the antibody is present as a sole specificity. If present in combination, antigen-negative blood may be provided by the blood centre to prevent wastage of phenotyped units.

serological test, an assessment of ABO compatibility may be based on a 'computer check,' usually referred to as 'electronic issue'. Some transfusion laboratories, where surgery takes place in a different hospital, have extended electronic issue to the selection of compatible units, as dictated by the transfusion laboratory, from a remote issue refrigerator.[42]

The process of crossmatching blood is to prevent the transfusion of incompatible red cells and a subsequent haemolytic transfusion reaction. The different types of crossmatch are outlined in the following paragraphs. Whichever crossmatch technique is chosen, it should be clear that all patients with known red cell antibodies of potential clinical significance, even if currently undetectable, should have an indirect antiglobulin crossmatch and are not suitable for electronic issue.[11,12]

CROSSMATCHING

Choice of Test

Indirect Antiglobulin Crossmatch

The arguments for retaining an indirect antiglobulin crossmatch are based on the failure to identify antibodies against low-frequency antigens in the antibody screen. However, there is evidence, summarized by Garratty,[31] that the likelihood of missing a clinically significant antibody is approx. 1 in 10 615 crossmatches if the indirect antiglobulin test component is omitted and antibody detection relies on a sensitive antibody screen alone. Moreover, the usual outcome of transfusion if an antibody is present but undetected by the antibody screen is limited to shortened red cell survival.

An indirect antiglobulin crossmatch should always be performed if the patient has red cell antibodies of likely clinical significance, even if currently undetectable. The reasons for this are as follows:

1. It acts as a double check that the donation has been correctly phenotyped and labelled as negative for the corresponding antigen(s)
2. It ensures serological compatibility even if the identification of the antibody(ies) is incorrect or incomplete
3. It allows detection of antibodies to low-frequency antigens not present on the screening cells, which may be more likely to be present in a patient who is clearly a 'responder' and which may be masked by other alloantibodies.

Other circumstances in which an indirect antiglobulin crossmatch should be performed include the following:

1. The patient has had an ABO-incompatible solid organ transplant and is being transfused within 3 months of the transplant. This is necessary to detect IgG antibodies that may be produced by passenger lymphocytes in the transplanted organ.[43]
2. The patient has an alloantibody of low clinical significance detectable in the routine antibody screen such as anti-C^w.
3. The patient has known cold antibodies. In this case blood may be issued if compatible in the antiglobulin crossmatch performed strictly at 37°C, without the need for antigen-negative blood.

Methods for indirect antiglobulin crossmatching are the same as those used for antibody screening. Crossmatching may be less effective than antibody screening at detecting incompatibility as a result of IgG antibodies. This is partly because the cells may only show heterozygous expression of an antigen to which the patient has an antibody, potentially leading to weaker or negative reactions, and also because the cell suspensions and other techniques (e.g. cutting pigtails from donations, labelling tubes, washing cells) are less likely to be standardized and present more opportunity for transposition errors than the screening processes.

Immediate Spin Crossmatch

The sole purpose of this technique is to detect ABO incompatibility. It can be used in order to issue blood for transfusion when the patient has a full blood group and negative antibody screen. It may be used to convert a group and save/screen when blood is required and is often used in addition to an antiglobulin crossmatch. The immediate spin crossmatch will ensure that the correct units have been selected and that the correct ABO group has been assigned to the unit of donor red cells. Clearly it is not a suitable test

to use for detection of ABO incompatibility if the reverse blood group reveals a very weak anti-A or anti-B or if the patient falls into one of the categories described in the previous section.

There is evidence of poor standardization of this technique,[44] but its sensitivity can be optimized by selecting the appropriate cell suspension, incubation time and serum: cell ratio. The following tube method is recommended:

Mix 2 volumes of plasma with 1 volume of 2–3% cells suspended in PBS or LISS (or EDTA saline if serum is used).

Incubate at room temperature for 2–5 min to enhance the detection of weak ABO antibodies.

Centrifuge at 100 g for 1 min.

Read the reaction carefully using a 'tip and roll' technique.

False-negative results (in immediate spin crossmatch)

Incompatibilities between A_2B donor cells and group B patient sera are not consistently detected with this technique.[45] Of more concern is the potential failure of agglutination with potent ABO antibodies[46,47] on account of rapid complement fixation with bound C1 interfering with agglutination if using serum. Red blood cells must therefore be suspended in saline containing EDTA.

False-positive results (in immediate spin crossmatch)

Cold reacting antibodies, other than anti-A and anti-B, may cause agglutination in an immediate spin crossmatch. This has the potential to cause delays to transfusion while further procedures are used to rule out ABO incompatibility.

Electronic Issue

In many countries electronic issue is a commonly used alternative to the immediate spin crossmatch for issuing blood for transfusion when the patient has had a full blood group, a current negative antibody screen and no history of clinically significant antibodies. ABO and D compatible units are selected and issued through a computer system, which contains logic rules to prevent the issue of ABO and D incompatible blood.

BCSH guidelines[12] and AABB standards[48] require that there be concordant determinations of the patient's ABO and D type either on two separate samples, at least one of which must be a current sample or on one current sample tested twice, depending on the security present in the system. In addition, there must be no clinically significant antibodies detected and no record of any having been detected previously. The AABB recommends that the group of donor units is rechecked, but the BCSH accepts written verification by the supplying transfusion service of the accuracy of the donor unit label. It is strongly recommended by the BCSH that ABO and D grouping procedures are automated with positive sample identification (e.g. barcodes) and electronic transfer of results from the analyser to the transfusion laboratory computer, whereas the AABB does not have such a requirement. Ideally, computer algorithms should direct the procedure, only allowing issue if all the criteria are fulfilled. For example, issue of red cells for transfusion will be prevented if only one ABO and D group is on file or if the previous and current groups do not agree. Any manually controlled part of this process increases the risk of error. Electronic issue, based on fully validated systems, has been in place in several countries for some time and has proved to be clinically safe, providing the recommendations are rigidly adhered to.[49–51]

EMERGENCY BLOOD ISSUE

In clinical emergencies in which immediate red cell support is required, there may not be time for full compatibility testing. Either abbreviated testing is employed and rapid techniques are used or group O red cells are issued. There must be a documented procedure for dealing with emergencies. Local policies on this should be formally assessed for risk and adequate training should be given to staff, particularly those providing the service out of routine laboratory hours. Out-of-hours staff should be included in internal proficiency testing as well as external quality assessment exercises designed to test emergency tests and techniques.[3,11]

The transfusion laboratory should be involved in the development of emergency procedures within the hospital, including massive haemorrhage protocols and the major accident plan. All staff should receive regular training and should take part in emergency practice drills. Clear and effective communication is key to the success of provision of blood components in an emergency and the transfusion laboratory needs to be fully informed about the current status of the patient or patients, so as to provide an efficient and timely service.

Rapid ABO and D Typing

In an emergency, a sample *should* be obtained prior to transfusion and the patient's ABO and D type should be determined as rapidly as possible using the techniques already described. Tube and slide tests are most convenient.

Confirmation

A reverse group, a repeat cell group or an immediate spin crossmatch should be carried out on the sample before issuing blood of an appropriate ABO group. The ABO and D group must always be confirmed by a further test on a second aliquot from the sample. If an inadequately labelled sample is provided, group O units should be issued until a further sample can be tested.

Selection of Units

Some hospitals provide one or two units of O D negative red cells for use by clinicians pending the availability of ABO and D specific compatible red cells. Because of the relatively short supply of O D negative red cells (only 8% of Caucasian blood donors are O D negative in the UK) the National Blood Transfusion Committee has issued guidance to hospitals about the restrictions on the use of O D negative red cells in patients of another blood group.[52]

Compatibility Testing

Group-specific red cells can be issued following an immediate spin crossmatch to check for ABO incompatibility or a LISS antiglobulin crossmatch and antibody screen can be done if more time is available. If no matching procedure is performed, the red cell units must be group-checked unless the supplier has indicated confidence in the validity of the donor unit labelling. Units issued following abbreviated testing must be labelled as such (e.g. 'Selected for patient . . . but not crossmatched'). Cells from the donor units should be removed before issuing the units to enable retrospective crossmatch although a crossmatch is only necessary if the antibody screen is subsequently found to be positive.

Antibody Screening

Good practice requires a simultaneous crossmatch and antibody identification if the antibody screen is positive. If group-specific units have been issued without an indirect antiglobulin test crossmatch, an antibody screen must be performed as soon as possible. If the antibody screen is negative, it is not necessary to carry out a retrospective crossmatch. It is not acceptable to perform a crossmatch and not carry out an antibody screen. If the antibody screen is found to be positive, then contact the clinicians responsible for the patient to discuss how to proceed regarding the issue of potentially incompatible blood. Always follow agreed local procedure. Any untransfused incompatible units should be withdrawn from issue as soon as possible.

Massive Transfusion

Massive transfusion is defined as more than one blood volume within 24 h and is usually taken to mean 8 or 10 units for an adult.[53] After this volume of transfusion, it is no longer necessary to undertake an antiglobulin crossmatch, but immediate spin crossmatch or electronic issue is recommended to check for ABO compatibility. If ABO non-identical blood is given initially, blood of the same group as the patient should be used as soon as possible after the first transfusion. In some situations the recipient's need for red cell transfusion may necessitate the use of incompatible units, but this is a clinical decision based on the need for blood balanced against the known clinical significance of the red cell antibody detected.

Selection of Platelets and Plasma

In patients with hypotensive shock and/or large volume red cell replacement, a coagulopathy develops that requires replacement of other blood components. The use of platelets, fresh frozen plasma and cryoprecipitate may initially be determined by clinical evaluation of the patient's haemostatic state including observation of diffuse microvascular bleeding. Massive haemorrhage protocols should be developed to enable release of these coagulation factors at the request of the clinicians, in advance of the results of laboratory tests. Ongoing management of the patient can be guided by the results of these initial full blood count and coagulation screen tests, combined with frequent re-evaluation of both the laboratory tests and clinical evaluation of the haemostatic state.[53]

Potential Errors

Errors leading to transfusion of incorrect blood components are more likely to occur out of routine laboratory hours; therefore it has been recommended that only genuine emergency transfusions should take place out of hours.[1,2] There may, however, be circumstances where patients with haemoglobinopathies receiving regular transfusion support are given blood overnight to minimize disruption of their education or employment.

ANTENATAL SEROLOGY AND HAEMOLYTIC DISEASE OF THE NEWBORN

Maternal ABO and D grouping and red cell antibody screening must be done early in pregnancy as a routine. This is the basis for the prevention, detection and, with antibody titration or quantification, the management of haemolytic disease of the fetus and newborn (HDFN).

Haemolytic Disease of the Fetus and Newborn

Haemolytic disease of the fetus and newborn is a haemolytic anaemia of the fetus and/or newborn infant that occurs when maternal alloantibody to fetal antigens crosses the placenta and causes haemolysis of fetal red cells or suppression of fetal red cell progenitors, the latter occurring with antibodies within the Kell system.[54,55]

As IgG is the only immunoglobulin that crosses the placenta, only red cell antibodies of this class are a potential cause of HDFN. Anti-D causes the most severe form of HDFN, but the success of prophylaxis with anti-D

immunoglobulin for potentially sensitizing events in pregnancy and after delivery of a D positive baby has reduced the number of cases and routine antenatal anti-D prophylaxis (RAADP) has reduced it even further. The relative proportion of HDFN due to other IgG red cell antibodies has thus increased.[56] Although HDFN resulting from anti-D is the most severe form of the disease, anti-c can give rise to significant haemolysis *in utero*, sufficient in some cases to result in intrauterine death and therefore to warrant intervention in pregnancy. Anti-K has a different mode of action[54,55] but can also result in a severely affected fetus. Other IgG antibodies (e.g. anti-E, anti-Ce, anti-Fy^a and anti -Jk^a) uncommonly give rise to fetal haemolysis of sufficient severity to merit antenatal intervention. Haemolytic disease of the newborn (HDN) as a result of ABO antibodies can also occur and is described later. For a detailed discussion of the investigation and management of HDFN, the reader is referred to the reviews by Kumar and O'Brien,[57] Bowman[58] and the textbook *Mollison's Blood Transfusion in Clinical Medicine*.[30]

Antenatal Serology

ABO and D Grouping and Antibody Screening

Maternal ABO and D grouping as well as antibody screening and identification are performed early in pregnancy (i.e. when first seen and 'booked in') and then at 28 weeks' gestation. All pregnant women, whether D positive or D negative, should be screened for red cell antibodies.[59] Further testing depends on the specificity of any antibodies detected, whether they are capable of causing HDFN and the obstetric history.

Follow-Up Antibody Screening

Protocols for antenatal screening and follow-up vary from country to country. In the United Kingdom, the following is recommended by the BCSH:[59]

1. All pregnant women have ABO, D and antibody screen in early pregnancy when 'booked-in' and at 28 weeks' gestation. If the antibody screen at 28 weeks is negative, no further routine testing is required.
2. Pregnant women with anti-D, antibodies to Kell-related antigens and anti-c should be tested monthly to 28 weeks and then every 2 weeks to delivery. The tests should include antibody quantification or titration as well as testing for additional red cell antibodies.
3. Pregnant women with other red cell antibodies should have a titration done when booked in and again at 28 weeks.
4. All pregnant women with a previous history of HDFN or those who have a significant increase in anti-D, antibodies to Kell-related antigens or anti-c should

be referred to a specialist fetal medicine unit for further assessment of the need for antenatal intervention.

5. Pregnant women who have red cell antibodies of other specificities, capable of giving rise to HDFN and which demonstrate a significant increase in titre over the course of the pregnancy, should have their condition discussed with their obstetrician. It is now appreciated that an increasing titre rather than an individual level is more predictive of an affected fetus.[60]

Prediction of Fetal Blood Group

Partner Testing

The father's blood group phenotype should be determined in all cases in which the mother has a clinically significant red cell alloantibody. If the father's red cells lack the corresponding antigen, the baby is not at risk. However, caution is advised because the assumed father may not be the biological father of the fetus. It is useful to predict whether the partner of a woman who is D negative and who has immune anti-D is homozygous or heterozygous for the D antigen. This helps to forecast the chances of having children affected by anti-D HDFN.

The zygosity of the D antigen is usually predicted from the results of tests with anti-c, anti-C, anti-e and anti-E and from the likelihood of the homozygous or heterozygous association with these antigens (Table 22.6, see also Table 22.3). These data have been compiled for different racial groups. It is important, therefore, to tell the specialist laboratory the ethnic origin of the patient. Because the genetic basis for the common D types is now known, DNA typing provides a better alternative for predicting the potential for haemolytic disease of the newborn.[61]

Testing Fetal DNA in the Maternal Circulation

It is now possible to detect fetal DNA in the maternal circulation and, using DNA amplification techniques (see Chapter 8), to obtain D, c, E and K types on these cells. This has proved to be accurate at predicting the D type and, in the UK, it is now offered as a clinical service at the beginning of the 2nd trimester.[62] This may replace more invasive tests and supplement partner typing. It can be especially helpful if the father is absent or unknown.

Fetal Blood Sampling

Using ultrasound guidance, it is possible to take a sample of fetal blood for blood grouping, but this carries some risks. Contamination by maternal blood can hinder analysis of the sample obtained, leading to false-negative results. In addition, the procedure itself can lead to fetomaternal haemorrhage (FMH) and hence further sensitization to fetal antigens. There is also a risk of miscarriage.[57]

Antenatal Assessment of the Severity of Haemolytic Disease of the Fetus and Newborn

There has been considerable change in antenatal assessment of the severity of haemolytic disease of the newborn with non-invasive techniques being routinely used to assess the degree of fetal anaemia, with fetal blood sampling and, if necessary, intrauterine transfusion only being considered in cases suspected of having severe anaemia but before development of hydropic changes on the ultrasound scan.

Antibody Titrations during Pregnancy

Techniques for antibody titration are described in Chapter 21, but these have variable reproducibility and sensitivity. In many laboratories tube techniques have been replaced by column agglutination technology. Figure 22.7 shows the range of reaction grades used in titrations. The role of the serologist is to carry out serial antibody measurements to determine changes in the titre or concentration of the antibody. It is recommended that the technique chosen for titration should be validated against the National Institute for Biological Standards and Control anti-D standard.[59] Hence, laboratories should ensure that titres obtained with the anti-D standard are within one doubling dilution when it is used as an internal control. In addition, antibody titrations performed in pregnancy should be performed in parallel with the previous sample. Increases in titres of more than one doubling dilution should be monitored in conjunction with obstetricians.

Antibody Quantitation

Individual hospital transfusion laboratories should work closely with reference laboratories and obstetricians. Automated quantification is considered to be a more accurate predictor of when to proceed to more active investigation of the fetus but is usually only available for anti-D and anti-c. Results in iu (or µg per ml) are used as part of clinical algorithms to proceed to the next step of fetal investigation.[57]

Assessment of Fetal Anaemia

In a mother with increasing antibody levels and a fetus suspected or known to carry the red cell antigen against which the antibody is directed, an assessment of the severity of haemolysis is required. Traditionally this was done using amniocentesis to measure the optical density of the amniotic fluid (Lilley's lines) using spectrophotometry.

Table 22.6 The possible genotypes and frequencies in an English population (accounting for >99% of all Rh genotypes in this population)[61]

REACTION WITH ANTI-					POSSIBLE GENOTYPES	FREQUENCY
D	C	c	E	e		
+	+	+	−	+	DCe/dce R^1r	32.68
					DCe/Dce R^1R^0	2.16
					Dce/dCe R^0r'	0.05
+	+	−	−	+	DCe/DCe R^1R^1	17.68
					DCe/dCe R^1r'	0.82
−	−	+	−	+	dce/dce rr	15.10
−	+	+	−	+	dCe/dce r'r	0.76
−	−	+	+	+	dcE/dce r''r	0.92
+	+	+	+	+	DCe/DcE R^1R^2	11.87
					DCe/dcE R^1r''	1.00
					DcE/dCe R^2r'	0.28
					DCE/dce R^zr	0.19
					Dce/DCE R^0R^z	0.01
					Dce/dCE R^0R^y	<0.01
+	−	+	+	+	DcE/dce R^2r	10.97
					DcE/Dce R^2R^0	0.73
					Dce/dcE R^0r''	0.06
+	−	+	−	+	Dce/dce R^0r	2.00
					Dce/Dce R^0R^0	0.07
+	−	+	+	−	DcE/DcE R^2R^2	1.99
					DcE/dcE R^2r''	0.34

This, however, is an indirect measurement, whereas direct fetal blood sampling by ultrasound-guided cordocentesis provides not only direct diagnostic information but also a new approach to fetal therapy by direct fetal intravascular transfusion. However, both of these procedures carry the risk of miscarriage and further fetomaternal haemorrhage.[57] It is now common practice for fetal medicine units to offer non-invasive tests to determine fetal anaemia; middle cerebral artery Doppler studies have been very useful in this regard.[63] The incidence and severity of HDFN is declining and the increasingly specialized management of severely affected pregnancies has meant that these women are now being referred early in pregnancy to fetal medicine units who specialize in dealing with this condition, thus decreasing the involvement of the routine transfusion laboratory in any but the early stages.

Tests on Maternal and Cord Blood at Delivery

In all pregnancies with red cell antibodies, blood samples should be collected at delivery for the following tests. There should be a local protocol for these procedures, especially noting the importance of labelling these samples to avoid misidentification errors.

Figure 22.7 Column agglutination technology showing reaction grades 4+ to 0. Box 1, 4+. Box 2, 3+. Box 3, 2+. Box 4, 1+. Box 5, 0. Box 6, blank.

1. *Cord blood* (this is preferable to a sample from the baby because of the quantity of blood required)
    a. ABO and D group and phenotype for the red cell antigen against which the antibody is directed
    b. Direct antiglobulin test
    c. Haemoglobin concentration
    d. Bilirubin.
2. *Maternal blood*
    a. Repeat ABO and D group
    b. Repeat antibody screen.

Prevention of Haemolytic Disease of the Fetus and Newborn as a Result of Anti-D

Correct identification of women in early pregnancy who are D negative offers the chance to give intramuscular anti-D immunoglobulin to prevent sensitization to the D antigen at times during the pregnancy when significant fetomaternal haemorrhage is likely to occur, known as 'potentially sensitizing events' (PSE).[64,65] Accuracy in D grouping is particularly important because women who are D negative, erroneously grouped as D positive, risk not receiving prophylactic anti-D immunoglobulin (or being transfused with D positive cells). Sensitization to the D antigen could then result in severe HDFN in subsequent pregnancies as a result of development of anti-D. Serious Hazards of Transfusion (SHOT) has a reporting category for anti-D errors which includes any adverse event relating to the prescription, administration or omission of anti-D immunoglobulin that has the potential to cause harm to the mother or fetus immediately or in the future (Fig. 22.8).[2]

Anti-D Prophylaxis

Anti-D immunoglobulin should be given routinely as soon as possible after delivery (but always within 72 h) to women who are D negative who deliver babies that are D positive. It should also be given at times during pregnancy when sensitization could occur, such as during medical or surgical therapeutic termination of pregnancy, chorionic villus sampling, amniocentesis and following any abdominal trauma. It should also be given for episodes of vaginal bleeding where the pregnancy remains viable.[64,65] At delivery and for potentially sensitizing events after 20 weeks' gestation, it is necessary to screen for fetomaternal haemorrhage (FMH) using an acid elution method and estimate the degree of FMH if fetal cells are seen. The BCSH guidelines recommend confirming any FMH >2 ml by flow cytometry so that additional anti-D immunoglobulin can be given if the standard dose in use does not cover the estimated bleed.[66]

It takes 125 iu of anti-D immunoglobulin to cover a bleed of 1.0 ml fetal cells and preparations containing 250 iu, 500 iu, 1250 iu and 1500 iu are in routine prophylactic use.

Because of the risk of silent fetomaternal haemorrhage in pregnancy, routine antenatal anti-D prophylaxis (RAADP) is being offered to women in some countries. In the UK, this has been the subject of an appraisal by the National Institute for Health and Clinical Excellence[67] which recommends that anti-D immunoglobulin should be given either as

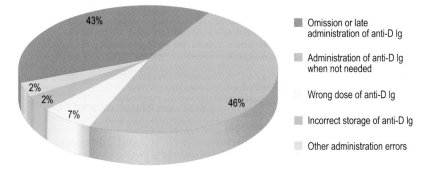

Figure 22.8 SHOT adverse events to anti-D immunoglobulin 2009.[2]

- Omission or late administration of anti-D Ig
- Administration of anti-D Ig when not needed
- Wrong dose of anti-D Ig
- Incorrect storage of anti-D Ig
- Other administration errors

two doses at 28 and 34 weeks or a single larger dose at 28 weeks, in addition to the postnatal dose and doses to cover any potentially sensitizing events during pregnancy. Women can decline RAADP, e.g. if they know the father is D negative or if they do not want any further pregnancies. The typing of fetal DNA in the maternal circulation may be used in the future to select women with fetuses that are D positive who would benefit from this additional prophylaxis, but, at the moment, it is not universally offered.[68]

The administration of prophylactic anti-D results in a positive maternal antibody screen due to passive anti-D. It may be difficult to distinguish between passive anti-D and low-level immune anti-D, particularly in the absence of a history of anti-D administration (this may have taken place at another institution). It is therefore important to take the 28-week sample for blood group and antibody screen *before* administration of anti-D. Although further antibody screens are not routinely required,[59] events in the 3rd trimester may result in a sample being sent to the transfusion laboratory. Laboratories need to have a strategy for dealing with these samples. Some implement screening against rr screening cells, whereas others proceed to full antibody identification on all samples.

Measurement of Fetomaternal Haemorrhage

The following tests are performed to estimate the quantity of fetal cells in the maternal circulation by the difference between fetal and maternal cells. Most commonly used is acid elution, also known as the Kleihauer test, which depends on the Hb F in fetal cells resisting the acid elution to a greater extent than the Hb A in maternal cells. The calculation of the volume of fetal cells is based on the work by Mollison,[30] which assumed that the maternal red cell volume is 1800 ml, fetal red cells are 22% larger than maternal cells and only 92% of fetal cells stain darkly (p. 338). Mollison's formula for calculating volume of fetomaternal haemorrhage is as follows:

Uncorrected volume of bleed =
$$\frac{1800 \times \text{fetal cells counted (F)}}{\text{Adult cells counted (A)}}$$

Corrected for fetal volume (1.22) =
$$\left(1800 \times \frac{F}{A}\right) \times 1.22 = J$$

Corrected for staining efficiency (1.09):

Volume of fetomaternal haemorrhage (ml fetal cells) = $J \times 1.09$.

Occasionally, the acid elution (or Kleihauer) test is used to investigate an intrauterine death or stillbirth where a large but silent fetomaternal haemorrhage is suspected as the cause of death. The D group of the mother is known but often not that of the fetus. In these circumstances, acid elution is the preferred test. Anti-D prophylaxis should be given to women who are D negative if the fetus is D positive or the D type of the fetus is unknown.

The flow cytometry method uses a fluorochrome-labelled anti-D antibody to measure a minority of D positive cells in the maternal D negative blood and is recommended for confirmation of a positive acid elution test where the estimated FMH exceeds 2 ml. However, flow cytometry may not always be available. Flow cytometric techniques using anti-Hb F have also been developed. The BCSH guidelines[66] give full details on performance and use of all these tests.

Recommended Action at Delivery (or Potentially Sensitizing Event)

All women who are D negative should be given a standard intramuscular dose (minimum of 500 iu after 20 weeks and 250 iu before 20 weeks' gestation) (into the deltoid muscle) of anti-D within 72 h of delivery (or potentially sensitizing event) unless the baby (or fetus) is known to be D negative.

On the basis of a confirmed FMH result, further anti-D immunoglobulin should be given if the FMH exceeds the volume covered by the standard anti-D immunoglobulin (Fig. 22.9). If the fetomaternal haemorrhage is more than 2 ml, the maternal sample, if possible, should be retested by a second technique such as flow cytometry; alternatively, the test should repeated on the same sample by a different operator.

A repeat sample for Kleihauer should be tested at 72 h (48 h if the anti-D immunoglobulin was given intravenously) to check for clearance of fetal cells. Further anti-D immunoglobulin may be required if fetal cells are present.

It is good practice to counsel women with a large fetomaternal haemorrhage about the risk of sensitization and an

---

Dosage of anti-D immunoglobulin to cover calculated fetomaternal haemorrhage[65]

125 iu anti-D immunoglobulin given intramuscularly is sufficient for a fetomaternal haemorrhage of 1 ml cells

500 iu will cover a FMH of less than 4 ml
1250 iu will cover a FMH of less than 10 ml
1500 iu will cover a FMH of less than 12 ml

Additional doses should be calculated using 125 iu for each 1 ml fetal cells and rounded to the nearest vial size.

Intravenous preparations are available for large bleeds. The dosage calculation for intravenous anti-D immunoglobulin is 100 iu for each 1 ml fetal cells.

Figure 22.9 Dosage of anti-D immunoglobulin to cover calculated fetomaternal haemorrhage.[65]

antibody screen 6-months postpartum can be arranged to see if sensitization to the D antigen has occurred although a negative antibody screen at this stage does not completely exclude sensitization.

ABO Haemolytic Disease of the Newborn

ABO incompatibility as a result of high-titre maternal IgG anti-A and anti-B antibodies can cause prolonged neonatal jaundice and anaemia associated with spherocytosis on the blood film in babies that are group A or B born to mothers that are group O. It should be distinguished from non-spherocytic haemolysis and from haemolytic disease of the newborn resulting from other red cell antibodies. Although confirmatory tests are best carried out on cord blood samples, it is often the case that babies have been discharged from hospital before the problem is detected. In Caucasian populations, about 15% of births are susceptible, but only about 1% are affected; even then the condition is mild and very rarely severe enough to need exchange transfusion. The condition is more common in other racial groups. A number of special factors combine to protect the fetus from the effects of ABO incompatibility. These include the relative weakness of A and B antigens on the fetal red cells and the widespread distribution of A and B glycoproteins in fetal fluids and tissues, which divert much of the maternal IgG antibody away from the fetal red cell 'target'. ABO haemolytic disease of the newborn may occur in a first pregnancy. Antenatal prediction of ABO haemolytic disease of the newborn is not essential for medical management because there is time to observe the baby after birth and treat according to the severity of the condition.

Serological Investigation

ABO haemolytic disease is difficult to diagnose, especially in Caucasians, because the direct antiglobulin test may be negative or weak even in a case of severe haemolytic disease. Furthermore, anti-A or anti-B is present in the mother's serum and special tests may be required to demonstrate high-titre IgG antibodies in the presence of IgM antibodies with the same specificity. The following are helpful pointers to diagnosis when ABO haemolytic disease of the newborn is suspected:

1. It is almost always confined to mothers who are group O because there are higher titres of IgG anti-A and anti-B in group O than in group A or B.
2. Because anti-A and anti-B are always present in mothers who are group O, evidence for ABO haemolytic disease of the newborn depends on demonstrating a high titre of IgG anti-A or anti-B by treating the mother's plasma to remove the IgM antibodies (p. 289) and then testing by the antiglobulin technique against adult A_1, B and O cells.

3. The direct antiglobulin test on the cord blood or baby's sample may be weak or negative; the latter at least reduces the likelihood of any other serological incompatibility.
4. The simplest evidence for the occurrence of ABO haemolytic disease of the newborn is obtained by testing plasma from the cord blood or baby's sample for anti-A or anti-B by the antiglobulin technique against adult A_1, B and O cells. The sooner after birth these tests are done, the better. Delays will lead to absorption of the antibody and the destruction of the red cells.
5. The best diagnostic test of ABO haemolytic disease of the newborn is to prepare an eluate from the baby's red cells and test it (together with the last wash supernatant as a control) by the antiglobulin test against adult A_1, B and O cells. In some cases reactions occur with both A_1 and B cells because of the presence of anti-A,B cross-reacting antibodies, although most severe cases of ABO haemolytic disease of the newborn contain separate specific anti-A and anti-B antibodies. The test with cells and the last wash control should be negative.

COMPATIBILITY TESTING IN SPECIAL TRANSFUSION SITUATIONS

Neonates and Infants within First 4 Months of Life

Infants younger than 4 months of age do not generally make alloantibodies but may have passively acquired maternal antibodies (see sections on haemolytic disease of the newborn and ABO and other red cell antigens).

Investigations on the Maternal Sample

ABO and D group
Antibody screen.

Investigations on the Infant Sample

ABO and D group (cell group only), repeated on the same sample if no historical group
Antibody screen if mother's sample not available
Direct antiglobulin test.

If the direct antiglobulin test is positive or any red cell antibodies are detected in the maternal or infant serum, the diagnosis of haemolytic disease of the newborn should be considered (see above).

Selection of Blood and Other Components

Where possible, the *cellular* component chosen should be ABO and D identical or an alternative compatible ABO group, taking into account the infant's blood group and maternal blood group (i.e. presence of maternal anti-A

Table 22.7 Choice of ABO group for blood components for administration to neonates and infants younger than age 4 months[69]

INFANTS ABO GROUP	ABO GROUP OF BLOOD COMPONENT TO BE TRANSFUSED		
	Red cells	Platelets	FFP[a]
O	O	O	O
A	A or O[b]	A	A or AB
B	B or O[b]	B[c] or A or O	B or AB
AB	AB or A or B or O[b]	AB[c] or A	AB

FFP, fresh frozen plasma.

[a]Only babies and infants who are blood group O should receive group O FFP because of anti-A and anti-B antibodies, whereas group AB FFP contains no naturally occurring antibodies.

[b]Group O components must be checked for high-titre anti-A and anti-B before being given to recipients that are not group O. This is particularly important for platelets because of the relatively large volumes of plasma.

[c]Group B or AB platelets may not be available.

and/or anti-B) (Table 22.7). Care should be taken when giving components containing group O plasma (containing anti-A and anti-B) to infants that are not group O. Despite high-titre anti-A and anti-B donors being excluded from donating components for this group, there have been reports of haemolysis of group A infants' red cells when given group O platelets.[1,2] Current production methods for fresh frozen plasma result in minimal red cell stroma which is not antigenic; therefore plasma components do not need to be D compatible. If the maternal and infant antibody screens are negative (including absent maternal IgG anti-A in the infant), ABO- and D-typed blood can be given with no serological crossmatch, even after repeated small volume transfusions, because formation of red cell antibodies is rare in infants younger than 4 months old. Repeat antibody screen is not necessary if repeat transfusions are required within the first 4 months of life.[69] In the case of haemolytic disease of the newborn (non-ABO or ABO) or maternal red cell antibodies, a crossmatch is required against maternal plasma using group O blood (which has been tested and shown to have low titres of anti-A and anti-B or 'HT negative') or other group compatible with red cell antibodies in the maternal serum. For neonates and infants, red cells for exchange transfusion should be <5 days old, negative for CMV antibodies, plasma reduced (or washed), Hb S negative, leucodepleted, K negative and irradiated.

Intrauterine (Fetal) Transfusion

Intrauterine (fetal) transfusion is usually carried out in a fetal medicine unit where local protocols should be in place. It is important for maternity units and associated neonatal units to have information about previous intrauterine transfusion because it may influence the selection of appropriate blood components if transfusion is required after delivery (see above). This is particularly important when the clinical care takes place in different institutions which are serviced by different transfusion departments. Shared-care protocols are one way of ensuring effective communication. When providing red cells for intrauterine transfusion, an antiglobulin crossmatch should be performed using maternal plasma and this must be repeated with a fresh maternal sample with every transfusion. Intrauterine transfusion can result in fetomaternal haemorrhage and hence sensitization to new antigens, so antibody identification and quantification or titration must be performed on all maternal samples. Red cells selected should be group O D negative (except where mother has made anti-c, when it will be necessary to give D positive, c-negative blood) and K negative. Further selection of phenotyped blood will depend on the maternal red cell antibody profile. In addition to the stipulations listed earlier for selection of blood for infants and neonates, blood for intrauterine transfusions should also be leucodepleted, K negative and irradiated to prevent transfusion-associated graft-versus-host disease and should be transfused within 24 h of irradiation.[69]

Patients Receiving Transfusions at Close Intervals

Patients who are acutely ill, particularly those on intensive care units and those undergoing intensive chemotherapy for haematological malignancy, may require frequent blood transfusions. This section does not include transfusions to neonates and infants within the first 4 months of life (see above) and other special considerations are necessary for recipients of a stem cell transplant (see below).

Alloantibodies can develop quickly following a transfusion. Therefore, a sample should be obtained for compatibility testing before each transfusion if they are separated by an interval of 3 days or more. There is no need for daily samples, but an antibody screen at least every 72 h is recommended as being practical and safe.

Chronic Transfusion Programmes

Examples of patients in whom a decision has been made that regular transfusions are required include those with β thalassaemia major, some patients with sickle cell anaemia and congenital or acquired bone marrow failure. It is important to establish a treatment plan for each patient with clear triggers for transfusion and regular checks for the adverse effects of transfusion, including iron overload. The risk of developing alloantibodies to red cell antigens on transfused blood influences the timing of blood samples (Table 22.1). If a less rigorous approach is taken for patients in whom repeated transfusions have not led to alloantibody formation, a mutual decision should be made by the clinician and the transfusion department after careful consideration of the risks.

A pre-transfusion Rh phenotype allows matching for D, C, c, E and e. Some ethnic groups commonly have the phenotype cDe (R_o) and D positive blood negative for C and E may be difficult to find, particularly if there are other red cell antibodies. In this situation D negative (cde/cde) blood is selected. Additionally, patients with haemoglobinopathies should have an extended red cell phenotype before they are first transfused to include the antigens K, Jk^a, Jk^b, Fy^a, Fy^b, M, N, S and s.[70,71] This may be used to select blood but is also helpful when investigating antibodies formed as a result of repeated transfusions. Although provision of red cells with a matched extended phenotype is undertaken by some units treating haemoglobinopathies,[72] the degree of matching depends on local resources and should not impede the delivery of effective transfusion support. There is insufficient evidence to make this recommendation for other patients who have been chronically transfused.

Allogeneic Haemopoietic Stem Cell Transplantation

An allogeneic haemopoietic stem cell transplant may introduce a new blood group; an ABO antigen (major mismatch), ABO antibody (minor mismatch) or both. The recipient/donor pairs have different ABO and D groups in about 15–20% of sibling stem cell transplants and this is more common in unrelated donor stem cell transplants. If there is a major ABO mismatch and isoagglutinins persist in the recipient's plasma, engraftment may result in a positive direct antiglobulin test when substantial numbers of donor red cells start to enter the circulation and some haemolysis may occur.

A *minor ABO mismatch* is when the donor has antibodies to the recipient's red cells (e.g. donor O, recipient A). Transfuse red cells of the donor ABO group until the recipient's own red cells are no longer detectable.

A *major ABO mismatch* is when the recipient has antibodies to the donor red cells (e.g. donor A, recipient O). Transfuse red cells of the patient's own type until red cell antibodies are no longer detectable by the indirect antiglobulin test and the direct antiglobulin test is negative and then transfer to donor type.

A *major plus minor mismatch* is when there are antibodies to recipient and donor red cells (e.g. donor A, recipient B). Transfuse group O red cells until the recipient's red cell antibodies are no longer detectable by the indirect antiglobulin test and the direct antiglobulin test is negative.

Prior to the transplant, recipient type red cells, platelets and fresh frozen plasma are given, but following engraftment, the choice of blood components depends on the ABO and D mismatch between the donor/recipient pairs.[11] For a recipient who is D positive with a donor who is D negative, D negative components should be used.

From the time of conditioning therapy, throughout the period of prophylaxis, all cellular blood components should be irradiated to prevent transfusion-associated graft versus host disease. The stem cell processing laboratory will ensure that products for infusion in the allogeneic setting do not contain significant numbers/amounts of red cells/plasma if there is the potential for a haemolytic transfusion reaction.

INVESTIGATION OF A TRANSFUSION REACTION

Adverse events related to transfusion can be acute (within 24 h) or delayed (Table 22.8). Transfusion laboratories should immediately be informed of a suspected transfusion reaction, being ideally placed to coordinate investigation, to communicate with clinicians and transfusion services and to advise about appropriate choice of blood components for subsequent transfusions. Serious adverse events should be reported confidentially to the national haemovigilance scheme, the local blood centre and the Hospital Transfusion Team. Acute transfusion reactions are easier to attribute to the transfusion than delayed reactions, although, in patients who are already very ill, they can go undiagnosed. The symptoms and signs of acute transfusion reactions are similar regardless of the cause so treatment

Table 22.8 Types of transfusion reaction

ACUTE TRANSFUSION REACTIONS	DELAYED TRANSFUSION REACTIONS
Acute haemolytic reaction	Delayed haemolytic reaction
Anaphylaxis	Transfusion transmitted infection
Bacterial contamination of blood component	Transfusion-associated graft-versus-host disease
Transfusion-associated acute lung injury	Post-transfusion purpura
Transfusion-associated circulatory overload	Iron overload
Allergic reaction	Immunosuppression
Febrile non-haemolytic transfusion reaction	

and investigation of causes is, by necessity, simultaneous. It is easier to distinguish between the causes of delayed transfusion reactions, but it may be more difficult to recognize their relationship to the transfusion episode because of the delay in onset. The following scheme outlines the role of the laboratory in investigation and management of transfusion reactions and a very useful algorithm can be found in the *Handbook of Transfusion Medicine*.[73]

Acute Transfusion Reactions

Acute life-threatening transfusion reactions can result from the following:

1. Acute intravascular haemolysis as a result of ABO incompatibility:
   Acute intravascular haemolysis can occur, although rarely, as a result of other red cell antibodies that activate complement through to the membrane attack complex (e.g. anti-Vel and anti-PP_1P^k).
2. Anaphylaxis and severe acute allergic reactions:
   These reactions are more commonly associated with blood components containing large amounts of plasma where the recipient has been presensitized to an allergen in the donor plasma. Recipients with IgA deficiency can develop antibodies to IgA which is present in plasma-containing blood components.
3. Severe extravascular haemolysis:
   This may happen where a strong antibody, which does not bind complement, or only binds it to the C3 stage, is missed in pre-transfusion testing and causes rapid extravascular clearance of incompatible transfused red cells. These reactions are usually less severe than those caused by ABO incompatibilities.
4. Transfusion of a bacterially contaminated blood component:
   This is more likely with platelets because they are stored at room temperature but can also occur with red cells. If contamination is suspected, the blood centre must be informed immediately so that other components from the same donor can be traced and withdrawn if not already transfused.
5. Transfusion-associated acute lung injury:
   This is an acute respiratory disorder, with one mechanism being passive transfer of antibodies in the donor unit that react with the recipient's own white blood cells, resulting in non-cardiogenic interstitial pulmonary oedema.
6. Transfusion associated circulatory overload: The onset of breathlessness within 6 h of transfusion due to pulmonary oedema resulting from fluid overload.

Although rare, the onset of an acute transfusion reaction is usually very dramatic and the patient is acutely ill. Treatment is aimed at resuscitating the patient and elucidating the cause to try and prevent any further incidents (Table 22.9). In addition, there are unpleasant but not

Table 22.9 Immediate investigations in the case of an acute transfusion reaction

Check for haemolysis
Perform visual examination of patient's plasma and urine (plasma and urine haemoglobin can be checked but this is not essential).
Blood film may show spherocytosis.
Bilirubin and lactate dehydrogenase (LDH) levels will be raised.

Check for incompatibility
Check the documentation and the patient's identity.
Repeat ABO group of patient pre-transfusion and post-transfusion and of the donor unit(s).
Screen the patient for red cell antibodies pre-transfusion and post-transfusion.
Repeat crossmatch with pre-transfusion and post-transfusion samples.
Direct antiglobulin test (DAT) on pre- and post-transfusion samples
Eluate from patient's red cells.

Check for disseminated intravascular coagulation
Perform blood count and film, coagulation screen and fibrin degradation products (or D-dimers).

Check for renal dysfunction
Check blood urea, creatinine and electrolytes.

Check for bacterial infection
Take blood cultures from the patient and donor unit including immediate Gram stain.

Immunological investigations
Check immunoglobulin A (IgA) levels and anti-IgA antibodies.

life-threatening reactions that may occur during transfusion. They include the following:

Allergic reactions – the patient may experience mild urticaria or itching caused by a reaction to plasma proteins in the donor unit.

Febrile non-haemolytic transfusion reactions – antibodies in the recipient react to donor white cells and cause an increase in temperature of no more than 1°C; alternatively, cytokines released from white cells in the donor units can cause a similar reaction. These conditions usually settle on slowing the transfusion and administration of antipyretics and antihistamines. They do not require detailed investigation. They are less common where cellular blood components are leucodepleted.

Acute Intravascular Haemolysis

Transfused red cells react with the patient's own anti-A or anti-B, and the red cells are destroyed in the circulation, causing collapse, renal failure and disseminated intravascular coagulation. Transfusion of ABO-incompatible cells usually results from an identification error. This can occur at point of blood sampling and labelling (wrong blood in tube), laboratory testing (technical error), blood unit labelling (administrative error) and collection from the blood refrigerator or inadequate bedside checking. If red cells are mistakenly transfused to the wrong patient, there is approximately a 1 in 3 chance that ABO incompatibility will occur. The reaction is most severe if group A blood is transfused to a patient who is group O, and only a small volume of red cells is required to cause this reaction. Prompt action in recognizing this acute emergency and stopping the transfusion may lead to a better outcome because the severity depends on the volume of blood transfused. If an acute transfusion reaction is suspected, the laboratory must be informed immediately and the unit of blood and giving set must be returned to the laboratory with blood and urine samples from the patient (Table 22.9).

Documentation check

The patient's identification wristband, the compatibility form and the compatibility label attached to the blood unit should be checked again at the bedside. Any discrepancies must be notified to the transfusion laboratory immediately and the transfusion should not go ahead until the discrepancy has been resolved. If the wrong blood has been administered, the units intended for that patient must be withdrawn from issue to prevent another parallel error occurring with another patient who may have the same or a similar name.

Serological investigations

Serological investigations have a two-fold purpose: (1) to check for any laboratory errors in the pre-transfusion sample group and compatibility check and (2) to repeat the group and compatibility tests with the post-transfusion sample to see if the pre-transfusion sample was from the correct patient. Reactions in liquid-phase tests should be read microscopically to detect any mixed-field reaction.

Tests for haemolysis

Because not all acute transfusion reactions are the result of haemolysis, haematological and biochemical tests as well as visual inspection of the plasma and urine are required. Further tests may be required to manage the resuscitation of the patient and direct the use of blood components to treat disseminated intravascular coagulation.

Microbiological tests

If the cause of the acute transfusion reaction is suspected to be due to contamination, blood cultures should be taken from the unit and the patient. Blood centres issue guidance for the investigation of potentially contaminated units and often will carry out this investigation themselves.

Delayed Haemolytic Transfusion Reaction

A delayed haemolytic transfusion reaction occurs when the recipient has been immunized to a red cell antigen by a previous transfusion or during pregnancy but the antibody is present at low or undetectable levels and may have been missed by the antibody screen. A secondary immune response is mounted to the incompatible antigen that has been transfused. The IgG- and/or complement-coated red cells are destroyed in the spleen and/or liver. Kidd antibodies are often implicated in delayed transfusion reactions because they are difficult to detect, often displaying a dosage effect, fall rapidly to undetectable levels and are frequently present in combinations of antibodies.

Haematological Investigation

The following suggest a delayed haemolytic transfusion reaction:

Haemoglobin concentration falls more rapidly than would be expected after a red cell transfusion
Increase in haemoglobin concentration is less than expected for the number of units transfused
Blood film shows spherocytosis
Positive direct antiglobulin test
Unconjugated bilirubin raised.

Serological Investigation

It is desirable to have the pre-transfusion sample available to test in addition to a post-transfusion sample, but this is not always possible because of the delay between the time of the transfusion and the investigation. It has been recommended by some that plasma samples are saved on all patients who are transfused, but this is not always practical. Unless the reaction is acute, the units transfused will not be available for retesting. In the UK, the phenotype of each unit is provided by the National Blood Service and this information can help in the investigation of a delayed transfusion reaction. The following tests should be carried out, preferably using different or more sensitive techniques:

1. Confirm the ABO and D group of the patient on a pre-transfusion and post-transfusion sample.
2. Perform a direct antiglobulin test on the patient's pre-transfusion and post-transfusion washed red cells. In the event of a positive direct antiglobulin test, elution of the antibody may aid identification or confirm specificities in cases of non-ABO incompatibility. Consideration should be given to performing an eluate

even if the DAT is negative. Sometimes the causative antibody is only detectable in the eluate.[1]

3. Repeat the crossmatch, if possible, using pre-transfusion and post-transfusion samples.

4. Screen the pre-transfusion and post-transfusion samples for red cell antibodies and identify any antibodies. The immediate post-transfusion sample may have no detectable red cell antibodies, although

they may be eluted from the patient's red cells if the direct antiglobulin test is positive. It is also possible to have a delayed haemolytic transfusion reaction with a negative direct antiglobulin test because the antibody-coated red cells have been removed from the circulation. If the immediate post-transfusion investigation is inconclusive, repeat the tests 10 days later to allow antibody levels to increase.

REFERENCES

1. Serious Hazards of Transfusion (SHOT). *Annual Reports 1996–2009.* Available at: www.shotuk.org.

2. Serious Hazards of Transfusion. *Annual Report 2009.* July 2010. Available at: www.shotuk.org.

3. Chaffe B, Jones J, Milkins C, et al. Recommended minimum standards for hospital transfusion laboratories. UK Transfusion Laboratory Collaborative. *Transfus Med.* 2009; 19(4):156–158.

4. British Committee for Standards in Haematology (BCSH). *Guidelines.* Available at:. www.bcshguidelines. com.

5. AABB (previously American Association of Blood Banks). Available at: www.aabb.org.

6. *The European Blood Directive 2002 and associated directives.* Available at: www.transfusionguidelines.org.uk/docs/pdfs/directive_2002_98_ec.pdf.

7. The Blood Safety and Quality Regulations. 2005. Available at: www.opsi.gov.uk/si/si2005/20050050.htm; plus amendments at: www.opsi.gov.uk/si/si2005/20051098 htm and www.opsi.gov.uk/si/si2006/20062013 htm.

8. Medicines and Healthcare Products Regulatory Agency. Available at: www.mhra.gov.uk/Howweregulate/Blood/index.htm.

9. Department of Health. *Better blood transfusion – safe and appropriate use of blood Health Service Circulars 1998/224, 2002/009 and 2007/001.* Available at:. www.dh.gov.uk/en/Publicationsandstatistics/Lettersandcirculars/Healthservicecirculars/DH_080613.

10. *Personal communication based on Annual Reports of UK National External Quality Assessment Scheme (Blood Transfusion Laboratory Practice).*

Contact scheme available via: www.ukneqas.org.uk.

11. British Committee for Standards in Haematology. Guidelines for compatibility procedures in blood transfusion laboratories. *Transfus Med.* 2004;14:59–73.

12. British Committee for Standards in Haematology. *The specification and use of Information Technology (IT) systems in Blood Transfusion Practice* 2006. Available at: www.bcshguidelines.com/pdf/computer_guide_220506.pdf.

13. *MHRA guidance on electronic issue* May. 2010. Available at: www.mhra.gov.uk/Howweregulate/Blood/index.htm.

14. British Committee for Standards in Haematology. *Guideline on the Administration of Blood Components.* 2009. Available at: www.bcshguidelines.com/pdf/Admin_blood_ components050110.pdf.

15. Wagar EA, Stankovic AK, Raab S, et al. Specimen labeling errors: a Q-probes analysis of 147 clinical laboratories. *Arch Pathol Lab Med.* 2008;132(10):1617–1622.

16. Dzik WH, Murphy MF, Andreu G, et al; the Biomedical Excellence for Safer Transfusion (BEST) Working Party of the International Society for Blood Transfusion. An international study of the performance of sample collection from patients. *Vox Sang.* 2003;85(1):40–47.

17. Murphy MF, Stearn BE, Dzik WH. Current performance of patient sample collection in the UK. *Transfus Med.* 2004;14:113–121.

18. Guidance from the Royal College of Pathologists and the Institute of Biomedical Science. *The retention and storage of pathological records and specimens.* 4th ed. Available at: www.

rcpath.org/resources/pdf/g031retentionstorageaugust09.pdf; 2009.

19. *Information for patients needing irradiated blood components from NHS Blood and Transplant.* National Blood Service Hospitals and Science website at: http://hospital.blood.co.uk/library/pdf/INF_PCS_HL_005_01_Irradiated.pdf.

20. Cannon M, Pierce R, Taber EB, et al. Fatal hydrops fetalis caused by anti-D in a mother with partial D. *Obstet Gynecol.* 2003;102(5):1143–1145.

21. Scott ML, Voak D. Monoclonal antibodies to RhD: development and uses. *Vox Sang.* 2000;78(suppl 2):79–82.

22. Jones J, Scott ML, Voak D. Monoclonal anti-D specificity and Rh D structure: criteria for selection of monoclonal anti-D reagents for routine typing of donors. *Transfus Med.* 1995;5:171–184.

23. Yip SP. Sequence variation at the human ABO locus. *Ann Hum Genet.* 2002;66(1):1–27.

24. BCSH Blood Transfusion Task Force. Guidelines for microplate techniques in liquid-phase blood grouping and antibody screening: a joint publication of the British Society for Haematology and the British Blood Transfusion Society. *Clin Lab Haematol.* 1990;12:437–460.

25. Horn KD. The classification, recognition and significance of polyagglutination in transfusion medicine. *Blood Rev.* 1999;13:36–44.

26. Garratty G, Arndt P, Co A, et al. Fatal haemolytic transfusion reaction resulting from ABO mistyping of a patient with acquired B antigen detectable only by some monoclonal anti-B reagents. *Transfusion.* 1996;36:351–357.

27. Knowles SM, Milkins CE, Chapman JF, et al. The United Kingdom National External Quality Assessment Scheme (Blood Transfusion Laboratory Practice): trends in proficiency and practice between 1985 and 2000. *Transfus Med*. 2002;12:11–23.

28. Denomme GA, Wagner FF, Fernandes BJ, et al. Partial D, weak D types and novel RHD alleles among 33,864 multiethnic patients: implications for anti-D alloimmunization and prevention. *Transfusion*. 2005;45(10):1554–1560.

29. Guidelines for the Blood Transfusion Services in the UK. *The Red Book*. 7th ed. Available at: www. transfusionguidelines.org.uk/index. aspx?Publication=RB; 2005.

30. Klein HG, Anstee DJ. The Rh blood group system. In: *Mollison's Blood Transfusion in Clinical Medicine*. 11th ed. Oxford: Blackwell; 2005.

31. Garratty G. Screening for RBC antibodies – what should we expect from antibody detection RBCs. *Immunohaematology*. 2002;18: 71–77.

32. Issitt PD, Combs MR, Bredehoeft SJ, et al. Lack of clinical significance of 'enzyme-only' red cell alloantibodies. *Transfusion*. 1993;33:284–293.

33. Shirey RS, Boyd JS, Ness PM. Polyethylene glycol versus low-ionic-strength solution in pre-transfusion testing: a blinded comparison study. *Transfusion*. 1994;34:368–370.

34. Reis KJ, Chachowski R, Cupido A, et al. Column agglutination technology: the antiglobulin test. *Transfusion*. 1993;33 (8):639–643.

35. MDA Evaluation Report MDA/96/ 14. *Six systems for the detection of red cell antibodies*. Hannibal House, London: MHRA.

36. Bromilow IM, Eggington JA, Owen GA, et al. Red cell antibody screening and identification: a comparison of two column technology methods. *Br J Biomed Sci*. 1993;50:329–333.

37. Cummins D, Downham B. Failure of DiaMed-ID microtyping system to detect major ABO incompatibility. *Lancet*. 1994;343:1649–1650.

38. Phillips P, Voak D, Knowles S, et al. An explanation and the clinical significance of the failure of microcolumn tests to detect weak ABO and other antibodies. *Transfus Med*. 1997;7:47–53.

39. Voak D, Downie DM, Haigh T, et al. Improved antiglobulin tests to detect difficult antibodies: detection of anti-K by LISS. *Med Lab Sci*. 1982;39: 363–370.

40. Contreras M, Hazlehurst GR, Armitage SE. Development of 'auto-anti-A₁ antibodies' following alloimmunisation in an A2 recipient. *Br J Haematol*. 1983;55:657–663.

41. British Committee for Standards in Haematology. Guidelines for implementation of a maximum surgical blood order schedule. *Clin Lab Haematol*. 1990;12:321–327.

42. Staves J, Davies A, Kay J, et al. Electronic remote blood issue: a combination of remote blood issue with a system for end-to-end electronic control of transfusion to provide a 'total solution' for a safe and timely hospital blood transfusion service. *Transfusion*. 2008;48(3):415–424.

43. Ramsey G. Red cell antibodies arising from solid organ transplants. *Transfusion*. 1991;31(1):76–86.

44. O'Hagan J, White J, Milkins CE, et al. Direct agglutination crossmatch at room temperature (DRT): the results of a NEQAS (BTLP) questionnaire. *Transfus Med*. 1999;9(suppl 1):42.

45. Lamberson RD, Boral LI, Berry-Dortch S. Limitations of the crossmatch for detection of incompatibility between A2B red blood cells and B patient sera. *Am J Clin Pathol*. 1986;86:511–513.

46. Shulman IA, Odono V. The risk of overt acute hemolytic transfusion reaction following the use of an immediate-spin crossmatch. *Transfusion*. 1994;34:87–88.

47. Berry-Dortch S, Woodside CH, Boral LI. Limitations of the immediate spin crossmatch when used for detecting ABO incompatibility. *Transfusion*. 1985;25:176–178.

48. AABB. *American Association of Blood Banks. Guidelines for Implementing the Electronic Crossmatch*. Basel: Karger; 2003.

49. Säfwenberg J, Högman CF, Cassemar B. Computerized delivery control – a useful and safe complement to the type and screen compatibility testing. *Vox Sang*. 1997;72:162–168.

50. Chapman JF, Milkins C, Voak D. The computer crossmatch: a safe alternative to the serological crossmatch. *Transfus Med*. 2000;10: 251–256.

51. Judd WJ. Requirements for the electronic crossmatch. *Vox Sang*. 1998;74(suppl 2):409–417.

52. UK National Blood Transfusion Committee. *The appropriate use of group O RhD negative red cells*. Available at: www.transfusionguidelines.org.uk/ docs/pdfs/nbtc_bbt_o_neg_ red_cells_recs _09_04.pdf; 2009.

53. BCSH. BCSH guidelines on the management of massive blood loss. *Br J Haematol*. 2006;135 (5):634–641.

54. Vaughan JI, Warwick R, Letsky E, et al. Erythropoietic suppression in fetal anemia because of Kell alloimmunization. *Am J Obstet Gynecol*. 1994;171(1):247–252.

55. Daniels G, Hadley A, Green CA. Causes of fetal anemia in haemolytic disease due to anti-K. *Transfusion*. 2003;43:115–116.

56. Koelewijn JM, Vrijkotte TG, van der Schoot CE, et al. Effect of screening for red cell antibodies, other than anti-D, to detect hemolytic disease of the fetus and newborn: a population study in the Netherlands. *Transfusion*. 2008;48(5):941–952.

57. Kumar S, O'Brien A. Recent developments in fetal medicine. *Br Med J*. 2004;328:1002–1006.

58. Bowman J. The management of hemolytic disease in the fetus and newborn. *Semin Perinatol*. 1997;21: 39–44.

59. British Committee for Standards in Haematology. *Guideline for blood grouping and antibody testing in pregnancy*. Available at: www. bcshguidelines.com/pdf/ pregnancy_070606.pdf; 2006.

60. Van Dijk BA, Dooren MC, Overbeeke MA. Red cell antibodies in pregnancy: there is no 'critical titre'. *Transfus Med*. 1995;5:199–202.

61. Daniels G. *Human Blood Groups*. Oxford: Blackwell; 2002.

62. Finning K, Martin P, Daniels G. A clinical service in the UK to predict fetal Rh (Rhesus) D blood group using free fetal DNA in maternal

plasma. *Ann N Y Acad Sci.* 2004;1022:119–123.

63. Abdel-Fattah SA, Soothill PW, Carroll SG, et al. Middle cerebral artery Doppler for the prediction of fetal anaemia in cases without hydrops: a practical approach. *Br J Radiol.* 2002;75:726–730.

64. BCSH. *BCSH Guidelines for the use of prophylactic anti-D immunoglobulin.* Available at: www.bcshguidelines. com/pdf/Anti-D_070606.pdf; 2006.

65. RCOG. Rh Prophylaxis, Anti-D Immunoglobulin (Green-top 22). *Royal College of Obstetricians and Gynaecologists.* 2002. Available at: www.rcog.org.uk.

66. British Committee for Standards in Haematology. *The estimation of fetomaternal haemorrhage.* Available at: www.bcshguidelines.com/pdf/ BCSH_Fetomaternal_sept2009 pdf; 2009.

67. National Institute for Health and Clinical Excellence. Routine antenatal anti-D prophylaxis for women who are rhesus D negative. *Technology Appraisal.* 2008;156. Available at: www.nice.org.uk/TA156.

68. Finning K, Martin P, Summers J, et al. Effect of high throughput RHD typing of fetal DNA in maternal plasma on use of anti-RhD immunoglobulin in RhD negative pregnant women: prospective feasibility study. *Br Med J.* 2008;336 (7648):816–818.

69. British Committee for Standards in Haematology. Transfusion guidelines for neonates and older children. *Br J Haematol.* 2004;124: 433–453.

70. Sickle Cell Society. Standards for the clinical care of adults with Sickle Cell Disease in the UK, Chapter 6. *Blood Transfusion.* 2008; Available at: www. sicklecellsociety.org/pdf/CareBook. pdf.

71. UK Thalassaemia Society. Standards for the clinical care of children and adults with thalassaemia in the UK, Chapter 6. *Blood Transfusion.* 2008. Available at: www.ukts.org/ pdfs/awareness/ukts-standards-2008.pdf.

72. Vichinsky EP, Luban NL, Wright E, et al. Prospective RBC phenotype matching in a stroke-prevention trial in sickle cell anemia: a multicenter transfusion trial. *Transfusion.* 2001;41:1086–1092.

73. McClelland DB. *Handbook of Transfusion Medicine.* 4th ed. UK Blood Transfusion Services. The Stationery Office; 2007. Available at: www.transfusionguidelines.org/ index. asp?Publication=h1 &Section=9 &pageid=8.

Chapter | **23** |

Approach to the diagnosis and classification of blood diseases

Imelda Bates, Barbara J. Bain

COMMON PRESENTATIONS OF HAEMATOLOGICAL DISEASES

An abnormal blood count or blood cell morphology does not necessarily indicate a primary haematological problem because it may reflect an underlying non-haematological condition or may be the result of therapeutic interventions. Anaemia occurs in many conditions, but a primary blood disease should be considered when a patient has splenomegaly, lymphadenopathy, a bleeding tendency or thrombosis and/or nonspecific symptoms characteristic of leukaemias and lymphomas (malaise, sweats or weight loss).

As with any clinical problem, the first steps in determining the diagnosis include obtaining a careful clinical and drug history and thorough physical examination. The result of these, in combination with the patient's age, sex, ethnic origin, social and family history and knowledge of the locally prevalent diseases, will determine subsequent laboratory investigations.

INITIAL SCREENING TESTS

Although the range of haematological tests available to support clinical and public health services is broad, it is often the simplest investigations that are most useful in indicating the diagnosis. Even poorly-resourced laboratories are usually able to provide an initial panel of tests such as haemoglobin concentration (Hb), white blood cell count (WBC) and platelet count (Chapter 26) and examination of a peripheral blood film for a differential leucocyte count (Chapter 3) and cellular morphology (Chapter 5). These screening tests will often enable the underlying pathological processes to be suspected promptly and point to a few key diagnostic tests. The investigation of specific haematological problems is covered in detail in Chapters 9 (iron deficiency anaemia), 10 (megaloblastic anaemia), 11, 12 and 13 (haemolytic anaemias), 14 (haemoglobinopathies) and 18, 19 and 20 (coagulation disorders).

Interpretation of Screening Tests

Results of laboratory screening tests should always be interpreted with an understanding of the limitations of the tests and the physiological variations that occur with sex, age and conditions such as pregnancy and exercise. Physiological variations in cell counts are detailed in Chapter 2. Abnormalities of red cells, white cells or platelets may be quantitative (increased or reduced numbers) or qualitative (abnormal appearance and/or function).

Quantitative Abnormalities of Blood Cells

Increased Numbers of Cells

Increases affecting more than one cell line

A simultaneous increase in the cells of more than one cell line suggests overproduction of cells originating in an early precursor cell. This occurs in myeloproliferative neoplasms in which one cell type may predominate, e.g. platelets in essential thrombocythaemia and red cells in polycythaemia vera, but there are often increases in other cell lines. The diagnosis will depend on which cell line dominates.

Erythrocytosis

Patients with a persistently (e.g. >2 months) raised venous haematocrit (Hct) (>0.52 l/l males, >0.48 l/l females) should be assessed to determine the cause of the apparent polycythaemia. Erythrocytosis can be relative or absolute and, if absolute, primary or secondary.

Relative: normal total red cell volume with reduced plasma volume

Absolute: males and females with Hct values above 0.60 and 0.56 l/l, respectively, can be assumed to have an absolute erythrocytosis and do not require confirmatory studies.[1] However, the reason for the elevation must still be elucidated.

> *Primary*: this is usually polycythaemia vera (PV), part of the spectrum of myeloproliferative neoplasms. Rarely, it is inherited, due to mutation of genes involved with erythropoietin or its receptor.
> *Secondary*: to chronic hypoxia (e.g. chronic lung disease, congenital heart disease, high-affinity haemoglobins) or aberrant erythropoietin production.

Secondary polycythaemia can generally be excluded by the clinical history and examination, assessment of serum erythropoietin concentration and arterial oxygen saturation, haemoglobin electrophoresis plus oxygen dissociation curve and abdominal ultrasound examination. The presence of splenomegaly is suggestive of PV and this diagnosis can be confirmed by demonstrating the *JAK2* V617F mutation, which is present in 95% of patients.[2] Only if this mutation (or one of the much less common *JAK2* exon 12 mutations) is not detected is the measurement of total red cell and plasma volume necessary (Chapter 17).

Leucocytosis

Neutrophilia

Neutrophils are commonly increased during pregnancy and in acute infections, inflammation, alcohol intoxication, corticosteroid therapy and acute blood loss or red cell destruction. Neutrophilia with the neutrophils showing heavy cytoplasmic granulation ('toxic' granulation) is a common finding in severe bacterial infections. In the absence of any underlying cause, a high neutrophil count with immature myeloid cells suggests chronic myelogenous leukaemia (CML); cytogenetic and molecular studies to look for t(9;22) and the *BCR–ABL1* fusion gene are indicated (Chapter 8).

Lymphocytosis

Lymphocytosis is a feature of certain infections, particularly infections in children. It may be especially marked in pertussis, infectious mononucleosis, cytomegalovirus infection, infectious hepatitis, tuberculosis and brucellosis. Lymphocytosis is also a common transient reaction to severe physical stress. Elderly patients with lymphoproliferative disorders, including chronic lymphocytic leukaemia and lymphomas, often present with lymphadenopathy and a lymphocytosis. Morphology and immunophenotyping of the cells combined with histological examination of a bone marrow trephine biopsy specimen (and if necessary other tissue biopsy) are used to classify these disorders and to give an indication of management and prognosis.[3] It is occasionally difficult to differentiate between a reactive and a neoplastic lymphocytosis. In this situation, immunophenotyping, to provide evidence of light chain restriction and polymerase chain reaction for immunoglobulin or T-cell receptor gene rearrangements, may indicate the presence of a monoclonal population of lymphocytes, thereby supporting a diagnosis of neoplastic, rather than reactive, lymphoproliferation. If lymph nodes are enlarged, a lymph node biopsy for histology and immunohistochemistry may be helpful in diagnosis.

Monocytosis

A slight to moderate monocytosis may be associated with some protozoal, rickettsial and bacterial infections including malaria, typhus and tuberculosis. High levels of monocytes (monocyte count $>1 \times 10^9/l$) in an elderly patient suggest chronic myelomonocytic leukaemia or, sometimes, atypical chronic myeloid leukaemia. Because these conditions fall into the myelodysplastic/myeloproliferative neoplasm group of disorders,[4] the diagnosis would be supported by finding splenomegaly, quantitative and qualitative abnormalities in other cell lines or a clonal cytogenetic abnormality.

Eosinophilia

Eosinophilia is typically associated with allergic disorders including drug sensitivity, skin diseases and parasitic infections. In most cases, the cause is indicated by the clinical history, which should include details of all medications and foreign travel, and by examination of the stool and urine for parasites, cysts and ova. A diagnosis of chronic eosinophilic leukaemia is made if there is dominant eosinophilia with an increase in blast cells in the blood or marrow, or cytogenetic or molecular evidence of an abnormal myeloid clone.[5] If no other cause for eosinophilia is found it is important, because of the therapeutic implications (i.e. responsiveness to imatinib), to confirm or exclude a diagnosis of eosinophilic leukaemia related to rearrangement of *PDGFRA* or *PDGFRB* (see p. 559).[6] The idiopathic hypereosinophilic syndrome is an unusual cause of eosinophilia in which release of the contents of eosinophil granules results in damage to the heart, lungs and other tissues. It is defined by the presence of a peripheral blood eosinophil count of 1.5×10^9/l or greater for at least 6 months with resultant tissue damage. This is a diagnosis of exclusion, made only when detailed investigations exclude other possible causes of eosinophilia including systemic mastocytosis, eosinophilic leukaemia and eosinophilia associated with a phenotypically aberrant T-cell population or a neoplastic clone of T cells.

Basophilia

Basophilia as an isolated finding is unusual. However, it is a common feature of myeloproliferative neoplasms and basophils may be particularly prominent in chronic myelogenous leukaemia. In this condition, an increasing basophil count may be the first indication of accelerated phase disease.

Thrombocytosis

Thrombocytosis is often associated with infectious and inflammatory conditions such as osteomyelitis and rheumatoid arthritis. Haematological causes of thrombocytosis include chronic blood loss, red cell destruction, splenectomy and rebound following recovery from marrow suppression. Under these circumstances, a moderately increased platelet count (e.g. $400–800 \times 10^9$/l) does not usually have any pathological implications. Primary thrombocythaemia is usually the result of a myeloproliferative neoplasm; rarely, it is an inherited condition. When there is isolated persistent thrombocytosis in a myeloproliferative neoplasm the diagnosis is essential thrombocythaemia (as long as a *BCR–ABL1* fusion gene has been excluded). Thrombotic or haemorrhagic complications can occur but often the diagnosis is an incidental one.[7] A significant proportion of individuals with essential thrombocythaemia have the *JAK2* V617F mutation, which is associated with an increased risk of thrombosis.[8] The criteria for this diagnosis are discussed on p. 559.

Reduced Numbers of Cells

Reductions in more than one cell line

A reduction in cell numbers occurs because of increased destruction, reduced production or increased pooling in the spleen or other organs. Reduced production of cells may be the result of aplastic anaemia, a lack of haematinics such as folate or vitamin B_{12} or interference with normal haemopoiesis by infiltration (e.g. leukaemia, lymphoma, multiple myeloma, metastatic carcinoma – often with secondary myelofibrosis), infection (e.g. HIV infection, tuberculosis, leishmaniasis) or exposure to toxins (e.g. alcohol) or myelosuppressive drugs (e.g. hydroxycarbamide or methotrexate). Certain myeloid neoplasms, e.g. primary myelofibrosis and MDS, are characterized by cytopenias, which are at least in part the result of ineffective haemopoiesis. Cytopenia is also sometimes a feature of acute myeloid leukaemia (AML), when it is due both to ineffective haemopoiesis and to replacement of normal haemopoietic stem cells by leukaemic cells. A relatively common cause of a global reduction in circulating cells is pooling of the cells in a markedly enlarged spleen (hypersplenism), which may be secondary to conditions such as primary myelofibrosis and portal hypertension. Examination of a bone marrow aspirate and trephine biopsy specimen is often helpful in determining the cause of cytopenias for which no obvious cause is apparent

Anaemia

The mechanisms which result in anaemia are decreased production, reduced red cell lifespan, blood loss and splenic pooling. Anaemia is broadly divided into three types: microcytic (low MCV), macrocytic (high MCV) and normocytic (normal MCV). The choice of investigations is guided by the MCV and red cell morphology in addition to clinical features. Figures 23.1–23.3 are flow charts that provide an orderly sequence of investigations for the different types of anaemia on the basis of these indices. Examination of a blood film will usually suggest the quickest route to the diagnosis; confirmation may require the more specific tests, which are given in the text. The presence of basophilic stippling in a patient with microcytic red cells suggests thalassaemia trait or, much less often, lead poisoning. A dimorphic blood film is typical of congenital sideroblastic anaemia but is more often the result of iron deficiency responding to treatment. Pappenheimer bodies suggest that a microcytic anaemia is the result of sideroblastic erythropoiesis.

Microcytic Anaemia

The most common cause of anaemia worldwide is iron deficiency, which can be suspected from a low MCV (Fig. 23.1) and the presence of hypochromic, microcytic red cells. Laboratory confirmation of iron deficiency may

Figure 23.1 Investigation of a microcytic hypochromic anaemia. HbEP, Hb electrophoresis; HPLC, high-performance liquid chromatography.

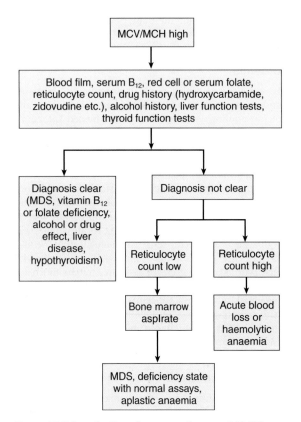

Figure 23.2 Investigation of a macrocytic anaemia. MDS, myelodysplastic syndrome.

be based on measurements of serum ferritin, serum iron plus either total iron-binding capacity or transferrin assay, red cell protoporphyrin and staining of bone marrow aspirates for iron (see Chapter 4). Assay of soluble transferrin receptors has good sensitivity and specificity for iron deficiency and may be useful in the presence of inflammation when interpretation of ferritin levels is difficult.[9] A diagnosis of iron deficiency must be followed by a search for the cause. This should include specific questions relating to blood loss and dietary insufficiency and may require stool examination for parasites and occult blood, endoscopic examination of the gastrointestinal tract to exclude occult malignancy and tests for coeliac disease. The differential diagnosis of iron deficiency anaemia includes anaemia of chronic disease. Clinical and laboratory features of inflammation or chronic infection may suggest this diagnosis, which is confirmed by demonstration of normal or high serum ferritin and reduced serum iron, transferrin and iron-binding capacity.

The thalassaemias also cause microcytosis, but both α and β thalassaemia trait are usually associated with an increased red blood cell count (RBC) and a normal or near-normal Hb despite a considerable reduction of the MCV and MCH. In contrast, in iron deficiency the MCV and MCH do not fall until the Hb is significantly reduced. Further investigations, such as high-performance liquid chromatography (HPLC) or haemoglobin electrophoresis supplemented by measurement of Hb A_2 and Hb F usually confirm the diagnosis of β thalassaemia trait. The diagnosis of α thalassaemia trait is more difficult; detection of infrequent Hb H inclusions is usually possible in α^0 thalassaemia trait, but definitive diagnosis requires DNA analysis.[10]

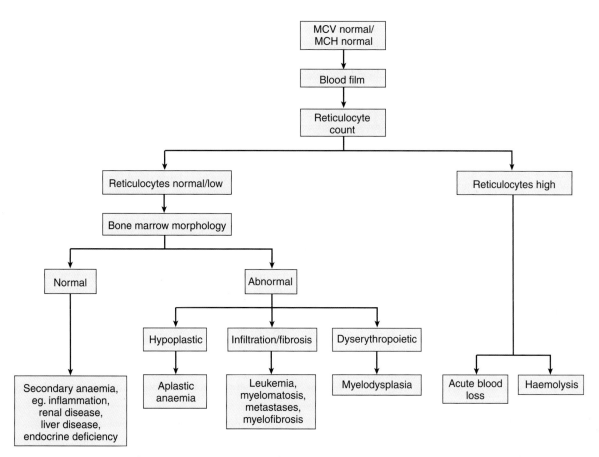

Figure 23.3 Investigation of a normocytic, normochromic anaemia.

A diagnosis of α^0 thalassaemia heterozygosity can be clinically important for prediction of haemoglobin Bart's hydrops fetalis since, if both parents have α^0 thalassaemia, this very serious condition can occur in a fetus. DNA analysis is therefore indicated when a pregnant woman of appropriate ethnic origin has an MCH of <25 pg. Hb H inclusions may not be detected in α^+ thalassaemia trait but this diagnosis is of less clinical importance and confirmation is thus not usually required.

Macrocytic Anaemia

A high MCV (Fig. 23.2) with oval macrocytes and hypersegmented neutrophils suggests folate or vitamin B_{12} deficiency and is an indication for assays of these vitamins (see Chapter 10); subsequent investigations could include malabsorption studies, tests for coeliac disease and tests for intrinsic factor and gastric parietal cell antibodies. In patients with these blood film findings and normal vitamin assays, haematinic deficiency is not completely excluded and further investigation is indicated. A Schilling test permits a definitive diagnosis of pernicious anaemia but currently this test is not available due to a lack of reagents.

In the absence of intrinsic factor antibodies, the diagnosis of pernicious anaemia may be presumptive. Pernicious anaemia is commonly associated with autoimmune thyroid disease and other autoimmune disorders, such as diabetes mellitus. A high MCV may also be associated with alcohol excess and liver disease or use of drugs such as hydroxycarbamide or zidovudine. Macrocytosis resulting from chronic haemolysis is associated with increased numbers of immature red cells, which appear slightly larger and bluer than normal red cells (polychromatic macrocytes) on a Romanowsky-stained peripheral blood film. Supravital staining of blood films (see p. 33) or an automated reticulocyte count can be used to confirm reticulocytosis. Untreated anaemia associated with polychromasia is likely to indicate blood loss or haemolysis. The combination of red cell fragments, thrombocytopenia and polychromasia indicates a microangiopathic haemolytic anaemia and should trigger further tests such as a platelet count, coagulation studies, assessment of renal function and a search for infection or neoplastic disease. This further assessment is urgent because these may be features of thrombotic thrombocytopenic purpura, which requires immediate treatment by plasma exchange.

Normocytic Anaemia

Normochromic, normocytic anaemia (Fig. 23.3) is frequently the result of an underlying chronic, non-haematological disease. Investigations should include screening for renal insufficiency, subclinical infections, autoimmune diseases and neoplasia. In the presence of anaemia, a lack of polychromasia, confirmed by reticulocytopenia, points toward a primary failure of erythropoiesis or lack of compensatory increased red cell production in blood loss or haemolysis. Examination of the bone marrow may be helpful in demonstrating haematological causes for a normochromic, normocytic anaemia such as aplastic anaemia or MDS.[11] Staining for iron may also show that there is a block in iron metabolism suggestive of anaemia associated with chronic inflammatory disease.

Leucopenia

Neutropenia

Once physiological variation, ethnicity and familial or cyclic neutropenia have been excluded (see p. 19), the non-haematological causes of isolated neutropenia to be considered include overwhelming infection, autoimmune disorders such as systemic lupus erythematosus, irradiation, drugs (particularly anticancer agents) and large granular lymphocyte leukaemia. Bone marrow examination may assist in determining whether the problem is the result of peripheral destruction (increased marrow myeloid precursors) or stem cell failure (lack of marrow myeloid precursors). Typical marrow appearances occur in drug-induced neutropenia, in which there is a relative paucity of mature neutrophils and in Kostmann's syndrome (infant genetic agranulocytosis) where there is maturation arrest at the promyelocytic stage.

Reduced numbers of lymphocytes, monocytes, eosinophils and basophils

Lymphocytes, eosinophils and basophils may all be reduced by physical stress such as surgery, trauma and infection. Lymphopenia with neutrophilia is a common combination of haematological abnormalities in severe acute respiratory syndrome and in many other patients with acute illness or trauma. Lymphopenia, especially affecting the CD4 cells, may occur in HIV infection and renal failure. Monocytopenia ($<0.2 \times 10^9/1$) is typically found in hairy cell leukaemia, which is also associated with pancytopenia, typical bone marrow histology and lymphocytes with a characteristic cytology and immunophenotype.

Thrombocytopenia

Thrombocytopenia is a common isolated finding and it is important to ensure that the laboratory result reflects a true reduction in platelet count before embarking on further diagnostic tests. Frequent causes of spurious thrombocytopenia include blood clots in the sample, platelet aggregation and platelet satellitism. Platelet aggregation, which is seen on the blood film, may occur *in vitro* as the result of a temperature-dependent or anticoagulant-dependent autoantibody or on slides that have been made directly from a finger prick sample. True thrombocytopenia is most frequently the result of autoantibodies (autoimmune 'idiopathic' thrombocytopenic purpura), HIV infection, anti-cancer chemotherapy, other drugs (such as thiazide diuretics), alcohol excess, hypersplenism and MDS (in the elderly). The blood film should be examined for giant or hypogranular platelets, red cell fragments, May–Hegglin inclusions in leucocytes and abnormal cells that might indicate leukaemia or lymphoma. The clinical circumstances, together with blood film and bone marrow examination, usually enable the various causes of thrombocytopenia to be differentiated. An association with thrombosis, disturbed renal or hepatic function and haemolytic anaemia, should prompt investigations for other diseases such as thrombotic thrombocytopenic purpura and, in a pregnant woman, the HELLP (haemolysis + elevated liver enzymes + low platelet count) syndrome. A bone marrow examination is often carried out early in the investigation of thrombocytopenia because it is helpful in excluding conditions such as acute leukaemia, which occasionally present with isolated thrombocytopenia.

Pancytopenia

Pancytopenia (reduction in the WBC, Hb and platelet count) is most often the result of anticancer chemotherapy, HIV infection, hypersplenism and bone marrow infiltration or failure. Careful examination of a blood film is important if the reason for the pancytopenia is not apparent from the clinical history. If this does not reveal the cause, bone marrow aspiration and trephine biopsy may be needed.

Qualitative Abnormalities of Blood Cells

In health, only the most mature forms of cells appear in the peripheral blood. Cells at various stages of immaturity, such as nucleated red blood cells, polychromatic red cells, myelocytes and metamyelocytes, may be released from the bone marrow in conditions where the bone marrow is overactive (e.g. acute haemolytic states or recovery from suppression) or functionally abnormal. Their presence in the peripheral blood indicates that active haemopoiesis is taking place.

Abnormalities of All Cell Lines

The combination of anisopoikilocytosis, mild macrocytosis, hypogranular neutrophils with abnormal nuclear morphology and platelet anisocytosis, often with quantitative abnormalities, is virtually pathognomonic of MDS. These features are reflected in the bone marrow with disturbance of the normal developmental pathway and sometimes nuclear:cytoplasmic asynchrony. Cytogenetic studies are helpful for confirming the diagnosis, especially when cytological abnormalities are minor, and can also assist in determining the prognosis.

Abnormalities of Individual Cell Lines

Red cells

Congenital abnormalities of the red cell affecting the structure (e.g. spherocytosis, elliptocytosis) and content (e.g. haemoglobinopathies, enzymopathies) often produce typical morphological changes (see Chapter 5). The type of changes will guide further investigations toward analysis of structural proteins, haemoglobin electrophoresis or HPLC, or enzyme assays. Acquired red cell abnormalities may also help to indicate underlying pathology. For example, target cells may prompt investigation of liver function, whereas increased rouleaux formation may indicate the need for investigations for multiple myeloma or inflammatory conditions.

White cells

Congenital abnormalities of neutrophils are unusual, but similar morphological abnormalities (e.g. Pelger–Huët cells) may be seen in acquired conditions such as MDS. Reactive changes in lymphocytes, including basophilic, faceted cytoplasm, are typically seen in infectious mononucleosis, which can be diagnosed using an appropriate serological screening test (see p. 105) or, if this is negative, by demonstration of immunoglobulin M (IgM) antibodies to the Epstein–Barr virus. These atypical lymphocytes can sometimes be difficult to differentiate from circulating lymphoma cells. Bone marrow histology, combined with immunophenotyping studies and determination of lymphocyte clonality by demonstration of light chain restriction or by gene rearrangement studies, may be needed to reach a firm conclusion.

Platelets

Platelets that function poorly may not necessarily appear morphologically abnormal, although sometimes they are hypogranular or larger than normal. A normal platelet count with an abnormal *in vitro* platelet function test is characteristic of a disorder of platelet function, but some patients with abnormal platelet function are also thrombocytopenic. Hereditary disorders of platelet function are uncommon and usually present as a bleeding diathesis. When a qualitative disorder of platelets is suspected, platelets should be examined to assess size and to detect the cytological features of the grey platelet syndrome. Qualitative disorders of platelets can broadly be divided into two categories: abnormalities of the platelet membrane (e.g.

Bernard–Soulier syndrome, Glanzmann's thrombasthenia) and abnormalities of platelet secretory function (e.g. storage pool diseases). Acquired disorders of platelet function are more common than inherited disorders. Haematological conditions associated with platelet dysfunction include myeloproliferative neoplasms, MDS and dysproteinaemias (in plasma cell neoplasms). Many widely prescribed drugs, including aspirin and non-steroidal anti-inflammatory agents, interfere with platelet function. Systemic conditions, particularly chronic renal failure and cardiopulmonary bypass, are also associated with a bleeding tendency as a result of qualitative platelet defects. Most of these acquired functional defects are not associated with any abnormality in platelet appearance but in MDS and, to a lesser extent, in the myeloproliferative neoplasms, there may be hypogranular and giant platelets.

SPECIFIC TESTS FOR COMMON HAEMATOLOGICAL DISORDERS

Common haematological disorders are outlined in the following sections with suggestions for investigations that may be helpful in confirming the diagnosis. The lists are not intended to be exhaustive because the range of tests provided locally will depend on the availability of expertise and technology. The investigations discussed are those that are likely to be available within a general haematology department.

Red Cell Disorders

Microcytic Hypochromic Anaemias

For more information, see Chapters 9 and 14.

- Measurement of serum ferritin or iron plus total iron-binding capacity or transferrin assay, red cell protoporphyrin or soluble transferrin receptors
- Bone marrow aspirate with staining for iron
- Stool examination for occult blood
- Gastrointestinal imaging and endoscopy, with biopsies if appropriate; rarely, blood loss studies with ^{51}Cr-labelled red cells
- Tests for malabsorption
- Serological tests for coeliac disease (e.g. endomysial antibodies, tissue transglutaminase antibodies)
- Serum lead (if lead poisoning is suspected)

If thalassaemia is suspected:

- Haemoglobin electrophoresis plus Hb A_2 and Hb F measurements or HPLC
- Haemoglobin H preparation
- Family studies
- DNA analysis (when the diagnosis is clinically important).

Macrocytic Anaemias

If macrocytic, megaloblastic erythroid maturation is demonstrated, further investigations should be undertaken as described in Chapter 10. If the blood film is typical of megaloblastic anaemia, relevant assays and further investigations can often indicate the diagnosis without the need for a bone marrow aspirate. Macrocytosis may also be secondary to conditions such as alcohol excess, liver disease, MDS, hydroxycarbamide administration and hypothyroidism. Reticulocytosis from any cause can also increase the MCV.

Aplastic Anaemia[11]

- Vitamin B_{12} and folate assays
- Viral studies, particularly for Epstein–Barr, HIV and hepatitis viruses
- Bone marrow aspirate and trephine biopsy including cytogenetic analysis
- Flow cytometry for glycosylphosphatidylinositol-anchored proteins* to detect a paroxysmal nocturnal haemoglobinuria (PNH) clone (urine examination for haemosiderin if positive)
- Peripheral blood gene mutation analysis for dyskeratosis congenita if there are relevant clinical features or lack of response to immunosuppressive therapy.

If Fanconi's anaemia is suspected:

- Studies of sensitivity of chromosomes to breakage by DNA cross-linking agents.

Haemolytic Anaemias

A haemolytic process may be suspected by the presence of a falling Hb, a reticulocytosis and jaundice with an increase in unconjugated bilirubin level (see Chapters 9, 10 and 11).

White Cell Disorders

The blood film is often of critical importance in the differential diagnosis of white cell disorders though it may sometimes be normal (e.g. in some patients with lymphoma or neutrophil functional defects). Changes in white cell numbers or morphology may occur rapidly in response to local or systemic disorders. In chronic leukaemias, bone marrow aspiration may add little to the diagnosis, but the pattern of infiltration of neoplastic cells seen on trephine biopsy can have diagnostic value or prognostic significance, e.g. in lymphoma and chronic lymphocytic leukaemia.

---

*The Ham test and sucrose lysis test are less sensitive and less quantitative than flow cytometry in the detection of PNH clones and when flow cytometry is available they have generally been abandoned as diagnostic tests for PNH.

Acute Leukaemia

- Full blood count and peripheral blood film
- Bone marrow aspirate (trephine biopsy if bone marrow aspirate is inadequate)
- Blood or marrow immunophenotyping, unless obviously myeloid, or in all patients if it is to be used for monitoring minimal residual disease (cytochemical stains can be used if immunophenotyping is not readily available)
- Cytogenetic analysis
- Molecular studies (e.g. fluorescence *in situ* hybridization – FISH – analysis) for detection of all patients with acute lymphoblastic leukaemia (ALL) with hyperdiploidy or *ETV6–RUNX1* fusion, detection of *BCR–ABL1* fusion in adults with ALL and detection of other mutations of specific oncogenes, e.g. *NPM1*, *CEBPA* and possibly *FLT3* in AML.

Neutropenia

- Vitamin B_{12} and folate assays
- Autoantibody screen including rheumatoid factor and investigations for systemic lupus erythematosus
- Serial neutrophil counts for cyclical neutropenia
- Tests for anti-neutrophil antibodies
- Bone marrow aspirate and trephine biopsy
- Flow cytometry for PNH (see aplastic anaemia above)
- Consider the need for investigation for an abnormal T-cell population.

Chronic Myelogenous Leukaemia

- Full blood count and peripheral blood film
- Bone marrow aspirate
- Cytogenetic analysis
- Molecular studies (e.g. real-time quantitative reverse transcriptase or FISH) for *BCR–ABL1* transcripts
- Neutrophil alkaline phosphatase score (only if cytogenetic and molecular genetic analysis are not available).

Chronic Lymphoproliferative Disorders/ Lymphadenopathy

Diagnosis may be made from various specimens including lymph nodes, bone marrow aspirates, trephine biopsy cores and peripheral blood and other fluids such as cerebrospinal fluid, ascitic fluid and pleural aspirates.[12]

- Full blood count and peripheral blood film
- Serum protein electrophoresis and immunoglobulin concentrations
- Plasma uric acid, calcium and lactate dehydrogenase (LDH)
- Serological screening for infectious mononucleosis, cytomegalovirus infection, HIV infection and

toxoplasmosis (if infectious cause suspected) and human T-cell leukaemia/lymphoma virus, when clinically relevant
- Bone marrow aspirate and trephine biopsy (to demonstrate the presence and distribution of abnormal lymphocytes) and/or lymph node or other tissue biopsy
- Flow cytometry immunophenotyping or immunohistochemistry of biopsy specimens
- Cytogenetic or molecular genetic analysis including investigation for immunoglobulin heavy chain or T-cell receptor gene rearrangement if the diagnosis of lymphoma is in doubt
- Imaging (plain radiographs, ultrasonography, computed tomography scan, magnetic resonance imaging).

Myelomatosis (Plasma Cell Myeloma)

- Full blood count and peripheral blood film[13]
- Serum protein electrophoresis, immunofixation and quantification of immunoglobulins and any paraprotein
- Urine electrophoresis and immunofixation for Bence–Jones protein (early morning urine sample and, if positive, quantification on 24 h collection)
- Serum free light chain quantification and ratio
- Serum albumin, tests of renal function, plasma uric acid, calcium, phosphate and alkaline phosphatase measurements
- β_2 microglobulin quantification
- Plasma viscosity
- Bone marrow aspirate (with cytogenetic or FISH analysis if results will influence treatment decisions, and flow cytometry immunophenotyping or DNA analysis if these analyses are to be used for monitoring minimal residual disease)
- Trephine biopsy
- Radiological skeletal survey.

Other Disorders

Myeloproliferative Neoplasms

- Full blood count and blood film
- Vitamin B_{12} (or B_{12}-binding capacity)
- Uric acid assay
- Serum erythropoietin assay
- *JAK2* mutation analysis if PV, ET or primary myelofibrosis is suspected
- Arterial oxygen saturation and carboxyhaemoglobin level (selected patients only)
- Abdominal ultrasound examination
- Bone marrow aspirate and trephine biopsy
- Cytogenetic analysis

- Neutrophil alkaline phosphatase (only if other more specific tests are unavailable)
- Red cell and plasma volume (selected patients only).

If splenectomy is contemplated:

- Ferrokinetic and red cell survival studies
- Spleen scan and red cell pool measurement.

Myelodysplastic syndromes

- Full blood count and blood film
- Bone marrow aspirate and trephine biopsy
- Cytogenetic analysis.

Pancytopenia with Splenomegaly

- Vitamin B_{12} and folate assays
- Serum rheumatoid factor and autoantibody screen
- Bone marrow aspirate and trephine biopsy
- Examination of bone marrow or splenic aspirate for amastigotes of *Leishmania donovani* and bacterial culture of marrow for infectious agents including *Mycobacterium tuberculosis*
- Biopsy of palpable lymph nodes
- Liver biopsy
- Tests for paroxysmal nocturnal haemoglobinuria (see p. 291).

The rationale behind these tests and details of specialized investigations can be found in comprehensive haematology textbooks, in electronic databases and on websites.

CLASSIFICATION OF HAEMATOLOGICAL NEOPLASMS

Previous classifications for haematological neoplasms have now been largely supplanted by the World Health Organization's Classification of Tumours of Haematopoietic and Lymphoid Tissues,[3] which outlines the international standards for assessment and diagnosis of haematological neoplasms. Application of the WHO criteria requires the results of history and physical examination, morphology (cytology or histology), immunophenotyping, cytogenetic analysis and, in some circumstances, molecular genetic analysis. The French–American–British (FAB) group classifications (see previous editions) continue to have a place (a) when these techniques are not all available and (b) in making a provisional morphological diagnosis, e.g. in acute leukaemia, while awaiting the results of further tests. Whichever classification is used the criteria should be strictly observed so that there is consistency between different centres and countries. To avoid confusion, FAB terminology (e.g. M1, M2) should not be applied if the WHO classification is being used. Details of the FAB classifications can be found in specialized textbooks.[14]

Table 23.1 WHO classification of myeloid neoplasms and acute leukaemias[15]

Myeloproliferative neoplasms (MPN)
Myeloid and lymphoid neoplasms associated with eosinophilia and abnormalities of *PDGFRA*, *PDGFRB* or *FGFR1*
Myelodysplastic/myeloproliferative neoplasms (MDS/MPN)
Myelodysplastic syndrome (MDS)
Acute myeloid leukaemia and related neoplasms
Acute leukaemias of ambiguous lineage
B lymphoblastic leukaemia/lymphoma
T lymphoblastic leukaemia/lymphoma

Table 23.2 WHO Classification of acute myeloid leukaemia and related neoplasms[15]

Therapy-related myeloid neoplasms
Acute myeloid leukaemia with recurrent genetic abnormalities 　AML with t(8;21)(q22;q22); *RUNX1-RUNX1T1* 　AML with inv(16)(p13.1q22) or t(16;16)(p13.1;q22); *CBFB-MYH11* 　APL with t(15;17)(q22;q12); *PML-RARA* 　AML with t(9;11)(p22;q23); *MLLT3-MLL* 　AML with t(6;9)(p23;q34); *DEK-NUP214* 　AML with inv(3)(q21q26.2) or t(3;3)(q21;q26.2); *RPN1-EVI1* 　AML (megakaryoblastic) with t(1;22)(p13;q13); *RBM15-MKL1* 　*Provisional entity: AML with mutated NPM1* 　*Provisional entity: AML with mutated CEBPA*
Acute myeloid leukaemia with myelodysplasia-related changes
Acute myeloid leukaemia, not otherwise specified 　AML with minimal differentiation 　AML without maturation 　AML with maturation 　Acute myelomonocytic leukaemia 　Acute monoblastic/monocytic leukaemia 　Acute erythroid leukaemia 　　Pure erythroid leukaemia 　　Erythroleukaemia, erythroid/myeloid 　Acute megakaryoblastic leukaemia 　Acute basophilic leukaemia 　Acute panmyelosis with myelofibrosis
Myeloid sarcoma
Myeloid proliferations related to Down syndrome 　Transient abnormal myelopoiesis 　Myeloid leukaemia associated with Down syndrome
Blastic plasmacytoid dendritic cell neoplasm

The WHO classification of haematological neoplasms has several major categories (Table 23.1)

Classification of Acute Myeloid Leukaemia

The WHO classification categorizes cases as AML (Table 23.2) if the following criteria are met:

1. There are at least 20% of blast cells of myeloid lineage in the blood or bone marrow *or*
2. If the erythroid cells are at least 50% of bone marrow cells, blast cells are at least 20% of non-erythroid cells *or*
3. Primitive erythroid cells constitute at least 80% of bone marrow cells *or*
4. There is a myeloid sarcoma (granulocytic sarcoma) *or*
5. One of a number of specified chromosomal rearrangements is present.

It should be noted that the WHO classification is hierarchical. If appropriate, cases are first assigned to the category of therapy-related leukaemia. Next, cases are assigned, if appropriate, to the category of AML with recurrent genetic abnormalities. Cases continue to be assigned to successive categories in the order shown in Table 23.2, with remaining cases finally being categorized as 'AML not otherwise specified.' This final group is further subdivided into categories resembling those of the FAB classification (but defined in quite a different manner). Blastic plasmacytoid dendritic cell neoplasm and myeloid neoplasms associated with Down syndrome are recognized as specific entities.

The WHO classification of acute leukaemia[15] lists cytogenetic abnormalities that, in combination with ≥20 blasts, indicate a diagnosis of AML with myelodysplasia-related changes; assignment to this category can also be based on a previous history of MDS or on morphological evidence of dysplasia.

Classification of the Myelodysplastic Syndromes

The WHO classification of MDS (Table 23.3) requires evidence for a myeloid neoplasm with ineffective and, generally, dysplastic haemopoiesis; blasts must be <20% in both

Table 23.3 WHO Classification of the myelodysplastic syndromes (MDS) (2008)

Refractory cytopenia with unilineage dysplasia
   Refractory anaemia
   Refractory neutropenia
   Refractory thrombocytopenia

Refractory anaemia with ring sideroblasts

Refractory cytopenia with multilineage dysplasia (with or without ring sideroblasts)

Refractory anaemia with excess blasts

Myelodysplastic syndrome with isolated del(5q)

Myelodysplastic syndrome, unclassifiable

Childhood myelodysplastic syndrome
   Provisional entity: refractory cytopenia of childhood

blood and bone marrow (Table 23.4). It will be noted that cytogenetic analysis is essential for the application of the WHO classification because cases of the 5q– syndrome cannot otherwise be recognized. Like the classification of AML, this is a hierarchical classification. Therapy-related MDS is categorized with therapy-related AML. Remaining cases are then assessed as to whether they meet the criteria for the 5q– syndrome. If they do not, they are assigned to the remaining categories, depending on the number of lineages showing dysplasia, the percentage of ring sideroblasts, the presence or absence of Auer rods and the percentage of blast cells in the blood and marrow. The WHO classification differs from the FAB classification in not regarding chronic myelomonocytic leukaemia as MDS; instead it assigns it to the MDS/MPN group.

Classification of Acute Lymphoblastic Leukaemia

The WHO classification requires that an acute leukaemia be positively shown to be lymphoid before it is categorized as ALL. This classification groups together ALL and lymphoblastic lymphoma, using the designations precursor B lymphoblastic leukaemia/lymphoblastic lymphoma and precursor T lymphoblastic leukaemia/lymphoblastic lymphoma. These designations are clearly too cumbersome to use in clinical practice and undoubtedly haematologists will continue to refer to 'acute lymphoblastic leukaemia.' The FAB classification of ALL is now redundant except that

FAB L3 morphology, i.e. the presence of 'blast cells' with basophilic cytoplasm and vacuolation, is of considerable clinical significance and should be recognized. In most, but not all, of these cases the cells are immunologically mature, expressing surface membrane immunoglobulin and the condition represents a leukaemic presentation of Burkitt lymphoma. The WHO categorization of such cases as lymphoma is more appropriate than their being categorized as ALL and is clinically important because the treatment, which is urgent, differs very considerably from the treatment of ALL.

Classification of Myeloproliferative Neoplasms and Related Conditions

The WHO classification of myeloproliferative neoplasms (previously called 'disorders') and related conditions (Table 23.5) is increasingly taking account of cytogenetic or molecular genetic analyses.

WHO criteria for a diagnosis of essential thrombocythaemia are: platelet count $\geq 450 \times 10^9$/l; megakaryocyte proliferation with large and mature megakaryocytes on examination of the bone marrow with little or no granulocyte or erythroid proliferation; not meeting WHO criteria for CML, PV, primary myelofibrosis, MDS or other myeloid neoplasm; demonstration of *JAK2* V617F or other clonal marker or no evidence of reactive thrombocytosis.[16]

WHO criteria for a diagnosis of primary myelofibrosis are divided into major criteria (e.g. megakaryocyte proliferation and atypical megakaryocytes accompanied by reticulin and/or collagen fibrosis; demonstration of *JAK2* V617F or other clonal marker; no evidence of reactive marrow fibrosis; not meeting WHO criteria for CML, PV, MDS or other myeloid neoplasm) and minor criteria (e.g. leukoerythroblastosis; increased serum LDH; anaemia; palpable splenomegaly).

WHO criteria for a diagnosis of systemic mastocytosis are highly complex.[3] A trephine biopsy with a mast cell tryptase stain is often crucial in the diagnosis. Molecular analysis for a *KIT* mutation can also be important.

Recognition of lymphoid and myeloid neoplasms associated with rearrangement of *PDGFRA*, *PDGFRB* or *FGFR1* requires cytogenetic analysis (for detection of translocations likely to indicate rearrangement of *PDGFRB* or *FGFR1*) and molecular analysis (for detection of the *FIP1L1−PDGFRA* fusion gene that results from a cryptic deletion at 4q12). Appropriate molecular analysis may be either FISH or reverse transcription polymerase chain reaction (RT-PCR). The diagnosis of chronic eosinophilic leukaemia, not otherwise specified, requires exclusion of rearrangement of these three specific genes.

The categorization of neoplasms with features of both myelodysplasia and myeloproliferation and their diagnostic criteria are listed in Table 23.6.

Table 23.4 WHO diagnostic criteria for the myelodysplastic syndromes (MDS)

DISEASE	BLOOD FINDINGS	BM FINDINGS
Refractory cytopenia with unilineage dysplasia (RCUD): (refractory anaemia [RA]; refractory neutropenia [RN]; refractory thrombocytopenia [RT])	Unicytopenia or bicytopenia[a] No or rare blasts (<1%)[b]	Unilineage dysplasia: ≥10% of the cells in one myeloid lineage <5% blasts <15% of erythroid precursors are ring sideroblasts
Refractory anaemia with ring sideroblasts (RARS)	Anaemia No blasts	≥15% of erythroid precursors are ring sideroblasts Erythroid dysplasia only <5% blasts
Refractory cytopenia with multilineage dysplasia (RCMD)	Cytopenia(s) No or rare blasts (<1%)[b] No Auer rods <1 × 10⁹/l monocytes	Dysplasia in ≥10% of the cells in ≥2 myeloid lineages (neutrophil and/or erythroid precursors and/or megakaryocytes) <5% blasts in marrow No Auer rods ±15% ring sideroblasts
Refractory anaemia with excess blasts-1 (RAEB-1)	Cytopenia(s) <5% blasts[b] No Auer rods <1 × 10⁹/l monocytes	Unilineage or multilineage dysplasia 5–9% blasts[b] No Auer rods
Refractory anaemia with excess blasts-2 (RAEB-2)	Cytopenia(s) 5–19% blasts[c] Auer rods ±[c] <1 × 10⁹/l monocytes	Unilineage or multilineage dysplasia 10–19% blasts[c] Auer rods ±[c]
Myelodysplastic syndrome – unclassified (MDS-U)	Cytopenias ≤1% blasts[b]	Unequivocal dysplasia in <10% of cells in one or more myeloid lineages when accompanied by a cytogenetic abnormality considered as presumptive evidence for a diagnosis of MDS (see Table 23.6) <5% blasts
MDS associated with isolated del (5q)	Anaemia Usually normal or increased platelet count No or rare blasts (<1%)	Normal to increased megakaryocytes with hypolobated nuclei <5% blasts Isolated del(5q) cytogenetic abnormality No Auer rods

Note: The blood findings for RAEB-1 state "<5% blasts[b]"; the subscripts and symbols (±, ≥, ≤) are rendered in LaTeX-equivalent plain form above. Superscript letters a, b, c are footnote markers.

[a]Bicytopenia may occasionally be observed. Cases with pancytopenia should be classified as MDS-U.
[b]If the marrow myeloblast percentage is <5% but there are 2–4% myeloblasts in the blood, the diagnostic classification is RAEB-1. Cases of RCUD and RCMD with 1% myeloblasts in the blood should be classified as MDS-U.
[c]Cases with Auer rods and <5% myeloblasts in the blood and <10% in the marrow should be classified as RAEB-2. Although the finding of 5–19% blasts in the blood is, in itself, diagnostic of RAEB-2, cases of RAEB-2 may have <5% blasts in the blood if they have Auer rods or 10–19% blasts in the marrow or both. Similarly, cases of RAEB-2 may have <10% blasts in the marrow but may be diagnosed by the other two findings, Auer rod + and/or 5–19% blasts in the blood.
From Vardiman et al (2009).[15]

Table 23.5 Myeloproliferative neoplasms (MPN) and related conditions[5,6,15,16]

Myeloproliferative neoplasms
    Chronic myelogenous leukaemia
    Polycythaemia vera
    Essential thrombocythaemia
    Primary myelofibrosis
    Chronic neutrophilic leukaemia
    Chronic eosinophilic leukaemia, not otherwise categorized
    Mast cell disease
    MPN, unclassifiable

Lymphoid and myeloid neoplasms associated with rearrangement of *PDGFRA*, *PDGFRB* or *FGFR1*
    Lymphoid and myeloid neoplasms associated with rearrangement of *PDGFRA*
    Myeloid neoplasms associated with rearrangement of *PDGFRB*
    Lymphoid and myeloid neoplasms associated with rearrangement of *FGFR1*

Table 23.6 Summary of the World Health Organization categories of myelodysplastic/myeloproliferative neoplasms

CATEGORY	CRITERIA
Chronic myelomonocytic leukaemia (CMML)	A Ph-negative, *BCR–ABL1*-negative disorder with monocyte count $>1 \times 10^9$/l Fewer than 20% blasts plus promonocytes in peripheral blood (PB) or bone marrow (BM) Either dysplasia of one or more myeloid lineages or alternative criteria met (acquired clonal cytogenetic abnormality or monocytosis persisting for at least 3 months and alternative causes of monocytosis excluded)
Atypical chronic myeloid leukaemia (aCML)	A Ph-negative, *BCR–ABL1*-negative disorder with leucocytosis resulting from an increase in neutrophils and their precursors, the precursors (promyelocyte to metamyelocytes) constituting a least 10% of PB white cells Basophils <2% of white cells Monocytes <10% of white cells Hypercellular BM with granulocytic hyperplasia and dysplasia, with or without dysplasia of other lineages Fewer than 20% blasts plus promonocytes in peripheral blood or bone marrow

Juvenile myelomonocytic leukaemia (JMML)	A Ph-negative, *BCR–ABL1*-negative disorder with monocyte count $>1 \times 10^9$/l
	Fewer than 20% blasts plus promonocytes in peripheral blood or bone marrow
	Plus two or more of the following
	    Haemoglobin F increased for age
	    Immature granulocytes in the PB
	    WBC $>10 \times 10^9$/l
	    Clonal chromosomal abnormality (monosomy 7 not excluded)
	    GM-CSF hypersensitivity of myeloid precursors *in vitro*

Myelodysplastic/myeloproliferative neoplasm, unclassifiable	A myelodysplastic/myeloproliferative disorder in which the criteria of one of the myelodysplastic syndromes are met There are prominent proliferative features (e.g. a platelet count of $\geq 450 \times 10^9$/l or a white cell count of $\geq 13 \times 10^9$/l) The condition has developed *de novo* The criteria for other MDS/MPD (CMML, aCML and JMML) are not met There is no Philadelphia chromosome, *BCR–ABL1* fusion gene, 5q−, inv(3)(q21q26) or t(3;3)(q21;q26)

REFERENCES

1. McMullin M, Bareford D, Campbell P, et al. Guidelines for the diagnosis, investigation and management of polycythaemia/erythrocytosis. *Br J Haematol*. 2005;130:174–195.

2. McMullin M, Reilly J, Campbell P, et al. Amendment to the guideline for diagnosis and investigation of polycythaemia/erythrocytosis. *Br J Haematol*. 2007;138:812–823.

3. Swerdlow S, Campo E, Harris N, et al. *WHO Classification of Tumours of Haematopoietic and Lymphoid Tissues*. 4th ed. WHO Classification of Tumours, Volume 2. IARC WHO Classification of Tumours, No 2. Lyon, France: IARC Press; 2008.

4. Orazi A, Germing U. The myelodysplastic/myeloproliferative neoplasms: myeloproliferative diseases with dysplastic features. *Leukemia*. 2008;22(7): 1308–1319.

5. Bain BJ, Gilliland DG, Vardiman JW, et al. Chronic eosinophilic leukaemia, not otherwise specified. In: Swerdlow SH, Campo E, Harris NL, et al., eds. *World Health Organization Classification of Tumours of Haematopoietic and Lymphoid Tissue*. 4th ed. Lyon, France: IARC Press; 2008:51–53.

6. Bain BJ, Gilliland DG, Horny H-P, et al. Myeloid and lymphoid neoplasms with eosinophilia and abnormalities of *PDGFRA*, *PDGFRB* and *FGFR1*. In: Swerdlow SH, Campo E, Harris NL, et al., eds. *World Health Organization Classification of Tumours of Haematopoietic and Lymphoid Tissue*. 4th ed. Lyon, France: IARC Press; 2008:68–73.

7. Harrison C, Green A. Essential thrombocythaemia. *Baillières Best Pract Clin Haematol*. 2006;19(3): 439–453.

8. Lussana F, Caberlon S, Pagani C, et al. Association of V617F Jak2 mutation with the risk of thrombosis among patients with essential thrombocythaemia or idiopathic myelofibrosis: a systematic review. *Thromb Res*. 2009;124(4):409–417.

9. Koulaouzidis A, Said E, Cottier R, et al. Soluble transferrin receptors and iron deficiency, a step beyond ferritin. A systematic review. *J Gastrointestin Liver Dis*. 2009;18(3): 345–352.

10. Ryan K, Bain B, Worthington D, et al. *Significant haemoglobinopathies: guidelines for screening and diagnosis. British Committee for Standards in Haematology*. Available at: www.bcshguidelines.com/pdf/significant_final_sept09.pdf; 2009 Accessed 3 3 2010.

11. Marsh J, Ball S, Cavenagh J, et al. *Guidelines for the diagnosis and management of aplastic anaemia. British Committee for Standards in Haematology*. Available at: www.bcshguidelines.com/pdf/AplasticAnaemia_010409.pdf; 2009 Accessed 3 3 2010.

12. Parker A, Bain B, Devereux S, et al. *Best Practice in Lymphoma Diagnosis and Reporting. British Committee for Standards in Haematology*. Available at: www.bcshguidelines.com/publishedHO.asp?tf=Haemato-Oncology&status=; 2008 Accessed 3 3 2010.

13. Smith A, Wisloff F, Samson D. *Guidelines on the diagnosis and management of multiple myeloma*. Available at: www.bcshguidelines.com/pdf/multiplemyeloma0206.pdf; 2005 Accessed 8 3 2010.

14. Bain BJ. *Leukaemia Diagnosis*. 4th ed. Oxford: Blackwell Publishing; 2010.

15. Vardiman J, Thiele J, Arber D, et al. The 2008 revision of the World Health Organization (WHO) classification of myeloid neoplasms and acute leukemia: rationale and important changes. *Blood*. 2009; 114(5):937–951.

16. Tefferi A, Vardiman J. Classification and diagnosis of myeloproliferative neoplasms: the 2008 World Health Organization criteria and point-of-care diagnostic algorithms. *Leukemia*. 2008;22:14–22.

Chapter | 24 |

Laboratory organization and management

S. Mitchell Lewis, Anne Bradshaw

CHAPTER CONTENTS

The essential functions of a haematology laboratory are (1) to provide clinicians with timely, unambiguous and meaningful reports to assist in the clinical diagnosis of disease and to monitor response to treatment; (2) to obtain reliable and reproducible data for health screening and epidemiological studies; and (3) to keep abreast with advancing technology as well as aspects of healthcare legislation that might be relevant to modern laboratory practice. The laboratory should also be involved in both the pre-analytical stage (i.e. test ordering, blood collection, specimen transport) and the post-analytical stage (i.e. preparing reports, transmission of results and maintaining a data file).

For good laboratory practice, it is essential to have a well-structured organization with competent direction and management. The principles outlined in this chapter apply to all laboratories, irrespective of their size, although large departments are likely to require the more complex arrangements that are described.

MANAGEMENT STRUCTURE AND FUNCTION

The management structure of a haematology laboratory should indicate a clear line of accountability of each member of staff to the head of department. In turn, the head of department may be managerially accountable to a clinical director (of laboratories) and thence to a hospital or health authority executive committee. The head of department is responsible for departmental leadership, for ensuring that the laboratory has authoritative representation within the hospital and for ensuring that managerial and administrative tasks are performed efficiently. Where the head of the department delegates managerial tasks to others, these responsibilities must be clearly defined and stated. Formerly, the director was usually a medically qualified haematologist, but nowadays in many laboratories, this role is being undertaken by appropriately qualified biomedical scientists, while medical haematologists serve as consultants. In that role, they should be fully conversant with the principles of laboratory practice, especially with interpretation and clinical significance of the various analytical procedures, so as to provide a reliable and authoritative link between laboratory and clinic. Furthermore, all medical staff, especially junior hospital doctors, should be invited to visit the laboratory, to see how it functions, how various tests are performed, their level of complexity, clinical utility and cost: this should give them confidence to order tests rationally, rather than automatically requesting all the tests listed on the laboratory request form.[1]

Management of the laboratory requires an executive committee answerable to the head of department. Under this executive, there should be a number of designated individuals responsible for implementing the functions of the department (Table 24.1).

The activities of the various members of staff clearly overlap and there must be adequate effective communication between them. There should be regular briefings at meetings of technical heads, with their section staff. The only way to avoid unauthorized 'leakage' of information from policy-making committees is to ensure that all members of staff are kept fully informed of any plans which might have a bearing on their careers, working practices and wellbeing.

In many countries, there are now requirements established by regulatory agencies for accreditation of laboratories and audit of their performance, as well as documents on laboratory management and practice from standards-setting authorities; there is also a plethora of guidelines from national and international professional bodies. These may indicate a need for a special sub-committee of the executive committee, whose duty it is to keep abreast of these matters, to be responsible for developing standard operating procedures (SOPs) and to inter-relate with the different sections in the same way as the safety officer.

Table 24.1 Example of components of a management structure

Executive committee
    Head of department
    Business manager
    Consultant haematologist
    Principal scientific officer

Safety officer

Quality control officer

Computer and data processing supervisor

Sectional scientific/technical heads
    Cytometry
    Blood film morphology
    Immunohaematology
    Haemostasis
    Blood transfusion
    Special investigations (haemolytic anaemias, haemoglobinopathies, cytochemistry, molecular techniques, etc.)

Clerical supervisor

Staff Appraisal

All members of staff should receive training to enhance their skills and to develop their careers. This requires setting of goals and regular appraisal of progress for both managerial and technical ability. The appraisal process should cascade down from the head of department and appropriate training must be given to those who undertake appraisals at successive levels. The appraiser should provide a short list of topics to the person to be interviewed, who should be encouraged to add to the list, so that each understands the items to be covered. Topics to be considered should include: quality of performance and accurate completion of assignments; productivity and dependability; ability to work in a team; and ability to relate to patients, clinicians and co-workers. It is not appropriate to include considerations relating to pay. An appraisal interview should be a constructive dialogue of the present state of development and the progress made to date; it should be open-ended and should identify future training requirements. Ideally, the staff members should leave the interviews with the knowledge that their personal development and future progress are of importance to the department; that priorities have been identified; that an action plan with milestones and a time scale has been agreed; and that progress will be monitored. Formal appraisal interviews (annually for senior staff and more often for others) should be complemented by less formal follow-up discussions to monitor progress and to check that suboptimal performance has been modified. Documentation of formal interviews can be limited to a short list of agreed objectives. Performance appraisal can have lasting value in the personal development of individuals, but the process can easily be mishandled and should not be started without training in how to hold an appraisal interview.[2]

Continuing Professional Development

Continuing professional development is a process of continuous systematic learning which enables health workers to be constantly brought up to date on developments in their professional work and thus ensure their competence to practice throughout their professional careers. Policies and programmes have been established in a number of countries and, in some, participation is a mandatory requirement for the right to practice.[3]

In the UK, clinical haematologists and clinical scientists who have the relevant qualifications awarded by the Royal College of Pathologists (RCPath) and are licenced to practice by the General Medical Council, are required to participate in a scheme organized by the College. This involves maintenance of a portfolio showing their participation in relevant educational and academic affairs and demonstrations of their professional skills.

The Institute for Biomedical Science undertakes a similar scheme for scientists/technologists working in the laboratory, which is mandatory for registration to practice by the UK Health Professions Council. The procedure is based on obtaining 'credits' for various activities that qualify, such as: attendance at specified lectures, workshops and conferences; giving lectures; writing books or journal articles; using computer or journal-based programmes; and taking part in peer review discussions.

Strategic and Business Planning

The head of department is responsible for determining the long-term (usually up to 5 years) strategic direction of the department. Strategic planning requires awareness of any national and local legislation that may affect the laboratory and of changes in local clinical practice that may alter workload. Expansion of a major clinical service, such as organ transplantation, or the opportunity to compete for the laboratory service of other hospitals and clinics, may pose an external opportunity, but may also be a threat to the laboratory, depending on its ability to respond to the consequential increase in workload. Technical or scientific expertise would be a strength, whereas a heavy workload, without adequate staffing or lack of automation for routine tests, is likely to preclude any additional developmental work and would, thus, be a weakness.

Increasingly, laboratories must meet financial challenges and the need for greater cost-effectiveness. This may require rationalization by eliminating unused laboratory capacity, avoiding unnecessary tests and ensuring more efficient use of skilled staff and expensive equipment. This may require centralization of multiple laboratory sites or, conversely, there may be advantages in establishing satellite centres for the benefit of patients and clinicians if these can be shown to be cost-effective. Account must also be taken of the role of the laboratory in supervision of the extra-laboratory point-of-care procedures that have become increasingly popular.

A business plan is primarily concerned with determining short-term objectives that will allow the strategy to be implemented over the next financial year or so. It requires prediction of future work level and expansion. Planning of these objectives should involve all staff because this will heighten awareness of the issues and will develop personal concern in the strategy. In all but the smallest laboratory, a business manager is required to coordinate such planning and to liaise with the equivalent business managers in other clinical and laboratory areas.

Workload Assessment and Costing of Tests

Laboratories should maintain accurate records of workload, overall costs and the cost per test in order to apportion resources to each section. Computerization of laboratories has greatly facilitated this process. In assessing workload, account must be taken of the entire cycle from test receipt to issue of a report, whether the test is by a manual or semi-automated method or by a high-volume multiple-analyte automated analyser. Apportioning of resources should also take account of the roles of biomedical scientists/senior technologists and junior technicians, supervised laboratory assistants, clerical staff and medical personnel responsible for reviewing the report. Out of hours service requires a different calculation of costs.

Methods were developed for determining the workload and costs for various laboratory tests taking account of test complexity, total number of tests performed, quality control procedures, cost of reagent and use of material standards so that laboratories could compare their operational productivity with a peer group of participating laboratories. A good example is given on the website Standards for Management Information Systems in the Canadian Health Service Organizations.

A similar workload recording method was published by the College of American Pathologists,[4] and the Welcan system was established in the UK.[5] However, more recently, benchmarking schemes have been established that take account of productivity, cost-effectiveness and utilization compared with a peer group. The College of American Pathologists created their Laboratory Management Index Program in which participants submit their laboratories operating data on a quarterly basis and receive peer comparison reports from similar laboratories around the country by which their own cost-effectiveness can be evaluated.

Financial Control

Full costing of tests includes all aspects of laboratory function (Table 24.2).

The amount allocated for staff salaries should include the cost of training and should take into account absences for annual leave or sickness. It needs also to take into account the extent to which staff of various levels, as described earlier, are involved. Indirect costs may be apportioned to different sections of a department who share common overhead costs.

Calculation of Test Costs

When preparing a budget, the following formula provides a reasonably reliable estimate of the total annual costs:

$$[L \times N] + [C \times N] + E + M + O + S + T + A$$

where

L = Labour costs for each test from estimate of time taken and the salary rate of the staff member(s) performing the tests
N = Number of tests in the year
C = Cost of consumables per test (including controls)
E = Annual equipment cost based on initial cost divided by expected life of the item or the annual cost of hire (see below)
M = Annual maintenance and servicing of equipment
O = Laboratory overheads (Table 24.2)
S = Supervision
T = Transport and communication

Table 24.2 Factors contributing to cost of laboratory tests

Direct costs
    Staff salaries
    Laboratory equipment purchases
    Reagents and other consumables
    Equipment maintenance
    Standardization and quality control
    Specific technical training on equipment

Indirect costs
    Capital costs and mortgage factor
    Depreciation
    Building repairs and routine maintenance
    Lighting, heating and waste disposal
    Personnel services
    Cleaning services
    Transport, messengers and porters
    Laundry services
    Computers and information technology
    Telephone and fax
    Postage
    Journals and textbooks

A = Laboratory administration, including salaries of clerical and other non-technical staff.

Efficient budgeting requires regular monitoring, at least monthly. Computer spreadsheets provide an easily comprehended view of the financial state and the likely responses in the running of the laboratory.

In general, staff cost is by far the largest component of the total costs of running a laboratory. Furthermore, many of the other costs are obligations outside the direct control of the laboratory. If financial savings become necessary, they can be achieved in a variety of ways, but large savings usually necessitate a reduction in staff because employment costs can account for three-quarters of total expenditure. Possible initiatives include the following:

- Rationalization of service with other local hospitals to eliminate duplication
- Restructuring within a hospital laboratory for cross-discipline working (usually between haematology and clinical chemistry)
- Subcontracting of labour-intensive tests to a specialist laboratory
- Greater use of automated instruments/methods
- Employment of part-time contract staff (e.g. for overnight and weekend emergency service or for the phlebotomy service) and sharing of emergency service between local hospitals
- Review of price setting on the basis of workload and calculated cost per test.

Increasingly, use of automated systems for routine screening tests allows the laboratory to consider staff reduction, although an estimate of savings must take account of capital, maintenance contracts and running costs of the equipment, especially the high cost of some reagents, and whether the system can be used to high capacity and throughout a 24 h service.

Purchasing expensive equipment outright adds to the capital assets of the laboratory, with the consequential cost of depreciation (usually 8–10% per annum). Leasing equipment can be a better alternative and, in many countries, most equipment is obtained in this way. Careful calculation of the lease cost is required because this can be up to 20% higher than outright purchase. An advantage of leasing is flexibility to upgrade equipment should workload increase or technology change. If maintenance and consumable costs are included in the same agreement, it may be possible to negotiate a reduction in charge for the consumables, but it is important to neither underestimate nor overestimate the annual requirements that will be included in the contract.

When automation is coupled with centralization of the service to another site, care must be taken to maintain service quality.[6] Failure to do so will encourage clinicians to establish independent satellite laboratories. Loss of contact between clinical users and laboratory staff may compromise the pre-analytical phase of the test process and may lead to inappropriate requests, excessive requests and test

samples that are of inadequate volume or are poorly identified. When services are centralized, attention must be paid
to all phases (pre-analytical, analytical and post-analytical)
of the test process, including the need for packaging the
specimens and the cost of their transport to the laboratory.[6]

TEST RELIABILITY

The reliability of a quantitative test is defined in terms of
the *uncertainty of measurement* of the analyte (sometimes
referred to in documents as 'measurand'). This is based
on its accuracy and precision.[7]

Accuracy is the closeness of agreement between the measurement that is obtained and the true value; the extent of
discrepancy is the *systematic error* or *bias*. The most important causes of systematic error are listed in Table 24.3. The
error can be eliminated or at least greatly reduced by using a
reference standard with the test, together with internal
quality control and regular checking by external quality
assessment (see Chapter 25, p. 594).

Precision is the closeness of agreement when a test is
repeated a number of times. Imprecision is the result of random errors; it is expressed as standard deviation (SD) and
coefficient of variation (CV%). When the data are spread
normally (Gaussian distribution), for clinical purposes,
there is a 95% probability that results that fall within a
range of +2SD to −2SD of the target value are correct
and a 99% probably if within the range of +3SD
to −3SD (see also Fig. 2.1).

Table 24.3 Systematic errors in analyses

Analyser calibration uncertain (no reference standard available)
Bias in instrument, equipment or glassware
Faulty dilution
Faults in the measuring steps (e.g. reagents, spectrometry, calculations)
Sampling not representative of specimen
Specimens not representative of *in vivo* status (Ch. 1, p. 3)
Incomplete definition of analyte or lack of critical resolution of analyser
Approximations and arbitrary assumptions inherent in analyser's function
Environmental effects on analyser
Pre-analytical deterioration of specimens

Some of the other factors listed in Table 24.3 can be
quantified to calculate the combined uncertainty of measurement. Thus, for example, when a calibration preparation is used, its uncertainty is usually stated on the label
or accompanying certificate. The standard uncertainty is
then calculated from the sum of the quantified uncertain-
ties as follows:

$$\sqrt{(SD_1)^2 + (SD_2)^2}$$

Expanded uncertainty of measurement takes account of non-
quantifiable items by multiplying the previous amount
by a 'coverage factor' (k), which is usually taken to be
×2 for 95% level of confidence.[7,8]

It may be necessary to decide by statistical analysis
whether two sets of data differ significantly. The *t*-test is
used to assess the likelihood of significant difference at various levels of probability by comparing the means or individually paired results. The *F*-ratio is useful to assess the
influence of random errors in two sets of test results (see
Appendix, p. 625).

Of particular importance are reports with 'critical laboratory values' that may be indicative of life-threatening conditions requiring rapid clinical intervention. Haemoglobin
concentration, platelet count and activated partial thromboplastin time have been included in this category.[9] The
development of critical values should involve consultation
with clinical services.

TEST SELECTION

It is important for the laboratory to be aware of the limits of
accuracy that it achieves in its routine performance each
day as well as day-to-day.[10] Clinicians should be made
aware of the level of uncertainty of results for any test
and the potential effect of this on their diagnosis and interpretation of response to treatment (see below).

To evaluate the diagnostic reliability and predictive value
of an individual laboratory test, it is necessary to calculate
test sensitivity and specificity.[11] *Sensitivity* is the fraction of
true positive results when a test is applied to patients
known to have the relevant disease or when results have
been obtained by a reference method. *Specificity* is the fraction of true negative results when the test is applied to
normals.

Diagnostic sensitivity = TP ÷ (TP + FN)
Diagnostic specificity = TN ÷ (TN + FP)
Positive predictive value = TP ÷ (TP + FP)
Negative predictive value = TN ÷ (TN + FN)

where TP = true positive; TN = true negative;
FP = false positive; FN = false negative.
Overall reliability can be calculated as:

$$\frac{TP + TN}{\text{Total number of tests}} \times 100\%$$

Sensitivity and specificity should be near 1.0 (100%) if the test is unique for a particular diagnosis. A lower level of sensitivity or specificity may still be acceptable if the results are interpreted in conjunction with other tests as part of an overall pattern. It is not usually possible to have both 100% sensitivity and 100% specificity. Whether sensitivity or specificity is more important depends on the particular purpose of the test. Thus, for example, if haemoglobinometry is required in a clinic for identifying patients with anaemia, sensitivity is important, whereas in blood donor selection, for selecting individuals who are not anaemic, specificity is more important.

Likelihood Ratio

The ratio of positive results in disease to the frequency of false-positive results in healthy individuals gives a statistical measure of the discrimination by the test between disease and normality. It can be calculated as follows:[12]

$$\frac{Sensitivity}{1 - Specificity}$$

The higher the ratio, the greater is the probability of disease, whereas a ratio <1 makes the possibility of the disease being correctly diagnosed by the test much less likely. Conversely, the likelihood of normality can be calculated as:

$$\frac{1 - Sensitivity}{Specificity}$$

An alternative method is that of Youden, which is obtained by calculating Specificity/(1 − Sensitivity).[13] Values range between −1 and +1. With a positive ratio rising above zero towards +1 there is an increasing probability that the test will discriminate the presence of the specified disease and there is decreasing likelihood that the test is valid when the ratio falls from 0 to −1.

Receiver–Operator Characteristic Analysis

The relative usefulness of different methods for the same test or of a new method against a reference method can also be assessed by analysing the receiver–operator characteristics (ROC).[12] This is demonstrated on a graph by plotting the true-positive rates (*sensitivity*) on the vertical axis against false-positive rates (1 − *specificity*) on the horizontal axis for a series of paired measurements (Fig. 24.1). Obviously, the ideal test would show high sensitivity (i.e. 100% on vertical axis), with no false positives (i.e. 0% on horizontal axis). Realistically, there would be a compromise between the two criteria, with test selection depending on its purpose, i.e. whether as a screening to exclude the disease in question or to confirm a clinical suspicion that the disease is present. In the illustrated case Test A is more reliable than Test B for both circumstances.

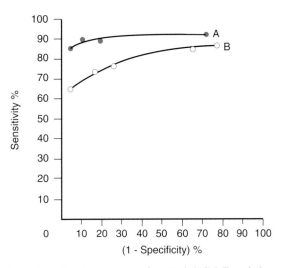

Figure 24.1 Receiver–operator characteristic (ROC) analysis. Graph shows curves relating true-positive rates (sensitivity) to false-positive rates (1 − specificity) for two tests A and B making the same measurements.

Test Utility

To ensure reliability of the laboratory service, tests with no proven value should be eliminated and new tests should be introduced only when there is independent evidence of technical reliability as well as cost-effectiveness.

For assessing cost-effectiveness of a particular test, account must be taken of (1) cost per test as compared with other tests that provide similar clinical information; (2) diagnostic reliability; and (3) clinical usefulness as assessed by the extent with which the test is relied on in clinical decisions, whether the results are likely to change the physician's diagnostic opinion and the clinical management of the patient, taking account of disease prevalence and a specified clinical or public health situation. This requires audit by an independent assessor to judge what proportion of the requests for a particular test are actually used intelligently and what percentage are unnecessary or wasted tests.[14,15] Information on the utility of various tests can also be obtained from benchmarking (see p. 579) and published guidelines. Examples of the latter are the documents published by the British Committee for Standards in Haematology (www.BCSHGuidelines.com). The realistic cost-effectiveness of any test may be assessed by the formula:

A/(B × C), where A = cost/test, as described on p. 566
B = diagnostic reliability, as described on p. 567
C = clinical usefulness, as described above.

Economic aspects should also be considered when providing an automated total screening programme for every patient, in contrast to specifically selected tests. Thus, while many clinicians may not be familiar with all of the 12 or more parameters included in the blood count as reported routinely by modern automated analysers and in most cases, some of these measurements are unlikely to be clinically useful, nevertheless the 'not-requested' information may be provided at no extra cost and even significant saving of time in the laboratory.

INSTRUMENTATION

Equipment Evaluation

Assessment of the clinical utility and cost-effectiveness of equipment to match the nature and volume of laboratory workload is a very important exercise. Guidelines for evaluation of blood cell analysers and other haematology instruments have been published by the International Council for Standardization in Haematology.[16] In the UK, appraisal of various items of laboratory equipment was formerly undertaken by selected laboratories at the request of the Department of Health's Medical Devices Agency, subsequently renamed Medicines and Healthcare products Regulatory Agency (MHRA) and now replaced by the Centre for Evidence-based Purchasing (CEP). (Their reports can be accessed from the website: www.pasa.nhs.uk/ceppublications.)

Principles of Evaluation

The following aspects are usually included in evaluations:

1. Verification of instrument requirements for space and services
2. Extent of technical training required to operate the instrument
3. Clarity and usefulness of instruction manual
4. Assessment of safety (mechanical, electrical, microbiological and chemical)
5. Determination of the following:
   a. Linearity
   b. Precision/imprecision
   c. Carryover
   d. Extent of inaccuracy by comparison with measurement by definitive or reference methods
   e. Comparability with an established method used in the laboratory
   f. Performance when used in an external quality control scheme
   g. Sensitivity (i.e. determination of the smallest change in analyte concentration that gives a measured result)
   h. Specificity (i.e. extent of errors caused by interfering substances)
6. Throughput time and number of specimens that can be processed within a normal working day
7. Reliability of the instrument when in routine use and adequacy of service and maintenance provided

8. Cost per test, including operating time, reagents, daily start-up procedure and regular (usually weekly) maintenance procedures
9. Staff acceptability, impact on laboratory organization and level of technical expertise required to operate the instrument
10. Any relevant authority label, e.g. CE mark on a device indicates that it conforms to defined specifications of the EU directive 98/79 for *in vitro* diagnostic medical devices (IVDD), as described in the Official Journal (OJ) of the EC: 7.12.98.

After an instrument has been purchased and installed, it is useful to undertake regular less extensive checks of performance with regard to precision, linearity, carryover and comparability.

Precision

Carry out appropriate measurements 10 times consecutively on three or more specimens selected in the pathological range so as to include a low, a high and a middle range concentration of the analyte. Calculate the replicate SD and CV as shown on p. 625. The degree of precision that is acceptable depends on the purpose of the test (Table 24.4). To check between-batch precision, measure three samples in several successive batches of routine tests; calculate the SD and CV in the same way.

Linearity

Linearity demonstrates the effects of dilution. Prepare a specimen with a high concentration of the analyte to be tested and, as accurately as possible, make a series of dilutions in plasma so as to obtain 10 samples with evenly spaced concentration levels between 10% and 100%. Measure each sample three times and calculate the means. Plot results on arithmetic graph paper. Ideally, all points

Table 24.4 Test precision for different purposes

PURPOSE OF TEST	EXPECTED CV% (AUTOMATED COUNTERS)		
	Hb	RBC	WBC
Scientific standard	<1	1	1–2
State of art:			
Best performance	1.5	2	3
Routine laboratories	2–3	3	5–6
Clinical needs	5–10	5	10–15

CV, coefficient of variation; Hb, haemoglobin concentration; RBC, red blood cell count; WBC, white blood cell count.

should fall on a straight line that passes through the zero of the horizontal and vertical axes. In practice, the results should lie within 2SD limits of the means calculated from the CVs, which have been obtained from analysis of precision (see earlier). Inspection of the graph will show whether there is linearity throughout the range or whether it is limited to part of the range.

Carryover

Carryover indicates the extent to which measurement of an analyte in a specimen is likely to be affected by the preceding specimen. Measure a specimen with a high concentration in triplicate, immediately followed by a specimen with a low concentration of the analyte:

$$Carryover(\%) = \frac{l_1 - l_3}{h_3 - l_3} \times 100$$

where l_1 and l_3 are the results of the first and third measurements of the samples with a low concentration and h_3 is the third measurement of the sample with a high concentration.

Accuracy and Comparability

Accuracy and comparability test whether the new instrument (or method) gives results that agree satisfactorily with those obtained with an established procedure and with a reference method. Test specimens should be measured alternately, or in batches, by the two procedures. If results by the two methods are analysed by correlation coefficient (r), a high correlation does not mean that the two methods agree. Correlation coefficient is a measure of relation and not agreement. It is better to use the limits of agreement method.[12] For this, plot the differences between paired results on the vertical axis of linear graph paper against the means of the pairs on the horizontal axis (Fig. 24.2); differences between the methods are then readily apparent over the range from low to high values. If the scatter of differences increases at high values, logarithmic transformed data should be plotted.

It is also useful to check for bias by including the instrument or method under test in the laboratory's participation in an external quality assessment scheme (see p. 594). Bias is expressed by:

$$\frac{R - M}{M} \times 100$$

where R = measurement by the device/method being tested and M = target result.

Another method to check for bias is by means of the variance index. For this, the coefficient of variation is established at an optimal chosen value (CCV) to ensure a reliable method and the variation index (VI%) is calculated as:

$$\frac{R - M}{M} \times \frac{100}{CCV} \times 100$$

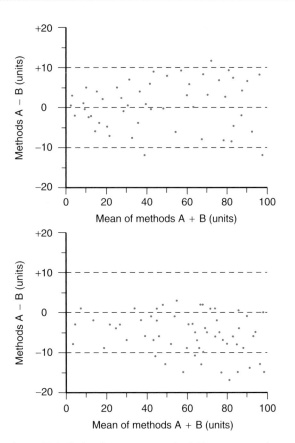

Figure 24.2 Limits of agreement method. Shows mean values for paired results by two methods A plus B (horizontal axis) plotted against the differences (A minus B) between the paired results (vertical axis). Horizontal lines represent equality with range of ±10 units (mean ±SD). Upper figure shows no bias between methods A and B, whereas lower figure shows false high results (negative values) for method B.

Maintenance logs

All laboratory equipment should be inspected regularly and specific maintenance procedures should be carried out. Each item of laboratory equipment should have a maintenance log to document what maintenance is required, the desired frequency and when it was last carried out. The log includes servicing and repairs by the manufacturer. Equipment used to test biological specimens must be cleaned thoroughly before a maintenance procedure is carried out to reduce the biohazard. The procedure for such cleaning must be documented (as a standard operating procedure), together with the name of the responsible worker and the date.

DATA PROCESSING

It is essential that accurate records of laboratory results are kept for whatever period is stipulated by national legislation. Computer-assisted data handling is essential for all but the smallest laboratory. For long-term storage of data, possibilities include a printed (hard) copy, a memory stick and external hard drive or a local server. Laboratory results are usually issued as numeric data with abnormal results highlighted for the clinician. Report forms should be reader friendly. Serial data are particularly useful to illustrate any trend with time and may be in the form of a cumulative tabulation or a graph. For the latter, an arithmetic scale should be used for haemoglobin concentration, red cell count and reticulocytes, whereas platelet and leucocyte counts are best displayed on a logarithmic scale (Fig. 24.3). A graph is particularly useful for displaying results in relation to target intervals because this facilitates adjustment of dosage of drugs that are likely to affect the blood. Furthermore, this method of archiving reduces the number of pages of laboratory reports in the patient's file.[17]

Laboratory Computers

Developments in computer technology have made available powerful microcomputers and sophisticated computer software at moderate prices. Such computers may be an integral part of an analytical instrument or interfaced to it by cable. A modem is required to link the computer to the telephone or broadband for access to the internet and electronic mail and also to interconnect within a local area network, so as to provide for data interchange and to enable multiple workers to use a common database. Such computers may be an integral part of an analytical instrument or interfaced to it. Because computers are developing at such a rate, it is essential to seek expert advice to ensure that the instrument being purchased is fit for purpose. Helpful advice on the applications of the internet for health professions is given in a monograph by Kiley.[18] Programmes that provide access to a vast amount of information include Google Scholar and the US National Library of Medicine PubMed and Medline, the latter being the primary component of PubMed especially on biomedical topics. Publishers of journals also provide internet access to citations and abstracts of articles, both current and archived, for a large number of medical journals. Access to the full journal articles usually requires a subscription fee for the full articles that can be read directly on the

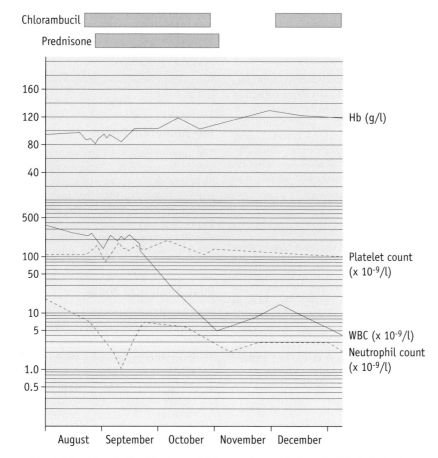

Figure 24.3 Haematological chart for plotting blood count data on a time-related graph. This illustrates the course in a patient with chronic lymphocytic leukaemia. Haemoglobin is recorded arithmetically; the other components are on a logarithmic scale. If reticulocytes are included, they should be recorded arithmetically.

571

computer or printed out, conveniently as a pdf file but in a scheme known as Health Inter-Network Access to Research Initiatives, an agreement was made between the World Health Organization and the world's leading publishers, whereby in more than 100 developing countries this access is available free of charge or at greatly reduced prices to staff and students of teaching hospitals, research and public health institutes, universities and professional colleges.

A comprehensive overview of various topics relating to life sciences is provided by the *Encyclopedia of Life Sciences* (ELS) published on the internet by Wiley-Blackwell. Many individual experts have their own websites for presenting dissertations and comments in their specialties, while manufacturers provide up-to-date information on their products.

It is impractical to provide a comprehensive index of all relevant websites; however, Table 24.5 lists some that are of particular interest for the haematology laboratory, including some that are also noted in the text. In any event, entering a key word or phrase is likely to provide access to a vast amount of information on virtually any topic as well as links to related items.

PRE-ANALYTICAL AND POST-ANALYTICAL STAGES OF TESTING

The haematology laboratory should be involved in the pre-analytical alstage (test requesting, blood sample collection and transport to the laboratory) as well as the post-analytical stage (return of results to the clinician). Account must also be taken of physiological variables (see Chapter 2) and endogenous variables, such as medicines and other substances taken by the patient.[19] Both variables have a significant impact on test reliability, laboratory performance and client satisfaction.

Test Requesting

There is considerable variation between clinicians in their test ordering patterns, and laboratory staff have historically exerted little influence on test request patterns, although sustained educational programmes may achieve more selective testing. Unnecessary requests often result from inappropriate request forms, such as those that permit clinicians to tick from a list instead of requesting specific tests. Modification of the requesting pattern might focus on specific needs, included use of problem-orientated request forms[20] and a computer-based ordering of tests using protocols written by specialist clinical teams.[21]

Specimen Collection and Delivery

It is essential to have positive identification of the patient as well as reliable sample identification and thus patient-sample and inter-sample identification must be checked

at all times. Failure to do so can result in delayed diagnosis, even misdiagnosis, resulting in incorrect treatment of the patient, and it may be a serious cause of error in blood transfusion. In one inter-laboratory Q-probe analysis in the USA (see p. 579), 0.1–5% of specimens were unacceptable due to mislabelling, incomplete label, illegible label and even specimens without any label.[22,23] Methods have been developed for electronic ordering of tests using the hospital's patient identification barcode for checking the patient's identity at the time of phlebotomy, printing the barcode onto the specimen containers and checking this by means of a hand-held scanner at all stages during processing in the laboratory until the report is issued.

After the blood has been collected, every effort must be made to ensure its delivery to the laboratory without delay. If this is not coordinated, samples may remain in clinical areas awaiting collection by porters who then follow a fixed circuit of other hospital areas before eventually reaching the laboratory. However, if responsibility for blood collection and transport is held by the laboratory, these separate activities can be coordinated. Alternative and faster means of specimen delivery to laboratories, with no significant effect of the specimens, include pneumatic tube conveyor or rail-track conveyor systems,[24,25] although there has been a report of lysed specimens due to a defect in the system.[26] Specimen transport from remote clinics to a central laboratories is referred to in Chapter 26 (see p. 614).

Pre-Analytical Phase

The time of receipt of the specimens in the laboratory should be registered.[19] The specimens must be checked to ensure that they are appropriate for the tests that are requested and that there has been no contamination by leakage on the outside of the tubes and/or the request forms. Requests should be registered and the specimens should be separated into 'routine' and 'urgent', the latter being handed directly to the appropriate staff member.

Post-Analytical Phase

After the tests have been carried out, the following procedures are required to ensure proficiency in the post-analytical phase:

1. Processing of results for transcription onto report forms
2. Immediate scrutiny of urgent results with issue of provisional report and its delivery to the requesting clinician
3. Assessment of the significance of results in the context of established reference values and decision for further tests. 'Critical laboratory values' for adults and for children should be established for life-threatening

Table 24.5 Selected www. internet sites of haematological interest

scholar.google.com	Access to an extensive bibliography on scientific and medical topics
who.int	World Health Organization[a]
international council for standardization in haematology	Lists publications from International Council for Standardization in Haematology – The acronym ICSH is inadequate – recent activities are also reported on www.islh (see below)
ish-world.org	Home page of International Society of Haematology
ifbls.org	International Federation of Biomedical Laboratory Science; arranges international congresses and educational resources
isth.org	International Society of Thrombosis and Haemostasis; includes bibliography and full reports of official communications from their scientific and standardization committees
islh.org	International Society for Laboratory Hematology; includes details of annual symposium and activities of the International Council for Standardization in Haematology
isbt-web.org	Home page of International Society of Blood Transfusion
rcpath.org.uk	General information from Royal College of Pathologists
ibms.org	General information from Institute of Biomedical Science, including various aspects of CPD
ifbls	International Federation of Biomedical Laboratory Science
ukneqas.org.uk	Home page of UK NEQAS; click onto Haematology for information on the various tests included in their surveys
ukas/cpa.co.uk	Clinical Pathology Accreditation, as authorized by UKAS, with details of its functions and the procedures for a laboratory applying for accreditation
pubmed.com	National Library of Medicine with access to MEDLINE
mhra.gov.uk	MDA reports of instrument and kits evaluations
bcshguidelines.com	Home page of the British Committee for Standards in Haematology, providing the full text of all current and past guidelines, whether published in book or journal format
transfusionguidelines	UK blood transfusion guideline documents
rph.wa.gov.au/labs	Malaria training programme from Royal Perth Hospital, Australia. For other sites on this topic: see www.Malariatraining.com
westgard.com	JO Westgard's 'Lesson of the Month' and other tutorials on quality assurance

[a]There are various items on the WHO website of particular interest for laboratory practice.
Note especially: /Essential health technology (EHT); /Diagnostics and laboratory technology (DLT); /Quality Management in Transfusion Medicine; /Medical devices.

conditions requiring rapid clinical intervention (e.g. haemoglobin concentration, platelet count, activated partial thromboplastin time)[27]

4. Transmission of final report without unreasonable delay to the location indicated on the request form. Computer-assisted reporting of results to linked monitors and printers located in clinical areas is very helpful,[28] but in some countries most hospitals rely on manual transport of result sheets and this can significantly prolong request completion times. Pneumatic tube and rail-track conveyor systems used for the pre-analytical stage can also be used for rapid return of results to wards and clinics.

Return of results is, of course, no guarantee that ward or clinic staff will react in a timely way to change a patient's treatment or even file report forms in the patient's medical record. It is the responsibility of the clinician to ensure that the reports of tests requested by them are received, noted and acted on. However, good laboratory practice includes speedy notification to the responsible clinical staff of a result that shows an apparently unexpected serious abnormality. A recent development has been the use of mobile cameraphones to transmit test results to the relevant clinician or even images (e.g. a stained blood film, from the laboratory) in order to obtain rapid authoritative support from an expert at a remote location.[29] In these situations, it may be necessary to comply with local or national regulations concerning confidentiality of patients records, including the use of encrypted memory sticks to store the information.

5. As an audit of utility of the laboratory, there should be regular contact with users to ensure that the reports arrive in due time for optimal use during clinical management and that the clinicians are satisfied that results are presented in a clear and unambiguous form; there should also be discussions on test selection, taking account of the clinical relevance of the tests that are undertaken, the introduction of new tests and evaluation of benefit versus cost, as discussed earlier.

Test Turnaround Time

As described above, it is essential to ensure that tests are carried out and results reported to clinicians as rapidly as possible. The usual measure of this is the test turnaround time, which takes account of work scheduling, selection of equipment and training.[30] It is most easily measured as the time lapse between arrival of a blood specimen in the laboratory and issue of the validated result. In a small unit, this can be undertaken manually, albeit tediously. In a computerized laboratory, however, it is relatively easy to record these times and then to calculate the median time, the 95th percentile for completing each test and the percentage of tests completed within a pre-selected time.[31] While this information is based on the performance of an individual laboratory, it should be possible to make comparisons with a peer group in benchmarking studies (see page 000).

It should, however, be noted that turnaround time as described above usually refers only to the analytical stage of testing and excludes the time delay of the pre-analytical and post-analytical stages of testing. When the laboratory has responsibility for all three stages, it becomes possible to extend the measurement of analytical turnaround time to the more meaningful parameter of request completion time (total time from initiation of the request to delivery of the result). The speed with which modern systems perform reduces the need for interrupting the routine specimens for urgent tests, but the laboratory should also have an efficient way to convey urgent results to the requesting clinician.[32] In critically ill patients, it is especially important to avoid any delay between receipt of

the test results by the ward staff and its relay to the relevant clinician for an active response. A report on this specific point by a College of American Pathologists Q-probe survey showed that while reports on tests from critically ill patients were generally received in the ward by computer link within less than 5 min, there was often a significant, and thus potentially serious, delay before they reached the relevant clinician.[33] The use of mobile camera phones as described above to transmit test results directly to the appropriate clinician could provide a solution, especially in an after-hours service.[29]

Point-of-Care Testing

Point-of-care testing (POCT), also known as *near-patient testing*, functions at two levels: either within a hospital as an adjunct to the laboratory or for primary healthcare outside the hospital.

Specialist clinical areas within hospitals have an increasing need for a customized laboratory service to meet their particular requirements. When rapid results are especially important, laboratory testing within the clinical area may be the best arrangement. Intensive care units have a long established need for near-patient monitoring of blood gases, but other clinicians use laboratory tests for monitoring ill patients and for making rapid decisions on treatment (e.g. in oncology outpatient clinics) and this has increased demand for a rapid results service. POCT may also be necessary when a test is performed on capillary (not anticoagulated) blood (e.g. for patients attending an anticoagulant control clinic).

Diagnostic laboratories are often located in areas of the hospital that are remote from critical care and outpatient areas. Rapid transit systems, including pneumatic tubes (see earlier), may be the preferred alternative to multiple satellite testing areas, particularly when the main laboratory already offers a rapid results service. Knowledge of test turnaround time in the laboratory (see above) is required in order to make an informed decision on the need for near-patient testing in satellite areas. When POCT equipment is the preferred option, the running of the satellite laboratory and maintenance of its equipment should be the responsibility of the appropriate pathology discipline. This is essential for quality control, safety and accreditation, whether the satellite is staffed by laboratory staff, as in busy locations or used by medical staff or nurses as a marginal activity. A designated member of laboratory staff should supervise this service, visiting each test location daily and ensuring that all results and quality control data are integrated into the main laboratory computer system. Some instruments designed for POCT will store quality-control data on a computer with a memory stick from which the data can subsequently be transferred to the main laboratory. Guidelines on the organization of a POCT service have been published by the British Committee for Standards in Haematology[34] and the UK Medical Devices

Agency,[35] in the USA by the Clinical and Laboratory Standards Institute[36] and internationally by the International Council for Standardization in Haematology[37] and the International Standard Organization.[38]

Point-of-Care Testing Beyond the Laboratory

POCT beyond the laboratory is increasingly popular in some countries and it is particularly useful when patients live a distance away from a hospital laboratory. Instrument manufacturers are now producing tabletop or hand-held devices that are simple to use, autocalibrated and require minimum maintenance. The haematology tests that are usually undertaken include haemoglobin concentration, blood cell counting by simple analysers, erythrocyte sedimentation rate and prothrombin time for oral anti-coagulation control.

Although this use of POCT is independent, the local hospital laboratory should encourage the doctors and clinics to seek advice and help with selection of appropriate instruments, their standardization/calibration and quality control, including a link into the external quality assessment scheme in which the laboratory participates. Harmonization of reports with laboratory records is helpful when a patient is referred to the hospital. Studies on the management of anti-coagulation control have shown that with appropriate training and cooperation from the laboratory, pharmacists are able to provide as reliable a service as the hospital-based one and, in general, with more convenience for the patient.[39]

A major source of error in POCT outside the hospital is faulty specimen collection, whether for venous or finger-prick samples. Clinic staff who undertake this procedure should be given supervised training (see Chapter 1, p. 3).

Patient Self-Testing

There is an increasing trend toward self-testing by patients, and simple portable pre-calibrated coagulometers, which use capillary blood to measure prothrombin time and the International Normalized Ratio, are now available. It has been shown that patients are able to use these instruments correctly and, once their treatment has been established, the individual patients can be relied on to maintain their anti-coagulation within the therapeutic range[40] (see also Chapter 20, p. 471). It is important that the selected instruments conform to national, European (CEN) or international (ISO) standards to ensure that they are reliable and that the instructions for their use are clear, unambiguous and written for the users.

Laboratory Services for General Practitioners

The customers of a haematology laboratory include not only hospital clinicians but also general practitioners/family doctors who have different priorities from hospital practitioners. They may have simple point-of-care screening tests on site, but appropriate service beyond that is outlined in the following sections.

Pre-Analytical Service

Provision of adequate information to the general practitioner is important. This may include a users' handbook or an encyclopedia listing all available tests, their utility and normal reference ranges, together with a wall chart to show the correct specimen container and volume of blood required, requirements for patient preparation (e.g. fasting), the timing of any medication that may affect the test result and the turnaround time for each test. The latter is important so that patients can be given a follow-up appointment to be told the result. Handbooks should be of loose-leaf format to facilitate updating. Education should cover safety aspects, such as how to deal with blood spillage or a needle-stick injury. A specimen transport system at an agreed time of day is particularly important so that patients can be given a suitable appointment for blood collection.

Post-Analytical Service

The general practitioner needs a fast report service for abnormal test results. Ideally, there should be an interfaced computer connection to the laboratory and to the duty haematologist or at least a direct e-mail address, telephone or fax number at the health centre. With transmission of results by fax or e-mail, confidentiality must be ensured by secure identification of the recipient and, when internet access is available, a secure password entry is essential. When there is no electronic link to the laboratory, it may prove economical to use the specimen transport service to return test results to general practitioners.

Standard Operating Procedures

Standard operating procedures are written instructions that are intended to maintain optimal consistent quality of performance in the laboratory. They should cover all aspects of work, with some relating to test procedures and others relating to specimen collection, laboratory safety, handling of urgent requests, data storage, telephone reporting policy, and so on. They may be based on standard textbook descriptions or an instrument manufacturer's instruction manual, but they should reflect daily practice and each laboratory must prepare its own individual set of SOPs. They should be reviewed regularly and any revisions must be highlighted with the date. Older versions must be archived and numbered copies of the new version must be distributed to authorized locations. A suggested format for an SOP is given in Table 24.6.

Table 24.6 Format for a standard operating procedure (SOP)

Cover page   Title, reference number, date of preparation, name of author, name of authorizer, distribution of the SOP and its availability
Scope   Purpose of the SOP; principles of procedure or test; grade(s) of staff permitted to undertake the task(s), responsibility for implementation of SOP, training requirement file
Specimen requirements   Type and amount; delivery arrangements; storage conditions, any time or temperature restrictions
Specimen reception   Registration and check of request form; criteria for rejecting a specimen

Health and safety precautions
    Obligatory protection requirements
    Handling and disposal of 'high-risk' samples, broken specimen containers and blood spillage

Equipment, materials and reagents   Lists of equipment, apparatus, reagents, controls, calibrators, forms and other stationery
Test procedure   Step-by-step details of sample processing, test procedure, quality control checks and use of standards, calculation of results
Reporting   Procedure for reporting results for routine and urgent requests; printed instructions to patient when relevant

Clinical significance
    An understanding of the clinical reason for the test and significance of abnormal results
    Reference range and confidence limits for healthy normal men, women and children

Test limitations   How to recognize errors and steps to avoid or correct them
Maintenance of equipment   List of schedule for routine in-house maintenance (daily, weekly) and servicing
Specimen storage post-test   Period of retention and conditions for storage: instructions for disposal of specimens and diluted subsamples
List of relevant literature
Date when SOP is due to be reviewed

LABORATORY AUDIT AND ACCREDITATION

Audit

Laboratory audit is the systematic and critical analysis of the quality of the laboratory service. The essence of audit is that it should be continuous and designed to achieve incremental improvement in quality of the day-to-day service. It should encompass the pre-analytical, analytical and post-analytical stages of laboratory practice; and should take account of five components:[41]

1. Solving problems associated with process or outcome
2. Monitoring workload in the context of demand control
3. Monitoring introduction of new tests or changes in practice
4. Monitoring adherence to guidelines and best practice
5. Monitoring of analytical quality.

Examples of specific aspects of laboratory practice requiring audit are given in Table 24.7.

The first stage of audit is to define the standard to be achieved; this may be in the form of a standard operating procedure for an analytical procedure, a protocol for test ordering, pre-surgery blood transfusion order schedule or a target turnaround time. These standards will have

Table 24.7 Examples of laboratory audit

Understanding of laboratory functions by users
Request forms: patient identity, clear indications of test(s) and relevant clinical information
Specimen labels with unambiguous identification of the patient
Appropriateness of test requests
Test menu in response to clinical needs
Appropriateness of blood samples (e.g. adequate volume, choice of anticoagulant)
Storage of reagents and specimens
Reference ranges and interpretation of abnormal results
Timeliness of reports
Internal quality control results
External quality assessment scheme performance
Cost-effectiveness of specialist tests
Precise and clear laboratory reports, especially highlighting abnormal results
Reporting methods (e.g. personal contact, computer, telephone, fax, camera phone)
Compliance with safety policies
Use of blood and blood products
Frequency and cause of transfusion reactions
Turnaround time for emergency requests
Satisfaction of outpatients undergoing venepuncture
Satisfaction of laboratory users on laboratory competence

been agreed within the laboratory and, whenever possible, in conjunction with relevant users of the laboratory. Clinical input is invaluable in relation to the clinical significance of analyser-generated results, test utility (see p. 568), appropriate laboratory utilization,[12] and the advantages and disadvantages of point-of-care tests (see p. 574). To monitor performance against the agreed standards, each laboratory section should form its own audit group or, if there is an audit group for the whole department, it should be open to all grades of staff to allow peer review and to take advantage of the educational value of audit. Laboratory staff should lead the audit process rather than having it imposed on them. It is good practice to make a short report of each audit meeting, recording attendance, the items identified for improvement and an action list.

In the UK, a national steering group monitors serious hazards of transfusion ('SHOT'). A large proportion of the incidents that have occurred have been the result of incorrect identification of patient–specimen link, with the wrong blood being collected from the hospital blood bank or satellite refrigerator, or failure in bedside checking procedures (see p. 519).

The audit process improves quality simply by examining and questioning established standards and guidelines. The ever-increasing need for cost-effectiveness is likely to forge closer working relationships between the different pathology disciplines, as well as between laboratories within the same discipline. This changing laboratory environment highlights the need for continuous training of haematology staff in good laboratory management and in the importance of audit.

Accreditation

The purpose of laboratory accreditation schemes is to allow external audit of a laboratory's organization, staffing, direction and management performance in an appropriate quality assurance programme and level of user satisfaction. The advantage to the accredited laboratory is that this indicates to clinical users that it has a demonstrable standard of practice with competence, impartiality and capability that has been independently confirmed by external peer review. Such review should include assessment of basic functional structure (laboratory facilities such as staff and equipment), processes (test analyses), outcome (quality of test results including timeliness and interpretation), interaction with clinical users and optimal use of resources.

In the UK, this proficiency testing function is undertaken by an independent organization, the UK Accreditation Service (www.ukas.com), which is the sole national body recognized by the UK Government and by the EU, with authority to validate specified tests that are undertaken by a laboratory, certifying that these tests are up to date, recognized as standard practice and comply with ISO and CEN standards (see p. 587). Previously, the majority of clinical laboratories in the UK were accredited by *Clinical Pathology Accreditation Ltd* (CPA), a body established by the Royal College of Pathologists and working in association with UKAS; however, as CPA has more recently been considered not to be independent of its participating laboratories, its function has been assumed directly by UKAS. For any specific test, reliability is judged by performance in the relevant surveys of the UK National External Quality Assurance Scheme (see Chapter 25).

In other countries, certification for accreditation may also be undertaken by government-authorized bodies. Thus, in the USA, control is undertaken mainly by the CAP Accreditation and Laboratory Improvement scheme in accordance with the Clinical Laboratories Improvement Amendments (CLIA 1988) regulations.[42,43] In Australia, control is maintained by a government authority, the National Pathology

Accreditation Advisory Council (NPAAC), which sets the standards for accreditation of laboratories. Descriptions of the requirements for national accreditation programmes are available on their websites.

An important component of all accreditation programmes is participation in proficiency testing/external quality assessment schemes (see Chapter 25). These schemes are expected to conform to standards that are specified by the *International Laboratory Accreditation Cooperation* (ILAC) and are described in ISO/IEC Guide 43. ISO 17043 (see Table 24.8) is an updated version of ISO Guide 43. Another useful document is *ILAC G22* ('Use of proficiency testing as a tool for accreditation in testing').

Some national schemes have established formal links with each other, such as the *Western European Laboratory Accreditation Cooperation*. The website of the European Proficiency Testing Information Service (*EPTIS*) lists a wide range of schemes worldwide in various sciences, including laboratory medicine.

INTERNATIONAL STANDARDS OF PRACTICE

The International Standards Organization (ISO) has established guidelines for laboratory practice. Of special importance are ISO 15189: 'Medical laboratories – particular requirements for quality and competence', which sets out the rules for laboratory management; ISO 9000 series: 'Quality management and quality systems' and ISO 17025: 'Competence of testing and calibration laboratories'. These and other relevant standards from ISO and the European authority CEN are listed in Table 24.8.

Table 24.8 ISO and European (EN) standards relating to medical laboratory practice	
ISO 9000	A series of standards and guidelines on selection and use of quality management systems and quality assurance (complementary aspects are specified in ISO 9001–9004)
ISO 22869	Guidance document on implementation of ISO 15189 (formerly ISO Guide 25)
ISO 15194	*In vitro* diagnostic medical devices: measurement of quantities in samples of biological origin; description of reference materials
EN 12286	*In vitro* diagnostic medical devices: presentation of reference measurement procedures
EN 13612	Performance evaluation of *in vitro* diagnostic medical devices
ISO 15198	Validation of manufacturers' recommendations for user quality control
ISO 25680	Calculation and expression of measurement uncertainty
ISO 22870	Point-of-care testing (POCT) – requirements for quality and competence
ISO/IEC 17043	Conformity assessment – general requirements for proficiency testing. This is update of ISO Guide 43–1 & 2
ISO/EN 17025	Competence of Testing and Calibration Laboratories; formerly ISO Guide 25 and EN45001
EN 375	Information supplied by manufacturers with *in vitro* diagnostic reagents
EN 591	Instructions for use of *in vitro* diagnostic instruments
EN 592	Instructions for use of *in vitro* diagnostic instruments for self-testing
EN 13532	General requirements for *in vitro* diagnostic medical devices for self-testing
ISO 17593	Requirements for *in vitro* monitoring systems for self-testing of oral anticoagulation therapy
EN 14136	Use of external quality assessment schemes in assessment of performance of *in vitro* diagnostic procedures
ISO 6710	Single-use containers for venous blood specimen collection
ISO 15190	Safety management for medical laboratories
ISO/EN 14971	Medical devices – application of risk management to medical devices
ISO, International Organization for Standardization; EN, Comité Européen de Normalization.	

BENCHMARKING

Benchmarking is now recognized as an essential technique for achieving continuous improvement in laboratory performance to ensure that it is effective and efficient with elimination of waste. It functions by providing a reference point for laboratories to assess their performance by comparison with their peers and the leaders in the field.[44] Departments are divided into several categories on the basis of their size, whether academic or non-teaching and whether responsible for special activities. Their responses to a lengthy annual questionnaire permit evaluation of various aspects of laboratory practice. By standardizing definitions of tests and requests, it is possible to establish an agreed method for estimating workload in a standard way and to provide the optimal criteria for staffing levels, skill-mix, productivity, reliability and cost-effectiveness, taking account of clinical needs and local patient population ('case-mix'). Thus, benchmarking judges the quality of service of a laboratory, by assessing whether it can be run more efficiently with improved cost-effectiveness and clinical effectiveness. It provides an assessment of the adequacy of staffing with realistic measure of workload parameters, how test throughput and reporting time might be improved, taking account of how variation in clinical practice might affect the laboratory service and whether cost-effectiveness and clinical benefit might be improved by decentralizing some components or conversely by eliminated satellite units. This has become an essential method for achieving continuous sustainable improvement based on evidence rather than intuition.

In the USA, the scheme known as 'Q-probe' was established in 1989 by the College of American Pathologists Laboratory Improvement Program, to facilitate implementation of CLIA '88 requirements by providing laboratories with continuing peer review and education with periodic on-site audit. Reports of various Q-probe studies are published regularly in the *Archives of Pathology and Laboratory Medicine*. In the UK, a similar scheme has been developed in keeping with the requirements of the Commission for Health Improvement (CHI). It is undertaken by the Clinical Benchmarking Company, which is a partnership established by the Clinical Management Unit of the Centre for Health Planning at Keele University with *Tribal Newchurch Limited* (www.newchurch.co.uk/consulting), an informatics service company specializing in working with healthcare organizations. For its laboratory services, it operates with a team of advisers appointed by the Royal College of Pathologists. Assessment of performance of an individual laboratory is based on comparison with best performance in a comparable peer cluster and performance in the UK National External Quality Assessment Scheme (see Chapter 25). Another organization with similar function is *DAWN Benchmarking*.

LABORATORY SAFETY

Principles of Safety Policy

Every laboratory worker should receive instructions on the potential hazards in their workplace, from specimen collection to waste disposal, and including sites where point-of-care tests are carried out, reagent stores and satellite storage refrigerators that hold blood and blood products. There should be a procedure to protect the health and wellbeing of all members of the staff and legitimate visitors, taking account of mandatory rules and regulations as well as local practices.

There should be a designated safety officer of sufficient seniority, with authority to implement departmental safety policy in all sections of the laboratory. The safety officer should be responsible for day-to-day management of safety issues and should be directly accountable to the head of department. There must be an established protocol for handling needle-stick injury to a member of staff, with immediate referral to the appropriate hospital department of occupational health, which should provide a 24 h advisory service. All incidents must be recorded, safety protocol reviewed and measures taken to prevent recurrence.

The safety officer must have the training and time to do the job well and provide ongoing training for other staff who must not be allowed to handle potentially hazardous materials until they have completed training in accordance with the safety requirements. The safety officer should represent the laboratory on relevant safety committees and work closely with hospital occupational health, control of infection and radiation protection officers. Within the department, a safety committee should be established as a useful forum for safety audit.

Departmental safety policy should be documented as a booklet which is readily accessible in each section of the laboratory. A loose-leaf format facilitates updating. It must provide a comprehensive account of departmental safety policy (Table 24.9). Attention must be drawn to known and potential hazards in relation to infection, toxic substances, fire, radiation and mechanical injury. Where a hazard cannot be eliminated, the risk should be reduced so far as is reasonably practicable (e.g. by reducing the frequency and period of exposure). The safety booklet should refer to relevant local, national and international safety legislation.

In addition to the safety booklet which sets out laboratory safety policy, SOPs should also include information on handling reagents which are classified by relevant authorities as *hazardous to health* (see below), together with relevant safety and decontamination protocols (see p. 582).

The standard for safety management in medical laboratories has been established by the International Organization for Standardization (ISO 14971 and 15190; Table 24.8). This

Table 24.9 Items to be included in laboratory safety policy document

Blood collection
Labelling, transport and reception of specimens
Handling of specimens and containment of high-risk specimens
Location of protective equipment
Managing and reporting needle-stick injury
Management of eye-splash
Disposal of used needles, syringes and lancets
Procedure for blood spillage
Hazard risk assessment for all substances in the laboratory
Safety in near-patient testing
Protective clothing
Health records of staff, including immunization
Laboratory security, out-of hours working and visitors to the department
Waste disposal
Electrical equipment testing
Recording of accidents
Safety cabinet monitoring
Laboratory cleaning policies
Policy for receiving and sending postal specimens
Radiation protection
Fire precautions
Staff training programmes
Safety inspections
Schedule for safety committee meeting

provides rules for a safe working environment in the laboratory and includes a comprehensive list of items to be checked when auditing safety practice. A similar document on safety of electrical equipment used in the laboratories has been established by the International Electrotechnical Commission (IEC).[45]

WHO has also published comprehensive manuals on safety in healthcare laboratories,[46,47] and there is a WHO website linked to the Safe Injection Global Network (www.who.int/injection_safety), which describes strategies for safe handling of blood intended for transfusion. This includes (a) selection of blood donors, testing of blood units, appropriate clinical use of blood and, when applicable, viral inactivation of human material for therapeutic use; (b) safe and appropriate use of injections, sharps waste management and prevention of cross-infection; and (c) procedures conducted according to universal precautions. Proposals for best practices and global activities are reviewed at: www.who.int/sign.

At a national level, in many countries there are mandatory requirements for safety at work and these include hospitals and clinical laboratories. In the UK, the authority for this is the Health and Safety Executive, which has established procedures for prevention of infections in clinical laboratories.[48] The toxicity of all chemical reagents used in the laboratory, including those incorporated into kits, is governed by the Health and Safety Executive (HSE), which is responsible for the Control of Substances Hazardous to Health (COSHH) regulations and requires that any substances hazardous to health should be categorized and certified by COSHH with regard to degree of physical and biological hazard, safety measure for use, handling of spillage and waste disposal (see www.hse.gov.uk/pubns/chindex.htm).

Other essential sets of regulations for the laboratory concern the use of radioactive materials. These are described in the Ionizing Radiations Regulations 1999 (No. 3232). The management of these various regulations and methods for investigation of accidents are described by Holt.[49]

The specific safety requirements to be considered in laboratory practice are described below. They include design of premises, electrical and radiation safety, fire hazard, toxic and carcinogenic reagents, handling of biohazardous material and waste disposal.

Design of Laboratory

The area where work is carried out should be sufficiently large to easily accommodate items of equipment, all of which should be installed on fixed surfaces or stable trolleys. If possible, equipment which produces excessive noise should be kept separate from the general working area. Optimal lighting should be ensured and there should be adequate ventilation with protection from dust as well as a comfortable ambient temperature for workers and for optimal functioning of equipment. There should be appropriate storage facilities for chemicals (see below). Fire extinguishers and first-aid cabinets should be placed in easily accessible sites. The laboratory working area must meet design standards for 'level 2 containment' and there should be restricted access, which should be enforced where possible.

Electrical and Radiation Safety

All electrical equipment used should be certified by its manufacturer to comply with the national or international safety standards. Electrical equipment should not interfere electrically with *in vivo* medical devices (e.g. pacemakers) unless clearly marked with an appropriate caution. Before installation, all electrical devices should be inspected by someone trained in portable appliance testing, who must ensure that all plugs, fuses and electrical cables are appropriate and functional and that the plugs and cables are not adjacent to water taps. There should be a planned programme of preventive maintenance for each item of electrical equipment. All equipment should be decontaminated before inspection or repair.

Protection when handling radioactive material and using equipment for measuring radioactivity is described in Chapter 17, p. 374.

Fire Hazard

Most fires result from accidents with flammable substances such as alcohol and solvents. All manipulations of such substances must be carried out away from naked flames. Bulk stocks should be kept in flame-protected bins in a storage area separated from the laboratory and clearly marked as 'FIRE RISK'. Not more than 400 ml should be kept on an open bench or shelf. In many countries, gas burners are no longer available, but where they are used, they must never be left unattended and pilot lights must never be left on overnight. The burners should be as close as possible to the gas source and lengthy connecting tubes must be avoided.

Fire blankets and fire extinguishers, especially those suitable for dealing with electrical and chemical fires, should be placed near to doors of rooms and at strategic points in corridors. They should be inspected regularly.

Chemical Safety

Dangerous chemicals such as strong acids and alkalis must be stored at floor level; chemicals which are likely to react with each other must be stored well apart; poisons should be stored in locked cabinets. Manufacturers' product safety data sheets must be checked for advice on safe handling of any potentially toxic or carcinogenic substances. Such reagents must be stored in a secure place with restricted access; they should be handled only by experienced staff wearing protective clothing and weighing should be carried out in an air-flow cabinet at face velocity of around 0.8 m/s.

Eyewash Facilities

An eyewash station should be conveniently located where hazardous chemicals or biological materials are handled. This should consist of a spray device attached to the water supply by a flexible hose. If access to plumbing is not available, the alternative is an ample supply of easy-to-open containers of water.

Biohazardous Specimens

When handling blood, the most commonly encountered pathogens are HIV and hepatitis viruses. All specimens of human origin should be regarded as potentially infectious and must be handled appropriately by means of *universal precautions* in order to minimize exposure of skin and mucous membranes to the hazard. Special precautions are necessary with highly infectious specimens (see below).

Universal Precautions

1. Personal hygiene precautions to be adopted in areas where blood is collected, specimens are handled and analytical work is carried out:
   a. Eating, drinking and the application of cosmetics are absolutely forbidden.
   b. Staff should not wear jewellery and ideally, watches and rings should be removed.
   c. Disposable latex rubber or plastic gloves should be worn during sample handling and analytical work.*
   d. An outer protective gown or coat should be worn and personal clothing should not be allowed to protrude beyond the sleeves of the protective clothing.
   e. Any exposed cuts or abrasions must be kept covered with waterproof dressings.
   f. Hands must be washed when leaving analytical areas.
2. Venepuncture should be performed wearing disposable thin plastic or rubber latex gloves. Care must be taken to prevent injuries when handling syringes and disposing of the needles. Do not recap used needles by hand; do not detach the needle from the syringe or break, bend or otherwise manipulate used needles by hand. Used disposable syringes and needles, lancets and other sharp items such as glass slides, must be placed in a puncture-resistant plastic 'sharps' container for disposal. Care must be taken to avoid blood contamination of tourniquets as a potential cause of cross-infection. If necessary, they should be washed with soap and water.
3. As far as possible, only disposable syringes, needles and lancets should be used. Disposable syringes and lancets must never be reused on a different person.

---

*Irritant reactions to latex rubber or plastic gloves may be due to mechanical friction of the skin from poor fitting, prolonged use without changing the gloves, perspiration or a specific allergy. Handwashing with a mild antiseptic soap and application of an anti-inflammatory hand cream may be helpful. It may also be helpful to wear powder-free gloves and to wear a larger-sized glove to increase air circulation until the hands heal. In the event of a specific allergy to the chemical ingredients within the gloves, it may be worthwhile trying a different type or brand of glove.

4. Specimens should be sent to the laboratory in individual closed plastic bags, separated from the request forms to prevent their contamination should there be any leakage from the specimens. Ideally, the plastic bag should be placed inside another container. Tubes which minimize the risk of leakage are available.
5. Mouth pipetting is absolutely prohibited.
6. Centrifugation must be performed in sealed centrifuge buckets.
7. Blood and bone marrow slides must be handled in the same way as blood samples until they are fixed in methanol, stained and covered with a cover glass.
8. Used material must be placed in designated biohazard plastic bags awaiting disposal (see below).
9. Protective laboratory clothing (e.g. white coats) must never be worn outside the laboratory.
10. Additional precautions with infectious or potentially infectious material:
    a. Only experienced staff should perform procedures.
    b. Specimens should be handled in a microbiological safety cabinet (if the procedure involves generation of an aerosol) or in a clearly segregated and designated area of the laboratory.
    c. Specimens should be handled using protective clothing (close-fitting disposable gloves, disposable plastic apron, glasses or goggles, face mask).
    d. Disposable plastic should be used instead of glassware; sharp-pointed instruments (e.g. scissors) should not be used.
    e. There should be special arrangements for waste disposal (see p. 583).

Disinfectants

There are several types of chemical which have been used as germicides, including aldehydes, phenols, halogens, alcohols and hypochlorites. However, some of these are no longer available in laboratories. Those that are now used are indicated in Table 24.10. No single disinfectant is effective against all pathogens and their effectiveness depends on the nature of the organism.[47,50]

Sodium hypochlorite (chlorine)

This is the most commonly used disinfectant in the laboratory as it is very active against all microorganisms, although less active against fungi. Its disadvantage is that it is corrosive to metal. As hypochlorite solutions gradually lose their strength, fresh dilutions must be made daily. For general use, a concentration of 1 g/l (1000 ppm) as available chlorine is required; a stronger solution containing 5 g/l (5000 ppm) is necessary for dealing with blood spillage.

Household bleaches usually contain 50 g/l as available chlorine and should thus be diluted 1:50 for general use and 1:10 for blood contamination. Other chlorine-containing compounds which can be used are prepared as follows:

Calcium hypochlorite. (70% available chlorine) 1.4 g/l; 7 g/l for blood contamination.
Sodium dichloroisocyanurate (NaDCC). (60% available chlorine) 1.7 g/l; 20 g/l for blood contamination
Chloramine. (25% available chlorine) 20 g/l in all conditions.

Alcohols

Ethanol and isopropyl alcohol have similar disinfectant properties at a concentration of 70–80% in water; higher or lower concentrations reduce their germicidal effectiveness. They are active against vegetative bacteria and lipid viruses

Table 24.10 Properties of common disinfectants

REAGENT	CONCENTRATION (SEE TEXT)	ACTIVE AGAINST					
		Fungi	Bacteria	Myco-bacteria	Spores	Lipid-coated viruses	Non-lipid-coated viruses
A: Hypochlorites	1–10%	+	+++	++	++	+	+
B: Ethanol	70–80%	0	+++	+++	0	+	±
C: Isopropanol	70%	0	+++	+++	0	+	±
D: Iodoform	0.1–2%	+++	+++	+++	+	+	+

+, ++ and +++, Extent of effectiveness; ±, Variable, dependent on virus; 0, Not effective.
The disinfectants must be handled as toxic substances; all are eye irritants while A and D are also skin irritants and corrosive.

but not against spores or fungi. Their effect on non-lipid viruses is variable. Alcohol is especially effective when mixed with other agents (e.g. 80% alcohol with 100 g/l of formaldehyde or with 2 g/l (2000 ppm) available chlorine).

Applications of Disinfectants

Routinely, on completion of the day's work, the working area should be wiped with a freshly prepared 1% w/v sodium hypochlorite solution (chlorine bleach). Reusable pipettes should be soaked in a 2.5% solution for 30 min or longer. A 10% solution must be used for cleaning up blood spillage. The diluted sodium hypochlorite solution should be freshly made each day. It is helpful to add detergent to the solution as disinfectants are most active on clean surfaces. A stabilized blend of peroxide with surfactant and organic acids in a buffer system is available as a commercial product, 'Virkon' (*Antec-DuPont*). It appears to be effective as a general disinfectant for all hard surfaces, plastic and stainless steel laboratory equipment, medical instruments and laundry and also for absorbing spilled blood or other body fluids.

Automated equipment

Some automated equipment can be disinfected by flushing several times with 10% w/v sodium hypochlorite, followed by several flushes with water. Hypochlorite causes corrosion of metal surfaces. Other instruments have special requirements for decontamination; always refer to the manufacturer's instructions.

Centrifuges

Laboratory centrifuges require particular attention. They should never be cleaned using hypochlorite solution or other metal corrosives. Any spillage of blood should be dealt with immediately and the bowl, head and buckets (including rubber pads) should be disinfected regularly (e.g. with 2% Virkon) and then rinsed with a detergent

(e.g. Decon 90) or 70% ethanol. Special care is required when a glass or plastic tube breaks in a centrifuge (Table 24.11).

Syringes and needles

Although single-use disposable syringes and needles are strongly recommended, circumstances may require re-usables. These must be washed thoroughly in running water to remove all traces of blood. Syringes are then soaked for at least 30 min and needles overnight in 10% hypochlorite bleach. They are then rinsed under running tap water and soaked in two changes of distilled or deionized water. Finally, before reuse, they must be sterilized by heating in an oven at 120°C for 30 min.

Gloves

Disposable gloves must not be reused as they may retain contaminated material and may deteriorate when cleaned. Rubber household gloves may be washed and decontaminated by soaking in 1% hypochlorite solution for 30 min, but they must be discarded if they have punctures or tears or if they show signs of deterioration such as peeling or cracking.

Laundry

Soiled laundry must be placed in leak-proof labelled bags for transport to the laundry where the items should be washed in hot water (>70°C) with detergent for 25–30 min before being rinsed or alternatively soaked in 1% w/v sodium hypochlorite solution (see above) before being washed by hand.

Waste Disposal

The safe disposal of laboratory waste is of prime importance. Laboratory waste and contaminated materials presents a health hazard both to laboratory workers and to

---

Table 24.11 Procedure for decontaminating a centrifuge after breakage of a tube

1.	Switch off centrifuge motor and do not open lid for 1 h to allow aerosols to settle. Inform the safety officer.
2.	When breakage involves a known high-risk specimen in a sealed bucket, strong gloves, goggles and a protective apron must be worn and the bucket opened in a safety cabinet.
3.	If the leakage was confined to a sealed bucket, manually open the centrifuge and, using forceps to remove broken tubes and any solid debris, discard the contents of the bucket into 2% Virkon.
4.	Decontaminate the inside of the lid, bowl and external surfaces of the buckets with 2% Virkon, rinse with Microsol 3+ (*Analis, Belgium*) or a detergent such as Decon 90 or 70% ethanol and leave to dry.
5.	Buckets, rotors and other small centrifuge items may be autoclaved where appropriate. Alternatively, more delicate items (e.g. whole microfuges) may be fumigated within a safety cabinet.
6.	All contaminated disposable material must be placed in appropriate bags for autoclaving.

the community. The careless dumping of solid and liquid chemical and biological waste is also a threat to the environment. WHO has a useful website (www.healthcarewaste-management.org) which provides up-to-date information on various aspects of waste management, including country-specific and region-specific problems and legal requirements.

Laboratory waste is classified under the following headings:

- Infectious materials
- Pathological materials
- Radioactive materials
- Genotoxic substances
- Sharps
- Chemicals, including analyser effluents
- Pharmaceuticals
- Heavy metals, including batteries, broken thermometers
- Pressurized containers
- General, non-clinical waste.

Blood and other potentially infected body fluids can be poured down a drain safely only if it is connected to a sanitary sewer. The drain should then be immediately flushed with water, followed by 250 ml of 10% hypochlorite and finally again flushed with water. In the absence of a sewer system, the material should be ducted into holding tanks for steam heating or chemical treatment before final discharge to the public sewers. Specimen containers, used syringes, swabs and tissues should be collected in special colour-coded bags for subsequent incineration or autoclaving before being disposed of in a rubbish dump. 'Sharps' containers should be incinerated without opening.

Highly infectious specimens require special management:

- They should be segregated from other potentially infectious waste and placed immediately in a leak-proof bag or container.
- If possible, they should be disinfected immediately by autoclaving or by chemical treatment; the waste can then be handled alongside other clinical waste.
- If not immediately disinfected, they should be placed in identifiable (e.g. yellow) bags, labelled with the biohazard symbol and marked as 'HIGHLY INFECTIOUS WASTE'. The bags should then be taken immediately to a central storage point for disposal.

Information about the disposal of specific chemicals is usually given in the manufacturer's safety data sheet and a waste control strategy should be established, taking account of toxic and carcinogenic materials, corrosive substances, flammable substances and reactive chemicals with risk of explosion. Analyser effluents which do not contain chemicals that potentially react with metal waste piping can be discharged directly into a main sewer.

Pressurized containers must not be punctured or incinerated. They should be carefully discharged in the open air away from people and then discarded in non-hazardous waste containers.

General waste includes office and domestic material, paper and packaging and other substances not hazardous to human health. This may either be incinerated or disposed of according to local facilities.

SPECIMEN SHIPPING

There are strict national and international regulations about packaging and shipment of patients' specimens and other biological material by post or air transport; these also apply to courier services.[51,52] The International Air Transport Association (IATA) requires that specimens must be packaged in accordance with requirements described on their website.

The following is a summary of the requirements:

1. A primary sealed, leak-proof container for the specimen
2. Absorbent material surrounding the primary container; if several primary containers are packed together they must be individually wrapped to prevent contact with each other and to ensure a tight packing
3. Secondary protecting container (e.g. rigid plastic tube, corrugated fibre-board or polystyrene box). If being sent by air, this container must be capable of withstanding a 95 kPa pressure differential without leakage
4. Outer packaging, such as a secure rigid cardboard or fibre-board box or a bubble-wrap mailing envelope
5. The outer package must be clearly labelled 'BIOHAZARD' together with the universal biohazard symbol. It is also advisable to add a warning that the parcel must only be opened by an authorized person, preferably in the laboratory. If sent by air, the label must state 'Packed in Compliance with IATA Packing Instruction 650'.

When plasma or serum must be maintained in a frozen state, the packed specimen should be placed in an insulated container surrounded by dry ice. Conversely, care must be taken to prevent freezing of whole blood specimens. The container must also permit release of CO_2 gas to prevent build-up of pressure. Specific airline regulations should be checked to ensure that dry ice is not deemed to be a hazardous material.

REFERENCES

1. Stanfliet JC, Macauley J, Pillay TS. Quality of teaching in chemical pathology; ability of interns to order and interpret. *J Clin Pathol*. 2009;62: 664–666.

2. Stuart J, Hicks JM. Good laboratory management: an Anglo-American perspective. *J Clin Pathol*. 1991;44: 793–797.

3. Delost MD, Miller WG, Chang GA, et al. Influence of credentials of clinical pathology professionals on proficiency testing performance. *Am J Clin Pathol*. 2009;132:550–554.

4. College of American Pathologists Workload and Personnel Management Committee. *Workload Recording Method and Personnel Management Manual*. College of American Pathologists. Northfield, IL: USA; 1992.

5. Bennett CH. Welcan UK: its development and future. *J Clin Pathol*. 1991;44:617–620.

6. Macdonald AJ, Bradshaw AE, Holmes WA, et al. The impact of an integrated haematology screening service on laboratory practice. *Clin Lab Haematol*. 1996;18:271–276.

7. International Organization for Standardization. *Accuracy (trueness and precision) of measurement, methods and results. ISO 5725 Parts 1–4*. Geneva: ISO; 1994.

8. Ellison SLR, Rosslein M, Williams A. *Quantifying uncertainty in analytic measurement*. Download from Eurachem-CITACGuide. 2007.

9. Wagar EA, Friedberg RC, Souers R, et al. Critical values comparison: A College of American Pathologists Q-probes survey of 163 clinical laboratories. *Arch Pathol Lab Med*. 2007;131:1769–1775.

10. Viljoen A, Twomey PJ. True or not: uncertainty of laboratory results. *J Clin Pathol*. 2007;60:587–588.

11. Galen RS, Gambino S. *Beyond Normality: the Predictive Value and Efficiency of Medical Diagnoses*. New York: Wiley; 1975.

12. Griner PF, Nayawski RJ, Mushlin AI, et al. Selection and interpretation of diagnostic tests and procedures: principles and applications. *Ann Intern Med*. 1981;94:553–592.

13. Youden WJ. Index for rating diagnostic tests. *Cancer*. 1950;3:32–35.

14. Hernandez JS. Cost-effectiveness of laboratory testing. *Arch Pathol Lab Med*. 2003;127:440–445.

15. van Walraven C, Naylor CD. Do we know what inappropriate laboratory utilization is? A systematic review of laboratory clinical audits. *J Am Med Assoc*. 1998;280:550–558.

16. International Council for Standardization in Haematology. Guidelines for the evaluation of blood cell analysers including those used for differential leucocyte and reticulocyte counting and cell marker applications. *Clin Lab Haematol*. 1994;16:157–174.

17. Henry JB, Kelly KC. Comprehensive graphic-based display of clinical laboratory data. *Am J Clin Pathol*. 2003;119:330–336.

18. Kiley R. *Medical Information on the Internet: a Guide for Health Professionals*. 3rd ed. Edinburgh: Churchill Livingstone; 2003.

19. Narayanan S. The preanalytic phase: an important component of laboratory medicine. *Am J Clin Pathol*. 2000;113:429–452.

20. Fraser CG, Woodford FP. Strategies to modify the test-requesting patterns of clinicians. *Ann Clin Biochem*. 1987;24:223–231.

21. Mutimer D, McCauley B, Nightingale P, et al. Computerised protocols for laboratory investigation and their effect on use of medical time and resources. *J Clin Pathol*. 1992;45:572–574.

22. Wagar EA, Stankovic AK, Raab S, et al. Specimen labeling errors: A Q-probes analysis of 147 clinical laboratories. *Arch Pathol Lab Med*. 2008;132: 1617–1622.

23. Lippi G, Blanckaert N, Bonini P, et al. Causes, consequences, detection and prevention of identification errors in laboratory diagnostics. *Clin Chem Lab Med*. 2009;47:143–153.

24. Kratz A, Salem RO, Van Cott EM. Effects of a pneumatic tube system on routine and novel hematology and coagulation parameters in healthy volunteers. *Arch Pathol Lab Med*. 2007;131:293–296.

25. Wallin O, Söderberg J, Grankvist K, et al. Preanalytical effects of pneumatic tube transport on routine haematology, coagulation parameters, platelet function and global coagulation. *Clin Chem Lab Med*. 2008;46:1443–1449.

26. Graham E. An episode of increased hemolysis due to a defective pneumatic air tube delivery system. *Clin Biochem*. 2009;42:1265–1269.

27. Wagar EA, Friedberg RC, Souers R, et al. Critical values comparison: A College of American Pathologists Q-probe survey of 163 clinical laboratories. *Arch Pathol Lab Med*. 2007;131:1769–1775.

28. Piva E, Sciacovelli M, Laposata M, et al. Evaluation of effectiveness of a computerized notification system for reporting critical values. *Am J Clin Pathol*. 2009;131:432–441.

29. McLean R, Jury C, Bazeos A, et al. Application of camera phones in telehaematology. *J Telemed Telecare*. 2009;15:339–343.

30. Winkelman JW, Tansijevic MJ, Wynbenga DR, et al. How fast is fast enough for clinical laboratory turnabout time? Measurement of the interval between result entry and inquiries for reports. *Am J Clin Pathol*. 1997;108:400–405.

31. Valenstein PN. Laboratory turnaround time. *Am J Clin Pathol*. 1996;105:676–688.

32. Hillbourne L, Lee H, Cathcart P. STAT testing? A guideline for meeting clinician turnaround time requirements. *Am J Clin Pathol*. 1996;105:671–675.

33. Valenstein PN, Wagar EA, Stankovic AK, et al. Notification of critical results: A College of American Pathologists Q-probes study of 121 institutions. *Arch Pathol Lab Med*. 2008;132:1862–1867.

34. Briggs C, Guthrie D, Hyde K, et al. Guidelines for point-of-care testing: Haematology. *Br J Haematol*. 2008;142:904–915.

35. Briggs C, Carter J, Lee S-H, et al. ICSH guidelines for worldwide point-of-care testing in haematology with special reference to the complete blood count. *International Journal of*

Laboratory Hematology. 2008;30: 105–116.

36. Medical Devices Agency. *Management and Use of IVD Point-of-Care Test Devices.* London: MDA, UK Department of Health; 2002.

37. Clinical and Laboratory Standards Institute. *Point-of-Care in vitro Diagnostic (IVD) Testing; Approved Guidelines.* 2nd ed. Vol 26. No 30. Wayne, PA, USA: CLSI; 2006.

38. International Standards Organization. *ISO 22870: Point-of-care testing (POCT) – requirements for quality and competence.* Geneva: ISO; 2006.

39. Rose PE, Fitzmaurice D. New approaches to the delivery of anticoagulant services. *Blood Rev.* 1998;12:84–90.

40. Ansell JE, Patel N, Ostrovsky D, et al. Long-term patient self-management of oral anticoagulation. *Arch Intern Med.* 1995;155:2185–2189.

41. Erasmus RT, Zemlin AE. Clinical audit in the laboratory. *J Clin Pathol.* 2009;62:593–597.

42. Clinical Laboratory Improvement Amendments (CLIA'88). *Code of Federal Regulations: Laboratory Requirements.* Federal register 10/2004 Part 493, p. 967. Atlanta, GA, USA: CDC.

43. College of American Pathologists. *Standards for laboratory accreditation.* Northfield, IL, USA: College of American Pathologists; 1998.

44. Galloway M, Nadin L. Benchmarking and the laboratory. *J Clin Pathol.* 2001;54:590–1559.

45. International Electrotechnical Commission. *Safety Requirements for Electrical Equipment for Measurement, Control and Laboratory Use: Part 1: General Requirements IEC/ISO/EN 61010.* Geneva: ISO; 2001 [Other sections of this standard relate to particular requirements, e.g. Part 020: laboratory centrifuges; Part 081: semi-automated analysers; Part 101 in vitro diagnostic (IVD) medical equipment].

46. World Health Organization. *Safety in Health-care Laboratories.* Document LAB/97.1. Geneva: WHO; 1997.

47. World Health Organization. *Laboratory Biosafety Manual.* 3rd ed. Geneva: WHO; 2004.

48. United Kingdom Health and Safety Executive. *Safe Working and the Prevention of Infections in Clinical Laboratories.* Sudbury, Suffolk, UK: HSE Books; 1991.

49. Holt A. *Principles of Health and Safety at Work.* 6th ed. Wigston, UK: Institute of Occupational Safety and Health; 2002.

50. Gardner JF, Peel MM. *Sterilization, Disinfection and Infection Control.* 3rd ed. London: Churchill Livingstone; 1998.

51. Nations United. *Recommendations on the Transport of Dangerous Goods. Model Regulations.* 15th ed. New York and Geneva: United Nations; 2007.

52. European Committee for Standardization. *EN 829: Transport Packages for Medical and Biological Specimens – Requirements, Tests.* Brussels: CEN; 1996.

Chapter | **25** |

Quality assurance

Mary West, Joan-Lluís Vives Corrons

In the haematology laboratory it is essential to ensure that the right test is carried out on the right specimen and that the correct results are delivered to the appropriate recipient without delay. Quality assurance (QA) is defined as the overall programme for achieving these objectives. It must also ensure adequate control of the pre-analytical and post-analytical stages, i.e. from specimen collection to the timely despatch of an informative report. A QA programme should also include standardization of tests and of instrumentation in order to achieve acceptable levels of precision and accuracy. These objectives represent *good laboratory practice* (*GLP*); the mechanism for achieving GLP is encompassed in *Total Quality Management* (*TQM*) (Table 25.1).

STANDARDIZATION

Clinical laboratory errors lead to adverse effects on patient diagnosis, therapy and outcomes, also resulting in the inappropriate use of funds. Standardization plays an important role in patient care because it contributes to a decrease in the number of errors, thus improving the harmonization of procedures and comparability between different laboratories. The introduction of the International Standardization Organization (ISO) standards BS EN ISO 9001 (*Quality management systems – requirements*), BS EN ISO 17025 (*General requirements*), BS EN ISO 15189 (*Medical laboratories – particular requirements for quality and competence*) and BS EN ISO 22870 (*Point-of-care testing*) places quality at the heart of all activities (see also Table 24.8). In the UK, the focus for laboratory practice has been on Clinical Pathology Accreditation (UK) Ltd (CPA), which has evolved to reflect the way service delivery is perceived within pathology and is now linked to UK Accreditation Service. Quality management systems may also include requirements arising from regulations related to blood and tissues and the Good Manufacturing Practice (GMP) guide, while through the ISO standards, there is a move towards international harmonization.

Standardization of haematology laboratory practice plays a pivotal role in patient care and is essential for

Table 25.1 Definitions used in total quality management (TQM)

1.	Quality assurance (QA)	Overall programme that ensures that the final results reported are correct. QA includes an adequate control of the pre-analytical and post-analytical stages from specimen collection to the timely dispatch of an informative report. A QA programme also includes standardization of procedures and instrumentation.
2.	Quality control (QC)	Measures that must be included during each assay run to verify that the test is working properly.
3.	Proficiency testing (PT)	Procedure to determine the quality of the results generated by the laboratory. Accordingly, PT is a challenge to the effectiveness of the QA and QC programmes and it can be internal or external (also termed 'quality assessment').
4.	Internal quality control (IQC)	Monitoring the haematology test procedures to ensure continual evaluation of the reliability of the daily work of the laboratory with validation of tests before reports are released.
5.	External quality assessment (EQA)	Evaluation by an outside agency of the between-laboratory and between-method comparability. It can be organized nationally, regionally or internationally.
6.	Continuous quality improvement (CQI)	Philosophy and attitude for analysing capabilities and processes and improving them repeatedly to achieve the objective of customer satisfaction.
7.	Accreditation	Certification by a duly recognized authority of the facilities, capability, objectivity, competence and integrity of an agency.
8.	Non-compliance	A process which does not comply with a quality system.

certification and accreditation. It should include the following topics:

1. Evaluation and selection of instrumentation and procedures
2. Training and certification of personnel
3. Establishment of quality control protocols
4. Test protocols, equipment maintenance and troubleshooting records
5. Protocols for test requisitioning and result reporting and active review of results by laboratory director or other designated person
6. Setting up policies regarding instrument maintenance and supplies.

Standardization of procedures and devices used in the haematology laboratory are the concern of the international professional organizations, especially the International Council for Standardization in Haematology (ICSH). The International Organization of Standardization (ISO) and Comité Européen de Normalization (CEN) have also established standards for medical laboratory practice and for the use of *in vitro* diagnostic medical devices. At a national level, the British Committee for Standards in Haematology (BCSH) publishes guidelines in books, on websites or as journal articles, and in the USA, a wide range of practice guidelines have been published by the Clinical and Laboratory Standards Institute (CLSI) (formerly the National Committee for Clinical Laboratory Standards, NCCLS). Lists of published documents and catalogues from these various organizations can be found on their various websites (see Table 25.2; see also Tables 24.5 and 24.8).

External quality-assessment schemes have a role in identifying unsatisfactory performance by devices. Some of the terms and definitions generally used in laboratory practice are summarized in Table 25.3.

CONTROL MATERIALS AND REFERENCE STANDARDS

The main international authority concerned with material standards (reference preparations) for laboratory medicine is the World Health Organization (WHO). In the European Union, the Institute for Reference Materials and Measurements (IRMM) has established numerous 'certified reference materials' for haematology and clinical chemistry. International standards are not intended for routine use but serve as stable standards for assigning values to commercial (or laboratory-produced) 'secondary standards' or calibrators.

Control materials are available commercially and they can also be made locally, although there may be technical difficulties in preparing such 'homemade' materials. For example, stored plasma may become turbid; chemical or serological analysis may be affected by instability of enzymes; immunological reactions may be interfered with by added preservatives. With the blood count, there are especially difficult problems because of the need to ensure homogeneity in aliquot samples and due to the instability of blood cells, while procedures that enhance the stability of blood samples may also affect the behaviour of the cells. Thus, control material is not strictly analogous to fresh blood. Nonetheless,

Table 25.2 Some organizations involved in standardization and quality management systems

ABBREVIATION	ORGANIZATION	WEBSITE
AFNOR	Association Française de Normalization	www.afnor.org
AENOR	Asociación Española de Normalización y Certificación	www.aenor.es
INSTAND	Gesellschaft zur Förderung der Qualitätssicherung in medizinischen Laboratorien	www.instandev.de
WHO	WHO EQAS for Haematology	www.who.int/diagnostics_laboratory/quality/haematology/en/index.html
AMREF	African Medical and Research Foundation, Nairobi, Kenya	www.amref.org
ANCLSH	Asian Network for Clinical Laboratory Standardization and Harmonization	www.ancls.org
ASQ	American Society of Quality	www.asq.org
BCSH	British Committee for Standards in Haematology	www.bcshguidelines.com
CAP	College of American Pathologists	www.cap.org
CEN	The European Committee for Standardization	www.cen.eu
CLSI	Clinical and Laboratory Standards Institute	www.clsi.org
ICSH	International Council for Standardization in Haematology	www.islh.org
IRMM	Institute of Reference Materials and Measurements	Irmm.jrc.ec.europa.eu
ISO	International Organization for Standardization	www.iso.org
JCAHO	Joint Commission for the Accreditation of Healthcare Organizations	www.jointcommission.org
PPTC	Pacific Paramedical Training Centre New Zealand	www.pptc.org.nz
RCPA	Royal College of Pathologists Australia	www.rcpaqap.com.au
UK NEQAS	United Kingdom National External Quality Assessment Scheme	www.ukneqas.org.uk
EQALM	European Committee of External Quality Assurance Programmes in Laboratory Medicine	www.eqalm.org

provided attention is paid to these difficulties, preserved or stabilized blood provides suitable material for internal quality control procedures for haemoglobin concentration, red cell counts, platelet counts and leucocyte counts (see p. 599: Preparation of extended-life material for QA).

Reference Standards

International reference materials relevant to haematology are held at designated institutions (Table 25.4), the relevant websites should be checked for availability of any particular one.

The accessibility of an international reference preparation of haemiglobincyanide (HiCN), first developed by the International Council for Standardization in Haematology (ICSH), has provided improved accuracy of haemoglobin measurement. In some countries, preparations that conform to the international standard are certified by the appropriate national authorities. An important feature of this material is that it is stable for at least several years. A limited quantity of the international standard can be obtained from WHO; a comparable certified reference material is available from IRMM (Table 25.4) and ICSH has recently produced a new preparation with similar specifications.[1] Where the use of cyanide reagent for routine haemoglobinometry is prohibited, the haemiglobincyanide standard can still be used to assign a haemoglobin value to a lysate or a whole blood preparation, which is then used as the local secondary

Table 25.3 Terms relating to quality control in clinical laboratory practice

Precision	Can be controlled by replicate tests and by repeated tests on previously measured specimens
Accuracy	Can be checked only by the use of reference materials that have been assayed by reference methods
Standardization	Encompasses both materials and methods. *Material standard* or *reference preparations* are used to calibrate analytical instruments and to assign quantitative values to calibrators. Where possible they must be traceable to defined physical or chemical measurement based on the metrological units of length (metre), mass (kilogram), amount of substance (mole) and time (seconds)
Reference method	Is an exactly defined technique that is used in association with a reference preparation, when available, to provide sufficiently precise and accurate data for scientific purposes and for assessing the validity of other methods
Selected method	Is one that is directly comparable with and traceable to the international reference method; it serves as an alternative to the reference method when an international reference material is not available; it should be used for evaluation and validation of a proposed routine (working) method
Working (or recommended) method	Is intended for use in routine practice, taking account of economy of labour and materials and ease of performance and having been shown by a validation study with a reference method to be sufficiently reliable for its intended purpose
Controls	Are preparations that are used for either internal quality control or external quality assessment. Some control preparations have assigned values but they should not be used as standards because the assigned values are usually only approximations and they are often stable for a limited time only
True value	This is an ideal concept which in general cannot be achieved
Accepted true value	The value approximating the true value, the difference between the two values is negligible
Error	The discrepancy between the result of a measurement and the true (or accepted true) value
Random error	An error which varies in an unpredictable manner, in magnitude and sign, when a large number of measurements of the same quantity are made under effectively identical conditions
Systematic error	An error which, in the course of a number of measurements of the same value of a given quantity, remains constant when measurements are made under the same conditions or varies according to a definite law when conditions change

standard after appropriate dilution. However, many laboratories are unable to make use of this reference preparation as they no longer have suitable instruments on which to use it. Undiluted lysate is usually stable for up to 6 months, or frozen for several years. Whole blood is stable for about 3 weeks, but for only a few days after dilution. Both whole blood and lysates are useful for quality assurance of haemoglobinometry; whole blood reference samples should be introduced into batches of blood samples and all the samples should be assayed together. This applies to both automated and manual methods.

Assigning Values to Reference Materials

Methods used for assigning values to reference materials must be as accurate and precise as is practical. Standardized reference methods have been described for haemoglobin concentration, red blood cell count, white blood cell count and packed cell volume/haematocrit (see Chapter 3).

QUALITY ASSURANCE PROCEDURES

The procedures that should be included in a quality assurance programme vary with the tests undertaken, the instruments used and (especially if these include a fully automatic counting system) the size of the laboratory and the numbers of specimens handled. Also, the computer facilities available and the amount of time that can be devoted to the quality control assurance must be taken into account. At least some form of internal quality control must be undertaken and there must be participation in an external quality assessment scheme where one is available. Some control procedures should be performed daily and other performance checks should be done at appropriate intervals. The latter is particularly important when there is a change

Table 25.4 Standard materials available internationally

General haematology	Erythropoietin, human, urinary Erythropoietin, recombinant DNA-derived Ferritin, human, recombinant Hb A$_2$ Hb F Folate, whole blood C-reactive protein Human serum for immunoassay	WHO/NIBSC
	Haemiglobincyanide Haemoglobin Reference Standard	WHO/NIBSC BCR/IRMM ICSH
Immunohaematology	Anti-A blood typing serum, anti-B blood typing serum, anti-RhD incomplete blood typing serum, RhD complete blood typing serum, E complete blood typing serum	WHO/CLB
Immunology	Human serum immunoglobulin Immunoglobulin G (IgG), A, M, E Antinuclear factor, homogeneous Horseradish peroxidase-conjugate sheep antihuman IgG Human serum complement components C1q, C4, C5, factor B and functional CH$_{50}$	WHO/NIBSC
Coagulation	Ancrod, antithrombin plasma, antithrombin concentrate, factor VIII and von Willebrand factor plasma, II, VII, IX, X, VIII, IXa concentrate, plasma fibrinogen, plasmin, plasminogen activator inhibitor, tissue plasminogen activator recombinant, streptokinase, alpha-thrombin, beta-thromboglobulin, antihuman platelet antigen 1a, platelet factor 4, proteins S and C plasma, urokinase high molecular weight, von Willebrand factor concentrate, von Willebrand factor antigen	WHO/NIBSC
	Thromboplastin bovine combined, thromboplastin human recombinant, thromboplastin rabbit plain	BCR/IRMM WHO/CLB
WHO/NIBSC	National Institute for Biological Standards and Control, South Mimms EN6 3QH, UK. E-mail: standards@nibsc.ac.uk; www.NIBSC/Catalogue list/Reference standards. See also: World Health Organization/biological standards	
BCR/IRMM	Institute for Reference Materials and Measurements, Retieseweg B2440, Geel, Belgium. E-mail: bcr.sales@irmm.jrc.be; www.irmm/reference materials	
WHO/CLB	Central Laboratory of Netherlands Red Cross Blood Transfusion Service, 125 Plesmanlaan, 1066 AD Amsterdam, Netherlands. Netherlands Blood Transfusion Service/Central Laboratory	

in staff and after maintenance service or repair has been carried out on equipment. A comprehensive protocol is summarized in Table 25.5.

During the last 20 years, automation, standardization and technological advances have significantly improved the analytical reliability of laboratory results with a high level of accuracy and decreased error rates in the blood count assay.

Quality design must begin with *analytical* quality, as it is the essential quality characteristic of any laboratory test. Analytical variations may arise from unsuspected abnormal binding protein(s) in patients, such as heterophile antibodies, anti-animal antibodies and anti-idiotypic antibodies. The exact effect will depend on the site of the interaction with the reaction, leading to falsely raised or lowered measurements.[2] More recent data underline the importance of analytical accuracy due to the frequent calibration error that leads to analytical bias affecting the number of patients passing decision thresholds in practice guidelines. The effects of this medically and economically have been demonstrated.[3] To ensure reliability in the analytical phase, procedures are required for internal quality control, external quality assessment and standardization. All laboratory staff require training in these various aspects of quality assurance. A useful training manual from WHO* describes

---

*Available on request to the Department of Essential Health Technology, WHO, 1211 Geneva 27, Switzerland.

Table 25.5 Schedule for quality control procedures	
1. Calibration with reference standards	
Instruments	6-month intervals or more frequently if control chart or EQA indicates bias or fluctuation in results and after any repair/service
Others: pipettes and scales	Calibration of equipment used for manual techniques should not be overlooked; these should be done annually
Diluting systems	Initially and at 1–2-week intervals
2. Control chart with control material	
Daily or more frequently with each batch of specimens	
Duplicate tests on two or three patients' samples: if control chart or delta check shows discrepancies	
3. Analysis of patients' results	
Daily to check constancy of mean values for MCV, MCH, MCHC: correlation assessment of test report	
Cumulative results: following previous tests and if changes in clinical state	
Blood film examination if unusual test results and/or counter flags appear	
4. EQAS performance	
Assessment monthly	

the principles and methods, together with practical exercises to illustrate these.[4] Another good teaching source is J.O. Westgard's website: www.westgard.com; this includes a 'Lesson of the Month' and other current topics that are regularly updated. The quality control of the analytical stage includes Internal Quality Control (IQC) and External Quality Assessment (EQA).

Internal Quality Control

IQC is based on monitoring the haematology test procedures that are performed in the laboratory and includes measurements on specially prepared materials and repeated measurements on routine specimens, together with daily statistical analysis of the data. IQC is primarily a demonstration of precision. It ensures continual checks that the established reliability of the laboratory's work does not fluctuate and that reports are validated before they are released. It is based on monitoring the procedures that are actually used for the tests in the laboratory.

IQC includes:

- Control charts with tests on control materials
- Duplicate tests on a proportion of the specimens
- Consistency of mean values of patient data
- Correlation check (e.g. blood film features or agreement with interrelated parameters).

Control Charts

These were first applied in clinical chemistry by Levey and Jennings.[5] They are now widely used in haematology for both automated and manual procedures. Samples of the control specimen are included in every batch of patients' specimens and the results are checked on a control chart. To check precision, it is not necessary to know the exact value of the control specimen. If, however, its value has been determined reliably by a reference method, the same material can also be used to check accuracy or to calibrate an instrument. If possible, controls with high, low and normal values should be used. It is advisable to use at least one control sample per batch, even if the batch is very small, also at set intervals during a large run, at least once for every 50 patient specimens. Because the controls are intended to simulate random sampling, they must be treated exactly like the patients' specimens. The results obtained with the control samples can be plotted on a chart as described below.

The mean value and standard deviation (SD) of the control specimen should first be established in the laboratory where the tests are performed. Using arithmetic graph paper, a horizontal line is drawn to represent the mean (as a base), and on an appropriate scale of quantity and unit, lines representing +2SD and −2SD are drawn above and below the mean. The results of successive control sample measurements are plotted. If the test is satisfactory, sequential results oscillate about the mean value and <5% of the results fall outside 2SD. Figure 25.1 illustrates a control chart from an automated system; a similar principle can be used for simple methods where the data are plotted manually (Fig. 25.2).

Any of the following indicates a fault in technique or in the instrument or reagent:

- One widely deviant result outside 3SD = a gross error or 'blunder'
- One or two results on or beyond the +2SD or −2SD limits = random error
- Several consecutive similar results on one side of the mean = calibration fault causing a consistent bias
- Consecutive fluctuating values, rising and falling by 2SD = imprecision.

The fault may be in the reagents or the laboratory-ware or it may be caused by incorrect adjustment/calibration of the instrument or other equipment, e.g. pipettes, technical error or even clerical error in transcribing the results. Before an intensive investigation, the test should be repeated with another sample and the possibility must also be considered that the inconsistency may be the result of deterioration or infection of the batch of reagent material or insufficient mixing of the sample. This control process is unlikely to detect an error in an individual specimen, which can only be detected by correlation checks. For haemoglobinometry, it may be useful to use both whole blood and lysate in a quality control check because differences in results

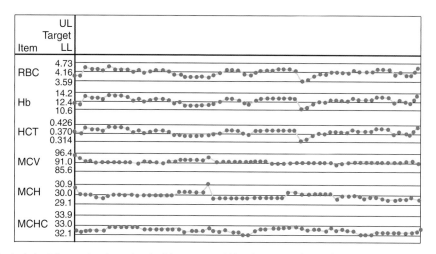

Figure 25.1 Control chart (Levey–Jennings chart) with automated blood count analyser. The mean value for each component of the blood count is shown, together with the upper limit (UL) and lower limit (LL) for satisfactory performance, which have been set at ± 2SD.

Figure 25.2 Control chart for haemoglobinometry by manual method. The limits for satisfactory performance have been set at ± 2SD.

obtained with these two preparations help to identify errors resulting from incorrect dilution, inadequate mixing or failure of a reagent to bring about complete lysis. If the control specimen is included with each batch of tests during the course of a day, their measurements should not differ by more than the established CV. A trend of sequentially increasing or decreasing values with the repeated measurements is indicative of drift.

Duplicate Tests on Patients' Specimens

Duplicate tests on patients' specimens provide another way of checking the precision of routine work.[6]

MCHC is used to identify any drift of the three indices and used to identify instrument faults; an increased SD signifies loss of precision. To ensure that each batch is representative, the samples should be randomized before analysis and, if possible, within batch of 20, no more than seven should come from one clinical source or from patients with the same clinical condition. In laboratories still using manual methods, a simple adaptation of the same principle can be applied, confined to MCHC and excluding results from any special clinic that are likely to be specifically biased. From the daily means for all measurements on 10 consecutive working days, an overall daily mean and SD are established. The mean MCHC is then calculated at the end of each day. If the test does not vary by more than ±2SD, it is considered satisfactory but this may be misleading if there is an error in the same direction in both haemoglobin and PCV. The results may be displayed graphically, as illustrated in Figure 25.3. It is useful in validating successive batches of calibrators. The method is now incorporated in many automated blood counters (Fig. 25.4). A similar instrument-specific procedure is used by some manufacturers who gather the data submitted through network links by users of their instruments. This enables them to maintain a constant check of performance of these instruments overall and to detect any that require recalibration or investigation of faults.

Correlation Check

Correlation check implies that any unexpected result of a test must be checked to see whether it can be explained on clinical grounds or whether it correlates with other tests.

Figure 25.3 Quality control based on patients' data. Control of manual blood counts using the mean cell haemoglobin concentration (MCHC) as an indicator.

Thus, for example, unexpectedly higher or lower haemoglobin might be explained, e.g. by a blood transfusion or by a haemorrhage, respectively. A low MCHC should be confirmed by demonstrating hypochromic red cells on a Romanowsky-stained blood film; a high MCV must correlate with macrocytosis. Similarly, the blood films should be examined to confirm marked leucocytosis or leucopenia or thrombocytosis or thrombocytopenia, to distinguish between platelets and red cell fragments or conversely between giant platelets and normal-sized red cells or to check an erroneously high leucocyte count as a result of incompletely lysed red cells in haemoglobinopathies or liver disease. This morphological procedure can only be used if the blood smear is correctly made and stained; otherwise, blood cell morphology may be misleading.

Recording blood count data on cumulative report forms or charts is good clinical practice and provides an inbuilt quality control system by making it easy to detect an aberrant result when compared with a previously determined baseline. This is especially useful in detecting the occasional wild errors caused by incorrect labelling of the specimen, inadequate suspension of the blood before sampling, partial clotting of a blood sample or deterioration on storage. A discrepant result without apparent clinical reason must be suspect until confirmed by a repeat test on a fresh specimen. The occurrence of a contrasting discrepancy in two different specimens on the same day would suggest that two specimens have been mixed up. It is worthwhile emphasizing the importance of the blood film for quality control, especially as it may tend to be considered obsolete with the increasingly automated blood count systems. Any obvious discrepancy between the count obtained by the analyser and subjective impression of morphology should always be checked. A blood film will confirm or refute an abnormally high or low leucocyte or platelet count. An important cause of artefactual leucopenia and thrombocytopenia is partial clotting of the specimen – this may be revealed by the presence, in the film, of fibrin strands with a mass of aggregated platelets. The film will also identify anomalies due to the presence of cold agglutinins, a high leucocyte count due to incomplete lysis of red cells in haemoglobinopathies, etc.

External Quality Assessment

EQA is based on the evaluation by an outside agency of the analytical performance on specially supplied samples by a number of laboratories. The objective is to achieve between-laboratory and between-method comparability and it does not necessarily guarantee accuracy unless the specimens have been assayed by a reference laboratory alongside a reference preparation of known value.

EQA complements internal quality control and is a basic requirement for clinical laboratory certification and accreditation. Certification is a procedure by which a third party gives written assurance that a product, process or service

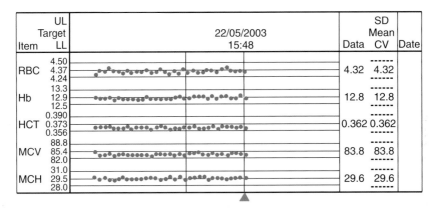

Figure 25.4 Quality control based on patients' data. Control of automated blood counts by mean results for RBC, Hb, HCT, MCV and MCH. The predetermined means are shown together with the upper limits (UL) and lower limits (LL) for satisfactory control.

conforms to specific requirements, whereas accreditation is a procedure by which an authoritative body gives formal recognition that a body or person is competent to carry out specific tasks. Accreditation standards related to clinical laboratories place emphasis on having an effective quality assurance system in place, with a commitment to meeting the needs of patients and their doctors as users of laboratory services and a need for continuous cycle of quality improvement at the centre of all policy-making operational decisions (see also Chapter 24, p. 579)

The term *EQA*, also known as proficiency testing (PT), was adopted in 1979 by a WHO working group on Quality Assurance of Health Laboratories. It is defined as: '*a system whereby a set of reagents and techniques are assessed by an external source and the results of the testing laboratory are compared with those of an approved reference laboratory or agency*'.[7] It allows an individual laboratory to compare its performance for one or more tests or techniques against that of other laboratories. Thus, even when all precautions are taken to achieve accuracy and precision in the laboratory, errors arise that are only detectable by objective EQA of the performance of a number of laboratories on material which has been supplied specially for the purpose. EQAS are usually organized, nationally or regionally, as one or PT programmes. National schemes are frequently termed NEQAS (National External Quality Assessment Scheme).

EQA analysis of performance is retrospective and, in addition to inter-laboratory comparability, its main objective is to achieve the harmonization of methods and procedures or educational purposes. EQAS is not necessarily intended to measure accuracy except when the control material is assayed by a reference laboratory alongside a standard reference. The principle is that the same material is sent from a national or regional centre to at least 20 participating laboratories. Results are returned to the EQAS organizer, statistically analysed and a target value with its range of variability (SD) calculated. This provides evaluation of the performance of each individual participant and identifies outliers. It is important that surveys should be performed at regular intervals, although their frequency may vary, depending on the diagnostic importance of the particular test, how frequently they are requested and their technical reliability. It is recommended that at least two specimens should be distributed together for each survey, a minimum of four times each year. Availability of survey material will always influence distribution timings, frequency and quality due to this (e.g. bone marrow films lacking particles).

The main purposes of EQA are to ensure continuous reliable performance by individual laboratories and to achieve harmonization or concordance between laboratories. However, some analysers handle preserved blood differently from routine specimens and, even if correctly calibrated, different types of counter may differ in their responses to EQA samples. It may thus be necessary to

analyse results separately for different groups of instruments. When there are unexplained differences in counts on EQA samples with different instruments in the same laboratory, counts should be made on fresh EDTA blood samples with the different instruments to ascertain their true comparability and, if necessary, recalibration of one should be undertaken to achieve concordance. Where appropriate, results from commercial kits and in-house methods should also be analysed in complementary groups. EQAS also have other additional complementary functions:

- Collecting information on the reliability of particular methods, materials and equipment
- Identifying problems with any *in vitro* diagnostic medical device (IVDMD) that requires reaction from the manufacturer and/or reporting to the responsible national authority as described in EN 14136
- Providing information on performance required for the purpose of licensing or accreditation and confirming competence in performance
- Improving performance
- Identifying laboratories whose performance provides a benchmarking standard and those with performance outside set levels
- Recommending state-of-the-art procedures for various analytical tests organizing workshops for education and training of laboratory staff and advising on best-practice guidelines
- Instilling confidence in staff, management and users of the laboratory services
- Providing laboratories with an extra level of risk management.

In summary, EQA is primarily intended to check the technical competence of individual laboratories, but it also provides an overview for assessing the state of the art and for identifying problems that have occurred in instruments, reagents or kits that may be affecting an entire group of users through no fault of their own. This provides a means for verification of manufacturers' conformity to their claimed specifications and for monitoring product performance in the laboratory, a requirement in Europe in the context of *the Directive on In-Vitro Diagnostic Medical Devices*.[8]

More information of this type would be useful for determining the priorities for national or international agencies engaged in developing standards. EQA should be used for highlighting shortcomings and for evaluating methods, technologies and reference/standard preparations. It is important for a clinical laboratory to participate in EQAS for accreditation or certification, as clearly stated in *ISO 9000, ISO Guides 25 and 58* and also in *ISO 15189*.[9]

Standardization of EQA Schemes

There are many such schemes for haematology based on the different laboratory diagnostic procedures. Many of these schemes are officially promoted or sponsored by national governments or local heath authorities. It is essential that participants in EQAS should have confidence in their efficiency and their effectiveness. ICSH has prepared guidelines for the organization and management of EQAS using proficiency testing. These guidelines are intended to help maintain a meaningful standard in the organization of EQAS and to harmonize the way in which they function. They include the following important principles and technical criteria:

1. Surveys should be sufficiently frequent to make sequential performance records meaningful and to identify participants who are persistently unsatisfactory as soon as possible.
2. Blood counts should be distributed at least monthly, other tests quarterly or more frequently depending on their clinical importance and reliability of analytical methods:
   a. There should be at least two specimens for every test, with values at diagnostically critical levels.
   b. To ensure that EQA relates to practice, survey samples should simulate natural specimens as closely as feasible and participants should be obligated to handle them in the same way as they handle routine specimens.
   c. The material used in surveys should be stable, at least until the closing date of the survey.
   d. The survey specimens must test negative for HIV antibody and hepatitis B and C antigens and must be labelled in accordance with national regulations for packaging and transport of biological material.
   e. Data processing must be as rapid as possible, with prompt reports to participants.
   f. Organizer/participant confidentiality must be maintained. Any information on an individual's results to a third party (e.g. a licensing authority) would be provided by the participant and must *not* be the responsibility or duty of the EQAS organizer.
   g. EQAS must be professionally led and should function independently of government health authorities.
   h. Industry may provide a useful service by organizing EQA surveys for users of their apparatus, but EQA schemes must always be independent of industry, both financially and operationally.
   i. Above all, EQAS itself must neither be a licensing authority nor a policing body – its primary major function is educational.

To analyse results on EQA specimens, it is first necessary to establish the target values. These might be 'truth' as determined by one or more reference centres or 'consensus' from the results of the participants. Referees should use reference methods which are traceable to a primary reference standard and the material should be tested on a minimum of five aliquots, five times on three different occasions and a mean value calculated from all the results. Consensus is based on the use of routine methods. As consensus may be biased by the most commonly used method or instrument group, it might be necessary to establish a different target value for each method or group. Consensus values should only be calculated when the number of results available is sufficient to allow statistically meaningful results. These are more convenient and practical to use than referees. Moreover, because of the absence of absolute metrological standards for most quantitative tests in haematology (haemoglobin concentration is an outstanding exception), the consensus mean or median is, in general, more likely to give a closer approximation of the true value. For qualitative tests, the correct result may be assumed as either that obtained as a consensus by 80% of the participants (as long as there is no clear division of results between methods) or by using results from a 'Gold Standard' (e.g. PCR).

Assessment of Participant Performance

Participant's performance evaluation with EQAS can be carried out by several procedures: quantitative tests, semi-quantitative tests and interpretative tests.

Quantitative Tests

Deviation index

From the results returned by the participants, the median or mean and SD are calculated. The deviation index (DI; also termed 'z-score') is used by many EQA schemes for assessing performance in quantitative tests. This is the amount of deviation from the mean ($\bar{X}$) or median (m) relative to a unit of 1 standard deviation (SD) (see below). The median is used when there is a non-Gaussian distribution of data with a wide range of results.[10] The SD is 'trimmed' to exclude any results outside ± 3SD. An individual laboratory can then compare its performance in the survey with that of other laboratories and with its own previous performance from the deviation index (DI) or z-score. This is calculated as the difference between the individual laboratory's result and the median or mean relative to the SD. Thus,

$$DI = \frac{[\text{Actual results for test} - \text{Adjusted mean or median}]}{\text{Trimmed SD}}$$

When results have a Gaussian distribution, the mean and SD are adjusted in a preliminary calculation by excluding all results in the highest and lowest 5%.

Instead of using a trimmed SD, as described earlier, the SD may be calculated from a constant or historical CV, which takes account of technical variance of the method, clinical utility of the test and the critical range of measurement for diagnostic discrimination in this method. A DI score of <0.5 denotes excellent performance; a score between 0.5 and 1.0 is satisfactory; and one between 1.0 and 2.0 is still acceptable. However, a score >2.0 suggests that the analyser calibration should be checked, whereas a DI >3.0 indicates a serious defect requiring urgent attention.

The DI provides a simple method for judging performance in a survey and it also indicates whether there have been changes in sequential surveys, thus distinguishing between casual errors and persistent unsatisfactory performance. A limitation of DI is that it is purely statistical. As the state of the art improves, some blood count parameters will have a CV of only 1–2%. Thus, the DI will indicate poor performance with unrealistically small deviations from the median. It may be better to use clinical relevance when determining the acceptable limits of percentage deviation from the target value. There are some differences in these limits as established in the USA for CLIA '88 requirements, those proposed by ICSH and those by an ISO panel.[9–11]

Consecutive monitoring

It is essential to monitor EQA results in consecutive surveys, noting any fluctuations in the DI. A convenient way for quantifying this is to add six recent DI scores (e.g. from the two samples in the last three surveys); any values >3.5 are rounded down to 3.5 to avoid an isolated very high value having an excessive effect on the calculation. The total is then multiplied by six. Failure to submit results in a survey gives a non-participation penalty of 50. A score of 100 or more indicates *persistent unsatisfactory performance*. It is, however, to be hoped that participants have corrected any problems before this stage is reached. When laboratories are unable to return results for persistent problems, they should ask to be 'suspended', until these can be resolved and full participation can be restored.

Out of consensus method

This is a refinement of the non-Gaussian procedure described earlier, which can be used, for example, for blood coagulation EQA. The median is calculated and all the participant results are then ranked in five grades as follows:

Group A: 25% of all results immediately adjacent to and above the median and 25% immediately adjacent to and below the median

Group B: The next 10% on each side of A
Group C: The next 5% on each side of B
Group D: The next 5% on each side of C
Group E: The final 5% on each side of D (and also no participation).

Performance in any particular test is assessed from the grades obtained in two consecutive exercises. Unsatisfactory performance is designated when the combination is D-D, E-C, E-D or E-E.

Target values and bias

The true value for a test can usually be assumed to be the result obtained by best performance of selected participants in the survey or by experts using reference methods or total participant consensus after trimming, as described earlier. This is the target value (TV) to be aimed for by all the participants. The percentage bias by an individual participant's result (R) can then be calculated as follows:

$$[(R - TV) \div TV] \times 100$$

The pattern of bias in successive surveys indicates whether there is a constant calibration error or a progressive fault or whether the original defect has been corrected.

Youden (xy) plot

The Youden plot is a useful method for relating measurements on two samples in a survey to provide a graphic display and, when a participant's results are unsatisfactory, for distinguishing between a consistent bias and random error. Results for the two samples are plotted on the horizontal (x) and the vertical (y) axis, respectively and the standard deviations (2SD or 3SD) for the two sets are drawn and interpreted as shown in outline in Figure 25.5.

Figure 25.5 Youden (*xy*) graph. The range of standard deviations (SDs) calculated from the overall results with sample *x* and sample *y*, respectively, are drawn on the *x* axis and the *y* axis; the individual paired results are then plotted on the graph. Results in the central square are satisfactory; those in B demonstrate a consistent bias with measurements that are too low (*B1*) or too high (*B2*), whereas results in other areas indicate random errors (inconsistency) in the two samples.

Methodology check

It is sometimes useful to check separate components of a method. Thus, appropriate samples can be used to check adequacy of mixing to ensure sample homogeneity, the reliability of the dilution procedure and how an instrument is used. As an example, a survey might include a pair of identical whole blood samples and lysates from the same specimen for measuring haemoglobin concentration, together with a pre-diluted haemoglobin solution.

Clinical significance

In assessing performance, the use of limits based on the SD is too rigid in some cases and too lenient in others. To ensure that results are clinically reliable, they should be within a certain percentage of the assigned value. This must take account of unavoidable imprecision of the method and normal diurnal variations. In practice, the following limits are adequate to meet these requirements:

Hb and RBC (by cell counter)	3–4%
PCV, MCV, MCH, MCHC	4–5%
Leucocyte count	8–10%
Platelet count	10–15%
Vitamin B_{12}, folate, iron, ferritin	20%
Hb A_2 and Hb F quantitation	5%

Semi-Quantitative Tests

Reactions such as lysis, agglutination or colour change are recorded as 0, 1+, 2+, 3+ or 4+. Assessment of performance should be based on extent of divergence from the target value, which might be a consensus of participant results or a referee's results. Account must be taken of the diagnostic and clinical significance of an incorrect or confusing result.

EQA schemes should assess not only technical reliability but also professional competence in interpretation of the measurements. Thus, participants should be required to report on the technical significance of their results (i.e. whether within normal reference values for the specified method) and also on the clinical significance, taking account of any clinical information provided. Incorrect interpretation of a correct quantitative result is often due to lack of understanding of the concept of reference values and to the use of inappropriate reference ranges. It is important in the post-analytical phase of quality management for each laboratory to establish its own reference values for normal and for specific groups (e.g. smokers, pregnancy). With qualitative tests, too, account must be taken of the clinical significance of the answer. For each test it is necessary to decide if it is as serious to err by reporting a feature which does not exist as to miss an abnormality

which is present and to penalize the score accordingly. Scoring may be either as a credit for correct answers or as a penalty for an incorrect answer. Thus, using the penalty method in G6PD screening, a correct answer scores zero, while an error will be graded depending on the implications of misclassification for the subsequent management of the patient: it is more serious to report a low level as normal (score 5) than a normal value as low (score 3), and when the true value is intermediate, it is more serious to report it as normal in a female (score 3) than in a male (score 1).

Interpretive Tests

In assessing qualitative or interpretive tests (e.g. stained blood smears for morphology), participant results are compared with the consensus obtained from a panel of referees or by concordance of at least 80% of the participants. Some schemes may use a panel of experts to produce a 'Comments' section in the report. The features reported are graded on their clinical significance, taking account of the specific medical condition, as follows:

- Essential for diagnosis: 5 points
- Likely to influence diagnostic decision: 2–3 points
- Might be helpful as a secondary consideration, but not essential, in reaching a diagnosis: 1 point
- Provides no useful information: 0 points.

All correct observations are given a positive score and false-positive observations are subtracted in accordance with the grading. The result is expressed as a percentage of the total possible score established by the referees. The more stringent limits have been proposed to provide greater sensitivity in diagnostic discrimination, but they may be impractical, resulting in an overestimate of the numbers of poor performers.[12,13]

Similarly, scores on parasite films will depend on clinical significance; a negative result on a film containing *Plasmodium falciparum* or a microfilaria, will be penalized more than a *Plasmodium ovale*, reported as a *Plasmodium malariae*.

While few EQA schemes provide a bone marrow slide on a regular basis, due to the difficulties of producing large numbers of films from the same donor, the introduction of digital morphology EQAS may be useful in the future. Preparation and reporting on these films should be standardized from conception using guidelines.[14]

INTERNAL AUDIT FOR TOTAL QUALITY MANAGEMENT

Internal audit provides evidence that the quality management system (QMS) has been effectively established, implemented and maintained. Systems of internal audit should be established and audits conducted according to a schedule and against agreed criteria. Audits are performed by individuals with appropriate training and, if possible, by those who are independent of the work being audited. A record of internal audit activities is logged within the audit document, which includes details of any non-compliances, corrective action(s) and/or preventative action(s). The results of internal audit should be regularly evaluated and any decisions taken to alter/improve the QMS should be documented and should be subject to monitoring and review.

Internal Audit of Examination Processes

The pre-examination, examination and post-examination processes should be subjected to internal audit. Audits should be conducted according to agreed criteria and performed by individuals with appropriate training. Details of internal audit activities that should be kept include any non-compliance noted and/or corrective and preventative actions. The results of these internal audits should be regularly evaluated and the decisions that are made should be documented and subject to monitoring and review.

Continuous Quality Improvement

The process for continuous quality improvement includes both preventative and corrective action. *Preventative action* is taken to reduce non-compliances, including:

- Investigation of the basic causes of potential non-compliances
- Implementation of preventative action required within an agreed timescale
- Ensuring that the action taken is recorded, seen to be effective and is submitted for management review.

Corrective action includes identification and elimination of the causes of non-compliance and monitoring of corrective actions that are implemented within an agreed time scale.

Control of Non-Compliance

When non-compliance has been detected, it is essential to ensure the reliability of the laboratory service. This requires the following steps:

1. The clinical consequence is considered and, if appropriate, the relevant users are informed.
2. The results of any tests already released are recalled or identified.
3. The responsible person is defined for the resumption of examinations.
4. Each episode of non-compliance is documented and reviewed.

PREPARATION OF EXTENDED-LIFE MATERIAL FOR USE IN QUALITY ASSESSMENT

Commercial products are available but, with appropriate expertise, control materials can also be made locally. All such preparations will require to have in-house values assigned for the relevant parameters.

Preparation of Preserved Whole Blood

Method[4,15]

1. Collect blood into a sterile container (e.g. a blood transfusion donor bag) with ACD or CPD anticoagulant (see p. 619). Leave for 2–3 days at 4°C.
2. Centrifuge the blood for 20 min at approximately 2000 *g*. Separate (and keep) the supernatant plasma but discard the buffy coat. Transfer the red cell concentrate into 500 ml bottles.
3. Mix 3 volumes of the red cells with 1.5 volumes of 9 g/l NaCl, centrifuge for 20 min at approximately 2000 *g* and remove the supernatant and upper layer of the red cells by suction.
4. Repeat step 3.
5. Dilute 5 volumes of the plasma with 2 volumes of 9 g/l NaCl and add broad-spectrum antibiotic, e.g. 1 mg penicillin and 5 mg gentamicin per 100 ml.
6. Add the diluted plasma from step 5 to the red cell concentrate at an appropriate ratio to obtain a preparation suitable for use as a red cell count control.
7. Mix well and, with continuous mixing, dispense in aliquot volumes into clean sterile vials,* and cap tightly. Store at 4°C.

Preparation of Haemolysate

Method

1. Collect blood as described earlier (e.g. into a blood transfusion donor bag). Blood unsuitable for transfusion, such as an underweight donor pack, can be used providing that the blood is not lysed. Remove blood to containers suitable for use with toluene and carbon tetrachloride. Centrifuge at approximately 2000 *g* for 20 min and discard the plasma and buffy coat.

---

*A mixing-dispensing unit is recommended for large-scale dispensing. A suitable one can be constructed using standard glassware, etc., except for the specially manufactured flask head which is not commercially available and needs to be made by a company specializing in Medical Engineering. (See Ward PG, Chappel DA, Fox JG, et al 1975 Mixing and bottling unit for preparing biological fluids used in quality control. *Laboratory Practice*. 24:577–583.)

2. Wash with equal volumes of 9 g/l NaCl, 3 times to ensure complete removal of the plasma, leucocytes and platelets. Mix well between washes.

3. Ensure the last centrifugation packs the red cells well, remove saline and to each 10 ml volumes of the washed cells, add 2 volumes of water and 2 volumes of toluene or carbon tetrachloride (in some countries carbon tetrachloride is not available). Cap and shake vigorously on a mechanical shaker or vibrator for 1 h. Then store at 4°C for 24–48 h to allow the lipid/cell debris to form a semisolid surface between the toluene/carbon tetrachloride and lysate.

4. On the following day, centrifuge at approximately 2000 g for 20 min, remove the lysate layers and pool them in a clean bottle.

5. Centrifuge the lysate at 2000 g for 1 h, remove the top 90% (leaving any debris); and then bottle in a clean container.

6. To each 70 ml of lysate, add 30 ml of glycerol and broad-spectrum antibiotic (see previous section). Haemoglobin values can be adjusted using 30% glycerol in saline, when the lysate is used. Mix well, dispense into sterile containers and cap tightly.

Stored at 4°C, the product should retain its assigned value for at least several months or for 1–2 years if kept at −20°C.

Preparation of Stabilized Whole Blood Control Material

Method

1. Obtain whole blood in CPD or ACD.[16] This should be as fresh as possible and never more than 3 days old. Filter through a 40 μm blood filter into a series of plastic bottles.

2. If an increased red cell count is required, centrifuge the blood and remove part of the plasma; if a lower red cell count is required, dilute the blood with an appropriate amount of that plasma. If paired bottles are gently centrifuged (approx. 1500 g) for 15 min to produce buffy coats, these can then be manipulated in a similar way to provide different levels of leucocyte and platelet counts. As many blood transfusion services now only provide leucodepleted blood and usually platelet and plasma poor, to enhance platelet counts platelet concentrate can be added. Similarly, to raise a white cell count, buffy coat packs can be used. Add broad-spectrum antibiotic (see above) to each sample.

3. Mix well and add 1 volume of fixative (6.75 ml formaldehyde 37–40% + 0.75 ml glutaraldehyde 50% + 26 g trisodium citrate to 100 ml water) to 50 volumes of the cell suspension. Mix on a mechanical mixer for 1 h at room temperature and leave at 4°C for 24 h.

4. With continuous mixing, dispense into sterile containers; cap tightly and seal with plastic tape.

Refrigerate at 4°C until required. Unopened vials should remain in good condition for several months if stored at this temperature.

Simple Method for Producing QC Preparations for Individual Types of Blood Cell Material

The following method for control material preparation provides a suitable procedure for red blood cell, leucocyte and platelet counting by some semi-automated blood cell counters, but is not suitable for more complex automated systems. If kept at 4°C, this material is stable for a maximum of 3 weeks.

Method

1. Collect a unit of human blood into CPD anticoagulant (see p. 620). Carry out the subsequent procedure within 1 day after collection.

2. Filter the blood through a blood transfusion recipient set into a 500 ml glass bottle.

3. Add 1 ml of fresh 40% formaldehyde. Mix well by inverting and then leave on a roller mixer for 1 h.

4. Leave at 4°C for 7 days, mixing by inverting a few times each day. At the end of this period of storage, mix well on a roller mixer for 20 min and, with constant mixing by hand, dispense in 2 ml volumes into sterile containers.

Preparation of Stable Control Material for EQAS

Preparation of Surrogate Leucocytes

Chicken and turkey red blood cells are nucleated and, when fixed, their size is within the human leucocyte range as recognized on electronic cell counters. They are thus suitable to serve as surrogate leucocytes.[4] This material may not be suitable for counting systems that are based on technologies other than impedance cell sizing.

Method

1. Centrifuge anticoagulated blood (any can be used) at approx. 2000 g for 20 min and remove the plasma aseptically.

2. Add an equal volume of 0.15 mol/l phosphate buffer, pH 7.4 (see p. 622); mix and transfer to a sterile centrifuge bottle; recentrifuge and discard the supernatant and buffy coat.

3. Repeat the wash and centrifugation twice. To the washed cells, add 10 times their volume of glutaraldehyde fixative (0.25% in 0.15 mol/l phosphate buffer, pH 7.4). Mix for 1 h on a mechanical mixer. Then leave overnight at 4°C.

To check that fixation has been complete, centrifuge 2–3 ml of the suspension, discard the supernatant and add water to the deposit. If lysis occurs, the cells are not fixed and the stock glutaraldehyde requires replacement.

4. When fixation is complete, centrifuge the suspension at approximately 2000 g for 10 min and discard the supernatant. Wash and centrifuge at approximately 2000 g for 10 min twice.

5. Resuspend the fixed cells to approximately 30% concentration in 9 g/l NaCl. Mix well with vigorous shaking. Add antibiotic (see above), cap tightly, seal with a plastic seal and store at 4°C.

Preparation of QC Material for Platelet Count

Reagent

Alsever's solution. (A) Trisodium citrate, 16 g; NaCl, 8.2 g to 1 litre with water; (B) dextrose, 41 g to 1 litre with water. Store at 4°C. Immediately before use, mix equal volumes of A and B; filter through 0.2 μm micropore filter. *EDTA solution.* 100 g/l of K_2 EDTA in the Alsever's solution; stable for 6 months at 4°C.[4]

Method

1. Collect a unit of blood into ACD or CPD anticoagulant. Centrifuge for 10 min at 200 g and collect the platelet suspension into a plastic container; alternatively, obtain a unit of pooled platelet concentrate prepared by a Blood Transfusion Service.

2. Add 1 ml of 100 g/l EDTA solution (100 g/l of K_2 EDTA in the Alsever's solution). Mix well and leave at 37°C for 2 h to allow the platelets to disaggregate.

3. Add 200 ml of glutaraldehyde fixative (0.25% in 0.15 mol/l phosphate buffer, pH 7.4). Shake vigorously by hand to ensure complete platelet distribution and leave for 48 h at room temperature with occasional shaking.

4. Centrifuge for 30 min at 3500 g. Wash the deposit twice in Alsever's solution and finally resuspend in 15–20 ml of Alsever's solution and broad-spectrum antibiotics.

5. Cap and seal. At 4°C, the preparation should have a shelf life of at least 6 months. Before use, resuspend by thorough shaking by hand, followed by mechanical mixing for approximately 15 min.

A simpler method for preserving platelets by adding prostaglandin E_1 to blood in ACD has been reported to provide a control preparation with stability of about 14 days.[17]

REFERENCES

1. Davis BH, Jungerius B. International Council for Standardization in Haematology technical report 1–2009: new reference material for haemiglobincyanide for use in standardization of blood haemoglobin measurements. *International Journal of Laboratory Hematology.* 2010;32: 139–141.

2. Kazmierczak SC, Catrou PG. Analytical interference. More than just a laboratory problem. *Am J Clin Pathol.* 2000;113:9–11.

3. Klee GG, Schryver PG, Kisabeth RM. Analytical bias specifications based on the analysis of effects on performance of medical guidelines. *Scand J Clin Lab Invest.* 1999;59: 509–512.

4. Lewis SM. *Quality Assurance in Haematology Document LAB/98.4.* Geneva: World Health Organization; 1998.

5. Levey S, Jennings ER. The use of control charts in the clinical laboratory. *Am J Clin Pathol.* 1950;20: 1059–1066.

6. Cembrowski GS, Lunetsky ES, Patrick CC, et al. An optimized quality control procedure for hematology analyzers with the use of retained patient specimens. *Am J Clin Pathol.* 1988;89:203–210.

7. World Health Organization. *EURO report 36: External quality assessment of health laboratories.* Copenhagen: WHO Regional Office for Europe; 1981.

8. Directive 98/79/EC of the European Parliament and of the Council on in vitro Diagnostic Medical Devices. October 1998.

9. International Standard ISO 15189 2007 Medical Laboratories. *Particular Requirements for Quality and Competence.*

10. International Council for Standardization in Haematology. Guidelines for organization and management of external quality assessment using proficiency testing. *International Journal of Haematology.* 1998;68:45–52.

11. International Organization for Standardization. *Guide 43–41 proficiency testing by interlaboratory comparisons. Development and Operation of Proficiency Testing Schemes.* Geneva: ISO; 1997.

12. Vives Corrons JL, Albarede S, Flandrin G, et al. Guidelines for blood smear preparation and staining procedure for setting up an external quality assessment scheme for blood smear interpretation. Part I: Control Material. *Clin Chem Lab Med.* 2004;42(8):922–926.

13. Vives Corrons JL, Blerk M Albarede S, et al. Guidelines for setting up an External Quality Assessment Scheme for blood smear interpretation. Part II: Survey Preparation, Statistical Evaluation and Reporting. *Clin Chem Lab Med.* 2006;44(8):1039–1043.

14. Lee H, Erbert WN, Porvit A, et al. ICSH guidelines for standardization of bone marrow specimens and reports: International Council for Standardization in Haematology. *International Journal of Laboratory Hematology.* 2008;30: 349–363.

15. Deom A, El Aouad R, Heick CC, et al. *Requirements and Guidance for External Quality Assurance Programmes for Health Laboratories: Document LAB/2000.* Geneva: World Health Organization; 2000.

16. Reardon DM, Mack D, Warner B, et al. A whole blood control for blood count analysers and source material for an external quality assessment scheme. *Med Lab Sci.* 1991;48:19–26.

17. Zhang Z, Tatsumi N, Tsuda I, et al. Long-term preservation of platelet count in blood for external quality control surveillance using prostaglandin E1. *Clin Lab Haematol.* 1999;21:71.

Chapter 26

Haematology in under-resourced laboratories

Imelda Bates, Jane Carter

INTRODUCTION: TYPES OF LABORATORIES

In most countries, there are likely to be some laboratories with limited resources, but in under-resourced countries, the majority of laboratories face chronic shortages of trained staff, low morale, inadequate equipment and erratic supplies of reagents. These have a major impact on the range and quality of services offered. Many laboratories lack the highly sophisticated equipment found in more wealthy settings and still operate using manual techniques. Smaller laboratories tend to be multifunctional, performing a range of haematology, parasitology, clinical chemistry and microbiology tests. A blood transfusion service is usually available at larger institutions and, unless there is access to a national blood service, laboratory staff are responsible for donor selection, blood collection and issuing of blood. If there is no separate system of public health laboratories, clinical laboratories may also be required to provide reliable health surveillance data for epidemiological and public health monitoring and to investigate disease outbreaks and refer samples for confirmation.

In under-resourced countries, these difficulties are compounded by the high burden of infectious diseases such as HIV/AIDS, tuberculosis and malaria. There are also additional pressures from external agencies for diagnostic and monitoring services which may not accurately reflect local public health priorities. Parasitological diagnosis of malaria is now recommended in all age groups to prevent the over-diagnosis and misuse of new anti-malarial combination drugs. Although it is currently the subject of much debate, WHO guidelines state that the only exception to the requirement for parasitological diagnosis is children aged under 5 years living in stable high-transmission settings where the likelihood of malaria as a cause for fever is high.[1] Occasionally, in tertiary centres, the diagnosis of tuberculosis requires aspiration and culture of the bone marrow and trephine biopsy examination, especially in patients who are HIV positive, in whom sputum tests for acid-fast organisms are frequently negative.[2] The decision to initiate antiretroviral therapy and the monitoring of therapy require regular haemoglobin concentration (Hb) estimations, CD4-positive lymphocyte counts (or percentages for paediatric care) and, ideally, plasma viral load determinations, although the maintenance of equipment for some of these tests is challenging for low-income countries.[3,4]

The purpose of this chapter is to provide guidance for an effective haematology service at the different levels of the healthcare system in resource-limited countries. In planning such services, it is necessary to determine what tests are needed at each level and to identify the relevant referral networks for clinical haematology. For example, successful management of haematological malignancies in countries with limited resources might involve partnerships between local institutions and those in more wealthy countries to adapt treatment protocols, to provide training or diagnostic services or to improve local supportive care facilities.[5,6]

ORGANIZATION OF CLINICAL LABORATORY SERVICES

In under-resourced countries clinical laboratory services may be considered at three levels according to their size, staffing and services offered. These are levels: (A) subdistrict facilities

Level of Laboratory	Haematology Services Performed
Health Centres	Simple haemoglobin estimation
	Screening for malaria
	HIV testing
District Hospitals	Haemoglobin measurement
	Examination of blood films (morphology and differential white cell count)
	Total platelet and white cell counts
	Screening for sickle haemoglobin (when appropriate)
	Malaria rapid test
	CD4 count
Central/Regional Hospitals	Automated blood count
	G6PD screen
	Haemoglobin electrophoresis
	Immunophenotyping
	HIV viral load estimation
	Basic clotting tests
	Oral anticoagulant control
	Processing of bone marrow aspirates
	Cross matching and antibody screening
	Preparation of some blood components
National Reference Centre	All relevant tests

Figure 26.1 Network of laboratories.

including health centres; (B) district and referral hospitals; and (C) central reference and teaching hospitals (Fig. 26.1).

Level A: Sub-District Facilities Including Health Centres

The level A laboratory provides basic diagnostic services to support patient management on-site and determine when a patient requires referral. In some countries, there may be no formal laboratory and some diagnostic tests are carried out at the point-of-care by nurses, assistants or orderlies with no technical qualifications. Haematology equipment at this level includes a method for estimating Hb and a microscope for examining slides for tuberculosis and malaria. However, maintenance of equipment in rural areas is often difficult and technical work may not be properly supervised, which can significantly compromise the quality of results.

Level B: District Hospitals

District hospital laboratories are usually multipurpose, performing microbiological and biochemical as well as haematological tests. Laboratory staff may comprise one or two qualified biomedical scientists supported by assistants who often have little or no formal training but have learnt various techniques at the bench. Equipment available for haematology may include a microscope and centrifuge and possibly a basic colorimeter for measurement of Hb. In some district hospitals, donor funds have provided more sophisticated equipment such as automated haematology and clinical chemistry analysers, predominantly to support HIV services. In the absence of a national blood service, district hospitals are responsible for blood transfusion services so the laboratory will be expected to perform blood grouping and cross-matching as well as screening for at least HIV, hepatitis B virus and possibly hepatitis C virus.

Level C: Central and Teaching Hospitals

At this level, the laboratory staff have usually received multidisciplinary training and some of the senior staff have received postgraduate training in a specialist laboratory discipline. Each laboratory usually has a specialist technical head who works closely with the clinical pathologist. Equipment available includes centrifuges, colorimeters, microscopes, haemoglobin electrophoresis equipment and possibly blood bank centrifuges for the separation of blood components. Automated haematology analysers are usually found in such laboratories. In many cases, these have been supplied by donor agencies, but long-term funding to support maintenance of these systems is often lacking and, consequently, they may be unreliable or not used at all owing to a shortage of appropriate reagents and inadequate maintenance.

AVAILABILITY OF TESTS AT EACH LEVEL

In under-resourced countries, the haematology tests available at the different levels of healthcare vary widely and depend on local clinical needs as well as availability of equipment and qualified technical laboratory personnel. The following is a general description of the tests that are likely to be required at each level.

Level A

- Haemoglobin estimation by a manual method (see p. 608)
- Malaria testing on peripheral blood thick and thin films (see p. 109) or rapid diagnostic test for *Plasmodium falciparum* and other species (see p. 110)
- Testing for HIV infection.

Level B

- Haemoglobin measurement (see p. 24)
- Peripheral blood morphology, especially to identify the cause of anaemia (Chapter 5)*
- Total white blood cell counts (see p. 610)
- Differential white cell count (see p. 31)
- Platelet estimates (usually from blood film)
- CD4 lymphocyte count (see p. 614)
- Malaria testing by thick and thin peripheral blood films (see p. 109) or rapid diagnostic test for *Plasmodium falciparum* and other species (see p. 110)
- Screening test for sickle haemoglobin in areas where this is relevant (see p. 314)
- Blood grouping and compatibility testing (Chapter 21)
- Some larger laboratories may have automated (Hb concentration), mean cell volume (MCV), mean cell haemoglobin (MCH), mean cell haemoglobin concentration (MCHC), white blood cell total and differential counts, platelet counts (see p. 36).

Level C

In addition to tests carried out at level B, the haematology services offered by level C may include the following:

- Automated Hb, MCV, MCH, MCHC, white blood cell total and differential counts, platelet counts (see p. 36)
- Haemoglobin electrophoresis or high-performance liquid chromatography (Chapter 12)
- Haemoglobin A_2 and haemoglobin F measurements (see pp. 322 and 325)
- Glucose-6-phosphate dehydrogenase screen (by fluorescent spot or methaemoglobin reduction method) (see p. 255)
- Flow cytometry immunophenotyping (Chapter 14)
- Polymerase chain reaction (PCR) or other method for diagnosis of mutations associated with haematological malignancies (Chapter 21)
- HIV plasma viral load estimations
- Staining of bone marrow smears for morphological assessment (see p. 59) and estimation of iron status (see p. 333)
- Bone marrow trephine biopsy examination (see p. 123)
- Identification of blood group antibodies (Chapter 19)
- Basic clotting screen (prothrombin time, thrombin time and activated partial thromboplastin time) (see p. 409)
- Oral anticoagulant control (see p. 467)

---

*A bench-aid on morphology is available from Tropical Health Technology.[7]

- Separation of whole blood into packed cells, plasma and, occasionally, platelets.

MICROSCOPES

The microscope is the most important piece of laboratory equipment in under-resourced countries and is essential for the diagnosis of anaemia, malaria and other blood parasitic infections and for performing total and differential white blood cell counts. Reliable assessment of morphological features requires a microscope that is clean and correctly set up with aligned lenses and an electric light source (either inbuilt or reflected light) to ensure clear images, especially at high magnification. Failure to maintain microscopes to a high standard by routine user maintenance or, ideally, with regular professional servicing, can lead to inaccurate diagnoses and inefficient use of technician time.[8,9] Routine maintenance of the microscope is described on p. 52.

Care of the Microscope

In hot, humid climates, if no precautions are taken, fungus may develop on the microscope – particularly on the surface of the lenses, in the grooves of the screws and under the paint – and the instrument will soon be useless. This can be prevented by placing the microscope every evening in an airtight dust cover together with silica gel. Dry the silica as necessary and reuse it. An alternative method is to place the microscope in a warm cupboard with a tight-fitting door, heated by a 40-watt light bulb. Check that the temperature inside the cupboard is at least $5°C$ warmer than that of the laboratory, but take care that it does not overheat.

In hot, dry climates, the main problem is dust. Fine particles work their way into the threads of the screws and under the lenses. This can be avoided as follows:

1. Always keep the microscope under a dustproof plastic cover when not in use.
2. At the end of the day's work, clean the microscope thoroughly by blowing air onto the lenses and moving parts using a rubber bulb.
3. Finish cleaning the lenses with a lens brush or fine paintbrush. If dust particles remain on the surface of the objectives, remove with clean lens paper.

'ESSENTIAL' HAEMATOLOGY TESTS

Despite the relatively high cost of running a laboratory service and the low *per capita* healthcare budget in under-resourced countries, there are few data available on which to base rational decisions about 'essential' laboratory tests.[10,11] In many of these countries, decisions are made at central level by healthcare planners without adequate consultation with laboratory managers and experts. The selection of 'essential' tests at each level should be based on the clinical and public health needs of the local community and the availability of qualified clinical and laboratory staff, as well as on the availability of funds. Essential test packages are usually defined as part of national policy and standards, taking into consideration medium- and long-term trends and the requirements of disease control programmes.

To ensure cost-effectiveness of the laboratory service, tests with no proven value should be eliminated and new tests for which there is independent evidence of clinical usefulness should be introduced,[12] as described in Chapter 24, p. 567. Tests that provide objective qualitative or quantitative information are preferred. Although it is not possible to draw up a list of essential tests that will be applicable to all countries, or even to different regions within a country, the following aspects should be considered.

Cost per Test

Often the cost of a test is calculated from the price of reagents divided by the number of tests performed. However, this oversimplifies the situation and is not accurate enough to form the basis for national policy decisions and budget allocation.[11] The factors that need to be taken into account when calculating the total annual costs for a laboratory are given in Chapter 24.

Diagnostic Reliability

It is important to know the sensitivity and specificity of a test and its predictive values (as calculated on p. 567) when selecting a laboratory test for clinical use. This information may be provided by manufacturers but it may not be locally applicable and, in many under-resourced countries, local test evaluation data are not available. In some countries, the 'gold standard' diagnostic services needed to determine 'true positive' and 'true negative' data in the local context are also lacking.

The quality of all tests carried out by a laboratory should be regularly monitored; systems for doing this are well-established (see Chapter 24) but are not easily implemented in under-resourced settings. The quality of a test influences its usefulness as well as its utilization by clinicians and community members. For example, if the result of a test in routine practice is correct only 80% of the time, then one in five tests will be wasted, reducing the effectiveness of the test by 20%. Furthermore, the inaccurate test may result in a patient receiving inappropriate treatment. Clinicians and the general public are increasingly aware of the need for accurate diagnosis. Clinicians may not order tests or use the results in patient management decisions if they do not trust the quality of the laboratory results[13] and poor quality healthcare may deter patients from using health facilities.

Clinical Usefulness

An assessment of the clinical usefulness of a test should be carried out by an independent clinician who is familiar with local diseases and the diagnostic support services that are available. This assessor needs to compare actual clinical practice with locally agreed 'best practice' or, if available, local guidelines.[12] From observation of a range of clinical interactions, the percentage of times that ideal practice is followed can be calculated. For example, transfusion guidelines may recommend that transfusions are given routinely to children with an Hb of <5 g/dl. The assessor can record how many children with Hb below this level failed to receive a transfusion and how many transfusions were given without waiting for the Hb result or at an inappropriate Hb level. For each test, the assessor needs to judge whether the test has been appropriately requested and is used to influence patient management or public health decisions. The percentage of tests that are not used to guide clinical decisions will provide a figure for 'clinical wastage' of the test that can be entered into the formula (Chapter 24).

MAINTAINING QUALITY AND RELIABILITY OF TESTS

Paradoxically, it is in under-resourced laboratories, where equipment and supplies are limited and training and supervision may be minimal, that the level of skills and motivation required to maintain a good-quality service need to be highest. Even the most basic of laboratories should ensure that procedures are in place to monitor quality (see Chapter 25). In addition to monitoring the technical quality of each test, the quality of the whole service must be ensured both within the laboratory and between laboratories. Standard operating procedures (see p. 575) should be drafted for every method performed in the laboratory; these can be adapted from existing standard operating procedure 'models'. In addition to providing standardized techniques, standard operating procedures are excellent teaching resources and adherence to these procedures will minimize errors. Standard operating procedures need to be regularly reviewed and updated to keep pace with technical developments and changes in local circumstances (e.g. non-availability of reagents, technical limitations).

Quality Control of a Test Method (Technical Quality)

Methods for the control of various haematology tests are described in Chapter 25 but some may need to be adapted to specific local circumstances in resource-poor countries. For example, if commercial controls are not affordable, each batch of sickle cell screening tests should include known positive and negative samples from a previous batch of tests; for monitoring constancy of Hb estimations, a high and a low value sample can be re-tested several times during the day.

Internal Quality Control

Internal quality control is a system within an individual laboratory for ensuring that the technical elements of the test are of acceptable quality. Monitoring of quality by processing control samples and plotting a control chart (see p. 593) will highlight major problems with the system. For example, an inaccurate differential white cell count may be due to problems with sample collection and handling, slide preparation, fixing and staining, morphological interpretation and microscope quality as well as inadequate microscopy technique. Measures such as the introduction of standard operating procedures, in-service training and equipment maintenance schedules can help to improve performance and reduce inaccuracies.

External Quality Assessment

The principles of external quality assessment (EQA) are described on p. 595. Poor communications and transport facilities make it difficult, but not impossible, to establish EQA in under-resourced laboratories. Among its other functions, EQA is used to identify poorly performing laboratories that require assistance and to detect the use of inaccurate techniques. Although participation in international, national or local external quality assessment schemes may be beyond the resources of a small rural laboratory, it should be possible for them to exchange samples and results with neighbouring facilities. Rural laboratories can also take advantage of supervisory visits by district officers to exchange samples, including external quality assessment materials and results with other laboratories. Accreditation schemes (see p. 577), either national or local, can be set up to formally recognize laboratories that are performing well and to assist those that are not.[14] Step-wise, rather than pass/fail, accreditation schemes provide a better measure of performance and motivate laboratories to improve their services.

BASIC HAEMATOLOGY TESTS

Haemoglobinometry

Various methods for the measurement of Hb are given in Chapter 3. The most accurate method that may be available in under-resourced laboratories is the hemoglobin-cyanide (cyanmethaemoglobin) method. However, this requires a power source and considerable technical expertise to carry out accurate dilutions and to prepare the standard curve. Use of pre-set haemoglobinometers removes the need for calibration curves, but the machine may still need to be set correctly.

Methods for measuring Hb that are robust, accurate and can be used by health workers in peripheral settings are described below.

Direct Reading Haemoglobinometers

HemoCue Blood Hemoglobin System*

HemoCue Blood Hemoglobin System (see Chapter 3) is a battery- or mains-operated portable, direct read-out machine that uses disposable dry chemistry cuvettes. Measurements are precise and accurate (provided that only the specified cuvettes are used and the reading surfaces are kept clean) and, unlike most other systems, it does not require pre-dilution of the sample. Although the use of the unique disposable cuvettes makes this method relatively expensive, the cuvettes for the new Hb 301 version are cheaper than

those for the Hb 201 and are designed for adverse climatic conditions. It is fast and very simple to use so that the cost may be offset by savings on training and supervision time.

Haemoglobin Colour Scale[†]

Many colour comparison methods have been developed in the past but these have become obsolete because the colours were not sufficiently comparable with blood or were not durable. The haemoglobin colour scale has been developed for anaemia screening where there is no laboratory.[15] It consists of a set of printed colour shades representing haemoglobin levels between 4 and 14 g/dl (i.e. 40 and 140 g/l). The colour of a drop of blood collected onto a specific type of paper matrix is compared with that on the chart (Fig. 26.2). It is intended for detecting the presence of anaemia and estimating its severity in 2 g/dl

Figure 26.2 Haemoglobin colour scale. The stained test-strip being read on the right indicates a severe anaemia with a haemoglobin value of about 60 g/l (6 g/dl).

---

*Available from HemoCue AB, Angelholm, Sweden; www.hemocue.com (Accessed 25 January 2010).

†Available from Teaching Aids at Low Cost; www.talcuk.org/accessories/ haemoglobin-colour-scale.htm (Accessed 25 January 2010).

(20 g/l) increments. The scale has been tested in resource-poor settings but more studies are needed to demonstrate whether it is superior to clinical diagnosis.[16–18] The instructions should be followed carefully because poor lighting, allowing the blood spot to dry out, and using the incorrect type of paper matrix for the test strips, can have detrimental effects on the results.

Packed Cell Volume

Although the packed cell volume (PCV) can be used as a simple screening test for anaemia and as a rough guide to the accuracy of haemoglobin measurements, it is not a substitute for a well-performed haemoglobin measurement. In addition to the technical problems (outlined on p. 28) there are particular problems with this method in resource-poor settings that may lead to errors in estimating the PCV. The lack of a mechanical mixing device means that specimens may not be adequately mixed before being introduced into the microhaematocrit tube. Poor-quality sealant means that the tubes often leak during centrifugation. Because the microhaematocrit tubes are difficult to label, samples may get mixed up in the centrifuge, especially when pressure of work is high and supervision is poor. Erratic power supplies, lack of devices for measuring g forces and poor equipment maintenance result in inadequate centrifugation with incomplete packing of the red cells.

Manual Cell Counts Using Counting Chambers

Visual counting of blood cells is an acceptable alternative to electronic counting for white blood cells but it is not recommended for routine red blood cell counts because the number of cells that can be counted within a reasonable time in the routine laboratory (e.g. about 400) will be too few to ensure a sufficiently precise result (see below). Although manual counting is recommended for platelet counts,[19] in practice, it is often easier to detect gross reductions or increases in platelet counts from examination of the peripheral blood film.

Counting Chambers

The visibility of the rulings in the counting chamber[19] is as important as the accuracy of calibration, so that chambers with a 'metallized' surface and Neubauer or Improved Neubauer rulings are recommended. These have nine 1 × 1 mm ruled areas, which, when covered correctly with the special thick coverglass, each contain a volume of 0.1 μl diluted blood (Figs 26.3, 26.4). Coverslips designed for mounting of microscopy preparations must not be used with counting chambers. The sample is introduced between the chamber and the coverglass using a pipette or capillary tube and the preparation is viewed using ×40 objective and ×6 or ×10 eyepieces. With Neubauer

and Improved Neubauer chambers, the cells in 4 or 8 horizontal rectangles of 1 × 0.05 mm (80 or 160 small squares) or in 5 or 10 groups of 16 small squares are counted, including the cells that touch the bottom and left-hand margins of the small squares.

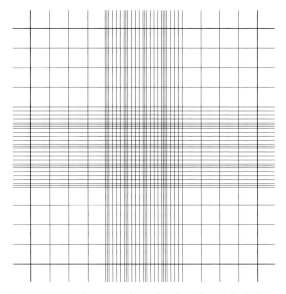

Figure 26.3 Neubauer counting chamber. The total ruled area is 3 × 3 mm; the central ruled area is 1 × 1 mm. In the central area, 16 groups of 16 small squares are separated by triple rulings.

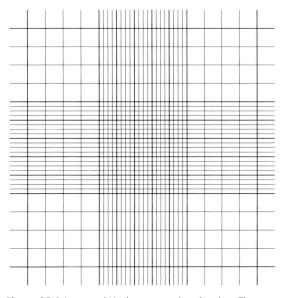

Figure 26.4 Improved Neubauer counting chamber. The central area consists of 25 groups of 16 small squares separated by closely ruled triple lines (which appear as thick black lines in the illustration).

Total White Blood Cell Count

To make the counting of white cells easier, diluted whole blood is mixed with a fluid to lyse the red cells and stain the white cell nuclei deep violet-black.

Diluent

The diluent is 2% (20 ml/l) acetic acid coloured pale violet with gentian violet.

Method

Make a 1 in 20 dilution of blood by adding 0.1 ml of *well-mixed* blood (lack of adequate mixing is a major source of error) to 1.9 ml of diluent* in a 75 × 10 mm plastic (or glass) tube. After sealing the tube with a lid or tightly fitting bung, mix the diluted blood in a mechanical mixer or by hand for at least 2 min by tilting the tube to an angle of about 120° combined with rotation, thus allowing the air bubble to mix the suspension. Fill a clean dry counting chamber, with its coverglass already in position, without delay. This is simply accomplished with the aid of a plastic Pasteur pipette or a length of stout capillary glass tubing that has been allowed to take up the suspension by capillarity. Take care that the counting chamber is filled in one action and that no fluid flows into the surrounding moat.

Leave the chamber undisturbed on a bench for at least 2 min for the cells to settle, but not much longer, because drying at the edges of the preparation initiates currents that cause movement of the cells after they have settled. The bench must be free of vibrations and the chamber must not be exposed to draughts or to direct sunlight or other sources of heat. It is important that the coverglass should be of a special thick glass and perfectly flat, so that when laid on the counting chamber, diffraction rings are seen. The coverglass should be of such a size that when placed correctly on the counting chamber, the central ruled areas lie in the centre of the rectangle to be filled with the cell suspension.

If any of the following filling defects occur, the preparation must be discarded and the filling procedure must be repeated using another clean dry chamber:

- Overflow into moat
- Chamber area incompletely filled
- Air bubbles anywhere in chamber area
- Any debris in chamber area.

To obtain a coefficient of variation of 5%, it is necessary to count about 400 cells (Table 26.1); in practice, it is reasonable to count 100 white cells. To minimize distribution errors, count the cells in the entire ruled area (i.e. 9 × 0.1 μl areas in an Improved Neubauer counting chamber). In practice, the 100 cell count can be achieved by counting the cells in the four larger corner squares.[19]

---

*Or a proportionately smaller volume: 0.02 ml (20 μl) of blood in 0.38 ml of lysing fluid.

Calculation

White blood cell count per litre (WBC/l)

$$= \frac{\text{No. of cells counted} \times \text{Dilution} \times 10^6}{\text{Volume counted } (\mu l)}$$

Thus, if N cells are counted in 0.1 μl, then the WBC/l is as follows:

$$\frac{N \times 20 \times 10^6}{0.1} = N \times 200 \times 10^6$$

(e.g. if 115 cells are counted, the WBC is $115 \times 200 \times 10^6/l = 23 \times 10^9/l$).

Range of white blood cell count in health

See Chapter 2, Tables 2.1, 2.2 and 2.3.

Platelet Count

Automated full blood counters produce platelet counts with a precision that is much superior to that of manual platelet counts. Manual platelet counts may occasionally be needed for blood samples with a significant proportion of giant platelets. Manual platelet counts are best performed on ethylenediaminetetra-acetic acid (EDTA) anticoagulated blood that has been obtained by clean venipuncture. Skin-prick samples are associated with platelet clumping so platelet counts are significantly lower and less constant than those performed on venous blood. Manual platelet counts are performed by visual examination of diluted, lysed whole blood using a Neubauer or Improved Neubauer counting chamber as for total white cell counts.[20,21]

Method

The diluent consists of 1% aqueous ammonium oxalate in which the red cells are lysed. This method is recommended in preference to using formal-citrate as diluent, which leaves the red cells intact and is more likely to give incorrect results when the platelet count is low.

Before diluting the blood sample, examine it carefully for the presence of blood clots. If these are present, a fresh specimen should be requested because clots will cause the platelet count to be artificially low. Make a 1 in 20 dilution of well-mixed blood in the diluent by adding 0.1 ml of blood to 1.9 ml of ammonium oxalate diluent (10 g/l). Not more than 500 ml of diluent should be made at a time, using scrupulously clean glassware and fresh glass-distilled or deionized water. If possible, the solution should be filtered through a micropore filter (0.22 μm) and kept at 4°C. For use, a small part of the stock is refiltered and dispensed in 1.9 ml volumes in 75 × 12 mm tubes.

Mix the suspension on a mechanical mixer for 10–15 min. Fill a Neubauer counting chamber with the suspension, using a stout glass capillary or Pasteur pipette. Place the counting

Table 26.1 Variance of haemocytometry count

NO. OF AREAS	TOTAL NO. OF CELLS COUNTED	√	σ	UNCERTAINTY OF TOTAL COUNT	RANGE PER 1 mm² AREA	CALCULATED COUNT/μl
1	50	7	14	36–64	36–64	7.2–12.8
2	100	10	20	80–120	40–60	8.0–12.0
4	200	14	28	172–228	43–57	8.6–11.4
6	300	17	34	266–334	44–56	8.9–11.1
8	400	20	40	360–440	45–55	9.0–11.0
10	500	22	44	456–544	46–54	9.2–10.8
16	800	28	56	744–856	47–53	9.4–10.6
20	1000	32	64	936–1064	47–53	9.4–10.6
30	1500	39	78	1422–1578	47–52	9.4–10.4
200	10 000	100	200	9800–10 200	49–51	9.8–10.2

The inherent error of a cell count results from the random way in which the cells are distributed in the counting chamber. This is known as the count variance (σ); it is calculated as $\sqrt{n} \div n$, where n = number of cells actually counted and variance is expressed as a percentage. The uncertainty of the count is in the range $n \pm \sigma$. In this theoretical example the final (calculated) count is based on the number of cells in a 1 mm² area at a dilution of 1:20. There were approximately 50 cells in each 1 mm² area. For convenience, results have been rounded to the nearest whole number. Counting in only one or two fields results in a wide variance that is reduced as more cells are counted. However, high precision is achieved only when thousands of cells are counted, which is only possible with automated cell counters.

chamber in a moist Petri dish and leave untouched for at least 20 min to give time for the platelets to settle.

Examine the preparation with the ×40 objective and ×6 or ×10 eyepieces. The platelets appear under ordinary illumination as small (but not minute), highly refractile particles if viewed with the condenser racked down; they are usually well separated and clumps are rare if the blood sample has been properly collected. To avoid introducing dirt particles into the chamber which might be mistaken for platelets, all equipment must be scrupulously clean. Platelets are more easily seen with the phase contrast microscope. A special, thin-bottomed (1 μm) counting chamber is best for optimal phase contrast effect. The number of platelets in one or more areas of 1 mm² should be counted. The total number of platelets counted should always exceed 200 to ensure a coefficient of variation of 8–10%.

Calculation

$$\text{Platelet count per litre} = \frac{\text{No. of cells counted} \times \text{Dilution} \times 10^6}{\text{Volume counted } (\mu l)}$$

Thus, if N is the number of platelets counted in an area of 1 mm² (0.1 μl in volume), the number of platelets per litre of blood is:

$$N \times 10 \times 20 \,(\text{dilution}) \times 10^6 = N \times 200 \times 10^6$$

Range of platelet counts in health

See Chapter 2, Tables 2.1, 2.2 and 2.3.

Errors in Manual Cell Counts

The errors associated with manual cell counts are *technical* and *inherent*.

Technical errors can be minimized by avoiding the following:

- Poor technique in obtaining the blood specimen
- Insufficient mixing of the blood specimen
- Inaccurate pipetting and the use of badly calibrated pipettes or counting chambers
- Inadequate mixing of the cell suspension
- Faulty filling of the counting chamber
- Careless counting of cells within the chamber.

Standardized Counting Chambers

To reduce errors, it is important to have a good-quality counting chamber. The exact chamber depth depends on the coverglass, which should be free from bowing and sufficiently thick so as not to bend when pressed on the chamber. The coverglass must be free from scratches and even the smallest particle of dust may cause unevenness in its lie on the chamber. The specifications described by WHO[19] outline a tolerance of dimensions for counting chambers that provides reasonable accuracy.

Accurate Dilutions

Bulb-diluting pipettes are not recommended; they are difficult to calibrate and easily broken. The volumes of blood used are unnecessarily small and it is difficult to fill the counting chamber so that the exact amount of fluid is delivered. Pipettes of 0.1 ml and 0.02 ml (20 µl) are relatively inexpensive and easy to calibrate. With a 2 ml volume in a glass or plastic tube provided with a tightly fitting rubber or plastic bung, a suspension is obtained that is easy to label and handle, and with a little practice, perfect filling of the counting chamber can regularly be accomplished with the aid of a fine plastic Pasteur pipette or stout glass capillary tube. Automatic diluter units are useful. These consist of a dual metering system that enables a volume of diluent and the appropriate volume of blood to be dispensed consecutively into a tube (see p. 632). A variety of automatic diluting systems are now available that have good accuracy and precision but a regular supply of disposable tips may be too expensive and difficult for smaller laboratories to maintain. Pipetting errors apply to all tests that involve dilution of the blood sample and they also occur with autodiluters (especially with viscid fluids) and when the delivery volume of the unit is not correctly adjusted.

Microscopy Artefacts

Dirt or clumped red cell debris may be mistaken for white cells or platelets. Clumping of white cells occurs particularly in heparinized blood, especially when the concentration of heparin exceeds 25 iu/ml of blood. The clumps are most frequently seen in blood that has been allowed to stand for several hours before undertaking the count. For this reason, EDTA is the anticoagulant of choice for blood count examinations.

Inherent errors result from uneven distribution of cells in the counting chamber and no amount of mixing will minimize this inherent variation in numbers between areas. Inherent error can only be reduced by counting more cells in a preparation. In theory, the count varies in proportion to the square root of the number of cells counted, i.e. if four times the number of cells are counted, the variation is halved (Table 26.1). For example, when performing a manual white cell count, 95% of the observed counts in a sample of true value 5.0×10^9 cells/l would lie within the range 4.0–6.0. In practice, the difference between 5.0 and 6.0×10^9 cells/l for a white cell count is of little clinical significance.

It is also important for the observer not to bias the count by foreknowledge of what result might be expected or by selecting certain areas in the chamber for counting.[22]

Peripheral Blood Morphology

Examination of the peripheral blood film is one of the most important and useful examinations in the peripheral laboratory but it requires a great deal of skill and experience as well as a good-quality microscope (see Chapter 5). In addition to providing information about quantitative changes in blood cells, careful analysis of the qualitative changes may help in elucidating the underlying reasons for clinical problems. These observations may identify the cause of anaemia or undiagnosed fever or the presence of a haemoglobinopathy (see Chapter 14). Problems that might occur when preparing blood films relate to the slides themselves and to the quality of fixing of the films and the quality of staining reagents. When glass slides are in short supply, laboratories sometimes find it necessary to wash and reuse slides (see p. 623). Traces of detergent can result in misleading appearances of the red cells (Fig. 26.5), as can residual stain and scratches on the slide. In humid conditions, particularly during the rainy season, water may be absorbed by the methanol used for fixing slides and this can cause gross artefactual changes in red cell appearance (see Fig. 4.2). To avoid this problem, stock bottles of methanol should be kept tightly closed after use; small amounts should be aliquoted into a bottle with a tightly fitting cap for daily use and replaced regularly from the stock bottle.

Modified (One-Tube) Osmotic Fragility Test

This simple and inexpensive test for screening for β thalassaemia trait is useful when quantification of haemoglobin A_2 is not possible and standardized automated analysers are not available for accurate measurement of MCV and MCH.

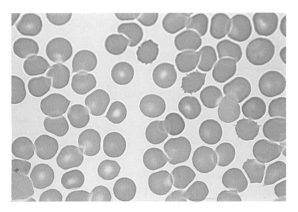

Figure 26.5 Red cell appearances on detergent washed slide.

A variety of concentrations of buffered saline have been used. A concentration of 0.36% in buffered saline (see p. 622 for preparation) is recommended to ensure a high sensitivity with an acceptable specificity.[23] Because the false-positive rate is around 10%, confirmation of a positive result requires referral of a sample to a laboratory able to quantitate haemoglobin A_2. The test can also be used to screen for α^0 thalassaemia trait, with positive samples being referred to a reference centre for DNA analysis. About 50% of samples containing haemoglobin E also give a positive result; this is an advantage rather than a disadvantage because detection of haemoglobin E is important in predicting the possibility of thalassaemia major or intermedia in compound heterozygotes with β thalassaemia.

Haemoglobin E Screening Test

Ideally, the diagnosis of haemoglobin E heterozygosity or homozygosity should be by haemoglobin electrophoresis at alkaline pH or high-performance liquid chromatography with a second method being used to confirm the provisional identification (see Chapter 14). When these facilities are not available, a screening test using the blue dye 2,6-dichlorophenolindophenol (DCIP), can be used. Samples containing haemoglobin E become faintly turbid when incubated with DCIP.[24,25]

Tests for Paroxysmal Nocturnal Haemoglobinuria

When facilities permit, flow cytometry for glycosylphosphatidylinositol-anchored proteins is the test of choice to detect paroxysmal nocturnal haemoglobinuria (PNH) clone. If positive, a sample of urine should be examined for haemosiderin. The Ham test and sucrose lysis test (see Chapter 13) can be used as tests for PNH. They are less sensitive and less quantitative than flow cytometry, but nevertheless are clinically useful.

Reagents for Prothrombin Time (PT) and Activated Partial Thromboplastin Time (APTT)

Rabbit Brain Thromboplastin for Prothrombin Time

Freeze-dried rabbit brain thromboplastins for use in the PT are now widely available commercially, with a shelf-life of 2–5 years or longer. Usually, they are calibrated against the World Health Organization (WHO) International Reference Preparation of thromboplastin and are supplied with an International Sensitivity Index (ISI) and a table converting prothrombin times to International Normalized Ratios (INR).

If a commercial preparation is not available, it is possible to prepare a homemade substitute using rabbit brain that does not require freeze drying and that is relatively stable.

Acetone-dried brain powder

Strip the membrane off freshly collected rabbit brain, wash free from blood and place in about three times its volume of cold acetone. Macerate for 2–3 min and then filter through absorbent lint (BP or USP grade) on a Büchner funnel. Repeat the extraction seven times; after two extractions, increase the time of exposure to acetone to c 20 min for each subsequent extraction. The material should become 'gritty' by the fourth or fifth extraction. After the last extraction, spread the acetone-dried brain on a piece of paper and allow to dry in air for 30 min. Rub through a 1 mm mesh nylon sieve to produce a coarse powder. Dispense into a batch of screw-capped bottles and dry over phosphorus pentoxide in a vacuum desiccator. After drying, screw down the caps tightly and store at 4°C or −20°C. At −20°C, the material should be stable for at least 5 years. A total of 100 g of whole brain yields c 15 g of dried powder.

Preparation of liquid suspension

Dissolve 0.9 g of NaCl and 0.9 g of phenol in 100 ml of water. Suspend 3.6 g of the acetone-dried brain in 100 ml of the phenol–saline solution at 15–20°C and allow to stand at this temperature for 4–5 h, mixing at 30-min intervals. Transfer to a 4°C refrigerator for 24 h and occasionally mix it. Thereafter, leave undisturbed at 4°C for 3 h and then decant the supernatant carefully through fine muslin or similar material. The ISI should be not more than 1.4 (see p. 469) and the mean normal prothrombin time should be 12–13 s. Store the suspension at 4°C. At this temperature, it will be stable for at least 6 months; at room temperature it will be stable for at least 7 days. It must not be allowed to freeze because freezing results in flocculation of the smooth suspension with deterioration of thromboplastic activity.

Phospholipid Reagent for Activated Partial Thromboplastin Time

Acetone-dried rabbit brain is suitable for preparing an APTT reagent. Bovine brain may also be used.

Prepare acetone-dried brain powder as described above. Suspend 5 g of the powder in 20 ml of chloroform (analytic grade) in a covered beaker for 1–2 h. Filter through filter paper to obtain a clear filtrate. Wash the brain deposit on the filter paper with 20 ml of chloroform and pool the clear filtrate with the previous filtrate. Evaporate the filtrate to dryness in a beaker of known weight in a waterbath at 60–70°C and weigh the residual deposit: 5 g of dried brain should yield c 1.5 g of phospholipid deposit. Emulsify in saline to give a 5% emulsion; 1.5 g of deposit should provide 30 ml of emulsion. Distribute the emulsion in small volumes in stoppered tubes. At −20°C it should be stable for at least 1 year.

For use, dilute 1 in 100 in saline and mix with an equal volume of 2.5 mg/ml kaolin suspension in imidazole buffer.

LABORATORY SUPPORT FOR MANAGEMENT OF HIV/AIDS: CD4-POSITIVE T-CELL COUNTS

The WHO recommends that district hospitals and higher level facilities should be able to provide a CD4+ cell count to aid identification of patients who would benefit from antiretroviral drugs and to monitor their progress. Several methods are available but their effectiveness in developing country settings is very variable.[26] Some of the low-cost methods that have good correlation with flow cytometric enumeration of CD4+ cells include the FACS count system (Becton Dickinson Sciences, CA), the Guava Easy CD4 assay (Guava technologies, Hayward, CA), Cyflow (Partec, Germany) and the panleucogating (PLG) CD4 technique. Manual methods such as Dynabeads (Dynal) and Cytospheres (Coulter) can also be used to measure CD4+ T-cell count but the cost, time and skill required make them unsuitable in many settings when other options are available.[27] Dried spots of serum or blood can be used to assess HIV-1 viral load and for resistance genotyping.[28]

LABORATORY MANAGEMENT

Interlaboratory Communication

A well-planned infrastructure is necessary to facilitate flow of communication (e.g. about specimens, results, patient management) between remote clinics and referral or central laboratories. Cell telephones and e-mail using mobile telephone networks are now widely available and are being used to transmit health-related information. In more remote stations, voice and e-mail messages can be transmitted using high-frequency (HF) or satellite radio systems. Alternative power sources such as generators, solar energy and batteries are used to support communication facilities in remote rural clinics.

Digital wireless data communications systems such as the Global System of Mobile (GSM) network are being increasingly used for routine laboratory reporting. The data volume required for text-based laboratory reports is extremely modest and their transmission is low cost. Result reporting can either be incorporated into the mainstream laboratory information system or by individual handsets for smaller independent laboratories.

Specimen Transport

The need to ensure appropriate conditions for keeping specimens after they have been collected and other aspects of specimen transport to the laboratory are described in Chapter 1. The special problem of transporting specimens from remote clinics to laboratories and reference centres in low-resource countries requires further consideration. Peripheral laboratories can assist in rural development initiatives by creating employment opportunities for bicycle riders, motorcyclists, taxi operators and formal and informal courier companies. Commercial or private air services can be used to deliver samples to referral centres. The location of clinics is helped if Global Positioning System (GPS) coordinates are available for each clinic.[29]

Staff Training

In poorer countries, there is often no system for regular supervision of individual laboratory staff and many staff do not receive continuing professional development. Monitoring standards of practice should continue for the whole professional life of laboratory staff to ensure high-quality results. For under-resourced countries, training may be provided in association with vertical health programmes such as HIV or tuberculosis control, but the need for training in basic haematological techniques is often overlooked because tests such as haemoglobin estimation and white cell counts are usually not linked to specific diseases and are therefore not incorporated into vertical programmes. However, because anaemia is the most prevalent disorder worldwide and is often the first sign of underlying disease, the importance of reliable haemoglobin measurements cannot be overemphasized. The need for integrated training programmes is becoming increasingly recognized, especially for peripheral laboratories. Continuing education needs to include the whole range of tests offered by the laboratory and not only tests that are used to support the diagnosis of specific diseases.

Individuals need to keep their own training records, perhaps in the form of a log book and to have their training achievements and plans regularly reviewed by their line managers. Central records of all training should also be maintained for monitoring purposes and to ensure equitable and appropriate distribution of training between different levels of staff. One of the most effective forms of continuing staff development is through regular on-site visits by trained supervisors, who stay for a sufficient length of time to be able to work with the resident staff, and are able to check equipment, supplies, records and attend to other administrative issues. Supervisors themselves need to be trained and monitored to ensure their own proficiency.

Regular monitoring of the quality of results from individual laboratories enables specific problems to be identified. Integrated External Quality Assurance (EQA) programmes tailored for peripheral laboratories are an excellent way to monitor laboratory performance across a wide range of tests. In addition, this quality monitoring allows discrete training needs to be identified, enabling limited teaching resources to be specifically targeted. Systems need to be established to report issues such as equipment failures, discontinuity of supplies and communication breakdowns to the local or regional management teams.

Access to up-to-date information is important for adapting and enhancing laboratory performance. Many medical and technical journals now publish their articles in full on the internet and by an arrangement between the main international publishers and WHO, they can be accessed free of charge or at a significantly discounted cost in most under-resourced countries (see www.who.int/hinari/en).

Clinical Staff Interaction

A major delay in test turnaround time (see p. 574) and the failure of clinicians to use test results is often due to the slow delivery of reports within the health facility after the test has been performed. Appropriate clinical use of the laboratory has a direct impact on the cost-effectiveness of the service.[12] Laboratory tests may be initiated by nurses, health field workers and public health officers, as well as doctors. Many of these individuals have little or no training in how to request appropriate tests, how to provide timely and suitable samples and how to use the results for maximal benefit to patients. Training for laboratory users needs to be incorporated into laboratory training programmes and be closely monitored. In poorer countries, there is often a dearth of clinicians with both clinical and laboratory experience who are qualified to provide such training. However, the relationship between the laboratory and clinical staff can be enhanced and use of the laboratory can be optimized by using a clinician/scientist team to provide joint training in both disciplines. Various publications are now available to guide laboratory users on which test to select, how to interpret the results and how to select and collect the correct samples.

Health Management Teams

Local health management teams are often responsible for ensuring that their laboratories are provided with the necessary tools to deliver a high-quality service. As a rule, these teams do not include members of the laboratory profession, who are often represented by other allied professionals such as pharmacists. Staff in under-resourced laboratories are therefore not always responsible for purchasing supplies and equipment for the laboratory, and this can result in the purchase of inappropriate or poor-quality equipment and reagents. In addition to encouraging adequate representation of laboratory professionals at management level, it is important to ensure that non-laboratory personnel responsible for making procurement decisions for the laboratory are aware of the needs of their laboratory service and seek advice from laboratory professionals.

Health and Safety

Details of laboratory safety issues are described in Chapter 24. Awareness of these issues should be constantly promoted within all laboratories,[30] and the working environment needs to be made as safe as possible. A 'Code of Safe Laboratory Practice' should be prepared that is affordable and relevant to the local circumstances. It should include the following:

- Risk assessment to identify potential workplace hazards and the risk they pose to individuals working or visiting the laboratory
- Education on safe working practices
- Provision of appropriate and adequate safety items such as white coats, gloves and pipetting devices
- Monitoring of adherence to health and safety regulations
- Prompt reporting and investigation of laboratory accidents
- Addressing medical waste disposal practices including use of sharps containers and waste bags and disposal of items in incinerators or deep pits.

Disposable syringes (see p. 2) are intended for single-use only. They cannot withstand sterilization and should never be reused. Similarly, disposable lancets for skin puncture must never be reused. The practice of using a single lancet on several patients consecutively and cleaning it with alcohol between use is unacceptable.

REFERENCES

1. WHO. *Guidelines for the Treatment of Malaria*. Available at: www.who.int/ malaria/publications/atoz/ 9241546948/en/index.html; Accessed 25 01 2010.
2. Akpek G, Lee SM, Gagnon DR, et al. Bone marrow aspiration, biopsy and culture in the evaluation of HIV-infected patients for invasive mycobacteria and histoplasma infections. *Am J Hematol*. 2001;67: 100–106.
3. Larsen C. The fragile environment of inexpensive CD4+ T-cell enumeration in the least developed countries: strategies for accessible support. *Clinical Cytometry Society*. 2008;74B(Suppl 1):S1007–S1116.
4. WHO. *Consultation on Laboratory Services for Monitoring HIV Antiretroviral Therapy in Resource-limited Settings*. Available at: www.who.int/ diagnostics_laboratory/ events_hivlab/en/; 2004 Accessed 25 01 2010.
5. Magrath I Shanta V, Advani S, et al. Treatment of acute lymphoblastic

leukaemia in countries with limited resources; lessons from use of a single protocol in India over a twenty year period. *Eur J Cancer.* 2005;41: 1570–1583.

6. Parkins E, Owen RG, Bedu-Addo G, et al. UK-based real-time lymphoproliferative disorder diagnostic service to improve the management of patients in Ghana. *Journal of Hematopathology.* 2009;2 (3):143–149.

7. WHO. *Learning Bench Aids Series 1–9.* 3rd ed. 2008 Available at: www.tht. ndirect.co.uk/2009orderform.htm; 2008 Accessed 25 01 2010.

8. Mundy C, Ngwira M, Kadawele G, et al. Evaluation of microscope condition in Malawi. *Transactions of the Royal Society of Medicine and Hygiene.* 2000;94:583–584.

9. Opoku-Okrah C, Rumble R, Bedu-Addo G, et al. Improving microscope quality is a good investment for under-resourced laboratories. *Transactions of the Royal Society of Medicine and Hygiene.* 2000;94:582.

10. World Health Organization. *Laboratory Services for Primary Heath Care: Requirements for Essential Clinical Laboratory Tests.* Document: LAB/98.1. Geneva: WHO; 1998.

11. Mundy CJ, Bates I, Nkhoma W, et al. The operation, quality and costs of a district hospital laboratory service in Malawi. *Trans R Soc Trop Med Hyg.* 2003;97:403–408.

12. Mepham S, Squire SB, Chisuwo L, et al. Utilization of laboratory services by health workers in a district hospital in Malawi. *J Clin Pathol.* 2009;62:935–938.

13. Bates I, Mundy C, Pendame R. Use of clinical judgement to guide administration of blood transfusions in Malawi. *Trans R Soc Trop Med Hyg.* 2001;95:510–512.

14. WHO. *Guidelines for the Establishment of Accreditation of Health Laboratories.* Available at: www.searo.who.int/ LinkFiles/Publications_SEA-HLM-394.pdf; Accessed 24 01 2010.

15. Lewis SM, Stott GJ, Wynn KJ. An inexpensive and reliable new haemoglobin colour scale for assessing anaemia. *J Clin Pathol.* 1998;51:21–24.

16. Critchley J, Bates I. Haemoglobin colour scale for anaemia diagnosis where there is no laboratory. *Int J Epidemiol.* 2005;34:1425–1434.

17. Van den Broek NR, Ntonya C, Mhanga E, et al. Diagnosing anaemia in pregnancy in rural clinics: assessing the potential of the haemoglobin colour scale. *Bull World Health Organ.* 1999;77:15–21.

18. Montresor A, Ramsan M, Khalfan N, et al. Performance of the haemoglobin colour scale in diagnosing severe and very severe anaemia. *Trop Med Int Health.* 2003;8:1–6.

19. WHO. *Recommended Methods for the Visual Determination of White Blood Cell Count and Platelet Count.* Document WHO/DIL/00.3. Geneva: World Health Organization; 2000.

20. Brecher G, Cronkite EP. Morphology and enumeration of human blood platelets. *J Appl Physiol.* 1950;3: 365–377.

21. Lewis SM, Wardle J, Cousins S, et al. Platelet counting – development of a reference method and a reference preparation. *Clin Lab Haematol.* 1979;1:227–237.

22. Sanders C, Skerry DW. The distribution of blood cells on haemocytometer counting chambers with special reference to the amended British Standards Specification 748 (1958). *J Clin Pathol.* 1961;48:298–304.

23. Chow J, Phelan L, Bain BJ. The role of a single-tube osmotic fragility for thalassemia screening in under-resourced laboratories. *Am J Hematol.* 2005;79:198–201.

24. Fucharoen G, Sanchaisuriya K, Sae-ung N, et al. A simplified screening strategy for thalassaemia and haemoglobin E in rural communities in south-east Asia. *Bull World Health Organ.* 2004;82: 364–372.

25. Chapple L, Harris A, Phelan L, et al. Reassessment of a simple chemical method using DCIP for screening for haemoglobin E. *J Clin Pathol.* 2005;59:74–76.

26. Kimmel AD, Losina E, Freedberg KA, et al. Diagnostic tests in HIV management: a review of clinical and laboratory strategies to monitor HIV-infected individuals in developing countries. *Bull World Health Organ.* 2006;84: 581–588.

27. Taiwo BO, Murphy RL. Clinical applications and availability of CD4+ T cell count testing in sub-Saharan Africa. *Cytometry B. Clin Cytom.* 2008;74(suppl 1):S11–S18.

28. Hamers RL, Smit PW, Stevens W, et al. Dried fluid spots for HIV type-1 viral load and resistance genotyping: a systematic review. *Antivir Ther.* 2009;14:619–629.

29. Medical Research Council of South Africa . *Geographic Information Systems in Health.* Available at: www.mrc.ac. za/mrcnews/june2001/ geoinformation.htm.

30. WHO. 2011 Laboratory Quality Management System Training Toolkit. http://www.who.int/ihr/ training/laboratory_quality/en/.

FURTHER USEFUL PUBLICATIONS

Laboratory Organization and Management

Houng L, El-Nageh MM. *Principles of management of health laboratories.* WHO Regional Publications; Eastern Mediterranean Series No. 3. 1993.

World Health Organization. *Selection of basic laboratory equipment for laboratories with limited resources.* In: Johns WL, El-ageh MM, eds. Regional Office for the Eastern Mediterranean; 2000.

World Health Organization. *Health laboratory services in support of primary healthcare in South East Asia.* WHO South East Asia Regional Office (SEARO); Publication No. 24. 2nd ed. 1999.

World Health Organization. *Health laboratory facilities in emergency and disaster situations.* WHO Regional Publications; Eastern Mediterranean Series No. 6. 1994.

World Health Organization. *Maintenance and repair of laboratory, diagnostic imaging and hospital equipment*. Geneva: WHO Distribution and Sales; 1994.

Practical Methods

Carter JY, Lema OE. *Practical laboratory manual for health centres in Eastern Africa*. PO Box 31025. Nairobi, Kenya: African Medical and Research Foundation; 1994.

Cheesbrough M. *District Laboratory Practice in Tropical Countries: Vols 1 and 2*. Cambridge: Cambridge University Press; 2006.

World Health Organization. *Manual of basic techniques*. Revised 2nd ed. Geneva: WHO Distribution and Sales; 2000.

World Health Organization. *Production of basic diagnostic laboratory reagents*. WHO Regional Publications; Eastern Mediterranean Series No. 2. 1995.

World Health Organization. *Methods Recommended for Essential Clinical Chemical and Haematological Tests for Intermediate Hospital Laboratories*. WHO/LAB/86.3. Geneva: WHO; 1986.

Quality Assurance

Lewis SM. *Quality Assurance in Haematology*. WHO Document: LAB/98.4. Geneva: WHO; 1998.

World Health Organization. *Quality Systems for Medical Laboratories: Guidelines for Implementation and Monitoring*. WHO Regional Publications; Eastern Mediterranean Series No. 14. 1995.

World Health Organization. *Quality Assurance Related to Health Laboratory Technology*. Geneva: WHO; 1993.

Training for Laboratories

Abbott FR. *Teaching For Better Learning: a Guide for Teachers of Primary Healthcare Staff*. Geneva: WHO; 1992.

World Health Organization. *Technical Training Requirements: Report of Meeting on Development of Appropriate Technology to Support Primary Healthcare*. Geneva: WHO; 1992.

SOURCES OF TEACHING MATERIAL AND EQUIPMENT FOR UNDER-RESOURCED LABORATORIES

Developing Health Technology
Bridge House, Worlington Road,
Barton Mills, IP28 7DX, UK
Tel: +44 (0) 1603 416058;
Fax: +44 (0) 1603 416066;
e-mail: dht@gordon-keeble.co.uk;
www.dht-online.org

Tropical Health Technology
PO Box 50, Fakenham,
Norfolk NR21 8XB, UK

Tel: +44 (0) 1328 855805;
Fax: +44 (0) 1328 853799;
e-mail: thtbooks@tht.ndirect.co.uk;
http://www.tht.ndirect.co.uk/

Teaching Aids at Low Cost (TALC)
PO Box 49, St Albans, Herts AL1 5TX, UK
Tel: +44 (0) 1727 853869;
Fax: +44 (0) 1727 846852;
e-mail: Info@talcuk.org;
www.talcuk.org

TALC Library/Resource Centre
Institute of Child Health,
30 Guilford Street,
London WC1N 1EH, UK
Tel: +44 (0) 207 242 9789,
ext. 2424.

Appendix

Barbara J. Bain, S. Mitchell Lewis

PREPARATION OF COMMONLY USED REAGENTS

Water

For most purposes, still-prepared distilled water or de-ionized water is equally suitable. Throughout this text, this is implied when 'water' is referred to. When doubly distilled or glass-distilled water is required, this has been specially indicated and when tap water is satisfactory or indicated, this, too, has been stated.

Anticoagulants and Preservative Solutions

Acid–Citrate–Dextrose (ACD) Solution – NIH-A

Trisodium citrate, dihydrate (75 mmol/l)	22 g
Citric acid, monohydrate (42 mmol/l)	8 g
Dextrose (139 mmol/l)	25 g
Water to 1 litre	

Sterilize the solution by autoclaving at 121°C for 15 min. Its pH is 5.4. For use, add 10 volumes of blood to 1.5 volumes of solution. For use in red cell survival studies, see p. 383.

Acid–Citrate–Dextrose (Alsever's) Solution

Dextrose (114 mmol/l)	20.5 g
Trisodium citrate, dihydrate (27 mmol/l)	8.0 g
Sodium chloride (72 mmol/l)	4.2 g
Water to 1 litre	

Adjust the pH to 6.1 with citric acid (*c* 0.5 g) and then sterilize the solution by micropore filtration (0.22 μm) or by autoclaving at 121°C for 15 min.

For use, add 4 volumes of blood to 1 volume of solution.

Citrate–Phosphate–Dextrose (CPD) Solution, pH 6.9

Trisodium citrate, dihydrate (102 mmol/l)	30 g
Sodium dihydrogen phosphate, monohydrate (1.08 mmol/l)	0.15 g
Dextrose (11 mmol/l)	2 g
Water to 1 litre	

Sterilize the solution by autoclaving at 121°C for 15 min. After cooling to c 20°C, it should have a brown tinge and its pH should be 6.9.

Citrate–Phosphate–Dextrose (CPD) Solution, pH 5.6–5.8

Trisodium citrate, dihydrate (89 mmol/l)	26.30 g
Citric acid, monohydrate (17 mmol/l)	3.27 g
Sodium dihydrogen phosphate, monohydrate (16 mmol/l)	2.22 g
Dextrose (142 mmol/l)	25.50 g
Water to 1 litre	

Sterilize the solution by autoclaving at 121°C for 15 min. For use as an anticoagulant preservative, add 7 volumes of blood to 1 volume of solution.

Citrate–Phosphate–Dextrose–Adenine (CPD-A) Solution, pH 5.6–5.8

Trisodium citrate, dihydrate (89 mmol/l)	26.30 g
Citric acid, monohydrate (17 mmol/l)	3.27 g
Sodium dihydrogen phosphate, monohydrate (16 mmol/l)	2.22 g
Dextrose (177 mmol/l)	31.8 g
Adenine (2.04 mmol/l)	0.275 g
Water to 1 litre	

Sterilize the solution by autoclaving at 121°C for 15 min. For use as an anticoagulant preservative, add 7 volumes of blood to 1 volume of solution.

Low Ionic Strength Solution (LISS)[1]

Sodium chloride (NaCl) (30.8 mmol/l)	1.8 g
Disodium hydrogen phosphate (Na_2HPO_4) (1.5 mmol/l)	0.21 g
Sodium dihydrogen phosphate (NaH_2PO_4) (1.5 mmol/l)	0.18 g
Glycine (NH_2CH_2COOH) (240 mmol/l)	18.0 g
Water to 1 litre	

Dissolve the sodium chloride and the two phosphate salts in c 400 ml of water; dissolve the glycine separately in c 400 ml of water; adjust the pH of each solution to 6.7 with 1 mol/l NaOH. Add the two solutions together and make up to 1 litre. Sterilize by Seitz filtration or autoclaving. The pH should be within the range of 6.65–6.85, the osmolality 270–285 mmol and conductivity 3.5–3.8 mS/cm at 23°C.

EDTA

Ethylenediaminetetra-acetic acid (EDTA), dipotassium salt	100 g
Water to 1 litre	

Allow appropriate volumes to dry in bottles at c 20°C so as to give a concentration of 1.5 ± 0.25 mg/ml of blood.

Neutral EDTA, pH 7.0, 110 mmol/l

EDTA, dipotassium salt	44.5 g
or disodium salt	41.0 g
1 mmol/l NaOH	75 ml
Water to 1 litre	

Neutral Buffered EDTA, pH 7.0

EDTA, disodium salt (9 mmol/l)	3.35 g
Disodium hydrogen phosphate (Na_2HPO_4) (26.4 mmol/l)	3.75 g
Sodium chloride (NaCl) (140 mmol/l)	8.18 g
Water to 1 litre	

Saline (Normal Ionic Strength)

Sodium chloride (NaCl) (154 mmol/l)	9.0 g
Water to 1 litre	

Trisodium Citrate ($Na_3C_6H_5O_7.2H_2O$), 109 mmol/l

Dissolve 32 g (*or* 38 g of $2Na_3C_6H_5O_7.11\ H_2O$) in 1 litre of water. Distribute convenient volumes (e.g. 10 ml) into small bottles and sterilize by autoclaving at 121°C for 15 min.

Heparin

Powdered heparin (lithium salt) is available with an activity of *c* 160 iu/mg. Dissolve it in water at a concentration of 4 mg/ml. Sodium heparin is available in 5 ml ampoules with an activity of 1000 iu/ml. Add appropriate volumes of either solution to a series of containers and allow to dry at *c* 20°C so as to give a concentration not exceeding 15–20 iu/ml of blood.

Buffers

Barbitone Buffer, pH 7.4

Sodium diethyl barbiturate ($C_8H_{11}O_3N_2Na$) (57 mmol/l)	11.74 g
Hydrochloric acid (HCl) (100 mmol/l)	430 ml

Barbitone Buffered Saline, pH 7.4

NaCl	5.67 g
Barbitone buffer, pH 7.4	1 litre

Before use, dilute with an equal volume of 9 g/l NaCl.

Barbitone Buffered Saline, pH 9.5

Sodium diethyl barbiturate ($C_8H_{11}O_3N_2Na$) (98 mmol/l)	20.2 g
Hydrochloric acid (HCl) (100 mmol/l)	20 ml
NaCl	5.67 g

Before use, dilute the buffer with an equal volume of 9 g/l NaCl.

Barbitone–Bovine Serum Albumin Buffer, pH 9.8

Sodium diethyl barbiturate ($C_8H_{11}O_3N_2Na$) (54 mmol/l)	10.3 g
NaCl (102 mmol/l)	6.0 g
Sodium azide (31 mmol/l)	2.0 g
Bovine serum albumin (BSA)	5.0 g
Water to 1 litre	

Dissolve the reagents in *c* 900 ml of water. Adjust the pH to 9.8 with 5 mol/l HCl. Make up the volume to 1 litre with water. Store at 4°C.

Citrate–Saline Buffer

Trisodium citrate ($Na_3C_6H_5O_7.2H_2O$) (5 mmol/l)	1.5 g
NaCl (96 mmol/l)	5.6 g
Barbitone buffer, pH 7.4	200 ml
Water	800 ml

Glycine Buffer, pH 3.0

Glycine (NH_2CH_2COOH) (82 mmol/l)	6.15 g
NaCl (82 mmol/l)	4.80 g
Water	820 ml
0.1 mol/l HCl	180 ml

HEPES Buffer, pH 6.6

N-2-hydroxyethylpiperazine-N′-2-ethanesulfonic acid (100 mmol/l)	23.83 g
NaOH (1 mol/l)	*c* 1 ml
Dimethyl sulphoxide	25 ml
Water to 1 litre	

Dissolve in *c* 100 ml of water. Add a sufficient volume of 1 mol/l NaOH (*c* 1 ml) to adjust the pH to 6.6. If the buffer is intended for use with Romanowsky staining (see p. 61), then add 25 ml of dimethyl sulphoxide (DMSO). Make up the volume to 1 litre with water.

HEPES–Saline Buffer, pH 7.6

HEPES (20 mmol/l)	4.76 g
NaCl	8.0 g
NaOH (1 mol/l)	
Water to 1 litre	

Dissolve in c 100 ml of water. Add a sufficient volume of 1 mol/l NaOH to adjust the pH to 7.6.

Make up volume to 1 litre with water.

Imidazole Buffered Saline, pH 7.4

Imidazole (50 mmol/l)	3.4 g
NaCl (100 mmol/l)	5.85 g
Water to 1 litre	

Dissolve in c 500 ml of water. Add 18.6 ml of 1 mol/l HCl and make up the volume to 1 litre with water. Store at room temperature ($18–25°C$).

Phosphate Buffer, Iso-Osmotic

(A) $NaH_2PO_4.2H_2O$ (150 mmol/l)	23.4 g/l
(B) Na_2HPO_4 (150 mmol/l)	21.3 g/l

pH	SOLUTION A	SOLUTION B
5.8	87 ml	13 ml
6.0	83 ml	17 ml
6.2	75 ml	25 ml
6.4	66 ml	34 ml
6.6	56 ml	44 ml
6.8	46 ml	54 ml
7.0	32 ml	68 ml
7.2	24 ml	76 ml
7.4	18 ml	82 ml
7.6	13 ml	87 ml
7.7	9.5 ml	90.5 ml

Normal human serum has an osmolality of 289 ± 4 mmol. Hendry[2] recommended slightly different concentrations of the stock solution: namely, 25.05 g/l $NaH_2PO_4.2H_2O$ and 17.92 g/l Na_2HPO_4 for an iso-osmotic buffer.

Phosphate Buffered Saline

Equal volumes of iso-osmotic phosphate buffer and 9 g/l NaCl.

Phosphate Buffer, Sörensen's

Stock solutions:

	66 mmol/l	100 mmol/l	150 mmol/l
(A) KH_2PO_4	9.1 g/l	13.8 g/l	20.7 g/l
(B) Na_2HPO_4	9.5 g/l	14.4 g/l	21.6 g/l
or $Na_2HPO_4.2H_2O$	11.9 g/l	18.0 g/l	27.1 g/l

To obtain a solution of the required pH, add A and B in the indicated proportions:

pH	A	B
5.4	97.0	3.0
5.6	95.0	5.0
5.8	92.2	7.8
6.0	88.0	12.0
6.2	81.0	19.0
6.4	73.0	27.0
6.6	63.0	37.0
6.8	50.8	49.2
7.0	38.9	61.1
7.2	28.0	72.0
7.4	19.2	80.8
7.6	13.0	87.0
7.8	8.5	91.5
8.0	5.5	94.5

This buffer is not iso-osmotic with normal plasma (see earlier).

Tris–HCl Buffer (200 mmol/l)

Tris (hydroxymethyl) aminomethane (24.23 g/l)	250 ml

To obtain a solution of the required pH, add the appropriate volume of 1 mol/l HCl and then make up the volume to 1 litre with water.

pH	VOLUME
7.2	44.5 ml
7.4	42.0 ml
7.6	39.0 ml
7.8	33.5 ml
8.0	28.0 ml
8.2	23.0 ml
8.4	17.5 ml
8.6	13.0 ml
8.8	9.0 ml
9.0	5.0 ml

100 mmol/l, 150 mmol/l, 300 mmol/l and 750 mmol/l stock solutions may be similarly prepared with an appropriate weight of Tris and volume of acid.

Tris–HCl Bovine Serum Albumin (BSA) Buffer, pH 7.6, 20 mmol/l

Tris (hydroxymethyl) aminomethane (20 mmol/l)	2.42 g
EDTA, disodium salt (10 mmol/l)	3.72 g
NaCl (100 mmol/l)	5.85 g
Sodium azide (3 mmol/l)	0.2 g
HCl (10 mol/l)	
Bovine serum albumin	10 g
Water to 1 litre	

Dissolve the reagents in c 800 ml of water. Adjust the pH to 7.6 with 10 mol/l HCl. Add 10 g of BSA and make up to 1 litre with water.

Buffered Formal Acetone

Dissolve 20 mg Na_2HPO_4 and 100 mg KH_2PO_4 in 30 ml distilled water. Add 45 ml acetone and 25 ml of 40% formalin. Mix well and store at $4°C$. Use cold. Make up new fixative every 4 weeks.

PREPARATION OF GLASSWARE

Siliconized Glassware

Use c 2% solution of silicone (dimethyldichlorosilane) in solvent. Immerse the clean glassware or syringes to be coated in the fluid and allow to drain dry. (Rubber gloves should be worn and the procedure should be performed in a fume cupboard provided with an exhaust fan.) Then rinse the coated glassware thoroughly in water and allow to dry in an oven at $100°C$ for 10 min or overnight in an incubator.

Cleaning Slides

New Slides

Boxes of clean, grease-free slides are available commercially. If these are not available, the following procedure should be carried out. Leave the slides overnight in a detergent solution. Then wash well in running tap water, rinse in distilled or deionized water and store in 95% ethanol or methanol until used. Dry with a clean linen cloth and carefully wipe free from dust before they are used.

Dirty Slides

When discarded, place in a detergent solution; heat at $60°C$ for 20 min; and then wash in hot, running tap water. Finally, rinse in water before being dried with a clean linen cloth.

Cleaning Glassware

Wash in running tap water. Then boil in a detergent solution; rinse in acid; and wash in hot, running tap water, as described above. Alternatively, the apparatus can be soaked in 3 mol/l HCl.

For the removal of deposits of protein and other organic matter, 'biodegradable' detergents are recommended. Decon 90 (Decon Laboratories Ltd, Hove BN3 3LY, UK) is suitable, but a number of similar preparations are also available.

Iron-free Glassware

Wash in a detergent solution, then soak in 3 mol/l HCl for 24 h; finally, rinse in deionized, double-distilled water.

SIZES OF TUBES

The sizes of tubes recommended in the text have been chosen as being appropriate for the tests described. The dimensions given are the length and external diameter (in mm). The equivalent in inches, as given in some catalogues and certain corresponding internal diameters, are as follows:

75 × 10 mm (internal diameter 8 mm) = 3 × ⅜ inch
75 × 12 mm (internal diameter 10 mm) = 3 × ½ inch

65×10 mm $= 2\frac{1}{2} \times \frac{3}{8}$ inch
38×6.4 mm $= 1\frac{1}{2} \times \frac{1}{4}$ inch ('precipitin tubes')
100×12 mm $= 4 \times \frac{1}{2}$ inch
150×16 mm $= 6 \times \frac{5}{8}$ inch
150×19 mm $= 6 \times \frac{3}{4}$ inch.

SPEED OF CENTRIFUGING

Throughout the book, the unit given is the relative centrifugal force (g). Conversion of this figure to rpm (rev/min) depends on the radius of the centrifuge; it can be calculated by reference to the nomogram illustrated in Figure A.1 or from the formula for relative centrifugal force (RCF):

$$RCF = 118 \times 10^{-7} \times r \times N^{-2}$$

where r = radius (cm) and N = speed of rotation (rpm). The following centrifugal forces are recommended:

'Low-spun' platelet-rich plasma	150–200 g (for 10–15 min)
'High-spun' plasma	1200–1500 g (for 15 min)
Packing of red cells	2000–2300 g (for 30 min)

STATISTICAL PROCEDURES

Mean ($\bar{x}$) is the sum of all the measurements (Σ) divided by the number of measurements (n).

Median (m) is the point on the scale that has an equal number of observations above and below.

Mode is the most frequently occurring result.

Gaussian distribution describes events or data that occur symmetrically about the mean (see Fig. 2.1, p. 12); with this type of distribution, mean, median and mode will be approximately equal. The extent of spread of measurements about the mean is expressed as the standard deviation (SD) and its calculation is described below. This means that 68% of the measurement will be within the ±1SD range, 95% will be within ±2SD and 99% will be within ±3SD.

Confidence intervals (CI) of any calculation on a sample indicate the upper and lower limits between which a specified proportion of results (e.g. 95%) on the population from which the sample is derived may be expected to occur.

Log normal distribution describes events that are asymmetrical (skewed) with a larger number of observations towards the lower end. The mean will thus be nearer that end; the mean, median and mode may differ from each other. To calculate geometric mean and SD, the data are first converted to their logarithms, and after calculating the mean and SD of the logarithms, the results are reconverted to the antilog.

Poisson distribution describes events that are random in their occurrence. This will be the case, for example, when blood cells are counted in a diluted suspension. The number of cells that are counted in a given volume will vary on each occasion; this count variation (σ) is $0.92\sqrt{\lambda}$, where λ = the total number of cells counted (see p. 611). It is an estimate of the standard deviation of the entire population, whereas SD denotes the standard deviation of the items that were actually measured.

Figure A.1 Nomogram for computing relative centrifugal forces.

Coefficient of variation (CV) is another way of indicating standard deviation, related to the actual measurement, so that variation at different levels can be compared. It is expressed as a percentage.

Standard error of mean (SEM) is a measure of dispersion of the mean of a set of measurements. It is used to compare means of two sets of data.

Calculations

Variance (s²)

$$\frac{\sum (x - \bar{x})^2}{n - 1}$$

Standard deviation (SD)

$$\sqrt{s^2}$$

Coefficient of variation (CV) as percentage

$$\frac{SD \times 100\%}{\bar{x}}$$

Standard error mean (SEM)

$$\frac{SD}{\sqrt{n}}$$

Standard deviation of paired results

$$\sqrt{\frac{\sum d^2}{2n}}$$

where d = differences between paired measurements and n = number of paired measurements.

Standard deviation of median

$$\frac{Central\ 50\%}{1.35} \text{ (betweeen 25\% and 75\%)}$$

Confidence interval

Decide on required confidence interval (e.g. 95% or 99%).

From the t-test Table (see p. 626) find the number at $n - 1$ degrees of freedom.

Calculate SD and SEM as above.

Then the confidence interval will be between $\bar{x}$ (t × SEM) and $\bar{x} + (t \times SEM)$.

When the original data are log normal, convert to their logs, use these figures throughout the calculation and convert the final results to their antilogs.

Analysis of Differences by *t*-Test

Analysis of differences by t-test is a method for comparing two sets of data (e.g. to assess the accuracy of a new method against a reference method).

Calculation

Determine the difference in each pair of tests (d) and the mean difference $(\bar{d})$

$$\text{Variance is obtained from } \frac{(d - \bar{d})^2}{n - 1}; \ t = \bar{d} \div \frac{s^2}{n}$$

From the t-test chart (Table A.1), read the value of t for the appropriate degree of freedom (i.e. $n - 1$). Express results as the level of probability (p) that there is no significant difference between the sets of data that are being compared.

Analysis of Variation by *F*-Ratio

Analysis of variation by F-ratio is a method to assess the relative precision of two sets of measurements.

Calculation

Determine variance (s^2) as described above for each set. Because the ratio must not be less than 1, use the higher variance as the numerator. Then, from the charts (Tables A.2A, A.2B), read the value at either 95% or 99% probability (i.e. p = 0.05 or p = 0.01) for the appropriate degrees of freedom (i.e. $n - 1$) for the two sets of data.

Interpretation

There is a significant difference in variation between the two sets when the calculated ratio is greater than the value read from the chart.

ANOVA

ANOVA is another method for sum of squares analysis of variation when comparing two sets of data (e.g. two different methods for doing a test or results from two individuals, A and B, doing the same test).

	SET A	SET B
Number of measurements	n	n
Add all results from each of the two sets	ΣA	ΣB
Square each sum	$(\Sigma A)^2$	$(\Sigma B)^2$

Combine the sets and divide by number of measurements:

$$\frac{(\Sigma A)^2 + (\Sigma B)^2}{n}$$

Subtract correction factor:

$$(\Sigma A + \Sigma B)^2 \div (\text{Total } n \text{ of } A + B)$$

Compare this measurement with the values given in the F-distribution tables at 95% or 99% for the appropriate degree of freedom. If the calculated sum is greater than the table reading, it can be concluded that there is a 95% (or 99%) probability that the differences between the sets are significant and are not the result of chance alone.

Table A.1 Critical values of *t*-test

df	% PROBABILITY LEVEL						
	50 (0.5)	40 (0.4)	30 (0.3)	20 (0.2)	10 (0.1)	5 (0.05)	1 (0.01)
1	1.000	1.376	1.963	3.078	6.314	12.706	63.657
2	0.816	1.061	1.386	1.886	2.920	4.303	9.925
3	0.765	0.978	1.250	1.638	2.353	3.182	5.841
4	0.741	0.941	1.190	1.533	2.132	2.776	4.604
5	0.727	0.920	1.156	1.476	2.015	2.571	4.032
6	0.718	0.906	1.134	1.440	1.943	2.447	3.707
7	0.711	0.896	1.119	1.415	1.895	2.365	3.499
8	0.706	0.889	1.108	1.397	1.860	2.306	3.355
9	0.703	0.883	1.100	1.383	1.833	2.262	3.250
10	0.700	0.879	1.093	1.372	1.812	2.228	3.169
11	0.697	0.876	1.088	1.363	1.796	2.201	3.106
12	0.695	0.873	1.083	1.356	1.782	2.179	3.055
13	0.694	0.870	1.079	1.350	1.771	2.160	3.012
14	0.692	0.868	1.076	1.345	1.761	2.145	2.977
15	0.691	0.866	1.074	1.341	1.753	2.131	2.947
16	0.690	0.865	1.071	1.337	1.746	2.120	2.921
17	0.689	0.863	1.069	1.333	1.740	2.110	2.989
18	0.688	0.862	1.067	1.330	1.734	2.101	2.878
19	0.688	0.861	1.066	1.328	1.729	2.093	2.861
20	0.687	0.860	1.064	1.325	1.725	2.086	2.845
21	0.686	0.859	1.063	1.323	1.721	2.080	2.831
22	0.686	0.858	1.061	1.321	1.717	2.074	2.819
23	0.685	0.858	1.061	1.321	1.717	2.074	2.819
24	0.685	0.857	1.059	1.318	1.711	2.064	2.797
25	0.684	0.856	1.058	1.316	1.708	2.060	2.787

Table A.1 Critical values of t-test – cont'd

df	% PROBABILITY LEVEL						
	50 (0.5)	40 (0.4)	30 (0.3)	20 (0.2)	10 (0.1)	5 (0.05)	1 (0.01)
26	0.684	0.856	1.058	1.315	1.706	2.056	2.779
27	0.684	0.855	1.057	1.314	1.703	2.052	2.771
28	0.683	0.855	1.056	1.313	1.701	2.048	2.763
29	0.683	0.854	1.055	1.311	1.699	2.045	2.756
30	0.683	0.854	1.055	1.310	1.697	2.042	2.750
40	0.681	0.851	1.050	1.303	1.684	2.021	2.704
50	0.680	0.849	1.048	1.299	1.676	2.008	2.678
60	0.679	0.848	1.046	1.296	1.671	2.000	2.660
120	0.677	0.845	1.041	1.289	1.658	1.980	2.617
∞	0.674	0.842	1.036	1.282	1.645	1.960	2.576

AUTOMATED (MECHANICAL) PIPETTES

Accurate pipetting is an essential requirement for all quantitative tests. A variety of automated hand-held pipettes are available, many of which incorporate a disposable tip with an ejector mechanism, which allows the user to remove it without hand contact. Some pipettes have a fixed capacity; in others a range of volumes can be obtained by means of an adjusting screw and the delivery volume is displayed on a digital readout.

Because the designs are varied, the specific manufacturer's instructions must be carefully followed. The following important points are common to all:

1. Always use the specified tip.
2. Washing and reusing tips is not recommended.
3. Ensure that the tip is fitted firmly to the pipette.
4. Keep the pipette clean of dirt and grease.
5. Always pipette in a vertical position.
6. Never leave the pipette on its side with liquid in the tip.
7. Return the pipette to its stand after use.
8. Operate by a slow, smooth, consistent procedure, avoiding bubbles or foaming.
9. Use 'reverse pipetting' for plasma, high-viscosity fluids and/or very small volumes. With the plunger pressed all the way down (2nd stop), dip the tip well below the surface of the fluid and release the plunger knob slowly. Remove the pipette; wipe the outside of the tip carefully with a tissue; and then, with the tip against the inside wall of the receiving container, deliver its contents by depressing the plunger knob to the 1st stop. Then discard the tip with its residual contents.
10. For blood dilution, fill and empty the tip with the blood 2–3 times, then depress the plunger to the 1st stop. With the tip well below the surface of the specimen, release the plunger to fill the tip with blood. Withdraw the pipette from the specimen, wipe the outside of the tip carefully with a tissue, dip the tip into the diluent well below the surface and press the plunger knob repeatedly to fill and empty the tip until the interior wall is clear. Then depress the plunger to the 2nd stop to empty the tip completely.
11. At intervals, monitor the reliability of the pipette by checking its accuracy and precision.

Quality control of pipette reliability involves the following:

1. Ensure that all the items to be used are at ambient room temperature.
2. Record the weight of a weighing beaker using a precision balance sensitive to 0.1 mg.
3. Record the temperature of a tube of distilled water, fill the pipette with the water, wipe the outside of the tip and dispense the water into the weighing beaker with the tip touching the side of the beaker.
4. Record the weight of the beaker plus water and calculate the weight of the water.
5. Calculate the volume (in μl) from the weight (in mg) ÷ the ambient temperature factor (Table A.3).
6. Repeat the procedure 10 times, changing the tip each time.

(continued on p. 632)

Table A.2A F distribution table: 99% probability (p = 0.01)

df NUMERATOR

	1	2	3	4	5	6	7	8	9	10	12	15	20	24	30	40	60	120	∞
1	4052	4999.5	5403	5625	5764	5859	5928	5981	6022	6056	6106	6157	6209	6235	6261	6287	6313	6339	6366
2	98.50	99.00	99.17	99.25	99.30	99.33	99.36	99.37	99.39	99.40	99.42	99.43	99.45	99.46	99.47	99.47	99.48	99.49	99.50
3	34.12	30.82	29.46	28.71	28.24	27.91	27.67	27.49	27.35	27.23	27.05	26.87	26.69	26.60	26.50	26.41	26.32	26.22	26.13
4	21.20	18.00	16.69	15.98	15.52	15.21	14.98	14.80	14.66	14.55	14.37	14.20	14.02	13.93	13.84	13.75	13.65	13.56	13.46
5	16.26	13.27	12.06	11.39	10.97	10.67	10.46	10.29	10.16	10.05	9.89	9.72	9.55	9.47	9.38	9.29	9.20	9.11	9.02
6	13.75	10.92	9.78	9.15	8.75	8.47	8.26	8.10	7.98	7.87	7.72	7.56	7.40	7.31	7.23	7.14	7.06	6.97	6.88
7	12.25	9.55	8.45	7.85	7.46	7.19	6.99	6.84	6.72	6.62	6.47	6.31	6.16	6.07	5.99	5.91	5.82	5.74	5.65
8	11.26	8.65	7.59	7.01	6.63	6.37	6.18	6.03	5.91	5.81	5.67	5.52	5.36	5.28	5.20	5.12	5.03	4.95	4.86
9	10.56	8.02	6.99	6.42	6.06	5.80	5.61	5.47	5.35	5.26	5.11	4.96	4.81	4.73	4.65	4.57	4.48	4.40	4.31
10	10.04	7.56	6.55	5.99	5.64	5.39	5.20	5.06	4.94	4.85	4.71	4.56	4.41	4.33	4.25	4.17	4.08	4.00	3.91
11	9.65	7.21	6.22	5.67	5.32	5.07	4.89	4.74	4.63	4.54	4.40	4.25	4.10	4.02	3.94	3.86	3.78	3.69	3.60
12	9.33	6.93	5.95	5.41	5.06	4.82	4.64	4.50	4.39	4.30	4.16	4.01	3.86	3.78	3.70	3.62	3.54	3.45	3.36
13	9.07	6.70	5.74	5.21	4.86	4.62	4.44	4.30	4.19	4.10	3.96	3.82	3.66	3.59	3.51	3.43	3.34	3.25	3.17
14	8.86	6.51	5.56	5.04	4.69	4.46	4.28	4.14	4.03	3.94	3.80	3.66	3.51	3.43	3.35	3.27	3.18	3.09	3.00
15	8.68	6.36	5.42	4.89	4.56	4.32	4.14	4.00	3.89	3.80	3.67	3.52	3.37	3.29	3.21	3.13	3.05	2.96	2.87
16	8.53	6.23	5.29	4.77	4.44	4.20	4.03	3.89	3.78	3.69	3.55	3.41	3.26	3.18	3.10	3.02	2.93	2.84	2.75

17	8.40	6.11	5.18	4.67	4.34	4.10	3.93	3.79	3.68	3.59	3.40	3.31	3.16	3.08	3.00	2.92	2.83	2.75	2.65
18	8.29	6.01	5.09	4.58	4.25	4.01	3.84	3.71	3.60	3.51	3.37	3.23	3.08	3.00	2.92	2.84	2.75	2.66	2.57
19	8.18	5.93	5.01	4.50	4.17	3.94	3.77	3.63	3.52	3.43	3.30	3.15	3.00	2.92	2.84	2.76	2.67	2.58	2.49
20	8.10	5.85	4.94	4.43	4.10	3.87	3.70	3.56	3.46	3.37	3.23	3.09	2.94	2.86	2.78	2.69	2.61	2.52	2.42
21	8.02	5.78	4.87	4.37	4.04	3.81	3.64	3.51	3.40	3.31	3.17	3.03	2.88	2.80	2.72	2.64	2.55	2.46	2.36
22	7.95	5.72	4.82	4.31	3.99	3.76	3.59	3.45	3.35	3.26	3.12	2.98	2.83	2.75	2.67	2.58	2.50	2.40	2.31
23	7.88	5.66	4.76	4.26	3.94	3.71	3.54	3.41	3.30	3.21	3.07	2.93	2.78	2.70	2.62	2.54	2.45	2.35	2.26
24	7.82	5.61	4.72	4.22	3.90	3.67	3.50	3.36	3.26	3.17	3.03	2.89	2.74	2.66	2.58	2.49	2.40	2.31	2.21
25	7.77	5.57	4.68	4.18	3.85	3.63	3.46	3.32	3.22	3.13	2.99	2.85	2.70	2.62	2.54	2.45	2.36	2.27	2.17
26	7.72	5.53	4.64	4.14	3.82	3.59	3.42	3.29	3.18	3.09	2.96	2.81	2.66	2.58	2.50	2.42	2.33	2.23	2.13
27	7.68	5.49	4.60	4.11	3.78	3.56	3.39	3.26	3.15	3.06	2.93	2.78	2.63	2.55	2.47	2.38	2.29	2.20	2.10
28	7.64	5.15	4.57	4.07	3.75	3.53	3.36	3.23	3.12	3.03	2.90	2.75	2.60	2.52	2.44	2.35	2.26	2.17	2.06
29	7.60	5.42	4.54	4.04	3.73	3.50	3.33	3.20	3.09	3.00	2.87	2.73	2.57	2.49	2.41	2.33	2.23	2.14	2.03
30	7.56	5.39	4.51	4.02	3.70	3.47	3.30	3.17	3.07	2.98	2.84	2.70	2.55	2.47	2.39	2.30	2.21	2.11	2.01
40	7.31	5.18	4.31	3.83	3.51	3.29	3.12	2.99	2.80	2.80	2.66	2.52	2.37	2.29	2.20	2.11	2.02	1.92	1.80
60	7.08	4.98	4.13	3.65	3.34	3.12	2.95	2.82	2.72	2.63	2.50	2.35	2.20	2.12	2.03	1.94			
120	6.85	4.79	3.95	3.48	3.17	2.96	2.79	2.66	2.56	2.47	2.34	2.19	2.03	1.95	1.86	1.76	1.66	1.53	1.38
∞	6.63	4.61	3.78	3.32	3.02	2.80	2.64	2.51	2.41	2.32	2.18	2.04	1.88	1.79	1.70	1.59	1.47	1.32	1.00

Table A.2B *F* distribution table: 95% probability (p = 0.05)

df NUMERATOR																			
	1	2	3	4	5	6	7	8	9	10	12	15	20	24	30	40	60	120	∞
1	161.4	199.5	215.7	224.6	230.2	234.0	236.8	238.9	240.5	241.9	243.9	245.9	248.0	249.1	250.1	251.1	252.2	253.3	254.3
2	18.51	19.00	19.16	19.25	19.30	19.33	19.35	19.37	19.38	19.40	19.41	19.43	19.45	19.45	19.46	19.47	19.48	19.49	19.50
3	10.13	9.55	9.28	9.12	9.01	8.94	8.89	8.85	8.81	8.79	8.74	8.70	8.66	8.64	8.62	8.59	8.57	8.55	8.53
4	7.71	6.94	6.59	6.39	6.26	6.16	6.09	6.04	6.00	5.96	5.91	5.86	5.80	5.77	5.75	5.72	5.69	5.66	5.63
5	6.61	5.79	5.41	5.19	5.05	4.95	4.88	4.82	4.77	4.74	4.68	4.62	4.56	4.53	4.50	4.46	4.43	4.40	4.36
6	5.99	5.14	4.76	4.53	4.39	4.28	4.21	4.15	4.10	4.06	4.00	3.94	3.87	3.84	3.81	3.77	3.74	3.70	3.67
7	5.59	4.74	4.35	4.12	3.97	3.87	3.79	3.73	3.68	3.64	3.57	3.51	3.44	3.41	3.38	3.34	3.30	3.27	3.23
8	5.32	4.46	4.07	3.84	3.69	3.58	3.50	3.44	3.39	3.35	3.28	3.22	3.15	3.12	3.08	3.04	3.01	2.97	2.93
9	5.12	4.26	3.86	3.63	3.48	3.37	3.29	3.23	3.18	3.14	3.07	3.01	2.94	2.90	2.86	2.83	2.79	2.75	2.71
10	4.96	4.10	3.71	3.48	3.33	3.22	3.14	3.07	3.02	2.98	2.91	2.85	2.77	2.74	2.70	2.66	2.62	2.58	2.54
11	4.84	3.98	3.59	3.36	3.20	3.09	3.01	2.95	2.90	2.85	2.79	2.72	2.65	2.61	2.57	2.53	2.49	2.45	2.40
12	4.75	3.89	3.49	3.26	3.11	3.00	2.91	2.85	2.80	2.75	2.69	2.62	2.54	2.51	2.47	2.43	2.38	2.34	2.30
13	4.67	3.81	3.41	3.18	3.03	2.92	2.83	2.77	2.71	2.67	2.60	2.53	2.46	2.42	2.38	2.34	2.30	2.25	2.21
14	4.60	3.74	3.34	3.11	2.96	2.85	2.76	2.70	2.65	2.60	2.53	2.46	2.39	2.35	2.31	2.27	2.22	2.18	2.13
15	4.54	3.68	3.29	3.06	2.90	2.79	2.71	2.64	2.59	2.54	2.48	2.40	2.33	2.29	2.25	2.20	2.16	2.11	2.07
16	4.49	3.63	3.24	3.01	2.85	2.74	2.66	2.59	2.54	2.49	2.42	2.35	2.28	2.24	2.19	2.15	2.11	2.06	2.01
17	4.45	3.59	3.20	2.96	2.81	2.70	2.61	2.55	2.49	2.45	2.38	2.31	2.23	2.19	2.15	2.10	2.00	2.01	1.96

18	4.41	3.55	3.16	2.93	2.77	2.66	2.58	2.51	2.46	2.41	2.34	2.27	2.19	2.15	2.11	2.06	2.02	1.97	1.92
19	4.38	3.52	3.13	2.90	2.74	2.63	2.54	2.48	2.42	2.38	2.31	2.23	2.16	2.11	2.07	2.03	1.98	1.93	1.88
20	4.35	3.49	3.10	2.87	2.71	2.60	2.51	2.45	2.39	2.35	2.28	2.20	2.12	2.08	2.04	1.99	1.95	1.90	1.84
21	4.32	3.47	3.07	2.84	2.68	2.57	2.49	2.42	2.37	2.32	2.25	2.18	2.10	2.05	2.01	1.96	1.92	1.87	1.81
22	4.30	3.44	3.05	2.82	2.66	2.55	2.46	2.40	2.34	2.30	2.23	2.15	2.07	2.03	1.98	1.94	1.89	1.84	1.78
23	4.28	3.42	3.03	2.80	2.64	2.53	2.44	2.37	2.32	2.27	2.20	2.13	2.05	2.01	1.96	1.91	1.86	1.81	1.76
24	4.26	3.40	3.01	2.78	2.62	2.51	2.42	2.36	2.30	2.25	2.18	2.11	2.03	1.98	1.94	1.89	1.84	1.79	1.73
25	4.24	3.39	2.99	2.76	2.60	2.49	2.40	2.34	2.28	2.24	2.16	2.09	2.01	1.96	1.92	1.87	1.82	1.77	1.71
26	4.23	3.37	2.98	2.74	2.59	2.47	2.39	2.32	2.27	2.22	2.15	2.07	1.99	1.95	1.90	1.85	1.80	1.75	1.69
27	4.21	3.35	2.96	2.73	2.57	2.46	2.37	2.31	2.25	2.20	2.13	2.06	1.97	1.93	1.88	1.84	1.79	1.73	1.67
28	4.20	3.34	2.95	2.71	2.56	2.45	2.36	2.29	2.24	2.19	2.12	2.04	1.96	1.91	1.87	1.82	1.77	1.71	1.65
29	4.18	3.33	2.93	2.70	2.55	2.43	2.35	2.28	2.22	2.18	2.10	2.03	1.94	1.90	1.85	1.81	1.75	1.70	1.64
30	4.17	3.32	2.92	2.69	2.53	2.42	2.33	2.27	2.21	2.16	2.09	2.01	1.93	1.89	1.84	1.79	1.74	1.68	1.62
40	4.08	3.23	2.84	2.61	2.45	2.34	2.25	2.18	2.12	2.08	2.00	1.92	1.84	1.79	1.74	1.69	1.64	1.58	1.51
60	4.00	3.15	2.76	2.53	2.37	2.25	2.17	2.10	2.04	1.99	1.92	1.84	1.75	1.70	1.65	1.59	1.53	1.47	1.39
120	3.92	3.07	2.68	2.45	2.37	2.17	2.09	2.02	1.96	1.91	1.83	1.75	1.66	1.61	1.55	1.50	1.43	1.35	1.25
∞	3.84	3.00	2.60	2.37	2.21	2.10	2.01	1.94	1.88	1.83	1.75	1.67	1.57	1.52	1.45	1.39	1.32	1.22	1.00

Table A.3 Ambient temperature factor for correction of weight:volume ratio

TEMP (°C)	VOLUME FACTOR
18	0.9986
19	0.9984
20	0.9982
21	0.9980
22	0.9978
23	0.9976
24	0.9973
25	0.9971
26	0.9968
27	0.9965
28	0.9963
29	0.9960
30	0.9957

7. Calculate the mean, SD and CV of the dispensed volume. From the mean, calculate the percentage deviation from the expected volume by the formula:

$$\frac{\text{Expected volume} - \text{Delivered volume}}{\text{Expected volume}} \times 100.$$

For routine purposes, this should not differ by more than 1.5%. The CV should be <1%.

AUTODILUTERS

Autodiluter systems provide a constant dilution of blood in reagent by a single process. To check their accuracy, a calibrated 0.2 ml pipette and 50 ml volumetric flask are required. Equipment certified as conforming to these measurements in accordance with national standards is available commercially, or their accuracy can be checked by the procedure described above.

Mix well a 2–3 ml specimen of anticoagulated fresh whole blood and lyse (see p. 310). Then dilute manually 1:251 in haemiglobincyanide reagent (see p. 26) using the calibrated pipette and volumetric flask. At the same time, dilute a sample of the lysed blood in haemiglobincyanide solution, in duplicate, by means of the autodiluter. Read the absorbance of each solution at 540 nm in a spectrophotometer. The dilution by the autodiluter is obtained from the formula:

$$A_1 \times \frac{\text{Dilution}}{A_2} \text{ (i.e. 1 : 251)}$$

where A_1 = absorbance at 540 nm of manual dilution and A_2 = absorbance at 540 nm of autodiluted sample.

If indicated, an appropriate adjustment should be made to the autodiluter in accordance with the manufacturer's instructions or a correction factor should be applied whenever the autodiluter is used.

REFERENCES

1. Moore HC, Mollison PL. Use of a low-ionic-strength medium in manual tests for antibody detection. *Transfusion.* 1976;16:291.

2. Hendry EB. Osmolarity of human serum and of chemical solutions of biological importance. *Clin Chem.* 1961;7:156.

Index

Page numbers ending in 'f' and 't' refer to Figures and Tables respectively

A

Abbott system
  Axsym substrates, 217, 218
  Cell-Dyn 4000, 46f, 47
  Sapphire, 44
ABC (Antigen Binding Capacity), 359
ABH substance secretion, testing for, 504
ABO grouping, 483, 535
  causes of discrepancies, 526–528
  false-negative reactions, 527–528
  false-positive reactions, 526–527
  haemolytic disease of the foetus and newborn, 76, 77f, 540
  rapid typing, 534
  reagents, 524
  system, 283, 485–488
Absorbance values, haemoglobin, 26–27
Absorption spectroscopy, 240
Acanthocytosis, 81–82
Accreditation, laboratory, 577–578
Accuracy, 567, 570
ACD (acid-citrate-dextrose), 6, 7, 260, 277–278, 619
Acetic acid, 232, 233
Acetone-dried brain powder, 613
Acetylphenylhydrazine, 266
Acid phosphatase reaction, 342–343
Acid/alcohol fixative, 430
Acid-citrate-dextrose (ACD), 6, 7, 260, 277–278, 619
Acidified glycerol lysis-time test (AGLT), 251–252
Acidified-serum lysis (Ham) test, 293–294

Acidified-serum test lysis with additional magnesium (modified Ham test), 294–295
Acquired B antigen, 527
Acquired immune deficiency syndrome *see* HIV/AIDS
Activated clotting time (ACT), 474
Activated partial thromboplastin time (APTT), 396, 410–412
  assays based on, 419–420
  circulating inhibitor screen based on, 421–422
  correction tests using, 416
  heparin monitoring, 473
  normal and abnormal clot waveforms, 408
  prolonged, 421
  reagents, 613–614
  thrombolytic therapy, 479
Activated PC resistance (APCR), 404, 456–457
Acute blood transfusion reactions, 543–544
Acute intravascular haemolysis, 543–544
Acute leukaemia
  acute lymphoblastic *see* Acute lymphoblastic leukaemia (ALL)
  acute myeloid *see* Acute myeloid leukaemia (AML)
  bone marrow aspiration, 128–129
  classification, 362–364, 363t
  immunological markers, 361–364
  mixed phenotype, 363–364
  monoclonal antibodies, 361t
  multiparametric flow cytometry, data analysis strategies, 357
  specific tests, 556
Acute lymphoblastic leukaemia (ALL), 94, 97f, 341, 350, 559
  classification, 361–362

Acute myeloid leukaemia (AML), 168–171, 349, 361–362, 558
Acute-phase response tests, 101–105
Adenosine 5-diphosphate, 434, 435
Adenosine triphosphate (ATP), 253, 267
Adenosylcobalamin, 202
Adrenaline, 19, 435, 436
Adsorption techniques, 283
AET cells, 296
Afibrinogenaemia, suspected, 424
African trypanosomiasis, 116, 117f
Agarose gel electrophoresis, 143, 313–314
Agglutinins, 6
Aggregation, platelets, 396, 432–438, 554
Agkistrodon contortrix contortrix, 454
Agkistrodon rhodostoma, 417
Alcohols, 582–583
Alder-Reilly anomaly, 90–91, 92f
Alkaline phosphatase antialkaline phosphatase (APAAP), 359–361
Allele-specific oligonucleotide hybridization, 145
Alloadsorbed sera, testing, 284
Alloantibodies, 492–493, 504–506, 507, 526
  red cell, 492, 493t
Allogeneic haemopoietic stem cell transplantation, 542
Alsever's solution, 6, 7, 619
Altitude, and blood count, 18
Amastigotes, 116
American Association for Molecular Pathology, 140
American trypanosomiasis, 116
Amidolytic assays, 401
Amino acids, 302

633

Index

Index

Index

Index